CLINICAL PHARMACY

Volume 11, Number 1
January 1992

Transdermal fentanyl

Rabies

Antiarrhythmics and cardiac devices

AMERICAN SOCIETY OF HOSPITAL PHARMACISTS

SELECT TUBEX.
A COLLEAGUE'S LIFE MAY DEPEND ON IT.

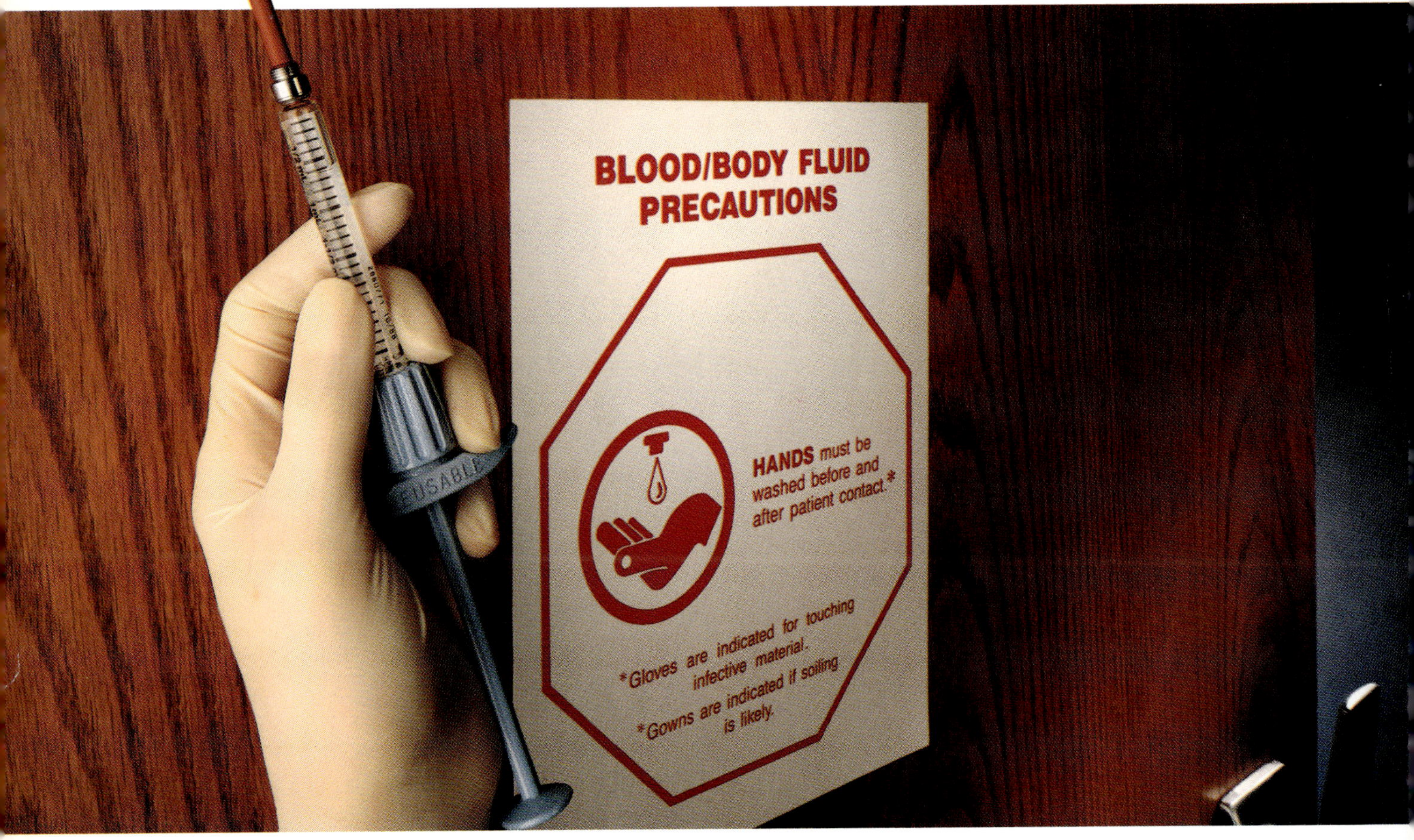

THE BEST SELF-DEFENSE INJECTION SYSTEM AGAINST NEEDLESTICK INJURIES

Although the risk of seroconversion is low, to date 60% of the reported seroconverted healthcare workers had occupational HIV exposure from needlestick injuries.[1] As AIDS cases escalate, so does the need for on-the-job self-defense. In addition, an estimated 200 healthcare workers die each year from hepatitis B viruses.[2]

IMPROVED TUBEX® INJECTOR SECURELY GRIPS CARTRIDGE

Now, the TUBEX Injector has been improved to provide a more secure grip on the cartridge within the Injector. And it's faster and easier than ever to load. The improved TUBEX Injector still offers the same safety advantages: it puts nurses farther from the needle and cartridge than any other injector system. There's no need to touch, shake, manipulate, or angle the needle or cartridge upon disposal.

For the best self-defense injection system against needlestick injuries, select the improved TUBEX Injector... a colleague's life may depend on it.

IMPROVED

INJECTOR Tubex®

(closed injection system) Ayerst

FARTHER FROM THE POINT OF DANGER

References
1. Centers for Disease Control. Update: Acquired immunodeficiency syndrome and human immunodeficiency virus infection among health-care workers. *MMWR*. 1988;37:229-234, 239.
2. US Dept of Labor. Occupational Safety and Health Administration. Worker exposure to AIDS and hepatitis B. 1987.

WYETH-AYERST LABORATORIES
Philadelphia, PA 19101

January 1992 Volume 11, Number 1 Coden: CPHADV ISSN: 0278-2677

CLINICAL PHARMACY

4 **News**

Didanosine and foscarnet marketed for use by patients with AIDS . . . Working group issues report on aluminum contamination of parenteral nutrient solutions, Christine A. Mowatt-Larssen . . . United Kingdom suspends sales of triazolam; FDA to review safety data . . . Felodipine marketed as antihypertensive agent

13 **Letters**

Beta-adrenergic agonists in asthma, Chris Nee, Jeff Herzfeld; Shannon L. Coonce, Christine M. Murphy, Pamela A. Simon

14 **Corrections**

Drug Review

22 **Transdermally administered fentanyl for pain management**
Karim Anton Calis, David R. Kohler, and Diane M. Corso

Therapy Review

37 **Features and treatment of rabies**
Maureen L. Frenia, Suzanne M. Lafin, and Joseph A. Barone

Grand Rounds

48 **Interference by antiarrhythmic agents with function of electrical cardiac devices**
Deborah A. Tworek, José Nazari, Marilyn Ezri, and Jerry L. Bauman

Drug Experience

57 **Muscle spasms associated with intrathecal morphine therapy: Treatment with midazolam**
Robert A. Littrell, L. Douglas Kennedy, William E. Birmingham, and W. David Leak

ASHP Reports

60 **Procedure for submission of manuscripts to journals published by the American Society of Hospital Pharmacists**

62 **Instructions for submitting computer disks with revised manuscripts**

DUE Criteria

63 **Criteria for use of zidovudine in adult and pediatric inpatients and outpatients**
S. Diane Goodwin and Kenneth W. Shipp

77 **CP Continuing Education**

85 **FDA Adverse Reaction Report Form and Instructions**

87 **Current Literature**

Drug Reaction Alerts . . . Book Review: *Advances in Pain Research and Therapy, Volume 18: The Design of Analgesic Clinical Trials (Max, Portenoy, Laska)*, Celeste Lindley

92 **Advertising Index**

Notice to readers: Starting with this issue of *Clinical Pharmacy*, the FDA Adverse Reaction Report form will appear in the January and July issues only, instead of in every issue.

Editorial Office
4630 Montgomery Avenue
Bethesda, MD 20814
301-657-3000
Fax 301-657-1615

Advertising Representative
William McCausland Associates, Inc.
P.O. Box 189
Pitman, NJ 08071
609-589-5454
Fax 609-582-7611

Printed on acid-free paper effective with Volume 8, January 1989.

Instructions to Authors

Clinical Pharmacy, a forum for the drug therapeutics information that pharmacists need to perform their clinical roles, gives priority to (1) studies that objectively evaluate drug effects in human trials, (2) evaluative review articles on the clinical uses of new drugs, and (3) evaluations of the current status of drug therapy in selected diseases. Contributions to the following sections are invited.

Drug Reviews: Detailed, analytical reviews on the clinical use of specific drugs, with preference given to new drugs and to evaluative rather than descriptive literature reviews.

Therapy Reviews: Articles that focus primarily on a disease state and its treatment.

Therapy Update: Concise analytical reviews of narrowly defined, important topics in pharmacotherapy.

Clinical Frontiers: Articles that review important, ongoing research on disease processes, drug mechanisms, or new technologies and project the likely implications for therapy.

Research: Reports of well-conducted original research on drug effects in humans.

Research Notes: Short research reports, such as updates on previously published work, confirmations of previous findings, or original research of modest scope.

Grand Rounds: Patient case reports and literature reviews combined in a way that gives them high educational value.

Drug Experience: Straightforward reports, with selected literature references, of unusual drug experiences.

Therapy Consultation: Brief advice, in a question-and-answer format, on how to handle specific drug-therapy problems. Readers are invited to submit questions, which the editor will forward to consultants for answering.

Letters: Short comments on previously published work or about potential problems, apparent trends, or controversies in drug therapy or clinical research.

Commentaries: Well-reasoned expressions of opinion on drug-therapy or clinical-research issues.

The editors have the sole authority to decide in which section to publish an accepted manuscript.

Manuscripts are subject to review by qualified outside reviewers, as well as by the editors, and will be accepted for publication only if they are believed to represent an important contribution to the literature. All papers submitted for publication must be accompanied by a completed copy of a manuscript checklist. The checklist, which generally conforms to the Uniform Requirements for Manuscripts Submitted to Biomedical Journals, appears on pages 60-61 of the January 1991 issue. Authors of especially important original work may request "fast-track" review of their papers. Authors may suggest appropriate reviewers for their papers.

Accepted materials become the permanent and sole property of ASHP and may not be published or reprinted elsewhere without written permission from both the author and the editor.

The editors reserve the right to revise all materials submitted, if necessary. The publisher assumes no responsibility for the statements and opinions advanced by contributors to Clinical Pharmacy.

Under the terms of the Copyright Revision Act of 1976 (Public Law 94-553) it is necessary to have the rights of the authors transferred to the publisher in order to provide for the widest possible dissemination of professional and scientific literature. Accordingly, all transmittal letters accompanying manuscripts submitted for publication, including contributions for the Letters column, must contain the following language: "In consideration of the American Society of Hospital Pharmacists (ASHP) taking action in reviewing and editing my (our) submission, the author(s) undersigned hereby transfer(s), assign(s), or otherwise convey(s) all ownership rights in the submission and all copyright ownership to ASHP. In the event that such work is not published by ASHP, all said rights shall be released." We regret that we cannot consider manuscripts for publication that are not accompanied by transmittal letters containing the above language signed by all authors.

Authors must certify in their letter of transmittal that none of the material in their manuscript has been published previously nor is under consideration or been accepted for publication elsewhere. If this certification cannot be made, suitable explanation must be offered.

Eight copies of all manuscripts should be submitted. Manuscripts should be typewritten with double spacing (including tables) on one side of good-quality, 21.6 x 27.9-cm white paper, and with margins of at least 2.5 cm. For guidance on style, authors should consult the manuscript checklist, recent issues of Clinical Pharmacy, and the *Council of Biology Editors Style Manual, fifth edition. The American Heritage Dictionary of the English Language and the AMA's Manual of Style* contain helpful advice on correct usage.

Galley proofs or final edited manuscripts are sent to authors for inspection against the original manuscript and for correction. Unnecessary alterations at this stage must be avoided. An order form for reprints is sent to the corresponding author at the time of publication.

Clinical Pharmacy (ISSN 0278-2677) is published monthly by the American Society of Hospital Pharmacists, 4630 Montgomery Avenue, Bethesda, MD 20814. Joseph A. Oddis, Executive Vice President. Second-class postage is paid at Bethesda, MD, and at additional mailing offices. **Postmaster: Send address changes to: *Clinical Pharmacy*, 4630 Montgomery Avenue, Bethesda, MD 20814.**

Annual Subscription Rate:	*USA*	*Non-USA*
ASHP Members	$45	$60
ASHP Student Members and Residents	$35	$50
Institutions and Nonmembers	$80	$95

The cost of single copies is $10. Airmail delivery outside the continental United States is available for an additional charge of $90 per year. Requests to replace missing issues free of charge are honored only up to six months after date of issue.

Payments to ASHP are not deductible as charitable contributions for federal income tax purposes. However, they may be deductible under other provisions of the Internal Revenue Code.

Advertising for Clinical Pharmacy is accepted in accordance with the Statement of Advertising Policy of the American Society of Hospital Pharmacists (see *Am J Hosp Pharm*. 1987; 44:1146). For additional information, contact the Advertising Representative (William McCausland Associates, Inc., P.O. Box 189, Pitman, NJ 08071. Phone 609-589-5454, Fax 609-582-7611).

All articles published, including editorials, letters, and book reviews, represent the opinions of the authors and do not reflect the official policy of the American Society of Hospital Pharmacists or the institution with which the author is affiliated, unless this is specified.

Microfilm and microfiche editions are available for purchase. Contact University Microfilms, 300 N. Zeeb Road, Ann Arbor, MI 48106.

Articles in Clinical Pharmacy are abstracted and indexed in *Current Contents, Clinical Sciences, Current Awareness in Biologic Sciences, Excerpta Medica, Index Medicus, Inpharma, International Pharmaceutical Abstracts*, and *Reactions*.

March 1992 Volume 11, Number 3 Coden: CPHADV ISSN: 0278-2677

CLINICAL PHARMACY

208 **News**

Review of 1991 shows 30 new drugs, several important biologics cleared for marketing . . . Pfizer delays marketing azithromycin . . . FDA warns of overdose risk from dosage cups . . . FDA seizes cold sterilizing solution . . . Pamidronate released for management of hypercalcemia of malignancy . . . Quinapril marketed as antihypertensive agent . . . False-positive viral antibody test results reported in influenza vaccine recipients

222 **Letters**

Diffuse rash associated with transdermal fentanyl, Cheryl A. Stoukides, Mary Stegman

Therapy Reviews

223 **Gram-negative sepsis, the sepsis syndrome, and the role of antiendotoxin monoclonal antibodies**
Steven L. Barriere and B. Joseph Guglielmo

236 **Treatment of preeclampsia and eclampsia**
Janet McCombs

Therapy Update

246 **Systemic absorption of intraperitoneal antimicrobials in continuous ambulatory peritoneal dialysis**
Maureen A. O'Brien and Nancy A. Mason

Editorial

255 **Who should receive antiendotoxin monoclonal antibody therapy?**
Thomas C. Hardin and Joseph T. DiPiro

DUE Criteria

257 **Criteria for use of antiendotoxin monoclonal antibodies (HA-1A and E5) in adult and pediatric inpatients**
Michele F. Shepherd

261 **CP Continuing Education**

273 **Current Literature**

Drug Reaction Alerts . . . Book Reviews: *Guide to Clinical Trials* (*Spilker*), James E. Tisdale . . . *Pharmacokinetics and Pharmacodynamics, Volume 3: Peptides, Peptoids, and Proteins* (*Garzone, Colburn, Mokotoff*), C. Lindsay DeVane

280 **Advertising Index**

Instructions to Authors

CLINICAL PHARMACY, a forum for the drug therapeutics information that pharmacists need to perform their clinical roles, gives priority to (1) studies that objectively evaluate drug effects in human trials, (2) evaluative review articles on the clinical uses of new drugs, and (3) evaluations of the current status of drug therapy in selected diseases. Contributions to the following sections are invited.

Drug Reviews: Detailed, analytical reviews on the clinical use of specific drugs, with preference given to new drugs and to evaluative rather than descriptive literature reviews.

Therapy Reviews: Articles that focus primarily on a disease state and its treatment.

Therapy Update: Concise analytical reviews of narrowly defined, important topics in pharmacotherapy.

Clinical Frontiers: Articles that review important, ongoing research on disease processes, drug mechanisms, or new technologies and project the likely implications for therapy.

Research: Reports of well-conducted original research on drug effects in humans.

Research Notes: Short research reports, such as updates on previously published work, confirmations of previous findings, or original research of modest scope.

Grand Rounds: Patient case reports and literature reviews combined in a way that gives them high educational value.

Drug Experience: Straightforward reports, with selected literature references, of unusual drug experiences.

Therapy Consultation: Brief advice, in a question-and-answer format, on how to handle specific drug-therapy problems. Readers are invited to submit questions, which the editor will forward to consultants for answering.

Letters: Short comments on previously published work or about potential problems, apparent trends, or controversies in drug therapy or clinical research.

Commentaries: Well-reasoned expressions of opinion on drug-therapy or clinical-research issues.

The editors have the sole authority to decide in which section to publish an accepted manuscript.

Manuscripts are subject to review by qualified outside reviewers, as well as by the editors, and will be accepted for publication only if they are believed to represent an important contribution to the literature. All papers submitted for publication must be accompanied by a completed copy of a manuscript checklist. The checklist, which generally conforms to the Uniform Requirements for Manuscripts Submitted to Biomedical Journals, appears on pages 60-61 of the January 1992 issue. Authors of especially important original work may request "fast-track" review of their papers. Authors may suggest appropriate reviewers for their papers.

Accepted materials become the permanent and sole property of ASHP and may not be published or reprinted elsewhere without written permission from both the author and the editor.

The editors reserve the right to revise all materials submitted, if necessary. The publisher assumes no responsibility for the statements and opinions advanced by contributors to CLINICAL PHARMACY.

Under the terms of the Copyright Revision Act of 1976 (Public Law 94-553) it is necessary to have the rights of the authors transferred to the publisher in order to provide for the widest possible dissemination of professional and scientific literature. Accordingly, all transmittal letters accompanying manuscripts submitted for publication, including contributions for the Letters column, must contain the following language: "In consideration of the American Society of Hospital Pharmacists (ASHP) taking action in reviewing and editing my (our) submission, the author(s) undersigned hereby transfer(s), assign(s), or otherwise convey(s) all ownership rights in the submission and all copyright ownership to ASHP. In the event that such work is not published by ASHP, all said rights shall be released." We regret that we cannot consider manuscripts for publication that are not accompanied by transmittal letters containing the above language signed by all authors.

Authors must certify in their letter of transmittal that none of the material in their manuscript has been published previously nor is under consideration or been accepted for publication elsewhere. If this certification cannot be made, suitable explanation must be offered.

Eight copies of all manuscripts should be submitted. Manuscripts should be typewritten with double spacing (including tables) on one side of good-quality, 21.6 x 27.9-cm white paper, and with margins of at least 2.5 cm. For guidance on style, authors should consult the manuscript checklist, recent issues of CLINICAL PHARMACY, and the *Council of Biology Editors Style Manual, fifth edition. The American Heritage Dictionary of the English Language and the AMA's Manual of Style* contain helpful advice on correct usage.

Galley proofs or final edited manuscripts are sent to authors for inspection against the original manuscript and for correction. Unnecessary alterations at this stage must be avoided. An order form for reprints is sent to the corresponding author at the time of publication.

CLINICAL PHARMACY (ISSN 0278-2677) is published monthly by the American Society of Hospital Pharmacists, 4630 Montgomery Avenue, Bethesda, MD 20814. Joseph A. Oddis, Executive Vice President. Second-class postage is paid at Bethesda, MD, and at additional mailing offices. **Postmaster: Send address changes to: *Clinical Pharmacy*, 4630 Montgomery Avenue, Bethesda, MD 20814.**

Annual Subscription Rate:	*USA*	*Non-USA*
ASHP Members	$45	$60
ASHP Student Members and Residents	$35	$50
Institutions and Nonmembers	$80	$95

The cost of single copies is $10. Airmail delivery outside the continental United States is available for an additional charge of $90 per year. Requests to replace missing issues free of charge are honored only up to six months after date of issue.

Payments to ASHP are not deductible as charitable contributions for federal income tax purposes. However, they may be deductible under other provisions of the Internal Revenue Code.

Advertising for CLINICAL PHARMACY is accepted in accordance with the Statement of Advertising Policy of the American Society of Hospital Pharmacists (see *Am J Hosp Pharm.* 1987;44:1146). For additional information, contact the Advertising Representative (William McCausland Associates, Inc., P.O. Box 189, Pitman, NJ 08071. Phone 609-589-5454, Fax 609-582-7611).

All articles published, including editorials, letters, and book reviews, represent the opinions of the authors and do not reflect the official policy of the American Society of Hospital Pharmacists or the institution with which the author is affiliated, unless this is specified.

Microfilm and microfiche editions are available for purchase. Contact University Microfilms, 300 N. Zeeb Road, Ann Arbor, MI 48106.

Articles in CLINICAL PHARMACY are abstracted and indexed in *Current Contents, Clinical Sciences, Current Awareness in Biologic Sciences, Excerpta Medica, Index Medicus, Inpharma, International Pharmaceutical Abstracts*, and *Reactions*.

April 1992 Volume 11, Number 4

Coden: CPHADV ISSN: 0278-2677

CLINICAL PHARMACY

287 **News**

Benzodiazepine antagonist approved by FDA . . . Acellular pertussis vaccine approved by FDA . . . Third HMG-CoA reductase inhibitor marketed for cholesterol reduction . . . Cefprozil enters oral antibiotic market . . . FDA seeks changes in benzodiazepine packaging and labeling . . . EPA seeks information on efficacy of sterilants and disinfectants . . . Expert panel issues guidelines on asthma management . . . Guidelines address systemic glucocorticosteroid use for infection management

308 **Letters**

Topical capsaicin for osteoarthritis, Patrice L. Flynn and Dennis West

308 **Correction**

Special Feature

309 **Acute pain management: Operative or medical procedures and trauma, part 1**
Agency for Health Care Policy and Research

Therapy Updates

332 **New considerations for *Haemophilus influenzae* type b vaccination**
Julianne B. Pinson and C. Wayne Weart

337 **β-Adrenergic antagonists for primary prevention of gastrointestinal hemorrhage in patients with cirrhosis and esophageal varices**
Cheryl A. Elder and Maryann S. Reynolds Restino

Research Notes

342 **Multicenter evaluation of a patient-controlled analgesia device for the treatment of postoperative pain**
Daniel P. Wermeling, Stan A. Greene, Bradley A. Boucher, Mark E. Lehman, Gerald G. Briggs, Edward R. Bezarro, and Thomas S. Foster

347 **Effect of lidocaine–prilocaine cream on pain from subcutaneous injection**
Anna Taddio, Isabelle Robieux, and Gideon Koren

Commentary

350 **Treating ischemic stroke: Is nimodipine the answer?**
Edzard Ernst

Drug Experience

352 **Simultaneous concentrations of ciprofloxacin in breast milk and in serum in mother and breast-fed infant**
Debra K. Gardner, Steven G. Gabbe, and Chris Harter

DUE Criteria

355 **Criteria for use of colfosceril (Exosurf Neonatal) in neonates**
Varsha Bhatt-Mehta and Robert E. Schumacher

357 **Criteria for use of beractant (Survanta) in neonates**
Rebecca Rogers Prevost, Robert Mirro, and Sheldon B. Korones

368 **Current Literature**

Drug Reaction Alerts . . . Book Review: *Data Collection Forms in Clinical Trials (Spilker, Schoenfelder)*, Karen J. Schoenbrun . . . Books Received

374 **Advertising Index**

Instructions to Authors

Clinical Pharmacy, a forum for the drug therapeutics information that pharmacists need to perform their clinical roles, gives priority to (1) studies that objectively evaluate drug effects in human trials, (2) evaluative review articles on the clinical uses of new drugs, and (3) evaluations of the current status of drug therapy in selected diseases. Contributions to the following sections are invited.

Drug Reviews: Detailed, analytical reviews on the clinical use of specific drugs, with preference given to new drugs and to evaluative rather than descriptive literature reviews.

Therapy Reviews: Articles that focus primarily on a disease state and its treatment.

Therapy Update: Concise analytical reviews of narrowly defined, important topics in pharmacotherapy.

Clinical Frontiers: Articles that review important, ongoing research on disease processes, drug mechanisms, or new technologies and project the likely implications for therapy.

Research: Reports of well-conducted original research on drug effects in humans.

Research Notes: Short research reports, such as updates on previously published work, confirmations of previous findings, or original research of modest scope.

Grand Rounds: Patient case reports and literature reviews combined in a way that gives them high educational value.

Drug Experience: Straightforward reports, with selected literature references, of unusual drug experiences.

Therapy Consultation: Brief advice, in a question-and-answer format, on how to handle specific drug-therapy problems. Readers are invited to submit questions, which the editor will forward to consultants for answering.

Letters: Short comments on previously published work or about potential problems, apparent trends, or controversies in drug therapy or clinical research.

Commentaries: Well-reasoned expressions of opinion on drug-therapy or clinical-research issues.

The editors have the sole authority to decide in which section to publish an accepted manuscript.

Manuscripts are subject to review by qualified outside reviewers, as well as by the editors, and will be accepted for publication only if they are believed to represent an important contribution to the literature. All papers submitted for publication must be accompanied by a completed copy of a manuscript checklist. The checklist, which generally conforms to the Uniform Requirements for Manuscripts Submitted to Biomedical Journals, appears on pages 60-61 of the January 1992 issue. Authors of especially important original work may request "fast-track" review of their papers. Authors may suggest appropriate reviewers for their papers.

Accepted materials become the permanent and sole property of ASHP and may not be published or reprinted elsewhere without written permission from both the author and the editor.

The editors reserve the right to revise all materials submitted, if necessary. The publisher assumes no responsibility for the statements and opinions advanced by contributors to Clinical Pharmacy.

Under the terms of the Copyright Revision Act of 1976 (Public Law 94-553) it is necessary to have the rights of the authors transferred to the publisher in order to provide for the widest possible dissemination of professional and scientific literature. Accordingly, all transmittal letters accompanying manuscripts submitted for publication, including contributions for the Letters column, must contain the following language: "In consideration of the American Society of Hospital Pharmacists (ASHP) taking action in reviewing and editing my (our) submission, the author(s) undersigned hereby transfer(s), assign(s), or otherwise convey(s) all ownership rights in the submission and all copyright ownership to ASHP. In the event that such work is not published by ASHP, all said rights shall be released." We regret that we cannot consider manuscripts for publication that are not accompanied by transmittal letters containing the above language signed by all authors.

Authors must certify in their letter of transmittal that none of the material in their manuscript has been published previously nor is under consideration or been accepted for publication elsewhere. If this certification cannot be made, suitable explanation must be offered.

Eight copies of all manuscripts should be submitted. Manuscripts should be typewritten with double spacing (including tables) on one side of good-quality, 21.6 x 27.9-cm white paper, and with margins of at least 2.5 cm. For guidance on style, authors should consult the manuscript checklist, recent issues of Clinical Pharmacy, and the *Council of Biology Editors Style Manual, fifth edition. The American Heritage Dictionary of the English Language and the AMA's Manual of Style* contain helpful advice on correct usage.

Galley proofs or final edited manuscripts are sent to authors for inspection against the original manuscript and for correction. Unnecessary alterations at this stage must be avoided. An order form for reprints is sent to the corresponding author at the time of publication.

Clinical Pharmacy (ISSN 0278-2677) is published monthly by the American Society of Hospital Pharmacists, 4630 Montgomery Avenue, Bethesda, MD 20814. Joseph A. Oddis, Executive Vice President. Second-class postage is paid at Bethesda, MD, and at additional mailing offices. **Postmaster: Send address changes to: *Clinical Pharmacy*, 4630 Montgomery Avenue, Bethesda, MD 20814.**

Annual Subscription Rate:	*USA*	*Non-USA*
ASHP Members	$45	$60
ASHP Student Members and Residents	$35	$50
Institutions and Nonmembers	$80	$95

The cost of single copies is $10. Airmail delivery outside the continental United States is available for an additional charge of $90 per year. Requests to replace missing issues free of charge are honored only up to six months after date of issue.

Payments to ASHP are not deductible as charitable contributions for federal income tax purposes. However, they may be deductible under other provisions of the Internal Revenue Code.

Advertising for Clinical Pharmacy is accepted in accordance with the Statement of Advertising Policy of the American Society of Hospital Pharmacists (see *Am J Hosp Pharm.* 1987;44:1146). For additional information, contact the Advertising Representative (William McCausland Associates, Inc., P.O. Box 189, Pitman, NJ 08071. Phone 609-589-5454, Fax 609-582-7611).

All articles published, including editorials, letters, and book reviews, represent the opinions of the authors and do not reflect the official policy of the American Society of Hospital Pharmacists or the institution with which the author is affiliated, unless this is specified.

Microfilm and microfiche editions are available for purchase. Contact University Microfilms, 300 N. Zeeb Road, Ann Arbor, MI 48106.

Articles in Clinical Pharmacy are abstracted and indexed in *Current Contents, Clinical Sciences, Current Awareness in Biologic Sciences, Excerpta Medica, Index Medicus, Inpharma, International Pharmaceutical Abstracts*, and *Reactions*.

May 1992 Volume 11, Number 5 Coden: CPHADV ISSN: 0278-2677

CLINICAL PHARMACY

378 **News**

HDL testing should be routine part of assessments of coronary heart disease risk, says consensus panel . . . Oral temafloxacin approved for U.S. market . . . Sertraline cleared for marketing as antidepressant . . . Nabumetone marketed for osteoarthritis, rheumatoid arthritis . . . FDA warns quality of underground zalcitabine is poor; Roche expands premarketing access programs . . . Tacrine made available under treatment IND protocol

386 **Letters**

Asthma in children, Dennis M. Williams; Pamela A. Simon, Christine M. Murphy, Shannon L. Coonce . . . Use of succimer, Steven M. Marcus, Bruce Ruck; Katherine V. Mann, John D. Travers; William Banner, Jr.

Special Feature

391 **Acute pain management: Operative or medical procedures and trauma, part 2**
Agency for Health Care Policy and Research

Drug Review

415 **Doxazosin: A new α_1-adrenergic antagonist**
Kenneth S. Babamoto and William T. Hirokawa

Research Notes

428 **Absolute bioavailability of aminophylline liquid administered enterally in adults requiring mechanical ventilation**
Karen F. Shalansky, Leigh M. Vaughan, Cristina Ustad, Martin G. Tweeddale, and Steven A. Sahn

432 **Possible ganciclovir-induced hepatotoxicity in patients with AIDS**
Helen L. Figge, George R. Bailie, Laurie L. Briceland, and Steven F. Kowalsky

DUE Criteria

435 **Criteria for use of pancuronium bromide, vecuronium bromide, atracurium besylate, tubocurarine chloride, metocurine iodide, pipecuronium bromide, and doxacurium chloride**
Andrew J. Donnelly, Julie A. Golembiewski, Richard Skupski, and Jeffrey E. Wojtynek

442 **CP Continuing Education**

448 **Current Literature**

Drug Reaction Alerts . . . Books Received

454 **Advertising Index**

Editorial Office
4630 Montgomery Avenue
Bethesda, MD 20814
301-657-3000
Fax 301-657-1615

Advertising Representative
William McCausland Associates, Inc.
P.O. Box 189
Pitman, NJ 08071
609-589-5454
Fax 609-582-7611

Printed on acid-free paper effective with Volume 8, January 1989.

Instructions to Authors

Clinical Pharmacy, a forum for the drug therapeutics information that pharmacists need to perform their clinical roles, gives priority to (1) studies that objectively evaluate drug effects in human trials, (2) evaluative review articles on the clinical uses of new drugs, and (3) evaluations of the current status of drug therapy in selected diseases. Contributions to the following sections are invited.

Drug Reviews: Detailed, analytical reviews on the clinical use of specific drugs, with preference given to new drugs and to evaluative rather than descriptive literature reviews.

Therapy Reviews: Articles that focus primarily on a disease state and its treatment.

Therapy Update: Concise analytical reviews of narrowly defined, important topics in pharmacotherapy.

Clinical Frontiers: Articles that review important, ongoing research on disease processes, drug mechanisms, or new technologies and project the likely implications for therapy.

Research: Reports of well-conducted original research on drug effects in humans.

Research Notes: Short research reports, such as updates on previously published work, confirmations of previous findings, or original research of modest scope.

Grand Rounds: Patient case reports and literature reviews combined in a way that gives them high educational value.

Drug Experience: Straightforward reports, with selected literature references, of unusual drug experiences.

Therapy Consultation: Brief advice, in a question-and-answer format, on how to handle specific drug-therapy problems. Readers are invited to submit questions, which the editor will forward to consultants for answering.

Letters: Short comments on previously published work or about potential problems, apparent trends, or controversies in drug therapy or clinical research.

Commentaries: Well-reasoned expressions of opinion on drug-therapy or clinical-research issues.

The editors have the sole authority to decide in which section to publish an accepted manuscript.

Manuscripts are subject to review by qualified outside reviewers, as well as by the editors, and will be accepted for publication only if they are believed to represent an important contribution to the literature. All papers submitted for publication must be accompanied by a completed copy of a manuscript checklist. The checklist, which generally conforms to the Uniform Requirements for Manuscripts Submitted to Biomedical Journals, appears on pages 60-61 of the January 1992 issue. Authors of especially important original work may request "fast-track" review of their papers. Authors may suggest appropriate reviewers for their papers.

Accepted materials become the permanent and sole property of ASHP and may not be published or reprinted elsewhere without written permission from both the author and the editor.

The editors reserve the right to revise all materials submitted, if necessary. The publisher assumes no responsibility for the statements and opinions advanced by contributors to Clinical Pharmacy.

Under the terms of the Copyright Revision Act of 1976 (Public Law 94-553) it is necessary to have the rights of the authors transferred to the publisher in order to provide for the widest possible dissemination of professional and scientific literature. Accordingly, all transmittal letters accompanying manuscripts submitted for publication, including contributions for the Letters column, must contain the following language: "In consideration of the American Society of Hospital Pharmacists (ASHP) taking action in reviewing and editing my (our) submission, the author(s) undersigned hereby transfer(s), assign(s), or otherwise convey(s) all ownership rights in the submission and all copyright ownership to ASHP. In the event that such work is not published by ASHP, all said rights shall be released." We regret that we cannot consider manuscripts for publication that are not accompanied by transmittal letters containing the above language signed by all authors.

Authors must certify in their letter of transmittal that none of the material in their manuscript has been published previously nor is under consideration or been accepted for publication elsewhere. If this certification cannot be made, suitable explanation must be offered.

Eight copies of all manuscripts should be submitted. Manuscripts should be typewritten with double spacing (including tables) on one side of good-quality, 21.6 x 27.9-cm white paper, and with margins of at least 2.5 cm. For guidance on style, authors should consult the manuscript checklist, recent issues of Clinical Pharmacy, and the *Council of Biology Editors Style Manual, fifth edition. The American Heritage Dictionary of the English Language and the AMA's Manual of Style* contain helpful advice on correct usage.

Galley proofs or final edited manuscripts are sent to authors for inspection against the original manuscript and for correction. Unnecessary alterations at this stage must be avoided. An order form for reprints is sent to the corresponding author at the time of publication.

Clinical Pharmacy (ISSN 0278-2677) is published monthly by the American Society of Hospital Pharmacists, 4630 Montgomery Avenue, Bethesda, MD 20814. Joseph A. Oddis, Executive Vice President. Second-class postage is paid at Bethesda, MD, and at additional mailing offices. **Postmaster: Send address changes to: *Clinical Pharmacy*, 4630 Montgomery Avenue, Bethesda, MD 20814.**

Annual Subscription Rate:	*USA*	*Non-USA*
ASHP Members	$45	$60
ASHP Student Members and Residents	$35	$50
Institutions and Nonmembers	$80	$95

The cost of single copies is $10. Airmail delivery outside the continental United States is available for an additional charge of $90 per year. Requests to replace missing issues free of charge are honored only up to six months after date of issue.

Payments to ASHP are not deductible as charitable contributions for federal income tax purposes. However, they may be deductible under other provisions of the Internal Revenue Code.

Advertising for Clinical Pharmacy is accepted in accordance with the Statement of Advertising Policy of the American Society of Hospital Pharmacists (see *Am J Hosp Pharm.* 1987;44:1146). For additional information, contact the Advertising Representative (William McCausland Associates, Inc., P.O. Box 189, Pitman, NJ 08071. Phone 609-589-5454, Fax 609-582-7611).

All articles published, including editorials, letters, and book reviews, represent the opinions of the authors and do not reflect the official policy of the American Society of Hospital Pharmacists or the institution with which the author is affiliated, unless this is specified.

Microfilm and microfiche editions are available for purchase. Contact University Microfilms, 300 N. Zeeb Road, Ann Arbor, MI 48106.

Articles in Clinical Pharmacy are abstracted and indexed in *Current Contents, Clinical Sciences, Current Awareness in Biologic Sciences, Excerpta Medica, Index Medicus, Inpharma, International Pharmaceutical Abstracts,* and *Reactions.*

June 1992 Volume 11, Number 6 Coden: CPHADV ISSN: 0278-2677

CLINICAL PHARMACY

458 **News**

Heavy use of inhaled β agonists associated with increased risk of fatal or near-fatal asthma, study shows . . . Lomefloxacin reaches U.S. market . . . Warnings about use of angiotensin-converting-enzyme inhibitors in advanced pregnancy strengthened . . . New labeling and patient insert for triazolam approved by FDA . . . Cognitive enhancers illegal, says FDA . . . Call for applications to conduct research on patient outcomes associated with pharmaceutical therapy in ambulatory-care setting

Special Feature

483 **ASHP therapeutic guidelines on antimicrobial prophylaxis in surgery**
ASHP Commission on Therapeutics

Drug Review

514 **Mesalamine and olsalazine: 5-Aminosalicylic acid agents for the treatment of inflammatory bowel disease**
Larry W. Segars and Barry J. Gales

Therapy Update

529 **Methotrexate for treatment of unruptured ectopic pregnancy**
Rebecca Rogers Prevost, Thomas G. Stovall, and Frank W. Ling

Research

533 **Effect of a single dose of lactase on symptoms and expired hydrogen after lactose challenge in lactose-intolerant subjects**
Steven W. Sanders, Keith G. Tolman, and Donald P. Reitberg

539 **Bioequivalence of verapamil hydrochloride extended-release pellet-filled capsules when opened and sprinkled on food and when swallowed intact**
Gary D. Kozloski, Joseph M. De Vito, Jerry B. Johnson, Gregory B. Holmes, Margaret A. Adams, and Thomas L. Hunt

543 **Complications of home parenteral nutrition**
Eric T. Herfindal, Linda R. Bernstein, Alvin F. Wong, Valerie W. Hogue, and Jeanne A. Darbinian

Commentary

549 **New calcium-channel blockers: Improved therapy?**
Edmund V. Capparelli

DUE Criteria

553 **Criteria for use of agents for extrapyramidal adverse effects in adult, adolescent, and child inpatients and outpatients**
Patricia A. Marken and Jeanne R. Ezell

559 **CP Continuing Education**

561 **ASHP Journal Continuing-Education Instructions and Enrollment Form**

562 **Current Literature**

Drug Reaction Alerts . . . Book Reviews: *Combined Modality Cancer Therapy: Radiation and Infusional Chemotherapy* (*Lokich, Byfield*), Richard Slimowitz . . . Drugs in Gastroenterology (*Braga, Guslandi, Tittobello*), Curtis E. Haas . . . *Self-study Materials: Concepts in Oncology Therapeutics: A Self-Instructional Course* (*Finley*), Robert J. Ignoffo . . . Books Received

570 **Advertising Index**

Editorial Office
4630 Montgomery Avenue
Bethesda, MD 20814
301-657-3000
Fax 301-657-1615

Advertising Representative
William McCausland Associates, Inc.
P.O. Box 189
Pitman, NJ 08071
609-589-5454
Fax 609-582-7611

Printed on acid-free paper effective with Volume 8, January 1989.

Instructions to Authors

Clinical Pharmacy, a forum for the drug therapeutics information that pharmacists need to perform their clinical roles, gives priority to (1) studies that objectively evaluate drug effects in human trials, (2) evaluative review articles on the clinical uses of new drugs, and (3) evaluations of the current status of drug therapy in selected diseases. Contributions to the following sections are invited.

Drug Reviews: Detailed, analytical reviews on the clinical use of specific drugs, with preference given to new drugs and to evaluative rather than descriptive literature reviews.

Therapy Reviews: Articles that focus primarily on a disease state and its treatment.

Therapy Update: Concise analytical reviews of narrowly defined, important topics in pharmacotherapy.

Clinical Frontiers: Articles that review important, ongoing research on disease processes, drug mechanisms, or new technologies and project the likely implications for therapy.

Research: Reports of well-conducted original research on drug effects in humans.

Research Notes: Short research reports, such as updates on previously published work, confirmations of previous findings, or original research of modest scope.

Grand Rounds: Patient case reports and literature reviews combined in a way that gives them high educational value.

Drug Experience: Straightforward reports, with selected literature references, of unusual drug experiences.

Therapy Consultation: Brief advice, in a question-and-answer format, on how to handle specific drug-therapy problems. Readers are invited to submit questions, which the editor will forward to consultants for answering.

Letters: Short comments on previously published work or about potential problems, apparent trends, or controversies in drug therapy or clinical research.

Commentaries: Well-reasoned expressions of opinion on drug-therapy or clinical-research issues.

The editors have the sole authority to decide in which section to publish an accepted manuscript.

Manuscripts are subject to review by qualified outside reviewers, as well as by the editors, and will be accepted for publication only if they are believed to represent an important contribution to the literature. All papers submitted for publication must be accompanied by a completed copy of a manuscript checklist. The checklist, which generally conforms to the Uniform Requirements for Manuscripts Submitted to Biomedical Journals, appears on pages 60-61 of the January 1992 issue. Authors of especially important original work may request "fast-track" review of their papers. Authors may suggest appropriate reviewers for their papers.

Accepted materials become the permanent and sole property of ASHP and may not be published or reprinted elsewhere without written permission from both the author and the editor.

The editors reserve the right to revise all materials submitted, if necessary. The publisher assumes no responsibility for the statements and opinions advanced by contributors to Clinical Pharmacy.

Under the terms of the Copyright Revision Act of 1976 (Public Law 94-553) it is necessary to have the rights of the authors transferred to the publisher in order to provide for the widest possible dissemination of professional and scientific literature. Accordingly, all transmittal letters accompanying manuscripts submitted for publication, including contributions for the Letters column, must contain the following language: "In consideration of the American Society of Hospital Pharmacists (ASHP) taking action in reviewing and editing my (our) submission, the author(s) undersigned hereby transfer(s), assign(s), or otherwise convey(s) all ownership rights in the submission and all copyright ownership to ASHP. In the event that such work is not published by ASHP, all said rights shall be released." We regret that we cannot consider manuscripts for publication that are not accompanied by transmittal letters containing the above language signed by all authors.

Authors must certify in their letter of transmittal that none of the material in their manuscript has been published previously nor is under consideration or been accepted for publication elsewhere. If this certification cannot be made, suitable explanation must be offered.

Eight copies of all manuscripts should be submitted. Manuscripts should be typewritten with double spacing (including tables) on one side of good-quality, 21.6 x 27.9-cm white paper, and with margins of at least 2.5 cm. For guidance on style, authors should consult the manuscript checklist, recent issues of Clinical Pharmacy, and the *Council of Biology Editors Style Manual, fifth edition. The American Heritage Dictionary of the English Language and the AMA's Manual of Style* contain helpful advice on correct usage.

Galley proofs or final edited manuscripts are sent to authors for inspection against the original manuscript and for correction. Unnecessary alterations at this stage must be avoided. An order form for reprints is sent to the corresponding author at the time of publication.

Clinical Pharmacy (ISSN 0278-2677) is published monthly by the American Society of Hospital Pharmacists, 4630 Montgomery Avenue, Bethesda, MD 20814. Joseph A. Oddis, Executive Vice President. Second-class postage is paid at Bethesda, MD, and at additional mailing offices. **Postmaster: Send address changes to: *Clinical Pharmacy*, 4630 Montgomery Avenue, Bethesda, MD 20814.**

Annual Subscription Rate:	*USA*	*Non-USA*
ASHP Members	$45	$60
ASHP Student Members and Residents	$35	$50
Institutions and Nonmembers	$80	$95

The cost of single copies is $10. Airmail delivery outside the continental United States is available for an additional charge of $90 per year. Requests to replace missing issues free of charge are honored only up to six months after date of issue.

Payments to ASHP are not deductible as charitable contributions for federal income tax purposes. However, they may be deductible under other provisions of the Internal Revenue Code.

Advertising for Clinical Pharmacy is accepted in accordance with the Statement of Advertising Policy of the American Society of Hospital Pharmacists (see *Am J Hosp Pharm.* 1987; 44:1146). For additional information, contact the Advertising Representative (William McCausland Associates, Inc., P.O. Box 189, Pitman, NJ 08071. Phone 609-589-5454, Fax 609-582-7611).

All articles published, including editorials, letters, and book reviews, represent the opinions of the authors and do not reflect the official policy of the American Society of Hospital Pharmacists or the institution with which the author is affiliated, unless this is specified.

Microfilm and microfiche editions are available for purchase. Contact University Microfilms, 300 N. Zeeb Road, Ann Arbor, MI 48106.

Articles in Clinical Pharmacy are abstracted and indexed in *Current Contents, Clinical Sciences, Current Awareness in Biologic Sciences, Excerpta Medica, Index Medicus, Inpharma, International Pharmaceutical Abstracts*, and *Reactions*.

July 1992 Volume 11, Number 7 Coden: CPHADV ISSN: 0278-2677

CLINICAL PHARMACY

574 **News**

FDA announces four initiatives for drug approval system . . . Results of ISIS-3 published . . . Pediatrics academy issues new guidelines for acellular pertussis vaccine use

583 **Letters**

Use of surfactant products, Elizabeth M. Zola . . . Value of transdermal fentanyl, Dennis W. Joubert; David R. Kohler, Karim A. Calis, and Diane M. Corso

585 **Correction**

Drug Reviews

591 **Oxaprozin: A once-daily nonsteroidal anti-inflammatory drug**
Lucinda G. Miller

603 **Ticlopidine: A new platelet aggregation inhibitor**
Matthew K. Ito, Alden R. Smith, and Marisa L. Lee

Therapy Update

618 **Long-term dobutamine therapy for refractory congestive heart failure**
Kerry K. Pickworth

Research

625 **Influence of sucralfate on the detection of occult blood in simulated gastric fluid by two screening tests**
Jonathan S. Holman and Jill A. Shwed

Research Note

628 **Safety and tolerability of an intravenous immune globulin at various concentrations in 5% dextrose injection or sterile water for injection**
Kenneth B. Miller, David P. Schenkein, and Richard L. Wasserman

Grand Rounds

632 **Warfarin-induced intramural hematoma of the small intestine**
Minyon L. Avent, Bruce R. Canaday, and William T. Sawyer

Drug Experience

636 **Sucralfate-associated aluminum toxicity in a patient with renal failure: Treatment with deferoxamine**
David I. Min and John A. D'Elia

640 **CP Continuing Education**

649 **FDA Adverse Reaction Report Form and Instructions**

652 **Current Literature**

Drug Reaction Alerts . . . Book Review: *The Biochemical Basis of Neuropharmacology, Sixth Edition (Cooper, Bloom, Roth)*, Martha P. Fankhauser . . . Books Received

656 **Advertising Index**

Instructions to Authors

Clinical Pharmacy, a forum for the drug therapeutics information that pharmacists need to perform their clinical roles, gives priority to (1) studies that objectively evaluate drug effects in human trials, (2) evaluative review articles on the clinical uses of new drugs, and (3) evaluations of the current status of drug therapy in selected diseases. Contributions to the following sections are invited.

Drug Reviews: Detailed, analytical reviews on the clinical use of specific drugs, with preference given to new drugs and to evaluative rather than descriptive literature reviews.

Therapy Reviews: Articles that focus primarily on a disease state and its treatment.

Therapy Update: Concise analytical reviews of narrowly defined, important topics in pharmacotherapy.

Clinical Frontiers: Articles that review important, ongoing research on disease processes, drug mechanisms, or new technologies and project the likely implications for therapy.

Research: Reports of well-conducted original research on drug effects in humans.

Research Notes: Short research reports, such as updates on previously published work, confirmations of previous findings, or original research of modest scope.

Grand Rounds: Patient case reports and literature reviews combined in a way that gives them high educational value.

Drug Experience: Straightforward reports, with selected literature references, of unusual drug experiences.

Therapy Consultation: Brief advice, in a question-and-answer format, on how to handle specific drug-therapy problems. Readers are invited to submit questions, which the editor will forward to consultants for answering.

Letters: Short comments on previously published work or about potential problems, apparent trends, or controversies in drug therapy or clinical research.

Commentaries: Well-reasoned expressions of opinion on drug-therapy or clinical-research issues.

The editors have the sole authority to decide in which section to publish an accepted manuscript.

Manuscripts are subject to review by qualified outside reviewers, as well as by the editors, and will be accepted for publication only if they are believed to represent an important contribution to the literature. All papers submitted for publication must be accompanied by a completed copy of a manuscript checklist. The checklist, which generally conforms to the Uniform Requirements for Manuscripts Submitted to Biomedical Journals, appears on pages 60-61 of the January 1992 issue. Authors of especially important original work may request "fast-track" review of their papers. Authors may suggest appropriate reviewers for their papers.

Accepted materials become the permanent and sole property of ASHP and may not be published or reprinted elsewhere without written permission from both the author and the editor.

The editors reserve the right to revise all materials submitted, if necessary. The publisher assumes no responsibility for the statements and opinions advanced by contributors to Clinical Pharmacy.

Under the terms of the Copyright Revision Act of 1976 (Public Law 94-553) it is necessary to have the rights of the authors transferred to the publisher in order to provide for the widest possible dissemination of professional and scientific literature. Accordingly, all transmittal letters accompanying manuscripts submitted for publication, including contributions for the Letters column, must contain the following language: "In consideration of the American Society of Hospital Pharmacists (ASHP) taking action in reviewing and editing my (our) submission, the author(s) undersigned hereby transfer(s), assign(s), or otherwise convey(s) all ownership rights in the submission and all copyright ownership to ASHP. In the event that such work is not published by ASHP, all said rights shall be released." We regret that we cannot consider manuscripts for publication that are not accompanied by transmittal letters containing the above language signed by all authors.

Authors must certify in their letter of transmittal that none of the material in their manuscript has been published previously nor is under consideration or been accepted for publication elsewhere. If this certification cannot be made, suitable explanation must be offered.

Eight copies of all manuscripts should be submitted. Manuscripts should be typewritten with double spacing (including tables) on one side of good-quality, 21.6 x 27.9-cm white paper, and with margins of at least 2.5 cm. For guidance on style, authors should consult the manuscript checklist, recent issues of Clinical Pharmacy, and the *Council of Biology Editors Style Manual, fifth edition. The American Heritage Dictionary of the English Language and the AMA's Manual of Style* contain helpful advice on correct usage.

Galley proofs or final edited manuscripts are sent to authors for inspection against the original manuscript and for correction. Unnecessary alterations at this stage must be avoided. An order form for reprints is sent to the corresponding author at the time of publication.

Clinical Pharmacy (ISSN 0278-2677) is published monthly by the American Society of Hospital Pharmacists, 4630 Montgomery Avenue, Bethesda, MD 20814. Joseph A. Oddis, Executive Vice President. Second-class postage is paid at Bethesda, MD, and at additional mailing offices. **Postmaster: Send address changes to: *Clinical Pharmacy*, 4630 Montgomery Avenue, Bethesda, MD 20814.**

Annual Subscription Rate:	*USA*	*Non-USA*
ASHP Members	$45	$60
ASHP Student Members and Residents	$35	$50
Institutions and Nonmembers	$80	$95

The cost of single copies is $10. Airmail delivery outside the continental United States is available for an additional charge of $90 per year. Requests to replace missing issues free of charge are honored only up to six months after date of issue.

Payments to ASHP are not deductible as charitable contributions for federal income tax purposes. However, they may be deductible under other provisions of the Internal Revenue Code.

Microfilm and microfiche editions are available for purchase. Contact University Microfilms, 300 N. Zeeb Road, Ann Arbor, MI 48106.

Articles in Clinical Pharmacy are abstracted and indexed in *Current Contents, Clinical Sciences, Current Awareness in Biologic Sciences, Excerpta Medica, Index Medicus, Inpharma, International Pharmaceutical Abstracts*, and *Reactions.*

August 1992 Volume 11, Number 8 Coden: CPHADV ISSN: 0278-2677

CLINICAL PHARMACY

669 **News**

FDA approves release of recombinant interleukin-2 product . . . Federal task force revises recommendations for PCP prophylaxis

672 **Therapy Consultation**
Use of ursodiol in a patient with biliary cirrhosis

674 **Letters**

Use of cytomegalovirus immune globulin, David R. Snydman . . . Potential interaction between terfenadine and macrolide antibiotics, Linda M. Cortese, Darrel C. Bjornson

Drug Review

677 **Pravastatin: A new drug for the treatment of hypercholesterolemia**
Paul L. Jungnickel, Kimberly A. Cantral, and Pierre A. Maloley

Therapy Review

690 **Treatment of nonsteroidal anti-inflammatory drug-induced gastropathy**
Donald R. Miller

Therapy Update

705 **Endocrine complications associated with human immunodeficiency virus infection**
Joseph V. Etzel, Joseph M. Brocavich, and Michael Torre

Commentary

714 **Are antiarrhythmic drugs obsolete?**
James E. Tisdale and Charles R. Webb

DUE Criteria

727 **Criteria for use of adenosine in adults with paroxysmal supraventricular tachycardia**
Enid Morales and Patrick L. McCollam

731 **CP Continuing Education**

735 **Current Literature**

Drug Reaction Alerts . . . Book Review: *Manual of Antibiotics and Infectious Diseases, Seventh Edition* (*Conte, Barriere*), Kyle Vance-Bryan . . . Books Received

742 **Advertising Index**

Editorial Office
4630 Montgomery Avenue
Bethesda, MD 20814
301-657-3000
Fax 301-657-1615

Advertising Representative
William McCausland Associates, Inc.
P.O. Box 189
Pitman, NJ 08071
609-589-5454
Fax 609-582-7611

Printed on acid-free paper effective with Volume 8, January 1989.

Instructions to Authors

Clinical Pharmacy, a forum for the drug therapeutics information that pharmacists need to perform their clinical roles, gives priority to (1) studies that objectively evaluate drug effects in human trials, (2) evaluative review articles on the clinical uses of new drugs, and (3) evaluations of the current status of drug therapy in selected diseases. Contributions to the following sections are invited.

Drug Reviews: Detailed, analytical reviews on the clinical use of specific drugs, with preference given to new drugs and to evaluative rather than descriptive literature reviews.

Therapy Reviews: Articles that focus primarily on a disease state and its treatment.

Therapy Update: Concise analytical reviews of narrowly defined, important topics in pharmacotherapy.

Clinical Frontiers: Articles that review important, ongoing research on disease processes, drug mechanisms, or new technologies and project the likely implications for therapy.

Research: Reports of well-conducted original research on drug effects in humans.

Research Notes: Short research reports, such as updates on previously published work, confirmations of previous findings, or original research of modest scope.

Grand Rounds: Patient case reports and literature reviews combined in a way that gives them high educational value.

Drug Experience: Straightforward reports, with selected literature references, of unusual drug experiences.

Therapy Consultation: Brief advice, in a question-and-answer format, on how to handle specific drug-therapy problems. Readers are invited to submit questions, which the editor will forward to consultants for answering.

Letters: Short comments on previously published work or about potential problems, apparent trends, or controversies in drug therapy or clinical research.

Commentaries: Well-reasoned expressions of opinion on drug-therapy or clinical-research issues.

The editors have the sole authority to decide in which section to publish an accepted manuscript.

Manuscripts are subject to review by qualified outside reviewers, as well as by the editors, and will be accepted for publication only if they are believed to represent an important contribution to the literature. All papers submitted for publication must be accompanied by a completed copy of a manuscript checklist. The checklist, which generally conforms to the Uniform Requirements for Manuscripts Submitted to Biomedical Journals, appears on pages 60-61 of the January 1992 issue. Authors of especially important original work may request "fast-track" review of their papers. Authors may suggest appropriate reviewers for their papers.

Accepted materials become the permanent and sole property of ASHP and may not be published or reprinted elsewhere without written permission from both the author and the editor.

The editors reserve the right to revise all materials submitted, if necessary. The publisher assumes no responsibility for the statements and opinions advanced by contributors to Clinical Pharmacy.

Under the terms of the Copyright Revision Act of 1976 (Public Law 94-553) it is necessary to have the rights of the authors transferred to the publisher in order to provide for the widest possible dissemination of professional and scientific literature. Accordingly, all transmittal letters accompanying manuscripts submitted for publication, including contributions for the Letters column, must contain the following language: "In consideration of the American Society of Hospital Pharmacists (ASHP) taking action in reviewing and editing my (our) submission, the author(s) undersigned hereby transfer(s), assign(s), or otherwise convey(s) all ownership rights in the submission and all copyright ownership to ASHP. In the event that such work is not published by ASHP, all said rights shall be released." We regret that we cannot consider manuscripts for publication that are not accompanied by transmittal letters containing the above language signed by all authors.

Authors must certify in their letter of transmittal that none of the material in their manuscript has been published previously nor is under consideration or been accepted for publication elsewhere. If this certification cannot be made, suitable explanation must be offered.

Eight copies of all manuscripts should be submitted. Manuscripts should be typewritten with double spacing (including tables) on one side of good-quality, 21.6 x 27.9-cm white paper, and with margins of at least 2.5 cm. For guidance on style, authors should consult the manuscript checklist, recent issues of Clinical Pharmacy, and the *Council of Biology Editors Style Manual, fifth edition. The American Heritage Dictionary of the English Language and the AMA's Manual of Style* contain helpful advice on correct usage.

Galley proofs or final edited manuscripts are sent to authors for inspection against the original manuscript and for correction. Unnecessary alterations at this stage must be avoided. An order form for reprints is sent to the corresponding author at the time of publication.

Clinical Pharmacy (ISSN 0278-2677) is published monthly by the American Society of Hospital Pharmacists, 4630 Montgomery Avenue, Bethesda, MD 20814. Joseph A. Oddis, Executive Vice President. Second-class postage is paid at Bethesda, MD, and at additional mailing offices. **Postmaster: Send address changes to: *Clinical Pharmacy*, 4630 Montgomery Avenue, Bethesda, MD 20814.**

Annual Subscription Rate:	*USA*	*Non-USA*
ASHP Members	$45	$60
ASHP Student Members and Residents	$35	$50
Institutions and Nonmembers	$80	$95

The cost of single copies is $10. Airmail delivery outside the continental United States is available for an additional charge of $90 per year. Requests to replace missing issues free of charge are honored only up to six months after date of issue.

Payments to ASHP are not deductible as charitable contributions for federal income tax purposes. However, they may be deductible under other provisions of the Internal Revenue Code.

Advertising for Clinical Pharmacy is accepted in accordance with the Statement of Advertising Policy of the American Society of Hospital Pharmacists (see *Am J Hosp Pharm.* 1987;44:1146). For additional information, contact the Advertising Representative (William McCausland Associates, Inc., P.O. Box 189, Pitman, NJ 08071. Phone 609-589-5454, Fax 609-582-7611).

All articles published, including editorials, letters, and book reviews, represent the opinions of the authors and do not reflect the official policy of the American Society of Hospital Pharmacists or the institution with which the author is affiliated, unless this is specified.

Microfilm and microfiche editions are available for purchase. Contact University Microfilms, 300 N. Zeeb Road, Ann Arbor, MI 48106.

Articles in Clinical Pharmacy are abstracted and indexed in *Current Contents, Clinical Sciences, Current Awareness in Biologic Sciences, Excerpta Medica, Index Medicus, Inpharma, International Pharmaceutical Abstracts*, and *Reactions*.

September 1992 Volume 11, Number 9 Coden: CPHADV ISSN: 0278-2677

CLINICAL PHARMACY

747 **News**

Zalcitabine approved under accelerated drug review policy . . . Adverse effects prompt withdrawal of temafloxacin . . . Talley to succeed Zellmer as editor of *AJHP* and *Clinical Pharmacy*

750 **Correction**

751 **Therapy Consultation**

Diabetes control during bowel cleansing with PEG–electrolyte solution

Drug Review

753 **Lomefloxacin and temafloxacin: Two new fluoroquinolone antimicrobials**
William T. Symonds and David E. Nix

Therapy Review

767 **Treatment of adult acute leukemia**
Dayna L. McCauley

Commentary

797 **White clot syndrome and thrombocytopenia: Reasons to abandon heparin i.v. lock flush solution**
James C. Garrelts

Grand Rounds

800 **Dapsone-induced methemoglobinemia and hemolytic anemia**
Brian L. Erstad

Drug Experience

806 **Apparent potentiation of warfarin activity by tetracycline**
Erica A. Danos

DUE Criteria

809 **Criteria for use of amphotericin B bladder irrigation in adult inpatients**
Patricia A. Montgomery, Patricia S. Woster, and Pamala A. Jacobson

811 **CP Continuing Education**

819 **Current Literature**

822 **Advertising Index**

Editorial Office
4630 Montgomery Avenue
Bethesda, MD 20814
301-657-3000
Fax 301-657-1615

Advertising Representative
William McCausland Associates, Inc.
P.O. Box 189
Pitman, NJ 08071
609-589-5454
Fax 609-582-7611

Printed on acid-free paper effective with Volume 8, January 1989.

Instructions to Authors

Clinical Pharmacy, a forum for the drug therapeutics information that pharmacists need to perform their clinical roles, gives priority to (1) studies that objectively evaluate drug effects in human trials, (2) evaluative review articles on the clinical uses of new drugs, and (3) evaluations of the current status of drug therapy in selected diseases. Contributions to the following sections are invited.

Drug Reviews: Detailed, analytical reviews on the clinical use of specific drugs, with preference given to new drugs and to evaluative rather than descriptive literature reviews.

Therapy Reviews: Articles that focus primarily on a disease state and its treatment.

Therapy Update: Concise analytical reviews of narrowly defined, important topics in pharmacotherapy.

Clinical Frontiers: Articles that review important, ongoing research on disease processes, drug mechanisms, or new technologies and project the likely implications for therapy.

Research: Reports of well-conducted original research on drug effects in humans.

Research Notes: Short research reports, such as updates on previously published work, confirmations of previous findings, or original research of modest scope.

Grand Rounds: Patient case reports and literature reviews combined in a way that gives them high educational value.

Drug Experience: Straightforward reports, with selected literature references, of unusual drug experiences.

Therapy Consultation: Brief advice, in a question-and-answer format, on how to handle specific drug-therapy problems. Readers are invited to submit questions, which the editor will forward to consultants for answering.

Letters: Short comments on previously published work or about potential problems, apparent trends, or controversies in drug therapy or clinical research.

Commentaries: Well-reasoned expressions of opinion on drug-therapy or clinical-research issues.

The editors have the sole authority to decide in which section to publish an accepted manuscript.

Manuscripts are subject to review by qualified outside reviewers, as well as by the editors, and will be accepted for publication only if they are believed to represent an important contribution to the literature. All papers submitted for publication must be accompanied by a completed copy of a manuscript checklist. The checklist, which generally conforms to the Uniform Requirements for Manuscripts Submitted to Biomedical Journals, appears on pages 60-61 of the January 1992 issue. Authors of especially important original work may request "fast-track" review of their papers. Authors may suggest appropriate reviewers for their papers.

Accepted materials become the permanent and sole property of ASHP and may not be published or reprinted elsewhere without written permission from both the author and the editor.

The editors reserve the right to revise all materials submitted, if necessary. The publisher assumes no responsibility for the statements and opinions advanced by contributors to Clinical Pharmacy.

Under the terms of the Copyright Revision Act of 1976 (Public Law 94-553) it is necessary to have the rights of the authors transferred to the publisher in order to provide for the widest possible dissemination of professional and scientific literature. Accordingly, all transmittal letters accompanying manuscripts submitted for publication, including contributions for the Letters column, must contain the following language: "In consideration of the American Society of Hospital Pharmacists (ASHP) taking action in reviewing and editing my (our) submission, the author(s) undersigned hereby transfer(s), assign(s), or otherwise convey(s) all ownership rights in the submission and all copyright ownership to ASHP. In the event that such work is not published by ASHP, all said rights shall be released." We regret that we cannot consider manuscripts for publication that are not accompanied by transmittal letters containing the above language signed by all authors.

Authors must certify in their letter of transmittal that none of the material in their manuscript has been published previously nor is under consideration or been accepted for publication elsewhere. If this certification cannot be made, suitable explanation must be offered.

Eight copies of all manuscripts should be submitted. Manuscripts should be typewritten with double spacing (including tables) on one side of good-quality, 21.6 x 27.9-cm white paper, and with margins of at least 2.5 cm. For guidance on style, authors should consult the manuscript checklist, recent issues of Clinical Pharmacy, and the *Council of Biology Editors Style Manual, fifth edition. The American Heritage Dictionary of the English Language and the AMA's Manual of Style* contain helpful advice on correct usage.

Galley proofs or final edited manuscripts are sent to authors for inspection against the original manuscript and for correction. Unnecessary alterations at this stage must be avoided. An order form for reprints is sent to the corresponding author at the time of publication.

Clinical Pharmacy (ISSN 0278-2677) is published monthly by the American Society of Hospital Pharmacists, 4630 Montgomery Avenue, Bethesda, MD 20814. Joseph A. Oddis, Executive Vice President. Second-class postage is paid at Bethesda, MD, and at additional mailing offices. **Postmaster: Send address changes to: *Clinical Pharmacy*, 4630 Montgomery Avenue, Bethesda, MD 20814.**

Annual Subscription Rate:	*USA*	*Non-USA*
ASHP Members	$45	$60
ASHP Student Members and Residents	$35	$50
Institutions and Nonmembers	$80	$95

The cost of single copies is $10. Airmail delivery outside the continental United States is available for an additional charge of $90 per year. Requests to replace missing issues free of charge are honored only up to six months after date of issue.

Payments to ASHP are not deductible as charitable contributions for federal income tax purposes. However, they may be deductible under other provisions of the Internal Revenue Code.

Advertising for Clinical Pharmacy is accepted in accordance with the Statement of Advertising Policy of the American Society of Hospital Pharmacists (see *Am J Hosp Pharm.* 1987;44:1146). For additional information, contact the Advertising Representative (William McCausland Associates, Inc., P.O. Box 189, Pitman, NJ 08071. Phone 609-589-5454, Fax 609-582-7611).

All articles published, including editorials, letters, and book reviews, represent the opinions of the authors and do not reflect the official policy of the American Society of Hospital Pharmacists or the institution with which the author is affiliated, unless this is specified.

Microfilm and microfiche editions are available for purchase. Contact University Microfilms, 300 N. Zeeb Road, Ann Arbor, MI 48106.

Articles in Clinical Pharmacy are abstracted and indexed in *Current Contents, Clinical Sciences, Current Awareness in Biologic Sciences, Excerpta Medica, Index Medicus, Inpharma, International Pharmaceutical Abstracts*, and *Reactions*.

October 1992 Volume 11, Number 10 Coden: CPHADV ISSN: 0278-2677

CLINICAL PHARMACY

825 **News**

Finasteride approved for treatment of benign prostatic hyperplasia . . . Terfenadine and astemizole pose cardiovascular risks to certain patients, health professionals warned

829 **Correction**

830 **Therapy Consultation**

Transdermal scopolamine for hyperemesis gravidarum

Drug Review

834 **Recombinant interferon gamma for treatment of chronic granulomatous disease and other disorders**
Ann M. Bolinger and Mary A. Taeubel

Therapy Review

851 **Management of psychotropic-induced hyperprolactinemia**
Patricia A. Marken, Radwan F. Haykal, and Joseph N. Fisher

Therapy Update

857 **Oral anticoagulant therapy in patients undergoing dental surgery**
Robert T. Weibert

Clinical Frontiers

865 **The postantibiotic effect**
J. Michael Spivey

Commentaries

876 **Characterization of the postantibiotic effect**
Steven C. Ebert

877 **Regularly scheduled versus as-needed use of inhaled β agonists in the treatment of asthma**
Malcolm R. Hill and Kathryn V. Blake

Drug Experience

880 **Colfosceril in an infant with adult respiratory distress syndrome**
C. Y. Jennifer Chan, Terri L. Barton, and Deborah K. Rasch

883 **Fluconazole failure in a child with burns and candidemia**
Dean C. Wilson

DUE Criteria

885 **Criteria for use of didanosine in adult and pediatric patients**
Linda M. Cortese and Darrel C. Bjornson

892 **CP Continuing Education**

895 **Current Literature**

Drug Reaction Alerts . . . Book Reviews: *Applied Therapeutics: The Clinical Use of Drugs, Fifth Edition* (*Koda-Kimble, Young*), Vincent F. Mauro and Laurie S. Mauro . . . *Clinical Immunotoxicology* (*Newcombe, Rose, Bloom*), Daniel P. Healy . . . *Handbook of Basic Pharmacokinetics . . . including Clinical Applications, Fourth Edition* (Ritschel), Larry E. Patterson . . . *Neoplastic Diseases: Fundamentals of Clinical Oncology* (*Rosenthal*), Bud J. Kane and John G. Kuhn . . . Books Received

904 **Advertising Index**

Editorial Office
7272 Wisconsin Avenue
Bethesda, MD 20814
301-657-3000
Fax 301-657-1258

Advertising Representative
William McCausland Associates, Inc.
P.O. Box 189
Pitman, NJ 08071
609-589-5454
Fax 609-582-7611

Printed on acid-free paper effective with Volume 8, January 1989.

Instructions to Authors

Clinical Pharmacy, a forum for the drug therapeutics information that pharmacists need to perform their clinical roles, gives priority to (1) studies that objectively evaluate drug effects in human trials, (2) evaluative review articles on the clinical uses of new drugs, and (3) evaluations of the current status of drug therapy in selected diseases. Contributions to the following sections are invited.

Drug Reviews: Detailed, analytical reviews on the clinical use of specific drugs, with preference given to new drugs and to evaluative rather than descriptive literature reviews.

Therapy Reviews: Articles that focus primarily on a disease state and its treatment.

Therapy Update: Concise analytical reviews of narrowly defined, important topics in pharmacotherapy.

Clinical Frontiers: Articles that review important, ongoing research on disease processes, drug mechanisms, or new technologies and project the likely implications for therapy.

Research: Reports of well-conducted original research on drug effects in humans.

Research Notes: Short research reports, such as updates on previously published work, confirmations of previous findings, or original research of modest scope.

Grand Rounds: Patient case reports and literature reviews combined in a way that gives them high educational value.

Drug Experience: Straightforward reports, with selected literature references, of unusual drug experiences.

Therapy Consultation: Brief advice, in a question-and-answer format, on how to handle specific drug-therapy problems. Readers are invited to submit questions, which the editor will forward to consultants for answering.

Letters: Short comments on previously published work or about potential problems, apparent trends, or controversies in drug therapy or clinical research.

Commentaries: Well-reasoned expressions of opinion on drug-therapy or clinical-research issues.

The editors have the sole authority to decide in which section to publish an accepted manuscript.

Manuscripts are subject to review by qualified outside reviewers, as well as by the editors, and will be accepted for publication only if they are believed to represent an important contribution to the literature. All papers submitted for publication must be accompanied by a completed copy of a manuscript checklist. The checklist, which generally conforms to the Uniform Requirements for Manuscripts Submitted to Biomedical Journals, appears on pages 60-61 of the January 1992 issue. Authors of especially important original work may request "fast-track" review of their papers. Authors may suggest appropriate reviewers for their papers.

Accepted materials become the permanent and sole property of ASHP and may not be published or reprinted elsewhere without written permission from both the author and the editor.

The editors reserve the right to revise all materials submitted, if necessary. The publisher assumes no responsibility for the statements and opinions advanced by contributors to Clinical Pharmacy.

Under the terms of the Copyright Revision Act of 1976 (Public Law 94-553) it is necessary to have the rights of the authors transferred to the publisher in order to provide for the widest possible dissemination of professional and scientific literature. Accordingly, all transmittal letters accompanying manuscripts submitted for publication, including contributions for the Letters column, must contain the following language: "In consideration of the American Society of Hospital Pharmacists (ASHP) taking action in reviewing and editing my (our) submission, the author(s) undersigned hereby transfer(s), assign(s), or otherwise convey(s) all ownership rights in the submission and all copyright ownership to ASHP. In the event that such work is not published by ASHP, all said rights shall be released." We regret that we cannot consider manuscripts for publication that are not accompanied by transmittal letters containing the above language signed by all authors.

Authors must certify in their letter of transmittal that none of the material in their manuscript has been published previously nor is under consideration or been accepted for publication elsewhere. If this certification cannot be made, suitable explanation must be offered.

Eight copies of all manuscripts should be submitted. Manuscripts should be typewritten with double spacing (including tables) on one side of good-quality, 21.6 x 27.9-cm white paper, and with margins of at least 2.5 cm. For guidance on style, authors should consult the manuscript checklist, recent issues of Clinical Pharmacy, and the *Council of Biology Editors Style Manual, fifth edition. The American Heritage Dictionary of the English Language and the AMA's Manual of Style* contain helpful advice on correct usage.

Galley proofs or final edited manuscripts are sent to authors for inspection against the original manuscript and for correction. Unnecessary alterations at this stage must be avoided. An order form for reprints is sent to the corresponding author at the time of publication.

Clinical Pharmacy (ISSN 0278-2677) is published monthly by the American Society of Hospital Pharmacists, 7272 Wisconsin Avenue, Bethesda, MD 20814. Joseph A. Oddis, Executive Vice President. Second-class postage is paid at Bethesda, MD, and at additional mailing offices. **Postmaster: Send address changes to: *Clinical Pharmacy*, 7272 Wisconsin Avenue, Bethesda, MD 20814.**

Annual Subscription Rate:	*USA*	*Non-USA*
ASHP Members	$49	$64
ASHP Student Members and Residents	$39	$39
Institutions and Nonmembers	$89	$104

The cost of single copies is $10. Airmail delivery outside the continental United States is available for an additional charge of $90 per year. Requests to replace missing issues free of charge are honored only up to six months after date of issue.

Payments to ASHP are not deductible as charitable contributions for federal income tax purposes. However, they may be deductible under other provisions of the Internal Revenue Code.

Advertising for Clinical Pharmacy is accepted in accordance with the Statement of Advertising Policy of the American Society of Hospital Pharmacists (see *Am J Hosp Pharm.* 1987;44:1146). For additional information, contact the Advertising Representative (William McCausland Associates, Inc., P.O. Box 189, Pitman, NJ 08071. Phone 609-589-5454, Fax 609-582-7611).

All articles published, including editorials, letters, and book reviews, represent the opinions of the authors and do not reflect the official policy of the American Society of Hospital Pharmacists or the institution with which the author is affiliated, unless this is specified.

Microfilm and microfiche editions are available for purchase. Contact University Microfilms, 300 N. Zeeb Road, Ann Arbor, MI 48106.

Articles in Clinical Pharmacy are abstracted and indexed in *Current Contents, Clinical Sciences, Current Awareness in Biologic Sciences, Excerpta Medica, Index Medicus, Inpharma, International Pharmaceutical Abstracts*, and *Reactions*.

November 1992 Volume 11, Number 11 Coden: CPHADV ISSN: 0278-2677

CLINICAL PHARMACY

912 **News**

FDA approves treatment IND protocol for taxol

917 **Therapy Consultation**

Erythromycin, motilin, and gastroparesis

Drug Reviews

919 **Sumatriptan: A new drug for vascular headache**
Van Doren Hsu

930 **Paroxetine, sertraline, and fluvoxamine: New selective serotonin reuptake inhibitors**
Sara R. Grimsley and Michael W. Jann

Research Notes

958 **Intrathecal administration of morphine followed by patient-controlled intravenous administration for postoperative analgesia**
Robert W. Wetmore, Mark A. Kalt, John W. Sybert, and Earl T. Hecker

961 **Pharmacokinetics and safety of intramuscular injection of concentrated ceftriaxone in children**
John S. Bradley, Lisa S. Compogiannis, William E. Murray, Mark A. Acosta, and Gloria L. Tsu

965 **Nausea and vomiting after abdominal surgery**
John M. Benson, Joseph T. DiPiro, Cathy L. Coleman, Jan D. Hirsch, L. Deane Donnigan, Johnny A. Stanfield, and Talmadge A. Bowden, Jr.

Commentary

968 **Lowering the plasma fibrinogen concentration with drugs**
Edzard Ernst

DUE Criteria

972 **Criteria for use of sumatriptan in adult inpatients and outpatients**
Van Doren Hsu

976 **CP Continuing Education**

978 **Current Literature**

Drug Reaction Alerts

988 **Advertising Index**

Editorial Office
7272 Wisconsin Avenue
Bethesda, MD 20814
301-657-3000
Fax 301-657-1258

Advertising Representative
William McCausland Associates, Inc.
P.O. Box 189
Pitman, NJ 08071
609-589-5454
Fax 609-582-7611

Printed on acid-free paper effective with Volume 8, January 1989.

Instructions to Authors

CLINICAL PHARMACY, a forum for the drug therapeutics information that pharmacists need to perform their clinical roles, gives priority to (1) studies that objectively evaluate drug effects in human trials, (2) evaluative review articles on the clinical uses of new drugs, and (3) evaluations of the current status of drug therapy in selected diseases. Contributions to the following sections are invited.

Drug Reviews: Detailed, analytical reviews on the clinical use of specific drugs, with preference given to new drugs and to evaluative rather than descriptive literature reviews.

Therapy Reviews: Articles that focus primarily on a disease state and its treatment.

Therapy Update: Concise analytical reviews of narrowly defined, important topics in pharmacotherapy.

Clinical Frontiers: Articles that review important, ongoing research on disease processes, drug mechanisms, or new technologies and project the likely implications for therapy.

Research: Reports of well-conducted original research on drug effects in humans.

Research Notes: Short research reports, such as updates on previously published work, confirmations of previous findings, or original research of modest scope.

Grand Rounds: Patient case reports and literature reviews combined in a way that gives them high educational value.

Drug Experience: Straightforward reports, with selected literature references, of unusual drug experiences.

Therapy Consultation: Brief advice, in a question-and-answer format, on how to handle specific drug-therapy problems. Readers are invited to submit questions, which the editor will forward to consultants for answering.

Letters: Short comments on previously published work or about potential problems, apparent trends, or controversies in drug therapy or clinical research.

Commentaries: Well-reasoned expressions of opinion on drug-therapy or clinical-research issues.

The editors have the sole authority to decide in which section to publish an accepted manuscript.

Manuscripts are subject to review by qualified outside reviewers, as well as by the editors, and will be accepted for publication only if they are believed to represent an important contribution to the literature. All papers submitted for publication must be accompanied by a completed copy of a manuscript checklist. The checklist, which generally conforms to the Uniform Requirements for Manuscripts Submitted to Biomedical Journals, appears on pages 60-61 of the January 1992 issue. Authors of especially important original work may request "fast-track" review of their papers. Authors may suggest appropriate reviewers for their papers.

Accepted materials become the permanent and sole property of ASHP and may not be published or reprinted elsewhere without written permission from both the author and the editor.

The editors reserve the right to revise all materials submitted, if necessary. The publisher assumes no responsibility for the statements and opinions advanced by contributors to CLINICAL PHARMACY.

Under the terms of the Copyright Revision Act of 1976 (Public Law 94-553) it is necessary to have the rights of the authors transferred to the publisher in order to provide for the widest possible dissemination of professional and scientific literature. Accordingly, all transmittal letters accompanying manuscripts submitted for publication, including contributions for the Letters column, must contain the following language: "In consideration of the American Society of Hospital Pharmacists (ASHP) taking action in reviewing and editing my (our) submission, the author(s) undersigned hereby transfer(s), assign(s), or otherwise convey(s) all ownership rights in the submission and all copyright ownership to ASHP. In the event that such work is not published by ASHP, all said rights shall be released." We regret that we cannot consider manuscripts for publication that are not accompanied by transmittal letters containing the above language signed by all authors.

Authors must certify in their letter of transmittal that none of the material in their manuscript has been published previously nor is under consideration or been accepted for publication elsewhere. If this certification cannot be made, suitable explanation must be offered.

Eight copies of all manuscripts should be submitted. Manuscripts should be typewritten with double spacing (including tables) on one side of good-quality, 21.6 x 27.9-cm white paper, and with margins of at least 2.5 cm. For guidance on style, authors should consult the manuscript checklist, recent issues of CLINICAL PHARMACY, and the *Council of Biology Editors Style Manual, fifth edition. The American Heritage Dictionary of the English Language and the AMA's Manual of Style* contain helpful advice on correct usage.

Galley proofs or final edited manuscripts are sent to authors for inspection against the original manuscript and for correction. Unnecessary alterations at this stage must be avoided. An order form for reprints is sent to the corresponding author at the time of publication.

CLINICAL PHARMACY (ISSN 0278-2677) is published monthly by the American Society of Hospital Pharmacists, 7272 Wisconsin Avenue, Bethesda, MD 20814. Joseph A. Oddis, Executive Vice President. Second-class postage is paid at Bethesda, MD, and at additional mailing offices. **Postmaster: Send address changes to: *Clinical Pharmacy*, 7272 Wisconsin Avenue, Bethesda, MD 20814.**

Annual Subscription Rate:	*USA*	*Non-USA*
ASHP Members	$49	$64
ASHP Student Members and Residents	$39	$39
Institutions and Nonmembers	$89	$104

The cost of single copies is $10. Airmail delivery outside the continental United States is available for an additional charge of $90 per year. Requests to replace missing issues free of charge are honored only up to six months after date of issue.

Payments to ASHP are not deductible as charitable contributions for federal income tax purposes. However, they may be deductible under other provisions of the Internal Revenue Code.

Advertising for CLINICAL PHARMACY is accepted in accordance with the Statement of Advertising Policy of the American Society of Hospital Pharmacists (see *Am J Hosp Pharm.* 1987;44:1146). For additional information, contact the Advertising Representative (William McCausland Associates, Inc., P.O. Box 189, Pitman, NJ 08071. Phone 609-589-5454, Fax 609-582-7611).

All articles published, including editorials, letters, and book reviews, represent the opinions of the authors and do not reflect the official policy of the American Society of Hospital Pharmacists or the institution with which the author is affiliated, unless this is specified.

Microfilm and microfiche editions are available for purchase. Contact University Microfilms, 300 N. Zeeb Road, Ann Arbor, MI 48106.

Articles in CLINICAL PHARMACY are abstracted and indexed in *Current Contents, Clinical Sciences, Current Awareness in Biologic Sciences, Excerpta Medica, Index Medicus, Inpharma, International Pharmaceutical Abstracts,* and *Reactions.*

December 1992 Volume 11, Number 12 Coden: CPHADV ISSN: 0278-2677

CLINICAL PHARMACY

991 News

CDC advises on management of persons exposed to multiple-drug-resistant tuberculosis . . . Three studies examine angiotensin-converting-enzyme-inhibitor prevention of heart failure . . . Cefpodoxime marketing approved by FDA . . . Free drug programs for indigent patients should be more accessible, says Senate committee on aging

Therapy Review

1005 **Antipyretic therapy in the febrile child**
Laureen A. Drwal-Klein and Stephanie J. Phelps

Research Notes

1022 **Toxicity of rapidly infused concentrated intravenous immune globulin**
Cindy Ippoliti, Loretta Ann Williams, and Steven Huber

1026 **Pharmacokinetics of ondansetron in patients receiving cisplatin therapy**
Michael D. Parr, William J. McIntyre, Lisa M. Henderson, John S. MacDonald, and Mary H. H. Chandler

Drug Experience

1030 **Removal of ethosuximide and phenobarbital by peritoneal dialysis in a child**
Eric D. Marquardt, Denis Y. Ishisaka, Kumar K. Batra, and Barbara Chin

ASHP Report

1032 **Acknowledgment to reviewers—October 1, 1991, to September 30, 1992**

DUE Criteria

1033 **Criteria for use of theophylline (aminophylline) in inpatients and outpatients with pulmonary disease**
Marjorie Shaw Phillips

CP Continuing Education

1039 **ASHP journal continuing-education instructions and enrollment form**

1040 Current Literature

Drug Reaction Alerts . . . Books Received

1042 Advertising Index

1043 Annual Index

Editorial Office
7272 Wisconsin Avenue
Bethesda, MD 20814
301-657-3000
Fax 301-657-1258

Advertising Representative
William McCausland Associates, Inc.
P.O. Box 189
Pitman, NJ 08071
609-589-5454
Fax 609-582-7611

Printed on acid-free paper effective with Volume 8, January 1989.

Instructions to Authors

Clinical Pharmacy, a forum for the drug therapeutics information that pharmacists need to perform their clinical roles, gives priority to (1) studies that objectively evaluate drug effects in human trials, (2) evaluative review articles on the clinical uses of new drugs, and (3) evaluations of the current status of drug therapy in selected diseases. Contributions to the following sections are invited.

Drug Reviews: Detailed, analytical reviews on the clinical use of specific drugs, with preference given to new drugs and to evaluative rather than descriptive literature reviews.

Therapy Reviews: Articles that focus primarily on a disease state and its treatment.

Therapy Update: Concise analytical reviews of narrowly defined, important topics in pharmacotherapy.

Clinical Frontiers: Articles that review important, ongoing research on disease processes, drug mechanisms, or new technologies and project the likely implications for therapy.

Research: Reports of well-conducted original research on drug effects in humans.

Research Notes: Short research reports, such as updates on previously published work, confirmations of previous findings, or original research of modest scope.

Grand Rounds: Patient case reports and literature reviews combined in a way that gives them high educational value.

Drug Experience: Straightforward reports, with selected literature references, of unusual drug experiences.

Therapy Consultation: Brief advice, in a question-and-answer format, on how to handle specific drug-therapy problems. Readers are invited to submit questions, which the editor will forward to consultants for answering.

Letters: Short comments on previously published work or about potential problems, apparent trends, or controversies in drug therapy or clinical research.

Commentaries: Well-reasoned expressions of opinion on drug-therapy or clinical-research issues.

The editors have the sole authority to decide in which section to publish an accepted manuscript.

Manuscripts are subject to review by qualified outside reviewers, as well as by the editors, and will be accepted for publication only if they are believed to represent an important contribution to the literature. All papers submitted for publication must be accompanied by a completed copy of a manuscript checklist. The checklist, which generally conforms to the Uniform Requirements for Manuscripts Submitted to Biomedical Journals, appears on pages 60-61 of the January 1992 issue. Authors of especially important original work may request "fast-track" review of their papers. Authors may suggest appropriate reviewers for their papers.

Accepted materials become the permanent and sole property of ASHP and may not be published or reprinted elsewhere without written permission from both the author and the editor.

The editors reserve the right to revise all materials submitted, if necessary. The publisher assumes no responsibility for the statements and opinions advanced by contributors to Clinical Pharmacy.

Under the terms of the Copyright Revision Act of 1976 (Public Law 94-553) it is necessary to have the rights of the authors transferred to the publisher in order to provide for the widest possible dissemination of professional and scientific literature. Accordingly, all transmittal letters accompanying manuscripts submitted for publication, including contributions for the Letters column, must contain the following language: "In consideration of the American Society of Hospital Pharmacists (ASHP) taking action in reviewing and editing my (our) submission, the author(s) undersigned hereby transfer(s), assign(s), or otherwise convey(s) all ownership rights in the submission and all copyright ownership to ASHP. In the event that such work is not published by ASHP, all said rights shall be released." We regret that we cannot consider manuscripts for publication that are not accompanied by transmittal letters containing the above language signed by all authors.

Authors must certify in their letter of transmittal that none of the material in their manuscript has been published previously nor is under consideration or been accepted for publication elsewhere. If this certification cannot be made, suitable explanation must be offered.

Eight copies of all manuscripts should be submitted. Manuscripts should be typewritten with double spacing (including tables) on one side of good-quality, 21.6 x 27.9-cm white paper, and with margins of at least 2.5 cm. For guidance on style, authors should consult the manuscript checklist, recent issues of Clinical Pharmacy, and the *Council of Biology Editors Style Manual, fifth edition. The American Heritage Dictionary of the English Language and the AMA's Manual of Style* contain helpful advice on correct usage.

Galley proofs or final edited manuscripts are sent to authors for inspection against the original manuscript and for correction. Unnecessary alterations at this stage must be avoided. An order form for reprints is sent to the corresponding author at the time of publication.

Clinical Pharmacy (ISSN 0278-2677) is published monthly by the American Society of Hospital Pharmacists, 7272 Wisconsin Avenue, Bethesda, MD 20814. Joseph A. Oddis, Executive Vice President. Second-class postage is paid at Bethesda, MD, and at additional mailing offices. **Postmaster: Send address changes to: *Clinical Pharmacy*, 7272 Wisconsin Avenue, Bethesda, MD 20814.**

Annual Subscription Rate:	*USA*	*Non-USA*
ASHP Members	$49	$64
ASHP Student Members and Residents	$39	$39
Institutions and Nonmembers	$89	$104

The cost of single copies is $10. Airmail delivery outside the continental United States is available for an additional charge of $90 per year. Requests to replace missing issues free of charge are honored only up to six months after date of issue.

Payments to ASHP are not deductible as charitable contributions for federal income tax purposes. However, they may be deductible under other provisions of the Internal Revenue Code.

Advertising for Clinical Pharmacy is accepted in accordance with the Statement of Advertising Policy of the American Society of Hospital Pharmacists (see *Am J Hosp Pharm.* 1987; 44:1146). For additional information, contact the Advertising Representative (William McCausland Associates, Inc., P.O. Box 189, Pitman, NJ 08071. Phone 609-589-5454, Fax 609-582-7611).

All articles published, including editorials, letters, and book reviews, represent the opinions of the authors and do not reflect the official policy of the American Society of Hospital Pharmacists or the institution with which the author is affiliated, unless this is specified.

Microfilm and microfiche editions are available for purchase. Contact University Microfilms, 300 N. Zeeb Road, Ann Arbor, MI 48106.

Articles in Clinical Pharmacy are abstracted and indexed in *Current Contents, Clinical Sciences, Current Awareness in Biologic Sciences, Excerpta Medica, Index Medicus, Inpharma, International Pharmaceutical Abstracts*, and *Reactions*.

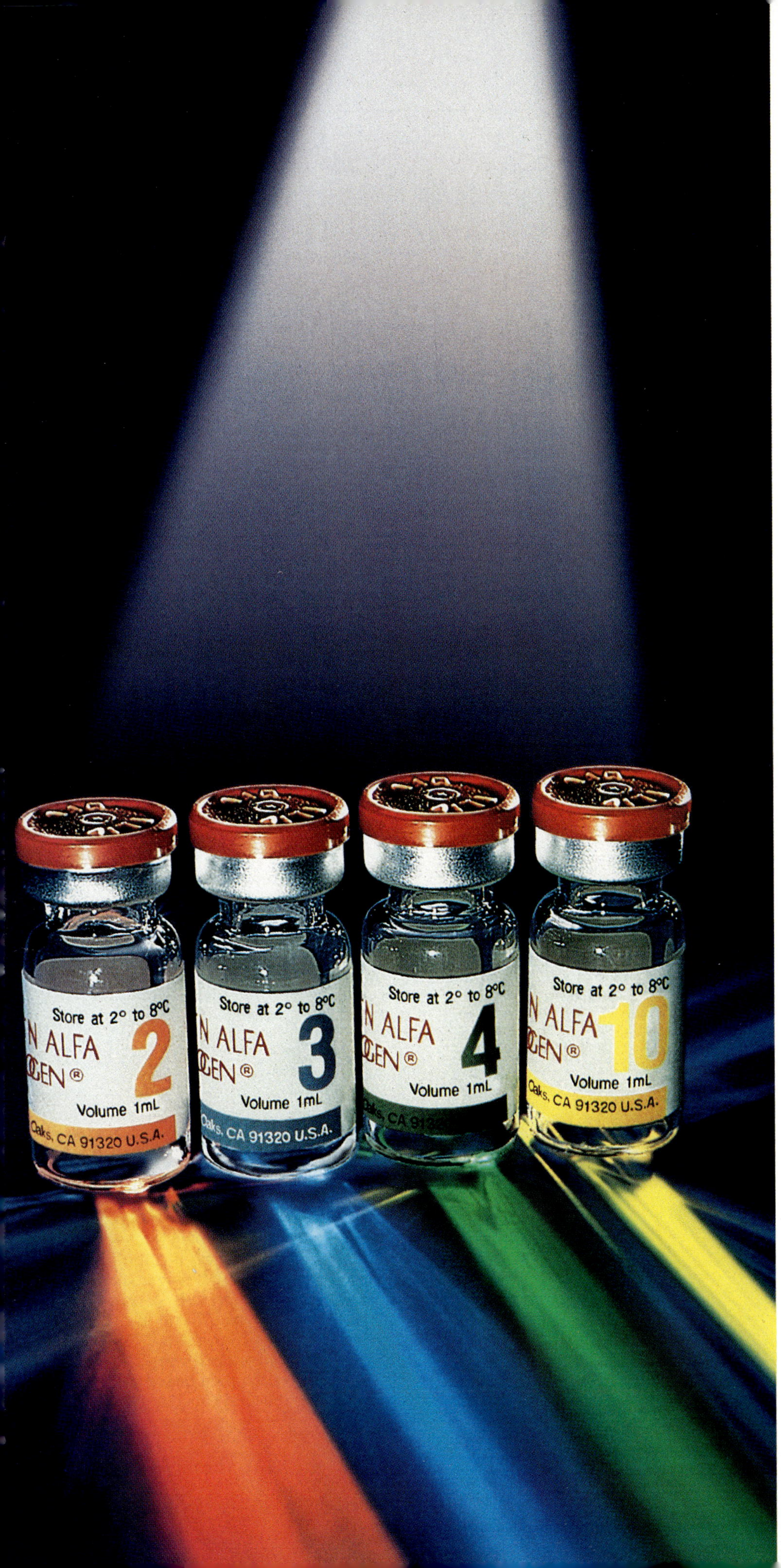
Store at 2° to 8°C
2
Volume 1mL
Store at 2° to 8°C
3
Volume 1mL
Store at 2° to 8°C
4
Volume 1mL
Store at 2° to 8°C
10
Volume 1mL
CA 91320 U.S.A.

News

Didanosine and foscarnet marketed for use by patients with AIDS 4

Working group issues report on aluminum contamination of parenteral nutrient solutions 6
Christine A. Mowatt-Larssen

United Kingdom suspends sales of triazolam; FDA to review safety data 9

Felodipine marketed as antihypertensive agent 9

News Briefs 9

Upcoming Specialty Meetings 9

Didanosine and foscarnet marketed for use by patients with AIDS

FDA has approved marketing of two drugs for use by patients with AIDS—foscarnet for treatment of cytomegalovirus (CMV) retinitis and didanosine for use by patients with advanced stages of human immunodeficiency virus (HIV) infection.

Didanosine. Didanosine (ddI, Videx, Bristol-Myers Squibb Company) is labeled for the treatment of adults and children older than six months with advanced HIV infection who cannot tolerate zidovudine therapy or who have demonstrated clinical or immunologic deterioration during zidovudine therapy. The approval was based largely on Phase I studies showing an increase in the CD4 cell count during therapy. These results were compared with historical data. Information on CD4 cell counts obtained from an ongoing trial comparing didanosine with zidovudine were also reviewed. Evidence that didanosine affects clinical endpoints such as survival or the incidence of opportunistic infections is currently lacking. Reliance on surrogate endpoints permitted earlier approval of the drug but means less information about long-term safety and efficacy.

The major adverse effects are pancreatitis and peripheral neuropathy, which occurred in 9% and 34%, respectively, of the Phase I study participants who received didanosine at dosages equal to or less than the recommended dosage.

Didanosine is rapidly degraded at an acidic pH. Oral absorption may be reduced by up to 50% if didanosine is administered with food. Bioavailability is 20–25% higher with the chewable tablet than with the oral solution.

Twice daily administration is recommended. The starting dosage is based on the patient's weight (adults) or body surface area (children). Videx is supplied as 25-, 50-, 100-, or 150-mg tablets that can be chewed or dispersed in water, single-dose foil packets of buffered powder (containing 100, 167, 250, or 375 mg of didanosine) for oral solution, or bottles containing 2 or 4 g of didanosine for oral solution (for pediatric use). The pediatric formulation is constituted and then mixed with antacid before being dispensed; the final concentration is 10

Continued on page 6

News *Continued from page 4*

mg/mL. When the oral tablets are used by adults or children older than one year, two tablets must be given to ensure adequate acid neutralizing capacity for drug absorption.

The cost to the wholesaler for a one-year supply of didanosine tablets taken at a dosage of 200 mg twice daily is $1745.

Foscarnet. Foscarnet sodium (Foscavir, Astra Pharmaceutical Products, Inc.) provides an alternative to ganciclovir in the treatment of CMV retinitis in patients with AIDS. Direct comparative data for the two drugs have not been published.

An induction regimen followed by daily maintenance doses has been shown to slow the progression of CMV retinitis. Efficacy for other manifestations of CMV disease has not been proved.

About 80–90% of an i.v. dose of foscarnet is excreted unchanged in the urine. Clearance is decreased in patients with renal impairment.

Most patients treated with foscarnet experience some nephrotoxicity. Renal function must be assessed regularly, and dosage adjustments must be made for changes in renal function. Foscarnet use is also associated with electrolyte imbalances. In five controlled studies, seizures occurred in 10% of patients receiving foscarnet therapy. About one third of patients treated in U.S. clinical trials received foscarnet and zidovudine concomitantly. No evidence of additive myelosuppression was seen, but effects on anemia may have been additive. A possible interaction between foscarnet and intravenous pentamidine (hypocalcemia) has been reported.

Foscarnet sodium solution may be given undiluted through a central venous line or diluted to 12 mg/mL and administered through a peripheral venous line. The recommended initial dosage for patients with normal renal function is 60 mg/kg infused over at least one hour every eight hours for two to three weeks. This induction regimen is followed by maintenance therapy with 90–120 mg/kg/day infused intravenously over two hours. Both induction and maintenance dosages should be adjusted in patients with renal impairment.

Foscavir is supplied as a 24-mg/mL solution in 250- and 500-mL bottles packaged in cases of 12.

Working group issues report on aluminum contamination of parenteral nutrient solutions

In response an FDA notice of intent and request for information concerning aluminum content of injectable drug products, a working group appointed by the American Society for Clinical Nutrition and the American Society for Parenteral and Enteral Nutrition has reviewed issues relating to aluminum content of parenteral nutrient solutions. The working group's report was published recently in the *Journal of Parenteral and Enteral Nutrition.*[1] FDA's intention is to set an upper limit of 25 μg/L for aluminum content of large-volume infusion solutions and to require manufacturers of small-volume

Continued on page 8

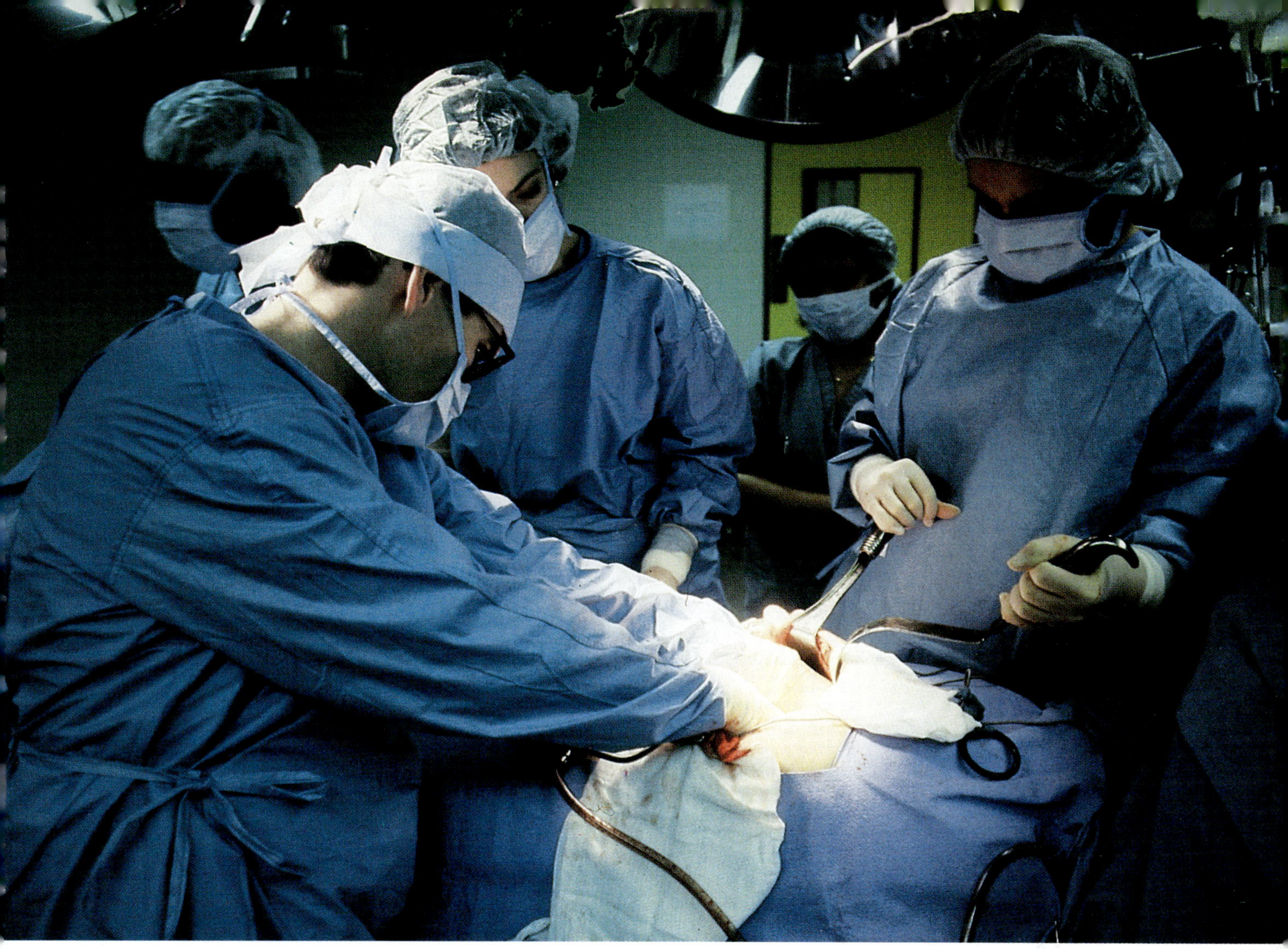

Continued from page 6

injections (e.g., calcium and phosphate salts) to measure and report aluminum content on the package label. Aluminum is present as a contaminant in certain infusion solutions and small-volume injections and may accumulate in serum, tissue, and bone.

Recommendations of the Working Group. The working group supports FDA's notice of intent but suggested several additional considerations. The working group strongly recommended that cumulative amounts of aluminum intake be reported as the quantity of aluminum per kilogram of body weight, particularly in infants, so body burden of aluminum is normalized. The working group also suggested that the terms safe, unsafe, and toxic be defined in terms of quantity of aluminum per kilogram of body weight and that these definitions be made known to physicians and pharmacists. An additional concern of the working group was that FDA's notice of intent did not take into account the maximal concentration of aluminum in small-volume injections. The working group suggested that the maximum allowable aluminum content of these products be set soon. Use of a standardized unit of measurement in product labeling was another recommendation: µmol/L should be the primary unit, with µg/L given in parentheses. Last, the working group suggested that package inserts of infusion solutions and small-volume injections containing aluminum should state in appropriate warning language that the accumulation of aluminum in bone may contribute to the pathogenesis of bone disease and that the use of aluminum-contaminated products in uremic patients may result in aluminum accumulation and cause encephalopathy as well as bone disease.

Risks Associated with Aluminum Accumulation. Over the past 12 years several published reports have related aluminum accumulation to various toxicities.

Initially, reports dealt with dialysis patients who developed osteomalacia and dementia secondary to aluminum contamination of dialysate.[2] The removal of aluminum from dialysis fluids did not eliminate the problem, since patients with chronic renal failure frequently are hyperphosphatemic and receive oral aluminum hydroxide to bind phosphorus.[3] Calcium carbonate is now recommended as an alternative to aluminum hydroxide in patients with chronic renal failure.

Patients receiving long-term parenteral nutrition and infants receiving parenteral nutrition also are at increased risk for aluminum accumulation, which has been shown to be a causative factor in metabolic bone disease.

Early reports of metabolic bone disease involved patients receiving long-term parenteral nutrition with protein supplied as casein hydrolysate, which was highly contaminated with aluminum.[4,5] Although currently available crystalline amino acid solutions contain less aluminum (<50 µg/L), other components of nutrient solutions—calcium and phosphate salts, vitamins, and albumin—have been shown to contain high amounts of aluminum (>500 µg/L).[6] Studies using crystalline amino acids have demonstrated less accumulation of aluminum in plasma and bone than did studies using casein hydrolysate and have reaffirmed that metabolic bone disease in patients receiving long-term parenteral nutrition is multifactorial.[7,8] Yet, a recent study in France involving children receiving long-term parenteral nutrition found a high aluminum content (mean ± S.D., 232 ± 89 µg/L) in parenteral nutrient solutions; the result was elevated plasma and urine aluminum concentrations and accumulation of aluminum in bone.[9] Variations in study design and differences in nutrient solution composition make it difficult to draw conclusions from studies involving this patient population. Monitoring the aluminum content of nutrient solutions administered to patients requiring long-term parenteral nutrition support will help minimize one confounding variable in the development of metabolic bone disease.

Infants are also at risk for aluminum accumulation. Parenteral nutrient solutions prepared for infants may have higher aluminum concentrations because infants require larger amounts of calcium and phosphorus on a milligram per kilogram basis. The primary route for aluminum elimination is renal; therefore, premature neonates with lower glomerular filtration rates and patients with renal insufficiency are at greater risk for aluminum accumulation. Infants receiving parenteral nutrition have been found to have elevated concentrations of aluminum in plasma and urine and accumulation of aluminum in bone.[10] It is difficult to define the contribution of aluminum to the development of metabolic bone disease in infants because multiple risk factors exist, the most common being insufficient intake of calcium and phosphorus.

Implications for Pharmacists. It is foreseeable that pharmacists involved in the provision of parenteral nutrition will be responsible for monitoring the amount of aluminum in parenteral nutrient solutions. For patients who are at risk for aluminum accumulation, pharmacists may be involved in the monitoring and pharmacologic management of aluminum accumulation in serum and bone.

1. Klein GL, Alfrey AC, Shike M et al. Parenteral drug products containing aluminum as an ingredient or a contaminant: response to the Food and Drug Administration notice of intent and request for information. *J Parenter Enter Nutr.* 1991; 15:194-8.
2. Parkinson IS, Ward MK, Feest TG et al. Fracturing dialysis osteodystrophy and dialysis encephalopathy: an epidemiological survey. *Lancet.* 1979; 1:406-9.
3. Salusky IB, Foley J, Nelson P et al. Aluminum accumulation during treatment with aluminum hydroxide and dialysis in children and young adults with chronic renal disease. *N Engl J Med.* 1991; 324:527-31.
4. Klein GL, Alfrey AC, Miller NL et al. Aluminum loading during total parenteral nutrition. *Am J Clin Nutr.* 1982; 35:1425-9.
5. Ott SM, Maloney NA, Klein GL et al. Aluminum is associated with low bone formation in patients receiving chronic parenteral nutrition. *Ann Intern Med.* 1983; 98:910-4.
6. Koo WWK, Kaplan LA, Horn J et al. Aluminum in parenteral nutrition solution—sources and possible alternatives. *J Parenter Enter Nutr.* 1986; 10:591-5.
7. Shike M, Shils ME, Heller A et al. Bone disease in prolonged parenteral nutrition: osteopenia without mineralization defect. *Am J Clin Nutr.* 1986; 44:89-98.
8. Lipkin EW, Ott SM, Klein GL. Heterogeneity of bone histology in parenteral nutrition patients. *Am J Clin Nutr.* 1987; 46:673-80.
9. Larchet M, Chaumont P, Galliot M et al. Aluminum loading in children receiving long-term parenteral nutrition. *Clin Nutr.* 1990; 9:79-83.
10. Sedman AB, Klein GL, Merritt RJ et al. Evidence of aluminum loading in infants receiving intravenous therapy. *N Engl J Med.* 1985; 312:1337-43.

Christine A. Mowatt-Larssen, Pharm.D.
ASHP Foundation Fellow in Nutrition Support
University of Tennessee, Memphis

United Kingdom suspends sales of triazolam; FDA to review safety data

On October 2, the United Kingdom's Committee on the Safety of Medicines suspended sales of triazolam (Halcion, The Upjohn Company) after concluding that the frequency of psychiatric adverse effects was higher with triazolam than with other hypnotic agents. Upjohn officials contend that the safety data requested and reviewed by the drug regulatory agency in the United Kingdom support the original decision to approve marketing of the product. FDA plans to examine the basis for this decision and will consider whether any changes are needed in the regulatory status or labeling requirements of triazolam in the United States.

Felodipine marketed as antihypertensive agent

An extended-release formulation of felodipine (Plendil, Merck Sharp & Dohme) has been marketed for the treatment of hypertension.

Felodipine, a dihydropyridine calcium-channel blocker, is almost completely absorbed after oral administration. The drug undergoes extensive first-pass metabolism. Felodipine is more than 99% bound to plasma proteins. A negligible amount of intact felodipine is recovered in urine. Six metabolites have been identified; none has substantial vasodilating activity.

Felodipine was studied as monotherapy or in combination with other antihypertensive agents over a dosage range of 2.5–20 mg/day. The most common adverse effects reported during clinical trials were peripheral edema (22.3%) and headache (18.6%).

The recommended starting dosage is 5 mg once daily. A maximum daily dosage of 20 mg is recommended. Lower dosages (maximum, 10 mg/day) are generally recommended for elderly persons and patients with impaired hepatic function because drug clearance is reduced in these patient populations.

Plendil is available as extended-release tablets containing 5 or 10 mg of felodipine. The tablets are supplied in unit dose packages of 100 and unit-of-use bottles of 30 or 100.

News Briefs

- Warner-Lambert Company has received FDA approval to market **pentostatin** (Nipent) for the treatment of hairy cell leukemia in patients who do not respond to standard therapy. Pentostatin, a structural analogue of adenosine, was previously available under a treatment IND protocol to patients with hairy cell leukemia who had not responded to or had not tolerated interferon alfa therapy.

- The investigational agent **oxandrolone** (Oxandrin, Gynex, Inc.) has been designated an orphan drug as adjunctive therapy for patients with human immunodeficiency virus (HIV) wasting syndrome.

- Copies of a 1991 report on **biotechnology medicines under development** can be obtained by writing to Editor, Biotechnology Medicines in Development, Communications Division, Pharmaceutical Manufacturers Association, 1100 15th Street, N.W., Washington, DC 20005. For each drug, the manufacturer, indication, and stage of development are listed. The information is based on PMA-sponsored surveys of government and industry sources.

Upcoming Specialty Meetings

10th Annual Practical Update on Infectious Disease. Sacramento, CA, February 7–8; $100 registration fee; contact Office of Continuing Medical Education, University of California, Davis, Medical Center, 2701 Stockton Boulevard, Sacramento, CA 95817; 916-734-5390, (fax) 916-736-0188.

American Burn Association. Salt Lake City, UT, April 1–4; contact A. W. Munster, M.D., Baltimore Regional Burn Center, Francis Scott Key Medical Center, 4940 Eastern Avenue, Baltimore, MD 21224.

American College of Cardiology. Dallas, TX, April 12–16; contact ACC, 9111 Old Georgetown Road, Bethesda, MD 20814; 301-897-5400.

American College of Obstetricians and Gynecologists. Las Vegas, NV, April 26–30; contact ACOG, 409 12th Street S.W., Washington, DC 20024; 202-638-5577.

Letters

Beta-adrenergic agonists in asthma 13
Chris Nee, Jeff Herzfeld
Shannon L. Coonce, Christine M. Murphy,
Pamela A. Simon

Corrections 14

The Letters *column is a forum for rapid exchange of ideas among readers of* Clinical Pharmacy. *Liberal criteria are applied in the review of submissions to encourage contributions to this column.*

The Letters *column includes the following types of contributions: (1) comments, addenda, and minor updates on previously published work, (2) alerts on potential problems related to drug therapy or clinical research, (3) observations or comments on trends in drug therapy or clinical research, and (4) brief expressions of opinion about controversies in drug therapy or clinical research.*

Letters need not be submitted with the journal's manuscript checklist. The following conditions, however, must be adhered to: (1) the body of the letter must be no longer than two typewritten pages, (2) the use of references, tables, and illustrations should be minimized, (3) the authors' names, affiliations, and mailing addresses must be typed at the end of the letter in the format used by Clinical Pharmacy, *and (4) the entire letter (including references, tables, and authors' names) must be typed double-spaced on plain white paper (not letterhead). Following acceptance of a letter, the authors are required to sign an exclusive publication statement and a copyright transferal form.*

Beta-adrenergic agonists in asthma

Murphy et al.[1] stated in the September issue of *Clinical Pharmacy* that β_2-adrenergic agonists are first-line agents for the treatment of asthma. Their statement needs to be qualified in terms of the overall asthma-management strategy, which is related to the onset and severity of the disease.

Current research emphasizes the importance of the biphasic response of the airways that leads to symptoms characterized as asthma.[2,3] Bronchospasm occurs in the immediate phase of acute asthma exacerbation; an inflammatory response in the late phase dictates the severity of asthma.[4] Appreciation of this sequence of airway responses will direct the pharmacotherapeutic management of asthma toward a stepped-care approach.[5]

Important points in the treatment of asthma are to (1) avoid asthma-precipitating stimuli, (2) consider inhalation to be the preferred route of medication administration, (3) reserve antimicrobials for appropriate indications rather than routine use, and (4) recognize the need for education and continuity of care.[6] Although pharmacologic intervention plays a major role in the treatment of asthma, patient-specific treatment and education should be integrated into stepped-care therapy.[5-7]

It is important to realize that asthma is a chronic inflammatory condition. The emphasis on rescue with β_2 agonists (bronchodilators) may actually mask the underlying cause of asthma.[7] The appropriateness of using β_2 agonists as first-line agents must also be questioned because the mortality and morbidity from asthma has increased internationally. Thus, concern about overuse of inhaled bronchodilators and underuse of anti-inflammatory agents has redirected and refocused the approach to asthma therapy.[5,8]

The use of anti-inflammatory agents, such as inhaled corticosteroids and cromolyn sodium, as first-line, maintenance treatment may lessen the need for bronchodilators and reduce asthma-associated morbidity and mortality.[7,8] Treatment with β_2 agonists should be reserved mainly for the bronchospastic phase of asthma; these drugs should be used on an as-needed basis, not as first-line agents in all patients.

1. Murphy CM, Coonce SL, Simon PA. Treatment of asthma in children. *Clin Pharm.* 1991; 10:685-703.
2. Larsen GL. New concepts in the pathogenesis of asthma. *Clin Immunol Immunopathol.* 1989; 53:S107-18.

3. Hangreave FE. Late-phase asthmatic responses and airway inflammation. *J Allergy Clin Immunol.* 1989; 83:525-7.
4. Busse WW. The role of inflammation in asthma: a new focus. *J Respir Dis.* 1989; 10(Nov):72-80.
5. Bone RC. A step care strategy for asthma management. *J Respir Dis.* 1988; 9(Nov):104-17.
6. Hargreave FE, Dolovich J, Newhouse MT. The assessment and treatment of asthma: a conference report. *J Allergy Clin Immunol.* 1990; 85:1098-111.
7. Barnes PJ. A new approach to the treatment of asthma. *N Engl J Med.* 1990; 321:1517-27.
8. Haahtela T, Jarvinen M, Kava T et al. Comparison of a β_2-agonist, terbutaline, with an inhaled corticosteroid, budesonide, in newly detected asthma. *N Engl J Med.* 1991; 325:388-92.

Chris Nee, Pharm.D., Clinical Pharmacist
Jeff Herzfeld, Pharm.D., Manager, Clinical Pharmacy Services
PacifiCare Inc.
5856 Corporate Avenue
Cypress, CA 90630

We thank Drs. Nee and Herzfeld for reemphasizing the fact that cromolyn and inhaled corticosteroids have become first-line agents in the management of chronic asthma. We believe, however, that all patients with asthma, regardless of their symptom classification (e.g., intermittent, chronic) need to have access to an inhaled β_2 agonist for relief of acute symptoms.

Clinicians have indeed become concerned about β_2 agonists because regularly scheduled use of these agents in the management of chronic asthma is implicated in the international rise in asthma-related morbidity and mortality.[1] We do not recommend regular use of these drugs but suggest that they be used on an as-needed basis only. If patients are using β_2 agonists regularly (more than twice a week), a long-term prophylactic medication should be added.

When inhalation of a β_2 agonist fails to control acute symptoms, prompt treatment with high-dose oral corticosteroids is indicated. If a patient has chronic symptoms, prophylactic therapy should be instituted with either cromolyn or inhaled corticosteroids. Theophylline is an alternative to these agents.[2]

1. Sears MR, Taylor DR, Print CG et al. Regular inhaled beta-agonist treatment in bronchial asthma. *Lancet.* 1990; 336:1391-6.
2. Murphy CM, Coonce SL, Simon PA. Treatment of asthma in children. *Clin Pharm.* 1991; 10:685-703.

Shannon L. Coonce, Pharm.D., Clinical Pharmacist
University Medical Center of Southern Nevada
1800 West Charleston Boulevard
Las Vegas, NV 89102

Christine M. Murphy, Pharm.D., Clinical Assistant Professor
Pamela A. Simon, Pharm.D., Clinical Assistant Professor

Department of Pharmacy Practice
The University of Illinois at Chicago
833 South Wood Street, Room 244 (M/C 886)
Chicago, IL 60612

Corrections

American Academy of Pediatrics issues recommendations on treatment of Lyme disease (October 1991, News). On page 738, the article should state that the recommended therapy for early-stage Lyme disease in children older than nine years is tetracycline hydrochloride 250 mg four times daily or doxycycline 100 mg twice daily.

Advances in the treatment of unstable angina pectoris (November 1991, Therapy Review). On page 831, Table 3 should indicate the following results for reference 52: 8% decr. in MI or cardiac death at 5 days, 11% decr. at 30 days, 6% decr. at 90 days (all NS).

Retreatment with digoxin immune Fab (November 1991, Letter). On page 824, the second sentence of the first full paragraph should indicate that the release of digoxin from digoxin–antibody complexes is only one possible explanation for a rebound in the free digoxin concentration.

EXOSURF® Neonatal™
(COLFOSCERIL PALMITATE, CETYL ALCOHOL, TYLOXAPOL)
For Intratracheal Suspension / 10 mL vials

PLEASE CONSULT FULL PRODUCT INFORMATION BEFORE PRESCRIBING.

INDICATIONS AND USAGE: Exosurf Neonatal is indicated for:

1. **Prophylactic** treatment of infants with birth weights of less than 1350 grams who are at risk of developing RDS (see PRECAUTIONS).
2. **Prophylactic** treatment of infants with birth weights greater than 1350 grams who have evidence of pulmonary immaturity, and
3. **Rescue** treatment of infants who have developed RDS.

CONTRAINDICATIONS: There are no known contraindications to treatment with Exosurf Neonatal.

WARNINGS: Intratracheal Administration Only: Exosurf Neonatal should be administered only by instillation into the trachea. **General:** The use of Exosurf Neonatal requires expert clinical care by experienced neonatologists and other clinicians who are accomplished at neonatal intubation and ventilatory management. Adequate personnel, facilities, equipment, and medications are required to optimize perinatal outcome in premature infants. Instillation of Exosurf Neonatal should be performed **only** by trained medical personnel experienced in airway and clinical management of unstable premature infants. Vigilant clinical attention should be given to all infants prior to, during, and after administration of Exosurf Neonatal. **Acute Effects:** Exosurf Neonatal can rapidly affect oxygenation and lung compliance. **Lung Compliance:** If chest expansion improves substantially after dosing, peak ventilator inspiratory pressures should be reduced immediately, without waiting for confirmation of respiratory improvement by blood gas assessment. Failure to reduce inspiratory ventilator pressures rapidly in such instances can result in lung overdistention and fatal pulmonary air leak. **Hyperoxia:** If the infant becomes pink and transcutaneous oxygen saturation is in excess of 95%, FiO_2 should be reduced in small but repeated steps (until saturation is 90 to 95%) without waiting for confirmation of elevated arterial pO_2 by blood gas assessment. Failure to reduce FiO_2 in such instances can result in hyperoxia. **Hypocarbia:** If arterial or transcutaneous CO_2 measurements are <30 torr, the ventilator rate should be reduced at once. Failure to reduce ventilator rates in such instances can result in marked hypocarbia, which is known to reduce brain blood flow. **Pulmonary Hemorrhage:** In the single study conducted in infants weighing <700 grams at birth, the incidence of pulmonary hemorrhage (10% vs 2% in the placebo group) was significantly increased in the Exosurf Neonatal group. None of the five studies involving infants with birth weights >700 grams showed a significant increase in pulmonary hemorrhage in the Exosurf Neonatal group. In a cross-study analysis of these five studies, pulmonary hemorrhage was reported for 1% (14/1420) of infants in the placebo group and 2% (27/1411) of infants in the Exosurf Neonatal group. Fatal pulmonary hemorrhage occurred in three infants; two in the Exosurf Neonatal group and one in the placebo group. Mortality from all causes among infants who developed pulmonary hemorrhage was 43% in the placebo group and 37% in the Exosurf Neonatal group. Pulmonary hemorrhage in both Exosurf Neonatal and placebo infants was more frequent in infants who were younger, smaller, male, or who had a patent ductus arteriosus. Pulmonary hemorrhage typically occurred in the first 2 days of life in both treatment groups. In more than 7700 infants in the open, uncontrolled study, pulmonary hemorrhage was reported in 4%, but fatal pulmonary hemorrhage was reported rarely (0.4%). In the controlled clinical studies, Exosurf Neonatal treated infants who received steroids more than 24 hours prior to delivery or indomethacin postnatally had a lower rate of pulmonary hemorrhage than other Exosurf Neonatal treated infants. Attention should be paid to early and aggressive diagnosis and treatment (unless contraindicated) of patent ductus arteriosus during the first 2 days of life (while the ductus arteriosus is often clinically silent). Other potentially protective measures include attempting to decrease FiO_2 preferentially over ventilator pressures during the first 24 to 48 hours after dosing, and attempting to decrease PEEP minimally for at least 48 hours after dosing. **Mucous Plugs:** Infants whose ventilation becomes markedly impaired during or shortly after dosing may have mucous plugging of the endotracheal tube, particularly if pulmonary secretions were prominent prior to drug administration. Suctioning of all infants prior to dosing may lessen the chance of mucous plugs obstructing the endotracheal tube. If endotracheal tube obstruction from such plugs is suspected, and suctioning is unsuccessful in removing the obstruction, the blocked endotracheal tube should be replaced immediately.

PRECAUTIONS:

General: In the controlled clinical studies, infants known prenatally or postnatally to have major congenital anomalies, or who were suspected of having congenital infection, were excluded from entry. However, these disorders cannot be recognized early in life in all cases, and a few infants with these conditions were entered. The benefits of Exosurf Neonatal in the affected infants who received drug appeared to be similar to the benefits observed in infants without anomalies or occult infection. **Prophylactic Treatment–Infants <700 Grams:** In infants weighing 500 to 700 grams, a single prophylactic dose of Exosurf Neonatal significantly: improved FiO_2 and ventilator settings, reduced pneumothorax, and reduced death from RDS, but increased pulmonary hemorrhage (see WARNINGS). Overall mortality did not differ significantly between the placebo and Exosurf Neonatal groups (see Table 1 in full product information). Data on multiple doses in infants in this weight class are not yet available. Accordingly, clinicians should carefully evaluate the potential risks and benefits of Exosurf Neonatal administration in these infants. **Rescue Treatment–Number of Doses:** A small number of infants with RDS have received more than two doses of Exosurf Neonatal as rescue treatment. Definitive data on the safety and efficacy of these additional doses are not available. **Carcinogenesis, Mutagenesis, Impairment of Fertility:** Exosurf Neonatal at concentrations up to 10,000 μg/plate was not mutagenic in the Ames Salmonella assay. Long-term studies have not been performed in animals to evaluate the carcinogenic potential of Exosurf Neonatal. The effects of Exosurf Neonatal on fertility have not been studied.

ADVERSE REACTIONS:

General: Premature birth is associated with a high incidence of morbidity and mortality. Despite significant reductions in overall mortality associated with Exosurf Neonatal, some infants who received Exosurf Neonatal developed severe complications and either survived with permanent handicaps or died.

In controlled clinical studies evaluating the safety and efficacy of Exosurf Neonatal, numerous safety assessments were made. In infants receiving Exosurf Neonatal, pulmonary hemorrhage, apnea and use of methylxanthines were increased. A number of other adverse events were significantly reduced in the Exosurf Neonatal group, particularly various forms of pulmonary air leak and use of pancuronium. Tables 3 and 4 summarize the results of the major safety evaluations from the controlled clinical studies.

Table 3: Safety Assessments[a]—Prophylactic Treatment

Number of Doses:	Single Dose		Single Dose		Single Dose		1 vs 3 Doses	
Birth Weight Range:	500 to 700 grams		700 to 1350 grams		700 to 1100 grams		700 to 1100 grams	
Treatment Group:	Placebo (Air)	EXOSURF	Placebo (Air)	EXOSURF	Placebo (Air)	EXOSURF	EXOSURF 1 Dose	EXOSURF 3 Doses
Number of Infants:	N=108	N=107	N=193	N=192	N=222	N=224	N=356	N=360
	% of Infants		% of Infants		% of Infants		% of Infants	
Intraventricular Hemorrhage (IVH)								
Overall	51	57	31	27	36	36	38	35
Severe IVH	26	25	10	8	13	14	9	9
Pulmonary Air Leak (PAL)								
Overall	52	48	16	11	32	25	29	27
Pneumothorax	23	10*	5	6	19	11*	14	12
Pneumopericardium	1	4	2	0	<1	1	1	1
Pneumomediastinum	2	1	2	3	7	1**	3	2
Pulmonary Interstitial Emphysema	43	44	13	7*	26	20	23	22
Death from PAL	4	6	<1	<1	2	1	2	1
Patent Ductus Arteriosus	49	53	66	70	50	55	59	57
Necrotizing Enterocolitis	2	4	11	13	3	4	6	2*
Pulmonary Hemorrhage	2	10**	2	4	1	4	4	6
Congenital Pneumonia	4	4	2	4	2	2	1	1
Nosocomial Pneumonia	10	10	2	4	4	7	14	15
Non-Pulmonary Infections	33	35	34	39	28	29	35	34
Sepsis	30	34	30	34	23	24	30	27
Death From Sepsis	4	4	3	3	1	2	3	2
Meningitis	4	6	3	1	2	3	1	2
Other Infections	7	4	5	3	6	10	10	11
Major Anomalies	3	1	2	4	7	4	4	4

Table 3: Safety Assessments[a]—Prophylactic Treatment (Cont.)

Number of Doses:	Single Dose		Single Dose		Single Dose		1 vs 3 Doses	
Birth Weight Range:	500 to 700 grams		700 to 1350 grams		700 to 1100 grams		700 to 1100 grams	
Treatment Group:	Placebo (Air)	EXOSURF	Placebo (Air)	EXOSURF	Placebo (Air)	EXOSURF	EXOSURF 1 Dose	EXOSURF 3 Doses
Number of Infants:	N=108	N=107	N=193	N=192	N=222	N=224	N=356	N=360
	% of Infants		% of Infants		% of Infants		% of Infants	
Hypotension	70	77	52	47	59	62	54	50
Hyperbilirubinemia	22	21	63	61	27	31	20	21
Exchange Transfusion	4	3	1	2	2	2	3	1
Thrombocytopenia[b]	21	25	not available		9	8	12	10
Persistent Fetal Circulation	0	1	1	1	0	2*	1	<1
Seizures	11	8	2	2	11	9	6	5
Apnea	34	33	76	73	55	65*	62	68
Drug Therapy								
Antibiotics	96	99	98	96	98	99	>99	99
Diuretics	55	60	39	37	59	63	64	65
Anticonvulsants	14	18	23	24	20	16	9	8
Inotropes	46	40	20	20	26	20	28	27
Sedatives	62	71	65	64	63	57	52	52
Pancuronium	19	11	22	14*	19	13*	15	11
Methylxanthines	38	43	77	77	61	72*	75	82*

[a] All parameters were examined with "as-treated" analyses. * p<0.05
[b] Thrombocytopenia requiring platelet transfusion. ** p<0.01

Table 4: Safety Assessments[a]—Rescue Treatment

Number of Doses:	Two Doses		Two Doses	
Birth Weight Range:	700 to 1350 grams		1250 grams and above	
Treatment Group:	Placebo (Air)	EXOSURF	Placebo (Air)	EXOSURF
Number of Infants:	N=213	N=206	N=622	N=615
	% of Infants		% of Infants	
Intraventricular Hemorrhage (IVH)				
Overall	48	52	23	18*
Severe IVH	13	9	5	4
Pulmonary Air Leak (PAL)				
Overall	54	34***	30	18***
Pneumothorax	29	20*	20	10***
Pneumopericardium	4	1	1	2
Pneumomediastinum	8	4	5	2**
Pulmonary Interstitial Emphysema	48	25***	24	13***
Death from PAL	7	3	<1	1
Patent Ductus Arteriosus	66	57	54	45*
Necrotizing Enterocolitis	3	3	1	2
Pulmonary Hemorrhage	3	1	<1	1
Congenital Pneumonia	2	3	2	2
Nosocomial Pneumonia	5	7	2	2
Non-Pulmonary Infections	19	22	13	13
Sepsis	15	17	8	8
Death From Sepsis	<1	<1	1	<1
Meningitis	1	<1	1	<1*
Other Infections	5	8	5	6
Major Anomalies	3	3	4	4
Hypotension	62	57	50	39**
Hyperbilirubinemia	17	19	12	10
Exchange Transfusion	3	4	1	2
Thrombocytopenia[b]	10	11	4	<1**
Persistent Fetal Circulation	1	1	6	2**
Seizures	10	10	6	3*
Apnea	48	65**	37	44*
Drug Therapy				
Antibiotics	100	99	98	98
Diuretics	60	65	45	34***
Anticonvulsants	17	17	10	5**
Inotropes	36	31	27	16***
Sedatives	72	68	76	64***
Pancuronium	34	17**	33	15***
Methylxanthines	62	74**	49	53

[a] All parameters were examined with "as-treated" analyses. * p<0.05 *** p<0.001
[b] Thrombocytopenia requiring platelet transfusion. ** p<0.01

Pulmonary Hemorrhage: See WARNINGS. **Abnormal Laboratory Values:** Abnormal laboratory values are common in critically ill, mechanically ventilated, premature infants. A higher incidence of abnormal laboratory values in the Exosurf Neonatal group was not reported. **Events During Dosing:** Data on events during dosing are available from more than 8800 infants in the open, uncontrolled clinical study (Table 5).

Table 5: Events During Dosing in the Open, Uncontrolled Study[a]

Treatment Type:	Prophylactic Treatment	Rescue Treatment
Number of Infants:	N=1127	N=7711
	% of Infants	% of Infants
Reflux of Exosurf	20	31
Drop in O_2 saturation (≥20%)	6	22
Rise in O_2 saturation (≥10%)	5	6
Drop in transcutaneous pO_2 (≥20 mm Hg)	1	8
Rise in transcutaneous pO_2 (≥20 mm Hg)	2	5
Drop in transcutaneous pCO_2 (≥20 mm Hg)	<1	1
Rise in transcutaneous pCO_2 (≥20 mm Hg)	1	3
Bradycardia (<60 beats/min)	1	3
Tachycardia (>200 beats/min)	<1	<1
Gagging	1	5
Mucous Plugs	<1	<1

[a] Infants may have experienced more than one event.
Investigators were prohibited from adjusting FiO_2 and/or ventilator settings during dosing unless significant clinical deterioration occurred.

Reflux: Reflux of Exosurf Neonatal into the endotracheal tube during dosing has been observed and may be associated with rapid drug administration. If reflux occurs, drug administration should be halted and, if necessary, peak inspiratory pressure on the ventilator should be increased by 4 to 5 cm H_2O until the endotracheal tube clears. ***>20% Drop in Transcutaneous Oxygen Saturation:*** If transcutaneous oxygen saturation declines during dosing, drug administration should be halted and, if necessary, peak inspiratory pressure on the ventilator should be increased by 4 to 5 cm H_2O for 1 to 2 minutes. In addition, increases of FiO_2 may be required for 1 to 2 minutes. ***Mucous Plugs:*** See WARNINGS.

DOSAGE AND ADMINISTRATION: See full product information.

BURROUGHS WELLCOME CO., Research Triangle Park, NC 27709

Wellcome Printed in U.S.A. EX-Y01228

Drug Review

Transdermally administered fentanyl for pain management

Karim Anton Calis, David R. Kohler, and Diane M. Corso

Abstract: The physicochemical properties, pharmacology, pharmacokinetics, serum concentrations and clinical effects, adverse effects and contraindications, and dosage of transdermally administered fentanyl are described, and clinical studies evaluating the use of a transdermal fentanyl system in the treatment of postoperative pain and chronic cancer-associated pain are reviewed.

After application of a transdermal system, fentanyl is absorbed into the skin beneath the patch, where a depot forms in the upper skin layers. Plasma fentanyl concentrations are barely detectable for about two hours after patch placement. Eight to 12 hours after patch placement, concentrations approximate those achieved with equivalent i.v. doses of fentanyl. Some studies comparing transdermally administered fentanyl with placebo in postoperative patients showed that the patients who received fentanyl required fewer supplementary analgesics and reported less pain than the patients who received placebo. However, the overall efficacy and safety of the transdermal fentanyl system for the treatment of postoperative pain have not been adequately evaluated. Studies of cancer patients showed that transdermally administered fentanyl appears to be effective in the management of chronic, cancer-related pain. Dermatological reactions to the fentanyl patch are generally transient and mild. Other adverse effects are those that are commonly associated with narcotic analgesics. The 25-µg/hr patch should be used for initial treatment in patients not previously treated with narcotics. The dosage may be gradually increased until effective analgesia is obtained.

Although experience with the product is limited, transdermally administered fentanyl appears to be effective for the long-term management of cancer-related pain.

Index terms: Analgesics and antipyretics; Blood levels; Dosage forms; Drug administration routes; Fentanyl; Patches transdermal; Pharmacokinetics; Topical preparations; Toxicity
Clin Pharm. 1992; 11:22-36

Fentanyl is a potent synthetic narcotic that was first introduced into clinical practice in the early 1960s. It possesses strong analgesic properties and is a useful component of general anesthesia regimens.

Although injections and oral doses of narcotic analgesics can generally provide adequate pain control, these routes are not always ideal. We summarize the clinical experience with a recently marketed transdermal fentanyl delivery system for the management of acute and chronic pain.

Physicochemical Properties

Fentanyl is a synthetic phenylpiperidine derivative and a chemical congener of the reversed ester of meperidine.[1] This tertiary amine has the chemical name *N*-phenyl-*N*-(1-2-phenylethyl-4-piperidyl) propanamide. It is extremely lipid soluble, as demonstrated by

Karim Anton Calis, Pharm.D., is Coordinator, Drug Information Service, and Endocrinology Clinical Pharmacy Specialist, Department of Pharmacy, Warren G. Magnuson Clinical Center (WGMCC), National Institutes of Health, Bethesda, MD, and Clinical Assistant Professor, School of Pharmacy, University of Maryland, Baltimore. David R. Kohler, Pharm.D., is Oncology Clinical Pharmacy Specialist, Department of Pharmacy, WGMCC. At the time of this writing Diane M. Corso, was a pharmacy resident, Department of Pharmacy, WGMCC.

Address reprint requests to Dr. Calis at the Drug Information Service, Warren G. Magnuson Clinical Center, National Institutes of Health, Building 10, Room 1N-257, Bethesda, MD 20892.

The assistance of Mitchell B. Max, M.D., Greg Susla, Pharm.D., and Joseph F. Gallelli, Ph.D., in reviewing the manuscript and the secretarial assistance of Cori DeGraff are acknowledged.

This is article **680-204-9202** in the **ASHP Continuing-Education System**; it qualifies for 1.0 hour of continuing-education credit. See page 77 for learning objectives and test questions.

its n-octanol:water partition coefficient of 860:1.[2]

Fentanyl base has a molecular weight of 336.46, a melting point of 84 °C, and a pKa of 8.4.[3] At physiologic pH, fentanyl is 91% ionized.[4]

Fentanyl's high lipid solubility, potency, and low molecular weight make it a suitable candidate for transcutaneous delivery.[5,6]

Pharmacology

Fentanyl's pharmacologic effects are similar to those of morphine and meperidine.[7] On a weight basis, fentanyl is 50 to 100 times more potent than morphine and has a shorter duration of analgesic action after a single dose.[8]

Fentanyl exerts its pharmacologic effects by direct agonistic effects predominantly at the opiate mu receptor. Mu receptors are distributed in the central nervous system and in other tissues. In addition to analgesia, these receptors produce sedation, euphoria, dysphoria, drowsiness, alterations in mood, and mental clouding, but little hypnotic activity.[7]

Like other narcotic agents, fentanyl depresses the respiratory centers in the brain stem and may decrease respiratory rate, tidal volume, minute ventilation, and the ventilatory response to carbon dioxide. Additionally, fentanyl produces miosis, depresses the cough reflex, and may produce nausea and vomiting at analgesic doses by stimulating the chemoreceptor trigger zone and, possibly, by increasing vestibular sensitivity.

Fentanyl and other narcotics increase gastrointestinal tone, decrease propulsive contractions of gastrointestinal smooth muscle, and prolong gastrointestinal transit time. Gastric, biliary, and pancreatic secretions are decreased, resulting in delayed digestion. Biliary spasm and an increase in biliary tone may occur. Pressure in the common bile duct may rise because of constriction of the sphincter of Oddi. The tone of urinary smooth muscle can also be increased, resulting in ureteral spasm, dysuria, and even urinary urgency. Fentanyl preserves cardiac stability and has no major cardiovascular effects at therapeutic dosages, although orthostatic hypotension and postural syncope may occur as a result of peripheral vasodilation. Skeletal muscle rigidity may be seen at high doses. Fentanyl has minimal effects on uterine smooth muscle. Unlike other narcotics, fentanyl does not produce histamine release even at anesthetic doses.[9] Histamine assays and skin wheal testing in human subjects indicate that clinically important histamine release rarely occurs with fentanyl administration.[2]

Transdermal Drug Delivery

Transdermal therapeutic systems are a relatively new dosage form. When applied to an area of intact skin, they deliver a medication systemically at a controlled rate over a specified period of time.[10]

The transdermal absorption rate of a drug is determined by the delivery system and by the skin area on which the system is applied. A rate-controlling membrane in the transdermal system limits the release rate of the drug to a fraction of its permeation rate through the least permeable skin surface. This membrane allows the transdermal delivery system to control the rate at which the drug reaches the skin.[10-11] Therefore, drug absorption does not depend on the widely variable permeability of the stratum corneum, which would otherwise act as the rate-limiting step for drug absorption through the skin.[12]

The process of drug release and absorption from transdermal systems has been reviewed extensively.[13-20] Release of a drug from a transdermal system is characterized by an initial phase during which the drug present in the contact adhesive is rapidly absorbed through the skin, followed by a plateau phase with constant, sustained release of the drug from the reservoir.[12]

The drug penetrates the keratinous layers of the stratum corneum by passive diffusion and proceeds through the epidermis to the dermis, where it is absorbed into the systemic circulation.[21-24]

Not all drugs are suitable for transcutaneous administration. The skin has excellent barrier properties and exhibits physicochemical characteristics that limit which molecules will readily permeate. In general, compounds with low molecular weights (<1000) and adequate lipophilic and hydrophilic properties readily penetrate the skin. Other essential characteristics that make transdermal absorption feasible include a high apparent partition coefficient, high potency (to minimize the contact area of the delivery system), low volume of distribution, minimal binding to cutaneous tissue, and insignificant cutaneous metabolism. Ideally, drugs chosen for transdermal delivery should have a short elimination half-life and be nonirritating and nonsensitizing.[10,22]

Transdermal drug delivery offers several potential advantages over more conventional routes of administration. Because the drug is absorbed slowly and released in a sustained manner, relatively constant serum drug concentrations mimicking the concentrations obtained with constant-rate intravenous infusions can be achieved over long periods of time. This characteristic allows for less frequent administration of drugs with short half-lives, avoids invasive methods of drug delivery, and may decrease adverse effects associated with fluctuations in serum concentrations of the drug.

Transdermal systems circumvent erratic gastrointestinal absorption and first-pass metabolism and are effective alternatives when swallowing is difficult. Because they are more convenient than most other methods of drug delivery, transdermal systems also offer the potential to improve patients' compliance.

Possible disadvantages of transdermal drug delivery include the potential for local irritation, hypersensitivity reactions to components of the delivery system, and drug tolerance.

Transdermal Fentanyl Delivery Systems

Fentanyl is available in a transdermal therapeutic system (TTS, Alza Corporation, Palo Alto, CA) that provides continuous systemic delivery of the drug for 72 hours. The transdermal system, marketed in the United States by Janssen Pharmaceutica (Piscataway, NJ), is a rectangular, transparent unit composed of a protective liner and four functional layers (Figure 1). Beginning with the outermost layer, these include a polyester film backing; a drug reservoir of fentanyl base and alcohol, USP, gelled with hydroxyethyl cellulose; an ethylene-vinyl acetate copolymer membrane; and a silicone adhesive.[2] Alcohol (0.1 mL/10 sq cm) is used to increase the permeability of the skin to fentanyl and to enhance the rate of drug flow through the rate-limiting membrane. Only a small amount of alcohol (<0.1 mL per 10 sq cm) is actually released from the system during a 72-hour application period.

The impermeable outer layer prevents the loss of drug from the system and the entry of water into the drug reservoir. A three-day supply of fentanyl is contained within a sealed reservoir (form–fill–seal design).[10] The next layer is composed of a membrane that controls the rate of drug release from the reservoir.

A fentanyl-saturated silicone adhesive layer holds the system in place and effectively administers a "bolus" of fentanyl after the initial application of a patch.[12,25]

Another fentanyl transdermal delivery system (FTDS, Cygnus Therapeutic Systems, Redwood City, CA) is currently in Phase III clinical trials in the United States.[26] This system is being developed in conjunction with Anaquest, Inc., (Madison, WI) as a 24-hour system for the management of postoperative pain. Unlike Alza's TTS, FTDS is an unsealed, multilaminate system containing a solid matrix in which the drug is trapped.[a]

Because published clinical data were unavailable for the FTDS at the time of this writing, this review pertains only to the Alza system.

Pharmacokinetics

The clinical pharmacokinetics of transdermally administered fentanyl have not been extensively evaluated. Pharmacokinetic data for transdermal fentanyl are primarily derived from surgical patients undergoing various orthopedic or abdominal procedures. Patients with hepatic, renal, neurologic, or respiratory impairment and those with a history of drug abuse or regular narcotic use were generally excluded.

Additional pharmacokinetic data derived from surgical patients and healthy adult volunteers receiving intravenously administered fentanyl also are presented. It should be noted, however, that substantial variability in intravenous fentanyl pharmacokinetics has been reported.[8,27] Such variability may be due to differences in analytical methods or the combined effects of premedication, anesthesia, and surgery on the cardiovascular system.[8]

Differences in the pharmacokinetics and pharmacodynamics of transdermally administered fentanyl related to patients' weight, age, or sex or the duration of surgery have not been reported. Such differences, if they exist, are difficult to detect from available studies because of limitations in the study methodologies (short-term studies and small sample sizes).

Absorption. Michaels et al.[28] were the first to demonstrate fentanyl's potential for in vitro skin permeability. Roy and Flynn[6] later determined the in vitro penetration rates of several representative narcotics through human cadaver skin sections. Their work indicated that fentanyl and sufentanil could be successfully delivered percutaneously, whereas morphine, codeine, and hydromorphone could not. Further in vitro study by these investigators revealed that the free base form of fentanyl penetrates the skin more readily than the ionized form and that permeability coefficients are adequate through diverse skin sites, such as the sole of the foot, chest, thigh, and abdomen.[29] Using radiolabeled fentanyl (citrate and base), Sebel et al.[22] demonstrated that fentanyl is absorbed through human skin by measuring urine recovery of fentanyl and its metabolites in healthy volunteers. In general, drug permeation through human skin at a selected skin site, expressed as the coefficient of variation, can vary from 46% to 66% among individuals.[30] Variations in drug penetration between skin regions in an individual can vary 20–40%.[30]

Transdermal absorption of fentanyl appears to be generally characterized by a zero-order process.[31] After application of a transdermal system, fentanyl is absorbed into the skin beneath the patch, where a depot

Figure 1. Illustration of the fentanyl transdermal system. Provided courtesy of Alza Corporation.

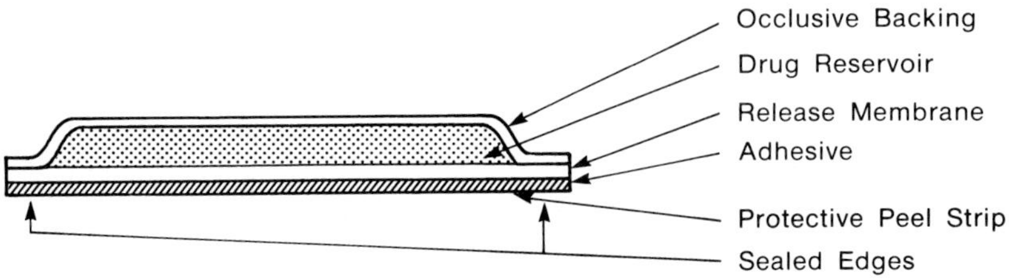

forms in the upper skin layers. Fentanyl is absorbed from the depot into the systemic circulation. Serum fentanyl concentrations remain relatively undetectable for approximately two hours after placement of the transdermal system because of formation of the skin depot.[31] Serum fentanyl concentrations rise gradually during the first 12–14 hours after application of the system and remain relatively constant until removal at 24 hours.[12]

The absorption of transdermally administered fentanyl was examined extensively in a well-designed study by Varvel et al.[12] The distribution and elimination characteristics of fentanyl were determined from a pharmacokinetic study of intravenous fentanyl in eight patients undergoing surgery and were used to define the absorption profile of transdermally administered fentanyl in the same group of patients. The amount of fentanyl delivered was determined as the difference between the initial content of the transdermal system (10 mg) and the residual content as measured by high-performance liquid chromatography (HPLC) after removal of the system. A three-compartment method (Loo-Riegelman) was used to determine the transdermal fentanyl absorption profile for each patient. The rate of fentanyl absorption from a transdermal system with a predicted nominal delivery rate of 100 μg/hr appeared to be relatively constant at 91.9 ± 25.7 μg/hr (mean ± S.D.) starting 4 to 8 hours after placement of the transdermal system until removal of the system at 24 hours. The mean ± S.D. dose of fentanyl delivered during the 24-hour period was 3.41 ± 0.88 mg, indicating that nearly 65% of the drug remained in the system. The amount of fentanyl actually absorbed through the skin was 2.97 ± 0.76 mg, yielding a systemic bioavailability of approximately 92%. An estimated 1.07 ± 0.43 mg of fentanyl (36% of the absorbed dose) remained in the skin depot after removal of the system at 24 hours and would be expected to be absorbed into the systemic circulation at a gradually declining rate.

Gourlay et al.[32] also evaluated the accuracy of the hourly fentanyl delivery rates by comparing the initial and residual fentanyl content of the transdermal systems. The assayed difference divided by the duration of the patch application provided a method for comparing the accuracy and uniformity of the transdermal fentanyl systems. Analysis of the data demonstrated considerable variability in hourly delivery rates, both within and among patients, but the actual mean delivery rates were within 10% of the nominal rates. The difference between mean actual delivery rates and nominal rates was even greater in an earlier study reported by the same investigators.[33] The studies by Gourlay et al., however, may not reflect the actual absorption characteristics of the transdermal fentanyl system because the investigators failed to evaluate the distribution and elimination of fentanyl in their subjects. Assessment of these variables is necessary to accurately evaluate the rate and extent of percutaneous drug absorption.

Vigorous exercise may transiently increase the cutaneous absorption of drugs from the skin reservoir sites by increasing blood flow to the skin and increasing drug removal from the skin.[22] Other factors that may affect permeability of the stratum corneum and influence drug absorption include the type of vehicle in which the drug is delivered, use of permeation enhancers, and skin site. Factors that can increase the rate or extent, or both, of drug absorption through the skin include excessive skin hydration, occlusion of the skin surface, skin damage (because of disease, chemicals, or overexposure to the sun), hyperfunction of the sweat glands, elevated cutaneous temperature, and increased vascular perfusion, which can vary with exercise and sleep.[22,23,34]

Distribution. Like other highly lipid soluble drugs, fentanyl is widely distributed throughout mammalian organs and tissues.[35,36] After intravenous injection in the rabbit, high fentanyl concentrations are quickly achieved in well-perfused tissues, including the lung, kidney, spleen, heart, and brain. The drug also is distributed to the intestines, liver, and skeletal muscles.

As expected, fentanyl is distributed into adipose tissues, which comprise a slowly equilibrating compartment.[8,35,37-39] This property accounts for fentanyl's brief duration of action after a single intravenous dose (analgesia persists for 30 to 60 minutes) and for potential accumulation of the drug and exaggeration of its pharmacologic effects with repeated or continuous administration.[8]

In three studies, fentanyl was administered intravenously to surgical patients or healthy adult volunteers.[12,40,41] The mean rapid distributional half-life ranged from 1 to 1.65 minutes, and the mean slow distributional half-life ranged from 12.7 to 24.7 minutes. The central compartment had a mean distribution volume of 12.7–26.6 L, whereas the steady-state volume of distribution was 311–398 L.

Variability in the range of distribution volumes reported for fentanyl has been large. This variability may be due in part to perioperative influences in surgical patients (e.g., the effects of anesthesia, surgery, or other medications on hemodynamics) and to differences in analytical methods (assay sensitivity or type).[8,27]

Fentanyl is 79–87% bound to plasma proteins at physiologic pH.[8] This relationship is not affected by wide variations of plasma fentanyl concentrations.[41] The unbound fraction increases with small reductions in pH in the region of pH 6 to 8.[4]

An estimated 3–4% of an intravenous fentanyl dose may be secreted into gastric juice.[42] However, Lehmann et al.[43] observed that plasma fentanyl concentrations were barely detectable after the administration of fentanyl by nasogastric tube to anesthetized patients, indicating that reabsorption of fentanyl previously secreted into the stomach contributes minimally to the ultimate disposition of fentanyl.

Metabolism. The metabolism of fentanyl in humans has not been completely elucidated.[8] Fentanyl is eliminated from the body predominantly by biotransformation in the liver and is metabolized primarily by *N*-dealkylation to norfentanyl.[44] Norfentanyl and fentanyl also undergo hydroxylation to hydroxypropionyl derivatives. Concentrations of fentanyl metabolites are equal to those of the parent compound within 30 minutes of intravenous fentanyl administration.[41] Metabolite concentrations subsequently exceed fentanyl concentrations and remain higher because of their slower elimination. All known fentanyl metabolites are believed to be pharmacologically inactive or minimally active.[41]

Piperidine ring hydroxylation, aromatic hydroxylation, and amide hydrolysis also may contribute to the metabolism of fentanyl.[39,45] Although metabolism or degradation by the skin's bacterial flora can occur with topical or transdermal drug application,[17,46-48] bioavailability data indicate that these events are unlikely with percutaneously administered fentanyl.[12]

Clearance and Elimination. Renal clearance of unchanged fentanyl accounts for less than 8% of an intravenously administered dose in healthy volunteers[41] and surgical patients.[49,50] Approximately 85% of a fentanyl dose is recovered in the urine, mostly as metabolites, within 72 hours of intravenous administration.[41] A small amount (approximately 9%) is recovered in the feces, predominantly as metabolites.

After an intravenous dose, fentanyl is rapidly and extensively distributed to tissues, and 98.6% of the dose is eliminated from the plasma in 60 minutes.[41]

The duration of action of fentanyl is limited by redistribution rather than clearance.[37] The clearance of fentanyl at doses used clinically does not appear to be dose dependent.[41,51]

Variability in the range of clearance values reported for fentanyl has been large.[8,27] This variability may be due in part to disparities of assay sensitivity and the methodologies used by different investigators and to coexistent confounding hemodynamic effects associated with surgery, anesthesia, and other medications in subjects undergoing surgery. In three studies involving both surgical patients and healthy adult volunteers, the mean clearance of fentanyl after intravenous administration was reported to range from 34 to 53 L/hr.[12,40,41]

Duthie et al.[52] measured fentanyl clearance after a 24-hour transdermal application in 19 patients (mean age of 49 years) undergoing abdominal surgery. One group received transdermal fentanyl (nominal rate of 100 μg/hr) after a 100-μg intravenous bolus, whereas the other group received the same transdermal fentanyl dose after a 200-μg intravenous dose. The amount of fentanyl delivered was determined as the difference between the initial content of the transdermal system and the residual content as measured by HPLC after removal of the system from the patient at 24 hours. A mean clearance of 27 L/hr was reported for the first group, and a mean clearance of 39 L/hr was reported for the second group. A third group (13 patients, mean age of 49 years) received 100 μg of fentanyl (as the citrate salt) per hour by continuous intravenous infusion and had a mean clearance of 43 L/hr. Clearance values reported for patients receiving transdermally administered fentanyl may have been affected by inaccuracies in the estimates of transdermal fentanyl absorption. The absorption profile from a transdermal study can be accurately determined only from the distribution and elimination characteristics obtained from a preceding pharmacokinetic study with intravenously administered drug in the same group of patients.

Fentanyl's elimination is limited by redistribution from poorly perfused tissues.[8] Mean terminal half-lives of 2 to 4 hours have been reported in healthy volunteers after single intravenous doses of fentanyl, whereas values of 2.5 to 7 hours have been observed in surgical patients.[8] More recent studies have indicated that the half-life of fentanyl in surgical patients after single intravenous doses is approximately six to eight hours.[12,40,53,54] Apparent terminal elimination half-life values in surgical patients after removal of the transdermal fentanyl system have ranged from 14 to 25 hours.[12,31,33,52,53,55,56] These values are far in excess of those observed after a single intravenous fentanyl bolus and are a consequence of continued absorption from a skin depot beneath the patch.[12,31,33,53,55] Systemic absorption from this site continues at a gradually decreasing rate, contributing to an attenuated decline in serum concentrations and giving the appearance of prolonged elimination. Varvel et al.[12] evaluated the pharmacokinetics of transdermally administered fentanyl in eight patients (mean age of 45 years) undergoing orthopedic surgery and reported a terminal elimination half-life of 6.1 hours after a single intravenous fentanyl dose and an apparent terminal elimination half-life of 17 hours after removal of the transdermal system in the same group of patients.

The effects of surgery or renal, hepatic, cardiac, or pulmonary disease on the disposition of fentanyl have not been adequately evaluated. Hyperventilation and accompanying hypocarbia have been reported to decrease the clearance of fentanyl.[57] Elderly patients are known to be more sensitive to the pharmacologic effects of narcotics owing to apparent alterations in protein binding, distribution, and elimination.[58-60] Bentley et al.[61] reported a prolonged terminal elimination half-life and markedly decreased fentanyl clearance (3.5-fold) in patients over the age of 60 years who received single intravenous fentanyl doses, compared with younger patients (mean age of 36 years) who received the same dose. The volume of distribution was reported to be similar in both groups. Conversely, Singleton et al.[62] observed that the clearance of fentanyl was similar in "elderly" and "younger" patients receiving single intravenous doses of fentanyl. These investigators reported a smaller steady-state distribution volume and higher plasma fentanyl concentrations immediately after intravenous administration to elderly patients. Variability in the results of these studies was attributed in part to differences in surgical procedures. All patients in the first study underwent abdominal surgery, whereas patients in the latter study underwent unspecified extra-abdominal procedures. Because abdominal surgery produces a substantial decrease in hepatic blood flow,[63] Singleton et al. suggested that the clearance of fentanyl (a drug with a high hepatic extraction ratio) may have been substantially decreased in Bentley et al.'s study population.[62] Scott and Stanski,[40] however, in a simultaneous pharmacokinetic and pharmacodynamic study, observed that fentanyl dosage requirements decrease with increasing age.

Serum Concentrations and Clinical Effects

Studies of fentanyl administered by continuous intravenous infusion for postoperative analgesia indicate that doses of approximately 1.5 µg/kg/hr appear to be effective and generally well tolerated in adult patients.[52,53,64-67] Such doses have typically produced mean serum or plasma fentanyl concentrations ranging from 1 to 2 ng/mL.

Gourlay et al.[68] observed that 0.693 ng/mL was the minimum effective blood fentanyl concentration for the treatment of postoperative pain. This figure represents the mean fentanyl concentration at which analgesia was attained in postoperative patients who regulated their own fentanyl doses using patient-controlled analgesia (PCA) infusion devices.

Plasma fentanyl concentrations of 1–3 ng/mL have been considered to be the minimum effective analgesic concentrations in surgical patients,[69-73] but wide interpatient variability may be seen.[12,73,74] Although marked respiratory depression has been reported at these concentrations when large initial doses were given for anesthesia,[75-77] a predictable correlation between arterial carbon dioxide pressure and plasma fentanyl concentrations has not yet been defined.[43]

A radioimmunoassay (RIA) method with adequate sensitivity has been used extensively to determine fentanyl concentrations in biological fluids.[78,79] More recently, sensitive assays that use gas–liquid chromatography (GLC) with nitrogen–phosphorus and mass spectroscopy detection methods have been developed.[80]

Kowalski et al.[81] reported that earlier RIA techniques resulted in overestimates of fentanyl concentrations. They developed a sensitive fentanyl GLC methodology with a lower limit of detection of 0.1 ng/mL. A comparison of the fentanyl RIA to a GLC method specific for the parent drug confirmed the validity of the RIA for the routine determination of fentanyl concentrations in human serum samples.[82]

Fentanyl concentrations in surgical patients after application of a transdermal fentanyl system are shown in Table 1. Serum fentanyl concentrations measured after application of a fentanyl patch reflect the net effects of absorption, distribution, and elimination. Although intrapatient variability in serum fentanyl concentrations appears to be low after placement of a transdermal fentanyl system, interindividual variability in serum concentrations is substantial during single[12] and multiple[2] applications in surgical patients.

If current estimates of fentanyl's elimination rate are accurate (six to eight hours), serum fentanyl concentrations observed at the end of a 24-hour transdermal administration period would theoretically approach steady-state levels.[31]

Serum, plasma, and blood fentanyl concentrations 8 to 12 hours after application of a fentanyl patch were generally similar to those achieved with equal doses of fentanyl administered by continuous intravenous infusion.[52,53] Transdermally delivered fentanyl produces relatively constant plasma concentrations in the postoperative patient[12,31,52] that are maintained throughout a 72-hour patch application period.[55,56] The slow change in serum fentanyl concentrations is due to the accumulation and depletion of fentanyl in the skin depot.[83] Fentanyl concentrations typically reach a plateau 14 to 20 hours after the initial 24-hour application of the transdermal system.[12,53,55,84]

The relationship between fentanyl concentration and analgesic response in postoperative patients who receive transdermal fentanyl appears to be similar to that reported in patients who receive postoperative intravenous infusions of fentanyl. However, the small sample size common to all of the published trials, the lack of controls in some studies, and the routine use of supplementary narcotic analgesics obscure this relationship.

Therapeutic Efficacy for Postoperative Pain

To date, efficacy of the transdermal fentanyl system has been evaluated in 357 postoperative patients with acute pain. Patients with acute pain were studied for periods of 24 to 48 hours.

Bell et al.[56] evaluated the perioperative safety and efficacy of multiple, sequentially applied fentanyl TTSs in 11 consecutive patients scheduled to undergo colorectal surgery. Patients received preoperative medication including transdermal fentanyl 75 µg/hr applied two hours before surgery. An additional 300 µg of fentanyl was administered during induction of anesthesia and during the first hour of the operative procedure. Patches were replaced every 24 hours for a total of three applications. Supplementary analgesia with intravenous and intramuscular morphine was available.

Analgesic efficacy was serially assessed by a 10-point visual analogue scale (VAS) for pain intensity until 84 hours after the initial patch application. Patients' VAS scores varied most widely during the first 24 hours and decreased over the succeeding 48 hours. The amount of morphine required for supplemental analgesia declined similarly. TTS-fentanyl patches were well tolerated, and patients' satisfaction with the quality of pain control was uniformly good.

Caplan et al.[83] conducted a double-blind, parallel-group, comparative evaluation of transdermally administered fentanyl given concomitantly with regional anesthesia in patients undergoing shoulder surgery. Forty patients were randomly assigned to receive either a 75-µg/hr fentanyl patch (n = 22) or an identical placebo patch (n = 20). Transdermal systems were applied immediately before interscalene block anesthesia and were worn for 24 hours. Patients also received fentanyl (as the citrate salt) 100 µg by intravenous bolus injection concurrently with the application of fentanyl patches. Intravenous and intramuscular morphine was available to both groups for supplemental analgesia during the first 24 hours. During the 12-hour period after removal of fentanyl patches, patients were offered their choice of supplemental analgesia with either intramuscular morphine or orally administered acetaminophen 300 mg with codeine phosphate 30 mg.

Patients who received transdermal fentanyl required significantly fewer supplemental analgesics throughout the 36-hour study period compared with patients treated with placebo. The mean ± S.D. rates of morphine sulfate use were 0.8 ± 0.61 mg/hr and 1.3 ± 0.64 mg/hr during the period of active drug administration and 0.3 ± 0.36 mg/hr and 0.5 ± 0.32 mg/hr during the 12-hour period after patch removal for the fentanyl-treated and placebo-treated groups, respectively. Likewise, patients who received fentanyl indicated significantly less pain by 100-mm VAS evaluations of pain intensity than patients who received placebo.

The incidence and severity of all adverse reactions were similar in both groups, with the exception of patients' ventilatory rates and the incidence of vomiting. Fentanyl-treated patients had significantly lower respiratory rates compared with placebo-treated patients (14 ± 3 versus 16 ± 2 breaths/minute, respectively). Three patients who received transdermal fentanyl sustained ventilatory rates of five to seven breaths/minute during sleep, which increased in response to arousal.

Seventy-nine percent of the fentanyl-treated pa-

Table 1.
Fentanyl Concentrations in Surgical Patients after Application of a Transdermal Fentanyl System

Reference	No. Patients	Mean Age or Age Range (yr)	Mean Weight or Weight Range (kg)	Sampled Fluid[a]	Assay Method[b]	I.V. Fentanyl Dose (µg)[c]	Nominal TTS Fentanyl Dosage (µg/hr)	Duration of Patch Application (hr)[d]	Mean ± S.D. Concentration after Patch Application (ng/mL)
52	6 M/4 F	49	70	P	RIA	100	100[e]	24	0.3 ± 0.1 at 2 hr, 0.7 ± 0.2 at 4 hr, 1.3 ± 0.2 at 8 hr, 1.6 ± 0.2 at 12 hr, 2.0 ± 0.2 at 24 hr[f]
	5 M/4 F	49	74	P	RIA	200	100[e]	24	0.3 ± 0.1 at 2 hr, 1.1 ± 0.2 at 4 hr, 1.2 ± 0.3 at 8 hr, 1.5 ± 0.2 at 12 hr, 1.3 ± 0.1 at 24 hr[f]
85	7 M/15 F	52	69	P	RIA	200	100[e]	24	1.5 ± 0.1 at 12 hr, 2.0 ± 0.2 at 24 hr[f]
83	16 M/6 F	41.2	81.2	S	RIA	100[g]	75[g]	24	0.96 ± 1.02 at 8 hr, 1.46 ± 0.97 at 24 hr
84	20 M/8 F	18–65	72	S	RIA	None	75[e]	24	1.9 ± 0.9 at 24 hr[h]
55	5 M/5 F	56–72	≤100	P	RIA	300	75[e]	72	1.5 ± 0.5 between 0 and 72 hr
56	5 M/6 F	29–67	50–100	P	RIA	300	75[e]	72[i]	2.7 ± 2.05 between 0 and 72 hr
31	5 M/3 F[j]	21–70	50–97	P	RIA	None	75[e]	24	1 ng/mL peak concentration at mean of 21 hr after a mean lag time of 2 hr
53	8 M	58	80	S	RIA	300	100[e]	24	2.15 ± 0.93 between 15 and 24 hr
12	3 M/5 F	45	68	S	GLC/MS	Mean of 778	100[k]	24	1.8 ± 0.8 between 14 and 24 hr
33	5 M/8 F	44	71	B	GLC/NP	Mean of 170	75[c,l]	48[m]	1.25 ± 0.78 between 12 and 24 hr 1.85 ± 0.72 between 36 and 48 hr

[a]P=plasma, S=serum, B=blood.
[b]RIA=radioimmunoassay, GLC/MS=gas–liquid chromatography with mass spectroscopic detection, GLC/NP=gas–liquid chromatography with nitrogen–phosphorus detection.
[c]Given during or immediately before induction of general anesthesia.
[d]Patch applied to upper anterior chest wall.
[e]Approximately two hours before surgical incision.
[f]Reported as mean ± S.E.
[g]Given before regional anesthesia.
[h]Estimated from serum concentration–time plot.
[i]Old patch removed and new patch applied to different site at 24 and 48 hours.
[j]Five patients completed the blood sampling schedule.
[k]24 hours after i.v. fentanyl dose.
[l]Dosage individualized by using equation derived from a previous study.
[m]Old patch removed and new patch applied to different site at 24 hours.

tients and 44% of the placebo-treated patients expressed overall satisfaction with their levels of pain control, which constituted a significant difference in favor of fentanyl. Thirty-seven percent of patients who received fentanyl, but none of the patients who received placebo, provided unsolicited expressions of satisfaction with the "constant" quality of analgesia.

The investigators concluded that transdermal delivery of fentanyl produces analgesia that is quantitatively superior to that produced by intermittently administered morphine and provides a more consistent quality of analgesia. Patients in this study received only regional anesthesia, thereby eliminating the potentially confounding systemic effects of general anesthetics.

Holley and Van Steennis[53] monitored patients' serum fentanyl concentrations during and after surgery in a trial comparing TTS-fentanyl (100 μg/hr) with fentanyl administered at four different dosages by continuous intravenous infusion, and with placebo. They observed a slow increase in patients' serum fentanyl concentrations after application of the TTS-fentanyl patch and a correspondingly slow decline in these concentrations after patch removal. In providing recommendations for the perioperative use of TTS-fentanyl, they acknowledged the delayed onset of adequate analgesia (attributable to the delayed systemic availability of fentanyl from the transdermal delivery system) and the potential for persistence of toxicity (attributable to the attenuated elimination of fentanyl from the body). They recommended a conservative choice in selecting a dosage strength of TTS-fentanyl to provide a base or background level of analgesia and concomitant administration of a more rapidly acting agent.

Rowbotham et al.[85] studied the safety and efficacy of TTS-fentanyl as postoperative analgesia in 40 patients in a double-blind, placebo-controlled trial. Patients were randomly assigned to receive either TTS-fentanyl 100 μg/hr or TTS-placebo patches, applied two hours before upper abdominal surgery. Additional analgesic prophylaxis included intravenous fentanyl (as the citrate salt) 200 μg given preoperatively and morphine administered postoperatively by PCA, which was continued until 48 hours after application of the fentanyl patches.

Pain intensity was assessed by a 10-point VAS. The investigators also compared the degree of central nervous system depression produced by the two regimens on indices of patients' respiratory function. Patients' ventilatory efforts were evaluated by spirometry for peak expiratory flow rate (PEFR), and blood oxygenation and carbon dioxide retention were measured serially by arterial blood gas (ABG) analyses.

Notably, two patients who received TTS-placebo, but none who received TTS-fentanyl, demanded the maximum amount of morphine available by PCA at 90 minutes postoperatively. Patients who received fentanyl had a significantly lower mean requirement for morphine than placebo-treated patients throughout active treatment and for 24 hours after removal of the TTS-fentanyl patch. The range of scores and the median VAS values for pain intensity were significantly lower for patients treated with fentanyl than for patients who received placebo at each interval during the first 24 hours.

The combined effects of narcotic analgesics and general anesthesia on ventilation and perfusion also differed between the groups. The mean PEFR at 12 and 24 hours was significantly greater in patients who received fentanyl. Although the mean ventilatory rate for patients treated with fentanyl was lower than that for placebo-treated patients at the same points in time, no patient sustained a ventilatory rate sufficiently low (i.e., fewer than eight breaths/minute for longer than five minutes) to require their withdrawal from the study. Despite the difference in ventilatory rates, ABG tensions were similar in both groups.

The investigators concluded that fentanyl produced a substantial background analgesia that provided superior pain relief. Patients treated with TTS-fentanyl experienced fewer adverse effects as a result of their lower requirement for supplemental morphine postoperatively. However, the investigators cautioned that supplementary analgesic therapy would probably be necessary if a transdermal delivery system capable of delivering no more than 100 μg of fentanyl per hour were used.

Gourlay et al.[32] reported a double-blind, placebo-controlled study of TTS-fentanyl for postoperative analgesia. Forty patients were randomly assigned to receive dermal patches containing either fentanyl or placebo. The rate of delivery of transdermally administered fentanyl approximated a dosage strength calculated from an equation previously developed by the investigators. The dosage strength of TTS-fentanyl most commonly used was 50 μg/hr (range = 25–75 μg/hr). Patients treated with fentanyl patches received additional intravenous fentanyl (as the citrate salt) 2 μg/kg administered intraoperatively. Patients treated with placebo patches received intraoperative analgesia with intravenously administered meperidine hydrochloride 1 mg/kg. Patch systems were replaced at 24 hours after the initial application with an identical drug-containing or placebo-containing system. Both groups of patients were given supplementary postoperative analgesia with meperidine.

Patients evaluated the intensity of the pain they experienced postoperatively by means of a 100-mm VAS. Additionally, their level of postoperative sedation was graded by a five-point descriptive scale. There were no significant differences between groups in terms of VAS pain intensity or sedation rating scores. Three patients treated with fentanyl sustained at least one episode of bradypnea (fewer than 10 breaths/minute), and although one patient developed pulmonary edema, the etiological contribution of fentanyl was not clear.

The difference between the groups' mean requirements for supplemental meperidine was significant only during the three 12-hour periods of assessment from 12–48 hours after surgery. In contrast, patients who were treated with TTS-fentanyl required substantially, albeit not significantly, greater amounts of supplementary meperidine during the first 12 hours after surgery. The investigators postulated that either the long and variable delay in attaining effective systemic concentrations of fentanyl after application of the transdermal system or fentanyl's relatively short duration of action may have accounted for the increased requirement in fentanyl-treated patients for supplemental meperidine within the first 12 hours. Overall, there was no difference between groups in the total mean supplementary amount of meperidine required over the 48-hour study period.

Latasch and Lüders[84] evaluated the analgesic efficacy of TTS-fentanyl in a double-blind, placebo-controlled study in 60 patients undergoing knee arthrotomy. Patients received a combination of medications intramuscularly, including meperidine hydrochloride 50 mg, promethazine hydrochloride 50 mg, and atropine sulfate 1 mg, administered before induction of anesthesia. Arthroscopic evaluation, under spinal anesthesia induced by bupivacaine, preceded arthrotomy. The investigators chose to study the time delay after application of the TTS-fentanyl patch until patients had adequate analgesic levels of fentanyl. To satisfy that objective, patches delivering fentanyl 75 μg/hr transdermally were not applied until after arthroscopy and before arthrotomy. Patches remained in place for 24 hours after application. Piritramide 12.5 mg by intramuscular injection was available to both groups for breakthrough pain.

Patients who received TTS-fentanyl required significantly less piritramide than those who received placebo ($p < 0.001$). Patients' requirements for supplemental analgesia demonstrated that the period of greatest need occurred after cessation of spinal anesthesia, during the first five to eight hours after arthrotomy. These data are consistent with the observation that serum concentrations of fentanyl did not reach steady-state levels until approximately 15 hours after patch application. The investigators did not identify a target serum analgesic concentration, but concluded that earlier application of fentanyl patches may more optimally control breakthrough pain.

Six hours after application of TTS-fentanyl, one patient had markedly diminished arterial oxygen and carbon dioxide tensions of 8.6 kPa and 6.8 kPa (65 and 51 mm Hg), respectively, concurrent with markedly elevated serum concentrations of fentanyl (between 5 and 6 ng/mL). Additionally, the patient had a mean respiratory rate of more than 9 breaths/minute, and although moderately sedated, he remained arousable. The investigators correlated the serum fentanyl concentrations with the patient's low body weight and recommended that fentanyl patches delivering ≥75 μg/hr be limited to patients whose body weight exceeds 60 kg.

The incidence and severity of graded levels of sedation were significantly greater for patients who received TTS-fentanyl. Although patients were to have been evaluated by verbal rating scales for pain and adverse effects and by a global assessment of pain, the results of these evaluations were not presented.

TTS-fentanyl has been reported to be safe when used concomitantly with other central nervous system depressants (e.g., benzodiazepines, barbiturates, nitrous oxide, halogenated volatile anesthetics, and neuromuscular blocking agents) in patients receiving regional anesthesia and during induction and administration of general anesthesia.

Therapeutic Efficacy for Cancer-Related Pain

Efficacy of the transdermal fentanyl system has been evaluated in 153 cancer patients with chronic pain. Patients were evaluated for periods of 30 days to more than one year.

Miser et al.[86] studied five consecutive patients who experienced chronic pain related to their malignant disease, their treatment, or both. Before treatment, all patients indicated a level of pain intensity greater than 35 mm as scored by a 100-mm VAS. Patients received a continuous intravenous infusion of fentanyl that was individually adjusted to provide the lowest rate of drug administration consistent with an adequate level of pain relief (defined by a VAS score of <35 mm). Once an adequate level of analgesia had been achieved, a fentanyl patch was applied to the patient's chest wall, back, or upper arm at a dose and delivery rate within 25 μg/hr of the intravenous dosage. Intravenous infusion of fentanyl was tapered over six hours after application of the patch and then discontinued. TTS-fentanyl patches were changed every 24 hours, and skin application sites were rotated to avoid local irritation. The dosage strength of the fentanyl patch was adjusted after a minimum of 12 hours at the previous dosage to maintain good to excellent pain control (i.e., a VAS score of <35 mm). The median dosage strength of fentanyl administered transdermally was 225 μg/hr (range = 75–350 μg/hr).

All patients had good or better pain control with the transdermal delivery system for periods ranging from 3 to 156 days (mean = 45 days). One of the five patients required concomitant administration of a nonsteroidal anti-inflammatory drug to maintain adequate analgesia.

Simmonds et al.[87] provided preliminary data from an uncontrolled study evaluating the long-term efficacy and safety of TTS-fentanyl patches in patients with cancer-related pain. Thirty-nine patients received orally administered doses of morphine adjusted to establish their individual analgesic requirements. Once the dosages of morphine were stabilized, morphine was replaced by fentanyl and administered via a TTS-fentanyl patch that was reapplied every three days. The median fentanyl dosage at the time of first application was 50 μg/hr (range = 25–255 μg/hr). The median dosage of fentanyl at the conclusion of the study, including final doses at the time of withdrawal from the study, was 100 μg/hr (50–525 μg/hr). Twenty-three patients (59%) required a ≥50% escalation of their dosage.

Analgesic efficacy was indicated by a decrease in patients' mean VAS pain scores from 46 mm at the time that oral morphine dosages were stabilized to 41 mm one month after initial use of the transdermal system. Although the decrease in VAS scores indicated a general improvement in analgesic effect, pain relief could not be wholly attributed to fentanyl or to the delivery system used. Some unspecified percentage of patients continued to require up to 720 mg/day of supplementary prompt-release oral morphine sulfate for breakthrough pain. Patients' compliance and acceptance of the patch system, however, were excellent. The practicability of TTS-fentanyl for safe and effective long-term analgesia was supported by the duration of patients' study participation (5–365 days [median = 84 days]) and the variety of events that occurred concurrently with the study (e.g., surgery, herpes zoster eruption, antineoplastic drug administration). Notably absent was information regarding the incidence of adverse effects associated with therapy.

Zech et al.[88] studied 13 inpatients with severe cancer-related pain who received fentanyl on demand for 24 hours via PCA. Subsequently, the initial dosage strength for transdermally administered fentanyl, applied at hour 24, was based on the patients' PCA dose titration. Supplementary intravenously administered fentanyl was continued from hours 24 through 96. Patches were replaced every 72 hours, and the fentanyl dosage was adjusted at hour 96 based on each patient's total analgesic requirement for intravenous plus transdermally administered drug.

The initial mean ± S.D. dosage of fentanyl was 65.4 ± 30 μg/hr (range = 25–125 μg/hr). After 72 hours the mean dosage had escalated to 77.1 ± 37.5 μg/hr (range = 25–150 μg/hr).

Analgesic efficacy was assessed by VAS pain intensity scores and by a 4-point "percentage of pain relief" scale. Patients' mean ± S.D. VAS pain scores improved, falling from 45.9 ± 18.6 mm to 34.9 ± 15.2 mm after the initial 24-hour PCA fentanyl titration, and subsequently to 23.4 ± 15.5 mm 24 hours after application of fentanyl patches. Patients' mean ± S.D. pain relief scores improved 57.7 ± 25.8% (range = 25–100%) over baseline. Supplementary subcutaneously administered morphine was available on an as-needed basis, and an unspecified standardized adjuvant medication was provided. The usual supplementary daily dosage of morphine sulfate was reported as approximately 90 mg. The investigators did not provide data detailing the number of patients who required supplementary analgesia, nor did they describe whether the standardized adjuvant medication(s) may have included nonnarcotic analgesics.

None of the patients experienced severe adverse effects, and patient compliance and acceptance of therapy were reported to be excellent. However, based on their observations on day 7 that patients' VAS scores and the number of supplementary morphine doses increased while plasma fentanyl concentrations simultaneously decreased, the investigators suggested that fentanyl patches may need to be changed more frequently in some patients.

Levy et al.[89] reported preliminary data from a double-blind, placebo-controlled, crossover trial that focused on the safety and analgesic efficacy of transdermally administered fentanyl and on patients' quality of life. Fifty-six inpatients with chronic cancer-related pain received TTS-fentanyl. Dosages were adjusted over three to five days to establish patients' individual analgesic requirements. Patients were then discharged from the hospital with TTS-fentanyl patches to ensure the stability of their analgesic requirements for one week. Subsequently, patients were randomly assigned to continue to receive either TTS-fentanyl or TTS-placebo for one week, after which they were crossed over to receive the alternate treatment for an additional seven days.

The investigators reported significant differences between baseline data and measurements made during the two study periods with respect to pain, the use of supplemental oral morphine, and patients' feelings of tension and anger. However, statistical comparisons of the same variables between groups during the two study periods revealed no significant differences.

The investigators observed that patients' total narcotic intake (i.e., fentanyl and morphine) was significantly lower during the placebo treatment period, but they did not specify whether the basis for their comparison was supplemental morphine use during the alternate treatment period or general narcotic use before entry into the study. The study design was flawed by the investigators' apparent disregard for the distribution and elimination phenomena associated with fentanyl and the well-described delay in achieving effective serum fentanyl concentrations with transdermal administration. All patients in the study received fentanyl during a 10- to 15-day period of dose titration and maintenance stabilization immediately before the test period; patients initially assigned to receive fentanyl also had an additional seven days of TTS-fentanyl administration. Neither group was subjected to an intervening period of drug washout before receiving fentanyl or placebo or at the time of treatment crossover. One may predict that the continued absorption of fentanyl from the skin underlying the site of patch placement and its redistribution from adipose tissues may have resulted in systemic concentrations that were sufficient to provide a persistent and confounding analgesic effect. Therefore, it is not remarkable that patients would have required less supplemental morphine, at least initially, during the placebo treatment period.

Transdermal delivery eliminates the need for repeated injections and the attendant discomfort they produce, the cyclic waxing and waning of effects that directly correlate with fluctuations in systemic concentrations of an analgesic after intermittent administration, and the infectious risks associated with maintaining indwelling vascular access or subcutaneous infusion devices for patients receiving long-term analgesics by intermittent or continuous infusion.

Adverse Effects

Complications of fentanyl treatment that are unique to transdermal administration may be predicted to result from either local irritation or variations in the kinetics of drug release from the delivery system. The latter category of adverse effects may be expected to vary directly with systemic drug concentrations.

Dermatological reactions to the TTS-fentanyl patch have been characterized as transient and mild, typical of skin occlusion and local irritation rather than an allergic contact dermatitis, although sensitization has occurred with other transdermally administered drugs.[90,91] Various investigators have reported transient asymptomatic or pruritic erythematous reactions involving the area of skin occluded by the transdermal systems. The reported incidence varies from none in some series to approximately 60% of patients.[32,83,85,86] Erythema generally resolves within 6 to 24 hours after patch removal.[32,83] Similar dermatological manifestations have appeared on the skin of patients treated with placebo patches, indicating that the reaction is more likely attributable to the contact adhesive rather than to fentanyl.[83] Chronic local irritation may be minimized by rotating the sites of patch application. Because skin occlusion creates a favorable environment for bacterial and fungal overgrowth, pretreatment of the patch application site with topical chlorhexidine solution has been recommended to diminish the incidence of bacterial overgrowth.[90]

Other adverse effects that are independent of the drug delivery system are those that are commonly associated with narcotic analgesics.

Nausea and vomiting due to transdermal fentanyl may be difficult to assess in some clinical situations because of the numerous factors that may elicit or contribute to an emetic response. Three of five patients studied by Miser et al.[86] experienced nausea and vomiting that had preceded use of the TTS-fentanyl patch. Notably, patients' symptoms did not worsen during TTS-fentanyl use. Eighteen fentanyl-treated and 15 placebo-treated patients received metoclopramide for nausea in the trial reported by Gourlay et al.[32] Neither the incidence of nausea nor the mean dosage of metoclopramide administered over the 48-hour study period was significantly different between the fentanyl and the placebo groups. By comparison, treated and control patients had similar incidences of nausea in the study reported by Caplan et al.[83]; however, the incidence of emesis was significantly greater in fentanyl-treated patients (73% versus 30%).

The central nervous system depressant effects of narcotics may compromise optimal protection or relief from pain and at least temporarily require diminishing or discontinuing analgesic therapy until the untoward effects abate. Various degrees of somnolence are reported in more than 10% of patients receiving TTS-fentanyl. The effects of medical conditions or therapies that depress the sensorium (e.g., infection and sepsis, dehydration, azotemia, hepatic encephalopathy, and therapy with other drugs that have depressant effects on the central nervous system) may also be exacerbated by narcotics such as fentanyl, with a resultant obtundation or further diminution in patients' mental acuity requiring reduction or temporary interruption of analgesic therapy.[86] Alternatively, analeptic agents (e.g., dextroamphetamine) may be used as adjuvants to maintain an acceptable level of mentation.[86]

As with other opioid agonists, the acceptable level of respiratory depression may constrain the amount of fentanyl that can be administered and consequently the level of analgesia that can be achieved. The manufacturer reports that, overall, hypoventilation was seen in 4% of postoperative patients and 2% of cancer patients who received transdermal fentanyl. Plezia et al.[92] reported that the postoperative course of two patients was complicated by failure to recover spontaneous respirations immediately after extubation. Both patients subsequently responded to administration of naloxone. Two patients in the study conducted by Miser et al.[86] experienced respiratory depression during the period of maintenance dose titration. The investigators attributed the effect to the two-compartment distribution characteristics of fentanyl and its physiological correlate, the prolonged period that is required to eliminate fentanyl from the tissues underlying the site of patch application and from adipose tissues.[53,86] They further described fentanyl's contribution to the exacerbation of central nervous system depression associated with medical complications, an additional potential hazard related to attenuated fentanyl clearance from adipose tissues.[86]

Nine percent of patients withdrew from the clinical trials because of intolerable adverse effects. According to the manufacturer, 10% or more of cancer patients receiving transdermal fentanyl in clinical trials experienced nausea, vomiting, constipation, dry mouth, somnolence, confusion, asthenia, and sweating. Abdominal pain, headache, anorexia, diarrhea, dyspepsia, dizziness, restlessness, hallucinations, anxiety, depression, euphoria, dyspnea, apnea, pruritus, and urinary retention were reported in 3–10% of the patients. Although many of the adverse effects reported can be expected to occur with all narcotics, a causal relationship with transdermally administered fentanyl was not always established. Some of the adverse symptoms may have been attributable to patients' underlying disease or to the combined use of fentanyl with other supplementary analgesics. Nausea and vomiting can generally be managed by using antiemetic agents. The routine liberal use of stool softeners is recommended for patients receiving narcotics and may prevent the development of constipation in those receiving fentanyl. Other adverse effects may respond to dosage reductions or other pharmacologic interventions, or they may require the discontinuation of treatment.

Contraindications and Precautions

Transdermally administered fentanyl is contraindicated in patients who have known hypersensitivity to fentanyl and should be used cautiously in patients with a history of hypersensitivity to contact adhesives. The drug should be used with caution in elderly and debilitated patients because the distribution and clearance of fentanyl can be altered. As with other narcotics, hypoventilation can occur in patients receiving fentanyl. Therefore, the drug should be administered cautiously in patients with respiratory disorders and other patients whose conditions or treatments may predispose them to respiratory depression or otherwise potentiate the effects of fentanyl. The management of hypoventilation should include the usual supportive care to ensure maintenance of a patent airway. Immediate removal of the transdermal system and administration of naloxone are recommended in the presence of serious respiratory depression. Close observation of the patient and repeated or continuous administration of naloxone may be necessary despite removal of the patch because the drug continues to be absorbed from the skin depot for a period that may be expected to exceed the duration of response to naloxone. Serum fentanyl concentrations typically decline by 50% approximately 14 to 25 hours after removal of the transdermal system.

Transdermal fentanyl should be avoided in patients with head injuries and increased intracranial pressure because it may obscure the patient's clinical course. Fentanyl may also cause bradycardia and should therefore be used cautiously in patients with bradyarrhythmias. Because the release of fentanyl from the delivery system may be increased with elevations in body temperature, febrile patients and theoretically those in warm surroundings should be closely monitored for narcotic adverse effects. The manufacturer states that absorption of fentanyl can theoretically increase by nearly 35% when the body temperature increases to 40 °C.

Because adequate controlled studies in pregnant women are lacking, fentanyl should be used during pregnancy only when the potential benefit outweighs the potential risk to the fetus (FDA pregnancy category C). Because fentanyl is excreted in human milk, its use by nursing mothers also should be avoided. Studies performed by the manufacturer indicate that fentanyl has low genotoxic potential and presents minimal mutagenic risk at usual therapeutic dosages. The manufacturer also reports that the silicone adhesive used in the fentanyl transdermal system shows no evidence of mutagenic activity.

Dosage and Administration

The lowest dosage strength of transdermal fentanyl (25 μg/hr) should generally be used for the initial treatment of chronic pain in patients who have not received other narcotics. The dosage may be gradually increased until adequate analgesia is attained. According to the manufacturer, most of the clinical trials with transdermal fentanyl in the management of chronic pain involved patients who had previously received other narcotics and in whom some degree of tolerance was likely. Typically, a conservative conversion method was used to switch such patients to transdermal fentanyl. Briefly, the patient's analgesic requirements from the previous 24 hours were calculated, and the total was converted to an equianalgesic dosage of oral morphine as described by Foley.[93] The daily dosage of morphine was then equated to a transdermal fentanyl dose such that 90 mg of oral morphine sulfate per day (or 15 mg of injectable morphine sulfate per day) was considered approximately equivalent to 25 μg of fentanyl per hour. The analgesic activity ratio of 10 mg of morphine sulfate administered intramuscularly to 100 μg of i.v. fentanyl (as the citrate salt) was used by the manufacturer to derive this conversion factor. The method provides only an estimate of patients' analgesic requirements. The manufacturer reports that nearly 50% of patients who are switched to fentanyl patches require an increase in dosage after initial application. Because clinical experience with the systematic dosing of transdermal fentanyl for chronic pain management is limited, low initial dosages should also be used for opioid-tolerant patients. The full analgesic effects of transdermal fentanyl may not be achieved for several days after initial application. The dosage should be increased slowly (i.e., not more frequently than every four to six days) until adequate pain relief is attained. The manufacturer recommends that after the first dosage adjustment patients wear a higher-dose patch through two consecutive 72-hour applications before further dosage increases are made. Supplementary doses of short-acting, prompt-release analgesics may be necessary during dosage titration, and some patients may require additional doses thereafter for breakthrough pain.

The dosage of fentanyl, as with other narcotics, must be carefully adjusted according to the individual needs of each patient. The lowest effective dosage should be used. The manufacturer recommends that elderly and debilitated patients receive reduced initial dosages of transdermal fentanyl because the clearance of the drug in such patients may be markedly reduced. It is not yet known whether the dosage of fentanyl should be adjusted in patients with renal or hepatic impairment. However, because the drug is metabolized by the liver and largely excreted by the kidneys, accumulation of fentanyl and its metabolites is possible. The safety and efficacy of transdermal fentanyl in children has not been evaluated; therefore, pediatric dosage recommendations are not available at this time.

The transdermal fentanyl system is typically worn continuously for 72 hours. When analgesia is required for more than 72 hours, a new patch should be applied to an alternate site. This allows the skin depot below the first patch to be gradually depleted of fentanyl (as a result of continued systemic absorption) while the drug concentrates in the skin layers below the new patch application site. Serum fentanyl concentrations during the transition from one patch to another would not be expected to fluctuate substantially if a different skin site is used. Fentanyl concentrations, however, may rise markedly if the application site is not rotated because the existing skin depot site is already replete with drug deposited by the previous patch. Replacing the fentanyl system more frequently than every 72 hours (e.g., every 24 hours) has resulted in significantly higher mean serum fentanyl concentrations[56] and is not generally recommended. According to the manufacturer, however, a small number of patients may require application of the system every 48 hours. For delivery rates in excess of 100 μg/hr, multiple systems may be applied simultaneously over different areas of the skin. Gradual tapering of fentanyl may prevent the precipitation of acute withdrawal symptoms.

Patient Instruction

Patients should be instructed in the proper use of the transdermal fentanyl delivery system. Immediately after removal from the sealed package, the transdermal fentanyl system should be applied to a nonhirsute area of intact skin on the upper torso. A flat, nonirritated site should be selected, and excess hair should be carefully clipped to avoid injury to the skin. The skin surface must be dry and free of any substance that may produce irritation or otherwise alter the absorption of the drug (e.g., alcohol, soaps, lotions). Once applied, the patch should be pressed evenly and firmly in place for approximately 20 seconds to ensure that the pressure-sensitive adhesive is in full contact with the skin surface and that the edges are completely sealed. The patient or provider of care should minimize touching of the adhesive surface to avoid absorption of fentanyl through the skin surface of the hand. Although vigorous rubbing of the patch may lead to inadvertent removal of the system, bathing, showering, and swimming with the patch in place are acceptable. Patients must be reminded to rotate the skin site when applying a new patch.

To prevent the potential diversion of fentanyl for illicit use, the manufacturer suggests that used transdermal patches be carefully folded so that the system adheres to itself and discarded in the toilet. Although the components of the transdermal system are not biodegradable, the manufacturer suggests that their disposal into the public sewer system would not add substantially to solid waste.

Availability, Cost, and Approved Labeling

Fentanyl transdermal system (Duragesic, Janssen Pharmaceutica) is a schedule II controlled substance indicated for the management of chronic pain in patients requiring narcotic analgesia. The system is available in four sizes with a delivery rate per hour proportional to the patch surface area.

The 10 sq cm, 20 sq cm, 30 sq cm, and 40 sq cm patches contain 2.5 mg, 5 mg, 7.5 mg, and 10 mg of fentanyl and have nominal delivery rates of 25 μg/hr, 50 μg/hr, 75 μg/hr, and 100 μg/hr, respectively. Fentanyl is provided continuously at the selected rate for three days. The transdermal fentanyl system is supplied in cartons containing five individually packaged systems. The average wholesale price per patch is $8.08 (10 sq cm), $12.11 (20 sq cm), $18.50 (30 sq cm), and $23.04 (40 sq cm).[94]

Assuming that 360 mg of oral morphine sulfate per day equals 100 μg of transdermal fentanyl per hour for 24 hours, the cost for a single day of therapy would be $10.57 for MS Contin (Purdue Frederick),[95] $6.47 for Roxanol SR (Roxane),[95] and $7.68 for the fentanyl system. That indicates that the cost of transdermal fentanyl therapy may be comparable to that of the oral extended-release morphine products currently marketed in the United States.

Conclusion

Fentanyl is the first narcotic to be incorporated into a transdermal drug delivery system for the management of pain. The transdermal system delivers fentanyl to the skin continuously at a controlled rate and, after a delay of nearly 12 hours, produces relatively constant therapeutic plasma concentrations for up to 72 hours. Plasma concentrations 8 to 12 hours after application of a fentanyl patch may vary substantially among patients but are generally similar to those achieved with equal doses of fentanyl administered by continuous intravenous infusions.

Although experience with the product is limited, transdermally administered fentanyl appears to be effective in the long-term management of cancer-related pain. The efficacy and safety of the transdermal fentanyl system in the treatment of postoperative pain have not been adequately evaluated, and the transdermal fentanyl system cannot generally be recommended for this indication. Transdermally administered fentanyl may be particularly appropriate for outpatients or institutionalized individuals with relatively constant chronic pain who are medically stable and require opioid analgesics but who are unable to ingest oral agents because of vomiting or dysphagia. The transdermal route of fentanyl administration may also be appropriate for patients who would otherwise require placement of a vascular, subcutaneous, or spinal access device for effective long-term pain control.

Patients receiving transcutaneously administered fentanyl should be assessed for their response to the therapeutic effects of the analgesic and closely monitored for signs of toxicity throughout therapy and for several days after removal of the transdermal system.

[a]Farber MA, Cygnus Therapeutic Systems. Personal communication. 1991 Apr 5.

References

1. Soudijn W. The pharmacology and the pharmacokinetics of fentanyl. In: Wood C, ed. Stress-free anaesthesia. London: Royal Society of Medicine; 1978:4-10.
2. Janssen Pharmaceutica. Duragesic package insert. Piscataway, NJ; 1991 Jan.
3. Roy SD, Flynn GL. Solubility and related physicochemical properties of narcotic analgesics. *Pharm Res*. 1988; 5:580-6.
4. Meuldermans WEG, Hurkmans RMA, Heykants JJP. Plasma protein binding and distribution of fentanyl, sufentanil, alfentanil, and lofentanil in blood. *Arch Int Pharmacodyn Ther*. 1982; 257:4-19.
5. Flynn GL, Stewart B. Percutaneous drug penetration: choosing candidates for transdermal development. *Drug Dev Res*. 1988; 13:169-85.
6. Roy SD, Flynn GL. Transdermal delivery of narcotic analgesics: comparative permeabilities of narcotic analgesics through human cadaver skin. *Pharm Res*. 1989; 6:825-32.
7. The pharmacologic basis of therapeutics. 8th ed. Gilman AG, Rall TW, Nies AS et al., eds. New York: Pergamon; 1990.
8. Mather LE. Clinical pharmacokinetics of fentanyl and its newer derivatives. *Clin Pharmacokinet*. 1983; 8:422-46.
9. Rosow CE, Moss J, Philbin DM et al. Histamine release during morphine and fentanyl anesthesia. *Anesthesiology*. 1982; 56:93-6.
10. Yum SI. Transdermal therapeutic systems and rate controlled drug delivery. *Med Prog Technol*. 1989; 15:47-52.
11. Fara JW. Short and long term transdermal drug delivery systems. Paper presented at the International Two-Day Conference on Drug Delivery Systems. Paris, Jan 31–Feb 1, 1983.
12. Varvel JR, Shafer SL, Hwang SS et al. Absorption characteristics of transdermally administered fentanyl. *Anesthesiology*. 1989; 70:928-34.
13. Moore L, Chien YW. Transdermal drug delivery: a review of pharmaceutics, pharmacokinetics, and pharmacodynamics. *CRC Crit Rev Ther Drug Carrier Syst*. 1988; 4:285-349.
14. Brown L, Langer R. Transdermal delivery of drugs. *Annu Rev Med*. 1988; 39:221-9.
15. Shaw JE. Transdermal drug delivery: potentials and limitations. In: Lemberger L, Reidenberg MM, ed. Proceedings of the Second World Conference on Pharmacology and Therapeutics. Bethesda, MD: American Society for Pharmacology and Experimental Therapeutics; 1984:444-58.
16. Shaw JE, Theeuwes F. Transdermal dosage forms. In: Prescott LF, Nimmo WS, eds. Rate control in drug therapy. Edinburgh: Churchill Livingstone; 1985:65-70.
17. Guy RH, Hadgraft J, Bucks DA. Transdermal drug delivery and cutaneous metabolism. *Xenobiotica*. 1987; 17:325-43.
18. Cleary GW. Transdermal controlled release systems. In: Langer RS, Wise DL, eds. Medical applications of controlled release. Vol. 1. Boca Raton, FL: CRC Press; 1985:205.
19. Merkle HP. Transdermal delivery systems. *Methods Find Exp Clin Pharmacol*. 1989; 11:135-53.
20. Kligman AM. Skin permeability: dermatologic aspects of transdermal drug delivery. *Am Heart J*. 1984; 108:200-6.
21. Caplan RA, Southam M. Transdermal drug delivery and its application to pain control. *Adv Pain Res Ther*. 1990; 14:233-40.
22. Sebel PS, Barrett CW, Kirk CJC et al. Transdermal absorption of fentanyl and sufentanil in man. *Eur J Clin Pharmacol*. 1987; 32:529-31.
23. Loth H. Skin permeability. *Methods Find Exp Clin Pharmacol*. 1989; 11:155-64.
24. Ridout G, Santus GC, Guy RH. Pharmacokinetic considerations in the use of newer transdermal formulations. *Clin Pharmacokinet*. 1988; 15:114-31.
25. Gale RM, Osborne J, Goetz V. In vitro functionality of a transdermal therapeutic system (Fentanyl). *Pharm Res*. 1987; 4(2 Suppl):S-70. Abstract.
26. Anon. Cygnus contraceptive patch licensed to Parke-Davis. *FDC Reports. Prescription and OTC pharmaceuticals*. 1991; 53(Jan 14):T&G4-5.
27. Reilly CS, Wood AJJ, Wood M. Variability of fentanyl pharmacokinetics in man. *Anaesthesia*. 1984; 40:837-43.
28. Michaels AS, Chandrasekaran SK, Shaw JE. Drug permeation through human skin: theory and in vitro experimental measurement. *Am Inst Chem Eng J*. 1975; 21:985-96.
29. Roy SD, Flynn GL. Transdermal delivery of narcotic analgesics: pH, anatomical, and subject influences on cutaneous permeability of fentanyl and sufentanil. *Pharm Res*. 1990; 7:842-7.
30. Southwell D, Barry B, Woodford R. Variations in permeability of human skin within and between specimens. *Int J Pharm*. 1984; 18:299-309.
31. Plezia PM, Kramer TH, Linford J et al. Transdermal fentanyl: pharmacokinetics and preliminary clinical evaluation. *Pharmacotherapy*. 1989; 9:2-9.
32. Gourlay GK, Kowalski SR, Plummer JL et al. The efficacy of transdermal fentanyl in the treatment of postoperative pain: a double-blind comparison of fentanyl and placebo systems. *Pain*. 1990; 40:21-8.
33. Gourlay GK, Kowalski SR, Plummer JL et al. The transdermal administration of fentanyl in the treatment of postoperative pain: pharmacokinetics and pharmacodynamic effects. *Pain*. 1989; 37:193-202.
34. Scheuplein RJ, Blank IH. Permeability of the skin. *Physiol Rev*. 1971; 51:702-47.
35. Hess R, Hertz A, Freidel K. Pharmacokinetics of fentanyl in rabbits in view of the importance for limiting the effect. *J Pharmacol Exp Ther*. 1971; 179:474-84.
36. Hess R, Stiebler G, Hertz A. Pharmacokinetics of fentanyl in man and the rabbit. *Eur J Clin Pharmacol*. 1972; 4:135-41.
37. Hug CC, Murphy MR. Tissue redistribution of fentanyl and termination of its effects in rats. *Anesthesiology*. 1981; 55:369-75.
38. Hug CC, Murphy MR. Fentanyl disposition in cerebrospinal fluid and plasma and its relationship to ventilatory depression in the dog. *Anesthesiology*. 1979; 50:342-9.
39. Hug CC, Murphy MR, Sampson JF et al. Biotransformation of morphine and fentanyl in anhepatic dogs. *Anesthesiology*. 1981; 55:A261.
40. Scott JC, Stanski DR. Decreased fentanyl and alfentanil requirements with age: a simultaneous pharmacokinetic and pharmacodynamic evaluation. *J Pharmacol Exp Ther*. 1987; 240:159-66.
41. McClain DA, Hug CC. Intravenous fentanyl kinetics. *Clin Pharmacol Ther*. 1980; 28:106-14.
42. Stoeckle H, Hengstmann JH, Schuttler J. Pharmacokinetics of fentanyl as a possible explanation for recurrence of respiratory depression. *Br J Anaesth*. 1979; 51:741-5.
43. Lehmann KA, Freier J, Daub D. Fentanyl-Pharmakokinetik und postoperative Atemdepression. *Anaesthesist*. 1982; 31:111-8.
44. Goromaru T, Futuia T, Baba S et al. Metabolism of fentanyl in rats and man. *Anesthesiology*. 1981; 55:A173.
45. Goromaru T, Matsura H, Furuta T et al. Identification of fentanyl metabolites in rat urine by gas chromatography-mass spectrometry with stable isotope tracers. *Drug Metab Dispos*. 1982; 10:542-6.
46. Denyer SP, Guy RH, Hadgraft J et al. The microbial degradation of topically applied drugs. *Int J Pharmaceut*. 1985; 26:89-97.
47. Kao J, Hall J. Skin absorption and cutaneous first pass metabolism of topical steroids: in vitro studies with mouse skin in organ culture. *J Pharmacol Exp Ther*. 1987; 241:482-7.
48. Pannatier A, Jenner P, Testa B et al. The skin as a drug-me-

tabolizing organ. *Drug Metab Rev*. 1978; 8:319-43.
49. Schleimer R, Benjamini E, Eisele J. Pharmacokinetics of fentanyl as determined by radioimmunoassay. *Clin Pharmacol Ther*. 1978; 23:188-94.
50. Bovill JG, Sebel PS. Pharmacokinetics of high-dose fentanyl. *Br J Anaesth*. 1980; 52:795-801.
51. Bower S, Hull CJ. The comparative pharmacokinetics of fentanyl and alfentanil. *Br J Anaesth*. 1982; 54:871-7.
52. Duthie DJR, Rowbotham DJ, Wyld R et al. Plasma fentanyl concentrations during transdermal delivery of fentanyl to surgical patients. *Br J Anaesth*. 1988; 60:614-8.
53. Holley FO, Van Steennis C. Postoperative analgesia with fentanyl: pharmacokinetics and pharmacodynamics of constant-rate i.v. and transdermal delivery. *Br J Anaesth*. 1988; 60:608-13.
54. Hudson RJ, Thomson IR, Cannon JE et al. Pharmacokinetics of fentanyl in patients undergoing abdominal aortic surgery. *Anesthesiology*. 1986; 64:334-8.
55. Larijani GE, Bell SD, Goldberg ME et al. Pharmacokinetics of fentanyl following transdermal application. *Anesthesiology*. 1988; 69:A363.
56. Bell SD, Larijani GE, Goldberg ME et al. Evaluation of transdermal fentanyl for multi-day analgesia in postoperative patients. *Anesthesiology*. 1988; 69:A362.
57. Cartwright P, Prys-Roberts C, Gill K et al. Ventilatory depression related to plasma fentanyl concentrations during and after anesthesia in humans. *Anesth Analg*. 1983; 62:966-74.
58. Kaiko RF. Age and morphine analgesia in cancer patients with postoperative pain. *Clin Pharmacol Ther*. 1980; 28:823-6.
59. Holmberg L, Odar-Cedarlof I, Boreus LO et al. Comparative disposition of pethidine and norpethidine in old and young patients. *Eur J Clin Pharmacol*. 1982; 22:175-9.
60. Kwentus JA, Harkins SW, Lignon N et al. Current concepts of geriatric pain and its treatment. *Geriatrics*. 1985; 40:48-54.
61. Bentley JB, Borel JD, Nenad RE et al. Age and fentanyl pharmacokinetics. *Anesth Analg*. 1982; 61:968-71.
62. Singleton MA, Rosen JI, Fisher DM. Pharmacokinetics of fentanyl in the elderly. *Br J Anaesth*. 1988; 60:619-22.
63. Gelman SI. Disturbances in hepatic blood flow during anesthesia and surgery. *Arch Surg*. 1976; 111:881-3.
64. Nimmo WS, Todd JG. Fentanyl by constant rate I.V. infusion for postoperative analgesia. *Br J Anaesth*. 1985; 57:250-4.
65. Duthie DJR, McLaren AD, Nimmo WS. Pharmacokinetics and fentanyl during constant I.V. infusion for the relief of pain after surgery. *Br J Anaesth*. 1986; 58:950-6.
66. Ellis DJ, Millar WL, Reisner LS. A randomized double-blind comparison of epidural versus intravenous fentanyl for analgesia after cesarean section. *Anesthesiology*. 1990; 72:981-6.
67. Rosenberg PH, Heino A, Scheinin B. Comparison of intramuscular analgesia, intercostal block, epidural morphine, and on-demand i.v. fentanyl in the control of pain after upper abdominal surgery. *Acta Anaesthesiol Scand*. 1984; 28:603-7.
68. Gourlay GK, Kowalski SR, Plummer JL et al. Fentanyl blood concentration-analgesic response relationship in the treatment of postoperative pain. *Anesth Analg*. 1988; 67:329-37.
69. Hug CC. Pharmacokinetics and dynamics of narcotic analgesics. In: Prys-Roberts C, Hug CC, eds. Pharmacokinetics of anaesthesia. Oxford: Blackwell; 1984:187-234.
70. Mather LE, Phillips GD. Opioids and adjuvants: principles of use. In: Cousins MJ, Phillips GD, eds. Acute pain management. New York: Churchill Livingstone; 1986:77-103.
71. Andrews CJH, Prys-Roberts C. Fentanyl—a review. In: Bullingham RES, ed. Opiate analgesia. Eastbourne, England: Saunders; 1983:97-122.
72. Cookson RF. Analgesic plasma concentrations. *Br J Anaesth*. 1980; 52:959-60.
73. Lehmann KA, Heinrich C, van Heiss R. Balanced anesthesia and patient controlled postoperative analgesia with fentanyl: minimum effective concentrations, accumulation, and acute tolerance. *Acta Anaesthesiol Belg*. 1988; 39:11-23.
74. Hill HF, Saeger L, Bjurstrom R et al. Steady-state infusions of opioids in human volunteers: I. Pharmacokinetic tailoring. *Pain*. 1990; 43:57-67.
75. Andrews CJH, Sinclair M, Dye A et al. The additive effect of nitrous oxide on respiratory depression in patients having fentanyl or alfentanil infusions. *Br J Anaesth*. 1982; 54:1129P.
76. Gill KJ, Cartwright DP, Scoggins A et al. Ventilatory depression related to plasma fentanyl concentrations during and after anaesthesia. *Br J Anaesth*. 1980; 52:63P.
77. Stoekel H, Schuttler J, Magnussen H et al. Plasma fentanyl concentrations and the occurrence of respiratory depression in volunteers. *Br J Anaesth*. 1982; 54:1087-95.
78. Henderson GL, Frincke J, Leung CY et al. Antibodies to fentanyl. *J Pharmacol Exp Ther*. 1975; 192:489-96.
79. Michiels M, Hendricks R, Heykants J. A sensitive radioimmunoassay for fentanyl. *Eur J Clin Pharmacol*. 1977; 12:153-8.
80. Gillespie TJ, Gandolfi AJ, Maiorino RM et al. Gas chromatographic determination of fentanyl and its analogues in human plasma. *J Anal Toxicol*. 1981; 5:133-7.
81. Kowalski SR, Gourlay GK, Cherry DA et al. A sensitive GLC method for the determination of fentanyl concentration in blood. *J Pharmacol Methods*. 1987; 18:347-55.
82. Woestenborghs RJ, Stanski DR, Scott JC et al. Assay methods for fentanyl in serum: gas-liquid chromatography versus radioimmunoassay. *Anesthesiology*. 1987; 67:85-90.
83. Caplan RA, Ready LB, Oden RV et al. Transdermal fentanyl for postoperative pain management. *JAMA*. 1989; 261:1036-9.
84. Latasch L, Lüders S. Transdermal fentanyl against postoperative pain. *Acta Anaesthesiol Belg*. 1989; 40:113-9.
85. Rowbotham DJ, Wyld R, Peacock JE et al. Transdermal fentanyl for the relief of pain after upper abdominal surgery. *Br J Anaesth*. 1989; 63:56-9.
86. Miser AW, Narang PK, Dothage JA et al. Transdermal fentanyl for pain control in patients with cancer. *Pain*. 1989; 37:15-21.
87. Simmonds MA, Payne R, Richenbacher J et al. TTS (fentanyl) in the management of pain in patients with cancer. *Proc Am Soc Clin Oncol*. 1989; 8:324. Abstract.
88. Zech D, Dauer HG, Stollenwerk B et al. PCA and TTS fentanyl in the treatment of cancer pain. *Pain*. 1990; (Suppl 5):S356. Abstract.
89. Levy S, Jacobs S, Johnson J et al. Transdermal fentanyl: pain and quality of life effects. *Proc Am Soc Clin Oncol*. 1988; 7:292. Abstract.
90. Hogan DJ, Maibach HI. Adverse dermatologic reactions to transdermal drug delivery systems. *J Am Acad Dermatol*. 1990; 22:811-4.
91. Holdiness MR. A review of contact dermatitis associated with transdermal therapeutic systems. *Contact Dermatitis*. 1989; 20:3-9.
92. Plezia PM, Linford J, Kramer TH et al. Transdermally administered fentanyl for postoperative pain: a randomized, double-blind, placebo-controlled trial. *Anesthesiology*. 1988; 69:A364.
93. Foley KM. The treatment of cancer pain. *N Engl J Med*. 1985; 313:84-95.
94. Drug Topics redbook annual pharmacists' reference. Cardinale VA, Thurlow RM, eds. Oradell, NJ: Medical Economics; 1991. April update.
95. Drug Topics redbook annual pharmacists' reference. Cardinale VA, Thurlow RM, eds. Oradell, NJ: Medical Economics; 1991.

Therapy Review

Features and treatment of rabies

MAUREEN L. FRENIA, SUZANNE M. LAFIN, AND JOSEPH A. BARONE

Abstract: The epidemiology, virology, transmission, pathology, clinical manifestations, diagnosis, and treatment of rabies infection are described.

The incidence of rabies is increasing. The virus is usually transmitted through the bite of an infected animal; however, corneal transplantation from an infected donor and viral inhalation may also result in infection.

The clinical course of rabies occurs in five stages. Stage I is the incubation period, stage II is the prodromal period, stage III is the neurological period, stage IV is coma, and stage V, which occurs infrequently, is recovery. Early in the disease, constitutional symptoms and signs of local wound healing may be present. During the later stages, a wide array of clinical manifestations may occur, including hydrophobia and aerophobia, which are pathognomonic for rabies.

Once inoculation with the rabies virus is suspected, prompt therapy, including appropriate wound care and rabies vaccination, is imperative, even in previously immunized individuals. Human diploid-cell vaccine and rabies vaccine adsorbed, which stimulate the production of antibodies, and human rabies immune globulin, which provides protective antibodies, are nearly 100% effective in preventing progression from stage I disease.

If left untreated, rabies is usually fatal. However, treatment with human diploid-cell vaccine or rabies vaccine adsorbed and with human rabies immune globulin is nearly always curative if initiated early in the incubation period.

Index terms: Immunization; Rabies; Rabies immune globulin; Rabies vaccines; Vaccines
Clin Pharm. 1992; 11:37-47

The recent increase in the number of rabies cases in the United States has attracted the attention of health-care professionals, the media, and the lay public. The number of rabid raccoons in the Mid-Atlantic and Southern states has grown, resulting in frequent exposure of residents in these areas. There is concern that other areas of the United States may be affected as the movement of rabid animals continues.

In the past, rabies was considered endemic; however, after vaccination requirements were implemented in 1940, a decline in the number of rabies cases caused by domestic animals was documented.[1-4] Rabies usually occurs through the bite of an infected animal, although it may occasionally be transmitted through a nonbite route.[1,5-10] Currently, wild animals transmit most rabies infections.[2] The oral vaccination of wild animals has shown some promise as a mechanism for limiting rabies in wildlife, although more research in this area is needed.[11-15]

If left untreated, rabies is almost always fatal. When inoculation is suspected, prompt therapy, including appropriate wound care[16] and vaccination,[17-20] is imperative.

Epidemiology

Wild animals are the main source of rabies; they have contributed to the recent increase in the number of humans infected with the disease.[2] Since the requirement for vaccination of domesticated animals was instituted, the incidence of rabies contracted from dogs and cats has declined.[1-3] However, vaccination of animals is not without problems, and failures have been documented in a limited number of vaccine recipients.[4,21] Laboratory animals also constitute a risk to workers, who may be exposed to rabies during experimentation.

Rabies is frequently a problem in children. The inci-

MAUREEN L. FRENIA, PHARM.D., is Emergency Medicine/Clinical Toxicology Fellow, Department of Pharmacy, University Medical Center, Jacksonville, FL; at the time this article was written, she was a Doctor of Pharmacy candidate, College of Pharmacy, Rutgers University, Piscataway, NJ. SUZANNE M. LAFIN, PHARM.D., is Emergency Medicine Clinical Pharmacist, Robert Wood Johnson University Hospital, New Brunswick, NJ, and Adjunct Clinical Professor, College of Pharmacy, Rutgers University. JOSEPH A. BARONE, PHARM.D., is Associate Professor and Chairman, Department of Pharmacy Practice and Administration, College of Pharmacy, Rutgers University, and Assistant Director for Academic Affairs, Robert Wood Johnson University Hospital.

Address reprint requests to Dr. Frenia, University Medical Center, Clinical Toxicology Service, 655 West Eighth Street, Jacksonville, FL 32209.

This is article **680-204-9204** in the **ASHP Continuing Education System;** it qualifies for 1.0 hour of continuing-education credit. See page 78 for learning objectives and test questions.

dence of rabies is highest in children younger than 15 years; of the 129 cases of rabies that occurred from 1950 to 1968 in the United States, 67 (52%) were in this age group. The amount of time that children spend outdoors and their desire to closely contact animals may contribute to the prevalence of rabies in this age group.[22]

In the United States, nine cases of rabies in humans (four of the nine exposures occurred abroad) were reported from 1963 to 1968, as opposed to 230 cases documented from 1946 to 1963.[23] From November 1989 to November 1991, 1377 cases of rabies in animals were confirmed (by examination of animal heads) in the state of New Jersey alone.[a] The number of persons exposed is expected to increase, reflecting the increased number of animals carrying the virus.

Virology

Rabies is a member of the Rhabdoviridae family of viruses. Rabies virus is a bullet-shaped, neurotropic virus that gains access to the central nervous system via peripheral nerves.[24] Rhabdoviruses affect not only mammals but plants and insects as well.[25,26] Those that infect mammals have been divided into two genera, *Lyssavirus* and *Vesiculovirus*. The lyssaviruses consist of six viruses but only three, Mokola, Duvenhage, and rabies, are known to cause disease in humans.[7,26] Infection with Mokola results in an encephalitis-like syndrome without the signs of rage commonly seen with rabies.[27] The other members of the genus *Lyssavirus* are the Lagos bat virus and the Kotonkan and Obodhiang viruses.[28]

The stability of the rabies virus in vitro is both pH- and temperature-dependent. Rabies virus is labile and is destroyed at a pH of <3 or >11. It has a half-life in vitro of 24 hours, 4 hours, 30 minutes, and 35 seconds at 4, 40, 54, and 60 °C, respectively.[29] The significance of these dependent variables after rabies transmission is unknown, because studies in humans are not available.

Modes of Transmission

Animal Bites. Infection with the rabies virus is one of the most serious complications that can result from an animal bite. Viral infection is common following direct inoculation of the virus into the flesh of the victim during confrontation with the animal. Raccoons, foxes, bats, skunks, wolves, llamas, and unvaccinated dogs and cats frequently carry the rabies virus.[30-40] On the other hand, bites from herbivores, lagomorphs (rabbits and hares), and rodents rarely require rabies prophylaxis.[33,41,42]

Bites inflicted during an unprovoked attack are more likely to result in transmission of rabies.[42] Animals carrying the virus tend to display inappropriate behavior and, in times of fury, may attack and infect a bystander for no apparent reason.[25] Penetration of the skin or contact with the mucous membranes of the victim is required for transmission of the virus from host to victim. Casual contact with rabid animals, such as petting, does not constitute exposure and does not require treatment.[43] The area of the body that has been exposed is another factor in the likelihood of rabies infection. Inoculation into areas that contain large amounts of nerve tissue (i.e., face and hands) will more frequently result in viral transmission since the virus gains access to the CNS through peripheral nerve tissue.[41] Risk of viral transmission is also related to the vaccination status of the animal, as well as the area in which the animal dwells, since some geographic locations are more frequently infested with animals carrying the virus.[4,22]

The animal involved in an attack should be observed and evaluated according to state and local health department procedures. Domestic animals that have bitten a person should be confined for 10 days. Animals that harbor the virus are likely to develop signs and symptoms of rabies within this period, although there are exceptions.[44] Animals carrying the rabies virus frequently demonstrate clinical manifestations similar to those in humans.[4,21,35] Eng and Fishbein[21] found that the most common clinical signs displayed by rabid dogs and cats are aggressive behavior (45%), ataxia (38%), irritability (29%), anorexia (28%), lethargy (27%), and excessive salivation (25%). Other signs in these animals included limb and jaw paralysis, seizures, and voice changes.[21] Hydrophobia and aerophobia have not been described in animals. Eng and Fishbein[21] reviewed 37 cases of rabies in dogs and cats and found that 95% of the animals died within seven days of the onset of illness. One dog died on the 8th day and one cat died on the 10th day of illness. If the animal exhibits behavior consistent with rabies during this time, it must be killed and decapitated. A period of confinement is not necessary for stray or wild animals; instead, these animals' heads should be removed immediately after the attack. The heads of the animals should be shipped in ice to the appropriate state or local health department for evaluation.[42]

Corneal Transplantation. Human fluids, including cerebrospinal fluid, tears, and saliva, have been shown to contain the rabies virus, but contact with these secretions has not resulted in disease transmission.[45] To date, corneal transplantation is the only form of horizontal transmission documented, and transmission by this route has occurred rarely.[10,46] Benefits to the recipients of corneal transplants are said to far outweigh the risks of the procedure, since morbidity and mortality are extremely low (if rabies is not transmitted).[46]

Houf et al.[47] reported a case of a 37-year-old woman who underwent corneal transplantation. The cornea was donated by a 39-year-old professional lumberman who died of a presumed case of Guillain-Barré syndrome. The recipient developed symptoms consistent with rabies five weeks after the transplantation, and she died two weeks later as a result of cardiovascular failure. Postmortem examinations confirmed the diagnosis of rabies in both the donor and the cornea recipient.[47,48]

Other cases have been reported.[49,50] Two patients who received corneal transplants from the same donor died within five weeks after the operation. The donor, a 16-year-old boy, had died of unknown causes. Before their deaths, the donor and the two recipients manifested clinical signs and symptoms consistent with rabies, including aerophobia and hydrophobia. Rabies was later confirmed in one recipient and the donor during postmortem examinations of brain tissue. An autopsy was not performed on the second recipient.

Another case of human-to-human transmission of rabies via corneal transplantation occurred in a 36-year-old male.[49] The organ donor had died of a flaccid quadriplegia syndrome. The recipient died six weeks after the transplantation. Postmortem examination, including viral detection by fluorescent antibody staining and examination of brain tissue, confirmed the diagnosis of rabies in the recipient.

Viral Inhalation. The second nonbite route for rabies transmission is direct inhalation of the virus. After a spelunking expedition in a cave known to contain bats carrying the rabies virus, two men developed signs and symptoms of rabies virus infection.[51] However, both men denied having been bitten by a bat while they were in the cave. Their symptoms eventually progressed, leading to death in both men. Their deaths were attributed to the inhalation of bat excretions containing the virus.

Experiments to confirm the hypothesis that it is possible to contract rabies by a nonbite route have been conducted.[51] Carnivores, including dogs, cats, raccoons, ringtails (cacomistles), coyotes, foxes, and skunks, were placed in screened cages that prevented direct contact with bats. Thirteen of them were exposed for seven days in a cave infested with bats carrying the rabies virus. After they were removed from the cave, four of the exposed animals died of confirmed rabies. Another 28 carnivores were placed in cages in the same location; however, this time, all bats were removed from the immediate area. None of those 28 carnivores contracted rabies. Twenty-two more carnivores were exposed to a bat-infested cave for 24–30 days. All of the 22 animals subsequently died of rabies. Researchers concluded that the most likely route of virus transmission was through an airborne medium, such as an aerosol from bat excretions.

A similar case of rabies transmission via inhalation has been reported.[8] The exposure occurred as a result of the inhalation of aerosolized virus during homogenization of rabid goat brains for the production of rabies vaccine. The victim, a 56-year-old laboratory worker, died of rabies 21 days after exposure to the virus. The virus was retrieved from brain tissue of the victim during a postmortem examination. The victim had received a rabies vaccination 13 years earlier, but serum antibodies to the virus never developed. To prevent such occurrences, immunization with subsequent documentation of immunity through serologic testing should be required for all persons who work in environments where the likelihood of rabies exposure is relatively high.

Pathogenesis

Viral invasion of the host animal's salivary glands and subsequent release through secretions allow transmission of the virus from host to victim. Upon entering the victim, the rabies virus first proliferates in muscle cells near the bite.[24,52] It has been proposed that the virus may remain in these muscle cells during long incubation periods. The reason for viral proliferation in this area has not been determined. The prolonged incubation period, ranging from 10 days to eight months, provides adequate time for treatment to be effective.[1,22,34] After the virus replicates within the muscle cells, it can be found in the neuromuscular spindles and, subsequently, in the peripheral nervous system.[24] From there, the virus gains access to the CNS. The period in which the virus spreads from the peripheral nervous system to the CNS may range from days to years.[52] Symptoms of rabies infection usually develop after the virus has reached the CNS.[24,52] Eventually, the limbic system becomes infected and signs and symptoms of madness or fury may be demonstrated by the infected individual.[7,52] (The limbic system is responsible for control of sexual behavior and emotions such as fear and rage.[24,53]) If exposure to the virus is suspected, treatment should be initiated as soon as possible because it is no longer effective once the rabies virus has entered the peripheral nervous system.

After rabies transmission through viral inhalation, neuroepithelial cells on the surface of the nasal mucosa become heavily coated with the virus. This leads to the eventual invasion of the nervous system and viral infection.[24]

Although the virus usually enters the CNS at the level of the spinal cord, transport to the brain is rapid, as demonstrated by sequential immunofluorescence studies.[7,24] In hamsters, Murphy[24] witnessed ascension of the virus from the spinal cord to the brainstem within hours.

Clinical Manifestations

Rabies is a systemic illness, frequently affecting many organ systems. It has been classified into two types, furious rabies and paralytic rabies, based on clinical manifestations.[7] Patients with furious rabies show signs of rage and hyperactivity, whereas patients with paralytic rabies develop a progressive flaccid paralysis often mistakenly diagnosed as Guillain-Barré syndrome.[54]

The number and variety of nonspecific clinical manifestations of rabies may easily result in misdiagnosis. It may not be until hydrophobia and aerophobia, two symptoms pathognomonic for rabies viral infections, are prominent that the diagnosis of rabies is made.

The clinical course of rabies infection occurs in five stages. Each stage is associated with specific signs and symptoms, although some overlap of the clinical manifestations may be seen between stages.[55]

Stage I: The Incubation Period. The incubation period of rabies is the time between inoculation and the manifestation of symptoms. This period usually ranges from 10 days to eight months, with an average of one to two months.[1,22,34] Although it is not fully understood, the variation in the incubation period may be attributed to the size of the inoculum or the severity of the bite.[39,56] Symptoms during this stage are minimal and are usually related to local wound healing.[37] These may include erythema and swelling in the area of the bite. As stated earlier, this period provides time for a vaccine, if given immediately after inoculation, to promote the development of antibodies, thereby protecting the patient before the virus is able to reach the nervous system.[22]

Stage II: The Prodromal Stage. The progression to stage II disease is associated with a very poor prognosis. Constitutional symptoms similar to an influenza infection signal the beginning of stage II. This prodromal stage may last for 2 to 10 days. Nonspecific symptoms during this stage include chills, fever, malaise, anorexia, nausea, vomiting, and headache.[1,6,22,34,57] These symptoms have been followed by swelling of the lips, drooling, and ulcerations of the mouth. Signs of apprehension and rage have also been described.[6]

Up to two thirds of patients may experience pain at the site of the wound.[7,34,58] This neuritic pain may be the patient's chief complaint at the time of initial presentation.[22,32,44,58] Itching also may occur in the area surrounding the bite.[7,36] The itching may be severe enough to provoke self-inflicted excoriation of the skin. Proliferation of the virus in the sensory nerves surrounding the area of the bite may be responsible for these local symptoms.[7]

Stage III: The Neurological Period. Manifestations of stage III disease include a wide array of systemic disorders. In no other stage are the symptoms as numerous or as varied. This is the stage in which aerophobia and hydrophobia, the hallmark symptoms of rabies infection, are usually seen.[7] Other symptoms, including hyperactivity, seizures, paralysis, and nuchal rigidity, are also frequently apparent.[32,44,55,58,59]

In a review of the presenting features in fatal rabies cases, the majority of patients (52%) showed signs of hyperexcitability, although hyperventilation and chest pain were also commonly seen. Seventeen percent of patients presented with hydrophobia as the initial feature.[44] Patients have also been tachypneic, tachycardic, and febrile at the time of admission.[6]

A distinct sign common to many patients with rabies infection is aerophobia, extreme fear associated with air in motion. This sign is elicited by blowing air across the face of the victim, which causes muscle spasms in the neck and pharyngeal regions.[44] Foaming at the mouth may also occur and is thought to be a result of a combination of hypersalivation and difficulty with swallowing.[54]

Hydrophobia, an abnormal fear of water, is also associated distinctly with rabies.[7,60,61] Studies in patients with rabies have revealed features of hydrophobia that were once misunderstood.[60] Hydrophobia, characterized by spasm of the muscles of inspiration and deglutition, may be provoked by the sight of liquids or during an attempt to drink liquids.[7,60] However, it is thought that airway obstruction does not occur during hydrophobia, as is evidenced by normal chest expansion. Although the specific pathophysiology of hydrophobia is not fully understood, it appears to exert a protective effect on the respiratory tract. Hydrophobia instills a powerful fear in patients and can prevent activities involving water, including showering and bathing.[59,60]

Because of the potential difficulties with swallowing fluids and with excess secretions, patients should be monitored closely for signs of malnutrition. Effects of rabies on the hypophyseal–hypothalamic–thymic axis have resulted in a wasting syndrome and, subsequently, failure to thrive.[62] Total parenteral nutrition should be instituted if necessary.

Mental status deterioration, with cycles of hyperactivity and unresponsiveness, have been documented. Hyperactivity or fury lasting from hours to days may be provoked by various stimuli or may occur spontaneously during the later stages of rabies. Frequently, periods of hyperactivity may alternate with periods of appropriate behavior.[6]

Many other symptoms, which may occur less frequently, have been described during stage III. Urogenital symptoms including penile pain and prolonged, intermittent priapism with ejaculation as the initial symptoms of rabies have been reported in the literature.[54,61,63,64] These penile symptoms are thought to be secondary to damage of the amygdaloid nucleus.[54,61]

Other neurological problems reported include a positive Babinski's sign, facial paralysis progressing to a total flaccid paralysis, opisthotonos, seizures, and apnea.[57,58,65,66] Paralysis has been reported as the most prominent manifestation during the course of rabies.[34] The acute neurological period usually lasts for one week; however, longer periods of these manifestations have been noted.[55] Death may occur during this stage.

Stage IV: Coma. During this late stage of rabies, prior signs of hydrophobia are replaced with irregular respiration, often with prolonged periods of apnea requiring respiratory assistance.[7] The duration of coma ranges from hours to months.[55] Respiratory arrest resulting in death may occur during this time.

Stage V: Recovery. The infrequency of recovery from a documented rabies virus infection cannot be overemphasized. Few patients have recovered from documented rabies, and reports in the literature are scarce.[25,67,68] Aggressive treatment and supportive care have been shown to prolong or improve the clinical course in a limited number of patients.[1,6,67,69]

One of the best-documented cases of recovery from rabies is that of a six-year-old boy bitten on his hand by a brown bat, *Eptesicus fuscus*.[67] Rabies was confirmed in the bat by the fluorescent antibody test. Four days after the attack, a 14-day course of duck embryo rabies vaccine was initiated. The patient developed symptoms of rabies two days after the vaccination series was completed. His clinical course progressed through stage IV. Signs and symptoms including lethargy, nuchal rigidity, abnormal behavior, incontinence, seizures, atrial arrhythmias, bradycardia, acidosis, aphasia, flaccid paralysis, elevated intracranial pressure, and coma were seen. Rabies was diagnosed by detection of antibodies in the serum, cerebrospinal fluid, and brain tissue of the boy. (Although an increase in antibodies may be seen following a course of duck embryo vaccine, the titers detected greatly exceeded those that would be expected after vaccination.) The victim's serum indirect fluorescent antibody titer and a test for rabies neutralization by fluorescent foci inhibition exceeded values that would result from immunization alone. Attempts to isolate the virus from brain tissue, cerebrospinal fluid, and saliva during his disease course were unsuccessful. Supportive treatment included anticonvulsant therapy, placement of an intraventricular shunt, and tracheostomy with frequent suctioning and supplemental oxygen to help treat hypoxia. The patient fully recovered four months after the onset of symptoms. It was thought that the aggressiveness of the supportive treatment was responsible for the favorable outcome.

Other Manifestations. In addition to the clinical manifestations described, other problems, usually associated with late-stage disease, may be detected. Any or all of the following complications can be present at various times during a rabies viral infection. The degree of severity and the order of presentation may vary widely.

Pituitary dysfunction may result in either diabetes insipidus or the syndrome of inappropriate antidiuretic hormone (SIADH), which would require treatment with vasopressin injections or fluid restriction, respectively.[6,61] Fluid balance and blood pressure maintenance may be complicated, since hypersecretion and hyposecretion of vasopressin may be seen during a patient's hospital course.[6]

Cardiovascular complications including myocarditis, ventricular fibrillation, arrhythmia, bradycardia, asystole, congestive heart failure, and superior vena cava obstruction have occurred.[6,60,61,70,71] Patients with rabies have required inotropic support and fluid therapy in the face of various cardiovascular complications.[6] If diabetes insipidus or SIADH is present, cardiovascular problems may be even more difficult to manage than usual.

Pulmonary complications leading to coma may also occur.[6] Periods of hypoventilation may progress to apnea and require oxygen supplementation and respiratory assistance.[69] Rales and rhonchi may be heard on auscultation.[6]

Diagnosis

The diagnosis of rabies can be difficult. Currently, there are no tests available to confirm rabies until the patient develops clinical symptoms.[6,44] The presence of hydrophobia and aerophobia strengthens a suspicion of rabies. Because of similarities with other disease states and the diversity in the clinical presentation of rabies, the differential diagnosis must include viral respiratory tract infections, Guillain-Barré syndrome, brain tumor or abscess, tetanus, myocarditis, viral encephalitis, and psychosis.[1,2,6,34,44,55,58,70] "Rabies hysteria" should also be considered. This occurs in a bite victim who is aware of the signs and symptoms of rabies but has not been bitten by a rabid animal. Patients with rabies hysteria, as opposed to patients with true rabies, have a shorter incubation phase, a longer duration of illness, and eventual recovery. Results of tests to confirm rabies in these patients are negative, but because of the long incubation time in true rabies and because some patients may have received medications that suppress antibody response (e.g., steroids), true rabies cannot be ruled out.[44]

There are two laboratory tests available to confirm a diagnosis of rabies: the rapid fluorescent focus inhibition test (RFFIT) and direct immunofluorescent rabies antibody staining of specific body tissues.[6] The more frequently used test in the United States is the RFFIT. This test is based on the comparison of a patient's antibody titer against the known standard (depending on the testing procedure, the standard titer measurement of 1.0 IU is approximately equal to the reciprocal titer of 1:30–1:140).[55] Results are available within 24 hours, and guidelines have been developed to evaluate the titer that is obtained. Both vaccinations and active disease will elicit the production of antibodies in 24–72 hours.

RFFIT titers can be correlated with the type of vaccination administered. After administration of duck embryo vaccine and nerve tissue vaccine, titers range from 10 IU to 50 IU (1:1000–1:5,000). Titers greater than this may indicate a different form of vaccination or the presence of active disease. Serum titers as high as 1:86,800 have been documented after administration of human diploid-cell vaccine.[72] Since serum titers are elevated, cerebrospinal fluid titers may be more specific in diagnosing disease following rabies prophylaxis with human diploid-cell vaccine.[67,73] Cerebrospinal fluid titers after vaccination will usually be less than 1:64, whereas titers produced by actual infection are usually more than 1:200.[54]

Immunofluorescent rabies antibody staining of brain tissue, neck skin, corneal impressions, serum, cerebrospinal fluid, and saliva has also been used in the diagnosis of rabies.[1,6,54,67,74] Immunofluorescence facilitates the location of an antigen or antibody in a tissue or smear.[6] After the specimen is exposed to a specific antibody or antigen that is labeled with fluorochrome, a diagnosis can be made by examining the pattern of fluorescence. Negative results should be confirmed with an additional test.[75] RFFIT is often the confirmatory test suggested to diagnose rabies infection.[76]

Rabies virus has also been isolated from neural tissue on autopsy.[67] Negri bodies (round or oval inclusion bodies seen in the cytoplasm and sometimes in the processes of neurons of rabid animals after death) may be detected on microscopic examination.[34,77] The rabies virus itself may be transiently detected in the cerebrospinal fluid or saliva; however, autosterilization of brain tissue has occurred in documented rabies cases.[1,67] This phenomenon is thought to result from a large increase in antirabies antibody.[54,67]

In animals, rabies is diagnosed by using direct fluorescent antibody tests. Examination of brain tissue for Negri bodies or the virus itself has also been used to diagnose rabies.[67] If an animal is suspected of carrying the rabies virus, it should be killed so the brain may be analyzed by an appropriate rabies diagnostic center. Since the virus is usually localized to the CNS, the brain is the most appropriate organ to be used for viral isolation.[55]

Biological Products in Treatment of Rabies

The development of rabies vaccines began in 1881 when Pasteur discovered that the virus could be obtained from the CNS of an infected animal.[25] Since then, numerous biological products have been investigated, including nerve tissue vaccine, duck embryo vaccine, rabies vaccine adsorbed, human diploid-cell vaccine, and human rabies immune globulin.[78,79] Currently, human diploid-cell vaccine or rabies vaccine adsorbed is used in the United States in conjunction with human rabies immune globulin for the prevention of rabies following exposure.[42] Nerve tissue vaccine and duck embryo vaccine are no longer used in the United States because of adverse effects and problems with efficacy.[17,18,23,78,80,81] Rabies vaccine adsorbed was recently made available in the United States; however, it is not yet widely used.[79]

The biological products that are currently used in the United States (human diploid-cell vaccine, rabies vaccine adsorbed, and human rabies immune globulin) are nearly 100% effective in preventing progression from stage I disease when they are administered appropriately after an attack by a rabid animal. Therapy with these agents has been shown to protect an exposed individual from the development of rabies by providing and inducing protective antibodies against the virus.[18] Treatment with both vaccine and rabies immune globulin should begin as soon as possible after exposure regardless of the amount of time lapsed since presumed viral transmission.[42] Treatment regimens aimed at curing the rabies virus infection after it has invaded the CNS have failed. Rabies is almost always fatal if left untreated, and the importance of prophylactic therapy cannot be overemphasized.

Although the morbidity and mortality associated with the disease are well documented, the controversy of whether treatment is being used excessively still exists.[21,82,83] In one study, it was estimated that only 4% of patients who receive rabies prophylaxis each year have truly been exposed to a rabid animal.[21] A second evaluation determined that postexposure therapy was overused in patients exposed to domestic animals, rodents, and lagomorphs, because these animals are rarely responsible for rabies transmission.[83] Practicing clinicians should contact state or local health departments for assistance in determining the need for rabies therapy. Most health departments require the initiation of the rabies vaccine within seven days of the attack. Often, this is not enough time to locate, isolate and test the animal for the virus, and this may contribute to the problem of overuse of rabies immunization.

Nerve Tissue Vaccine. In countries other than the United States, nerve tissue vaccine is used to provide protection following exposure.[81] Alternative therapies have been sought because of complications with this vaccine, including vaccine failures and neurological adverse effects.[17,18,78,81] Neurological complications, including encephalomyelitis and peripheral neuropathy, occur in approximately 0.08% of persons immunized with nerve tissue vaccine. Mortality results in one fourth of these cases.[23] The use of nerve tissue vaccine in countries other than the United States continues because those countries cannot produce human diploid-cell vaccine in quantities large enough to supply endemic areas, because of the low yield and high production cost.[7,81,84]

Duck Embryo Vaccine. Duck embryo vaccine is no longer used in the United States, although its use in other countries is not unusual. The vaccine is prepared from duck embryos that were previously infected with a fixed rabies virus. The resulting product is inactivated with β-propiolactone and administered to induce the production of antibodies to rabies virus.[85]

Treatment with duck embryo vaccine consists of 23 1-mL doses (along with a single dose of human rabies immune globulin). The first 21 doses of duck embryo vaccine are given daily for three weeks or twice daily for one week and then once daily for the second week. Two booster doses are then required 10 and 20 days after the 21st dose of duck embryo vaccine. The site of subcutaneous administration of the vaccine should be rotated; appropriate areas include the abdominal area, lower back, and thighs.[86] Many individuals in the United States continue to associate the treatment of rabies with the series of abdominal injections (of duck embryo vaccine) that were previously used. Healthcare professionals and the lay public need to become familiar with the current standards of rabies treatment.

Rabies Vaccine Adsorbed. Rabies vaccine adsorbed is produced and distributed by the Michigan Department of Public Health. The vaccine is produced in a diploid-cell culture of fetal rhesus monkey lung. The vaccine is subsequently inactivated with β-propiolactone and adsorbed to aluminum phosphate. The production of antibodies is stimulated after its administration. Rabies vaccine adsorbed should be administered i.m., concomitantly with human rabies immune globulin. The postexposure administration schedule of this vaccine is 1 mL on days 0 (first day of vaccination series), 3, 7, 14, and 28. Rabies vaccine adsorbed may also be given for primary pre-exposure immunization. A study evaluating pre-exposure immunization showed that the vaccine does result in acceptable antibody titers as defined by the Centers for Disease Control.[87] Minor adverse reactions may be seen in the majority of patients who receive the drug, and they are usually limited to pain and swelling at the site of injection. These adverse effects, however, do not require discontinuation of therapy.[79] Further information on rabies vaccine adsorbed may be obtained by contacting the Division of Biologic Products of the Michigan Department of Public Health (telephone number, 517-335-8120).

Human Diploid-Cell Vaccine. Human diploid-cell vaccine (Imovax Rabies, Merieux) is a source of inactivated rabies virus capable of promoting active immunity in an individual.[18,19] The resulting rabies antibodies will neutralize the rabies virus and prevent its progression. Human diploid-cell vaccine is used for pre-exposure immunization as well as for postexposure prophylaxis. The vaccine for i.m. use is available in single-dose vials that contain 1 mL of drug following reconstitution. Each milliliter of the vaccine contains ≥ 2.5 IU of rabies antigen.[19] The vaccines should be refrigerated and should be used immediately after reconstitution. (Dosage is described in the Pre-exposure Prophylaxis and Postexposure Prophylaxis sections.)

The immunogenicity of human diploid-cell vaccine may be partially determined by the site of its administration.[88] The vaccine should be administered i.m. into the deltoid muscle, since fatal cases of rabies encephalitis have occurred following injection into the gluteal muscle.[9,88-90] This form of vaccine failure may be due to the inadvertent administration of the vaccine into fat instead of muscle, resulting in impaired drug uptake. After the initiation of immunization, the development of antibodies to the vaccine can be detected in 7–10 days and can be expected to peak in one to two months.[18,19]

Intradermal human diploid-cell vaccine (Imovax Rabies I.D., Merieux), which is a different product from that intended for i.m. use, is also available for pre-exposure prophylaxis, but it is not recommended for postexposure immunization. Intradermal administration is effective for pre-exposure immunization and may be economical, since its dose (0.25 IU/0.1 mL) is only one tenth of the i.m. dose.[91] When compared with i.m. administration, intradermal administration has resulted in earlier production of antibodies. Although antibody titers with the intradermal vaccine were sufficient for protection, titers following i.m. administration were higher after the first two weeks, and equivalent titers between the intradermal and i.m. administration may not be seen for up to 28–56 days.[91,b] It is therefore recommended that the three-dose series of intradermal vaccine used for pre-exposure prophylaxis be completed 30 days before potential exposure to the virus.

Mild adverse reactions following vaccination with human diploid-cell vaccine have been documented.[18] Five percent to 20% of patients experience syncope, nausea, vomiting, diarrhea, headache, low-grade fever, or prodromal symptoms, which can be expected to subside within 24–72 hours.[19] Rarely, hypersensitivity reactions have occurred. It is proposed that most hypersensitivity reactions following the administration of human diploid-cell vaccine are secondary to the β-propiolactone used for viral inactivation during production.[17] Although uncommon, neuroparalytic complications following the administration of the vaccine have also been documented. Bernard et al.[92] reported a case of an 11-year-old boy who developed signs and symptoms consistent with a Guillain-Barré-like syndrome three days after the completion of a rabies immunization series with human diploid-cell vaccine and human rabies immune globulin. The illness was presumed to result from the vaccine, but no definite relationship was established. A full recovery occurred three months after the onset of symptoms.

Human Rabies Immune Globulin. Human rabies immune globulin (Hyperab, Cutter; Imogam Rabies, Merieux), which is obtained from the plasma of hyperimmunized human donors, is administered after rabies exposure to provide passive immunity against the rabies virus.[20,43] This product contains antibodies to the rabies virus, which protect the victim until a natural immune response is mounted. Since the virus proliferates around the site of the bite, it is thought that administration of drug near the wound will neutralize the antigen present (dosage is described in Postexposure Prophylaxis). Human rabies immune globulin should not be administered i.v.[20,42] Treatment failures, although infrequent, have occurred when the drug was administered inappropriately.

After the administration of human rabies immune globulin, antibodies may be detected in 24 hours and will peak after 48–72 hours. Adverse effects associated with human rabies immune globulin occur infrequently and may include local tenderness, stiffness, and muscle soreness at the injection site.[42]

Pre-exposure Prophylaxis

Pre-exposure prophylaxis with human diploid-cell vaccine or rabies vaccine adsorbed may be beneficial to persons at high risk of viral contact.[93] This group includes veterinarians, laboratory workers, taxidermists, spelunkers, and other personnel who work in proximity to the virus. It is controversial whether travelers to endemic areas should receive pre-exposure vaccination. The decision should be based on the incidence of rabies in the area, the length of stay, and the availability of postexposure immunization should transmission occur.[17]

Pre-exposure immunization simplifies, but does not negate the need for, postexposure prophylaxis if exposure to the virus is suspected.[2,33] The treatment of a previously immunized individual following exposure to the virus is simplified in two ways: (1) human rabies immune globulin is not required and (2) the number of doses of human diploid-cell vaccine or rabies vaccine adsorbed is decreased from five to two.[33,93]

The pre-exposure rabies immunization series consists of one injection of human diploid-cell vaccine (1 mL of the i.m. injection or 0.1 mL of the intradermal injection) on days 0, 7, and 21 or 28.[42] When there is continued risk of exposure, booster doses (also 1 mL i.m. or 0.1 mL intradermally) should be administered every two years, unless serologic testing shows low quantities of antibodies and the need for additional boosters to maintain an acceptable titer.[19] For pre-exposure prophylaxis, the i.m. dosage of rabies vaccine adsorbed is identical to that of the human diploid-cell vaccine regimen. However, rabies vaccine adsorbed should not be given intradermally. Routine testing to determine the development of antibodies following vaccination is recommended only for immunosuppressed individuals and persons who work directly with the virus during production or research (e.g., laboratory workers and veterinarians).[42] Measurements to determine development of antibodies are dependent on the laboratory technique and the assay used. The Centers for Disease Control determined that antibody titers that neutralize a 1:25 dilution of challenge virus two to four weeks after immunization, as measured by RFFIT, are acceptable.[42] The World Health Organization has predicted that a titer of 0.5 IU/mL is sufficient.[42] An antibody titer able to neutralize a 1:25 dilution of virus has been shown to be approximately equal to 0.5 IU/mL.[19]

Postexposure Prophylaxis

It is imperative that the rabies immunization series be started as soon as possible if transmission of the virus is suspected. Treatment should not be postponed while awaiting the results of the brain examination of the vector if the animal is suspected to carry the rabies virus.[2] If negative results are obtained, therapy may be discontinued.[2,33,42] The treatment regimen used after exposure depends on whether pre-exposure immunization was administered.

Treatment with both human rabies immune globulin and human diploid-cell vaccine or rabies vaccine adsorbed is necessary for postexposure prophylaxis in nonimmunized individuals.[42,94] Only one dose of human rabies immune globulin is required; it should be given at the beginning of the postexposure immunization series (day 0). When human rabies immune globulin is administered, one half of the dose should be infiltrated around the wound; the other half should be injected intramuscularly into the deltoid muscle (the anterolateral aspect of the thigh may be used in small children).[20,42] The usual total dose of human rabies immune globulin is 20 IU/kg. It must be given concomitantly with the first dose of human diploid-cell vaccine or rabies vaccine adsorbed; however, the two drugs should not be mixed in the same syringe or be administered into the same area, since neutralization may result.[20] In nonimmunized individuals, human diploid-cell vaccine or rabies vaccine adsorbed is administered intramuscularly in a series of five 1-mL injections given on days 0, 3, 7, 14, and 28 of treatment.[19,42]

Human rabies immune globulin is not required for postexposure prophylaxis in previously immunized individuals.[42] Passive immunization is not necessary because antibody titers from prior administration of human diploid-cell vaccine or rabies vaccine adsorbed should be adequate and administration of human rabies immune globulin may interfere with the development of antibodies for active immunity.[43] Only two 1-mL doses of human diploid-cell vaccine or rabies vaccine adsorbed, given i.m. on days 0 and 3, are required. It should be reemphasized that pre-exposure prophylaxis does not negate the need for postexposure treatment if transmission of the virus is thought to have occurred.

No treatment failures have occurred in the United States after appropriate immunization with the combination of human rabies immune globulin and human diploid-cell vaccine or rabies vaccine adsorbed.[17] Guidelines for administration of these biological products must be followed, since deviation may result in therapeutic failures.[1,17,94-97] It may take up to 30 days to develop protective levels of antibodies after the administration of human diploid-cell vaccine, re-emphasizing the importance of early administration of human rabies immune globulin. A short incubation period, resulting in inadequate time for antibody production, may potentially result in a treatment failure.[81]

Drug Interactions

Reported drug interactions involving human rabies immune globulin and human diploid-cell vaccine are minimal. It has been documented that coadministration of chloroquine and human diploid-cell vaccine may result in unexpectedly low antibody response to the virus. Caution should be emphasized in persons traveling to developing countries who are receiving both rabies and malarial prophylaxis.[17,98] Corticosteroids and other immunosuppressive agents also may hinder the response to rabies treatment. These agents should therefore be withheld if possible during the rabies immunization series.[42]

Treatment during Pregnancy

Administration of human diploid-cell vaccine and human rabies immune globulin during pregnancy has been reported in a woman who was bitten by a bat approximately eight months after conception.[99] Human diploid-cell vaccine and human rabies immune globulin 20 IU/kg were administered three days after the bite. Human diploid-cell vaccine was also administered on days 6, 10, 17, and 31 after exposure. The patient experienced myalgia, anorexia, and fatigue after the vaccinations. Delivery occurred after 35 weeks' gestation. The mother and child were both reported to be alive and well one year after treatment. Also reported is the case of a woman exposed to rabies during her seventh month of pregnancy.[100] Treatment with a full course (21 days) of duck embryo vaccine and human rabies immune globulin was initiated 31 hours after the attack. Delivery occurred nine weeks after exposure. No abnormalities in the child were noted at a nine-month follow-up visit. The literature supporting the use of rabies vaccines during pregnancy is limited. No studies have evaluated the use of rabies vaccine adsorbed during pregnancy. It is believed that pregnancy should not deter the clinician from administering human diploid-cell vaccine and human rabies immune globulin in appropriate situations since the benefits of treatment outweigh the risks.[42]

Wound Care and Antimicrobial Therapy

The likelihood of both bacterial infections (and the associated cellulitis, erythema, and tenderness) and rabies may decline if proper wound care and immunization therapy are instituted.[41,101] The wound should be washed immediately with soap and water; however, meticulous wound cleansing does not negate the need for postexposure prophylaxis with human rabies immune globulin and human diploid-cell vaccine or rabies vaccine adsorbed.[42] At the hospital, the area should be cleansed with 1–2% benzalkonium chloride and then rinsed with 0.9% sodium chloride solution.[101,102] Cleansing with benzalkonium chloride will kill the rabies virus locally and flush microorganisms out of the wound, thereby helping to prevent bacterial infection. Although only benzalkonium chloride has been proved efficacious (in guinea pigs), 1% povidone–iodine has also been recommended for the irrigation of wounds following exposure to the rabies virus.[102]

Prophylaxis against tetanus must also be ensured. Patients with previous tetanus immunization who have not received a booster within the past five years should receive tetanus toxoid. However, for persons with an uncertain or incomplete tetanus immunization history, tetanus immune globulin, which provides passive immunization, is required. A primary course of immunization should be started in previously unvaccinated individuals.[16,42]

Antibacterial therapy is often necessary after an animal bite.[16] Empirical therapy should be based on the following factors: the type of animal, the depth and site of the wound, the age of the patient, and the underlying condition of the patient (e.g., whether the patient is asplenic). Patients at high risk for bacterial wound infection include those under two years of age, elderly patients, those with wrist or finger bites, and those with bites from humans, primates, raccoons, and cats. Patients at low risk are those with face and scalp bites; clean, nonpuncture wounds; and bites from rodents.[101] Although the efficacy of prophylactic antibacterial therapy has not been thoroughly investigated, high-risk patients should be treated.

Since oral flora are species specific, the animal must be correctly identified. Bite wounds commonly result in infection from both aerobic and anaerobic organisms. Infection from one specific organism is rare. Brook[103] examined 21 children who had been bitten by various animals. Anaerobic, aerobic, and mixed (aerobic and anaerobic) infections were found in 10%, 24%, and 66% of the wounds, respectively. In these same patients, 59 different organisms, including 37 aerobes and 22 anaerobes, were recovered from bites inflicted by animals. In another study, Goldstein et al.[104] evaluated 26 patients with 27 dog bite wounds. Aerobic and anaerobic pathogens were cultured from 74% and 41% of patients, respectively. When anaerobes were present, a mixed infection of anaerobes and aerobes was always documented.

The most common organisms found in the domestic dog or cat bite are *Staphylococcus aureus* and *Pasteurella multocida*. These organisms can be treated with either penicillin or ampicillin but, because of increased resistance, amoxicillin–clavulanate potassium has recently been recommended.[103,105] Alternate choices may include oral tetracycline or i.v. ceftriaxone. For patients who are allergic to the penicillins, tetracycline is an alternative.[105] Some oral cephalosporins are effective against flora found in animal bites, although many clinicians believe that because these agents have not been studied in the treatment of animal bites they should be avoided when possible. Pregnant patients who are allergic to penicillin may warrant treatment with oral cephalosporins. In these cases, the clinician must remember the spectrum of activity of the selected cephalosporin and the microorganisms that are not covered.

Future Considerations

A vaccine produced by recombinant technology is under investigation to control rabies in wildlife. The vaccinia–rabies glycoprotein vaccine acts by inducing rabies-neutralizing antibody in animals, thereby protecting the animals and eliminating them as vectors in the transmission of rabies to humans.[106,107]

Benefits of interferon therapy in humans are also being evaluated. The production of interferon can be stimulated by viral infection, and it may have antiviral and immunoregulatory activity.[25] Libby and Meislin[59] reported a case of rabies (diagnosed by neck biopsy) in which interferon was administered 70 days after inoculation with the virus. This was the first report of a patient treated with interferon in the United States. The patient died on day 16 of hospitalization. Dosage regimens involving interferon need to be evaluated. The time delay between inoculation and administration of drug therapy may have been a factor in interferon therapy failure; however, other cases have also been treated unsuccessfully in this manner.[7,59,108]

Conclusion

Rabies infections in humans are fatal if untreated. Postexposure treatment with human diploid-cell vaccine or rabies vaccine adsorbed and human rabies immune globulin is almost always curative if initiated early in the incubation period.

[a]New Jersey Department of Public Health, Epizootic Hotline (recorded message; telephone number, 609-292-5769). 1991 Nov.

[b]Dukes C, Merieux Institute. Personal communication. 1991 Jul 1.

References

1. Anderson LJ, Nicholson KG, Tauxe RV et al. Human rabies in the United States, 1960 to 1979: epidemiology, diagnosis and prevention. *Ann Intern Med*. 1984; 100:728-35.
2. Fishbein DB, Baer GM. Animal rabies: implications for diagnosis and treatment. *Ann Intern Med*. 1988; 109:935-7.
3. Steele JH. Rabies in the Americas and remarks on global aspects. *Rev Infect Dis*. 1988; 10(Suppl 4):S585-97.
4. Kappus KD. Canine rabies in the United States, 1971-1973: study of reported cases with reference to vaccination history. *Am J Epidemiol*. 1976; 103:242-9.
5. Constantine DG, Emmons RW, Woodie JD. Rabies virus in nasal mucosa of naturally infected bats. *Science*. 1972; 175:1255-6.
6. Bhatt DR, Hattwick MA, Gerdsen R et al. Human rabies. *Am J Dis Child*. 1974; 127:862-9.
7. Warrell DA, Warrell MJ. Human rabies and its prevention: an overview. *Rev Infect Dis*. 1988; 10(Suppl 4):S726-31.
8. Winkler WG, Fashinell TR, Leffing L et al. Airborne rabies transmission in a laboratory worker. *JAMA*. 1973; 226:1219-21.
9. Lumbiganon P, Bunyahotra V, Pairojkul C et al. Human rabies despite treatment with rabies immune globulin and human diploid cell rabies vaccine—Thailand. *JAMA*. 1988; 259:25-6.
10. Gottesdiener KM. Transplanted infections: donor-to-host transmission with the allograft. *Ann Intern Med*. 1989; 110:1001-6.
11. Baer GM. Research towards rabies prevention: overview. *Rev Infect Dis*. 1988; 10(Suppl 4):S576-7.
12. Baer GM. Oral rabies vaccination: an overview. *Rev Infect Dis*. 1988; 10(Suppl 4):S644-8.
13. Wandler AI, Capt S, Kappeler A et al. Oral immunization of wildlife against rabies: concept and first field experiments. *Rev Infect Dis*. 1988; 10(Suppl 4):S649-53.
14. Debbie JG, Bogel K. Public health aspects of current oral rabies vaccines. *Rev Infect Dis*.1988; 10(Suppl 4):S670-1.
15. Baer GM, Abeelseth MK, Debbie JG. Oral vaccination of foxes against rabies. *Am J Epidemiol*. 1971; 93:487-90.
16. Brook I. Human and animal bite infections. *J Fam Pract*. 1989; 28:713-8.
17. Nicholson KG. Rabies. *Lancet*. 1990; 335:1201-5.
18. Bahmanyar M, Fayaz A, Nour-Salehi S et al. Successful protection of humans exposed to rabies infection. *JAMA*. 1976; 236:2751-4.
19. AHFS drug information 91. McEvoy GK, ed. Rabies vaccine. Bethesda, MD: American Society of Hospital Pharmacists; 1991:2053-8.
20. AHFS drug information 91. McEvoy GK, ed. Rabies immune globulin. Bethesda, MD: American Society of Hospital Pharmacists; 1991:1993-5.
21. Eng TR, Fishbein DB. Epidemiologic factors, clinical findings, and vaccination status of rabies in cats and dogs in the United States in 1988. *J Am Vet Med Assoc*. 1990; 197:201-9.
22. Cereghino JJ, Osterud HT, Pinnas JL et al. Rabies: a rare disease but a serious pediatric problem. *Pediatrics*. 1970; 45:839-44.
23. Rubin RH, Gregg MB, Sikes RK. Rabies in citizens of the United States, 1963-1968: epidemiology, treatment, and complications of treatment. *J Infect Dis*. 1969; 120:268-73.
24. Murphy FA. Rabies pathogenesis. *Arch Virol*. 1977; 54:279-97.
25. Kaplan MM, Koprowski H. Rabies. *Sci Am*. 1980; 242(Jan):120-34.
26. Matthews RE. Classification and nomenclature of viruses. *Intervirology*. 1982; 17:109-14.
27. Familusi JB, Osunkoya BO, Moore DL et al. A fatal human infection with mokola virus. *Am J Trop Med Hyg*. 1972; 21:959-63.
28. Brown F, Bishop DHL, Crick J et al. Rhabdoviridae. *Intervirology*. 1979; 12:1-7.
29. World Health Organization expert committee on rabies. Sixth report. Geneva: World Health Organization Technical Report Series No.523; 1973:12.
30. Arellano-Sota C. Biology, ecology, and control of the vampire bat. *Rev Infect Dis*. 1988; 10(Suppl 4):S615-9.
31. Jenkins SR, Perry BD, Winkler WG. Ecology and epidemiology of raccoon rabies. *Rev Infect Dis*. 1988; 10(Suppl 4):S620-5.
32. Hattwick MA, Hochberg FH, Landrigan PJ et al. Skunk associated human rabies. *JAMA*. 1972; 222:44-7.
33. Fishbein DB, Arcangeli S. Rabies prevention in primary care. *Postgrad Med*. 1987; 82:83-95.
34. Dupont JR, Earle KM. Human rabies encephalitis: a study of forty-nine fatal cases with a review of the literature. *Neurology*. 1965; 15:1023-34.
35. Centers for Disease Control. Rabies in a llama—Oklahoma. *MMWR*. 1990; 39:203-4.
36. Humphrey GL, Kemp GE, Wood EG. A fatal case of rabies in a woman bitten by an insectivorous bat. *Public Health Rep*. 1960; 75:317-26.
37. Blattner RJ. Rabies infection transmitted by insectivorous bats: human case with virus isolation from spinal fluid during life. *J Pediatr*. 1961; 58:433-7.
38. Irons JV, Eads RB, Grimes JE et al. The public health importance of bats. *Tex Rep Biol Med*. 1957; 15:292-8.
39. Gomez MR, Siekert RG, Herrmann EC. A human case of skunk rabies. *JAMA*. 1965; 194:101-3.
40. Kent JR, Finegold SM. Human rabies transmitted by the bite of a bat. *N Engl J Med*. 1960; 263:1058-65.
41. Jacobs R. Summer summary of bite wound care: tetanus and rabies. *Mod Med*. 1982; 50:94-112.
42. Centers for Disease Control. Rabies prevention—United States 1991. *MMWR*. 1991; 40(Suppl RR1):1-19.
43. Loofbourow JC, Cabasso VJ, Roby RE et al. Rabies immune globulin (human) clinical trials and dose determination. *JAMA*. 1971; 217:1825-31.
44. Wilson JM, Hettiarachchi J, Wijesuriya LM. Presenting features and diagnosis of rabies. *Lancet*. 1975; 2:1139-40.
45. Helmick CG, Tauxe RV, Vernon AA. Is there a risk to contacts of patients with rabies? *Rev Infect Dis*. 1987; 9:511-8.
46. O'Day DM. Diseases potentially transmitted through corneal transplantation. *Ophthalmology*. 1989; 96:1133-8.
47. Houff SA, Burton RC, Wilson RW et al. Human-to-human transmission of rabies virus by corneal transplant. *N Engl J Med*. 1979; 300:603-4.
48. Centers for Disease Control. Human-to-human transmission of rabies by a corneal transplant—Idaho. *MMWR*. 1979; 28:109-111.
49. Centers for Disease Control. Human-to-human transmission of rabies via corneal transplant—France. *MMWR*. 1980; 29:25-6.
50. Centers for Disease Control. Human-to-human transmission of rabies via corneal transplant—Thailand. *MMWR*. 1981; 30:473-5.
51. Constantine DG. Rabies transmission by nonbite route. *Public Health Rep*. 1962; 77:287-9.
52. Murphy FA. The pathogenesis of rabies virus infection. In:

Koprowski H, Plotkin SA, eds. World's debt to Pasteur. New York: Liss; 1985:153-69.
53. Ganong WF. Review of Medical Physiology. East Norwalk, CT: Appleton & Lange; 1989.
54. Corey L. Rabies and other rhabdoviruses. In: Wilson JD, Braunwald E, Isselbacher KJ, eds. Harrison's principles of internal medicine. New York: McGraw-Hill; 1987:712-7.
55. Bernard KW, Fishbein DB. Rabies virus. In: Mandell GL, Douglas RG, Bennett JE, eds. Principles and practice of infectious diseases. New York: Churchill Livingstone; 1990:1291-303.
56. Nikolitsch M. Virus concentration and length of incubation period. *Trop Dis Bull.* 1958; 55:395-7.
57. Ghosh S. A case of rabies in England. *Br Med J.* 1964; 2:167-8.
58. Chopra JS, Banerjee AK, Murthy JM et al. Paralytic rabies: a clinico-pathological study. *Brain.* 1980; 789-802.
59. Libby J, Meislin HW. Human rabies. *Ann Emerg Med.* 1983; 12:217-20.
60. Warrell DA, Davidson NM, Pope HM et al. Pathophysiologic studies in human rabies. *Am J Med.* 1976; 60:180-90.
61. Udwadia ZF, Udwadia FE, Rao PP et al. Penile hyperexcitability with recurrent ejaculations as the presenting manifestation of a case of rabies. *Postgrad Med.* 1988; 64:85-6.
62. Torres-Anjel MJ, Volz D, Torres MJ et al. Failure to thrive, wasting syndrome, and immunodeficiency in rabies: a hypophyseal/hypothalamic/thymic axis effect of rabies virus. *Rev Infect Dis.* 1988; 10(Suppl 4):S710-25.
63. Bhandari M, Kumar S. Penile hypersensitivity as the presenting symptom of rabies. *Br J Urol.* 1986; 58:224-33.
64. Bramley JE, Cudmore RE, Holland JW. Penile pain in rabies. *Br Med J.* 1965; 2:880. Letter.
65. Love SV. Paralytic rabies: review of the literature and report of a case. *J Pediatr.* 1944; 24:312.
66. Varma K, Maheshwari MC, Chawdhary C et al. Acute ascending motor paralysis due to rabies: a clinical pathological report. *Eur Neurol.* 1985; 24:160.
67. Hattwick MA, Weis TT, Stechschulte CJ et al. Recovery from rabies. *Ann Intern Med.* 1972; 76:931-42.
68. Porras C, Barboza JJ, Fuenzalida E et al. Recovery from rabies in man. *Ann Intern Med.* 1976; 85:44-8.
69. Rubin RH, Sullivan L, Summers R et al. A case of human rabies in Kansas; epidemiologic, clinical, and laboratory considerations. *J Infect Dis.* 1970; 122:318-22.
70. Cheetham HD, Hart J, Coghill NF et al. Rabies with myocarditis. *Lancet.* 1970; 1:921-2.
71. Ross E, Armentrout SA. Myocarditis associated with rabies. *N Engl J Med.* 1962; 266:1087-9.
72. Bahmanyar M, Faydy A, Nour-Salehi S et al. Successful protection of humans exposed to rabies infection: post-exposure treatment with the new human diploid cell vaccine and antirabies serum. *JAMA.* 1976; 236:2751.
73. Porras C, Barboza JJ, Fuenzalida E et al. Recovery from rabies in man. *Ann Intern Med.* 1976; 85:44.
74. Koch FJ, Sagartz JW, Davidson DE et al. Diagnosis of human rabies by the cornea test. *Am J Clin Pathol.* 1975; 63:509-15.
75. Sitthi-Amorn C, Jiratanavattana V, Keoyoo J et al. The diagnostic properties of laboratory tests for rabies. *Int J Epidemiol.* 1987; 16:602-5.
76. Smith JS, Yager PA, Baer GM. A rapid reproducible test for determining rabies neutralizing antibody. *Bull World Health Organ.* 1973; 48:535.
77. Sung JH, Hayano M, Mastri AR et al. A case of human rabies and ultrastructure of the Negri body. *J Neuropathol Exp Neurol.* 1976; 35:541.
78. Sureau P. History of rabies: advances in research towards rabies prevention during the last 30 years. *Rev Infect Dis.* 1988; 10(Suppl 4):S581-4.
79. Centers for Disease Control. Rabies vaccine, adsorbed: a new rabies vaccine for use in humans. *MMWR.* 1988; 37:217-8.
80. Perine PL, Harris D, Kirkpatrick CH. Immunological reactions to duck embryo rabies vaccine. *JAMA.* 1968; 205:559.
81. Vodopija I. Current issues in human rabies immunization. *Rev Infect Dis.* 1988; 10(Suppl 4):S758-63.
82. Remington PL, Shope T, Andrews J. A recommended approach to the evaluation of human rabies exposure in an acute-care hospital. *JAMA.* 1985; 254:67-9.
83. Helmick CG. The epidemiology of human rabies post-exposure prophylaxis, 1980–1981. *JAMA.* 1983; 250:1990-6.
84. Wilde H, Chomchey P, Prakongsri S, et al. Safety of equine rabies immune globulin. *Lancet.* 1987; 2:1275. Letter.
85. Peck FB, Powell HM, Culbertson CG. A new antirabies vaccine for human use. Clinical and laboratory results using rabies vaccine made from embryonated duck eggs. *J Lab Clin Med.* 1955; 45:679-83.
86. Greenberg M, Childress J. Vaccination against rabies with duck embryo vaccine and semple vaccine. *JAMA.* 1960; 173:333-7.
87. Berlin BS, Mitchell JR, Burgoyne GH et al. Rhesus diploid rabies vaccine (adsorbed): a new rabies vaccine. *JAMA.* 1982; 247:1726-8.
88. Fishbein DB, Sawyer LA, Weir EH. Administration of human diploid-cell rabies vaccine in the gluteal area. *N Engl J Med.* 1988; 318:124-5. Letter.
89. Shill M, Baynes RD, Miller SD. Fatal rabies encephalitis despite appropriate post-exposure prophylaxis. *N Engl J Med.* 1987; 316:1257-8.
90. Centers for Disease Control. Human rabies despite treatment with rabies immune globulin and human diploid cell rabies vaccine—Thailand. *MMWR.* 1987; 36:759-65.
91. Warrell MJ, Suntharasamai P, Sinhaseni A. An economical regimen of human diploid cell strain anti-rabies vaccine for post-exposure prophylaxis. *Lancet.* 1983; 2:301-4.
92. Bernard KW, Smith PW, Kader FJ et al. Neuroparalytic illness and human diploid cell rabies vaccine. *JAMA.* 1982; 248:3136-8.
93. Roumiantzeff M, Ajjan N, Vincent-Falquit JC. Experience with pre-exposure rabies vaccination. *Rev Infect Dis.* 1988; 10(Suppl 4):S751-7.
94. Devriendt J, Staroukine M, Costy F et al. Fatal encephalitis apparently due to rabies. *JAMA.* 1982; 248:2304-6.
95. Anon. Rabies vaccine failures. *Lancet.* 1988; 1:917-8. Editorial.
96. Wattanasri S, Boonthai P, Thongcharoen P. Human rabies after late administration of human diploid cell vaccine without hyperimmune serum. *Lancet.* 1982; 2:870. Letter.
97. Centers for Disease Control. Human rabies—Rwanda. *MMWR.* 1982; 31:135-6.
98. Pappaioanou M, Fishbein DB, Dreesen DW et al. Antibody response to pre-exposure human diploid-cell rabies vaccine given concurrently with chloroquine. *N Engl J Med.* 1986; 314:280-4.
99. Varner MW, McGuinness GA, Galask RP. Rabies vaccination in pregnancy. *Am J Obstet Gynecol.* 1982; 143:717-8.
100. Cates W. Treatment of rabies exposure during pregnancy. *Obstet Gynecol.*1974; 44:893-6.
101. Callaham ML. Critical decisions in emergency medicine: bite wounds. *Hosp Ther.* 1985; 10(Sep):48-50, 55-7.
102. Kaplan MM, Cohen D, Koprowski H et al. Studies on the local treatment of wounds for the prevention of rabies. *Bull World Health Organ.* 1962; 26:765-75.
103. Brook I. Microbiology of human and animal bite wounds in children. *Pediatr Infect Dis J.* 1987; 6:29-32.
104. Goldstein EJ, Citron DM, Finegold SM. Dog bite wounds and infection: a prospective clinical study. *Ann Emerg Med.* 1980; 9:508-12.
105. Goldstein EJ, Richwald GA. Human and animal bite wounds. *Am Fam Physician.* 1987; 36(Jul):101-9.
106. Koprowski H. Glimpses into the future of rabies research. *Rev Infect Dis.* 1988; 10(Suppl 4):S810-5.
107. Koprowski H. Rabies oral immunization. *Curr Top Microbiol Immunol.* 1989; 146:137-51.
108. Merigan TC, Baer GM, Winkler WG et al. Human leukocyte interferon administration to patients with symptomatic and suspected rabies. *Ann Neurol.* 1984; 16:82-7.

Interference by antiarrhythmic agents with function of electrical cardiac devices

DEBORAH A. TWOREK, JOSÉ NAZARI, MARILYN EZRI, AND JERRY L. BAUMAN

Abstract: The possible interference of drugs with the function of implanted electrical cardiac devices in two patients is described, and the literature on the interaction between these drugs and devices is reviewed.

A 59-year-old woman had a permanent pacemaker implanted after diagnosis of tachycardia–bradycardia syndrome, and her drug regimen of digoxin, verapamil, and warfarin was supplemented with flecainide to prevent paroxysmal atrial fibrillation. A Holter monitor recording performed after five days of flecainide therapy showed the pacemaker was sensing and pacing normally. Approximately three weeks after pacemaker implantation and initiation of flecainide therapy, a Holter monitor recording showed high-grade atrioventricular block and failure of the pacemaker to capture. A chest roentgenogram showed that the pacemaker lead was properly placed. The pacemaker's pulse amplitude and pulse width were increased, and the device again functioned reliably. Six months later the pacing threshold was noted to have returned to normal.

A 64-year-old man had a history of aborted sudden cardiac death from ventricular tachyarrhythmias. The patient received an automatic implanted cardioverter–defibrillator (AICD); at that time, a 15-J discharge was required to terminate induced ventricular fibrillation (VF). Three years later, the AICD was replaced; the energy required for VF termination with the new unit was 16 J. Seven months after implantation of the new unit, the patient had several episodes of ventricular tachycardia (VT). Moricizine therapy was initiated. An electrophysiologic study (EPS) three days later showed that a larger shock (28 J) was required to terminate VF and that the pacing threshold had increased. Soon after the EPS the patient developed intractable VT and died.

Antiarrhythmic agents can increase the pacing threshold and interfere with the ability of the pacemaker to sense native depolarizations. Antiarrhythmic drugs reported to interfere with pacemaker function include type IA, IB, and IC agents. Antiarrhythmic agents may also increase the energy needed to terminate VF and may interfere with the ability of the AICD to discriminate supraventricular from ventricular tachyarrhythmias. Antiarrhythmic agents reported to affect the defibrillation threshold in humans include mexiletine and amiodarone. The second case in this article appears to be the first report of the effect of moricizine on defibrillation threshold.

Antiarrhythmic agents can interfere with the function of cardiac pacemakers and AICDs.

Index terms: Cardiac drugs; Devices; Drug interactions; Flecainide; Implants; Moricizine; Toxicity
Clin Pharm. 1992; 11:48-56

Drug–drug and drug–nutrient interactions are well-documented in the medical literature. Often overlooked, however, is the interaction between drugs and implantable medical devices.

Antiarrhythmic agents are often used in patients with implanted antiarrhythmic devices. Specifically, pacemakers are usually implanted in patients with symptomatic tachycardia–bradycardia syndrome to prevent symptomatic bradycardia; concurrently, antiarrhythmic agents may be initiated to manage the symptomatic tachyarrhythmias associated with this disorder. Similarly, patients with malignant ventricular tachyarrhythmias receive automatic implanted cardioverter–defibrillators (AICDs) and are often concurrently treated with antiarrhythmic agents to decrease the frequency of the AICD discharges. Al-

DEBORAH A. TWOREK, PHARM.D., is Cardiovascular Fellow, Department of Pharmacy Practice; JOSÉ NAZARI, M.D., is Clinical Assistant Professor, Department of Medicine, Section of Cardiology; MARILYN EZRI, M.D., is Clinical Associate Professor, Department of Medicine, Section of Cardiology; and JERRY L. BAUMAN, PHARM.D., is Associate Professor, Departments of Pharmacy Practice and Medicine, Section of Cardiology, The University of Illinois at Chicago.

Address reprint requests to Dr. Bauman at The University of Illinois at Chicago, College of Pharmacy, Room 244 (M/C 886), 833 South Wood Street, Chicago, IL 60612.

This is article **680-204-9201** in the **ASHP Continuing Education System.** It qualifies for 1.0 hour of continuing-education credit. See page 79 for learning objectives and test questions.

though drug–device combinations are intended to be complementary, deleterious interactions can occur. The addition of an antiarrhythmic agent to pacemaker therapy may alter pacemaker function and result in failure of a pacemaker discharge to cause cardiac depolarization and contraction (i.e., failure to capture). Antiarrhythmic agents may interfere with AICD function by increasing the threshold for defibrillation. That is, the AICD delivers a discharge that was consistently effective in restoring a stable rhythm before antiarrhythmic therapy; after drug treatment, the discharge delivered by the AICD is ineffective.

Few reports in the literature address potential drug–device interactions despite their documentation as early as 1967.[1] We report two cases of possible drug–device interactions and review the literature on antiarrhythmic agents and their potential influence on pacemakers and AICDs. The first case illustrates a possible drug–pacemaker interaction, and the second case illustrates a possible drug–AICD interaction.

Case Report 1

A 59-year-old woman was admitted to the hospital with a six-month history of palpitations and dizziness. She had been diagnosed with atrial fibrillation eight years before admission. Treatment with quinidine and then disopyramide had been attempted and was subsequently discontinued because of gastrointestinal intolerance and economic reasons, respectively. The combination of propranolol hydrochloride 40 mg p.o. twice a day and digoxin 0.25 mg p.o. once a day controlled the patient's ventricular response and symptoms for the ensuing eight years. In addition, the patient was receiving warfarin sodium 1.25 mg/day p.o for a probable embolic stroke.

On admission, laboratory test results were within normal limits. The electrocardiogram (ECG) demonstrated sinus bradycardia (heart rate, approximately 40 beats/min) with frequent premature atrial contractions and a 3.2-second sinus pause. Discontinuation of propranolol therapy failed to result in a subsequent increase in heart rate. An episode of atrial fibrillation with a ventricular response of approximately 150 beats/min, during which the patient complained of dizziness and diaphoresis, was documented. During therapy with the combination of verapamil and digoxin, to control ventricular rate, a 24-hour Holter monitor recording documented periods of sinus bradycardia (heart rate, 20 beats/min), multiple episodes of atrial fibrillation (maximum ventricular response, 174 beats/min), and occasional ventricular ectopy (which produced no symptoms).

Tachycardia–bradycardia syndrome was diagnosed, and a permanent pacemaker was subsequently implanted and set in the ventricle-ventricle-inhibit (VVI) mode (the electrode senses in the ventricle, stimulates the ventricle, and is inhibited by native impulses). The pacing threshold (the minimum electrical energy required of the pacemaker to initiate an action potential and cause cardiac muscle contraction) at the time of implantation was 0.6 volts (V) at 0.5 milliseconds (msec). The pacemaker was programmed to the following settings: pulse (output) amplitude, 2.5 V; pulse width (duration), 0.5 msec; sensitivity (strength of a native depolarization above which the pacemaker will be inhibited), 2.5 millivolts (mV); and rate, 60 beats/min. A chest roentgenogram showed that the pacemaker lead was appropriately positioned.

Therapy with flecainide acetate 100 mg p.o twice daily was started the next day to prevent episodes of paroxysmal atrial fibrillation, and success was documented by telemetric continuous electrocardiography. A Holter monitor recording performed after five days of flecainide therapy showed the pacemaker to be sensing (not discharging when native depolarizations of sufficient strength and rate were present) and pacing normally (Figure 1), and there were no episodes of bradycardia or atrial fibrillation. Seven days after pacemaker implantation, the patient was discharged without complaints of palpitations or dizziness. Discharge medications were flecainide, verapamil, digoxin, and warfarin.

Two weeks after discharge, a follow-up Holter monitor recording demonstrated periods of high-grade atrioventricular block and failure of the pacemaker to capture the ventricles (Figure 2). This adverse event was attributed to flecainide and the patient was immediately called to the clinic. The patient was asymptomatic, all serum electrolyte concentrations were within the normal range, and a repeat chest roentgenogram to evaluate lead placement was unchanged. The pacemaker was found to be

Papers in the Grand Rounds *section are patient case reports and literature review combined in a way that gives them high educational value. The papers lead off with a well-documented case report of an unusual drug experience (e.g., adverse drug reaction or other unexpected drug response, experimental use of a drug). The case generally deals with a difficult therapeutic problem or dilemma that is commonly encountered but may be overlooked or misunderstood. (Esoteric or rare occurences of minor importance do not make good* Grand Rounds *material.) A literature review puts the case in perspective with previously reported similar cases and alternative treatments. The review is integrated with related discussion of the case being reported.*

CP *readers are encouraged to use* Grand Rounds *for educational group discussions. For this purpose, discussion questions are printed at the end of* Grand Rounds *papers.*

Figure 1. Holter monitor recording of ECG leads V_5 and V_1 five days after the start of flecainide therapy (six days after pacemaker implantation). The pacemaker is functioning appropriately; each pacemaker discharge (arrow) causes immediate ventricular depolarization and a resultant wide QRS complex. The pacemaker rate is 60 beats/min.

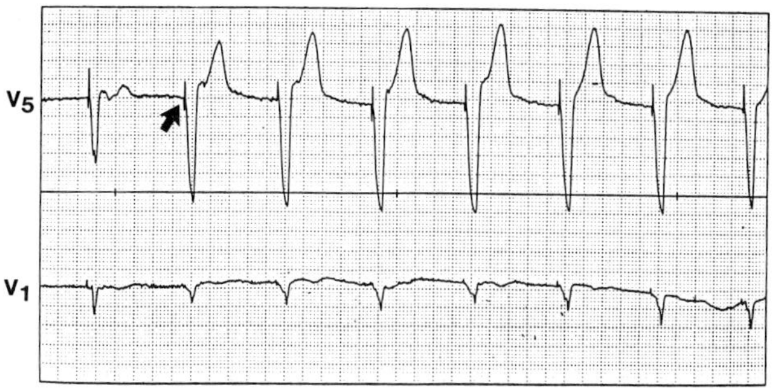

functioning according to the previously prescribed settings, but it was not capturing consistently. The following adjustments were made: (1) the pulse amplitude was increased from 2.5 V to 6.0 V and (2) the pulse width was increased from 0.5 msec to 0.7 msec. After these adjustments, the pacemaker functioned reliably for six months as shown by Holter monitor recordings. The pacing threshold was noted to have returned to normal, and maintenance of this low threshold was confirmed at a follow-up appointment six months later (Figure 3).

Figure 2. Holter monitor recording of ECG leads V_5 and V_1 approximately three weeks after the start of flecainide therapy and pacemaker implantation. The pacemaker is not capturing the ventricles; pacemaker discharges (visible only in V_5) are not followed by wide QRS complexes. Pacemaker discharge is appropriately inhibited by native ventricular depolarizations (narrow QRS complexes), which are a result of the patient's irregular sinus bradycardia. Consecutive noninhibited pacemaker discharges (the first is indicated by the arrow) show the pacemaker rate of 60 beats/min.

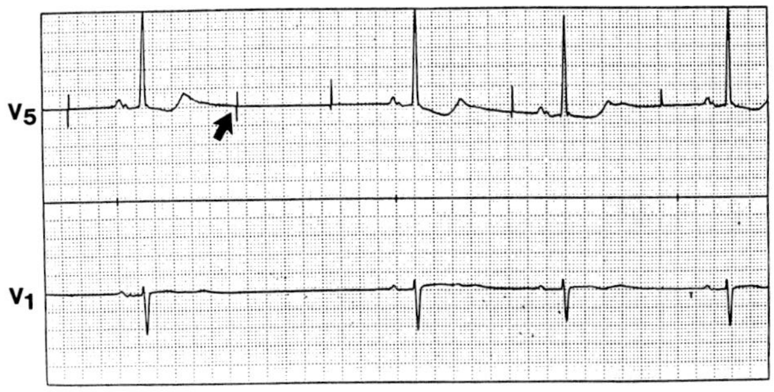

Figure 3. Pacing thresholds and pacemaker settings in a patient treated with flecainide. The white triangle shows the single pacing threshold (combination of pulse amplitude and pulse width needed to produce ventricular depolarization) determined at the time of pacemaker implantation. The white circle shows the amplitude–width combination initially set on the pacemaker; this setting was later shown to be inadequate to capture the ventricles. The pacemaker was reset to the combination indicated by the white square. The pacing thresholds measured approximately six months later (black circles) and one year later (black triangles) are suggestive of the initial value (white triangle). Dotted and solid lines indicate extrapolation between and beyond data points.

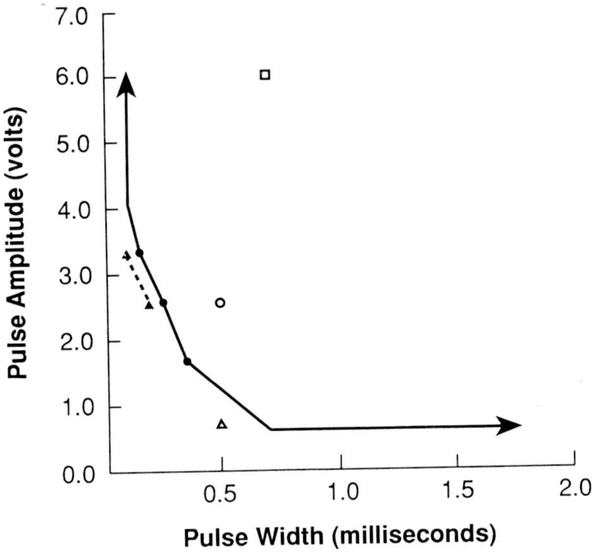

Pacemaker Function

Effective pacing from a pacemaker results from the transmission of electricity from a power source through a temporary or permanent lead to the myocardium. Pacing threshold is determined by (1) the lead–myocardium interface (contact between the surfaces of the lead and the excitable myocardium) and (2) electrical energy from the power source.

Contact between the lead and the myocardium is more likely to vary when a temporary, transvenous pacemaker is used. With a permanently implanted unit, the lead–myocardium interface becomes stable in the long term. Therefore, with permanent pacemakers, the determinants of threshold are the voltage (pulse amplitude) applied through a resistance (the impedance of the lead plus the lead–myocardium interface, which is stable through a narrow range) for a given period of time (pulse width). Pacing strength can be expressed as current (measured in milliamperes), voltage (measured in volts), or energy (measured in microjoules, μJ). Since resistance is relatively fixed unless the lead is fractured or damaged, pacing threshold, for practical purposes, is determined by the interaction between pacing strength and duration.

The programmable variable most often used for pacing strength is pulse amplitude (the height of the pacemaker impulse). Pulse width (the duration of the pacemaker impulse) is also generally a programmable variable in modern pacemakers. Pacing threshold is best expressed by a curve plotting pulse amplitude (volts) or current (milliamperes) versus duration or pulse width (milliseconds) (Figure 4). The greater the

Figure 4. Pacing threshold (strength–duration) curve. The vertical axis represents pacemaker pulse strength (or pulse amplitude, in volts), and the horizontal axis represents the pacemaker pulse duration (or pulse width, in milliseconds). The pacing threshold curve is determined by finding several combinations of the minimal pulse strength and duration required for capture (initiation of a cardiac action potential and contraction). A pacemaker will capture if its pulse amplitude and pulse width are above the curve; settings should be well above the curve to ensure an adequate margin of safety.

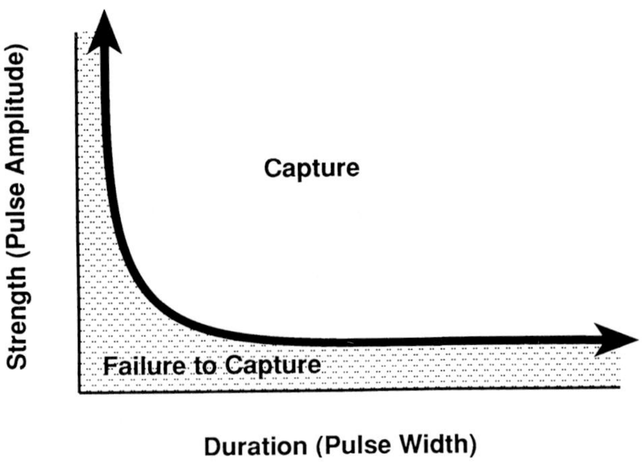

strength, the lesser the required duration (and vice versa). In practice, pacing threshold is determined at three or four voltage settings (current or energy can be used, but it is not commonly programmable) or pulse width settings to estimate the strength–duration curve.

Pacing threshold does not remain constant from the time of pacemaker implantation. Clinically important changes in pacing threshold may occur over time.[2] At implantation, a pacemaker usually has its lowest pacing threshold because the electrode is in direct contact with excitable myocardial tissue. Over a two- to six-week period, the pacing threshold rises to its highest level, at approximately three or four times the initial setting. During this time, edema and inflammation surround the metal tip of the electrode, and the electrical charge is dispersed before reaching the normal excitable tissue. After approximately six months, the pacing threshold falls and stabilizes to a level that is usually about twice the initial setting. Inflammation has subsided, and the electrode tip is surrounded by fibrous tissue.

At the time of implantation, cardiologists commonly identify the minimal voltage required to depolarize the ventricles and then set the pacemaker's pulse amplitude at 5 to 10 times this value to account for these influences. Later, settings are changed to those that provide an adequate pacing margin of safety: Usually, the pulse amplitude at the pacing threshold is doubled or the pulse width at threshold is tripled while staying away from the extremes of the strength–duration curve. At the extremes (asymptotes) of the threshold curve, small changes in either variable (attributable to electrolyte or circadian variation) can render pacemaker impulses unable to capture. Rate and sensitivity of the pacemaker are also programmed. An appropriate sensitivity setting allows the pacemaker to detect true intrinsic cardiac depolarizations (and to subsequently inhibit itself from discharging) and to ignore extraneous signals (noise).

Several physiological factors influence the threshold of a pacemaker once it has stabilized postoperatively. For example, in one small series, Preston et al.[1] documented a transient 30–40% increase in pacemaker threshold caused by sleeping and eating, while exercise-related increases in sympathetic tone resulted in an approximately 25% reduction in threshold. Electrolyte abnormalities and acid–base disorders can also alter the pacemaker stimulus required for impulse initiation.[1] In the same study,[1] an i.v. solution of potassium and insulin in glucose caused a significant rise of threshold in four patients with permanent pacemakers.

Effect of Antiarrhythmic Agents on Pacemaker Function

Antiarrhythmic agents can interfere with the ability of electrical devices to effectively depolarize the myocardial tissue. Although the exact mechanism remains unclear, this interference may simply be an extension of the therapeutic effects of these agents on cardiac conduction. Antiarrhythmic drugs probably do not affect the pacemaker per se but rather the conduction characteristics of the heart, influencing device function. Antiarrhythmic agents may increase refractoriness, decrease conduction velocity, and increase the excitability threshold by reducing membrane potential and depressing membrane responsiveness.[3] These actions could be expected to alter the ability of an external electrical impulse to initiate myocardial depolarization and contraction.

Antiarrhythmic agents may also interfere with the ability of a pacemaker to sense the patient's native rhythm, although this appears to be considerably less common than the failure to capture caused by these agents. Failure to sense when the pacemaker is set in the inhibitory mode would manifest as pacemaker-induced stimuli that occur despite the presence of the normal atrial or ventricular depolarizations. We could find only two reports of failure to sense attributed to antiarrhythmic drug therapy; in both reports, this interference occurred in the presence of relatively high serum procainamide concentrations (17 and 36 mg/L).[3,4]

Type IA Agents. Most of the literature regarding interactions between type IA antiarrhythmic agents and pacemakers consists of small studies and case reports. In one of the first studies on this topic, Preston and colleagues[1] evaluated two antiarrhythmic agents in addition to physiological activities and electrolyte alterations in patients with permanently implanted ventricular pacemakers. In three patients, digoxin 0.8 mg i.v. did not produce a significant percentage change in energy threshold. Procainamide hydrochloride 800 mg i.v. was tested in an additional three patients. Two did not experience significant alterations in threshold; however, the third had a 37% rise in threshold, which occurred two hours after administration.

Several other case reports address the effect of procainamide on pacemaker threshold. In one such report,[4] a 67-year-old man with a ventricular aneurysm received a permanent pacemaker (set at a rate of 90 beats/min) to prevent drug-refractory, recurrent ventricular tachycardia (VT). This mode of therapy proved unsuccessful and procainamide hydrochloride 750 mg p.o. every three hours was initiated. Renal function deteriorated, and the serum procainamide concentration was measured at 36 mg/L. The pacemaker latency (time between pacemaker stimulation of the myocardium and initiation of an impulse) increased and progressed until the pacemaker no longer captured. Once the serum procainamide concentration decreased to 0.3 mg/L, the ECG returned to the pretoxic pattern without an extended pacemaker latency. In another case, Moss and Goldstein[5] documented 2:1 pacemaker capture, which eventually led to complete failure to capture, in a patient being managed with intramuscular procainamide for multiformed ventricular ectopy. Normal pacemaker capture was reestablished once the current was increased from 2.8 mA to 5 mA.

Type IB Agents. Mohan et al.[6] studied the effects of lidocaine hydrochloride 2 mg/kg i.v. and mexiletine hydrochloride 5 mg/kg i.v. in a small number of patients who were being temporarily paced for a variety of conduction disorders. Both agents caused a significant increase in pacing threshold. Two instances of failure to capture occurred in elderly patients who had temporary transvenous pacemakers and required i.v. lidocaine therapy for management of VT. During lidocaine treatment, VT occurred and was unresponsive to overdrive suppression (directed through the pacemaker) because of loss of capture; direct cardioversion was needed to terminate the VT.[5]

Type IC Agents. The IC antiarrhythmic agents flecainide, encainide, and propafenone appear to have pronounced effects on pacemaker threshold. Walker et al.[7] reported failure to capture in an elderly woman with a permanent pacemaker programmed in the VVI mode. Four days after the initiation of therapy with flecainide acetate 200 mg p.o. twice daily, a maximum increase in pulse width (2.29 msec) and a voltage increase of approximately 12-fold (0.4 V to 5.0 V) was required to regain capture. Once flecainide was withdrawn, the voltage requirement fell over 24 hours to 1.2 V.

Hellestrand et al.[8] studied the immediate and long-term influence of flecainide on pacemaker threshold in 28 patients. The sample was composed of three subgroups, all of whom were receiving ventricular pacing: group 1 consisted of patients with a temporary pacemaker, group 2 consisted of patients with permanent leads of various types who were undergoing pacemaker generator changes, and group 3 consisted of patients with permanent multiprogrammable pacemakers in place for at least three months. The permanent leads in group 3 were all of uniform brand and model. The pacing threshold of the pacemakers used in groups 1 and 2 was determined by measuring pulse amplitude at the predetermined pulse widths of 0.5 msec and 1.0 msec. In group 3, pacing threshold was evaluated by measuring pulse width at the predetermined pulse amplitudes of 2.7 V and 4.9 V. All patients received 2 mg/kg of flecainide acetate i.v. over 10 minutes. Pacing thresholds were determined at five-minute intervals for 15 minutes starting at the point of flecainide administration. In group 1, the mean pulse amplitude increases were 0.78 and 0.59 V at pulse widths of 0.5 and 1.0 msec, respectively. The mean rise in pulse amplitude in group 2 at pulse widths of 0.5 and 1.0 msec were 0.54 and 0.43 V, respectively. In group 3, the mean increases in pulse width at pulse amplitudes of 2.7 and 4.9 V were 0.08 and 0.05 msec, respectively. All increases were statistically significant.

Five patients within group 3 participated in a three-week oral phase. Oral flecainide acetate was used in increasing weekly dosages (100, 200, then 400 mg/day), and pacing thresholds were determined at the end of each week. At the conclusion of the third week, the mean pacing threshold values increased from control values of 0.09 msec at 2.7 V and 0.06 msec at 4.9 V to 0.28 msec at 2.7 V and 0.16 msec at 4.9 V. These increases were statistically significant. The results of the oral phase suggest that the effects of flecainide on the pacing threshold may be dose-related. All serum flecainide concentrations determined during this phase were within the effective range.

Another study evaluated the influence of encainide on pacemaker threshold in 10 patients with permanent programmable pacemakers.[9] Increasing dosages of oral encainide hydrochloride (25 mg t.i.d., 50 mg t.i.d., and 75 mg t.i.d.) were administered during serial one-week periods. Single-blind placebo periods of one week preceded and followed treatment with encainide. Pacing thresholds were determined at the end of the first and last (exit) placebo periods and at the end of each encainide phase. Ambulatory 24-hour ECGs were used to detect failure to capture. Increasing doses of encainide produced statistically significant increases in median energy required for capture. The median energy thresholds were 5.3, 6.1, 6.9, 9.3, and 5.5 μJ for the initial placebo, 25 mg t.i.d., 50 mg t.i.d., 75 mg t.i.d., and exit placebo periods, respectively. Values returned to baseline at the conclusion of the study after drug washout. No symptomatic failure to capture occurred at any dosage. However, ECG recordings demonstrated an asymptomatic episode of failure to capture, three seconds in duration, in 1 of the 10 patients. Curiously, this patient experienced only small changes in energy requirement attributable to encainide during the weekly pacing threshold evaluations.

The effect of the remaining approved IC antiarrhythmic, propafenone, has been addressed in a case report.[10] A 58-year-old woman with tachycardia–bradycardia syndrome received a permanent multiprogrammable atrial pacemaker. Treatment with propafenone hydrochloride 150 mg p.o. three times daily was initiated for the prevention of new episodes of paroxysmal atrial fibrillation. Seven days later, the patient complained of fatigue and a slow pulse. A 12-lead ECG showed complete loss of atrial capture, resulting from a propafenone-related rise in pacing threshold. Complete 1:1 capture was regained after the pulse width was doubled from 0.5 msec to 1.0 msec.

Type III Agents. Few studies are available that evaluate the effects of type III antiarrhythmic agents on pacemaker function. One study, which evaluated the effects of long-term amiodarone therapy on pacing threshold both at the point of and one month after pacemaker implantation, showed no significant difference between amiodarone and control groups.[11] This lack of effect on pacing threshold was independent of the length of amiodarone treatment. Changes attributable to amiodarone in each patient cannot be determined from the report. Another study found that i.v. (total dose, 1.5 mg/kg) and oral (160 mg/day and 320 mg/day) sotalol hydrochloride did not significantly alter pacing thresholds of permanently implanted pacemakers.[12] Although more data are required, type III agents do not appear to alter pacing thresholds to the same degree as type I drugs.

Electrical versus Clinical Effects. There appears to be a poor correlation between the magnitude of observed changes in pacemaker function (e.g., pulse width, pulse amplitude, and latency) and clinical failure to capture. Relatively small antiarrhythmic-induced changes in pacemaker function may be associated with failure to capture, and large changes in pacemaker function may be associated with continued reliable pacemaker operation and a lack of significant clinical consequences.

As previously described in one study,[9] the only patient who experienced clinical failure to capture had minimal changes in pacemaker threshold after encainide treatment. The remaining patients, who had larger percentage changes in threshold, did not experience adverse clinical events (i.e., failure to capture). This observation can probably be attributed to the baseline settings of the pacemaker before antiarrhythmic drug therapy. If the pacemaker settings are programmed at levels far greater than the initial threshold to provide a large "margin of safety," relatively major drug-induced alterations are less likely to result in failure to capture. However, if the margin of safety is small, minor increases in threshold attributable to the drug may cause adverse clinical events.

Analysis of Case 1

In the case reported here, failure to capture of a permanent pacemaker was initially attributed to therapy with flecainide. Substantial alterations in both the voltage requirement and the pulse width were necessary to regain effectiveness of the pacemaker. We initially believed that flecainide caused this adverse effect because of the temporal relationship between initiation of treatment with this agent and the documented failure to capture and because of the exclusion of other potential factors (i.e., electrolyte disturbances, change in clinical status [besides rhythm abnormalities] or in lead placement). We suspected that the predischarge Holter monitor recording showing normal pacemaker function was performed before flecainide concentrations had reached steady state. Therefore, the full effects of this agent on the function of the pacemaker were believed not to have been evaluated.

Continued follow-up of the pacemaker's function has revealed a return to very low pacing thresholds (3.3 V at 0.5 msec) despite continued treatment with flecainide. The early increase in pacing threshold was most likely a marked exaggeration of the usual response that occurs after pacemaker implantation. It is unclear whether flecainide played a role in the marked increase in threshold, but it is clear that the drug was not responsible for an adverse long-term interaction.

Case Report 2

A 64-year-old man had a history of aborted sudden cardiac death (from ventricular tachyarrhythmias) and a remote myocardial infarction. His treatment course had included amiodarone followed by mexiletine; however, the drugs were discontinued because of pulmonary toxicity and ineffectiveness in arrhythmia suppression, respectively. The patient underwent implantation of an AICD, at which time a 15-joule (J) AICD discharge was required to terminate induced ventricular fibrillation (VF). Three years later, the AICD was replaced (with a unit with pacing capabilities) electively because of battery depletion (no changes were made in the pacing or defibrillation leads). With the newly implanted unit, the energy required for VF termination was approximately 16 J. The pacing threshold was 1 V (pulse amplitude) at 1 msec (pulse width). At two follow-up clinic visits (two weeks and six months after implantation), the energy required for VF termination remained below 16 J, and the pacing threshold was 2 V at 1 msec. However, seven months after implantation, the patient had a series of discharges from his AICD secondary to VT. Given his previous antiarrhythmic drug failures and the presence of extremely poor left ventricular systolic function, therapy with moricizine hydrochloride was initiated at 200 mg p.o. three times daily in an attempt to prevent frequent AICD discharges. After three days of therapy, it was noted that a 16-J shock was, for the first time, unsuccessful in terminating VF; a 28-J shock was required. In addition, the pacing threshold had risen to 4 V at 1 msec. Repeat testing in the absence of moricizine was impossible because the patient developed intractable VT and died during an exercise stress test immediately after his electrophysiologic study.

AICD Function

The AICD can terminate serious ventricular arrhythmias by automatic synchronized cardioversion and defibrillation. Newer-generation AICDs also may be programmed to terminate tachyarrhythmias by overdrive pacing and have back-up pacing abilities for bradyarrhythmias. Patients often receive an AICD if they experience one or more episodes of life-threatening ventricular arrhythmias and if their arrhythmias have not been controlled by one or more standard or investigational antiarrhythmic drugs. Defibrillation is accomplished by a series of shocks delivered through two patches that are sewn onto the myocardium or by a transvenous coil and a patch. The shocks are initiated by a generator implanted into the abdomen. One model of AICD is currently approved for use in the United States.[13] Its initial shock can be programmed between 0.1 and 30 J, followed by a second shock set between 12 and 30 J. Subsequent shocks (up to a total of six) are usually fixed at 30 J.

A successful defibrillation occurs when there is a relatively instantaneous depolarization of a critical mass of nonrefractory myocardial tissue, after which a stable rhythm resumes. One might assume that the minimal energy required for effective defibrillation can be easily measured and quantified as a "defibrillation threshold." However, this concept has been challenged, primarily because the term falsely implies a critical cutoff point between effective and ineffective shocks. Davy et al.[14] have introduced the concept of a defibrillation curve, which relates the delivered energy to the percentage of successful defibrillations. This curve incorporates the concept that high-energy failure or low-energy success may randomly occur. Defibrillation can be described statistically, with higher energies having greater probability of success and lower energies a lesser probability of success. Published studies and cases usually report single values for defibrillation threshold, which are generally measured as the minimum value that successfully defibrillates on at least three successive occasions.

Effect of Antiarrhythmic Agents on AICD Function

Antiarrhythmic agents may alter the energy required for an AICD to effectively defibrillate the myocardium. The mechanism of this effect has been explained by the influence of antiarrhythmic agents on transmembrane sodium and potassium currents.[15] In theory, drugs that increase potassium or decrease sodium conductances of the membrane will widen the zone between resting membrane and threshold potentials, thus increasing the energy required for defibrillation. Exact mechanisms require further study.

Available reports of this drug–device interaction consist predominantly of animal data and a few reports in humans.[16-32] In one case, a 64-year-old man received an AICD for recurrent sustained VT.[16] At the time of implantation, the energy required for successful defibrillation was determined to be 10–15 J. Mexiletine hydrochloride 100 mg p.o. four times daily was administered for the management of ventricular ectopy. Induced VF could not be terminated with shocks of 20 and 25 J, and a 40-J "rescue shock" was required to terminate the arrhythmia. Three weeks after the discontinuation of mexiletine, induced VF and VT were terminated with a 20-J and a 15-J shock, respectively. Another example occurred in a 56-year-old man who underwent AICD implantation while concurrently receiving amiodarone for the management of recurrent VT.[17] During implantation, unsuccessful defibrillation of the induced (by invasive programmed stimulation) ventricular flutter by means of the AICD was documented at 40 J. Three months after amiodarone therapy was discontinued, induced ventricular flutter and VF were terminated easily with a single 25-J shock. Guarnieri et al.[18] evaluated the change in defibrillation thresholds over time (at initial implantation and at the time of generator replacement [mean, 24 months]) and identified a substantial increase in threshold in the patients concurrently receiving amiodarone (mean increase, approximately 10 J). No correlation existed between total amiodarone dose (mean cumulative dose, 295.6 g) and defibrillation threshold. These results are consistent with those of Troup et al.,[19] who also found an association between amiodarone therapy and higher defibrillation thresholds.

Antiarrhythmic drugs are commonly given in combination with an AICD. Often, the addition of an antiarrhythmic drug will decrease the number of tachycardia episodes, thus decreasing the number of shocks to the patient (which saves discomfort and battery life). Antiarrhythmic agents may also abolish episodes of self-terminating VT that might otherwise (particularly with older devices) elicit unneeded shocks. The frequency of concurrent drug and device therapy varies; according to a recent report, 71% (40/56) of patients with AICDs were concurrently receiving antiarrhythmic drugs.[20] In this report, 16% (9/56) received type I antiarrhythmic drugs and 55% (31/56) received amiodarone.

Antiarrhythmic agents may also interfere with the ability of the AICD to disregard supraventricular tachyarrhythmias. Antiarrhythmic agents may widen the QRS complex of impulses of supraventricular origin and thus make it difficult for the AICD to discriminate between supraventricular and ventricular arrhythmias.[21] For example, a relatively benign supraventricular tachyarrhythmia, which would ordinarily produce narrow QRS complexes, might appear to the AICD to be a (dangerous) ventricular tachyarrhythmia if an antiarrhythmic has widened the QRS complex. The AICD might then attempt in vain to terminate the wide-complex supraventricular arrhythmia by delivering shocks to the ventricle.

The majority of the literature addressing AICD–antiarrhythmic drug interactions appears as studies in animals. The protocols and the methods of defibrillation measurements differ among the studies. Table 1 summarizes the influence of antiarrhythmic agents on the energy required for successful defibrillation.

Table 1.
Effect of Antiarrhythmic Agents on Energy Required for Successful Defibrillation

Drug	Effect
Animal Studies	
Quinidine	Increase[24] or no change[22,32]
Procainamide	No change[23,31]
Lidocaine	Increase[24,28]
Encainide	Increase[25]
O-demethylencainide	Increase[25]
3-Methoxy-*O*-demethylencainide	No change[25]
Flecainide	Increase[27] or no change[29]
Amiodarone	Decrease[26] or no change[26,30]
d-Sotalol	Decrease[22]
Digoxin	No change[23]
Case Reports in Humans	
Mexiletine	Increase[16]
Amiodarone	Increase[17,30]

Analysis of Case 2

This case suggests that moricizine increased both the defibrillation and pacing threshold in the same patient. To our knowledge, this is the first report of moricizine's effect on defibrillation threshold.

Discussion

The cases and literature reported here show how the addition of antiarrhythmic agents may alter the function of an implantable device and cause clinically significant and detrimental consequences. Many clinicians are accustomed to screening and detecting drug–drug and drug–nutrient interactions but may overlook drug–device interactions. The concurrent use of antiarrhythmic agents and implantable electrical devices is often desirable for management of arrhythmias. Thus, the potential for an adverse interaction between the antiarrhythmic drugs and the devices should be considered.

Our interpretation of the literature and our experience lead us to the following recommendations. Once baseline variables are recorded for an implanted pacemaker or AICD, the patient should have a 24-hour Holter monitor recording and assessment of thresholds after concentrations of the antiarrhythmic agent (and active metab ɛs) are thought to have reached steady state. Adjustments to the device should be based on these results. Because of amiodarone's delayed onset of action, threshold evaluation should occur three to four weeks after initiation of treatment.

Conclusion

Antiarrhythmic agents can interfere with artificial cardiac pacemakers by increasing the pacing threshold and, rarely, by decreasing the devices' ability to sense native depolarizations. These drugs can also influence the function of AICDs, most commonly by increasing the defibrillation threshold.

Discussion Questions

1. Name the pacemaker variables that are most commonly used to determine pacing threshold.
2. Describe the mechanism by which antiarrhythmic agents may interfere with pacemaker function.
3. List four antiarrhythmic agents reported to affect pacemaker function in humans.
4. Explain why the magnitude of antiarrhythmic-induced alterations in pacemaker function is not closely related to the frequency of meaningful clinical events.
5. Name two antiarrhythmic agents reported to affect the defibrillation threshold in humans.

References

1. Preston TA, Fletcher RD, Lucchesi BR et al. Changes in myocardial threshold: physiologic and pharmacologic factors in patients with implanted pacemakers. *Am Heart J.* 1967; 74:235-42.
2. Moses HW, Taylor GJ, Schneider JA et al. A practical guide to cardiac pacing. 2nd ed. Boston, MA: Little, Brown, and Company; 1987:43-57.
3. Dohrmann ML, Goldschlager NF. Myocardial stimulation threshold in patients with cardiac pacemakers: effect of physiologic variables, pharmacologic agents, and lead electrodes. *Clin Cardiol.* 1985; 3:527-37.
4. Gay J, Brown DF. Pacemaker failure due to procainamide toxicity. *Am J Cardiol.* 1974; 34:728-32.
5. Moss AJ, Goldstein S. Clinical and pharmacological factors associated with pacemaker latency and incomplete pacemaker capture. *Br Heart J.* 1969; 31:112-7.
6. Mohan JC, Kaul U, Bhatia ML. Acute effects of antiarrhythmic drugs on cardiac pacing threshold. *Acta Cardiol.* 1984; 39:191-201.
7. Walker PR, Papouchado M, James MA et al. Pacing failure due to flecainide acetate. *PACE.* 1985; 8:900-2.
8. Hellestrand KJ, Burnett PJ, Milne JR et al. Effect of the antiarrhythmic agent flecainide acetate on acute and chronic pacing thresholds. *PACE.* 1983; 6:892-9.
9. Salel AF, Seagren SC, Pool PE. Effects of encainide on the function of implanted pacemakers. *PACE.* 1989; 12:439-44.
10. Montefoschi N, Boccadamo R. Propafenone induced acute variation of chronic atrial pacing threshold: a case report. *PACE.* 1990; 13:480-3.
11. Nielson AP, Griffin JC, Herre JM et al. Effect of amiodarone on acute and chronic pacing thresholds. *PACE.* 1984; 7:462. Abstract.
12. Creamer JE, Nathan AW, Shennan A et al. Acute and chronic effects of sotalol and propranolol on ventricular repolarization using constant-rate pacing. *Am J Cardiol.* 1986; 57:1092-6.
13. Winkle RA. State-of-the-art of the AICD. *PACE.* 1991; 14:961-6.
14. Davy JM, Fain ES, Dorian MD et al. The relationship between successful defibrillation threshold in open-chest dogs: reappraisal of the defibrillation threshold concept. *Am Heart J.* 1987; 113:77-84.
15. Babbs CF. Alteration of defibrillation threshold by antiarrhythmic drugs: a theoretical framework. *Crit Care Med.* 1981; 9:362-3.
16. Marinchak RA, Friehling TD, Kline RA et al. Effect of antiarrhythmic drugs on defibrillation threshold: case report of an adverse effect of mexiletine and review of the literature. *PACE.* 1988; 11:7-11.
17. Fogoros RN. Amiodarone-induced refractoriness to cardioversion. *Ann Intern Med.* 1984; 100:699-700.
18. Guarnieri T, Levin JH, Veltri EP et al. Success of chronic defibrillation and the role of antiarrhythmic drugs with the automatic implantable cardioverter/defibrillator. *Am J Cardiol.* 1987; 60:1061-4.
19. Troup PJ, Chapman PD, Olinger GN et al. The implanted defibrillator: relation of defibrillation lead configuration and clinical variables to defibrillation threshold. *J Am Coll Cardiol.* 1985; 6:1315-21.
20. Epstein A, Kay GN, Dailey S et al. Incidence of antiarrhythmic drug use in AICD patients with high defibrillation thresholds. *J Am Coll Cardiol.* 1991; 17(Suppl A):352A. Abstract.
21. Gottlieb CD, Horowitz LN. Potential interactions between antiarrhythmic medication and the automatic implantable cardioverter defibrillator. *PACE.* 1991; 14:898-904.
22. Dawson AK, Steinberg MI, Shapland JE. Effect of class I and class III drugs on current and energy required for internal defibrillation. *Circulation.* 1985; 72(Suppl 3):384. Abstract.
23. Deeb GM, Hardesty RL, Thompson ME et al. Pharmacologic and pathologic effects of an automatic implantable defibrillator. *Trans Am Soc Artif Intern Organs.* 1981; 27:1-6.
24. Babbs CF, Yim GKW, Whistler SJ et al. Elevation of ventricular defibrillation threshold in dogs by antiarrhythmic drugs. *Am Heart J.* 1979; 98:345-50.
25. Fain ES, Dorian P, Davy JM et al. Effects of encainide and its metabolites on energy requirements for defibrillation. *Circu-*

lation. 1986; 73:1334-41.
26. Fain ES, Lee JT, Winkle RA. Effects of acute intravenous and chronic oral amiodarone on defibrillation energy requirements. *Am Heart J*. 1987; 114:8-17.
27. Hernandez R, Mann DE, Breckinreidge S et al. Effects of flecainide on defibrillation thresholds in the anesthetized dog. *J Am Coll Cardiol*. 1989; 14:777-81.
28. Dorian P, Fain ES, Davy JM et al. Lidocaine causes a reversible, concentration-dependent increase in defibrillation energy requirements. *J Am Coll Cardiol*. 1986; 8:327-32.
29. Szabo TS, Jones DL, McQuinn RL et al. Flecainide acetate does not alter the energy requirements for direct ventricular defibrillation using sequential pulse defibrillation in pigs. *J Cardiovasc Pharmacol*. 1988; 12:377-83.
30. Frame LH, Hoffman N, Kolenik SA et al. Oral loading with amiodarone increases ventricular defibrillation threshold with implanted electrodes in dogs. *J Am Coll Cardiol*. 1986; 7(Suppl A):82A. Abstract.
31. Marchlinski FE, Flores B. Effect of procainamide on the defibrillation threshold in man. *Circulation*. 1988; 78(Suppl 2):154. Abstract.
32. Dorian P, Fain ES, Davy JM et al. Effect of quinidine and bretylium on defibrillation energy requirements. *Am Heart J*. 1986; 112:19-25.

Drug Experience

Straightforward reports of unusual drug experiences are included in this section. These may be confirmations of previously reported drug experiences or brief apparent first reports. While selected references may be cited, the purpose of a Drug Experience *report is not to present an extensive review of the literature.*

A related section, Grand Rounds, *includes papers that are well-documented patient case reports with a thorough review of the important literature to help put the case in perspective.*

Muscle spasms associated with intrathecal morphine therapy: Treatment with midazolam

ROBERT A. LITTRELL, L. DOUGLAS KENNEDY, WILLIAM E. BIRMINGHAM, AND W. DAVID LEAK

Clin Pharm. 1992; 11:57-9

The introduction of intraspinal narcotic analgesia in the late 1970s was an important advancement in the treatment of cancer pain.[1,2] Intraspinal narcotics, however, may cause serious adverse effects. We report severe muscle spasms associated with intrathecal morphine therapy and the successful use of midazolam to control this reaction.

Case Report. A 36-year-old white woman had metastatic adenosquamous cervical carcinoma diagnosed in April 1988. Treatment with radiation implants, external radiation, and chemotherapy (cisplatin and fluorouracil) was inadequate. The patient also underwent a postirradiation total abdominal hysterectomy, bilateral salpingo-oophorectomy, and periaortic lymph node dissection in August 1988.

Although adequate analgesia was initially provided with acetaminophen–codeine tablets, the patient later required morphine sulfate extended-release tablets, ibuprofen, and acetaminophen–oxycodone. The patient was readmitted in November 1989 for severe pain in her left hip, thigh, and knee; she had been taking morphine sulfate extended-release tablets 30 mg every 12 hours and 10 acetaminophen–oxycodone tablets per day. A continuous i.v. morphine sulfate infusion was initiated and adjusted to a rate of 10 mg/hr for complete pain relief. Conversion to oral morphine sulfate therapy was attempted but failed despite doses of 150 mg every eight hours. An indwelling central venous catheter was placed to allow home infusion of the i.v. morphine sulfate at a rate of 10 mg/hr. Amitriptyline hydrochloride 50 mg p.o. every night was added, and the dosage of ibuprofen was increased from 800 mg every eight hours to 800 mg p.o. four times a day. The patient reported satisfactory pain control with outpatient adjustment of the i.v. morphine sulfate infusion until January 1990, when she was admitted for severe pain uncontrolled by a 30-mg/hr i.v. morphine sulfate infusion.

An epidural lumbar catheter was placed, and epidural administration of morphine and bupivacaine provided adequate analgesia. A long-term tunneled epidural catheter was placed at the L3–L4 interspace and an 18-cm length of catheter was threaded. A patient-controlled analgesia device was used to deliver the morphine–bupivacaine combination, and the patient was discharged. Adjustments of epidural analgesics were made on an outpatient basis.

The patient returned to the hospital in March 1990 with a complaint of severe left patellar and pelvic pain while receiving epidural morphine sulfate 4.4 mg/hr and bupivacaine hydrochloride 10 mg/hr with as-needed doses of morphine sulfate 0.8 mg and bupivacaine hydrochloride 2.5 mg (10-minute lockout interval). Roentgenographic studies of the left femur revealed multiple low-density, irregular, and ill-defined areas in the patella, with an overall moth-eaten pattern. Pain in the left patella was successfully treated over seven days with local radiation. Fluoroscopic evaluation confirmed the integrity of the epidural catheter, and an epidurogram revealed poor spread of contrast agent. Insertion of a new epidural catheter failed because of fibrosis of the epidural space.

An intrathecal catheter was placed on day 5 and an

ROBERT A. LITTRELL, PHARM.D., is Assistant Clinical Professor, College of Pharmacy, University of Kentucky (UK), Lexington. L. DOUGLAS KENNEDY, M.D., is Medical Director, Central Pain Management and Rehabilitation Center, Central Baptist Hospital, Lexington; at the time of manuscript preparation, he was Assistant Professor, College of Medicine, UK. WILLIAM E. BIRMINGHAM, PHARM.D., is Pharmacy Resident, Thomas Jefferson University Hospital, Philadelphia, PA; at the time of manuscript preparation, he was a Pharm.D. student, College of Pharmacy, UK. W. DAVID LEAK, M.D., is Medical Director, Pain Control Consultants, Westerville, OH.

Address reprint requests to Dr. Littrell at the College of Pharmacy, University of Kentucky, 800 Rose Street, Lexington, KY 40536-0084.

infusion of morphine sulfate 0.1 mg/hr and bupivacaine hydrochloride 0.67 mg/hr was initiated. Bupivacaine was discontinued on day 9 because of numbness of the left leg. The intrathecal morphine sulfate infusion was adjusted to provide complete analgesia. The patient was oriented and alert and was discharged on April 7, receiving intrathecal morphine sulfate 1 mg/hr.

The patient was readmitted on April 19 with intractable pelvic pain and vaginal and rectal spasms. Spasms were initially treated with diazepam 5 mg p.o. every six hours plus diazepam 5 mg i.v. every four to six hours as needed for breakthrough spasms. However, the spasms were completely relieved only when suppositories containing belladonna extract 15 mg and opium 60 mg were given intravaginally every six hours. Bupivacaine was added to the intrathecal drug solution, and the dosage of intrathecal analgesics was adjusted. At the time of discharge from the hospital on May 4, the patient was receiving one belladonna–opium suppository intravaginally four times a day and morphine sulfate 2 mg/hr and bupivacaine 1.25 mg/hr intrathecally.

On May 9, the patient was admitted to the hospital for exacerbation of pelvic pain and recurrence of severe myoclonic vaginal and rectal spasms despite belladonna–opium suppositories given four times a day. Morphine sulfate 10 mg i.v. was administered once for severe pain, and a single 1500-mg oral dose of methocarbamol was given with no effect on the spasms. Baclofen 20 mg p.o. three times a day was begun and i.v. midazolam 22 mg (as the hydrochloride salt) was administered incrementally over one hour with reduction of spasm severity.

In addition, 15 mg of hyperbaric (specific gravity greater than specific gravity of cerebrospinal fluid) bupivacaine hydrochloride administered intrathecally in increments over 15 minutes produced a T10 sensory-level blockade (sensory blockade extending from a line drawn laterally across the umbilicus to a line drawn laterally across the knees). The bupivacaine provided near-complete pain relief. A midazolam infusion of 5 mg/hr i.v. (as the hydrochloride salt) plus a patient-controlled component of 2 mg (of midazolam) with six-minute lockout provided sedation and controlled the spasms.

The patient remained comfortable and moderately sedated, and on May 18, the basal midazolam infusion was discontinued. The same day, the patient had episodes of severe pelvic pain. Intrathecal boluses of morphine sulfate did not relieve the pain. Intrathecal sufentanil 50 μg (as the citrate salt) given over one hour was effective and sufentanil was added to the intrathecal infusion solution. Hyperbaric bupivacaine hydrochloride 15 mg was administered intrathecally in divided doses, and the intrathecal rate was adjusted to deliver morphine sulfate 3 mg/hr, sufentanil 4.5 μg/hr, and bupivacaine hydrochloride 1.9 mg/hr. Patient-controlled i.v. midazolam and occasional i.v. midazolam boluses controlled the spasms. By May 31, the patient required no as-needed midazolam doses. Patient-controlled midazolam was discontinued and replaced with oral diazepam as needed.

On the day before planned discharge, the patient had increased pelvic pain and recurrent spasms. Intermittent doses of i.v. midazolam 2–5 mg relieved the spasms. Patient-controlled i.v. midazolam therapy was resumed at a dose of 1 mg with a 15-minute lockout interval. The intrathecal infusion rate was adjusted to obtain satisfactory analgesia, and the patient was discharged from the hospital on June 5 on ibuprofen 800 mg p.o. three times a day, amitriptyline hydrochloride 50 mg p.o. every night, baclofen 15 mg p.o. three times a day, diazepam 5 mg p.o. every eight hours as needed, and intrathecal morphine sulfate, sufentanil, and bupivacaine at 2.8 mg, 4.2 μg, and 3.5 mg per hour, respectively. The pain and spasms were satisfactorily relieved with this regimen until the patient died three months later.

Discussion. Intraspinal narcotic analgesia has become a valuable therapeutic tool in the treatment of cancer pain. Its use has been associated with relatively few serious adverse effects. The most common (pruritus, nausea and vomiting, sedation, and urinary retention) are usually self-limiting or treatable and infrequently result in discontinuation of therapy. Respiratory depression is a potentially life-threatening adverse effect most commonly observed in the postoperative patient and is rare in the opiate-tolerant cancer patient.[3,4] Our patient experienced none of these adverse effects while receiving intrathecal morphine sulfate but did develop a degree of tolerance and severe muscle spasms. Because of potentially confounding factors and the absence of a dechallenge, we can only suggest a relationship between intrathecal morphine administration and occurrence of spasms in our patient.

Some degree of tolerance occurs in most patients receiving long-term therapy with intraspinal narcotics, but it may be more common in those receiving intrathecal versus epidural agents.[4-10] Our patient developed a significant tolerance, and the morphine sulfate dosage was increased from 2.4 mg/day to 67.2 mg/day (plus sufentanil 100.8 μg/day) over a period of three months.

The occurrence of myoclonic-like spasms of the lower extremities has been reported by Krames et al.[9] in two cancer patients receiving intrathecal morphine sulfate 37 mg/24 hr and 21.4 mg/24 hr. The authors speculated but were unable to confirm that intraspinal spread of the malignancy resulted in distal sequestration of morphine in the cerebrospinal fluid. Sequestration possibly produced toxic morphine concentrations and resulted in lower-extremity spasms. Both patients' spasms were well controlled with oral baclofen and disappeared when intrathecal morphine administration was discontinued.

We report an additional case of spasticity, possibly related to doses of intrathecal morphine sulfate of 24 mg/24 hr, that was treated with continuous infusion, patient-controlled midazolam, and oral baclofen. Midazolam was chosen because its short half-life allows for safe administration by continuous infusion. To our knowledge, this is the first reported use of midazolam for treatment of severe muscle spasms. Interestingly, intrathecal bupivacaine resulting in complete motor blockade of the lower extremities and T10 sensory level blockade did not relieve the muscle spasms.

Continuous-infusion midazolam has been reported to be effective in the treatment of status epilepticus.[11] Patient-controlled anxiolysis with midazolam has also been reported.[12] We chose to allow patient-controlled midazolam boluses because several spasms occurred despite a constant i.v. midazolam infusion. The patient successfully controlled these spasms by self-administration of 1-mg midazolam boluses. The patient was moderately sedated, at her request, while receiving the continuous infusion; she became more alert when the infusion was discontinued and only patient-controlled midazolam was provided. The patient tolerated the midazolam well, and no adverse effects were apparent.

Conclusion. Rectovaginal spasms occurred in a patient receiving intrathecal morphine and were successfully controlled with i.v. midazolam.

References

1. Yaksh TL, Rudy TA. Analgesia mediated by a direct spinal action of narcotics. *Science.* 1976; 192:1257-8.
2. Wang JK, Nauss LA, Viars P. Pain relief by intrathecally applied morphine in man. *Anesthesiology.* 1979; 50:149-51.
3. Cousins MJ, Mather LE. Intrathecal and epidural administration of opioids. *Anesthesiology.* 1984; 61:276-310.
4. Ventafridda V, Spoldi E, Caraceni A et al. Intraspinal morphine for cancer pain. *Acta Anaesthesiol Scand Suppl.* 1987; 85:47-53.
5. Coombs DW, Maurer LH, Saungers RL et al. Outcomes and complications of continuous intraspinal narcotic analgesia for cancer pain control. *J Clin Oncol.* 1984; 2:1414-20.
6. Penn RD, Paice JA. Chronic intrathecal morphine for intractable pain. *J Neurosurg.* 1987; 67:182-6.
7. Greenberg HS, Taren J, Ensminger WD et al. Benefit from and tolerance to continuous intrathecal infusion of morphine for intractable cancer pain. *J Neurosurg.* 1982; 57:360-4.
8. Ali NMK, Hanna N, Hoffman JS. Percutaneous epidural catheterization for intractable pain in terminal cancer patients. *Gynecol Oncol.* 1989; 32:22-5.
9. Krames ES, Gershow J, Glassberg A et al. Continuous infusion of spinally administered narcotics for the relief of pain due to malignant disorders. *Cancer.* 1985; 56:696-702.
10. Ali NMK, Hoffman JS. Tolerance during long-term administration of intrathecal morphine. *Conn Med.* 1989; 53:266-8.
11. Crisp CB, Gannon R, Knauft F. Continuous infusion of midazolam hydrochloride to control status epilepticus. *Clin Pharm.* 1988; 7:322-4.
12. Loper KA, Ready LB. Patient controlled anxiolysis with midazolam. *Crit Care Med.* 1989; 17:200-1.

ASHP Reports

Procedure for submission of manuscripts to journals published by the American Society of Hospital Pharmacists

—Detach or copy these pages and mail with manuscript—

To expedite manuscript review, the American Society of Hospital Pharmacists requires that a copy of this form be completed and enclosed with each paper submitted for publication to the *American Journal of Hospital Pharmacy* (*AJHP*) or *Clinical Pharmacy*. Authors thereby certify that their papers comply with the major stylistic requirements of ASHP's journals, which are generally in conformance with the Uniform Requirements for Manuscripts Submitted to Biomedical Journals (*Ann Intern Med.* 1988; 108:258-65 and *Br Med J.* 1988; 296:401-5). ASHP exceptions to the Uniform Requirements are noted with an asterisk (*). Authors must comply with and check each point on the list (or mark "NA" for not applicable). If a manuscript is received without a completed form, the editor will mail a blank form to the author and will not process the paper until the form has been completed. *The procedure applies to all manuscripts except letters, book reviews, therapy consultations, management consultations, and similar column material. (For letters to the editor, see the instructions on the first page of the Letters column in most issues.)*

Authors are requested to include with each manuscript a letter of transmittal, the minimum content of which is noted in the checklist below. Authors are encouraged to suggest appropriate reviewers for a manuscript. For exceptionally important work, the editors will consider requests by the authors for expedited ("fast track") review.

Unsolicited manuscripts are acknowledged within one week of their receipt with a letter from the editors. The letter includes a code number that should be cited in all communications regarding the manuscript.

Manuscripts should be submitted to the editor of the appropriate journal at the following address: 4630 Montgomery Avenue, Bethesda, MD 20814.

Letter of Transmittal

_____Summarizes in no more than two sentences the nature of the manuscript.
_____Includes information on prior or duplicate publication or submission elsewhere of any part of the work.
_____Includes a statement of financial or other relationships (e.g., stock ownership, advisory board, speaker's bureau, honoraria) that might lead to a conflict of interests.

General

The corresponding author for this manuscript is

____

The preferred mailing address for the corresponding author is (please include a complete street address in case it is necessary for us to use overnight mail)

____

____

____

____

The corresponding author can be reached during business hours at the following telephone and fax numbers:

____

_____Eight complete copies (including photostatic copies of all figures) of the manuscript are submitted. One set of camera-ready figures is submitted. The authors understand that the editors are not obligated to return any of this material.
_____Manuscript is typed double-spaced *throughout* (including tables, references, footnotes, figure captions, and author identification) on 21.6 x 27.9-cm white paper with margins of at least 2.5 cm all around.
_____Manuscript is not typed using all upper-case letters.
_____All pages are numbered consecutively (in the upper right-hand corner), beginning with the title page and including tables.
_____Each of the following elements begins on a separate page, in this sequence: title page, author identification page, abstract, text, footnotes, references, tables, figure captions, and figures.*
_____Abbreviations are in accordance with the *CBE Style Manual*, 5th ed. (pages 241-68). No drug or chemical names are abbreviated.
_____Pharmacokinetic abbreviations agree with those given in the following article: Rowland M, Tucker G. Symbols in pharmacokinetics. *J Pharmacokinet Biopharm.* 1980; 8:497-507.
_____If the manuscript reports the results of a survey, three copies of the survey instrument should be sent for use in the review process (not for publication).
_____Manuscript is accompanied by copies of any permission to reproduce published material, to use illustrations of identifiable persons, or to name persons for their contributions.
_____A copy of any *closely related* manuscript that may aid in the review of the submitted paper (e.g., another paper that reports a separate portion of a study submitted to ASHP) is included.

Title Page

_____Contains concise, informative title and no other information.

Author Identification Page

_____Lists as authors only those individuals who have participated sufficiently in the work to take public responsibility for the content. (Participation solely in the collection of data does not justify authorship. See *Clin Pharm.* 1986; 5:33 for elaboration.)
_____Lists the authors near the top of the page, giving first name, middle initial, and last name of each.
_____Identifies each author in the format used in the author identification section of papers published in *AJHP* and *Clinical Pharmacy*, giving highest academic degree, position, department, and institution.
_____Denotes address for reprint requests.
_____Identifies in one or more paragraphs, as appropriate, (a) contributions that need acknowledging but do not justify authorship, (b) acknowledgments of technical help, (c) acknowledgments of material and financial support (including grant numbers), and (d) financial relationships that may constitute a conflict of interest.
_____If the paper was presented in whole or in part at a meeting, includes name of meeting, location, and date paper was presented.

Abstract (not required for Letters, Notes, Research Notes, Drug Experience, Commentaries, or Reflections)

_____Is less than 150 words.
_____For research reports, concisely states objectives, methods (procedures), main results (including specific data and their statistical significance, if possible), and principal conclusions.
_____For *AJHP* descriptive reports, concisely states purposes of program, how the program works, and conclusions.
_____For review articles and primers, concisely identifies main topics covered in the review, summary of major points, and conclusion.

Text

_____When reporting experiments on humans, indicates whether the procedures followed were in accord with the ethical standards of the institution's committee on human experimentation or in accord with the Helsinki Declaration of 1975.
_____Names of authors, institutions, or patients are not mentioned, except in descriptive reports where institution identification is essential to understanding the program.
_____For Drug Experience papers, patient's age, gender, race, weight, pertinent past medical history, and baseline laboratory values are included, as well as the generic names, manufacturers, trade names, formulations, and routes of administration of all drug products used.
_____Descriptive headings are used to identify major sections of the paper; subheadings also may be used.

_____For stability studies, complies with guidelines for such studies (see *Am J Hosp Pharm.* 1983; 40:1159-60 and *Am J Hosp Pharm.* 1988; 45:1569-71), including documentation that the assay used is stability indicating.
_____Identifies in the Methods section all statistical tests used and the a priori level of significance; unusual or complex statistical methods are explained briefly or referenced.
_____If more than one statistical test is used, the data evaluated by each test are clearly identified in the Methods section.
_____Mean values for study results are accompanied by some measure of variability or precision (e.g., standard deviations); the use of confidence intervals, when appropriate, is encouraged.
_____Identifies precisely all drugs and chemicals used by generic name (with salt, if applicable). Trade names are used only to identify that a specific brand of drug was used. For reports of clinical research, identification of drugs as being racemic mixtures of single isomers is encouraged.
_____Measurements are reported in the units in which they were made.
_____Volume, distance, and weight measurements should be expressed in metric units.*
_____For commercial products important to the paper, denotes, in parentheses, the trade name or model number; the manufacturer's name, city, state, and zip code; and the lot number. If such designations are numerous, they are listed as footnotes at the end of the text.
_____Every reference, figure, table, and appendix is cited in the text in numerical order. (Order of mention in text determines the number given to each.)
_____Footnotes are identified consecutively in the text by superscript, lower-case letters.*

References

_____Are identified in text, tables, and legends by superscript* Arabic numbers.
_____Are typed double-spaced on sheets separate from the text and numbered consecutively as they appear in the text. References that appear in tables should receive consecutive numbers based on the placement of the table in the text.
_____Do not include any "unpublished observations" and "personal communications." (References to written, not oral, communications may be inserted, in parentheses, in the text or included as footnotes.)
_____Have been verified by the author(s) against the original documents.
_____Abbreviations of journal titles conform to those used in *Index Medicus* (January issue).
_____Include inclusive page numbers.
_____Are in the style adopted by the U.S. National Library of Medicine and used in *Index Medicus* with the exception that only the first three authors (last name and two initials, if available) are ever listed. Examples of this style follow:

(a) Standard journal article—(list all authors when three or less; when four or more, list only first three and add et al.*):
1. Roberts LW, O'Donnell J, Matsuda T et al. Pharmacy-assisted burn unit skin bank program. Am J Hosp Pharm. 1977; 34:1353-4.

(b) Article from journal paginated by issue:
2. Goldschmidt L. Remodeling on a shoe-string improves pharmacy's efficiency. Hospitals. 1979; 53(May 1):115-6.

(c) Letter, editorial, or abstract:
3. Wightkin WT, Buckhammer CR. Simple method for intravenous-to-oral theophylline dose conversion. Clin Pharm. 1982; 1:300-1. Letter.
4. Zellmer, WA. Prescribing pharmacists. Am J Hosp Pharm. 1982; 39:1481. Editorial.
5. Bartle WR, Walker SE, Shapero T. Effect of cimetidine on phenytoin metabolism. Clin Pharmacol Ther. 1982; 31:202. Abstract.

(d) Book—personal author(s):
6. Osler AG. Complement: mechanisms and functions. Englewood Cliffs, NJ: Prentice-Hall; 1976.

(e) Chapter or article in a book:
7. Weinstein L, Swartz MN. Pathogenic properties of invading microorganisms. In: Sodeman WA Jr, Sodeman WA, eds. Pathologic physiology: mechanisms of disease. Philadelphia: Saunders; 1974:457-72.

(f) Editor, compiler, or chairman as author of book:
8. Wertheimer AI, Smith MC, eds. Pharmacy practice: social and behavioral aspects. 7th ed. Baltimore: University Park Press; 1981.

(g) Governmental agency publication:
9. National Center for Health Statistics. Acute conditions: incidence and associated disability, United States July 1968–June 1969. Rockville, MD: National Center for Health Statistics, 1972; DHEW publication no. (HSM) 72-1036. (Vital and health statistics; series 10: Data from the National Health Survey; no. 69.)

(h) Package insert:
10. Roche Laboratories. Accutane package insert. Nutley, NJ: 1982 May.

(i) Paper presented at a meeting:
11. Stern NB, Millburg WJ, Steckel SD. Managing proper disposal of antineoplastic agents. Paper presented at 17th Annual ASHP Midyear Clinical Meeting. Los Angeles, CA: 1982 Dec 7.

Tables

_____Are typed double-spaced, each (complete with title and footnotes) on a separate page (not submitted as photographs).
_____Are submitted in the original typed size, not photo-reduced.
_____Do not contain information duplicated in the text or figures.
_____Are in the style used in ASHP's journals.
_____Do not contain horizontal or vertical rules within the tabulated information.
_____Use superscript letters for footnote designations.*
_____If use data from another published or unpublished source, permission is obtained from the source (proof submitted with paper) and the source is acknowledged.

Figure Captions

_____Are typed double-spaced on a sheet separate from the text.
_____Are numbered consecutively as they are cited in the text.
_____All abbreviations and symbols used in the figure are defined; when appropriate, the measure of variability or precision represented is identified (e.g., do error bands represent standard deviation(s) or a confidence interval?).

Figures

_____Are professionally drawn and photographed. (Freehand or typewritten lettering is unacceptable.) Computer-generated figures are acceptable only if produced on letter-quality printers.
_____Are submitted as sharp, glossy, black-and-white photographic prints, usually 12.7 x 17.3 cm but no larger than 20.3 x 25.4 cm.
_____Are designed such that, when reduced to one-column width (8 cm), are legible and occupy no more than 10 cm of column length.
_____Axis labels appear outside the axes.
_____Titles and detailed explanations (including keys to symbols used) are in the captions, not the illustrations themselves.
_____If previously published, the original source is acknowledged, and written permission from the copyright holder to reproduce the material is submitted.
_____Each photographic print has a label pasted on its back indicating the figure number and title of the paper. (Do not note authors' names.*
_____Do not write on the back.)
Copies of all figures are included with each copy of manuscript.

Copyright and Authorship

_____The following copyright transferal and authorship statements are submitted on a separate sheet identified with the title of the paper and signed and dated by each author.

In consideration of the American Society of Hospital Pharmacists (ASHP) taking action in reviewing and editing my (our) submission, the author(s) undersigned hereby transfer(s), assign(s), or otherwise convey(s) all ownership rights in the submission and all copyright ownership to ASHP. In the event that such work is not published by ASHP, all said rights shall be released.

_____I have participated sufficiently in the conception, design, data analysis (where applicable), and writing of this manuscript to take public responsibility for the content. I have read the final version of the paper and find it suitable for publication.

_____If this paper has been presented at a meeting other than one sponsored by ASHP, a copy of a release from the sponsors of that meeting, permitting publication elsewhere, is enclosed.

Exclusive Publication Statement

_____I certify that none of the material in this manuscript has been previously published and none of this material or substantially similar material is under consideration or has been accepted for publication elsewhere, except as described in the attachment. This includes journal articles, letters to the editor, symposia, editorials, proceedings, transactions, books, articles published by invitation, news reports, and preliminary publication of any kind except an abstract of 400 words or less.

____

(Signature of Corresponding Author) (Date)

If you have not complied with the item immediately above, please include an explanation in your letter of transmittal.

Instructions for submitting computer disks with revised manuscripts

—Detach or copy this page and mail with revised manuscript—

After your paper has been accepted for publication in *AJHP* or *Clinical Pharmacy* and revised as requested, follow these specifications for preparing a word processing disk of the manuscript. Tables and figures do not need to be put on the disk, but all other parts of the manuscript, including captions, should be. Disks will not be returned to authors.

When you copy your manuscript to disk make sure that all of it is in one document or file and that it is in a "straight text" format, with **no headers, footers, or special formatting instructions.** Footnotes should be listed in one group at the end of the document, along with the references.

The following word processing software formats can currently be accepted:

ASCII text
DCA-RFT and FFT*
Displaywrite 3 and 4
Enable (WP)
Freestyle
Leading Edge WP
Lotus Manuscript
Microsoft Word for the PC*
Multimate (up to version 3.3)
Multimate Advantage I and II
Navy DIF Standard
NBI
Officewriter (up to version 4.0)
Palantir
PC-Write (up to version 2.6)
PeachText 5000
pfs: Write, Professional Write, and First Choice
PMate
Spellbinder
Volkswriter
WordPerfect, versions 4.1–5.1*
WordMarc Composer
Wordstar*
Writing Assistant
XyWrite

**Indicates word processing formats preferred by* AJHP *and* CP

If you have an IBM compatible system, but your word processing program is not listed, save your manuscript in the ASCII or generic text file format (same as printing to a file).

3.5" or 5.25" low- and high-density floppy disks are all acceptable. However, **only IBM compatible disks** can be accepted.

If you need further assistance, call ASHP headquarters, 301-657-3000, and ask for Carol Cavanaugh, ext. 225, or Yvonne Yirka, ext. 256.

Be sure to label the disk with the following information:

1. Manuscript reference code number
2. Name of corresponding author
3. Word processing file format (e.g., WordPerfect 5.1)
4. Date the disk was sent

Please use an appropriate protective container to mail your disk, and be sure to **include two printed copies of your manuscript as it appears on the disk.** It is important for the printed copies to be identical to the mansucript that is on the disk.

Below, list the name, phone number, and office hours of a contact person who can give specific information about how the disk was produced.

Name: ______________________

Phone: (_____) ______________________ ext. ______

Office hours: ______________ Days: ______________

Time zone: ______________________

By signing below, I certify that the revised manuscript has been prepared according to these specifications.

____

(Signature of Corresponding Author) (Date)

DUE Criteria

The DUE Criteria *section of* Clinical Pharmacy *features model drug-use evaluation criteria that may be employed as a component of a comprehensive quality assurance program. The criteria sets are presented in the format used in the ASHP book* Criteria for Drug Use Evaluation. *Some of the criteria sets will have been originally published in that book; others will be presented here for the first time and published in future volumes of the ASHP book. The practitioners who developed a criteria set are acknowledged.*

In selecting drug products for coverage in DUE Criteria, *priority is given to products that have been recently marketed, those that are frequently prescribed, those that have high potential risk associated with their use, and those that are expensive. When feasible, a criteria set will be linked with a* Drug Review *that appears in the same issue.*

These criteria sets are a starting point for the development of DUE Criteria for a specific practice setting. Readers are encouraged to modify the model criteria to fit their own circumstances.

Criteria for use of zidovudine in adult and pediatric inpatients and outpatients[a]

Element	Standard 100%	Standard 0%	Exception[b] or Critical Preventive/Responsive Measure[c]	Sources of Information
Justification for Use				
1. Treatment of human immunodeficiency virus (HIV)-infected adult with evidence of impaired immunity (T4 helper/inducer lymphocyte count of <500 cells/cu mm) or AIDS[1-11]	X		1A. None	1. History and physical (H&P), laboratory reports, progress notes, physician orders, infectious diseases (ID) consultation report
or				
2. Treatment of HIV-infected pediatric patient (age 3 months–12 years) with[1,12-14] a. Symptomatic HIV infection, or b. Asymptomatic HIV infection and laboratory evidence of significant immunosuppression	X		2A. None	2. H&P, laboratory reports, progress notes, physician orders, ID consultation report
or				
3. Treatment of HIV-related thrombocytopenia[15,16]	X		3A. None	3. H&P, laboratory reports, progress notes, physician orders, ID consultation report, hematology consultation report
Critical (Process) Indicators				
4. No history of hypersensitivity to zidovudine	X		4A. None	4. H&P, allergy record
5. Zidovudine not used in pregnant or lactating woman[1]	X		5A. Zidovudine used when benefits outweigh risks	5,5A. H&P, laboratory reports, physician orders, progress notes, ID consultation report
6. Positive enzyme-linked immunosorbent assay for HIV antibody with confirmatory Western blot before initiation of zidovudine therapy[17]	X		6A. Antibody-positive infant (<15 months of age) born to HIV-infected mother must also have: a. Virus isolated from blood or body tissues, or b. Evidence of immune impairment plus symptomatic	6,6A. H&P, laboratory reports, progress notes, physician orders

Prepared by S. Diane Goodwin, Pharm.D., Assistant Professor, Division of Pharmacy Practice, School of Pharmacy, University of Colorado Health Sciences Center, Denver, CO, and Kenneth W. Shipp, Clinical Pharmacist, Division of Infectious Diseases, Department of Medicine, Duke University Medical Center, Durham, NC.

Element	Standard 100%	Standard 0%	Exception[b] or Critical Preventive/Responsive Measure[c]	Sources of Information
			disease, or c. Clinical findings that meet Centers for Disease Control (CDC) definition for pediatric AIDS[18]	
7. Baseline laboratory tests obtained within two weeks preceding initiation of zidovudine therapy: a. Complete blood count (CBC) with differential b. Platelet count c. Serum creatinine (SCr) d. Serum creatine kinase e. T4 helper/inducer lymphocyte count (average of two measurements taken at least 72 hours apart)	X		7A. None	7. Laboratory reports, physician orders, progress notes
8. Zidovudine administered intravenously to patient with nothing-by-mouth orders[1]	X		8A. None	8. Physician orders, progress notes, nursing notes, medication administration record (MAR)
9. Appropriate oral dosage in adult with symptomatic HIV infection or AIDS: 200 mg every four hours around the clock for one month, then 100 mg every four hours[1,4,9,10]	X		9A. Maintain dose of 200 mg every four hours in patient with HIV-related neurologic disease[8] 9B. ID consultation recommendation for alternative dosing regimen	9. H&P, progress notes, physician orders, MAR 9A. Neurology consultation report, physician orders 9B. ID consultation report, physician orders
10. Appropriate oral dosage in adult with asymptomatic HIV infection: 100 mg every four hours while awake (five times daily)[1,5]	X		10A. ID consultation recommendation for alternative dosing regimen	10. H&P, progress notes, physician orders, MAR 10A. ID consultation report, physician orders
11. Appropriate oral dosage for pediatric patient (age 3 months–2 years): 180 mg/sq m every six hours around the clock, not to exceed 200 mg per dose[1,14]	X		11A. ID consultation recommendation for alternative dosing regimen	11. H&P, progress notes, physician orders, MAR 11A. ID consultation report, physician orders
12. Patient or caregiver counseled about proper drug administration and importance of drug compliance and laboratory follow-up	X		12A. None	12. Progress notes, nursing notes
13. Appropriate intravenous dosage for adult: 1–2 mg/kg every four hours around the clock (as one-hour infusion)[1]	X		13A. ID consultation recommendation for alternative dosing regimen	13. H&P, progress notes, physician orders, MAR 13A. ID consultation report, physician orders
14. Zidovudine dosage decreased in patient receiving concomitant probenecid therapy[19-21]	X		14A. None	14. H&P, physician orders, progress notes, MAR
15. CBC with differential and platelet count monitored every two weeks for two months, then monthly	X		15A. Monitoring performed more often in patient with renal or hepatic dysfunction 15B. Monitoring performed more often (every two weeks) in patient with unstable blood counts or on other bone-marrow-suppressive drugs 15C. Monitoring performed quarterly (every three months) in patient with stable blood counts after one year of zidovudine therapy	15, 15A. Laboratory reports, progress notes, physician orders 15B, C. Laboratory reports, progress notes, physician orders, MAR
16. Serum chemistry (e.g., SCr) monitored every two weeks for one month, then quarterly	X		16A. Monitoring performed more often in patient with renal or hepatic dysfunction 16B. Monitoring performed more	16, 16A, B. Laboratory reports, progress notes, physician orders

Element	Standard 100%	Standard 0%	Exception[b] or Critical Preventive/Responsive Measure[c]		Sources of Information
			often in patient with unstable values		
17. Serum creatine kinase monitored quarterly after six months of zidovudine therapy[22]	X		17A. Monitoring performed more often in patient with signs and symptoms of myositis or myopathy	17. 17A.	Laboratory reports, progress notes, physician orders Electromyogram (EMG) reports, muscle biopsy reports, physician orders
18. T4 helper/inducer lymphocyte count measured every six months	X		18A. T4 helper/inducer lymphocyte count measured every three months when approaching 200/cu mm 18B. If T4 helper/inducer lymphocyte count falls rapidly while on zidovudine therapy, consider alternative antiretroviral therapy	18, 18A, B.	Laboratory reports, progress notes, physician orders
19. Concomitant ribavirin therapy avoided during zidovudine treatment[23]	X		19A. None	19.	Physician orders, MAR, progress notes
Complications					
20. Anaphylaxis (difficulty breathing, hypotension, cardiac arrest)		X	20A. Identify other drug and nondrug causes 20B. Discontinue zidovudine 20C. Provide symptomatic and supportive care (re-establish airway, cardiopulmonary resuscitation)	20. 20A–C.	Progress notes, nursing notes Progress notes, physician orders, nursing notes, MAR
21. Rash or other dermatologic manifestation[1,24,25]		X	21A. Identify other drug and nondrug causes 21B. Treat mild reaction symptomatically (antihistamine, anti-inflammatory agent) 21C. If reaction severe, discontinue zidovudine and initiate didanosine therapy or enroll eligible patients in expanded-access trials (e.g., dideoxycytidine)	21. 21A–C.	Progress notes, nursing notes Progress notes, physician orders, nursing notes, dermatology consultation reports, MAR
22. Miscellaneous adverse effects (headache, insomnia, nausea, vomiting, diarrhea)[1,4,5,10,12,14,16,24,25]		X	22A. Identify other drug and nondrug causes 22B. Treat mild reaction symptomatically; provide supportive care 22C. If reaction severe, discontinue zidovudine and initiate didanosine therapy or enroll eligible patient in expanded access trials	22. 22A–C.	Progress notes, nursing notes Progress notes, physician orders, nursing notes, MAR
23. Anemia[1,4,5,9,12-15,24]		X	23A. Identify other drug and nondrug causes 23B. Re-evaluate need for concomitant bone-marrow-suppressive drugs 23C. When hemoglobin <7.5 g/dL (or ≥25% lower than baseline), transfuse patient or administer epoetin (100 units/kg i.v. or s.c. three times weekly; only in patient with endogenous serum erythropoietin concentration of ≤500 mU/mL)[26] 23D. If hemoglobin <7.5 g/dL (or ≥25% below baseline) on second occasion despite use of blood transfusions or epoetin, temporarily discontinue zidovudine and	23. 23A–E.	Laboratory reports, progress notes Laboratory reports, progress notes, nursing notes, MAR, transfusion records, physician orders

Element	Standard 100%	Standard 0%	Exception[b] or Critical Preventive/Responsive Measure[c]	Sources of Information
			restart at one half the original dose[1]	
			23E. If 23C–23D not successful, discontinue zidovudine and initiate didanosine therapy	
24. Neutropenia[1,4,5,9,12-15,24]		X	24A. Identify other drug and nondrug causes 24B. Re-evaluate need for concomitant bone-marrow-suppressive drugs 24C. When absolute neutrophil count <750/cu mm (or ≥50% below baseline), temporarily discontinue zidovudine; if absolute neutrophil count <750/cu mm (or ≥50% below baseline) on second occasion, temporarily discontinue zidovudine and restart at one half original dose[1] 24D. Discontinue zidovudine if patient requires ganciclovir therapy[27,28] 24E. Consider use of colony-stimulating factors[29] 24F. If 24C–24E not successful, discontinue zidovudine therapy and initiate didanosine therapy or enroll patient in expanded-access trial	24. Laboratory reports, progress notes 24A–F. Progress notes, physician orders, nursing notes, MAR, laboratory reports
25. Nail or mucocutaneous discoloration[1,24,30-34]		X	25A. Identify other drug and nondrug causes 25B. Reassure patient	25. Progress notes, nursing notes 25A. Physician orders, progress notes, MAR, nursing notes 25B. Progress notes, nursing notes
26. Neurologic effects (seizures, encephalopathy)[1,4,22,24]		X	26A. Identify other drug and nondrug causes 26B. Provide symptomatic and supportive care 26C. Discontinue zidovudine therapy and consider other antiretroviral agents	26. Progress notes, nursing notes 26A–C. Electroencephalogram (EEG) reports, progress notes, nursing notes, physician orders, MAR
27. Myositis/myopathy[1,4,22,24,35]		X	27A. Identify other drug and nondrug causes 27B. If patient symptomatic, decrease zidovudine dose 27C. If symptoms moderate or severe, temporarily discontinue zidovudine and restart at one half original dose[22,35] 27D. Treat severe symptoms with concomitant nonsteroidal anti-inflammatory agents or prednisone (40–60 mg daily, with tapering)[22,35] 27E. If severe symptoms fail to respond to above measures (27B–27D), discontinue zidovudine and initiate didanosine therapy or enroll eligible patient in expanded-access programs	27. Progress notes, nursing notes, EMG reports, muscle biopsy reports, laboratory reports 27A–E. Progress notes, nursing notes, physician orders, MAR, laboratory reports
28. Non-Hodgkin's lymphoma[36,37]		X	28A. Identify other drug and nondrug causes 28B. Administer appropriate treatment (according to lymphoma classification)	28. Progress notes, nursing notes, oncology consultation reports, biopsy reports 28A. Progress notes, nursing notes, physician orders, MAR 28B. Physician orders, MAR,

Element	Standard 100%	Standard 0%	Exception[b] or Critical Preventive/ Responsive Measure[c]	Sources of Information
				progress notes, oncology consultation report
29. Local reaction from i.v. therapy (phlebitis, pain, inflammation)[1]		X	29A. Identify other drug and nondrug causes 29B. Provide symptomatic and supportive care 29C. Decrease infusion rate 29D. Rotate i.v. sites	29, 29A–C. Progress notes, nursing notes Progress notes, physician orders, nursing notes, MAR
Outcome Measures				
30. Improvement in Karnofsky performance score[38]	X		30A. Patient died 30B. Patient failed to return for follow-up appointment 30C. Patient's baseline score was 100	30, 30A–C. Progress notes, nursing notes
31. Improvement in patient's and caregivers' subjective assessment of symptoms (decreased fatigue, increased appetite, etc.)[1-12,14]	X		31A, Patient died 31B. Patient failed to return for follow-up appointment 31C. Patient asymptomatic at initiation of therapy	31, 31A–C. Progress notes, nursing notes
32. Improvement in objective symptoms (weight gain, improvement/clearing of mild fungal infections, reduction in fever episodes)[1,12,14]			32A. Patient died 32B. Patient failed to return for follow-up appointment 32C. Patient asymptomatic at initiation of therapy	32, 32A–C. Progress notes, nursing notes, laboratory reports
33. HIV disease progression slowed or halted (patient did not develop severe opportunistic infection, neoplasm, or neurologic disease)[1-12,14,31]	X		33A. Patient died 33B. Patient failed to return for follow-up appointment	33, 33A–B. Progress notes, nursing notes, laboratory reports
34. Improvement in platelet count[15,16]			34A. Patient died 34B. Patient failed to return for follow-up appointment 34C. Platelet count was normal at initiation of therapy	34, 34A–C. Progress notes, laboratory reports
35. Patient alive at end of therapy (if zidovudine therapy discontinued because of toxicity or treatment failure)	X		35A. Patient failed to return for follow-up appointment	35, 35A. Progress notes

[a] Criteria address justification for use (indications), critical (process) indicators, complications of therapy, and patient outcome. Each criterion consists of an element, a standard, exceptions to the standard, and sources of information. The element is the minimum level of evidence needed to show that patient care was optimal. The standard defines the deviation from an element that is acceptable. If no deviation is acceptable, the standard is 100%. Exceptions are circumstances in which deviation is allowable. Sources of information listed are the most reliable sources. Sources pertaining to an element or exception are identified by the number assigned to the element or exception (e.g., 5, 5A).

[b] For justification for use and critical (process) indicators.

[c] For complications and outcome measures.

References

1. Burroughs Wellcome. Retrovir package insert. Research Triangle Park, NC; 1990 May.
2. Yarchoan R, Weinhold KJ, Lyerly HK et al. Administration of 3′-azido-3′-deoxythymidine, an inhibitor of HTLV-III/LAV replication, to patients with AIDS or AIDS-related complex. *Lancet.* 1986; 1:575-80.
3. Fischl MA, Richman DD, Grieco MH et al. The efficacy of azidothymidine (AZT) in the treatment of patients with AIDS and AIDS-related complex. *N Engl J Med.* 1987; 317:185-91.
4. Fischl MA, Richman DD, Hansen N et al. The safety and efficacy of zidovudine (AZT) in the treatment of subjects with mildly symptomatic human immunodeficiency virus type 1 (HIV) infection. *Ann Intern Med.* 1990; 112:727-37.
5. Volberding PA, Lagakos SW, Koch MA et al. Zidovudine in asymptomatic human immunodeficiency virus infection. *N Engl J Med.* 1990; 322:941-9.
6. Creagh-Kirk T, Doi P, Andrews E et al. Survival experience among patients with AIDS receiving zidovudine. *JAMA.* 1988; 260:3009-15.
7. Fischl MA, Richman DD, Causey DM et al. Prolonged zidovudine therapy in patients with AIDS and advanced AIDS-related complex. *JAMA.* 1989; 262:2405-10.
8. Schmitt FA, Bigley JW, McKinnis R et al. Neuropsychological outcome of zidovudine (AZT) treatment of patients with AIDS and AIDS-related complex. *N Engl J Med* 1988; 319:1573-8.
9. Collier AC, Bozzette S, Coombs RW et al. A pilot study of low-dose zidovudine in human immunodeficiency virus infection. *N Engl J Med.* 1990; 323:1015-21.
10. Fischl MA, Parker CB, Pettinelli C et al. A randomized controlled trial of a reduced daily dose of zidovudine in patients with the acquired immunodeficiency syndrome. *N Engl J Med.* 1990; 323:1009-14.
11. Schulman KA, Lynn LA, Glick HA et al. Cost effectiveness of low-dose zidovudine therapy for asymptomatic patients with human immunodeficiency virus (HIV) infection. *Ann Intern Med.* 1991; 114:798-802.
12. Pizzo PA, Eddy J, Falloon J et al. Effect of continuous intravenous infusion of zidovudine (AZT) in children with symptomatic HIV infection. *N Engl J Med.* 1988; 319:889-96.

13. McKinney RE Jr, Pizzo PA, Scott GB et al. Safety and tolerance of intermittent intravenous and oral zidovudine therapy in human immunodeficiency virus–infected pediatric patients. *J Pediatr.* 1990; 116:640-7.
14. McKinney RE Jr, Maha MA, Connor EM et al. A multicenter trial of oral zidovudine in children with advanced human immunodeficiency virus disease. *N Engl J Med.* 1991; 324:1018-25.
15. The Swiss Group for Clinical Studies on the Acquired Immunodeficiency Syndrome (AIDS). Zidovudine for the treatment of thrombocytopenia associated with human immunodeficiency virus (HIV). *Ann Intern Med* 1988; 109:718-21.
16. Oksenhelder E, Bierling P, Ferchal F et al. Zidovudine for thrombocytopenic purpura related to human immunodeficiency virus (HIV) infection. *Ann Intern Med.* 1989; 110:365-8.
17. Centers for Disease Control. Revision of the CDC surveillance case definition for acquired immunodeficiency syndrome. *MMWR.* 1987; 36:3s-15s.
18. Centers for Disease Control. Classification system for human immunodeficiency virus (HIV) infection in children under 13 years of age. *MMWR.* 1987; 36:225-36.
19. Kornhauser DM, Petty BG, Hendrix CW et al. Probenecid and zidovudine metabolism. *Lancet.* 1989; 2:473-5.
20. DeMiranda P, Good SS, Yarchoan R et al. Alteration of zidovudine pharmacokinetics by probenecid in patients with AIDS or AIDS-related complex. *Clin Pharmacol Ther.* 1989; 46: 494-500.
21. Hedaya MA, Elmquist WF, Sawchuk RJ. Probenecid inhibits the metabolic and renal clearances of zidovudine (AZT) in human volunteers. *Pharm Res.* 1990; 4:411-7.
22. Till M, MacDonell KB. Myopathy with human immunodeficiency virus type 1 (HIV-1) infection: HIV-1 or zidovudine? *Ann Intern Med.* 1990; 113:492-4.
23. Vogt MW, Hartshorn KL, Furman PA et al. Ribavirin antagonizes the effect of azidothymidine on HIV replication. *Science.* 1987; 235:1376-9.
24. Langtry HD, Campoli-Richards DM. Zidovudine: a review of its pharmacodynamic and pharmacokinetic properties, and therapeutic efficacy. *Drugs.* 1989; 37:408-50.
25. Richman DD, Fischl MA, Grieco MH et al. The toxicity of azidothymidine (AZT) in the treatment of patients with AIDS and AIDS-related complex. *N Engl J Med.* 1987; 317:192-7.
26. Fischl MA, Galpin JE, Levine JD et al. Recombinant human erythropoietin for patients with AIDS treated with zidovudine. *N Engl J Med.* 1990; 332:1488-93.
27. Jacobson MA, DeMiranda P, Gordon SM et al. Prolonged pancytopenia due to combined ganciclovir and zidovudine therapy. *J Infect Dis.* 1988; 158:489-90.
28. Hochster H, Dieterich D, Bozzette S et al. Toxicity of combined ganciclovir and zidovudine for cytomegalovirus disease associated with AIDS. *Ann Intern Med.* 1990; 113:111-7.
29. Groopman JE. Status of colony-stimulating factors in cancer and AIDS. *Semin Oncol.* 1990; 17(Suppl 1):31-7.
30. Fisher CA, McPoland PR. Azidothymidine-induced nail pigmentation. *Cutis.* 1989; 43:552-4.
31. Don PC, Fusco F, Fried P et al. Nail dyschromia associated with zidovudine. *Ann Intern Med.* 1990; 112:145-6.
32. Groark SP, Hood AF, Nelson K. Nail pigmentation associated with zidovudine. *J Am Acad Dermatol.* 1989; 21:1032-3.
33. Greenberg RG, Berger TG. Nail and mucocutaneous hyperpigmentation with azidothymidine therapy. *J Am Acad Dermatol.* 1990; 22:327-30.
34. Grau-Massanes M, Millan F, Febrer MI et al. Pigmented nail bands and mucocutaneous pigmentation in HIV-positive patients treated with zidovudine. *J Am Acad Dermatol.* 1990; 22:687-8.
35. Dalakas MC, Illa I, Pezeshkpour GH et al. Mitochondrial myopathy caused by long-term zidovudine therapy. *N Engl J Med.* 1990; 322:1098-105.
36. Pluda JM, Yarchoan R, Jaffe ES et al. Development of non-Hodgkin's lymphoma in a cohort of patients with severe human immunodeficiency virus (HIV) infection on long-term antiretroviral therapy. *Ann Intern Med.* 1990; 113:276-82.
37. Moore RD, Kessler HD, Richman DD et al. Non-Hodgkin's lymphoma in patients with advanced HIV infection treated with zidovudine. *JAMA.* 1991; 265:2208-11.
38. Karnofsky DA, Abelmann WH, Craver LF et al. The use of nitrogen mustards in the palliative treatment of carcinoma. *Cancer.* 1948; 1:634-56.

Current Literature

Drug Reaction Alerts 87

Book Review

Advances in Pain Research and Therapy, Volume 18: The Design of Analgesic Clinical Trials 92

Edited by Mitchell B. Max, Russell K. Portenoy, and Eugene M. Laska

Reviewed by Celeste Lindley

Drug Reaction Alerts

Drug Reaction Alerts focuses primarily on serious, unlabeled reactions to new chemical entities. The citations are compiled monthly from International Pharmaceutical Abstracts, which covers over 800 pharmacy and health-related journals worldwide. An address for reprints (when available) follows the name of the corresponding author in each citation.

Pharmacists may use the FDA Adverse Reaction Report form that appears in the January and July issues of Clinical Pharmacy for submitting reports of adverse drug reactions directly to FDA.

Abortifacients

Pons JC (Department of Obstetrics and Gynecology and Pathology, Antoine Beclere Hospital, Clamart 92141, France), Imbert MC, Elefant E et al. Development after exposure to **mifepristone** in early pregnancy. *Lancet*. 1991; 338:763. Cases. (two offspring whose mothers, aged 25 and 30 years, received mifepristone 400 mg as abortifacient then decided to continue pregnancy to term; in offspring of 25-year-old woman, ultrasound scan at 17 weeks gestation showed complete lack of amniotic sac, stomach, gallbladder, and urinary tract, and pregnancy was terminated at 18 weeks gestation by prostaglandin administration; in offspring of 30-year-old woman, ultrasound scan showed normal fetal morphology, and healthy, 3.03-kg boy was delivered at 41 weeks gestation; postnatal examination of infant showed no abnormality)

Aerosols

Berdy GJ (Library Eye Research Institute, 20 Staniford Street, Boston, MA 02114), Berdy SS, Odin LS et al. Angle closure glaucoma precipitated by aerosolized **atropine**. *Arch Intern Med*. 1991; 151:1658-60. Cases. (two women, aged 57 and 62 years, with steroid-dependent obstructive pulmonary disease and angle-closure glaucoma; received atropine 2 or 2.5 mg every 4 hours by aerosolization for three or four days; developed exacerbation of angle-closure glaucoma; concomitant aminophylline, corticosteroids, and metaproterenol; 62-year-old woman received topical pilocarpine and dipivefrin as maintenance therapy for glaucoma; in 57-year-old woman, therapy with topical pilocarpine hydrochloride led to resolution of symptoms; in 62-year-old woman, therapy with acetazolamide and mannitol by i.v. injection and topical pilocarpine hydrochloride, timolol, and prednisolone acetate led to resolution of symptoms)

Antifungals

Abbott M, Hughes DL, Patel R et al. (Kinghorn GR, Department of Genitourinary Medicine, Royal Hallamshire Hospital, Sheffield S10 2JF, England). Angio-edema after **fluconazole**. *Lancet*. 1991; 338:633. Case. (21-year-old woman; received fluconazole 150 mg twice monthly for seven doses as chemoprophylaxis for severe candidal vulvovaginitis; developed swollen tongue and buccal ulceration two days after dose 6; developed orbital and buccal swelling and paresthesia of

Continued on page 91

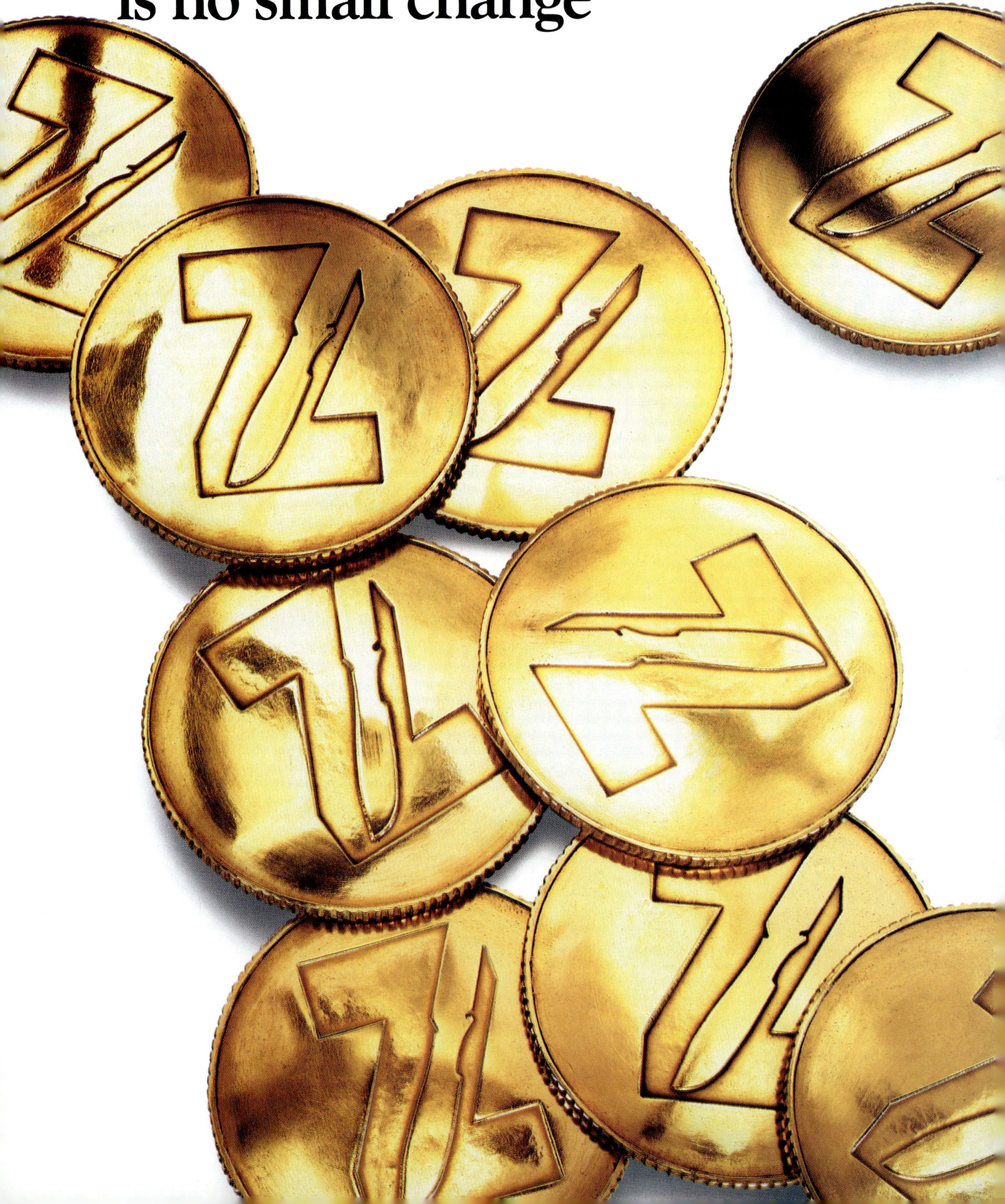

Continued from page 87

mouth and perineum within four hours after dose 7 and tongue swelling, difficulty breathing, and oral ulceration within 12 hours; withdrawal of fluconazole and therapy with nystatin pessaries and cream led to resolution of symptoms)

Antilipemic Agents

Ahmad S (Cardio-Diagnostic Clinique, 1000 Brookside Drive, Fairmont, VA 26554). **Lovastatin**-induced lupus erythematosus. *Arch Intern Med*. 1991; 151:1667-8. Cases. (64-year-old woman and 40-year-old man with hypercholesterolemia; received lovastatin 20 mg/day for two years and for unstated period of time, respectively; developed lupus erythematosus, which was confirmed by positive [1:640] fluorescent antinuclear antibody test; withdrawal of lovastatin and therapy with a tapering course of prednisone and aspirin as needed for relief of symptoms led to slow resolution of symptoms)

Vouillamoz D (CHU Vaudois, 1011 Lausanne, Switzerland), Schaller MD, Bianchi L et al. **Beclobrate** and fatal acute hepatitis. *Lancet*. 1991; 338:581. Case. (64-year-old man with hypercholesterolemia; received beclobrate 100 mg/day for 6.5 months; became anorexic and jaundiced; total serum bilirubin concentration, 304 μM [normal, <17 μM]; serum aminotransferase concentrations elevated; concomitant chondroitin sulfate for osteoarthritis of hip; admitted to hospital three weeks later; died seven days after admission; examination at autopsy showed panlobular hepatic necrosis with bridging)

Antivirals

Marcellin P, Colin JF, Boyer N et al. (Benhamou JP, Services of Hepatology and INSERM U 24, Immunohaematology, Anatomy, and Pathological Cytology, Hôpital Beaujon, 92100 Clichy, France). Fatal exacerbation of chronic hepatitis B induced by recombinant alpha-interferon. *Lancet*. 1991; 338:828. Case. (62-year-old man with chronic hepatitis B virus infection; received **interferon alfa-2b** 5 million units three times weekly for 10 weeks; serum alanine aminotransferase concentration began to increase above normally increased concentration after eight weeks; showed signs of jaundice and ascites after 11 weeks; examination of liver tissue obtained by transvenous liver biopsy showed cirrhosis and acute hepatitis with widespread necrosis; developed encephalopathy with coma; died three days later of septic shock due to *Pseudomonas putida*)

Corticosteroids

Connett G, Lenney W (Royal Alexandra Hospital for Sick Children, Brighton BN1 3JN, England). Inhaled **budesonide** and behavioral disturbances. *Lancet*. 1991; 338:634-5. Cases. (four children, aged 30 months to three years, with asthma; received budesonide 400 μg two to three times daily by inhalation; developed behavioral disturbances; reduction of budesonide dose to 200 μg two times daily in two-year-old boy led to improved behavior; change of therapy from budesonide to beclomethasone dipropionate in other patients led to resolution of behavioral symptoms; positive rechallenge for 32-month-old and three-year-old boys)

Drug Interactions

Metroka CE, McMechan MF, Andrada R (St. Luke's/Roosevelt Hospital Center, New York, NY 10019) et al. Failure of prophylaxis with **dapsone** in patients taking dideoxyinosine. *N Engl J Med*. 1991; 325:737. Study. (investigational-new-drug and open-label studies of **didanosine** with buffer packet; 66 patients with AIDS; received oral dapsone 25 mg four times daily, oral trimethoprim–sulfamethoxazole [1:5] 160 mg twice daily, or pentamidine 300 mg monthly by aerosolization as chemoprophylaxis for *Pneumocystis carinii* pneumonia [PCP]; 11 of 28 patients who received dapsone and 1 of 12 patients who received pentamidine developed PCP; mean time to development of PCP, 66 days (range, 10–130 days; $n = 12$); nine patients could not be evaluated because of noncompliance or development of adverse reactions to didanosine in first 30 days of study)

Richter WO, Jacob BG, Schwandt P (Medical Department II, University of Munich, Klinikum Grosshadern, D-8000 Munich 70, Germany). Interaction between fiber and **lovastatin**. *Lancet*. 1991; 338:706. Study. (case series; three women and one man, aged 49–61 years, with hypercholesterolemia; women received **pectin** 15 g/day with a lipid-lowering diet and man received **oat bran** 50–100 g/day and lovastatin 80 mg/day for four weeks; developed increased serum low-density lipoprotein concentration; withdrawal of pectin or oat bran led to return of serum low-density lipoprotein concentration to prestudy concentration)

Drugs, Adverse Reactions

Latov N (Department of Neurology, Black Building. [Room 3-323]), Columbia University, New York, NY 10032), Koski CL, Walicke PA. Guillain-Barré syndrome and parenteral **gangliosides**. *Lancet*. 1991; 338:757. Case. (70-year-old woman with symptoms of L-5 radiculopathy; received brain gangliosides daily by injection for 10 days; developed Guillain-Barré syndrome; weakness progressed to quadriparesis and areflexia; serum anti-G_{M1}, asialo-G_{M1}, and antiperipheral myelin antibody concentrations were increased; strength began to improve on day 9 in hospital; made slow but complete recovery)

Hypotensive Agents

Woodmansey P, Channer KS (Cardiology Department, Royal Hallamshire Hospital, Sheffield S10 2JF, England). **Nifedipine** and hypotension. *Lancet*. 1991; 338:763-4. Case. (52-year-old man with high blood pressure; received one extended-

Continued on page 92

release nifedipine 20 mg; awoke with dense right hemiparesis two hours after dose; concomitant atenolol and hydrochlorothiazide; computed tomography scan showed cerebral infarction; blood pressure was lower than at previous hospital admission)

Parasympatholytic Agents

Andrews NP, Bevan J (University Hospital of Wales, Cardiff CF4 4XW, Wales). Torsades de pointes and **terodiline**. *Lancet*. 1991; 338:632-3. Case. (64-year-old woman without previous heart disease; received terodiline 25 mg twice daily for three weeks; developed torsades de pointes; withdrawal of terodiline and treatment with ventricular pacing, magnesium, and atenolol led to improvement; serum terodiline concentration within therapeutic range six days after withdrawal of drug)

Preservatives

Noel I, Galloway A, Ive FA (Dryburn Hospital, Durham DH1 5TW, England). Hypersensitivity to **thiomersal** in hepatitis B vaccine. *Lancet*. 1991; 338:705. Case. (27-year-old man; received two doses of hepatitis B vaccine five months apart; developed local reaction that lasted for four weeks; results of patch testing showed delayed-type hypersensitivity to thimerosal, a preservative in vaccine formulation; discontinuation of vaccination schedule led to recovery and serum antibody to hepatitis B surface antigen titer >100 IU/L two months later)

Toxicity

Dwyer C, Chapman RS (Department of Dermatology, Stobhill General Hospital, Glasgow G21 3UW, Scotland). **Calcipotriol** and hypercalcemia. *Lancet*. 1991; 338:764-5. Case. (67-year-old woman with exfoliative psoriasis covering 40% of her body; instructed to apply calcipotriol ointment 50 µg/g twice daily for seven days; developed nausea, muscle weakness, and abdominal pain; adjusted serum calcium concentration, 3.51 mM [normal, 2.2–2.6 mM]; estimated that 200 g of ointment was applied over one week; withdrawal of calcipotriol and therapy with high fluid intake led to return of serum calcium concentration to normal)

Book Review

Advances in Pain Research and Therapy, Volume 18: The Design of Analgesic Clinical Trials

Edited by Mitchell B. Max, Russell K. Portenoy, and Eugene M. Laska.

Published by Raven Press, 1185 Avenue of the Americas, New York, NY 10036, 1991. xxi + 729 p. Price $122.

As stated by the editors in the preface, this book is intended to be used as a resource by both the novice and the experienced analgesic investigator. The first of the book's three parts, "Steps in the Clinical Evaluation of an Analgesic," is written for the investigator interested in studying basic properties and potential clinical applications of analgesic agents. Experimental pain models and methods of efficacy and toxicity assessment are described; more methods for assessing efficacy are provided than for assessing toxicity. Single- and multiple-dose trial designs and their advantages and limitations are described.

The second part, "Designing Analgesic Studies to Meet Specific Clinical Needs," is aimed at the clinical specialist interested in a particular patient population. Areas addressed include neuropathic pain syndromes, cancer pain, low back pain, sickle cell disease, headache, dysmenorrhea, oral surgery, orofacial pain, pain in children, and patient-controlled analgesia. Issues unique to each type of pain, specific barriers to performing analgesic trials, and potential strategies for solution are discussed.

The third part of the book, "Other Issues," addresses a variety of topics relevant to pain research, including pharmacokinetic and pharmacodynamic assessment, biostatistics, methods for evaluating interventions to improve analgesic prescribing practices, the Food and Drug Administration's regulation of clinical studies, and measurement and analysis of pharmacologic and nonpharmacologic treatment of pain.

Expert commentaries that highlight unresolved issues and ongoing controversies appear at the end of several chapters. Many of these commentaries are excerpts of discussions from a January 1990 meeting at which preliminary versions of a number of the chapters were presented to audiences of analgesic research experts.

The major focus of this book is the conduct of randomized controlled trials of analgesic agents; however, important basic information regarding pain measurement, study design, and elementary pharmacokinetics, pharmacodynamics, and biostatistics is also included. Each chapter has excellent references. The contributing authors constitute an impressive group of recognized pain research experts from academic, industrial, and federal regulatory and research bodies.

Reviewed by Celeste Lindley, Pharm.D., School of Pharmacy, Campus Box 7360, Beard Hall, The University of North Carolina at Chapel Hill, Chapel Hill, NC 27599-7360.

Advertising Index

Alpha Therapeutic Corporation
Venoglobulin–I, 15-16
American Society of Hospital Pharmacists
AHFS Drug Information 92, 56
Concepts in Immunology and Immunotherapeutics, 91
Criteria for Drug Use Evaluation, Volumes 1 and 2, 68
Handbook on Injectable Drugs, Sixth Edition, 59
IV-EASE, 14
Rx Triage, 9
Amgen Inc.
Epogen, 3
Neupogen, 69-76
Burroughs Wellcome Company
Exosurf Neonatal, 17-21
Epilepsy Foundation of America
Institutional, 80
Idaho State University
Positions Available, 81
Eli Lilly and Company
Hospital Division, 7
Roerig, A Division of Pfizer Pharmaceuticals
Diflucan, 10-12
Ross Laboratories
Survanta, 5-6
SmithKline Beecham
Timentin, inside back cover, outside back cover
Toledo Hospital
Positions Available, 81
The Upjohn Company
Zefazone, 88-90
Wyeth-Ayerst Laboratories, Inc.
Ativan Injection, 82-84
Tubex, inside front cover

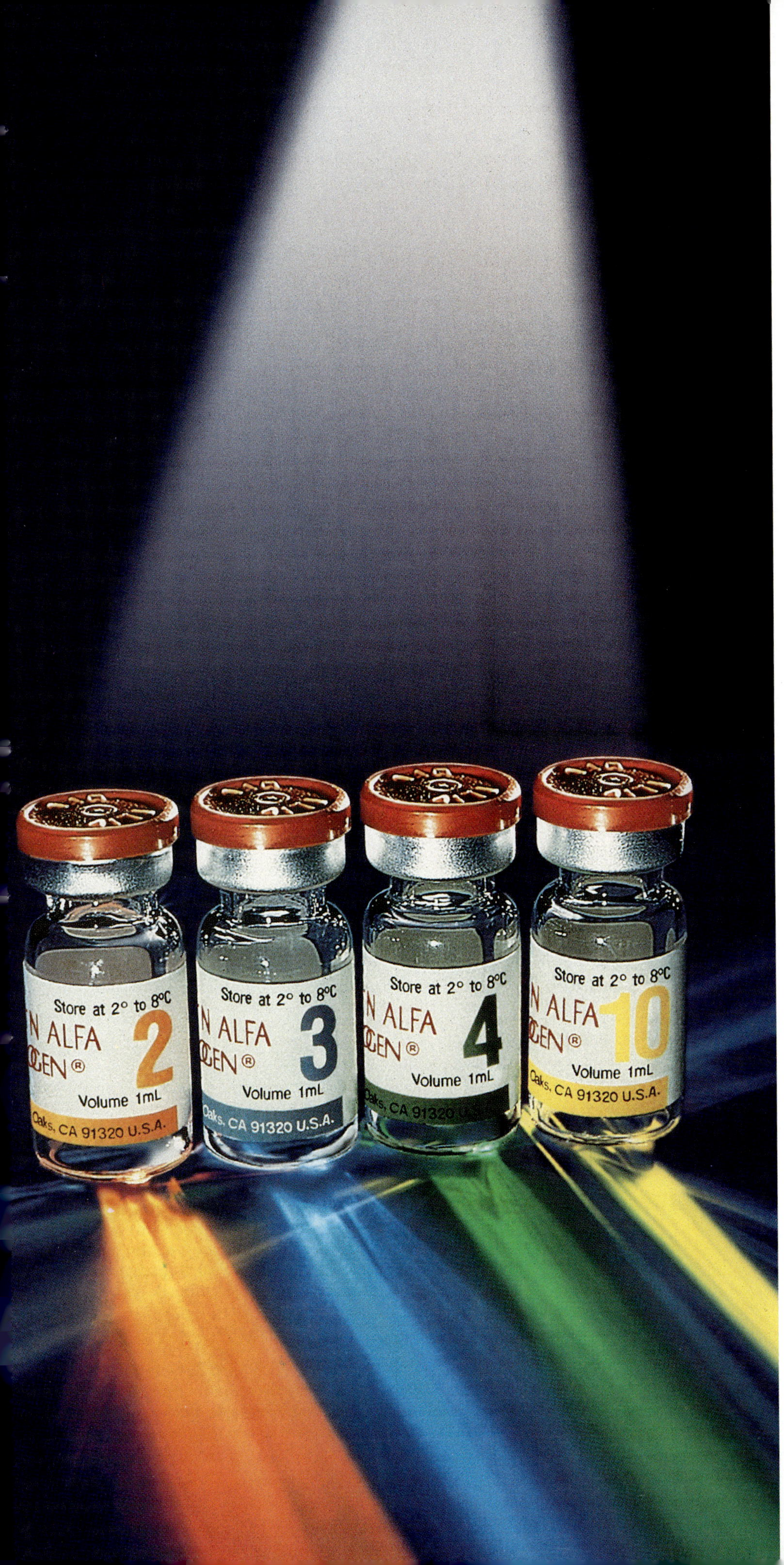
Store at 2° to 8°C
N ALFA
GEN ®
2
Volume 1mL
Oaks, CA 91320 U.S.A.
Store at 2° to 8°C
N ALFA
GEN ®
3
Volume 1mL
Oaks, CA 91320 U.S.A.
Store at 2° to 8°C
N ALFA
GEN ®
4
Volume 1mL
Store at 2° to 8°C
N ALFA
GEN ®
10
Volume 1mL
Oaks, CA 91320 U.S.A.

News

Review of 1991 shows 30 new drugs, several important biologics cleared for marketing 208

Pfizer delays marketing azithromycin 218

FDA warns of overdose risk from dosage cups 220

FDA seizes cold sterilizing solution 220

Pamidronate released for management of hypercalcemia of malignancy 220

Quinapril marketed as antihypertensive agent 220

False-positive viral antibody test results reported in influenza vaccine recipients 220

News Briefs 221

Upcoming Specialty Meetings 221

Review of 1991 shows 30 new drugs, several important biologics cleared for marketing

FDA's approval of 30 new drugs in 1991 matched the agency's 1985 record for most new drug approvals. The median time from NDA filing to FDA approval was 22 months, compared with 24 months in 1990 and 29 months in 1989. The mean approval time, which increased by 2.4 months in 1991, reflected an effort to reduce the backlog of products awaiting approval. Five of the newly approved drugs received FDA's 1A designation, indicating that the drug is a significant therapeutic gain; these drugs are ceredase, didanosine, fludarabine, histrelin, and pentostatin. The 30 new drugs and their indications are as follows:

- Alglucerase (Ceredase, Genzyme), an enzyme replacement therapy for patients with Gaucher's disease
- Azithromycin (Zithromax, Pfizer), a macrolide antibiotic
- Benazepril hydrochloride (Lotensin, Ciba-Geigy), an angiotensin-converting-enzyme inhibitor for treatment of hypertension
- Beractant (Survanta, Abbott), a modified natural surfactant for prevention and treatment of neonatal respiratory distress syndrome
- Cefprozil monohydrate (Cefzil, Bristol-Myers Squibb), an oral cephalosporin
- Clarithromycin (Biaxin, Abbott), a macrolide antibiotic
- Didanosine (Videx, Bristol-Myers Squibb), for treatment of adults and children with advanced human immunodeficiency virus infection who cannot tolerate zidovudine therapy or have demonstrated immunologic deterioration during zidovudine therapy
- Doxacurium chloride (Nuromax, Burroughs Wellcome), a nondepolarizing, long-acting neuromuscular blocking agent for use during surgery
- Enoxacin (Penetrex, Warner-Lambert), a fluoroquinolone antimicrobial
- Etodolac (Lodine, Wyeth-Ayerst), a nonsteroidal anti-inflammatory agent
- Felodipine (Plendil, Merck Sharp & Dohme), a calcium-channel blocker for treatment of hypertension
- Fludarabine phosphate (Fludara, Berlex), an anti-

Continued on page 218

EXOSURF® Neonatal™
(COLFOSCERIL PALMITATE, CETYL ALCOHOL, TYLOXAPOL)
For Intratracheal Suspension / 10 mL vials

PLEASE CONSULT FULL PRODUCT INFORMATION BEFORE PRESCRIBING.

INDICATIONS AND USAGE: Exosurf Neonatal is indicated for:

1. **Prophylactic** treatment of infants with birth weights of less than 1350 grams who are at risk of developing RDS (see PRECAUTIONS),
2. **Prophylactic** treatment of infants with birth weights greater than 1350 grams who have evidence of pulmonary immaturity, and
3. **Rescue** treatment of infants who have developed RDS.

CONTRAINDICATIONS: There are no known contraindications to treatment with Exosurf Neonatal.

WARNINGS: Intratracheal Administration Only: Exosurf Neonatal should be administered only by instillation into the trachea. **General:** The use of Exosurf Neonatal requires expert clinical care by experienced neonatologists and other clinicians who are accomplished at neonatal intubation and ventilatory management. Adequate personnel, facilities, equipment, and medications are required to optimize perinatal outcome in premature infants. Instillation of Exosurf Neonatal should be performed **only** by trained medical personnel experienced in airway and clinical management of unstable premature infants. Vigilant clinical attention should be given to all infants prior to, during, and after administration of Exosurf Neonatal. **Acute Effects:** Exosurf Neonatal can rapidly affect oxygenation and lung compliance. **Lung Compliance:** If chest expansion improves substantially after dosing, peak ventilator inspiratory pressures should be reduced immediately, without waiting for confirmation of respiratory improvement by blood gas assessment. Failure to reduce inspiratory ventilator pressures rapidly in such instances can result in lung overdistention and fatal pulmonary air leak. **Hyperoxia:** If the infant becomes pink and transcutaneous oxygen saturation is in excess of 95%, FiO_2 should be reduced in small but repeated steps (until saturation is 90 to 95%) without waiting for confirmation of elevated arterial pO_2 by blood gas assessment. Failure to reduce FiO_2 in such instances can result in hyperoxia. **Hypocarbia:** If arterial or transcutaneous CO_2 measurements are <30 torr, the ventilator rate should be reduced at once. Failure to reduce ventilator rates in such instances can result in marked hypocarbia, which is known to reduce brain blood flow. **Pulmonary Hemorrhage:** In the single study conducted in infants weighing <700 grams at birth, the incidence of pulmonary hemorrhage (10% vs 2% in the placebo group) was significantly increased in the Exosurf Neonatal group. None of the five studies involving infants with birth weights >700 grams showed a significant increase in pulmonary hemorrhage in the Exosurf Neonatal group. In a cross-study analysis of these five studies, pulmonary hemorrhage was reported for 1% (14/1420) of infants in the placebo group and 2% (27/1411) of infants in the Exosurf Neonatal group. Fatal pulmonary hemorrhage occurred in three infants; two in the Exosurf Neonatal group and one in the placebo group. Mortality from all causes among infants who developed pulmonary hemorrhage was 43% in the placebo group and 37% in the Exosurf Neonatal group. Pulmonary hemorrhage in both Exosurf Neonatal and placebo infants was more frequent in infants who were younger, smaller, male, or who had a patent ductus arteriosus. Pulmonary hemorrhage typically occurred in the first 2 days of life in both treatment groups. In more than 7700 infants in the open, uncontrolled study, pulmonary hemorrhage was reported in 4%, but fatal pulmonary hemorrhage was reported rarely (0.4%). In the controlled clinical studies, Exosurf Neonatal treated infants who received steroids more than 24 hours prior to delivery or indomethacin postnatally had a lower rate of pulmonary hemorrhage than other Exosurf Neonatal treated infants. Attention should be paid to early and aggressive diagnosis and treatment (unless contraindicated) of patent ductus arteriosus during the first 2 days of life (while the ductus arteriosus is often clinically silent). Other potentially protective measures include attempting to decrease FiO_2 preferentially over ventilator pressures during the first 24 to 48 hours after dosing, and attempting to decrease PEEP minimally for at least 48 hours after dosing. **Mucous Plugs:** Infants whose ventilation becomes markedly impaired during or shortly after dosing may have mucous plugging of the endotracheal tube, particularly if pulmonary secretions were prominent prior to drug administration. Suctioning of all infants prior to dosing may lessen the chance of mucous plugs obstructing the endotracheal tube. If endotracheal tube obstruction from such plugs is suspected, and suctioning is unsuccessful in removing the obstruction, the blocked endotracheal tube should be replaced immediately.

PRECAUTIONS:

General: In the controlled clinical studies, infants known prenatally or postnatally to have major congenital anomalies, or who were suspected of having congenital infection, were excluded from entry. However, these disorders cannot be recognized early in life in all cases, and a few infants with these conditions were entered. The benefits of Exosurf Neonatal in the affected infants who received drug appeared to be similar to the benefits observed in infants without anomalies or occult infection. **Prophylactic Treatment-Infants <700 Grams:** In infants weighing 500 to 700 grams, a single prophylactic dose of Exosurf Neonatal significantly: improved FiO_2 and ventilator settings, reduced pneumothorax, and reduced death from RDS, but increased pulmonary hemorrhage (see WARNINGS). Overall mortality did not differ significantly between the placebo and Exosurf Neonatal groups (see Table 1 in full product information). Data on multiple doses in infants in this weight class are not yet available. Accordingly, clinicians should carefully evaluate the potential risks and benefits of Exosurf Neonatal administration in these infants. **Rescue Treatment-Number of Doses:** A small number of infants with RDS have received more than two doses of Exosurf Neonatal as rescue treatment. Definitive data on the safety and efficacy of these additional doses are not available. **Carcinogenesis, Mutagenesis, Impairment of Fertility:** Exosurf Neonatal at concentrations up to 10,000 μg/plate was not mutagenic in the Ames Salmonella assay. Long-term studies have not been performed in animals to evaluate the carcinogenic potential of Exosurf Neonatal. The effects of Exosurf Neonatal on fertility have not been studied.

ADVERSE REACTIONS:

General: Premature birth is associated with a high incidence of morbidity and mortality. Despite significant reductions in overall mortality associated with Exosurf Neonatal, some infants who received Exosurf Neonatal developed severe complications and either survived with permanent handicaps or died.

In controlled clinical studies evaluating the safety and efficacy of Exosurf Neonatal, numerous safety assessments were made. In infants receiving Exosurf Neonatal, pulmonary hemorrhage, apnea and use of methylxanthines were increased. A number of other adverse events were significantly reduced in the Exosurf Neonatal group, particularly various forms of pulmonary air leak and use of pancuronium. Tables 3 and 4 summarize the results of the major safety evaluations from the controlled clinical studies.

Table 3: Safety Assessments[a]—Prophylactic Treatment

Number of Doses:	Single Dose		Single Dose		Single Dose		1 vs 3 Doses	
Birth Weight Range:	500 to 700 grams		700 to 1350 grams		700 to 1100 grams		700 to 1100 grams	
Treatment Group:	Placebo (Air)	EXOSURF	Placebo (Air)	EXOSURF	Placebo (Air)	EXOSURF	EXOSURF 1 Dose	EXOSURF 3 Doses
Number of Infants:	N=108	N=107	N=193	N=192	N=222	N=224	N=356	N=360
	% of Infants		% of Infants		% of Infants		% of Infants	
Intraventricular Hemorrhage (IVH)								
Overall	51	57	31	27	36	36	38	35
Severe IVH	26	25	10	8	13	14	9	9
Pulmonary Air Leak (PAL)								
Overall	52	48	16	11	32	25	29	27
Pneumothorax	23	10*	5	6	19	11*	14	12
Pneumopericardium	1	4	2	0	<1	1	1	1
Pneumomediastinum	2	1	2	3	7	1**	3	2
Pulmonary Interstitial Emphysema	43	44	13	7*	26	20	23	22
Death from PAL	4	6	<1	<1	2	1	2	1
Patent Ductus Arteriosus	49	53	66	70	50	55	59	57
Necrotizing Enterocolitis	2	4	11	13	3	4	6	2*
Pulmonary Hemorrhage	2	10**	2	4	1	4	4	6
Congenital Pneumonia	4	4	2	4	2	2	1	1
Nosocomial Pneumonia	10	10	2	4	4	7	14	15
Non-Pulmonary Infections	33	35	34	39	28	29	35	34
Sepsis	30	34	30	34	23	24	30	27
Death From Sepsis	4	4	3	3	1	2	3	2
Meningitis	4	6	3	1	2	3	1	2
Other Infections	7	4	5	3	6	10	10	11
Major Anomalies	3	1	2	4	7	4	4	4
Hypotension	70	77	52	47	59	62	54	50
Hyperbilirubinemia	22	21	63	61	27	31	20	21
Exchange Transfusion	4	3	1	2	2	2	3	1
Thrombocytopenia[b]	21	25	not available		9	8	12	10
Persistent Fetal Circulation	0	1	1	1	0	2*	1	<1
Seizures	11	8	2	2	11	9	6	5
Apnea	34	33	76	73	55	65*	62	68
Drug Therapy								
Antibiotics	96	99	98	96	98	99	>99	99
Diuretics	55	60	39	37	59	63	64	65
Anticonvulsants	14	18	23	24	20	16	9	8
Inotropes	46	40	20	20	26	20	28	27
Sedatives	62	71	65	64	63	57	52	52
Pancuronium	19	11	22	14*	19	13*	15	11
Methylxanthines	38	43	77	77	61	72*	75	82*

[a] All parameters were examined with "as-treated" analyses. * $p<0.05$

[b] Thrombocytopenia requiring platelet transfusion. ** $p<0.01$

Table 4: Safety Assessments[a]—Rescue Treatment

Number of Doses:	Two Doses		Two Doses	
Birth Weight Range:	700 to 1350 grams		1250 grams and above	
Treatment Group:	Placebo (Air)	EXOSURF	Placebo (Air)	EXOSURF
Number of Infants:	N=213	N=206	N=622	N=615
	% of Infants		% of Infants	
Intraventricular Hemorrhage (IVH)				
Overall	48	52	23	18*
Severe IVH	13	9	5	4
Pulmonary Air Leak (PAL)				
Overall	54	34***	30	18***
Pneumothorax	29	20*	20	10***
Pneumopericardium	4	1	1	2
Pneumomediastinum	8	4	5	2**
Pulmonary Interstitial Emphysema	48	25***	24	13***
Death from PAL	7	3	<1	1
Patent Ductus Arteriosus	66	57	54	45*
Necrotizing Enterocolitis	3	3	1	2
Pulmonary Hemorrhage	3	1	<1	1
Congenital Pneumonia	2	3	2	2
Nosocomial Pneumonia	5	7	2	2
Non-Pulmonary Infections	19	22	13	13
Sepsis	15	17	8	8
Death From Sepsis	<1	<1	1	<1
Meningitis	1	<1	1	<1*
Other Infections	5	8	5	6
Major Anomalies	3	3	4	4
Hypotension	62	57	50	39**
Hyperbilirubinemia	17	19	12	10
Exchange Transfusion	3	4	1	2
Thrombocytopenia[b]	10	11	4	<1**
Persistent Fetal Circulation	1	1	6	2**
Seizures	10	10	6	3*
Apnea	48	65**	37	44*
Drug Therapy				
Antibiotics	100	99	98	98
Diuretics	60	65	45	34***
Anticonvulsants	17	17	10	5**
Inotropes	36	31	27	16***
Sedatives	72	68	76	64***
Pancuronium	34	17**	33	15***
Methylxanthines	62	74**	49	53

[a] All parameters were examined with "as-treated" analyses. * $p<0.05$ *** $p<0.001$

[b] Thrombocytopenia requiring platelet transfusion. ** $p<0.01$

Pulmonary Hemorrhage: See WARNINGS. **Abnormal Laboratory Values:** Abnormal laboratory values are common in critically ill, mechanically ventilated, premature infants. A higher incidence of abnormal laboratory values in the Exosurf Neonatal group was not reported. **Events During Dosing:** Data on events during dosing are available from more than 8800 infants in the open, uncontrolled clinical study (Table 5).

Table 5: Events During Dosing in the Open, Uncontrolled Study[a]

Treatment Type:	Prophylactic Treatment	Rescue Treatment
Number of Infants:	N=1127	N=7711
	% of Infants	% of Infants
Reflux of Exosurf	20	31
Drop in O_2 saturation ($\geq 20\%$)	6	22
Rise in O_2 saturation ($\geq 10\%$)	5	6
Drop in transcutaneous pO_2 (≥ 20 mm Hg)	1	8
Rise in transcutaneous pO_2 (≥ 20 mm Hg)	2	5
Drop in transcutaneous pCO_2 (≥ 20 mm Hg)	<1	1
Rise in transcutaneous pCO_2 (≥ 20 mm Hg)	1	3
Bradycardia (<60 beats/min)	1	3
Tachycardia (>200 beats/min)	<1	<1
Gagging	1	5
Mucous Plugs	<1	<1

[a] Infants may have experienced more than one event.
Investigators were prohibited from adjusting FiO_2 and/or ventilator settings during dosing unless significant clinical deterioration occurred.

Reflux: Reflux of Exosurf Neonatal into the endotracheal tube during dosing has been observed and may be associated with rapid drug administration. If reflux occurs, drug administration should be halted and, if necessary, peak inspiratory pressure on the ventilator should be increased by 4 to 5 cm H_2O until the endotracheal tube clears. ***>20% Drop in Transcutaneous Oxygen Saturation:*** If transcutaneous oxygen saturation declines during dosing, drug administration should be halted and, if necessary, peak inspiratory pressure on the ventilator should be increased by 4 to 5 cm H_2O for 1 to 2 minutes. In addition, increases of FiO_2 may be required for 1 to 2 minutes. ***Mucous Plugs:*** See WARNINGS.

DOSAGE AND ADMINISTRATION: See full product information.

Wellcome
BURROUGHS WELLCOME CO., Research Triangle Park, NC 27709

Printed in U.S.A. EX-Y01228

Continued from page 208

neoplastic agent for use in patients with B-cell chronic lymphocytic leukemia who have not responded to standard therapy

- Flumazenil (Mazicon, Hoffmann-La Roche), a benzodiazepine antagonist
- Foscarnet sodium (Foscavir, Astra), for treatment of cytomegalovirus retinitis in patients with AIDS
- Fosinopril sodium (Monopril, Bristol-Myers Squibb), an angiotensin-converting-enzyme inhibitor for treatment of hypertension
- Gallium nitrate injection (Ganite, Fujisawa), for treatment of cancer-related hypercalcemia
- Histrelin acetate (Supprelin, Ortho), a synthetic luteinizing hormone-releasing hormone agonist for treatment of precocious puberty
- Isosorbide mononitrate (Ismo, Wyeth-Ayerst), for prevention of angina
- Loracarbef (Lorabid, Eli Lilly), a carbacephem antimicrobial
- Nabumetone (Relafen, SmithKline Beecham), a nonsteroidal anti-inflammatory drug
- Ondansetron hydrochloride injection (Zofran, Glaxo), a selective serotonin antagonist for prevention of nausea and vomiting associated with cancer chemotherapy
- Pamidronate disodium injection (Aredia, Ciba-Geigy), a biophosphonate for treatment of cancer-related hypercalcemia
- Pentostatin (Nipent, Warner-Lambert), for treatment of hairy cell leukemia that is refractory to interferon alfa therapy
- Pravastatin (Pravachol, Bristol-Myers Squibb), an inhibitor of 3-hydroxy-3-methylglutaryl coenzyme A (HMG CoA) reductase for use as an adjunct to diet for the reduction of cholesterol levels
- Quinapril hydrochloride (Accupril, Parke-Davis), an angiotensin-converting-enzyme inhibitor for treatment of hypertension
- Ramipril (Altace, Hoechst-Roussel and Upjohn), a calcium-channel blocker for treatment of hypertension
- Sertraline hydrochloride (Zoloft, Pfizer), a serotonin reuptake inhibitor for treatment of depression
- Simvastatin (Zocor, Merck Sharp & Dohme), an HMG CoA reductase inhibitor for use as an adjunct to diet for cholesterol reduction
- Succimer (Chemet, McNeil), an orally active heavy-metal chelating agent for the treatment of lead poisoning in children with blood lead concentrations greater than 45 μg/dL
- Ticlopidine hydrochloride (Ticlid, Syntex), for reducing the risk of thrombotic stroke in patients who have had stroke precursors or a completed stroke

Among the biologic licensing applications approved during 1991 were

- Antithrombin III (Thrombin III, Miles), a purified product for treatment of hereditary antithrombin III deficiency
- Diphtheria and tetanus toxoids and acellular pertussis vaccine adsorbed (Acel-imune, Lederle), for childhood immunizations as the fourth and fifth doses in the immunization series
- Filgrastim (Neupogen, Amgen), a recombinant granulocyte colony-stimulating factor for use in preventing infections associated with febrile neutropenia in patients with nonmyeloid malignancies who are receiving cancer chemotherapy
- Sargramostim (Leukine, Immunex; Prokine, Hoechst-Roussel), a recombinant granulocyte–macrophage colony-stimulating factor for use in patients with delayed or failed bone marrow engraftment and for use in accelerating myeloid recovery in patients with Hodgkin's disease, non-Hodgkin's lymphoma, or acute lymphoblastic leukemia who are undergoing autologous bone marrow transplantation.

The 1991 approvals included seven orphan drugs and two orphan biologics: alglucerase, antithrombin III, beractant, fludarabine, gallium, histrelin, pentostatin, sargramostim, and succimer.

Pfizer delays marketing azithromycin

Pfizer Pharmaceuticals has delayed marketing azithromycin until the FDA reviews information on 19 patients who received the drug and experienced serious adverse events including four patient deaths, a company spokesperson said. (Azithromycin was reviewed in the February issue of *Clinical Pharmacy.)*

All 19 patients had upper- or lower-respiratory-tract infections, Pfizer drug information pharmacist Joseph Gasperino said. The deaths occurred in the group of seven patients who had pneumonia.

Gasperino said the information came to the company's attention during the postapproval launch period. Azithromycin, an azalide antibiotic approved by the FDA on November 1, is licensed to Pfizer by the Yugoslavian company Pliva. Pfizer is responsible for reporting all available data on the drug to the FDA as soon as it is available, regardless of drug source.

Based on a preliminary review of the data, the 19 patients would not have received azithromycin in U.S. clinical studies, Gasperino said. The patients could have had microorganisms known not to be susceptible to azithromycin or could have had underlying diseases. "The fatalities were not azithromycin-related," he said.

FDA spokesperson Eva Kemper confirmed that the patients were too ill to have received azithromycin or erythromycin under normal circumstances.

After it received the new information, the company immediately contacted the FDA and offered not to market or promote the drug until after the FDA examined the data, Kemper said. "They (Pfizer) acted very responsibly."

[The symposium "The New Azalides: Pharmacology and Therapeutics," scheduled for December 11 at ASHP's Midyear Clinical Meeting, was cancelled, presumably as part of Pfizer's effort not to promote the drug.]

Gasperino said the company was ready to launch the drug, also known by the brand name Zithromax, when the new data arrived. Pfizer does not expect any changes to the already-approved label for azithromycin. The patient cases are being evaluated in the context of the approved labeling for upper- or lower-respiratory-tract in-

Continued on page 220

Continued from page 218

fections, he said. The company hopes to launch its product by March.

Kemper said the data review is being expedited; however, no firm date has been set for finalizing the review and issuing an opinion.

Details on the patients are considered confidential information by Pfizer and the FDA.

FDA warns of overdose risk from dosage cups

FDA has warned that a serious risk of accidental overdose exists for products packaged with drug delivery devices such as cups, spoons, or droppers that have misleading markings or markings that are incompatible with the directions for use. Problems cited by FDA include the provision of dosage cups with capacities that greatly exceed the recommended dosage, the use of abbreviations on dosage cups that are not used in the directions for use, and the provision of dosage cups with multiple graduated scales (e.g., scales for teaspoonfuls and tablespoonfuls, milliliters, and drams) when the dosage directions are given for one scale only (e.g., teaspoonfuls). According to FDA, numerous reports of accidental overdoses involving pediatric oral liquid acetaminophen products and cough and cold products have been attributed to problems such as these.

FDA has asked drug establishments to review the labeling of all drug products packaged with a drug delivery device to determine if incompatibilities exist and to make corrections where necessary.

FDA seizes cold sterilizing solution

The FDA, Environmental Protection Agency, and Federal Trade Commission have taken steps to begin a mandatory recall of Sporicidin cold sterilizing solution (Sporicidin Company, Rockville, MD), a product used to sterilize or disinfect medical instruments, equipment, and fiberoptics used in endoscopic surgery, anesthesiology, and respiratory therapy. The manufacturing firm failed to obtain FDA clearance to market the sterilizing solution, and subsequent investigations have shown that the product failed effectiveness tests. Sporicidin cold sterilizing solution and Sporicidin-HD are covered by the cease and desist order. These two products plus Sporicidin brand disinfectant solution, Sporicidin brand disinfectant spray, and Sporicidin disinfectant towelettes were involved in the seizure action.

Pamidronate released for management of hypercalcemia of malignancy

An intravenous formulation of pamidronate disodium (Aredia, Ciba-Geigy) has been approved by FDA for the management of moderate or severe hypercalcemia associated with malignancy. Pamidronate, a biphosphonate, inhibits bone resorption.

In one study, 64% of patients treated with pamidronate had decreases in serum calcium concentration by 24 hours after the start of therapy. About 61% of patients receiving a 60-mg dose had normal corrected serum calcium concentrations seven days after the start of therapy, and all of the patients receiving a 90-mg dose had normal concentrations at seven days. Pamidronate is effective in patients with or without bone metastases.

Transient, mild temperature elevations were noted in 27% of clinical trial participants who received pamidronate. Catheter-site reactions were reported in 18% of patients receiving a 90-mg dose.

The dosage should be determined on the basis of the serum calcium concentration: 60–90 mg if the corrected calcium concentration is 12–13.5 mg/dL and 90 mg if the corrected calcium concentration is >13.5 mg/dL. The dose should be infused intravenously over 24 hours.

Each vial of Aredia contains 30 mg of lyophilized pamidronate disodium with mannitol. The vials are packaged four to a carton.

Quinapril marketed as antihypertensive agent

Quinapril hydrochloride (Accupril, Parke-Davis), a once-a-day angiotensin-converting-enzyme inhibitor, has received FDA approval for the treatment of hypertension.

Quinapril is at least 60% absorbed after oral administration. It is converted to an active metabolite, quinaprilat, and other inactive compounds. Quinaprilat is eliminated primarily by renal excretion. Quinaprilat has an elimination half-life of about 2 hours, with a prolonged terminal half-life of 25 hours.

Therapy with quinapril is generally well tolerated. The adverse-effect profile is similar to those of other angiotensin-converting-enzyme inhibitors. Simultaneous administration of tetracycline and quinapril reduces the absorption of tetracycline by 28–37%.

The recommended starting dosage in patients not receiving diuretics is 10 mg once daily. A dosage of 20, 40, or 80 mg given once daily or in two divided doses is required by most patients. The starting dosage should be reduced in patients with renal insufficiency and those continuing diuretic therapy.

Accupril is available as 5-mg tablets in bottles of 90 and as 10- and 20-mg tablets in bottles of 90 and unit dose packages of 100.

False-positive viral antibody test results reported in influenza vaccine recipients

According to a statement released by FDA on December 18, approximately 90 blood donors at more than 20 blood establishments have reacted to tests used to screen for antibodies to human immunodeficiency virus type 1, hepatitis C, and human T-lymphotropic virus type 1. Subsequent tests showed these reactions to be false-positive results. According to FDA, preliminary investigations have shown that at least 60% of these prospective blood donors had recently been vaccinated against influenza, 2% denied having received influenza vaccine, and the vaccination history of the other donors was not known. FDA is working with the manufacturers of the influenza vaccine and the antibody test kits to determine the cause of the false-positive reactions.

News Briefs

• **An oral formulation of ketorolac tromethamine** (Toradol, Syntex) has been approved for marketing. The new product should be available in March.

• **Butorphanol tartrate** (Stadol, Mead Johnson) is now available as a nasal spray.

• Labeled indications for **cimetidine hydrochloride** (Tagamet, SmithKline Beecham) have been expanded to include use as a 50-mg/hr continuous intravenous infusion for prevention of upper gastrointestinal bleeding in critically ill hospitalized patients.

• Labeled indications for **leucovorin calcium** (Lederle) have been expanded to include use in combination with fluorouracil for therapy of advanced colorectal cancer; leucovorin is given to enhance the cytotoxic effects of fluorouracil.

• FDA has withdrawn approval for **nylidrin hydrochloride** (Arlidin, Rorer) because substantial evidence of efficacy for the drug's labeled indications (treatment of peripheral vascular disease and treatment of certain disturbances of the inner ear) is lacking.

Upcoming Specialty Meetings

Fifth National Forum on AIDS, Hepatitis, and Other Blood-Borne Diseases. Atlanta, GA, March 29–April 1; contact National Foundation for Infectious Diseases, 4733 Bethesda Avenue, Bethesda, MD 20814.

Malnutrition in the Hospitalized Patient: A New Era of Therapeutic Intervention. Boston, MA, May 6–8; contact Harvard Medical School, 641 Huntington Avenue, Boston, MA 02117; 617-432-1525.

Second Annual Review and Update Course in Cardiovascular Medicine. Chicago, IL, May 7–9; contact Svetlana Lisanti, Conference Administrator, Center for Bio-Medical Communication, Inc., 80 West Madison Avenue, Dumont, NJ 07628; 201-385-8080.

Pulsatile Drug Delivery—Current Applications and Future Trends. Königswinter/Bonn, Germany, May 20–22; contact APV, International Association for Pharmaceutical Technology, Hafenstrasse 23, D-6500 Mainz, Germany; 06131-677812, (fax) 06131-613391.

International Congress for Infectious Diseases. Nairobi, Kenya, June 7–11; contact International Society for Infectious Diseases, 180 Longwood Avenue, Boston, MA 02115; 617-432-2270, (fax) 617-731-1541.

American Diabetes Association. San Antonio, TX, June 18–23; contact ADA, 1660 Duke Street, Alexandria, VA 22314; 703-549-1500.

Endocrine Society. San Antonio, TX, June 24–27; contact A. Singer, 9650 Rockville Pike, Bethesda, MD 20814; 301-571-1802.

Letters

The Letters *column is a forum for rapid exchange of ideas among readers of* Clinical Pharmacy. *Liberal criteria are applied in the review of submissions to encourage contributions to this column.*

The Letters *column includes the following types of contributions: (1) comments, addenda, and minor updates on previously published work, (2) alerts on potential problems related to drug therapy or clinical research, (3) observations or comments on trends in drug therapy or clinical research, and (4) brief expressions of opinion about controversies in drug therapy or clinical research.*

Letters need not be submitted with the journal's manuscript checklist. The following conditions, however, must be adhered to: (1) the body of the letter must be no longer than two typewritten pages, (2) the use of references, tables, and illustrations should be minimized, (3) the authors' names, affiliations, and mailing addresses must be typed at the end of the letter in the format used by Clinical Pharmacy, *and (4) the entire letter (including references, tables, and authors' names) must be typed double-spaced on plain white paper (not letterhead). Following acceptance of a letter, the authors are required to sign an exclusive publication statement and a copyright transferal form.*

Diffuse rash associated with transdermal fentanyl

We present what we believe is the first report of diffuse rash associated with transdermal fentanyl.

A 57-year-old white woman with metastatic lung carcinoma complained of diffuse, unrelenting pain in the area of a pulmonary mass. Her medications included prochlorperazine rectal suppositories and levothyroxine, alprazolam, and dexamethasone oral tablets. Past use of codeine and meperidine had caused nausea, vomiting, and hyperactivity. Transdermal fentanyl was selected for pain control because of its convenient dosage interval (three days) and because the patient and her family were reluctant to have morphine prescribed.

Therapy was begun with one 25-μg/hr transdermal fentanyl patch (Duragesic-25, Janssen Pharmaceutica) applied every 72 hours. The application site alternated between the right and left anterior chest. The 25-μg/hr dosage was effective initially, but on the 17th day of fentanyl therapy the patient complained of increasing pain. The dosage was doubled by applying two 25-μg/hr patches (one next to the other). The morning after the dosage change, the patient awoke covered with nonpruritic reddish-purple macular papules; only her face and scalp were spared. The fentanyl patches were removed, and the patient was given 50 mg of diphenhydramine hydrochloride orally, followed by 25 mg orally every four hours. The rash disappeared over the next three days.

Adverse effects mentioned in the product information for transdermal fentanyl include rash, application-site reactions (erythema, papules, itching, edema), exfoliative dermatitis, and pustule formation.[1] To date, transdermal-fentanyl-associated skin reactions described in the medical literature have been limited to those occurring at the site of patch application. Gourley et al.[2] evaluated the use of transdermal fentanyl in 13 surgical patients. Eight patients had skin erythema that appeared one hour after patch removal at the application site, and two patients reported a rash at the vicinity of the patch margin closest to their surgical incision. The authors speculated that the rash resulted from prolonged contact of the patch with the iodophor solution used for skin disinfection. Caplan et al.[3] evaluated transdermal fentanyl for postoperative pain relief and reported that local erythema was evident one hour after patch removal in 13 of 22 patients.

Local skin reactions, such as contact dermatitis, are not uncommon with transdermal drug therapy and often appear several months after therapy is begun.[4-6] Systemic adverse reactions may also follow the application of transdermal dosage forms. Adverse reactions to such products have been attributed to the drug as well as to the patch adhesive and drug vehicle. We could not determine whether the reaction in our patient was caused by the increased drug dosage or by the increased exposure to nondrug constituents of the patches.

Clinicians should be aware that skin reactions to transdermal fentanyl may not be limited to the application site.

1. Janssen Pharmaceutica. Duragesic package insert. Piscataway, NJ; 1991 Jan.
2. Gourley GK, Kowalski SR, Plummer JL et al. The transdermal administration of fentanyl in the treatment of postoperative pain: pharmacokinetics and pharmacodynamic effects. *Pain.* 1989; 37:193-202.
3. Caplan RA, Ready LB, Oden RV et al. Transdermal fentanyl for postoperative pain management. *JAMA.* 1989; 261:1036-9.
4. Boekhorst JC. Allergic contact dermatitis with transdermal clonidine. *Lancet.* 1983; 1:1031-2.
5. Rosenfeld AS, White WB. Allergic contact dermatitis secondary to transdermal nitroglycerin. *Am Heart J.* 1984; 108:1061-2.
6. Schwartz BK, Clendenning WE. Allergic contact dermatitis from hydroxypropyl cellulose in a transdermal estradiol patch. *Contact Dermatitis.* 1988; 18:106-7.

CHERYL A. STOUKIDES, PHARM.D., Director
University of Rhode Island Drug Information Center

MARY STEGMAN, M.D.
Department of Oncology

Roger Williams Medical Center
825 Chalkstone Avenue
Providence, RI 02908

Therapy Reviews

Gram-negative sepsis, the sepsis syndrome, and the role of antiendotoxin monoclonal antibodies

STEVEN L. BARRIERE AND B. JOSEPH GUGLIELMO

Abstract: The incidence and mortality, pathogenesis, clinical manifestations, and management of sepsis and the sepsis syndrome are reviewed, and the use of antiendotoxin monoclonal antibodies to treat patients with sepsis is discussed.

The sepsis syndrome and septic shock are induced by the presence of endotoxin, a lipopolysaccharide found in the outer membrane of gram-negative bacteria. Proper management of gram-negative sepsis includes appropriate antimicrobial therapy, fluids and electrolytes, nutritional support, administration of vasopressors, and mechanical ventilation if necessary.

To date, two antiendotoxin monoclonal antibodies have been produced and subjected to extensive clinical testing. HA-1A, a human cell line-derived monoclonal immunoglobulin M (IgM) antibody that contains only a small fragment of murine protein, was tested in one trial. HA-1A significantly reduced mortality in patients with sepsis and gram-negative bacteremia and produced better resolution of major morbidities than placebo in those patients. E5, an IgM antibody produced entirely via murine monoclonal antibody technology, was evaluated in two trials. Results from the first trial showed that E5 significantly reduced mortality in patients with gram-negative infection who were not in refractory shock. In contrast, results from the second trial did not show any significant reduction in mortality among patients with gram-negative infection who received E5. However, resolution of major morbidities occurred more frequently among E5 recipients in both trials. HA-1A and E5 were both well tolerated in the trials. The cost of therapy is expected to be $3000–$4000 per treatment course.

The antiendotoxin monoclonal antibodies represent the next step along the path toward important reductions in morbidity and mortality from gram-negative infection. However, the financial implications of the use of HA-1A and E5 are enormous, and stringent patient selection criteria for administration of these products will have to be developed.

Index terms: Antibodies; Bacterial infections; HA-1A; Immunotherapy; Sepsis; Shock; Xomen-E5
Clin Pharm. 1992; 11:223-35

Sepsis, septicemia, the sepsis syndrome, and septic shock are terms often used interchangeably by clinicians. However, confusion arises when these terms are used in the context of management and outcome prognosis, because their meanings may be quite different. It has been proposed that "sepsis" be defined as clinical evidence of infection with tachypnea, tachycardia, and hyperthermia (or hypothermia).[1,2] Caution must be taken in evaluating these findings in a patient receiving antipyretics or β-adrenergic-blocking agents. Early recognition of sepsis is crucial so that appropriate management can be instituted to prevent the progression to frank septic shock. Once a patient has developed signs of decreased end organ perfusion, his or her condition is referred to as sepsis syndrome. In this setting, in the absence of other clinical conditions that may produce volume depletion (diarrhea, dehydration) or decreased blood pressure (antihypertensives), hypotension is referred to as septic shock.[1] Responsiveness to fluids or vasopressors, or both, may serve as a prognostic sign for the ultimate patient outcome.

In this article we review the incidence and mortality, pathogenesis, clinical manifestations, and man-

STEVEN L. BARRIERE, PHARM.D., FCCP, is Specialist in Infectious Diseases, Department of Pharmaceutical Services, and Adjunct Professor of Medicine and Pharmacology, School of Medicine, UCLA Center for the Health Sciences, Los Angeles, CA. B. JOSEPH GUGLIELMO, PHARM.D., is Professor of Clinical Pharmacy, School of Pharmacy, University of California, San Francisco, CA.

Address reprint requests to Dr. Barriere at the UCLA Medical Center, Room 16-131 CHS, Los Angeles, CA 90024-6984.

Dr. Guglielmo and Dr. Barriere have served on a hospital pharmacy advisory board for Centocor. Dr. Barriere has received honoraria from Centocor for lectures on the management of gram-negative sepsis.

This is **article 680-204-9209** in the **ASHP Continuing-Education System**; it qualifies for 1.0 hour of continuing-education credit. See page 263 for learning objectives and test questions.

agement of sepsis and the sepsis syndrome and discuss the use of antiendotoxin monoclonal antibodies to treat patients with sepsis.

Incidence and Mortality

Sepsis and related consequences are common complications of serious bacterial infection and occur occasionally in patients with viral or fungal infections (especially those caused by *Candida* species).

Serious bacterial infection is more common today than ever before.[3,4] Current estimates indicate that there are more than 450,000 blood stream infections (septicemia) in the United States every year. The incidence of sepsis or the sepsis syndrome appears to be rising as well. The Centers for Disease Control estimates that, in 1987, 176 of every 100,000 hospital discharge diagnoses included sepsis.[5] This figure represents an increase of nearly 140% over the incidence in 1979. The greatest increase was seen for persons over 65 years of age, in whom the incidence rose by more than 160%. Septicemia is the 13th leading cause of death in the United States and accounts for $5–10 billion in annual health care expenditures.[5]

Approximately 50% of the cases of septicemia are caused by gram-negative bacteria.[4] Septic shock is a complication of at least 50–60% of gram-negative bacteremias and 5–10% of gram-positive or fungal blood stream infections.[4] These incidence figures are expected to increase with larger numbers of immunocompromised patients, more frequent use of invasive devices or procedures, greater availability of life-sustaining technology, higher frequency of infections caused by antibiotic-resistant organisms, and the aging population.

Mortality due to gram-negative sepsis ranges from 10% to nearly 90% depending on the patient's underlying diseases, the organism producing the infection, the host response to the infection, and the antimicrobial therapy instituted.[6-14] Most studies report rates between 20% and 50%. Several recent investigations have focused on the risk factors for mortality in patients with gram-negative bacteremia.[11-14] The patient's underlying diseases, the presence of shock, and inappropriate antimicrobial therapy most often correlated with a poor prognosis. Hence, as noted above, early identification of patients with gram-negative sepsis and institution of appropriate therapy are essential to minimizing the mortality from the infection.

Pathogenesis

An explanation of the mechanisms and pathogenesis of sepsis and its consequences is essential for understanding the role of therapeutic modalities apart from antimicrobial agents. Moreover, interactions between antimicrobials and microorganisms may have an important effect on the evolution of the sepsis syndrome in infected patients.[15]

After establishment of a nidus of infection, the events that lead to sepsis are multifactorial and interrelated in a highly complex fashion (Figure 1). Certain structural components of the organism (lipopolysaccharide, peptidoglycan, teichoic acid, or various exotoxins) are capable of activating macrophages, neutrophils, and the complement and coagulation cascades.[4,16] In gram-negative bacteria, the substance responsible for this activation is the core or innermost region of cell membrane lipopolysaccharide (endo-

Figure 1. Sequence of events leading from release of endotoxin to establishment of sepsis syndrome. GM-CSF = granulocyte–macrophage colony-stimulating factor.

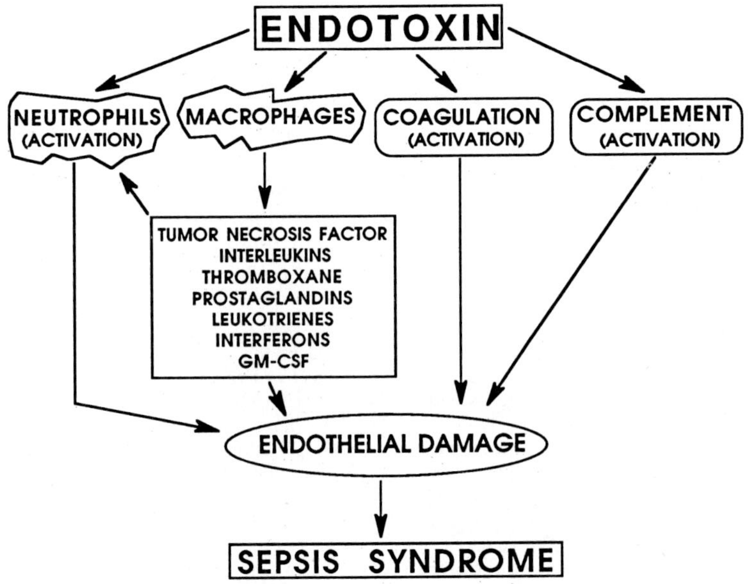

toxin).[3,4] This core is only one of the constituents of the outer cell membrane of gram-negative bacteria, which is made up of lipopolysaccharide and lipoproteins. Lipid A (the innermost region of lipopolysaccharide) is composed of a disaccharide and six long-chain fatty acids. Lipid A is the biologically active portion of the lipopolysaccharide molecule. It has direct effects on various cells, and it triggers the cascade of events that, unchecked, lead to septic shock and death.[16-18]

In response to the presence of endotoxin, macrophages produce tumor necrosis factor and various interleukins (particularly interleukin-1 and interleukin-6).[18] Additionally, there are numerous substances produced that can profoundly affect the cardiovascular system. These include platelet-activating factor, arachidonic acid metabolites, various kinins, myocardial depressant substance, endorphins, and histamine.[4] Endotoxin also may activate neutrophils, and it clearly can activate the classical complement pathway, as well as stimulate coagulation. This generalized inflammatory response is manifested as the signs and symptoms of the sepsis syndrome.

Much indirect evidence for the pathogenic role of endotoxin has been presented. When purified endotoxin is injected into animals, their response is similar to that seen in septic patients.[19] However, there is a lag period of recovery, supporting the concept that mediator activation is necessary for the initiation of the chain of events that leads to septic shock and death.

Injection of purified endotoxin into healthy humans results in metabolic and cardiovascular responses that mimic those seen in septic shock: decreased mean arterial pressure and systemic vascular resistance, increased cardiac index and heart rate, fever, arthralgias, myalgias, and headache.[4] Endotoxemia was found more than four times as frequently in patients with septic shock as those with nonseptic shock.[20] During septic shock, endotoxemia occurs frequently in the absence of gram-negative bacteremia, but multiple organ failure and myocardial depression occur 5–10 times more frequently in patients with endotoxemia.[20] Endotoxin (lipid A) directly stimulates release of tumor necrosis factor and can directly activate the classical pathway of complement.[4,21]

Although good data support the role of endotoxin in the pathogenesis of septic shock, some findings are contradictory. Mice, differing in their sensitivity to endotoxin by as much as 5000-fold, have demonstrated the same lethal response to challenge with identical doses of gram-negative bacteria.[4] Endotoxin-tolerant volunteers are not protected from clinical manifestations of experimental typhoid fever or tularemia.[22] Finally, although controversial, direct measurement of endotoxin in the blood stream does not consistently correlate with clinical manifestations and outcome of gram-negative septicemia.[20]

Danner et al.[20] attempted to clarify the incidence and importance of endotoxemia in humans. They collected serial samples of blood (every 4 hours for 24 hours) from 100 consecutive patients with septic shock who were admitted to an intensive-care unit. Endotoxin was measured with the chromogenic, limulus amoebocyte lysate (LAL) assay. Endotoxemia was detected by serial sampling in 43 patients but was detected on initial sampling in only 20 patients, underscoring the findings of inconsistency cited previously. These investigators found that the presence of endotoxemia was significantly associated with positive blood cultures (53%, endotoxemia; 25%, no endotoxemia), lactic acidemia (5.5 ± 0.8 mmol/L, endotoxemia; 3.0 ± 0.3 mmol/L, no endotoxemia); low systemic vascular resistance (456 ± 30 dyne · sec · cm^{-5}, endotoxemia; 582 ± 33 dyne · sec · cm^{-5}, no endotoxemia), and depressed left ventricular ejection fraction (34 ± 2%, endotoxemia; 45 ± 2%, no endotoxemia). Additionally, in the subset of patients with bacteremic septic shock, endotoxemia was associated with higher mortality (39%, endotoxemia; 7%, no endotoxemia). As was noted previously, endotoxemia may often be found without bacteremia; in this study only 26% of the endotoxemic patients had documented gram-negative bacteremia.[20]

At least as important as the effects of endotoxin are the effects of the numerous mediators elicited in response to endotoxin. Tumor necrosis factor and interleukins (especially interleukin-1 and interleukin-6) are the subjects of extensive research relating to the pathogenesis and management of septic shock.[21,23,24] Administration of tumor necrosis factor to animals and healthy humans results in a syndrome identical to that observed after administration of endotoxin.[19,25] It has been demonstrated that tumor necrosis factor and interleukin-1 administered concomitantly to animals are synergistic in their effects.[23] Blockade of the effects of these substances by antibodies, receptor antagonists, or soluble analogues is effective at reducing the mortality from sepsis in experimental animals.[26] Ongoing investigations are assessing the effectiveness of these modalities in infected humans who have the sepsis syndrome.

Clinical Manifestations

The diagnoses of sepsis and septic shock would be evident in a patient with fever, rigors, and hypotension. However, the manifestations of sepsis are protean, and in some patients the clinical clues may be subtle.[27]

Fever. Fever is the most common finding, although hypothermia may be present. Endotoxin and other bacterial substances stimulate monocytes and macrophages to produce the so-called endogenous pyrogens: tumor necrosis factor, interleukin-1, and alpha interferon.[4,16,17] Tumor necrosis factor may be directly pyrogenic and also induces the release of interleukin-1. These pyrogens elicit fever by stimulating prostaglandin E_2 synthesis in or near the hypothalamus. This results in a "reset" of the body's thermostat to a higher temperature. Although most patients are hyperthermic, some patients (especially very young, very old, or chronically debilitated individuals) may have hypothermia. The prognostic importance of low body temperature is unclear. Although experimentally elevated body temperature correlates with better outcome, there are few clinical studies to support this finding.[27]

Cardiac and Pulmonary Manifestations. There are many cardiac and pulmonary signs of sepsis, encompassing most of the telltale clinical manifestations by which the sepsis syndrome and septic shock are defined.

Hyperventilation may be the first sign of early sepsis. It is often accompanied by respiratory alkalosis (arterial P_{CO_2} of <30 mm Hg). Tachypnea may be caused by direct effects of endotoxin or by various other endogenous mediators such as kallikreins, bradykinin, or prostaglandins. Increased respiratory drive may be due to increased cardiac output or increased lung water from alveolar capillary permeability. Arterial oxygen falls in the preshock state, probably because of ventilation–perfusion mismatching, widening of the alveolar–arterial oxygen gradient, and eventually right-to-left shunting. All these effects may occur in the absence of overt adult respiratory distress syndrome (ARDS). Sepsis is a hyperdynamic state, and the increased cardiac output compensates for decreases in systemic vascular resistance. Generalized capillary leakage and intravascular volume depletion contribute substantially to the clinical manifestations of sepsis and septic shock.

In the early shock state (sepsis syndrome), systemic vascular resistance declines markedly. This decline is thought to result from endotoxin-induced release of interleukin-1 and tumor necrosis factor, which leads to increased prostaglandin production (cyclooxygenase mediated). Interleukin-1 also apparently can inhibit vascular smooth muscle contractions. In experimental animals, the amount of circulating interleukin-1 and especially the amount of tumor necrosis factor correlate with the degree of hypotension.[28] This correlation also has been demonstrated in some human trials.[29]

Although some increase in cardiac output is observed during this phase, it is insufficient to maintain adequate perfusion. Although low systemic vascular resistance (<400 dyne · sec · cm^{-5}) may be seen in patients with early shock, generally reported values are in the range of 800 dyne · sec · cm^{-5}. The magnitude of the fall in systemic vascular resistance has not been shown to be prognostic. Some patients who die of septic shock may have higher systemic vascular resistance (profound vasoconstriction),[27] although this is generally not the case because most patients succumb to persistently low systemic vascular resistance.

In patients with septic shock, cardiac output may fall into the normal range and systemic vascular resistance may, as previously noted, rise or stabilize. Parker et al.[30] found that continued elevation of cardiac output correlated with mortality. These investigators also noted that a return to normal systemic vascular resistance and heart rate within 24 hours also correlated strongly with survival.

The myocardial depression in patients with late shock is believed to be caused by either (1) coronary hypoperfusion due to altered flow and microembolisms from disseminated intravascular coagulation (DIC), leading to ischemic myocardial dysfunction; or (2) the presence of a circulating myocardial depressant substance, the role of which has only recently been elucidated.[4] However, cardiac dysfunction is clearly mutifactorial.

Lactate accumulation begins early in patients with shock. The pathogenesis of lactic acidosis is not well understood. At least as important as anaerobic metabolism in poorly perfused tissue is inadequate removal of lactate by the kidneys and liver. A more valuable prognostic indicator than lactate concentration alone may be the ratio of lactate to pyruvate, because high lactate concentrations may be accompanied by elevated concentrations of pyruvate. These elevated pyruvate concentrations generally are not found in septic patients, in whom the combination of elevated lactic acid concentrations and low pyruvate concentrations indicates a poor prognosis.[27]

In patients with late septic shock, decreased cardiac output (or rather, failure of ventricular function to return to normal) leads to worsened acidosis and end organ failure.

The most important pulmonary manifestation of sepsis and septic shock is ARDS. ARDS (or shock lung) is manifested by refractory hypoxemia and noncompliant lungs due to increased lung water. The increased lung water is caused by increased permeability of the vascular epithelial basement membrane, accumulation of neutrophils (and their products), and perfusion of nonventilated alveoli. It has been observed that approximately 80% of sepsis-induced ARDS is due to gram-negative infection and that the incidence of ARDS in patients with gram-negative bacteremia is nearly 25%.[31] A comprehensive discussion of the pathogenesis of ARDS is beyond the scope of this review. The reader is referred to other more complete reviews.[31]

Renal Dysfunction. Renal dysfunction, which may occur in the absence of shock-induced hypoperfusion, may have numerous causes. Frank renal failure is usually attributed to hypoperfusion and resultant acute tubular necrosis.

Hematologic Findings. Although sepsis generally produces a leukocytosis with "left shift," overwhelming infection may produce neutropenia, which is prognostic of poor outcome. Additionally, functional changes occur in leukocytes, resulting in increased phagocytic and cytotoxic activities. Tumor necrosis factor, interleukin-1, and gamma interferon appear to be responsible for these alterations, and their action may be blocked by pentoxifylline.[32]

Of interest is the decrease in serum iron concentrations during sepsis, caused by binding to lactoferrin, an iron-binding protein produced by phagocytic cells. The release of iron also appears to be blocked. That may be a host defense mechanism because bacterial growth (and virulence) is enhanced in the presence of iron.[33]

The most serious hematologic manifestation of sepsis is DIC. Sepsis is the most common cause of DIC. It is produced by generation of intravascular thrombin and fibrin deposition, consumption of clotting factors and platelets, and fibrinolysis. Laboratory tests reveal thrombocytopenia, increased prothrombin time, elevated fibrin degradation products, and decreased levels of fibrinogen. The complications may be both hemorrhagic and thrombotic. Endotoxin itself appears to activate clotting through the intrinsic pathway as well as the extrinsic pathway procoagulants, and tumor necrosis factor can induce endothelial cells to produce a procoagulant.[34]

Liver Dysfunction. Liver dysfunction is common in sepsis. It is usually manifested as cholestatic jaundice, mild hyperbilirubinemia, and elevated alkaline phosphatase. Endotoxin and other endogenous mediators or immune complexes appear to be able to produce hepatocellular dysfunction.

Mental Status Changes. Finally, one of the hallmarks of the sepsis syndrome is mental status changes, including confusion or mild disorientation, lethargy, agitation, and frank obtundation. These findings may be subtle, but they may be the only presenting signs of sepsis in the elderly. Although the pathogenesis of these mental status changes is unclear, they may be due to altered amino acid metabolism or decreased cerebral blood flow that alters the blood–brain barrier.[27]

Other Manifestations. The foregoing signs are not all inclusive and do not encompass the various other metabolic, gastrointestinal, or cutaneous manifestations of sepsis and septic shock. However, they are the most common clinical findings and serve to characterize the septic patient and differentiate sepsis from other causes of hypotension such as cardiogenic shock and anaphylaxis.

Management of Sepsis and Septic Shock

The overall management of the septic patient is beyond the scope of this review. However certain points need to be emphasized. Antiendotoxin monoclonal antibodies are adjunctive to antimicrobials, fluid and electrolyte management, and other supportive care. They are not a substitute for nutritional support, mechanical ventilation, vasoactive compounds (e.g., dopamine, dobutamine), and the appropriate management of other complications or predisposing conditions of gram-negative sepsis.[21,24]

Appropriate empirical antimicrobial therapy has repeatedly been shown to have an important impact on mortality in patients with gram-negative bacteremia. Kreger et al.[35] summarized the experience from the 1950s to the 1970s and showed that appropriate empirical therapy resulted in an average of 22% mortality, whereas in patients who received inappropriate antimicrobial therapy the mortality rate was more than 40%. These data were derived from an era when the potent, broad-spectrum bactericidal antimicrobials available today were nonexistent. However, recent findings from the University of Miami show that early administration of appropriate antimicrobials to patients with the sepsis syndrome produced important benefits compared with inappropriate or even delayed appropriate therapy.[36] These benefits included decreased mortality, reduced intensive-care-unit and hospital stay, and less morbidity. Thus, even in the 1990s it is essential that antimicrobials for the septic patient be carefully selected based on the likelihood of various causative organisms from the putative source of infection.

For nearly 20 years corticosteroids given in high doses were thought to be beneficial in patients with sepsis.[37] This belief was derived from experimental animal data that suggested that administration of corticosteroids before bacterial challenge resulted in blockade of the production of tumor necrosis factor and various interleukins by macrophages.[38] However, once these mediators and cytokines were produced, corticosteroids were of no benefit.

The question of whether corticosteroids are beneficial in patients with sepsis was resolved by the recently published results of two large-scale prospective investigations.[39,40] Both studies found that high-dose corticosteroids (dexamethasone or methylprednisolone) were of no benefit either in treating patients with septic shock or in preventing the development of shock in patients with sepsis. Moreover, in certain patients, high-dose corticosteroids were found to be detrimental in terms of increased morbidity and mortality.[40] Other subsequent investigations have shown similar results with regard to lack of effectiveness in resolving other complications of sepsis (e.g., ARDS).[41]

A number of other adjunctive therapies for sepsis are undergoing active clinical or animal investigation.[38] These include pentoxifylline, nonsteroidal anti-inflammatory agents (cyclo-oxygenase inhibitors), an interleukin-1 receptor antagonist, and monoclonal antibodies to tumor necrosis factor. Also being investigated is the role of soluble analogues of certain mediators and endogenous peptides (e.g., bactericidal permeability-increasing protein and "defensins"[42]) in the pathogenesis and resolution of sepsis and septic shock. Therefore, the treatment of this syndrome continues to evolve.

Early Attempts at Immunotherapy

It has long been recognized that elevated levels of circulating antiendotoxin antibody (immunoglobulin M [IgM] or IgG) correlated with survival in patients with gram-negative infection. A study published nearly 20 years ago reported that bacteremic patients with elevated titers of anti-O antibody or anti-Re antibody (antibodies directed at the outer [O] antigen or the core of lipopolysaccharide [rough endothelium]) had reduced mortality rates.[43] Pollack et al.[44] also showed that elevated amounts of circulating antiendotoxin IgG and IgM correlated significantly with decreased mortality rate from *Pseudomonas* sepsis.

One of the earliest attempts at immunotherapy was reported by Feingold and Oski[45] in 1965. A five-year-old boy with aplastic anemia developed a severe soft tissue infection and sepsis caused by *Pseudomonas aeruginosa* after a bone marrow biopsy and rapidly deteriorated. The patient was given serum harvested from another patient who had just recovered from an episode of *Pseudomonas* burn wound sepsis, with the hope that circulating antibodies to the organism might be present and beneficial. The serum was administered without major adverse effects, the patient promptly defervesced, and he went on to recover from the infection. Of course, it is unknown whether antiendotoxin antibody was responsible for the dramatic response, or whether the response was caused by one or more of a variety of substances present in this serum from the other patient. However, this case serves as an early example of the efforts to use antibodies in patients with gram-negative sepsis.

J5 Antiserum

In the first major trial of immunotherapy for the treatment of sepsis, Ziegler et al.[46] produced a vaccination-derived antiserum to gram-negative bacterial endotoxin. The antiserum was produced by vaccinating healthy men with a heat-inactivated mutant strain of *Escherichia coli* J5. This mutant lacks the enzyme uridine-5′-diphosphate-galactose-4-epimerase. The absence of this enzyme prevents attachment of side chains to core lipopolysaccharide. Thus, lipopolysaccharide from the J5 mutant consists of lipid A and the core determinants: *N*-acetylglucosamine, 2-keto-3-deoxyoctonate, heptose, and glucose. Importantly, the lipid A moiety of gram-negative bacilli is remarkably similar among most species of gram-negative bacteria. Therefore, antibody produced to the J5-mutant endotoxin core also binds endotoxin of other gram-negative bacteria. After vaccination with the J5 mutant, the serum of the volunteers was harvested for use in the clinical study.

Patients were included in the trial "if they were severely ill, with recent deterioration in the form of sudden high fever or hypothermia, hypotension, or unexplained respiratory distress; if there was either good clinical evidence of an infection usually caused by gram-negative bacteria or an underlying disease predisposing to gram-negative infection . . . ."[46] Patients were randomized to receive J5 antiserum or nonimmune serum intravenously over 30 minutes. A total of 304 patients were entered into the trial, of whom 191 were found to have gram-negative bacteremia. Gram-negative bacteria were isolated from infected foci in 21 other patients with presumed gram-negative bacteremia. Of the 212 patients included in the final analysis, 103 patients received J5 antiserum and 109 were given nonimmune serum.

Twenty-two of the 91 patients (24%) with positive blood cultures who received the J5 antiserum died, compared with 38 of 100 (38%) who were given normal human serum.[46] The observed decrease in mortality associated with the J5 antiserum was determined to be significant. Of note, the decrease in mortality was particularly pronounced in patients with gram-negative bacteremia and profound shock: the mortality rate was 46% in the J5 group, compared with 76% in the control group ($p < 0.01$).

Using the same J5 preparation, Baumgartner and colleagues[47] studied the prophylactic use of antiserum in surgical patients at high risk for the development of gram-negative infection. Patients initially were randomized to receive J5 immune serum (or plasma) or control serum (or plasma) within 24 hours of admission to the surgical intensive-care unit. Another unit of serum or plasma was administered every five days thereafter, as long as patients remained at high risk for infection or had evidence of serious infection. Additional control or J5 immune plasma also was given to patients requiring 2 L or more of blood or plasma as a result of blood loss. Use of the antiserum, particularly in patients undergoing abdominal surgery, significantly reduced the incidence of shock and death in these high-risk surgical patients with gram-negative infection (3 of 71 [4%], J5 group; 22 of 83 [27%], control group; $p = 0.01$). Not surprisingly, administration of the J5 antiserum did not benefit the 72 patients with gram-positive or fungal infection. These results suggested a potential role for the prophylactic use of antiendotoxin antibody in certain high-risk patients.

Calandra and colleagues[48] compared the efficacy of IgG antibody to J5 (J5-IVIG) with that of standard IgG in the treatment of septic shock. Mortality from septic shock was 50% in the J5-IVIG group, compared with 49% in the control patients. Additionally, no reduction in the incidence of sepsis-associated complications was observed in the J5-IVIG group. These results suggested that antibodies other than IgG (such as IgM or other endogenous substances in the antiserum) are important in the treatment of gram-negative sepsis.

Although the results of the above studies were encouraging, broad use of the antiserum was not feasible for a variety of reasons. First, vaccination of serum donors is associated with mild toxicity, and there is no booster response with subsequent vaccination; therefore, a person could donate only once. Second, the antibody content of antiserum varies, resulting in inconsistency from lot to lot. Last, the risk of transmission of infectious agents to patients is a concern.

Antiendotoxin Monoclonal Antibodies

Because of the problems associated with the production of J5 antiserum, monoclonal antibody technology has been used, resulting in the production of large quantities of antiendotoxin antibodies.[49,50] As a result of this methodology, interlot variation is minimized and the risk of infection is eliminated.[51] To date, two antiendotoxin monoclonal antibodies have been produced and subjected to extensive clinical testing. HA-1A (Centoxin, Centocor) is a human cell line-derived monoclonal IgM antibody that contains only a small fragment of murine protein (J chain) accounting for about 3% of the total molecular weight,[52] whereas E5 (Xomen-E5, Xoma) is an IgM antibody produced entirely via murine monoclonal antibody technology.[53]

Teng et al.[52] attempted to document the benefit and specificity of human monoclonal IgM antibodies directed against endotoxin in an animal model of gram-negative sepsis. Development of a positive dermal Schwartzman reaction in rabbits and immunoprotection against lethal gram-negative bacteremia in mice were investigated. Endotoxin used for this experiment was derived from two strains of bacteria: *E. coli* 0111:B4 and an isolate of *Klebsiella pneumoniae*. The former organism was the laboratory strain from which the J5 mutant was derived. The Schwartzman reaction was elicited by intradermal inoculation of rabbits with endotoxin, followed by a repeat intravenous dose 18 hours later. One group of rabbits received antiendotoxin monoclonal antibody two hours before the intravenous dose, and another group received a placebo. A positive reaction was skin necrosis at the site of the intradermal injection of endotoxin. Nearly all of the mice that received placebo developed a positive reaction (96.6%), compared with only 12% of those given the antibody. In the sepsis protection study, several organisms were tested: *Pseudomonas aeruginosa*, *E. coli* 0111:B4, *E. coli* 017, the isolate of *Klebsiella pneumoniae*, and *Streptococcus pneumoniae*.[54] A significant increase in the dose (number of organisms) required to produce death in 50% of the animals was observed in the antibody-treated group compared with control animals. As expected, no benefit was observed in the animals infected with *Strep. pneumoniae*. These data suggest a broad spectrum of activity for the antiendotoxin antibody with specificity for gram-negative bacteria.

In contrast to that study, other investigators have found that antisera and anti-lipid A monoclonal antibodies are ineffective in animal models of sepsis. Griesman and Johnston[54] found that the J5 antiserum failed to protect mice from a variety of wild-type, smooth, gram-negative organisms. These organisms included *E. coli* 0111:B4, *E. coli* 0127:B8, *Salmonella typhimurium*, *Salmonella minnesota*, and *Citrobacter freundii*. The antiserum was found to be protective only against the J5 core glycolipid of the *E. coli* parent strain. When O-specific antiserum was administered, consistent protection was observed. However, this effect was limited to the homologous endotoxin.[54]

Baumgartner and colleagues[55] performed a similar study using polyclonal J5 antiserum, as well as the monoclonal antibody HA-1A. Bacteria used for the experiment included the J5 parent strain of *E. coli*, its J5 mutant, and an isolate of *Ps. aeruginosa*. Endotoxemic mortality in mice and the Schwartzman reaction in rabbits were used to assess efficacy of the antibody preparations. As expected, J5 antiserum was protective against the J5 mutant strain of *E. coli*. However, neither J5 antiserum nor HA-1A was protective in animals with sepsis induced by the J5 parent strain, *E. coli* 0111:B4. Similarly, neither product was protective in animals with sepsis induced by *Ps. aeruginosa*. Equivalent numbers of positive Schwartzman reactions were observed in animals that received the antibody products and in controls. Neither antibody product prevented the production of tumor necrosis factor or interleukin-6, suggesting that the antibodies did not have the capability to prevent the interaction of endotoxin and target cells (e.g., macrophages). The latter two studies suggest that anti-lipopolysaccharide antibodies may not be cross-protective among gram-negative bacteria or various lipopolysaccharide idiotypes.[54,55]

Pharmacokinetics of HA-1A and E5

The pharmacokinetics of the antiendotoxin monoclonal antibodies have been determined in uninfected subjects and in patients suspected of having gram-negative sepsis. Wedel et al.[56] studied the disposition of E5 after a 2-mg/kg dose given intravenously to healthy subjects. Peak serum concentrations were found to be approximately 40 μg/mL, which declined to 8–9 μg/mL at 24 hours after the dose. The terminal elimination half-life was estimated to be 18 hours, and total body clearance was calculated to be 232–266 mL/hr. Harkonen et al.[57] administered a single dose of E5 to patients with suspected gram-negative sepsis and found a shorter half-life of 10.2 hours. The apparent volume of distribution in these patients ranged from 3.7 to 8.2 L, which is consistent with the expected distribution volume of IgM antibody (intravascular volume). No significant differences in half-life, volume of distribution, or clearance were observed in bacteremic patients compared with nonbacteremic patients.[57]

HA-1A was given to 15 uninfected patients with incurable malignant diseases.[58] Intravenous doses ranged from 0.05 to 100 mg. Mean elimination half-life was found to be 31.5 hours, and clearance was estimated to be 1.1 mL/kg/hr. Steady-state volume of distribution was 46 mL/kg (10–20% larger than intravascular volume). Fisher et al.[59] administered HA-1A to 34 patients with a clinical diagnosis of sepsis syndrome in whom gram-negative infection was suspected. After administration of a 100-mg dose, the steady-state volume of distribution was 48.2 mL/kg. However, total body clearance was 2.9 mL/kg/min, greater than that observed in uninfected patients, and the elimination half-life was only 16.2 hours. As was the case in the E5 studies, no differences in disposition were observed between patients with and without bacteremia.[59]

Clinical Trials of HA-1A and E5

HA-1A Study. In a prospective, double-blind, controlled study, Ziegler et al.[60] studied the effects of HA-1A in patients with presumed gram-negative bacteremia and sepsis. Criteria for diagnosis of sepsis included the following:

1. Fever (>38.3 °C) or hypothermia (<35.6 °C);
2. Tachycardia (>90 beats per minute in the absence of β-blockade) and tachypnea (respiratory rate of >20 breaths/min or mechanical ventilation required); and
3. Either hypotension (systolic blood pressure of <90 mm Hg or a sustained drop of >40 mm Hg in the presence of adequate fluid challenge and the absence of antihypertensive agents) or two of the following signs of systemic toxicity or peripheral hypoperfusion: unexplained metabolic acidosis, arterial hypoxemia, acute renal failure, DIC, sudden decrease in mental acuity, or high cardiac index with low systemic vascular resistance.

On the basis of these entry criteria, 543 patients were enrolled in the trial. The patients were randomized to receive a single 100-mg intravenous dose of HA-1A or human albumin placebo. Intention-to-treat analysis of data for all patients showed no reduction in mortality in those patients receiving the HA-1A compared with those receiving placebo. Of the 543 patients enrolled in the study, 200 patients had documented gram-negative bacteremia. HA-1A significantly reduced mortality in those patients with sepsis and gram-negative bacteremia but not in patients with nonbacteremic gram-negative infections. At 28 days after infusion, there were 45 deaths among the 92 placebo recipients (49%), compared with 32 deaths among the 105 patients receiving HA-1A (30%; $p = 0.014$). As was seen in the earlier J5 antiserum study, a significant reduction in mortality also was observed in those patients with septic shock (33% mortality with HA-1A versus 57% mortality with placebo; $p = 0.017$).

One or more of the major complications of sepsis (shock, DIC, acute renal failure, acute hepatic failure, ARDS) was present at the time of infusion in 123 of the 200 patients with gram-negative bacteremia. During the first seven days after treatment, all evidence of these complicating conditions resolved in 26 of 62 patients given placebo (42%) compared with 38 of 61 patients given HA-1A (62%). No reduction in morbidity or mortality was observed in patients with nonbacteremic gram-negative infection, gram-positive infection, fungal infection, or unidentified infection. The drug was well tolerated, with one patient having a transient episode of hives near the site of infusion and another patient having facial flushing and mild hypotension. No patient was found to have detectable antibody directed against HA-1A. In summary, HA-1A appeared to significantly reduce the morbidity and mortality in patients with gram-negative bacteremia and sepsis.

E5 Studies. The E5 antiendotoxin antibody also has been studied in patients with sepsis.[61] The inclusion criteria differed somewhat from the HA-1A trial and included any two of the following: (1) fever (>38 °C) or hypothermia (<35 °C), (2) a white blood cell count of >12,000/cu mm or <3,000/cu mm or >20% bands, (3) positive blood culture for a gram-negative rod within the preceding 48 hours, and (4) presence of a known or suspected site of gram-negative infection.

A septic response was considered to have occurred when, in addition to the suspected infection, at least one of the following was present: (1) hypotension (systolic blood pressure of <90 mm Hg or an acute drop of 30 mm Hg), (2) metabolic acidosis, (3) decreased systemic vascular resistance, (4) tachypnea (respiratory rate of >20 breaths/min or minute ventilation of >10 L/min if patient is receiving mechanical ventilation), (5) unexplained renal failure, (6) acutely altered sensorium, or (7) DIC.

Patients received a 2-mg/kg intravenous dose of E5 antiendotoxin antibody or an identical-appearing placebo within eight hours of meeting entry criteria. A second infusion was given approximately 24 hours after the first dose. Of 486 patients entered in the trial, 316 had confirmed gram-negative sepsis. Of those 316 patients, 171 had bacteremia. As was the case in the HA-1A trial, analysis of all patients with sepsis revealed no decrease in mortality. Additionally, no difference in mortality was observed in those patients in whom no gram-negative infection was documented. However, in those patients who had gram-negative sepsis but who were not in refractory shock, the 14-day mortality was significantly reduced in the E5 group (12%) compared with the placebo group (23%). This benefit was observed in patients with and without concomitant bacteremia.

As was the case in the HA-1A trial, major morbidities at study entry (e.g., DIC, ARDS) appeared more likely to resolve with antiendotoxin treatment. However, the evaluation was based on numbers of episodes of morbidity, not on numbers of patients with one or more morbidities, as in the HA-1A trial. No benefit of E5 was observed in those patients with gram-negative sepsis who were in refractory shock. It is not possible to compare that group of patients with a similar group from the HA-1A trial, because patients in shock that was unresponsive to fluids were not enumerated in the HA-1A study.

The E5 antibody was well tolerated, with two patients developing rashes, one developing hypotension, and one developing an anaphylactoid reaction.[61] Of note, 47% of those patients who received the E5 antibody developed detectable IgG human antimurine antibody (HAMA) titers. Considering that antiendotoxin monoclonal antibodies are foreign proteins, they may be immunogenic. Formation of antibodies to these products might be expected to result in allergic responses, lack of efficacy in patients previously exposed to murine monoclonal antibody products (e.g., muromonab-CD3), or diminished antiendotoxin effects with repeated doses.

The incidence and importance of a HAMA response to E5 were studied by Kunz et al.[62] They examined data on the HAMA response from four different E5 studies and noted a 48% incidence. When the magnitude of the response was evaluated, only 4% of the determinations were found to be high titer (higher than 1:10,000). Interestingly, 8% of placebo recipients were found to have developed a HAMA response. Among four patients who developed allergic reactions in the E5 trial, two had a HAMA response. It would appear that the HAMA response does not correlate with allergic reactions to E5. It is unknown whether a high-titer HAMA response would result in diminished effectiveness of repeated doses of E5. This diminished effectiveness, however, has been observed with muromonab-CD3 in cases of renal transplant rejection.[63] HA-1A is primarily a human monoclonal antibody product, and no human antihuman antibody response has been detected thus far.[60] It is unknown whether any human antimurine antibody develops against the J chain portion of HA-1A, which is the only murine segment of the molecule.

The sensitivity of the assays for detection of antibodies to HA-1A and E5 appears to differ markedly. Therefore, it is possible that a low-level antibody response to HA-1A may have occurred.

In a second multicenter trial assessing the efficacy of E5, Wenzel et al.[64] randomized 847 patients to receive E5 or placebo, using the same dosage regimen employed in the first trial, as well as similar enrollment criteria. In contrast to the first trial, however, patients in shock were excluded from the study, because this subset of patients did not benefit from E5. In this second trial, 811 patients were evaluable, and 530 were found to have gram-negative sepsis. Failure of one or more major organs was found in 139 patients at the time of enrollment. These included ARDS (n = 52), acute renal failure (n = 73), and DIC (n = 40). Of the 530 patients with gram-negative sepsis, no decrease in mortality was observed in the E5 group compared with the placebo group (30% versus 26%, respectively).[64] Similarly, the 139 patients with major organ failures and gram-negative sepsis did not benefit from E5 administration (E5, 41% mortality; placebo, 47% mortality). However, major organ failures were "cured" more frequently in the E5 recipients than in those who received placebo (48% versus 25%, respectively; p = 0.005). Trends favoring E5 were observed in patients with DIC and ARDS, but were significant only in cases of acute renal failure (63% response to E5 versus 29% response to placebo; p = 0.004).

E5 also was found to be effective in preventing the development of major organ failures in the 530 patients with gram-negative sepsis. Significantly fewer episodes of ARDS developed in the E5 recipients (3%) compared with the placebo recipients (9%). Similarly, sepsis-associated central nervous system dysfunction developed in only 10% of the E5 recipients compared with 19% of the placebo recipients.

These investigators also performed a meta-analysis of the effect of E5 in patients from the two trials (n = 188) who had gram-negative sepsis but not septic shock and who also had major organ failures.[64] They demonstrated a significant reduction in mortality (relative risk ratio = 1.6; p = 0.03) associated with E5 administration compared with placebo. Similarly, their analysis indicated significantly greater cure of organ failures in E5 recipients. As was observed in the first trial, E5 was well tolerated, with a 2.6% incidence of mild hypersensitivity reactions. The HAMA response was observed in 44% of the E5 recipients.

It is difficult to establish the reasons for the differing results in the three HA-1A and E5 trials. However, it should be noted that the APACHE II scores for patients in the three studies differed (although these scores are a controversial prognostic indicator). Of note, in the HA-1A trial the worst score in the 24-hour period before enrollment was used, whereas in the E5 trials, the APACHE II score calculated at study entry was used. In the first E5 trial the mean APACHE II score for all patients was 17, whereas in the HA-1A trial the score was approximately 25. These scores predict vastly different mortality rates of 10–25% and 35–50%, respectively.[65] This fact suggests that, on average, the patients in the HA-1A trial were more seriously ill.

Numerous questions remain unanswered regarding the monoclonal antiendotoxin antibodies. The products appear to reduce mortality in certain patient populations while maintaining an excellent safety profile, but they are expected to be costly (approximately $3000–4000 for a course of therapy). As a result, serious drug use and control problems may occur with these products.

Questions about Antiendotoxin Monoclonal Antibodies

What is the mechanism of action of the antiendotoxin monoclonal antibodies? As Baumgartner et al.[66] have noted, conflicting data exist regarding the benefit of the antibodies in animal models. Baumgartner et al. were unable to show that HA-1A reduced lipopolysaccharide-induced tumor necrosis factor production. In vitro, HA-1A was found to bind nonspecifically to a wide range of gram-positive bacteria and yeasts, gram-negative bacteria, and high-density lipoproteins and cardiolipin, as measured by an immunoassay.[66] As noted above, conflicting data exist regarding whether HA-1A protects animals with experimental gram-negative sepsis. Baumgartner et al. state that no data support the hypothesis that HA-1A exerts a protective effect by binding to and neutralizing the effects of endotoxin and preventing release of the mediators of septic shock. However, a subinvestigation of the HA-1A trial evaluated the presence of circulating endotoxin and the impact of this finding on patient outcome.[67] Of 82 patients tested for endotoxemia by using a variant of the chromogenic LAL assay, only 27 (33%) had detectable levels of circulating endotoxin. This value is consistent with previously reported data.[20] However, all of the observed benefit of HA-1A was in the endotoxemic patients, because mortality was 30% in those who received the antibody compared with 73% in those who received placebo.[67] These data suggest that HA-1A does somehow interact with endotoxin to exert beneficial effects. Further investigations are needed to more precisely elucidate the mechanism of action of these products.

Who should receive antiendotoxin antibody therapy? For unclear reasons, the results of the HA-1A and E5 trials suggest that the products are effective in different patient populations. Both products have demonstrated efficacy in patients with gram-negative bacteremia and sepsis who are not in shock. HA-1A appears to reduce mortality in patients with gram-negative bacteremia and shock (hypotension), whereas E5 does not appear to be beneficial in patients with shock (hypotension unresponsive to fluids or vasopressors, or both). Conversely, the first E5 trial suggested that the product was effective in patients who had gram-negative sepsis without positive blood cultures, whereas HA-1A was not shown to be effective in this group. In the second E5 trial, E5 was ineffective at reducing mortality in patients who were not in shock. These differences in observed efficacy may be due to the fact that HA-1A is primarily a human monoclonal antibody, whereas E5 is murine derived. The differing outcomes are more likely due to differences in study design and definitions among the three investigations. As outlined previously, important differences in patient inclusion criteria existed in the three studies. Furthermore, differences in the definition of shock may have existed between the two trials, making direct comparison difficult. In general, both trials required adequate fluid resuscitation attempts for the diagnosis of shock to be made. However, the definition of fluid volume, use of vasopressors, and magnitude of blood pressure decline differed between studies or could not be ascertained from the published data.

Based on the results of the studies, the HA-1A product may be used in patients with documented septic shock. At the present time, the E5 antibody cannot be recommended in this patient population (at least in those patients with refractory shock). In those patients who are not in shock and who are presumed to have sepsis, the decision of who to treat becomes more difficult. One potential solution is to treat only those patients who fit the inclusion criteria of the respective studies. The individual hospital's patient populations, incidence of gram-negative bacteremia, and incidence of sepsis and septic shock must be carefully assessed. This analysis will assist in the identification of patients who are most likely to benefit from treatment with one of the antibodies. Some institutions may elect to give these products only to patients with microbiologically documented infection who have the sepsis syndrome. Others may require more or less stringent criteria for use.

One confounding finding from the first E5 trial is that patients with sepsis but without positive blood cultures had an associated reduction in mortality, although the difference did not reach significance because of small numbers. This finding was observed in neither the HA-1A trial nor the second E5 trial. It is difficult to reconcile these discordant results.

Another potential solution for patients who are not in shock and are presumed to have gram-negative sepsis would be to reserve the use of the products for those patients with documented positive blood cultures. Certain microbiology laboratory systems (BacT/Alert Microbial Detection System, Organon Teknika) that use a carbon dioxide detection system are reported to detect approximately 85% of Enterobacteriaceae in blood culture within 12 hours.[68,a] However, only 30% of nonfermenters (e.g., *Pseudomonas, Acinetobacter*) are detected within this time frame.

Data from the HA-1A trial indicate that the median time from enrollment in the trial to actual administration of the product was approximately 14 hours.[60] It is unknown whether delay in antibody administration affects outcome. This information is confusing, considering the experimental data that suggest that the drug must be administered immediately for it to be beneficial. Nevertheless, the lack of correlation between outcome and time of administration in the HA-1A trial suggests that administration of the antiendotoxin antibody only after documentation of positive blood cultures may be a reasonable approach in patients who are not in shock. Many hospital microbiology laboratories do not have new detection systems or lack 24-hour microbiology laboratory services. Therefore, this potential solution may be rather limited. Moreover, given the pathogenesis of septic shock and the rapidity with which events develop, delay in administration of antiendotoxin antibody may be detrimental.

The putative optimal use of these products is in the patient who has signs and symptoms of sepsis and who is endotoxemic.[67] That suggests that serum endotoxin assays may be useful in patient selection. The problem is that commercially available LAL assays are not highly specific; other proteins and antigen–antibody complexes may produce positive test results. The other issue is the timing of sampling. Endotoxin rapidly disappears from the circulation. Therefore, a patient who is actually endotoxemic may have a negative LAL test because of sampling error. Until a more sensitive and specific assay becomes readily available and can be used at the bedside, results of the current assay must be evaluated with caution.[69]

Certain patient populations either are not likely to

benefit from the administration of either antibody or have not been adequately studied. Therefore, the utility of either product is unknown for these patients at the present time. They include bone marrow and organ transplant recipients, patients with the acquired immunodeficiency syndrome, neutropenic cancer patients, patients with burns, patients with massive hemorrhage requiring blood transfusions, and children. Finally, patients with underlying diseases that are likely to be fatal within the short term are not candidates to receive these products.

What is the appropriate dosage regimen of the antibody? The HA-1A trial used a single 100-mg dose of antiendotoxin antibody, and a two-dose (2 mg/kg each dose) regimen was used in the E5 studies. IgM antibody, including the antiendotoxins, primarily is distributed in the vascular space, with a volume of distribution of approximately 45–50 mL/kg.[70] Considering that little variation exists in plasma volume among patients, it probably is not critical to calculate the dose of HA-1A on the basis of body weight. It is unknown whether smaller doses are as effective as larger doses in reducing morbidity and mortality. It also is not known whether larger doses are more efficacious than the studied doses, although such trials are under way. As a result, doses other than those used in the clinical trials cannot be recommended in the treatment of patients with gram-negative sepsis. In addition, whereas experience with the J5 antiserum suggests potential benefit in high-risk surgical patients, prophylactic use of the monoclonal antibody products is not recommended at this time.

The half-life of normal IgM is approximately five days.[70] In stable cancer patients the documented half-life of HA-1A is 32 hours, whereas in septic patients the half-life of HA-1A is shorter, approximately 16 hours.[59] This observed reduction in half-life is due to an increase in clearance. As noted above, septic patients have a documented clearance of 2.8 mL/kg/hr, which contrasts with 1.1 mL/kg/hr in uninfected cancer patients.[58,59] The observed increased clearance and decreased half-life in septic patients suggest that repetitive dosing may be indicated. Moreover, administration of bactericidal antimicrobials that produce cell lysis (β lactams, aminoglycosides, fluoroquinolones) has been shown to dramatically increase free circulating endotoxin concentrations in experimental animal models of sepsis.[71,72] This result suggests that the antiendotoxin antibodies should be given before antimicrobials if possible and that in certain situations repeated doses may be indicated. However, until studies are performed that document the benefit of repeated doses of these products, additional doses (more than one 100-mg dose of HA-1A or two 2-mg/kg doses of E5) cannot be recommended.

How should the antiendotoxin monoclonal antibody products be controlled? Considering the potential benefit, lack of toxicity, and considerable expense, use of these agents will be difficult to control. It is clear that criteria for use need to be established for each individual hospital to determine which patients should receive antiendotoxin antibody therapy. These criteria need to be based on discussion with prescribers, including specialists in such areas as critical care, infectious diseases, surgery, oncology, and other services, as well as pharmacy, microbiology, and hospital administration. Once these criteria are established, control mechanisms need to be put in place. It is our opinion that control must be multidisciplinary, using a combined pharmacist–physician system. The difficulty in diagnosing a patient with sepsis, including noninfectious diagnoses (e.g., hypovolemia, cardiogenic shock), mandates physician evaluation before release of the drug. In addition, ongoing drug-use evaluation should take place to determine whether these agents are being used appropriately.

What is the likely cost impact of the antiendotoxin monoclonal antibody products? As stated previously, the cost of therapy is expected to be $3000–4000 per treatment course (one dose of HA-1A or two doses of E5). Thus, the fiscal impact is likely to be substantial, potentially resulting in expenditures of millions of dollars per year at some hospitals. However, it is possible that the reduction in major morbidity (DIC, acute renal failure, ARDS, liver failure) associated with antiendotoxin antibody therapy may result in decreased cost because of decreased time in the intensive-care unit, less drug use, decreased need for mechanical ventilation, less hemodialysis, and so forth. Until well-designed cost–benefit analyses are performed, it is impossible to speculate as to whether these drugs will actually result in reduced costs for the hospital.

Cost-effectiveness analyses have been performed for both products, but these data have not yet been published. Under the assumption that all lives would be valued equally, cost-effectiveness analysis should assist in deciding whether the expense of these products is justified in terms of years of life saved and other quality-of-life indicators. These analyses suggest that use of HA-1A or E5 results in an expenditure of $4000–24,000 for each year of life saved.[73,b] That contrasts favorably with previously reported data that document expenditures of approximately $14,000 for each year of life saved when β blockers are used to treat hypertension and in excess of $80,000 for each year of life saved when heparin is used to prevent deep venous thrombosis.[74]

Baumgartner and colleagues[66] stated: "It seems premature to rely entirely on the results of a single clinical study (of HA-1A) before embarking on the large-scale use of such an expensive form of therapy . . . when the basic understanding of the specificity and function of the product is incomplete . . . ," and when there are still unanswered questions about the appropriate use of these products.

Conclusion

Sepsis, the sepsis syndrome, and septic shock still

produce substantial morbidity and mortality despite advances in antimicrobial therapy and supportive care. The antiendotoxin monoclonal antibody products represent the next step along the path toward important reductions in morbidity and mortality from gram-negative infection. Although both products have been found to be effective in the management of gram-negative sepsis, they appear to benefit different populations, and substantial concerns have been raised regarding their lack of overall benefit in the patient who appears "septic" but in whom the causative organism is unknown or the presence of bacteremia or endotoxemia cannot be documented. Moreover, their precise mechanism(s) of action, dosage regimens, and long-term effects (particularly from repeated doses) also are not well understood.

The financial implications for the use of HA-1A and E5 are enormous, and stringent patient selection criteria for administration of these products will have to be developed. Finally, most authorities believe that these products are only the next step in the evolution of therapies directed at the various steps in the pathogenesis of sepsis. Monoclonal antibodies directed against tumor necrosis factor, an interleukin-1 receptor antagonist, and other biotechnology-derived products are currently undergoing large-scale clinical evaluations. The consensus appears to be that combinations of these various therapeutic modalities will be most effective in minimizing the morbidity and mortality associated with sepsis and septic shock. However, these products will also likely be extremely expensive. Although the concept of using combinations of antiendotoxin monoclonal antibodies and other biotechnology-derived products for treatment of sepsis and septic shock is exciting, it is also daunting from a financial point of view. It presents a challenge to hospital pharmacists, physicians, and administrators, who must determine the appropriate, optimal, and most cost-beneficial and cost-effective use of this new technology.

---

[a]Mann L, UCLA Clinical Microbiology Laboratories. Personal communication. 1991 Jun.

[b]Smith C, M.D., Centocor. Personal communication. 1990 Sep.

References

1. Balk RA, Bone RC. The septic syndrome—definitions and clinical implications. *Crit Care Clin*. 1989; 5:1-8.
2. Bone RC. Sepsis, the sepsis syndrome, multi-organ failure: a plea for comparable definitions. *Ann Intern Med*. 1991; 114:332-3.
3. Beutler B. The explosion of septic shock. *Curr Opin Infect Dis*. 1990; 3:623-7.
4. Parillo JE, Parker MM, Natanson C et al. Septic shock in humans—advances in the understanding of pathogenesis, cardiovascular dysfunction and therapy. *Ann Intern Med*. 1990; 113:227-42.
5. Centers for Disease Control. Increase in national hospital discharge survey rates for septicemia—United States. 1979–1987. *MMWR*. 1990; 39:31-4.
6. Gransden WR, Eykyn SJ, Phillips I et al. Bacteremia due to *Escherichia coli*: a study of 861 episodes. *Rev Infect Dis*. 1990; 12:1008-18.
7. Garcia de la Torre M, Romero-Vivas J, Martinez-Beltran J et al. *Klebsiella* bacteremia: an analysis of 100 patients. *Rev Infect Dis*. 1985; 7:143-50.
8. Drelichman V, Band JD. Bacteremias due to *Citrobacter diversus* and *Citrobacter freundii*. *Arch Intern Med*. 1985; 145:1808-10.
9. Bouza E, Garcia de la Torre M, Erice A et al. Enterobacter bacteremia—an analysis of 50 episodes. *Arch Intern Med*. 1985; 145:1024-7.
10. Gallagher P, Watanakunakorn C. Pseudomonas bacteremia in a community teaching hospital, 1980–84. *Rev Infect Dis*. 1989; 11:846-52.
11. Gatell JM, Trilla A, Latorre X et al. Nosocomial bacteremia in a large Spanish teaching hospital: analysis of factors influencing prognosis. *Rev Infect Dis*. 1988; 10:203-10.
12. Roberts FJ, Geere IW, Coldman A. A three year study of positive blood cultures, with emphasis on prognosis. *Rev Infect Dis*. 1991; 13:34-46.
13. Bisbe J, Gatell JM, Puig J et al. *Pseudomonas aeruginosa* bacteremia: univariate and multivariate analyses of factors influencing the prognosis in 133 episodes. *Rev Infect Dis*. 1988; 10:629-35.
14. Hilf M, Yu VL, Sharp J et al. Antibiotic therapy for *Pseudomonas aeruginosa* bacteremia: outcome correlations in a prospective study of 200 patients. *Am J Med*. 1989; 87:540-6.
15. Bone RC, Fisher CJ, Clemmer TP et al. Sepsis syndrome: a valid clinical entity. *Crit Care Med*. 1989; 17:389-93.
16. Luce JM. Pathogenesis and management of septic shock. *Chest*. 1987; 91:883-8.
17. Jacobs RF, Tabor DR. Immune cellular interactions during sepsis and septic injury. *Crit Care Clin*. 1989; 5:9-26
18. Calandra R, Glauser MP. Cytokines and septic shock. *Diagn Microbiol Infect Dis*. 1990; 13:377-81.
19. Natanson C, Eichenholz PW, Danner RL et al. Endotoxin and tumor necrosis factor challenges in dogs simulate the cardiovascular profile of human septic shock. *J Exp Med*. 1989; 169:823-32.
20. Danner RL, Elin RJ, Hosseini JM et al. Endotoxemia in human septic shock. *Chest*. 1991; 99:169-75.
21. Rackow EC, Astiz ME. Pathophysiology and treatment of septic shock. *JAMA*. 1991; 266:548-54.
22. Greisman SE, Hornick RB, Wagner HN Jr et al. The role of endotoxin during typhoid fever and tularemia in man: IV. The integrity of endotoxin tolerance mechanisms during infection. *J Clin Invest*. 1969; 48:613-29.
23. Calandra T, Gerain J, Heumann D et al. High circulating levels of interleukin-6 in patients with septic shock: evolution during sepsis, prognostic value, and interplay with other cytokines. *Am J Med*. 1991; 91:23-9.
24. Young LS, Proctor RA, Beutler B et al. University of California/Davis Interdepartmental Conference on Gram-Negative Septicemia. *Rev Infect Dis*. 1991; 13:666-87.
25. Schirmer WJ, Schirmer JM, Fry DE. Recombinant human tumor necrosis factor produces hemodynamic changes characteristic of sepsis and endotoxemia. *Arch Surg*. 1989; 129:445-8.
26. Hinshaw LB, Tekamp-Olson P, Chang ACK et al. Survival of primates in LD_{100} septic shock following therapy with antibody to TNF-alpha. *Circ Shock*. 1990; 30:279-92.
27. Harris RL, Musher DM, Bloom K et al. Manifestations of sepsis. *Arch Intern Med*. 1987; 147:1895-1906.
28. Cannon JG, Tompkins RG, Gelfand JA et al. Circulating interleukin-1 and tumor necrosis factor in septic shock and experimental endotoxin fever. *J Infect Dis*. 1990; 161:79-84.
29. Calandra T, Baumgartner JD, Grau GE et al. Prognostic values of TNF/cachectin, IL-1, interferon-alpha, and interferon-gamma in the serum of patients with septic shock. *J Infect Dis*. 1990; 161:982-7.
30. Parker MM, Suffredini AF, Natanson C et al. Responses of left ventricular function in survivors and non-survivors of septic shock. *J Crit Care*. 1989; 4:19-25.
31. Fein A, Lippman M, Holtzman M et al. The risk factors,

incidence, and prognosis of ARDS and septicemia. *Chest.* 1983; 83:40-2.

32. Sullivan GW, Carper HT, Novick WJ Jr et al. Inhibition of the inflammatory action of IL-1 and TNF-alpha on neutrophil function by pentoxifylline. *Infect Immun.* 1988; 56:1722-9.
33. Bullen JJ, Ward CG, Rogers HJ. The critical role of iron in some clinical infections. *Eur J Clin Microbiol Infect Dis.* 1991; 10:613-7.
34. Nawroth PP, Stern DM. Modulation of endothelial cell hemostatic properties by TNF. *J Exp Med.* 1986; 163:740-5.
35. Kreger BE, Craven DE, McCabe WR. Gram-negative bacteremia: IV. Reevaluation of clinical features and treatment of 612 patients. *Am J Med.* 1980; 68:344-55.
36. Kett DH, Pena MA, Quartin AA et al. Appropriate antibiotic therapy in the sepsis syndrome. *Crit Care Med.* 1991; 21:S100.
37. Sprung CL, Caralis P, Marcial EH et al. The effects of high dose corticosteroids in patients with septic shock—a prospective controlled study. *N Engl J Med.* 1984; 311:1137-43.
38. Boyd JL, Stanford GG, Chernow B. The pharmacotherapy of septic shock. *Crit Care Clin.* 1989; 5:133-50.
39. Bone RC, Fisher CJ, Clemmer TP et al. A controlled clinical trial of high-dose methylprednisolone in the treatment of severe sepsis and septic shock. *N Engl J Med.* 1987; 317:653-8.
40. Veterans Administration Systemic Sepsis Cooperative Study Group. Effect of high dose glucocorticoid therapy on mortality in patients with clinical signs of systemic sepsis. *N Engl J Med.* 1987; 317:659-65.
41. Luce JM, Montgomery AB, Marks JD et al. Ineffectiveness of high-dose methylprednisolone in preventing parenchymal lung injury and improving mortality in patients with septic shock. *Am Rev Respir Dis.* 1988; 138:62-8.
42. Lehrer RI, Barton A, Daher KA et al. Interaction of human defensins with *E. coli*: mechanism of bactericidal activity. *J Clin Invest.* 1989; 84:553-61.
43. McCabe WR, Kreger BE, Johns M. Type-specific and cross-reactive antibodies in gram-negative bacteremia. *N Engl J Med.* 1972; 287:261-7.
44. Pollack M, Huang AI, Prescott RK et al. Enhanced survival in *Pseudomonas aeruginosa* septicemia associated with high levels of circulating antibody to *Escherichia coli* endotoxin core. *J Clin Invest.* 1983; 72:1874-81.
45. Feingold DS, Oski F. *Pseudomonas* infection: treatment with immune human plasma. *Arch Intern Med.* 1965; 116:326-8.
46. Ziegler EJ, McCutchan AJ, Fierer J et al. Treatment of gram-negative bacteremia and shock with human anti-serum to a mutant *Escherichia coli. N Engl J Med.* 1982; 307:1225-30.
47. Baumgartner JD, Glauser MP, McCutchan AJ et al. Prevention of gram-negative shock and death in surgical patients by antibody to endotoxin core glycolipid. *Lancet.* 1985; 2:59-63.
48. Calandra T, Glauser MP, Schellekens J et al. Treatment of gram-negative septic shock with human IgG antibody to *Escherichia coli* J5: a prospective double-blind randomized trial. *J Infect Dis.* 1988; 158:312-9.
49. Milstein C. Monoclonal antibodies. *Sci Am.* 1980; 243:66-74.
50. Kohler G. Derivation and diversification of monoclonal antibodies. *Science.* 1986; 233:1281-6.
51. Tami J, Parr MD, Brown SA et al. Monoclonal antibody technology. *Am J Hosp Pharm.* 1986; 43:2816-25.
52. Teng NNH, Kaplan HS, Hebert JM et al. Protection against gram-negative bacteremia and endotoxemia with human monoclonal IgM antibodies. *Proc Natl Acad Sci USA.* 1985; 82:1790-4.
53. Young LS, Gascon R, Alam S et al. Monoclonal antibodies for treatment of gram-negative infections. *Rev Infect Dis.* 1989; 11(Suppl 7):S1564-S1571.
54. Greisman SE, Johnston CA. Failure of antisera to J5 and R595 rough mutants to reduce endotoxemic lethality. *J Infect Dis.* 1988; 157:54-64.
55. Baumgartner JD, Heumann D, Gerain J et al. Association between protective efficacy of anti-lipopolysaccharide (LPS) antibodies and suppression of LPS-induced tumor necrosis factor and interleukin-6. Comparison of O-side chain specific antibodies with core LPS antibodies. *J Exp Med.* 1990; 171:889-96.
56. Wedel NI, Gorelick KJ, Saria EA et al. Pharmacokinetics and safety of antiendotoxin antibody E5 in normal subjects. *Crit Care Med.* 1990; 25:S212.
57. Harkonen S, Scannon P, Mischak RP et al. Phase I study of a murine monoclonal anti-lipid A antibody in bacteremic and non-bacteremic patients. *Antimicrob Agents Chemother.* 1988; 32:710-16.
58. Khazaeli MB, Wheeler R, Rogers K et al. Initial evaluation of a human IgM monoclonal antibody (HA-1A) in humans. *J Biol Response Mod.* 1990; 9:178-84.
59. Fisher CJ, Zimmerman J, Khazaeli MB et al. Initial evaluation of human monoclonal anti-lipid A antibody (HA-1A) in patients with sepsis syndrome. *Crit Care Med.* 1990; 18:1311-5.
60. Ziegler EJ, Fisher CJ, Sprung CL et al. Treatment of gram-negative bacteremia and septic shock with HA-1A human monoclonal antibody against endotoxin. *N Engl J Med.* 1991; 324:429-36.
61. Greenman RL, Schein RMH, Martin MA et al. A controlled clinical trial of E5 murine monoclonal IgM antibody to endotoxin in the treatment of Gram-negative sepsis. *JAMA.* 1991; 266:1097-102.
62. Kunz AY, Wedel NI, Saria EA et al. Human anti-murine antibody (HAMA) response to murine monoclonal antiendotoxin antibodies: significance in the treatment of Gram-negative sepsis. *Crit Care Med.* 1990; 25:S212.
63. Norman DJ, Shield CF, Henell KR et al. Effectiveness of a second course of OKT3 monoclonal anti-T cell antibody for treatment of renal allograft rejection. *Transplantation.* 1988; 46:523-9.
64. Wenzel R, Bone R, Fein A et al. Results of a second double-blind, randomized, controlled trial of antiendotoxin antibody E5 in gram-negative sepsis. Program abstracts of the 31st Interscience Conference on Antimicrobial Agents and Chemotherapy. Washington, DC: American Society for Microbiology; 1991:294. Abstract 1170.
65. Knaus WA, Draper EA, Wagner DP et al. APACHE II: a severity of disease classification system. *Crit Care Med.* 1985; 13:818-29.
66. Baumgartner JD, Heumann D, Glauser MP. The HA-1A monoclonal antibody for gram-negative sepsis. *N Engl J Med.* 1991; 325:281. Letter.
67. Wortel CH, Sprung C, van Deventer SJH. Anti-endotoxin treatment with HA1A: possible mechanism of beneficial effects in patients with gram-negative septicemia. Presented at Third International Congress on Infectious Diseases. Montreal, Canada: 1990 Jul 18. Abstract.
68. Thorpe TC, Wilson ML, Turner JE et al. BacT/Alert: an automated colorimetric microbial detection system. *J Clin Microbiol.* 1990; 28:1608-12.
69. Mertsola J, Cope LD, Munford RS et al. Detection of experimental *Hemophilus influenzae* type B bacteremia and endotoxemia by means of an immunolimulus assay. *J Infect Dis.* 1991; 164:353-8.
70. Barth WF, Wochner RD, Waldmann TA et al. Metabolism of human macroglobulins. *J Clin Invest.* 1964; 43:1036-48.
71. Shenep JL, Mogan KA. Kinetics of endotoxin release during antibiotic therapy for experimental gram-negative bacterial sepsis. *J Infect Dis.* 1984; 150:380-8.
72. Shenep JL, Barton RP, Mogan KA. Role of antibiotic class in the rate of liberation of endotoxin during therapy for experimental gram-negative sepsis. *J Infect Dis.* 1985; 151:1012-8.
73. Chalfin DB, Carlon GC. Cost-effectiveness issues in the treatment of ICU patients with gram-negative sepsis. Paper presented at 19th Annual Society for Critical Care Medicine Education and Scientific Symposium. San Francisco, CA: 1990 May 30.
74. Oster G, Tuden RL, Colditz GA. Prevention of venous thromboembolism after general surgery. Cost-effectiveness analysis of alternative approaches to prophylaxis. *Am J Med.* 1987; 82:889-99.

Treatment of preeclampsia and eclampsia

JANET MCCOMBS

Abstract: The characteristics and treatment of preeclampsia and eclampsia are reviewed.

Risk factors for preeclampsia include (1) nulliparity, (2) a mother or sister(s) with a history of the disorder, (3) essential hypertension or renal disease, or (4) a twin or molar pregnancy. Preeclampsia is diagnosed when the systolic blood pressure (BP) increases by 30 mm Hg or the diastolic BP increases by 15 mm Hg after the 20th week of gestation and the BP rise is accompanied by edema, proteinuria, or both. Severe preeclampsia is diagnosed when the BP reaches or exceeds 160 mm Hg systolic or 110 mm Hg diastolic after bed rest. Eclampsia is the occurrence of seizures (in the preeclamptic patient) that cannot be attributed to other causes; it occurs in about 0.2% of preeclamptic patients.

Magnesium sulfate (in the injectable, hydrated form) is the agent used most often for seizure prophylaxis in the preeclamptic patient in the United States. It is also used widely to control seizures once they develop. In the United States, diazepam is used to supplement magnesium sulfate if necessary to control seizures, but its use is not routine. Among antihypertensive agents, i.v. hydralazine is preferred in this country to control blood pressure in the severely preeclamptic or eclamptic patient. Several studies provide promising evidence that low-dose aspirin (60–150 mg daily beginning at 28–30 weeks of gestation) prevents preeclampsia in women who are at risk for its development.

Until additional comparative studies are completed, magnesium sulfate and hydralazine will remain the standard of care for the treatment of preeclampsia in the United States.

Index terms: Anticonvulsants; Aspirin; Diazepam; Eclampsia; Hypotensive agents; Magnesium sulfate; Phenytoin; Preeclampsia
Clin Pharm. 1992; 11: 236-45

Preeclampsia and eclampsia are well recognized complications in patients with pregnancy-induced hypertension (PIH). PIH is defined as a blood pressure (BP) of ≥140/90 mm Hg during the latter half of pregnancy in a patient without a history of hypertension. Preeclampsia is PIH with accompanying proteinuria, edema, or both. Preeclampsia also may be superimposed over chronic hypertension and is identified by an increase in BP rather than a specific BP measurement. Eclampsia is the occurrence of seizures resulting from cerebral effects of the disease in a preeclamptic patient. All patients with even mild PIH should be considered at risk for development of preeclampsia and eclampsia because eclampsia can occur without development of proteinuria. This article reviews the characteristics and treatment of preeclampsia and eclampsia.

Occurrence

Preeclampsia occurs in about 7% of all pregnancies.[1] It is most common in young primigravidas; about 67% of the cases are diagnosed during the first pregnancy that extends past the first trimester. Most of these patients do not experience a recurrence in subsequent pregnancies. Multiparous patients who develop preeclampsia tend to be older, may have a recurrence in later pregnancies, and are more likely to develop essential hypertension later in life. Patients at higher risk for preeclampsia include those who (1) are nulliparous, (2) have a mother or sister(s) with a history of the disorder, (3) have essential hypertension or renal disease, or (4) have a twin or molar pregnancy.

Etiology and Pathophysiology

Three principal mechanisms are currently believed to play a part in the development of this disorder.[2] These are increased vasospasm, an abnormal immunologic reaction, and increased vasoactive prostaglandins. Preeclamptic women show more vascular reactivity to pressors than healthy pregnant women, and healthy pregnant women show much less vascular reactivity to pressors than nonpregnant women.[1] A possible immunologic factor is suggested by the fact that most cases of PIH occur during the first pregnancy.[2] This circumstance implies that exposure to fetal antigens provides protection in subsequent pregnancies. Abnormal prostaglandin production also has been noted in preeclamptic patients.[2] This abnormality is most likely related to an alteration in the relative amounts of prostacyclin (prostaglandin I_2) and thromboxane A_2 produced.

Although the underlying cause of preeclampsia and eclampsia is unclear, a great deal is known about the pathophysiology. The major pathological event is vasospasm. The hypertension in preeclamptic and eclamptic patients is caused by vasospasm and in-

JANET MCCOMBS, PHARM.D., is Clinical Pharmacy Associate, College of Pharmacy, University of Georgia, Athens, GA 30602.
The assistance of Cynthia A. Mercer, M.D., and Thomas L. Lyons, M.D., is acknowledged.
This is **article 680-204-9207** in the **ASHP Continuing-Education System**; it qualifies for 1.0 hour of continuing-education credit. See page 262 for learning objectives and test questions.

creased peripheral resistance. The cause of the vasospasm is unknown, but preeclamptic patients are more sensitive than healthy pregnant women to angiotensin II as well as to all other pressor agents.[3] BP rises, but there is no increase in cardiac output.[1] In severe preeclampsia, hemodynamics are altered and blood flow to maternal organs, including the uteroplacental unit and the fetus, is decreased.[4,5]

Recently several theories have been suggested about the role of prostaglandins in PIH.[4] Prostacyclin is a potent vasodilator and an inhibitor of platelet aggregation and uterine contractility. It is produced in endothelial cells and smooth muscle. During a normal pregnancy, production of prostacyclin increases fivefold. However, the prostacyclin concentration is lower in hypertensive pregnant women than in healthy pregnant women.[6,7] This decrease in prostacyclin increases the sensitivity of the pregnant patient to angiotensin II.[6] The increased sensitivity to angiotensin II occurs as early as the 18th week of gestation in women who develop preeclampsia, even though the clinical signs do not usually appear until after the 32nd week.[6] Another prostaglandin, thromboxane A_2, also is increased in women with normal pregnancies, but it has effects that oppose those of prostacyclin.[7] Thromboxane A_2 is a vasoconstrictor that stimulates platelet aggregation and increases uterine contractility. It is produced in the kidney, endometrium, placenta, and platelets.

The most recent theory suggests that there is an imbalance of prostacyclin and thromboxane A_2 in preeclamptic women.[7] This imbalance, which favors thromboxane A_2, could cause increased vasoconstriction, platelet aggregation, and decreased uteroplacental blood flow—all of which are reported in the preeclamptic patient.

Two methods have been described to evaluate the angiotensin II sensitivity of women believed to be at risk for preeclampsia.[8] The rollover test, described by Gant et al.,[9] has limited clinical usefulness. The patient, tested at 28–32 weeks of gestation, rolls from a lateral recumbent position to the supine position. If there is a rise of 20 mm Hg in the diastolic BP, the test is considered positive, and the patient supposedly is likely to develop PIH. The explanation for the BP response is that when the pregnant patient is in the supine position, there is compression of the inferior vena cava, which decreases cardiac output and renal blood flow and increases renin release.

The angiotensin sensitivity test, which is considered somewhat more specific, is based on evidence that healthy pregnant patients are resistant to the pressor effects of angiotensin II, whereas women who develop preeclampsia develop an increased sensitivity to angiotensin II as early as the 18th week of pregnancy.[10,11] Patients are given an i.v. infusion of angiotensin amide (a pressor [not marketed in the United States] related to human angiotensin II). A patient requiring less than 10 ng/kg/min to increase diastolic BP 20 mm Hg has a positive test. The test is usually performed between 28 and 32 weeks of pregnancy and requires 60–90 minutes.

In normal pregnancy, the glomerular filtration rate increases, but it has been found to be 62–84% lower in preeclampsia than in early normal pregnancy.[6] The proteinuria seen in most preeclamptic patients is probably due to glomeruloendotheliosis, a state in which the glomeruli are swollen and enlarged, thus allowing passage of protein molecules.[1] The fluctuation in the quantity of protein excreted may be related to renal vascular spasm.[1] Excretion of uric acid is decreased because of the reduced glomerular filtration rate, and the serum uric acid concentration is an indicator of the severity of the preeclampsia.[6] A serum uric acid concentration of more than 5.5 mg/dL is a strong indicator of preeclampsia, which can be considered severe if the concentration exceeds 6.0 mg/dL. Reversal of renal damage in a patient who does not have underlying renal disease may be expected within six weeks after delivery.[12]

The immunologic theories about the cause of PIH arise from the fact that PIH is 10 times more likely to occur in first pregnancies than in subsequent pregnancies.[13] The immunologic theories are further supported by observations that some of the protective effect (from exposure to fetal antigens) seems to be lost in subsequent pregnancies with a different father.[14] Pregnant women form antibodies to fetal antigens. This antibody formation tends to be decreased in women with PIH and when there is increased HLA compatibility with the father.[15] It has been suggested that when the maternal immune response to an influx of fetal antigen is adequate, immune complexes will be cleared by the reticuloendothelial system.[1] If the response is inadequate, these pathological immune complexes could cause vasculitis, glomerular damage, and alteration of the coagulation system.[2] There is not enough evidence to support or disclaim an immunologic etiology in the development of PIH.

Preeclamptic patients have decreased sodium excretion and a decreased plasma volume.[6,12] The reduction in plasma volume is not an indicator of volume depletion because the extracellular fluid is shifted from the vascular to interstitial space. It is tempting to use volume expanders in the management of preeclampsia, but pulmonary edema may be a life-threatening complication of preeclampsia, and additional fluids could be harmful.[6]

Diagnosis

Preeclampsia is diagnosed when the systolic BP increases by 30 mm Hg or the diastolic BP increases by 15 mm Hg after the 20th week of gestation and the BP rise is accompanied by edema, proteinuria, or both. An increase in BP is the earliest and most sensitive indicator of preeclampsia.[6] The usual BP in young women in their teens and twenties is 120/60 mm Hg, which tends to decrease soon after they become pregnant.[1] Some clinicians suggest that if the BP exceeds 130/80 mm Hg at any time during pregnancy, preeclampsia should be considered.[6] Proteinuria is defined as a urinary protein concentration of ≥0.1 g/L in a random urine specimen or ≥0.3 g/L in a 24-hour collection. Edema, especially of the hands and face, may be the first sign of preeclampsia in up to 85% of patients.[1,6] A sudden weight gain may be the first indication of substantial fluid retention even before edema is clinically evident.

Preeclampsia typically occurs late in pregnancy, after the 32nd week of gestation, but it can develop (1) earlier, (2) during labor and delivery, or (3) later (in the postpartum period).[6] Postpartum preeclampsia and eclampsia typically develop within 24–48 hours of delivery, but they have been reported up to several weeks after delivery.[1,12] Hypertension that is manifested before 20 weeks of gestation is considered to be essential hypertension unmasked by the pregnancy.[5]

Severe preeclampsia is diagnosed when the BP reaches or exceeds 160 mm Hg systolic or 110 mm Hg diastolic after bed rest. Proteinuria of 5 g or greater in 24 hours or a dipstick reading of 3–4+ is also indicative of severe preeclampsia. The patient with severe preeclampsia may have oliguria (urine output of ≤500 mL/24 hr), cerebral or visual disturbances, pulmonary edema, and epigastric pain.[1,6]

Eclampsia is the occurrence of seizures (in the preeclamptic patient) that cannot be attributed to other causes. About 0.2% of preeclamptic patients will develop seizures.[12] Aggressive management of preeclampsia can prevent progression to eclampsia.[3] This management includes prenatal care with careful attention to weight gain, BP monitoring, and detection of proteinuria. Before seizures, patients may experience headache, visual disturbances, epigastric pain, and apprehension.[6]

General Management

The primary goal in the treatment of patients with preeclampsia is prevention of eclampsia and intracranial hemorrhage. Patients at risk for development of preeclampsia should do daily measurements of blood pressure at home.[16] Those at great risk may be candidates for low-dose aspirin therapy (discussed in the Aspirin section).

The patient with mild preeclampsia who can be compliant with strict bed rest, home BP monitoring, and daily determinations of urinary protein concentration may be managed at home. These patients are typically evaluated twice weekly in the office. Sodium and fluid restriction are not recommended because they may reduce intravascular fluid volume, which could adversely affect the fetus.[1] A patient with preeclampsia must be hospitalized if she (1) has advanced disease, (2) cannot be compliant, or (3) has rapidly progressing disease. Severe preeclampsia always indicates hospitalization with prophylaxis against seizures and control of BP until delivery can be accomplished.

Although the etiology of preeclampsia and eclampsia remains unclear, the cure is well documented. Delivery of the fetus arrests the problem; however, preeclampsia and eclampsia occasionally develop after delivery because the hormonal milieu does not immediately return to normal on delivery.[1] Properly controlled preeclampsia is not a contraindication to vaginal delivery, use of oxytocin, or epidural anesthesia. BP may remain somewhat elevated for several days to weeks postpartum, and the patient may be discharged home while continuing to take an oral antihypertensive. This patient should be warned about hypotension and re-evaluated weekly because in some cases the BP normalizes rapidly.

Termination of the pregnancy must be considered when a patient with mild preeclampsia has a progression of the disease despite treatment or when a patient is severely preeclamptic or eclamptic. In each situation, maternal mortality is decreased when the mother is stabilized (BP and convulsions controlled) before delivery.[1,2] Induction of labor may be attempted with oxytocin or artificial rupture of the membranes, or both. A cesarean delivery may be considered if the trial of labor is unsuccessful or there are other obstetric indications for a surgical delivery. Delivery should be completed within 24–48 hours after the decision to terminate the pregnancy in severely preeclamptic patients. A magnesium sulfate infusion should be continued during labor and delivery to prevent convulsions.

Magnesium Sulfate

Magnesium sulfate is the agent used most often for seizure prophylaxis in the preeclamptic patient in the United States.[17] It is important to note that magnesium sulfate is given to control or prevent eclamptic seizures, not to treat hypertension. The magnesium sulfate used in patients with preeclampsia is the injectable, hydrated form($MgSO_4 \cdot 7H_2O$). Magnesium sulfate therapy is initiated when severe preeclampsia is diagnosed or seizures occur in a patient not previously recognized as being preeclamptic.

Magnesium sulfate is most commonly given as either (1) a 4-g i.v. dose over four to five minutes, immediately followed by 10 g i.m. and then by 5 g i.m. every four hours in alternating buttocks or (2) a 4-g i.v. dose diluted in 5% dextrose injection 250 mL and infused over 15 minutes, followed by a maintenance infusion of 1–2 g/hr by controlled infusion pump.[18] These are known as Pritchard's and Zuspan's regimen, respectively.

Pharmacokinetics. When given i.v., magnesium sulfate has an immediate onset of action, and its duration of activity is about 30 minutes.[19] The onset of action of i.m. magnesium sulfate is about one hour, and its duration of action is three to four hours.[19] After administration, magnesium sulfate is rapidly distributed throughout the extracellular fluid and remains unbound.[1] Magnesium is almost exclusively excreted in the urine, with 90% of the dose excreted during the first 24 hours after an i.v. infusion of magnesium sulfate is discontinued in a patient with normal renal function.[20] The half-life in patients with normal renal function is four hours; if the glomerular filtration rate is decreased, the half-life increases.[1] Magnesium does cross the placenta, and fetal and neonatal concentrations mimic maternal concentrations.[1] Amounts of magnesium excreted in breast milk also have been determined. During the first 24 hours after an i.v. infusion of magnesium sulfate was stopped, about 1.5 mg of magnesium was present in breast milk; this amount, although small, was significantly higher than that in the breast milk of control patients.[21] On the second postinfusion day, there was no significant difference, and by the third day, amounts were almost identical. Mothers who want to nurse and are medically stable may be allowed to do so after magnesium therapy without danger to the newborn.

Mechanism of Action. The mechanism of action of magnesium in controlling and preventing eclamptic seizures is not clearly understood. However, an increase in serum magnesium concentration does have an effect on cell membranes, and magnesium blocks neuromuscular and cardiac conduction.[1] Magnesium decreases the contractility of smooth muscle (as is evident when it is used to inhibit preterm labor), and it also decreases central nervous system irritability.[1] Magnesium crosses the blood–brain barrier in small but significant amounts.[22] Perhaps when the cause of preeclampsia and eclampsia is discovered, the mechanism by which magnesium prevents seizures will become evident.

Therapeutic Use. There is a great deal of controversy between obstetric and neurologic experts about the preferred management of eclamptic seizures. There is less debate about the prophylactic use of magnesium sulfate in the preeclamptic patient, but once seizures develop, the choice of drug varies widely. Obstetricians favor an increased dosage of magnesium sulfate if the patient was already receiving the drug, or initiation of a magnesium sulfate regimen if not. Seizures not controlled with magnesium sulfate are treated with short-acting barbiturates or diazepam and muscular paralysis if necessary. Neurologists and even obstetricians in other countries prefer phenytoin or benzodiazepines for treatment of eclamptic seizures.

Advocates of magnesium sulfate therapy note that the drug is easy to administer and monitor, rapidly effective, and reliable.[23] There is no clinically significant maternal or neonatal respiratory depression, which is often seen with barbiturates and diazepam.[2]

Even though the pharmacology of magnesium sulfate for the prevention and control of eclamptic seizures is unknown, there is no doubt among physicians in this country that it is effective and widely accepted. Several authors have noted that because magnesium sulfate is the standard of care in the United States, failure to use the drug could increase legal liability if seizures occur.[12,23] Convulsions are uncommon (occurring in about 1 of 300 patients) when magnesium sulfate is used correctly as prophylaxis in preeclampsia.[23] If treatment is not begun until after seizures occur, 10–15% of patients will have a recurrent seizure.[23] Because magnesium sulfate is used routinely (one survey indicated that 100% of U.S. obstetricians used it to treat preeclamptic patients[18]), it is not possible to determine what the incidence of eclampsia in untreated patients would be.

Physicians who favor phenytoin in preeclampsia and eclampsia note that it is the most widely used anticonvulsant and, as such, its pharmacology is well defined.[24] In a small study comparing phenytoin and magnesium sulfate for treatment of eclamptic seizures, Dommisse[24] found that 4 of 11 patients treated with appropriate dosages of phenytoin had recurrent seizures but patients treated with recommended dosages of magnesium sulfate had no further seizures.

Another study by Crowther[25] compared magnesium sulfate with diazepam. Diazepam was chosen because it is inexpensive, readily available, and easily administered, especially in underdeveloped countries. The disadvantages of benzodiazepines include prolonged and heavy sedation that increases the risk of aspiration pneumonia, neonatal respiratory depression, and hypotonia.[1,25] Few problems have been associated with magnesium sulfate and although cardiac and respiratory arrest have been reported, these are rare and avoidable.[23] Although Crowther[25] could not suggest that one drug is more efficacious than the other, she concluded that magnesium sulfate is preferable to diazepam because it is associated with less maternal morbidity.

Although normal serum magnesium concentrations are 1.5–2.5 meq/L, the dosage of magnesium sulfate should produce a therapeutic serum magnesium concentration. The ideal serum concentration prevents seizures and minimizes maternal and fetal toxicity. Although there is some debate about the precise concentration necessary to prevent seizures, most agree on 4–7 meq/L.[26,27]

Sibai et al.[28] found that the aforementioned i.m. regimen (Pritchard's) achieved higher serum concentrations in the first three hours than the aforementioned i.v. regimen (Zuspan's) when a 2-g/hr maintenance infusion was used. However, after 3 hours, there was no significant difference in serum magnesium concentrations. The initial difference may be explained by increased retention of magnesium after i.m. administration and the higher initial dose of 14 g compared with 4 g. These investigators noted that the i.m. regimen is painful, requiring two initial injections of 10 mL each, followed by additional injections every four hours. The authors suggested that the i.m. regimen may be preferred when i.v. infusion pumps are not available, continuous monitoring is not feasible, or when the patient must be transferred to another facility. The authors added that, because of the difference in serum concentrations during the first three hours, it may be advantageous to increase the i.v. infusion rate to 3 g/hr initially with careful monitoring to avoid toxicity.[28]

Another study has also suggested that an i.v. infusion of 1–2 g/hr may not be adequate.[17] In patients receiving 1 g/hr, 98% had subtherapeutic magnesium concentrations, and 50% of those receiving 2 g/hr had lower-than-expected magnesium concentrations. In this study, 10 of the 13 patients who had seizures did so before therapeutic concentrations were achieved.

Adverse Effects. Toxicity is rare when magnesium sulfate is carefully administered and monitored. The few deaths and serious complications reported in the literature were primarily due to inadvertent overdoses (e.g., a 20-g bolus because of infusion pump failure).[29,30]

Monitoring of the patient receiving magnesium sulfate is of utmost importance. Careful attention to the monitoring guidelines can prevent toxicities. Deep tendon reflexes, respiratory rate, urine output, and serum concentrations are the most commonly followed variables. At the therapeutic serum magnesium concentration of 4–7 meq/L, deep tendon reflexes may be hypoactive but remain present. They should be checked at least hourly. If deep tendon reflexes are present, magnesium concentrations are rarely toxic. On the other hand, hypoactive reflexes do not ensure adequate serum concentrations of magnesium and are also the first sign of toxicity.[26] Urine output should be at least 100 mL/4 hr. Oliguria can indicate deteriorating renal function and can cause magnesium toxicity because magnesium is excreted predominantly in the urine. It is generally accepted that deep tendon reflexes disappear at a serum magnesium concentration of 10 meq/L, respiratory paralysis occurs at 10–13 meq/L, cardiac conduction is altered at greater than 15 meq/L, and cardiac arrest can be expected when levels of magnesium exceed 25 meq/L.[18]

Calcium gluconate is the preferred antidote for hypermagnesemia, and a 10-mL ampul of 10% solution should be kept at the bedside of any preeclamptic or eclamptic patient receiving magnesium sulfate. The gluconate salt of calcium is less irritating to endothelial surfaces than is the chloride salt.[29]

In managing an overdose of magnesium sulfate, the first consideration should be support of respiration, followed by administration of calcium salts and cardiac monitoring. The administration of loop or osmotic diuretics is suggested to enhance the excretion of magnesium.[29] It is especially important to remember that increased magnesium concentrations are not anesthetic or amnestic.

Phenytoin

Few reports in the literature support the use of phenytoin to prevent or stop eclamptic seizures. Slater et al.[31] reported promising results; there were no seizures and no major maternal or neonatal adverse effects in 26 preeclamptic patients treated with phenytoin. Others have suggested that phenytoin sodium may be used when seizures appear to be imminent and that 1 g in 100 mL of 0.9% sodium chloride injection should be infused at 50 mg/min.[6] This dose produced an average serum concentration of 18 μg/mL (therapeutic range for anticonvulsant activity, 10–20 μg/mL). There is some concern that the dosages required to control seizures may be cardiotoxic, necessitating electrocardiographic monitoring. Serum albumin concentrations may affect serum concentrations of phenytoin and should be taken into account to avoid phenytoin toxicity.

Coyagi and Otiv[32] described the use of a single high dose of phenytoin sodium to stop eclamptic seizures. When a standard dose of 900 mg i.v. (given at 50 mg/min) was used, patients with mild eclampsia who achieved serum concentrations higher than 10 μg/mL had no further seizures; however, only 4 of the 10 patients with severe eclampsia who had therapeutic serum concentrations responded.

Phenytoin crosses the placenta and is teratogenic when given early in pregnancy.[33] Neonates born to mothers taking phenytoin often have bleeding problems related to a vitamin K deficiency.[6,33] When phenytoin is used i.v. for the short-term management of eclampsia to facilitate delivery, these problems should not occur.

Further studies, particularly comparing phenytoin with more accepted agents such as magnesium sulfate, will be necessary before a change in the standard treatment can be recommended.

Diazepam

Diazepam has long been recognized as the drug of choice for the termination of status epilepticus. In Britain, diazepam is routinely used (10 mg i.v. repeated as necessary, up to 30 mg) in eclamptic patients to stop seizures and prevent recurrence.[27] High doses (20–50 mg) cause both maternal and neonatal respiratory depression.[3] Heavy sedation in the mother increases the risk of aspiration pneumonia.[25] Diazepam also causes loss of beat-to-beat variability in the fetal heart rate.[23] In the neonate, diazepam-associated delay of breathing or apnea may result in hypotonia, cold stress, and poor sucking.[3]

In the United States, diazepam is used to supplement magnesium sulfate if necessary to control seizures, but it is not used routinely. Pritchard[30] described a young woman who was hypertensive and convulsing, was admitted to a nonobstetric service, and was given 50 mg of diazepam in an attempt to control her seizures. Although the seizures were controlled, respiratory arrest occurred, followed by successful intubation and ventilation. When it was discovered that the patient had recently delivered, therapy with magnesium sulfate was initiated and the seizures were controlled.

Antihypertensives

Antihypertensive medications are not routinely used in the management of preeclampsia and eclampsia because there is no evidence that such use improves fetal outcome except when the mother's BP is extremely high.[1] When a patient's BP increases so much that intracranial bleeding becomes a risk (usually a diastolic BP of 105 mm Hg or higher), antihypertensive drugs are used with few exceptions. Some clinicians believe that the use of these medications in patients with mild elevations of BP can mask progression of the preeclampsia. These drugs are most commonly used in patients with severe preeclampsia to control BP for a short time until delivery can be accomplished. There is another concern that aggressive therapy in the presence of the decreased plasma volume typically seen in these patients can decrease cardiac output and compromise uterine perfusion.

Concern about the direct effects of antihypertensive medication on the fetus is understandable. Because preeclampsia usually develops after the 32nd gestational week, there should be little risk of congenital malformations from these drugs. Indirect effects such as decreased uterine perfusion would be more likely, but the benefits of the medication in preventing maternal intracranial bleeding would usually outweigh the risks. Occasionally, a patient will develop severe preeclampsia earlier in pregnancy. This patient, usually between 25 and 30 weeks of gestation, may be hospitalized, given antihypertensive medications, and meticulously observed for progression of the disease. If the patient's BP can be controlled for several weeks, the fetus can develop further and neonatal outcome can be improved.

Many different medications—including hydralazine, diazoxide, β-adrenergic blockers, and trimethaphan—have been used. Administration by injection, particularly by the i.v. route, is preferred. Minute-to-minute dosage adjustment is impossible with i.m. therapy, and i.m. absorption may be erratic in patients with preeclampsia and eclampsia because of vasospasm.[34] The endpoint of therapy is a diastolic BP of 90–100 mm Hg.

Hydralazine. Hydralazine, a potent vasodilator, is the drug preferred in this country to control BP in the severely preeclamptic or eclamptic patient. When hydralazine is administered i.v., BP decreases and there is a reflex increase in cardiac output that may increase uterine perfusion. The reflex tachycardia with increased cardiac output may decrease the hypotensive effect. On one hand, this increased cardiac output would make it difficult to lower BP too much, but conversely, the decrease in BP might not be great enough. It has been suggested that the addition of a β blocker such as labetalol or propranolol would inhibit the reflex tachycardia and help control blood pressure.[6] Patients are given hydralazine hydrochloride 5–10 mg i.v. every 20 minutes. Small, intermittent boluses are preferred because the peak usually occurs 20 minutes after the dose, and severe hypotension could result from an infusion.

Maternal adverse effects include tachycardia, flushing, headache, and epigastric pain.[1,12,35] Close attention to headache and epigastric pain is warranted because these also are associated with an impending seizure. If BP is decreased too rapidly, fetal distress can occur because rapid vasodilation can decrease placental blood flow. Adequate hydration of the mother can minimize this risk. Adverse effects on the fetus are uncommon, but thermoregulatory problems have been reported in neonates exposed to hydralazine in utero.[18]

Diazoxide. Diazoxide, another potent vasodilator, lowers BP but is a poor choice during pregnancy because its effects may be unpredictable. It may, for example, lower systolic BP to less than 60 mm Hg after a single dose. Marked hypotension could cause decreased uterine perfusion, which could take several hours to correct. It is suggested that 30-mg miniboluses be used if it is necessary to administer the drug during pregnancy.[5,35] The drug crosses the placenta and has been associated with fetal and neonatal hyperbilirubinemia and thrombocytopenia.[18] Because diazoxide alters carbohydrate metabolism, hyperglycemia can develop in the mother and child.[12,18] Maternal adverse effects are tachycardia, flushing, palpitations, and headache, which are common to all vasodilators.[18] Diazoxide has a potent effect on uterine smooth muscle and causes cessation of labor in up to 50% of patients.[6] Oxytocin is usually required to reinstate contractions.

Diazoxide is best reserved for patients who do not respond to adequate doses of hydralazine or who have postpartum exacerbations of hypertension.

Nitroprusside. Concerns about the use of the vasodilator nitroprusside involve possible cyanide toxicity in the fetus.[5] Sodium nitroprusside is administered as a continuous infusion and effectively decreases BP. The duration of action of three to five minutes makes it easy to adjust the dosage to achieve the desired effect. Once administered, sodium nitroprusside combines with hemoglobin to produce methemoglobin and cyanide. The cyanide is metabolized in the liver to thiocyanate, which is excreted in the urine. Nitroprusside crosses the placenta, and cyanide accumulation could occur if substantial amounts of cyanide were not converted by the fetal liver after large doses or prolonged administration or when metabolism was decreased.

Shoemaker and Meyers[36] reported the use of sodium nitroprusside in a patient at 24 weeks of gestation with severe hypertension. She received 235 μg/kg/hr for 15 hours before delivery. The total dose was 3.5 mg/kg. The fetus was stillborn, but evaluation of its liver indicated cyanide concentrations of less than 10 μg/mL (toxic concentrations are 30–40 μg/mL). Fetal demise was attributed to maternal hypertension and seriously compromised cardiac function. Although caution is prudent, sodium nitroprusside may be considered in resistant cases.

Labetalol. Labetalol, a combination α-adrenergic and β-adrenergic blocking agent, has been suggested for management of severe hypertension in pregnancy. There are few reports of controlled studies with labetalol, but evidence looks promising.[37] Labetalol hydrochloride may be given in a dose of 50–100 mg i.v. every 20 to 30 minutes as necessary, up to 300 mg. Oral administration also has been used with an onset of 30 minutes. The recommended protocol is intermittent doses i.v. every three hours after BP is controlled.[35] Maternal adverse effects are flushing and tremulousness.[1,35] No adverse fetal or neonatal effects have been reported. Studies have not indicated any decrease in uteroplacental blood flow.[12]

Sibai et al.[38] conducted a large study to compare labetalol therapy and hospitalization with hospitalization alone in mildly preeclamptic patients. Labetalol was given orally to patients starting at 26–35 weeks of gestation and continuing until delivery. Although the medication did control BP, these patients had a higher incidence of fetal growth retardation, and there was no improvement in perinatal outcome.

Nifedipine. Several authors have suggested the use of nifedipine for acute hypertensive episodes associated with pregnancy.[35,39,40] When administered sublingually, nifedipine decreases BP in 10–20 minutes and rarely causes hypotension.[39] Reports indicate that there is no nifedipine-induced reduction in uteroplacental blood flow and that there are no fetal heart rate abnormalities.[39] Adverse effects in mothers are minimal and include flushing and headache.[35,39,40] Calcium-channel blockers, including nifedipine, have been studied for the inhibition of preterm labor, and results indicate possible usefulness; thus, administration of nifedipine to control BP could prevent or stop labor.[41]

In a recent study, Fenakel et al.[40] compared nifedipine with hydralazine in 49 preeclamptic patients. Nifedipine 20 mg was given sublingually to one set of patients and repeated at 20 and 40 minutes if necessary to reduce BP below 160/100 mm Hg. It was then given orally (10–20 mg) every six hours until delivery. Hydralazine hydrochloride 12.5 mg i.v. was given to the other patients at intervals necessary to decrease BP below 160/110 mm Hg. After BP was controlled, hydralazine hydrochloride 20–30 mg was administered orally every six hours until delivery. If necessary, oral methyldopa was added to control BP. All patients in both groups also received i.v. magnesium sulfate. Mothers in both groups had minor adverse effects. Dizziness and transient increases in heart rate were noted in the hydralazine group, and hot flushes and headache were common after nifedipine treatment. Fetal distress possibly associated with hydralazine was seen in 11 of 27 fetuses. The authors concluded that nifedipine was preferable to hydralazine because it was more effective at controlling BP, the response was more predictable and less drastic, and the administration was more convenient.

There are several reports of severe drug interactions between nifedipine and magnesium sulfate.[35,42] These include substantial hypotension and muscle weakness. If it becomes necessary to use both drugs in the same patient, extreme caution must be used.

Other Antihypertensives. Methyldopa and clonidine, antihypertensives that act by stimulation of central α-receptors, have been suggested for the treatment of exacerbations of hypertension in patients with severe preeclampsia. Methyldopa is used orally as the drug of choice to treat chronic hypertension in pregnancy.[18,35] Such use has not been associated with any serious adverse effects. Because of the large amount of experience with methyldopa in pregnancy, it would be a logical choice to treat acute exacerbations of hypertension, but even when it is administered i.v. (as methyldopate), the onset of action is four to six hours. This slow onset of action considerably decreases its usefulness in patients with acute exacerbations of hypertension.

Clonidine is unavailable in injectable form, but the onset of action is 30–60 minutes after oral administration.[6] Advantages include a gradual rather than abrupt decrease in BP and no reflex tachycardia. Disadvantages include rebound hypertension after discontinuation of the medication and little experience with use during pregnancy.

Trimethaphan is a short-acting ganglionic blocking agent that rapidly decreases BP but also decreases uterine perfusion.[1] It crosses the placenta and has the potential for causing meconium ileus in the fetus.[12] It is not recommended for use in pregnancy. Another concern about trimethaphan involves a potential drug interaction. Concurrent use of trimethaphan and succinylcholine has caused prolonged neuromuscular blockade and necessitated intubation after cesarean delivery.[5] Because it is impossible to predict which severely preeclamptic patients might require a surgical delivery, trimethaphan is not a good choice.

Diuretics are not recommended for the treatment of preeclampsia because of concern about the effects in a patient whose plasma volume is already depleted.[5] Diuretics are indicated only when preeclampsia is complicated by pulmonary edema.

The angiotensin-converting-enzyme inhibitors would seem to be a logical choice to treat exacerbations of hypertension in patients with severe preeclampsia because it is known that preeclamptic patients are more sensitive to angiotensin II than healthy pregnant patients. However, harmful fetal effects such as renal dysfunction and hypotension are associated with these drugs, and they are contraindicated in pregnancy.[5] They have no role in the treatment of preeclampsia.

Aspirin

The most recent development in the management of preeclampsia is the use of aspirin to prevent development of the disorder in patients at risk. Several studies have investigated the use of low-dose aspirin (60–150 mg/day) for the prevention of preeclampsia in women identified as being at risk for its development.[43-49] Low-dose aspirin has been shown to decrease platelet thromboxane A_2 synthesis to a greater degree than it decreases vascular prostacyclin synthesis.[43,44] The daily dose of 60–150 mg inactivates cyclo-oxygenase, preventing the synthesis of prostaglandin E, prostacyclin, and thromboxane A_2. Cyclo-oxygenase is rapidly resynthesized in endothelial cells, and prostacyclin production resumes. In platelets, the effect on cyclo-oxygenase is permanent, causing a greater decrease in thromboxane A_2 synthesis.

Walsh[7] evaluated tissue samples from healthy and preeclamptic women. The placentas from preeclamptic patients produced three times more thromboxane A_2 but only half as much prostacyclin as those from healthy women. The more dramatic finding was that placentas from preeclamptic patients produced seven times more thromboxane A_2 than prostacyclin. In a similar study involving human placental arteries, Thorp et al.[45] found that low-dose aspirin selectively inhibited placental thromboxane A_2 production in vitro—both alone and in the presence of vasoconstricting amounts of angiotensin II.

Beaufils et al.[46] conducted a trial involving women at risk for development of preeclampsia. They administered 150 mg of aspirin and 300 mg of dipyridamole to 52 women beginning at three months of gestation; 50 women were used as controls. The study group was randomized but not blinded. These investigators found that significantly more patients in the treatment group had normal pregnancies as defined by BP of ≤140/85 mm Hg, no proteinuria, and delivery of a live infant of normal weight at more than 36 weeks of gestation. A higher frequency of surgical deliveries in the control group was attributed to more fetal distress. One third of the patients receiving dipyridamole and aspirin reported headaches, which usually improved when dipyridamole was divided into four rather than two daily doses. No bleeding problems or fetal malformations were observed.

Low-dose aspirin alone was shown to prevent PIH and preeclampsia in 46 patients in a double-blind, randomized, placebo-controlled trial by Wallenburg and associates.[47] The patients were determined to be at risk by the angiotensin sensitivity test at 28 weeks of gestation. They were given aspirin 60 mg or placebo tablets to be taken once daily, and compliance was documented. Of the 23 patients in the placebo group, 4 developed PIH, 7 developed preeclampsia, and 1 developed eclampsia. In the aspirin-treated group, two patients developed mild PIH, but there were no cases of preeclampsia. There were no apparent adverse effects, including bleeding problems, in the mothers or neonates. This report indicates that low-dose aspirin begun at 28 weeks of gestation may decrease the frequency of preeclampsia in patients sensitive to angiotensin II.

Schiff et al.[48] reported that women with a positive rollover test who took 100 mg of aspirin daily had significantly less PIH than women who were given placebo. The patients were enrolled in the randomized, double-blind study at 28–29 weeks of gestation. Proteinuria developed in 22.6% of the patients receiving placebo but in only 2.9% of the patients receiving aspirin. Patients stopped taking the tablets five days before their estimated delivery date. No bleeding complications or adverse effects were noted.

In a similar study, Schiff et al.[49] treated patients hospitalized at 30–36 weeks of gestation for mild PIH with either 100 mg of aspirin daily or placebo. There were no significant differences in outcome between the two groups, leading the authors to conclude that treatment must begin weeks before clinical signs and symptoms occur to be effective.

Many risks have been associated with long-term aspirin use in pregnancy. These risks include maternal antepartum and postpartum bleeding, prolonged gestation, prolonged labor, neonatal bleeding, premature closure of the ductus arteriosus, and neonatal pulmonary hypertension.[44]

Another study of low-dose aspirin included investigation of the drug's effects on the production of 6-keto-prostaglandin $F_{1\alpha}$ (which reflects endothelial prostacyclin production) and thromboxane B_2 (a stable metabolite of thromboxane A_2), platelet aggregation, and neonatal transitional circulation. Sibai et al.[44] studied the effects of placebo and aspirin (20, 60, or 80 mg/day) in 40 normotensive, primigravid patients beginning at 37 weeks of gestation. Patients receiving 60 or 80 mg of aspirin daily had significantly decreased thromboxane concentrations after one week. Prostacyclin concentrations were not affected. All neonates had evidence of a patent ductus arteriosus, and there was no evidence of bleeding or other adverse effects. Compared with placebo, aspirin did not prolong gestation or labor.

These studies provide promising evidence that low-dose aspirin prevents the development of preeclampsia in women at risk (i.e., those who have a family history of preeclampsia, who have essential hypertension or renal disease, or who have a molar or twin pregnancy), but more studies are needed. Aspirin therapy is not recommended in patients whose only risk factor is nulliparity.

Recommendations

Obstetric patients who are at substantial risk for the development of preeclampsia (excluding those in whom nulliparity is the sole risk factor) should be given 60–150 mg of aspirin daily beginning at 28–30 weeks of gestation. Mild preeclampsia in a compliant patient may be managed conservatively with bed rest, frequent office visits, and close monitoring. A severely preeclamptic or eclamptic patient must be managed more aggressively. This patient should be hospitalized and given an i.v. infusion of magnesium sulfate to prevent seizures (usually 4 g over 15 minutes, followed by a constant infusion of 1–2 g/hr). The patient receiving magnesium sulfate must be closely monitored for development of toxicity. Monitoring variables include deep tendon reflexes, respiratory rate, urine output, and serum magnesium concentrations (goal, 4–7 meq/L). Calcium gluconate should be kept at the bedside of every patient receiving magnesium sulfate to reverse toxic effects if necessary.

If BP must be controlled to accomplish delivery, i.v. hydralazine hydrochloride is recommended. The dose is 5–10 mg every 20 minutes as needed.

Seizures occurring before initiation of magnesium sulfate therapy or those not responding to adequate concentrations of magnesium should be controlled with i.v. diazepam. Delivery is indicated as soon as the mother and fetus are stable.

Conclusion

Preeclampsia is a complication of pregnancy that may require drug therapy. Acute hypertensive episodes are usually treated with hydralazine, and magnesium sulfate is used to prevent or stop the occurrence of seizures (eclampsia). Low-dose aspirin may help prevent the development of preeclampsia in high-risk patients.

References

1. Roberts JM. Pregnancy-related hypertension. In: Creasy RK, Resnik R, eds. Maternal–fetal medicine. Philadelphia: Saunders; 1989:777-823.
2. Worley RJ. Pregnancy-induced hypertension. In: Danforth DN, Scott JR, eds. Obstetrics and gynecology. Philadelphia: Lippincott; 1986:446-66.
3. Villar MA, Sibai BM. Eclampsia. *Obstet Gynecol Clin North Am*. 1988; 15:355-77.
4. Friedman SA. Preeclampsia: a review of the role of prostaglandins. *Obstet Gynecol*. 1988; 71:122-37.
5. Silver HM. Acute hypertensive crisis in pregnancy. *Med Clin North Am*. 1989; 73:623-38.
6. Ferris TF. Toxemia and hypertension. In: Burrow GN, Ferris TF, eds. Medical complications during pregnancy. Philadelphia: Saunders; 1988:1-33.
7. Walsh SW. Preeclampsia: an imbalance in placental prostacyclin and thromboxane production. *Am J Obstet Gynecol*. 1985; 152:335-40.
8. O'Brien WF. Predicting preeclampsia. *Obstet Gynecol*. 1990; 75:445-52.
9. Gant NF, Chand S, Worley RJ et al. A clinical test for predicting the development of acute hypertension in pregnancy. *Am J Obstet Gynecol*. 1974; 120:1-7.
10. Gant NF, Daley GL, Chand S et al. A study of angiotensin II pressor response throughout primigravid pregnancy. *J Clin Invest*. 1973; 52:2682-9.
11. Oney T, Kaulhausen H. The value of the angiotensin sensitivity test in the early diagnosis of hypertensive disorders in pregnancy. *Am J Obstet Gynecol*. 1982; 142:17-20.
12. Mabie SC, Sibai BM. Hypertensive states of pregnancy. In: Pernoll ML, ed. Current obstetric and gynecologic diagnosis and treatment. Norwalk, CT: Appleton and Lange; 1991:373-87.
13. MacGillvray I. Some observations on the incidence of preeclampsia. *Br J Obstet Gynaecol*. 1958; 65:536-9.
14. Astin M, Scott JR, Worley RJ. Pre-eclampsia/eclampsia: a fatal father factor. *Lancet*. 1981; 2:533.
15. Jenkins DM, Need J, Rajah SM. Deficiency to specific HLA antibodies in severe pregnancy pre-eclampsia/eclampsia. *Clin Exp Immunol*. 1977; 27:485-6.
16. Zuspan FP, Rayburn WF. Blood pressure self-monitoring during pregnancy: practical considerations. *Am J Obstet Gynecol*. 1991; 164:2-6.
17. Sibai BM, Lipshitz J, Anderson GD et al. Reassessment of intravenous $MgSO_4$ therapy in preeclampsia–eclampsia. *Obstet Gynecol*. 1981; 57:199-202.
18. Zuspan FP, Zuspan KJ. Acute and chronic hypertension during pregnancy. In: Rayburn WF, Zuspan FP, eds. Drug therapy in obstetrics and gynecology. East Norwalk, CT: Appleton-Century-Crofts; 1986:73-92.
19. AHFS drug information 90. McEvoy GK, ed. Magnesium sulfate. Bethesda, MD: American Society of Hospital Pharmacists; 1990:1145-7.
20. Cruikshank DP, Pitkin RM, Donnelly E et al. Urinary magnesium, calcium and phosphate excretion during magnesium sulfate infusion. *Obstet Gynecol*. 1981; 58:430-4.
21. Cruikshank DP, Varner MW, Pitkin RM. Breast milk magnesium and calcium concentrations following magnesium sulfate treatment. *Am J Obstet Gynecol*. 1982; 143:685-8.
22. Thurnau GR, Kemp DB, Jarvis A. Cerebrospinal fluid levels of magnesium in patients with preeclampsia after treatment with intravenous magnesium sulfate: a preliminary report. *Am J Obstet Gynecol*. 1987; 157:1435-8.
23. Sibai BM. Magnesium sulfate is the ideal anticonvulsant in preeclampsia–eclampsia. *Am J Obstet Gynecol*. 1990; 162:1141-5.
24. Dommisse J. Phenytoin sodium and magnesium sulphate in the management of eclampsia. *Br J Obstet Gynaecol*. 1990; 97:104-9.
25. Crowther C. Magnesium sulphate versus diazepam in the management of eclampsia: a randomized controlled trial. *Br J Obstet Gynaecol*. 1990; 97:110-7.
26. Chao A. The patellar reflex in preeclamptic women with subtherapeutic and therapeutic serum magnesium levels. *J Reprod Med*. 1990; 35:678-81.
27. Van Assche FA, Spitz B, Vansteelant L. Severe systemic hypertension during pregnancy. *Am J Cardiol*. 1989; 63:22C-25C.
28. Sibai BM, Graham JM, McCubbin JH. A comparison of intravenous and intramuscular magnesium sulfate regimens in preeclampsia. *Am J Obstet Gynecol*. 1984; 150:728-33.
29. Bohman VR, Cotton DB. Supralethal magnesemia with patient survival. *Obstet Gynecol*. 1990; 76:984-6.
30. Pritchard JA. Magnesium sulfate in the treatment of eclampsia. *Arch Neurol*. 1989; 46:947-8. Letter.
31. Slater RM, Wilcox FL, Smith WD et al. Phenytoin infusion in severe preeclampsia. *Lancet*. 1987; 1:1417-20.
32. Coyagi KJ, Otiv SR. Single high dose of intravenous phenytoin sodium for the treatment of eclampsia. *Acta Obstet Gynecol Scand*. 1990; 69:115-8.
33. Briggs GE, Freeman RK, Yaffe SJ. Drugs in pregnancy and lactation. Baltimore: Williams & Wilkins; 1990:502-8.
34. Laros RK. Hypertensive disorders during pregnancy. In: Willson RJ, Carrington ER. Obstetrics and gynecology. St. Louis: Mosby; 1987:364-79.
35. Naden RP, Redman CWG. Antihypertensive drugs in pregnancy. *Clin Perinatol*. 1985; 12:521-38.
36. Shoemaker CT, Meyers M. Sodium nitroprusside for control of severe hypertensive disease of pregnancy: a case report and discussion of potential toxicity. *Am J Obstet Gynecol*. 1984; 149:171-3.
37. Mabie WC, Gonzalez AR, Sibai BM et al. A comparative trial of labetalol and hydralazine in the acute management of severe hypertension complicating pregnancy. *Obstet Gynecol*. 1987; 70:328-33.
38. Sibai BM, Gonzalez AR, Mabie WC et al. A comparison of labetalol plus hospitalization versus hospitalization alone in the management of preeclampsia remote from term. *Obstet Gynecol*. 1987; 70:323-7.
39. Lindow SW, Davies N, Davey DA et al. The effect of sublingual nifedipine on uteroplacental blood flow in hypertensive pregnancy. *Br J Obstet Gynaecol*. 1988; 95:1276-81.
40. Fenakel K, Fenakel G, Appelman Z et al. Nifedipine in the treatment of severe preeclampsia. *Obstet Gynecol*. 1991; 77:331-7.
41. Creasy RK. Preterm labor and delivery. In: Creasy RK, Resnik R, eds. Maternal–fetal medicine. Philadelphia: Saunders; 1989:477-504.

42. Waisman GD, Mayorga LM, Camera MI et al. Magnesium plus nifedipine: potentiation of hypotensive effect in preeclampsia. *Am J Obstet Gynecol.* 1988; 159:308-9.
43. Lubbe WF. Low-dose aspirin in prevention of toxaemia of pregnancy. Does it have a place? *Drugs.* 1987; 34:515-8.
44. Sibai BM, Mirro R, Chesney CM et al. Low-dose aspirin in pregnancy. *Obstet Gynecol.* 1989; 74:551-7.
45. Thorp JA, Walsh SW, Brath PC. Low-dose aspirin inhibits thromboxane, but not prostacyclin, production by human placental arteries. *Am J Obstet Gynecol.* 1988; 159:1381-4.
46. Beaufils M, Donsimoni R, Uzan S et al. Prevention of preeclampsia by early antiplatelet therapy. *Lancet.* 1985; 1:840-2.
47. Wallenburg HCS, Makovitz JW, Dekker GA et al. Low-dose aspirin prevents pregnancy-induced hypertension and preeclampsia in angiotensin-sensitive primigravidae. *Lancet.* 1986; 1:1-3.
48. Schiff E, Peleg E, Goldenberg M et al. The use of aspirin to prevent pregnancy-induced hypertension and lower the ratio of thromboxane A_2 to prostacyclin in relatively high risk pregnancies. *N Engl J Med.* 1989; 321:351-6.
49. Schiff E, Barkai G, Ben-Baruch G et al. Low-dose aspirin does not influence the clinical course of women with mild pregnancy-induced hypertension. *Obstet Gynecol.* 1990; 76:742-4.

Therapy Update

Systemic absorption of intraperitoneal antimicrobials in continuous ambulatory peritoneal dialysis

MAUREEN A. O'BRIEN AND NANCY A. MASON

Abstract: The factors that influence drug movement across the peritoneum are presented, and the feasibility of administering antimicrobials intraperitoneally to treat systemic infections in patients undergoing continuous ambulatory peritoneal dialysis (CAPD) is explored.

Antimicrobials are often administered intraperitoneally to treat peritonitis in patients undergoing CAPD. It would be advantageous to administer antimicrobials by the same route to treat systemic infections as well. Factors that determine the propensity of a drug to cross the peritoneal membrane include molecular weight, protein binding, volume of distribution, ionic charge, water or lipid solubility, the permeability and surface area of the peritoneum, blood flow rate, dialysate dwell time, and the concentration of dextrose in the dialysate. The bioavailability of i.p. drugs has been determined (1) by measuring the area under the plasma concentration–time curve (AUC) of an i.p. dose and comparing it with the AUC of the same dose given i.v. and (2) by estimating the residual drug content in the dialysate after a specified dwell period. Pharmacokinetic studies show that the bioavailabilities of antimicrobials given intraperitoneally in patients undergoing CAPD range from 50% to 92%. Vancomycin has been the agent most widely studied. Serum antimicrobial concentrations achieved by this route of administration are in many cases similar to those accomplished by the i.v. route and within the therapeutic range. Dosage regimens based on the pharmacokinetic data have been suggested; however, their efficacy has not been formally documented.

The intraperitoneal route may have a role in the treatment of systemic infections in peritoneal dialysis patients, but specific recommendations cannot be made until clinical studies have been performed.

Index terms: Absorption; Aminoglycosides; Antibiotics; Cephalosporins; Dialysis; Dosage; Drug administration routes; Pharmacokinetics; Vancomycin
Clin Pharm. 1992; 11:246-54

Antimicrobials are frequently administered via the intraperitoneal (i.p.) route to treat peritonitis in patients undergoing continuous ambulatory peritoneal dialysis (CAPD). In general, dosing guidelines for peritonitis specify an i.v. or i.p. loading dose followed by continuous i.p. administration of the antimicrobial in each exchange of dialysis solution (dialysate). CAPD typically consists of the instillation of 1 to 2.5 L of dialysate (1.5%, 2.5%, or 4.25% dextrose solution with electrolytes) into the peritoneal cavity. Each volume of dialysate exchanged dwells in the peritoneal cavity for some 4 hours during the day and up to 10 hours overnight. The dialysate is then drained by gravity, and another volume of solution is administered. Reviews of the treatment of peritonitis associated with CAPD have been published elsewhere.[1-4]

In addition to the treatment of peritonitis, i.p. administration of antimicrobials may provide concentrations in plasma sufficient to treat systemic infections. Therefore, in the patient undergoing CAPD, there would be no need to place an i.v. line. This could be advantageous, as it is not uncommon that patients in

MAUREEN A. O'BRIEN, PHARM.D., is Assistant Professor of Clinical Pharmacy, University of Southern California, Los Angeles; at the time this article was written she was Clinical Pharmacy Resident, University of Michigan Medical Center (UMMC), Ann Arbor, and Clinical Instructor of Pharmacy, College of Pharmacy, The University of Michigan (UM). NANCY A. MASON, PHARM.D., is Assistant Clinical Professor of Pharmacy, College of Pharmacy, UM, and Clinical Pharmacist–Nephrology, UMMC.

Address reprint requests to Dr. O'Brien at the College of Pharmacy, University of Southern California, 1985 Zonal Avenue, Los Angeles, CA 90033.

Adapted from an article that appeared in the September 1991 issue of *Michigan Drug Letter*, a publication of the Department of Pharmacy Services, University of Michigan Medical Center, Ann Arbor.

This is **article 680-204-9203** in the **ASHP Continuing Education System**; it qualifies for 1.0 hour of continuing-education credit. See page 261 for learning objectives and test questions.

end-stage renal failure have poor i.v. access. In patients undergoing CAPD who need systemic antimicrobial therapy, the i.p. route may be more familiar and less invasive. As the access is pre-existent, nursing assistance for the maintenance of peripheral i.v. access would be unnecessary.

Since therapeutic plasma concentrations of some antimicrobials can be achieved after i.p. administration, it may be possible to treat systemic infections with certain intraperitoneally administered antimicrobials. Reviews of i.p. administration of antimicrobials for the treatment of systemic infections have not been published. This article reviews the factors that determine drug movement in patients undergoing peritoneal dialysis and discusses the systemic absorption of specific antimicrobials administered by the i.p. route during CAPD. Some dosing guidelines based on the available pharmacokinetic data are suggested for a variety of commonly used antimicrobials.

The Therapy Update *section provides concise analytical reviews of narrowly defined, important topics in pharmacotherapy. Priority is given to articles that focus on new or emerging standards in drug therapy. Articles are not intended to be comprehensive reviews of drugs or of disease states and their treatment.*

The Peritoneum

The peritoneal cavity is lined with simple squamous mesothelium. The peritoneal membrane consists of the visceral peritoneum, which covers the visceral organs such as the kidneys and liver, and the parietal peritoneum, which lines the inner surface of the abdominal wall. The mesothelial cells secrete a surfactant that aides in lubrication. The lumenal sides of the cells have many cytoplasmic extensions, which increase the surface area of the peritoneum.[5] Underlying the mesothelial cells is a basement membrane. The interstitium between these two layers contains a reticular formation of collagen fibers and proteoglycan filaments. Fluid, electrolytes, nutrients, and oxygen are transported through this interstitium.

The blood supply to the visceral peritoneum is provided by the superior mesenteric artery, whereas the parietal peritoneum is supplied by the intercostal, lumbar, and epigastric arteries. Blood in the visceral and parietal peritoneum returns to the portal and caval circulation, respectively; thus drugs administered by the i.p. route are subjected to partial first-pass metabolism by the liver.[5]

The parietal peritoneum and visceral peritoneum are both drained by an extensive lymphatic network. The lymphatic drainage returns protein and excess lymph to the venous circulation by a one-way system. Macromolecules are absorbed through the subdiaphragmatic lymphatic system.[5] An increase in the rate of lymphatic absorption may decrease the amount of fluid removed from the systemic circulation during peritoneal dialysis because of a change in oncotic pressure.[6]

Drug Movement across the Peritoneal Membrane

Solutes move across the peritoneal membrane primarily through diffusion from the area of higher concentration to the area of lower concentration. Therefore, higher initial drug concentrations within the peritoneum may promote greater systemic absorption. The factors that determine the propensity of a drug to cross the peritoneal membrane include molecular weight, protein binding, volume of distribution, ionic charge, and water or lipid solubility.[7] Other factors include the permeability and surface area of the peritoneal membrane, blood flow rate, dialysate dwell time, and the concentration of dextrose in the dialysate.[8]

The movement of solutes across the peritoneal membrane is inversely related to particle size. Drugs with molecular weights of less than 5200 (the size of inulin) are able to cross the peritoneal membrane.[7]

Protein binding plays an important role in the movement of drug molecules across the peritoneum. In general, the unbound fraction of a drug is able to cross much more quickly than the bound fraction; therefore, drugs with less protein binding are more readily cleared by CAPD. High plasma protein binding encourages systemic absorption of intraperitoneally administered drugs because of the concentration gradient between the smaller free fraction in blood and the larger free fraction in the relatively protein-free dialysate.[7,9] The dialysate protein concentration may increase during peritonitis,[10,11] which hypothetically could reduce the systemic absorption of highly bound drugs. This effect may be offset by the enhanced drug absorption and increased permeability of the membrane caused by inflammation during peritonitis.[11,12] In addition, patients with end-stage renal disease undergoing CAPD have altered protein binding that is due to reduced serum albumin concentrations and uremia itself.[8] The reduction in serum albumin has been attributed to poor nutritional status and protein loss during CAPD, which averages 8.8 g in 24 hours.[8]

The systemic volume of distribution influences drug movement according to the properties of mass transport.[7] The rapid movement of a drug from the peritoneal space to the systemic circulation contrasts with the slow appearance of the same drug in the peritoneal dialysate when administered by the i.v. route. This apparent discrepancy has been labeled unidirectional drug transport[13] but is most likely explained by the difference between the small volume of the peritoneal cavity and the large volume of distribution of the body.[10] When a drug is added to the small volume of the peritoneal cavity, the initial i.p. concentration is much higher than the systemic concentration, facilitating absorption. After i.p. administration, drugs with larger volumes of distribution are theoretically absorbed more completely because the rapid systemic distribution maintains a steep concentration gradient between the two compartments.[10] In contrast, when a drug with a small volume of distribution (hence, an increased vascular concentration) is administered systemically, removal by CAPD is promoted. [7,10,12]

The passage of drug molecules through pores and intercellular channels of the peritoneal membrane is dependent on ionic characteristics, as well as lipid and water solubility.[14] Membrane pores are lined with lipophilic and charged protein groups that inhibit the passage of charged molecules. As ionization at physiological pH increases, absorption of molecules through the membrane decreases.[14] For example, i.p. administration of heparin, an electrostatically charged molecule, rarely affects systemic coagulation.[9] In contrast, water-soluble drugs travel through intercellular channels of the membrane, allowing for quick diffusion. Lipid-soluble drugs must diffuse through the cell membrane and are not removed by CAPD as efficiently as water-soluble drugs. The effect of lipid solubility on the movement of intraperitoneally administered drugs is not clear, since the absorption of intraperitoneally introduced barbiturates is quite rapid.[15]

Peritoneal blood flow also affects drug movement. The administration of vasodilating drugs such as dipyridamole and low-dose dopamine increases the clearance of solutes with higher molecular weights because vasodilation stretches capillary walls, making them more permeable.[16] However, vasodilators do not influence the movement of smaller solutes, as smaller particles depend on concentration gradient rather than pore size for diffusion across the peritoneal membrane.

The permeability of the membrane may be altered in several disease states. Peritoneal dialysis clearances are reduced in the presence of lupus erythematosus, malignant hypertension, and scleroderma because of decreased blood flow to the peritoneum.[8] Increased permeability is seen chronically in diabetes[17] and acutely during routine peritonitis, in which increased transport of glucose and other solutes has been demonstrated.[18] Prolonged or recurrent peritonitis may ultimately cause adhesions and sclerosis, reducing the surface area (normally 1.5 to 4.5 sq m[8]) available for drug transport.[7]

The effect of dialysate dwell time on the movement of a drug varies depending on the molecular weight of the drug. Drugs with low molecular weights equilibrate rapidly. Therefore, rapid absorption will occur even during short dialysate dwell times. Movement of high-molecular-weight drugs is influenced much less by a shorter dwell time. It may take longer than six hours for high-molecular-weight drugs to approach equilibrium. Therefore, increasing the frequency of dialysate exchanges does not greatly affect the absorption rate of high-molecular-weight drugs.[9]

Dextrose in the dialysate creates osmotic pressure that pulls water from the systemic circulation into the peritoneal cavity (ultrafiltration). Dialysis of low-molecular-weight drugs is enhanced by increasing the dextrose concentration because of the solute "drag" that carries dissolved drugs and other solutes along with the water during this process.[8] The comparative effects of different dextrose concentrations on the systemic absorption of i.p. drugs have not been reported.

Determination of Bioavailability

The bioavailability of drugs administered by the i.p. route has been determined by using two methods. The more precise method involves determining the area under the plasma concentration–time curve (AUC) of an i.p. dose and comparing it with the AUC of the same dose given intravenously ($AUC_{i.p.}/AUC_{i.v.}$).[7,9] In the second method, bioavailability is estimated from the original drug content and the residual drug content in the dialysate after a specified dwell period. This method may overestimate systemic drug absorption because of possible decomposition of the drug during the dwell time, incomplete drainage of the dialysate from the peritoneum, or adherence of drug to the plastic bag or lines.[9]

Vancomycin

Vancomycin is the most widely studied antimicrobial administered intraperitoneally during CAPD. Vancomycin is excreted, mainly unchanged, by the kidneys. It has a six-hour serum half-life in patients with normal renal function and a half-life of four to eight days in patients with severe renal failure.[18] Vancomycin is a large molecule (molecular weight, 1450) containing several ionizable groups. The agent is 52% to 60% protein bound.[19]

Bunke et al.[18] studied the disposition of single doses of i.v. and i.p. vancomycin (as the hydrochloride salt) in six patients without peritonitis undergoing CAPD. The administration of a single dose of vancomycin 10 mg/kg i.p. in a 2-L dialysate volume with a four-hour dwell time resulted in a mean peak concentration in plasma of 6 mg/L, with 65% of the vancomycin being absorbed systemically (determined by measuring the residual concentration in the dialysate). Using these data, the authors postulated that a 30-mg/kg i.p. loading dose followed by 7 mg/kg in one exchange per day could maintain a steady-state vancomycin concentration of 11 to 14.8 mg/L. Alternatively, a 30-mg/kg i.p. loading dose followed by 1.5 mg/kg in each subsequent exchange with a four-hour dwell time was postulated to maintain plasma concentrations above 10 mg/L. Studies by other investigators have shown similar bioavailabilities and peak serum concentrations.[20-22] Pancorbo and Comty[21] suggested that 10 to 20 mg/L could be added to each i.p. exchange to maintain serum concentrations above 10 mg/L. Morse et al.[23] proposed that a weekly 30-mg/kg i.p. dose administered in an exchange with a six-hour dwell time could provide adequate serum vancomycin concentrations.

From the data reviewed and pharmacokinetic extrapolation, dosage schedules that mimic the serum vancomycin concentrations observed with intermittent i.v. administration can be devised for i.p. administration. One such regimen is 30 mg/kg i.p. followed by 15 mg/kg i.p. at intervals of about one elimination half-life (two to five days). This regimen allows trough concentrations to reach 10 to 15 mg/L before the next dose. Alternatively, relatively constant serum concentrations are attainable by adding smaller quantities of vancomycin to each bag of dialysate.[18,21] Although many i.p. dosage schemes have been proposed for vancomycin, clinical trials assessing the efficacy of these regimens in the treatment of systemic infections have not been conducted.

Aminoglycosides

Aminoglycosides are complex polar molecules consisting of aminosugars with glycosidic linkages. They exhibit both low protein binding (less than 10% bound to plasma protein) and a low volume of distribution (0.25 L/kg in healthy subjects).[24] The aminoglycosides have molecular weights of 400 to 500. Excretion is primarily by glomerular filtration; prolonged elimination half-lives are seen in patients with renal insufficiency.

Smeltzer et al.[25] evaluated the pharmacokinetics of amikacin (as the sulfate salt) in five patients without peritonitis undergoing CAPD in a crossover study comparing single 7.5-mg/kg i.p. and i.v. doses. Dialysate dwell time was five hours. Both methods of administration produced a similar half-life, volume of distribution, and total body clearance. The mean ± S.D. peak plasma concentration achieved after the i.p. dose was 19.6 ± 6.1 mg/L, compared with a range of 30 to 45 mg/L achieved by i.v. administration. At 72 hours after i.p. or i.v. administration, mean serum amikacin concentrations were 5.4 and 12.0 mg/L, respectively. The fraction absorbed after i.p. administration was calculated to be 53% (determined by $AUC_{i.p.}/AUC_{i.v.}$).

Somani et al.[13] studied five patients without peritonitis who received a single 1-mg/kg i.p. dose of gentamicin (as the sulfate salt). The dwell time was six hours. After a washout period the patients received the same dose i.v. Eighty-four percent of the i.p. dose was absorbed systemically (determined by $AUC_{i.p.}/AUC_{i.v.}$ and measurement of residual concentration). The mean peak serum concentration was 3.5 mg/L after i.p. administration. In a study by De Paepe et al.,[26] one patient with peritonitis was treated continuously with gentamicin 7.5 mg/L in each exchange for 21 days and achieved a peak concentration of 5 mg/L.

Walshe et al.[27] administered tobramycin (as the sulfate salt) 2 mg/kg i.v. and i.p. in single doses to five patients without peritonitis in a crossover study. The i.v. route resulted in a mean peak serum tobramycin concentration of 9.8 mg/L. Mean concentrations remained above 1.8 mg/L for 48 hours. The i.p. treatment produced a mean peak serum concentration of 5.6 mg/L at the end of the six-hour dwell time. The mean serum concentration remained above 1.3 mg/L for more than 48 hours. The bioavailability of i.p. tobramycin was 73% (determined by $AUC_{i.p.}/AUC_{i.v.}$). In another phase of the study, four patients received a 1-mg/kg i.p. loading dose of tobramycin and then a maintenance dose of 0.6 mg/kg in one exchange per day for an unspecified time. Measured trough concentrations were 2 to 2.5 mg/L. Peak concentrations were not reported. By using computer-aided physiological modeling, the authors postulated that a 3-mg/kg i.p. loading dose plus 1.2 mg/kg in one exchange per day would yield a peak concentration between 6 and 8 mg/L. This would also allow a 40% decrease in plasma concentration between doses, which is desirable because of the possible ototoxicity of aminoglycosides. In a similar study by Bunke et al.,[28] tobramycin bioavailability was 52% after a four-hour dwell time as determined by an unspecified method. Computer modeling suggested that a 4-mg/kg loading dose followed by 1.5 mg/kg in one four-hour dialysate exchange per day would provide steady-state concentrations between 2.8 and 4.1 mg/L.

These studies of the pharmacokinetics of intraperitoneally administered aminoglycosides show that serum concentrations similar to those observed after i.v. administration are possible. In addition to the dosage recommendations suggested by these studies, a patient-specific approach may be considered. Serum antimicrobial concentrations can be used to calculate half-life and clearance to determine when the serum drug concentration will reach the trough range. The next dose can then be given when the concentration reaches the recommended trough range (<2 mg/L for gentamicin and tobramycin and <10 mg/L for amikacin). As with vancomycin, none of these i.p. regimens have been compared for efficacy in the treatment of systemic infections.

Cephalosporins

The pharmacokinetics of cephalothin,[29] cefazolin,[30,31] cefoxitin,[32] cefoperazone,[33,34] cefotaxime,[35-37] ceftazidime,[38] ceftizoxime,[39] ceftriaxone,[40] and moxalactam[41] have been investigated during i.p. administration in CAPD-treated patients (Table 1). Although all these drugs are absorbed during i.p. administration, treatment of systemic infections by this route has not been documented. Pharmacokinetic information may be limited because systemic concentrations of cephalosporins are not routinely analyzed in the clinical setting.

Cefazolin is active against gram-positive cocci, group D β-hemolytic streptococci, and group B streptococci; it has limited activity against gram-negative bacteria. *Staphylococcus aureus* and *Streptococcus pneumoniae* are susceptible to cefazolin at concentrations of 0.1 to 1 mg/L. *Escherichia coli* and *Klebsiella pneumoniae* are inhibited in vitro at concentrations of 0.8 to 12.5 mg/L. The average peak serum concentration after a

Table 1.
Pharmacokinetics of Antimicrobials Administered by Continuous Ambulatory Peritoneal Dialysis[a]

Drug	Reference	Dosage	Dwell Time (hr)	Duration of Study	Mean Peak Plasma Concentration (mg/L) I.P.	Mean Peak Plasma Concentration (mg/L) I.V.	Bioavailability (%)	Mean $t_{1/2}$ (hr)	*V*	No. Patients	I.P. Dosage Recommendation
Vancomycin (as the hydrochloride salt)	18	10 mg/kg	4	SD	6	10	65	66	1.2 L/kg	6	30-mg/kg LD and 7 mg/kg/day or 1.5 mg/kg per exchange
	20	1-g LD and 50 mg per exchange ×3	6	18 hr	9.1	. . .	73	. . .	1.2–1.8 L/kg	5	. . .
	21	1 g	6	SD	23.7	. . .	54	66.9	0.43 L/kg	4	1-g LD and 10–20 mg/L per exchange
	22	500 mg LD and 250 mg/day	6	10 days	10	. . .	83	. . .	. . .	6[b]	500 mg LD and 250 mg/day
	23	30 mg/kg	6	SD	30.4	57.1	52	91	0.56 L/kg	4	30 mg/kg/wk
			6	SD	24.5	. . .	. . .	104	. . .	4[b]	. . .
Amikacin (as the sulfate salt)	25	7.5 mg/kg	5	SD	19.6	30–45	53	42	0.17 L/kg	5	. . .
Gentamicin (as the sulfate salt)	13	1 mg/kg	6	SD	3.5	. . .	84	27.9	0.2 L/kg	5	. . .
	26	7.5 mg/L	6	SD	1.5	. . .	69	. . .	. . .	5	. . .
			6	SD	. . .	. . .	85	. . .	. . .	5[b]	. . .
			6	21 days	5	. . .	. . .	. . .	. . .	1	. . .
Tobramycin (as the sulfate salt)	27	2 mg/kg	6	SD	5.6	9.8	73	31	0.27 L/kg	5	3-mg/kg LD and 1.2 mg/kg/day
	27	1-mg/kg LD and 0.6 mg/kg/day	6	. . .	2.1	. . .	. . .	. . .	. . .	4	. . .
	28	1.5 mg/kg	4	SD	1.8	3	52	35	0.47 L/kg	12	4-mg/kg LD and 1.5 mg/kg/day
Cephalothin (as the sodium salt)	29	100 mg/L	6	MD	5.3	. . .	. . .	. . .	. . .	7	100 mg/L per exchange
Cefazolin (as the sodium salt)	30	10 mg/kg	4	SD	30–40	>50	73	33	0.189 L/kg	6	10-mg/kg LD and 5 mg/kg per exchange
	31	1 g in 2 L × 1 and 500 mg in 2 L	6	3 days	110.9	. . .	85	. . .	. . .	5[b]	. . .
Cefoxitin (as the sodium salt)	32	50 mg/L	6	24 hr	7	. . .	71	20	22 L	9	Neither cefoxitin concentration is suggested for the treatment of systemic infections
		100 mg/L	. . .	. . .	15	. . .	. . .	. . .	. . .	. . .	
Cefoperazone (as the sodium salt)	33	1 g	10	SD	33	104	81	. . .	14 L	7	1 g per exchange four times a day
	34	2 g	6	SD	38	280	61	. . .	. . .	6	. . .

Continued on next page

Table 1 *(continued)*

Drug	Reference	Dosage	Dwell Time (hr)	Duration of Study	Mean Peak Plasma Concentration (mg/L) I.P.	Mean Peak Plasma Concentration (mg/L) I.V.	Bioavailability (%)	Mean $t_{1/2}$ (hr)	V	No. Patients	I.P. Dosage Recommendation
Cefotaxime (as the sodium salt)	35	2 g	6	SD	30	323	47	...	0.17 L/kg	8	...
	36	1 g	9	SD	20	100	...	...	...	10	...
	37	1 g	4	SD	15	72	58	11	...	8	...
Ceftazidime	38	50 mg/L	6	12 days	11	...	...	...	...	11[b]	...
	38	50 mg/L	5	12 days	...	...	...	...	...	2[b]	...
Ceftizoxime (as the sodium salt)	39	500 mg	6	SD	16	29	78	10.2	0.27 L/kg	8	...
Ceftriaxone (as the sodium salt)	40	2 g	5	SD	104	...	74	12.7	...	6	200 mg per exchange
Moxalactam (as the disodium salt)	41	1 g	4	SD	34	>100	...	15.5	...	10	...
Aztreonam	22	2 g in 2 L	6	5 days	83	...	92	9.3	...	6[b]	3 g/day
	42	1 g in 2 L	8	SD	42.5	...	91	2.4	...	6	500 mg/L per exchange
Ciprofloxacin	43	50 mg/L	6	7 days	1.1	...	...	...	...	44[b]	...
	44	5 mg/kg	4	SD	1.9	...	84	5.6	...	6	...
	44	25 mg/L	4	32 hr	0.5	...	66	...	...	6	...
Clindamycin (as the phosphate salt)	45	300 mg/L	4–6	28 hr	5.75	...	...	...	...	5	...
Trimethoprim–sulfamethoxazole	46	320 mg (trimethoprim)	4	SD	2.4	3.8	84	5.6	...	6	...
		1600 mg (sulfamethoxazole)			46	68	66	5.6	...		...
Ampicillin–sulbactam (as the sodium salts)	47	2 g 1 g	6	SD	87.5 27.8	170.3 48.0	60 80	9.6 9.4	19 L 18 L	6	2 g ampicillin and 1 g sulbactam every 12 hr
Azlocillin (as the sodium salt)	48	500 mg	6	7 days	16	...	...	...	...	1[b]	...
Imipenem with cilastatin (as the sodium salt)	49	500 mg	6	SD	10	29	79	...	...	6	...
Piperacillin (as the sodium salt)	50	1 g	6	MD	...	...	83	...	...	4	...
	50	1 g	6	SD	...	...	68	...	...	3[b]	...

[a]SD = single dose, MD = multiple dose, LD = loading dose, V = volume of distribution, $t_{1/2}$ = half-life.
[b]Patient(s) had peritonitis.

1-g i.v. dose is 188 mg/L. Cefazolin is 74% to 86% plasma protein bound and is excreted unchanged in the urine.[19]

Bunke et al.[30] administered a single dose of cefazolin (as the sodium salt) 10 mg/kg i.p. or i.v. to 12 subjects (six in each group). Seventy-three percent of the i.p. dose was absorbed systemically (determined by an unspecified method). Computer-predicted plasma concentrations were determined for i.p. cefazolin. It was estimated that a 10-mg/kg i.p. loading dose followed by 5-mg/kg doses in each exchange the first day and 2.5-mg/kg doses in each exchange thereafter should maintain plasma cefazolin concentrations between 50 and 65 mg/L.

Cefoperazone inhibits *Staph. aureus* and *Staph. epidermidis* in vitro at a concentration of 4 mg/L and many Enterobacteriaceae at a minimum inhibitory concentration for 90% of organisms (MIC_{90}) of 0.5 to 8 mg/L. It is active against some anaerobes at concentrations of 1 to 8 mg/L, but it is less active than cefoxitin.[19] Protein binding is approximately 90%. The dosage administered to patients with renal failure does not require adjustment because cefoperazone is primarily eliminated in the bile.

Keller et al.[33] compared seven patients who received cefoperazone (as the sodium salt) 1 g i.p. (10-hour dwell time) and 1 g i.v. in a single-dose, crossover study. Systemic bioavailability after i.p. administration was 81% (determined by $AUC_{i.p.}/AUC_{i.v.}$). The authors anticipated that cefoperazone 1 g i.p. in each six-hour exchange may be adequate to treat systemic infections. Johnson et al.[34] reported a cefoperazone bioavailability after i.p. administration of only 61% ($AUC_{i.p.}/AUC_{i.v.}$), however.

Cefotaxime is 13% to 36% bound to plasma proteins and has a volume of distribution of 0.24 L/kg.[19] A concentration of 0.5 mg/L in vitro inhibits *Strep. pneumoniae* and *Strep. pyogenes*. The MIC_{90} for *Staph. epidermidis* is 4.8 to 16 mg/L. The *Haemophilus influenzae* MIC_{90} is 0.08 to 0.8 mg/L, whereas *Pseudomonas* species are inhibited at concentrations of 32 to 65 mg/L. Cefotaxime is also active against many other gram-negative aerobic bacteria.[19]

In a crossover study by Heim et al.,[35] eight patients received a single 2-g dose of cefotaxime (as the sodium salt) i.v. or i.p. (dwell time, six hours). The bioavailability of the i.p. dose was 47% (determined by $AUC_{i.p.}/AUC_{i.v.}$). Similar bioavailabilities have been reported by other investigators.[36,37]

Ceftizoxime is 28% to 31% plasma protein bound. Its volume of distribution is 0.29 to 0.34 L/kg. It is excreted, largely unchanged, in the urine.[19] A concentration of 4 mg/L in vitro inhibits most strains of *Staph. aureus* and *Staph. epidermidis*. Ceftizoxime is reported to be active against most Enterobacteriaceae; the MIC_{90} is less than 1.6 mg/L.[19]

Gross et al.[39] examined eight patients who received ceftizoxime (as the sodium salt) by both the i.p. and i.v. routes. Seventy-eight percent of a 500-mg i.p. dose was absorbed after six hours (determined from the residual concentration in the dialysate). The authors concluded that therapeutic plasma ceftizoxime concentrations are obtainable by i.p. administration. Further investigation is needed to determine the optimal dosage.

Ceftriaxone has activity against gram-positive organisms. The MIC_{90} for *Strep. pneumoniae* and *Strep. viridans* is below 1 mg/L. The MIC_{90} for *Neisseria* species and *H. influenzae* is also below 1 mg/L, and most Enterobacteriaceae are susceptible at concentrations below 4 mg/L.[19] Ceftriaxone is 58% to 96% plasma protein bound.

Koup et al.[40] administered single doses of ceftriaxone (as the sodium salt) 2 g i.p. to six patients without peritonitis who were being maintained on CAPD. After five hours, 74% of the i.p. dose was absorbed (determined from the residual amount in the dialysate). Physiological modeling predicted that administration of 200 mg in each five-hour exchange would maintain steady-state serum concentrations of 50 to 100 mg/L, well above the MIC for gram-negative organisms, *Streptococcus* species, and susceptible strains of *Staph. aureus*.

In summary, the bioavailability of the cephalosporins studied after i.p. administration ranged from 47% to 81%, and peak plasma concentrations were adequate for treating most susceptible organisms when doses of 1 to 2 g were given. It would be reasonable to administer these agents at intervals similar to those used in end-stage renal disease. Alternatively, smaller doses of selected cephalosporins (100 to 250 mg/L) could be added to each dialysate exchange (Table 1). As with the other antimicrobials, there are no studies documenting the efficacy of treating systemic infections with i.p. cephalosporins.

Other Antimicrobials

Aztreonam is mainly used against gram-negative aerobic bacteria; MICs for *E. coli* and *Serratia marcescens* are 0.06 to 4 mg/L and 0.39 to 6.3 mg/L, respectively.[19] The administration of 1 g i.v. produces a mean peak serum concentration of 204 mg/L at 10 minutes.[51] Aztreonam pharmacokinetics have been examined by several investigators.[22,42] Nikolaidis et al.[42] administered a single 1-g i.p. dose of aztreonam in 2 L of dialysate (dwell time, eight hours) to 10 uninfected patients undergoing CAPD. Bioavailability was 90.8%. The authors concluded that aztreonam 500 mg/L may penetrate the peritoneum sufficiently to treat systemic infections.

Ciprofloxacin is active against many gram-positive and gram-negative aerobic bacteria, with an MIC of less than 1 mg/L.[19] After a single 100-mg i.v. dose in healthy adults, the average peak serum concentration is 2.8 mg/L. After a single 250- or 1000-mg oral dose, peak serum concentrations average 0.8 to 1.5 mg/L and 3.4 to 5.4 mg/L, respectively. Oral bioavailability is 50% to 85%.[19] Ciprofloxacin pharmacokinetics have been studied in CAPD-treated patients with peritonitis[47] and without peritonitis.[44,52] Dharmasena et al.[44] examined ciprofloxacin pharmacokinetics in six patients without peritonitis. A single 5-mg/kg i.p. dose was administered in 2 L of dialysate (dwell time, four hours). Bioavailability was 84%, with mean peak serum concentrations reaching 1.9 mg/L. Since the bioavailabilities of oral and i.p. ciprofloxacin are similar and since the cost of the injectable form is so high, i.p. administration of this drug may not be a prudent choice for the treatment of a systemic infection unless oral administration is not an option.

Clindamycin is microbiologically inactive in vitro. It is metabolized to an active form by hydrolases in vivo.[53] Serum concentrations greater than 5 mg/L are considered adequate to treat gram-positive aerobes and gram-negative anaerobes. An i.m. or i.v. dose of 300 mg (as the phosphate salt) every eight hours results in an average peak serum concentration of 6 or 10 mg/L, respectively.[19] After oral administration of 150 mg (as the hydrochloride salt), peak serum concentrations of 1.9 to 3.9 mg/L are attained.[19] In a study by Schwartz et al.,[45] nine uninfected patients undergoing CAPD received a loading dose of 300 mg/L in a 2-L bag of dialysate. One group of five patients received four subsequent exchanges containing 300 mg/L, and the other four patients received four subsequent exchanges containing 30 mg/L. After the fifth four-hour dwell period, mean concentrations of active clindamycin in serum were 5.8 and 1.6 mg/L for the two groups, respectively. However, only 3% of the drug remaining in the peritoneal fluid was converted to the active form. Golper et al.[54] also found that clindamycin is incompletely activated in dialysate effluent and suggested that clindamycin be administered by both the i.v. and i.p. routes to treat peritonitis.[55] However, Schwartz et al.[45] concluded that i.p. clindamycin was a feasible therapy for nonperitonitis infections in CAPD-treated patients with poor i.v. access.

Walker et al.[46] described the pharmacokinetics of single-dose trimethoprim 320 mg with sulfamethoxazole 1600 mg after i.v., i.p., and oral administration in 10 subjects on three separate occasions. The bioavailability of trimethoprim was 73% and 98% after i.p. and oral administration, respectively. The bioavailability of sulfamethoxazole was 65% and 87% after i.p. and oral administration, respectively. Peak concentrations of trimethoprim and sulfamethoxazole in serum after i.p. administration were lower than peak concentrations reached after oral administration of comparable doses. Thus, it may be inadvisable to treat systemic infections with i.p. trimethoprim–sulfamethoxazole unless the patient is unable to receive medications orally.

Ampicillin–sulbactam is active against staphylococci, streptococci, and many gram-negative organisms. Blackwell et al.[47] conducted a crossover study in which six uninfected patients undergoing CAPD received a single 2-g dose of ampicillin–sulbactam i.p. or i.v.. The authors concluded that additional doses every 12 to 24 hours would probably maintain serum drug concentrations above the MIC for most susceptible organisms.

The pharmacokinetics of i.p. azlocillin,[48] imipenem–cilastatin,[49] and piperacillin[50,56] have also been examined (Table 1). Incidental data have been reported for erythromycin.[57] However, data on key pharmacokinetic variables such as bioavailability and mean peak concentration have not been reported.

Conclusion

Many factors determine the ability of a drug to cross the peritoneal membrane. The antimicrobials reviewed in this article appear to be substantially absorbed—generally greater than 50% absorbed. Potential i.p. regimens for vancomycin and the aminoglycosides are relatively easy to determine, as serum concentration data are readily available. For the cephalosporins, a 1- to 2-g i.p. dose given at intervals consistent with the manufacturers' recommended i.v. dosages for patients undergoing CAPD would be reasonable. Drugs for which the oral form provides good bioavailability, such as ciprofloxacin or trimethoprim–sulfamethoxazole, should be administered orally when possible for reasons of cost and convenience.

The i.p. route may have a role in the treatment of systemic infections. However, it is difficult to make specific recommendations based on the present literature. In many studies only single-dose i.p. administration was examined, and serum drug concentrations were not measured at serum–dialysate equilibrium. Some recommendations are based on computer modeling, with no in vivo data to substantiate them. Most important, the clinical efficacy of i.p. antimicrobials against systemic infections has not been formally reported, although there is anecdotal support.

References

1. Spenser RC. Infections in continuous ambulatory peritoneal dialysis. *J Med Microbiol.* 1988; 27:1-9.
2. Winton MD, Everett ED. Antimicrobial therapy for CAPD-associated peritonitis. *Blood Purif.* 1989; 7:115-25.
3. Horton MW, Deeter RG, Sherman RA. Treatment of peritonitis in patients undergoing continuous ambulatory peritoneal dialysis. *Clin Pharm.* 1990; 9:102-18.
4. Johnson CA, Zimmerman SW, Rogge M. The pharmacokinetics of antibiotics used to treat peritoneal dialysis-associated peritonitis. *Am J Kidney Dis.* 1984; 4:3-17.
5. Khanna R, Nolph KD. The physiology of peritoneal dialysis. *Am J Nephrol.* 1989; 9:504-12.
6. Maher J. Physiology of the peritoneum: implications for peritoneal dialysis. *Med Clin North Am.* 1990; 74:985-95.
7. Lameire N, Ringoir S. Pharmacokinetic aspects of drug transport in continuous ambulatory peritoneal dialysis. *Adv Exp Med Biol.* 1989; 260:105-16.
8. Paton TW, Cornish WR, Manuel MA et al. Drug therapy in patients undergoing peritoneal dialysis. *Clin Pharmacokinet.* 1985; 10:404-26.
9. Janknegt R, Koks CHW. Pharmacokinetic aspects during continuous ambulatory peritoneal dialysis: a literature review. *Pharm Weekbl.* 1984; 6:229-36.
10. Keller E, Reetze P, Schollmeyer P. Drug therapy in patients undergoing continuous ambulatory peritoneal dialysis: clinical pharmacokinetic considerations. *Clin Pharmacokinet.* 1990; 18:104-17.
11. Morse GD, Apicella MA, Walshe JJ. Absorption of intraperitoneal antibiotics. *Drug Intell Clin Pharm.* 1988; 22:58-61.
12. Raja RM, Kramer MS, Barber D. Solute transport and ultrafiltration during peritonitis in CAPD patients. *Trans Am Soc Artif Intern Organs.* 1984; 1:8-11.
13. Somani P, Shipiro R, Stockard H et al. Unidirectional absorption of gentamicin from the peritoneum during continuous ambulatory peritoneal dialysis. *Clin Pharmacol Ther.* 1982; 32:113-20.
14. Maher JF. Characteristics of peritoneal transport: physiological and clinical implications. *Miner Electrolyte Metab.* 1981; 5:201-11.
15. Torres IJ, Litterst CL, Guarino AM. Transport of model compounds across the peritoneal membrane in the rat. *Pharmacology.* 1978; 17:330-40.
16. Steinhauer HB. Pharmacological manipulation of peritoneal transport in CAPD. *Clin Nephrol.* 1988; 30(Suppl 1):S29-33.
17. Lamiere N, Bogart F, Belpare F et al. Vancomycin kinetics during continuous ambulatory peritoneal dialysis. In: Godel R, ed. Continuous peritoneal dialysis. London: Churchill Livingstone; 1986: 66.
18. Bunke CM, Arnoff GR, Brier ME et al. Vancomycin kinetics during continuous ambulatory peritoneal dialysis. *Clin Pharmacol Ther.* 1983; 34:631-7.
19. AHFS drug information 90. McEvoy GK, ed. Bethesda, MD: American Society of Hospital Pharmacists; 1990:51-335.
20. Rogge M, Johnson CA, Zimmerman SW et al. Vancomycin disposition during continuous ambulatory peritoneal dialysis: a pharmacokinetic analysis of peritoneal drug transport.

Antimicrob Agents Chemother. 1985; 27:578-82.

21. Pancorbo S, Comty C. Peritoneal transport of vancomycin in four patients undergoing continuous ambulatory peritoneal dialysis. *Nephron*. 1982; 31:37-9.
22. Brown J, Altmann P, Cunningham J et al. Pharmacokinetics of once daily intra-peritoneal aztreonam and vancomycin in the treatment of CAPD peritonitis. *J Antimicrob Chemother*. 1990; 25:141-7.
23. Morse GD, Farolino DF, Apicella MA et al. Comparative study of intraperitoneal and intravenous vancomycin pharmacokinetics during continuous ambulatory peritoneal dialysis. *Antimicrob Agents Chemother*. 1987; 31:173-7
24. Sande MA, Mandell GL. Chemotherapy of microbial diseases. In: Goodman and Gilman's the pharmacological basis of therapeutics. 8th ed. Gilman AG, Goodman LS, Rall TW et al., eds. New York: Pergamon; 1990:1098.
25. Smeltzer BD, Schwartzman MS, Bertino J. Amikacin pharmacokinetics during continuous ambulatory peritoneal dialysis. *Antimicrob Agents Chemother*. 1988; 32:236-40.
26. De Paepe N, Lameire N, Belpaire F et al. Peritoneal pharmacokinetics of gentamicin in man. *Clin Nephrol*. 1983; 19:107-9.
27. Walshe G, Morse GD, Janicke DM et al. Crossover pharmacokinetic analysis comparing intravenous and intraperitoneal administration of tobramycin. *J Infect Dis*. 1986; 153:796-9.
28. Bunke CM, Aronoff GR, Brier ME et al. Tobramycin kinetics during continuous ambulatory peritoneal dialysis. *Clin Pharmacol Ther*. 1983; 34:110-6.
29. Munch R, Steurer J, Luthy R et al. Serum and dialysate concentrations of intraperitoneal cephalothin in patients undergoing continuous ambulatory peritoneal dialysis. *Clin Nephrol*. 1983; 20:40-3.
30. Bunke CM, Arnoff GR, Brier ME et al. Cefazolin and cephalexin kinetics in continuous ambulatory peritoneal dialysis. *Clin Pharmacol Ther*. 1983; 33:66-72.
31. Paton TW, Manuel A, Cohen LB. The disposition of cefazolin and tobramycin following intraperitoneal administration in patients on continuous ambulatory peritoneal dialysis. *Perit Dial Bull*. 1985; 5:73-6.
32. Arvidsson A, Alvan G, Tranaeus A et al. Pharmacokinetic studies of cefoxitin in continuous ambulatory peritoneal dialysis. *Eur J Clin Pharmacol*. 1985; 28:333-7.
33. Keller E, Jansen A, Pelz K et al. Intraperitoneal and intravenous cefoperazone kinetics during continuous ambulatory peritoneal dialysis. *Clin Pharmacol Ther*. 1984; 35:208-13.
34. Johnson CA, Zimmerman SW, Reitberg DP et al. Pharmacokinetics and pharmacodynamics of cefoperazone–sulbactam in patients on continuous ambulatory peritoneal dialysis. *Antimicrob Agents Chemother*. 1988; 32:51-6.
35. Heim KL, Halstenson CE, Comty CM et al. Disposition of cefotaxime and desacetyl cefotaxime during continuous ambulatory peritoneal dialysis. *Antimicrob Agents Chemother*. 1986; 30:15-9.
36. Albin HC, Demotes-Mainard FM, Bouchet JL et al. Pharmacokinetics of intravenous and intraperitoneal cefotaxime in chronic ambulatory peritoneal dialysis. *Clin Pharmacol Ther*. 1985; 38:285-9.
37. Matousovic K, Moravek J, Vitko S et al. Pharmacokinetics of intravenous and intraperitoneal cefotaxime in patients undergoing CAPD. *Perit Dial Bull*. 1985; 4:33-5.
38. Gray HH, Goulding S, Eykyn SJ. Intraperitoneal vancomycin and ceftazidime in the treatment of CAPD peritonitis. *Clin Nephrol*. 1985; 23:81-4.
39. Gross ML, Somani P, Ribner BS et al. Ceftizoxime elimination kinetics in continuous ambulatory peritoneal dialysis. *Clin Pharmacol Ther*. 1983; 34:673-80.
40. Koup JR, Keller E, Neumann H et al. Ceftriaxone pharmacokinetics during peritoneal dialysis. *Eur J Clin Pharmacol*. 1986; 30:303-7.
41. Ragnaud JM, Albin H, Wone C. Pharmacokinetics of latamoxef (moxalactam) in patients on CAPD. *Perit Dial Bull*. 1985; 5:208.
42. Nikolaidis P, Dombros N, Panagiotis A et al. Pharmacokinetics of aztreonam administered i.p. in continuous ambulatory peritoneal dialysis (CAPD) patients. *Perit Dial Bull*. 1989; 9:57-9.
43. Ludlam HA, Barton I, White L et al. Intraperitoneal ciprofloxacin for the treatment of peritonitis in patients receiving continuous ambulatory peritoneal dialysis (CAPD). *J Antimicrob Chemother*. 1990; 25:843-51.
44. Dharmasena D, Roberts DE, Coles GA et al. Pharmacokinetics of intraperitoneal ciprofloxacin in patients on CAPD. *J Antimicrob Chemother*. 1989; 23:253-9.
45. Schwartz MT, Kowalsky SF, McCormick EM et al. Clindamycin phosphate kinetics in subjects undergoing CAPD. *Clin Nephrol*. 1986; 26:303-6.
46. Walker SE, Patin DN, Churchill B et al. Trimethoprim–sulfamethoxazole pharmacokinetics during continuous ambulatory peritoneal dialysis (CAPD). *Perit Dial Int*. 1989; 9:51-6.
47. Blackwell BG, Leggett JE, Johnson CA et al. Ampicillin and sulbactam pharmacokinetics and pharmacodynamics in continuous ambulatory peritoneal dialysis (CAPD). *Perit Dial Int*. 1990; 10:221-6.
48. Leung ACT, Orange G, Henderson IS et al. Successful use of combined intraperitoneal azlocillin and aminoglycoside in the treatment of dialysis associated pseudomonas peritonitis. *Perit Dial Bull*. 1984; 4:98-100
49. Somani P, Freimer EH, Gross ML et al. Pharmacokinetics of imipenem–cilastatin in patients with renal insufficiency undergoing continuous ambulatory peritoneal dialysis. *Antimicrob Agents Chemother*. 1988; 32:530-4.
50. Ryckelynck JP, Debruyne D, Hurault De Ligny B et al. Pharmacokinetics of piperacillin during continuous ambulatory peritoneal dialysis. *Pathol Biol*. 1988; 36:507-10.
51. Swabb EA. Clinical pharmacology of aztreonam in healthy recipients and patients: a review. *Rev Infect Dis*. 1985; 7:S605-12.
52. Mrhar A, Karba R, Drinovec J et al. Computer simulation of ciprofoxacin pharmacokinetics in patients on CAPD. *Int J Artif Organs*. 1990; 13:169-75.
53. DcHaan RM, Metzler CM, Schellegnerg D et al. Pharmacokinetic studies of clindamycin phosphate. *J Clin Pharm*. 1973; 13:190-209.
54. Golper TA, Sewell DL, Fisher PB et al. Incomplete activation of intraperitoneal clindamycin phosphate during peritoneal dialysis. *Am J Nephrol*. 1984; 4:38-42.
55. Golper TA, Bennett WM, Jones SR. Peritonitis associated with chronic peritoneal dialysis. A diagnostic and therapeutic approach. *Dial Transplant*. 1978; 7:1173-8.
56. Debruyne D, Ryckelynck JP, Hurault De Ligny B et al. Pharmacokinetics of piperacillin patients on peritoneal dialysis with and without peritonitis. *J Pharm Sci*. 1990; 79:99-102.
57. Wadhwa NK, Arkins H, Cabralda T. Intraperitoneal erythromycin for gastroparesis. *Ann Intern Med*. 1991; 114:912. Letter.

Editorial

Who should receive antiendotoxin monoclonal antibody therapy?

Nothing in recent memory has created as many questions among pharmacists, physicians, and health-care administrators as the pending availability of antiendotoxin monoclonal antibody therapy for use in gram-negative sepsis. What evidence exists to establish the efficacy of antiendotoxin monoclonal antibody therapy? Which patients should be treated? What are the medical and legal implications of limiting the use of such therapy? What approach should the pharmacy and therapeutics (P&T) committee take in defining appropriate use patterns? How should the prescribing of this therapy be monitored and evaluated?

In this issue of *Clinical Pharmacy*, Barriere and Guglielmo[1] present a detailed review of the sepsis syndrome associated with gram-negative infection and the use of antiendotoxin monoclonal antibodies. Data establishing the clinical efficacy of both the murine monoclonal antibody (E5) and the "humanized" HA-1A are limited to only two published studies.[2,3] Although the authors of both studies reported significant positive findings associated with antiendotoxin treatment, making clinically applicable conclusions based on the data presented is problematic. Because study design and patient entry criteria varied between the trials, comparison of the findings is questionable. Furthermore, in both reports the results were stratified after the data analysis began rather than a priori. In fact, when data from all patients enrolled are subjected to "intention to treat" analysis, even with the use of very stringent entry criteria, no significant differences in mortality are found with monoclonal antibody therapy in either trial. Reductions in mortality were observed only in patients with gram-negative sepsis who were not in shock on entry (E5) and in patients with gram-negative bacteremia with or without shock on entry (HA-1A). Possibly too much emphasis is being placed on reducing mortality. In both studies, patients treated with antiendotoxin monoclonal antibody therapy had significant reductions in associated comorbidities, such as adult respiratory distress syndrome, disseminated intravascular coagulation, and acute renal failure; these findings may represent the major benefits of such treatment.

If benefits are associated with the use of monoclonal antibodies against endotoxin, why not use this therapy for everyone with suspected gram-negative sepsis, just in case it might work? At an anticipated cost of between $3000 and $4000 per treatment, the health-care system cannot afford this approach. Ways must be found to ensure that the use of this therapy is limited to appropriate patients. But, at the time a decision must be made to initiate treatment, patients who might benefit from antiendotoxin monoclonal antibody therapy cannot be differentiated from others who will not benefit.

Selecting appropriate patients for treatment is problematic in many other ways. If the entry criteria that were used in the published clinical trials are adapted to serve as guidelines for patient selection, many patients who do not need or will not benefit from therapy will be treated, leading to overuse of the product and needless expense. Furthermore, the entry criteria from those trials do not address the potential use of antiendotoxin monoclonal antibody therapy in children or in patients with AIDS, burns, organ transplants, or severe neutropenia. Should patients in these categories be considered for antiendotoxin monoclonal antibody therapy? The need for a rapid test for endotoxemia has been suggested, but such a test is not currently available and, even if it were, endotoxemia is a variable finding in patients with gram-negative infections. What about waiting until gram-negative bacteremia is documented? This would be one way to limit use to patients who might truly benefit from therapy, but many patients who stand to gain from treatment would not receive it, since fewer than 50% of patients with gram-negative sepsis develop culture-proven bacteremia. Additionally, there is no evidence that waiting until culture results are available before giving monoclonal antibody therapy will produce the same degree of efficacy reported with treatment initiated earlier in the course of illness. Therefore, it seems that proven gram-negative bacteremia should not be used as the only criterion. Persistent hypotension, refractory to fluids and requiring vasopressor therapy, in patients with known or suspected gram-negative infections might be an important criterion for patients who might benefit from HA-1A but not from E5.

Currently, it is not possible to arrive at concise and widely acceptable guidelines for selecting patients to receive antiendotoxin monoclonal antibody therapy. However, each facility should develop some initial guidelines for use. In some settings, it is probably advisable for neighboring hospitals to collaborate in developing uniform guidelines or criteria for use, so that availability of the products and restrictions on their use are consistent within the community. The guidelines and criteria that are developed and adopted initially should be continually evaluated and revised as new information becomes available.

Withholding therapy from some patients can be unset-

The idea for this editorial was suggested by the ASHP Commission on Therapeutics.

 0278-2677/92/0301-0255$00.50.

tling, but this will be a result when criteria for use of this therapy are stringently applied. Few would find fault with prohibiting use in patients who are not critically ill or those with infections that readily respond to antimicrobial therapy alone. It may also be appropriate to exclude use in patients, such as those with "do not resuscitate" orders, for whom there is already a lack of commitment to aggressive treatment. Unfortunately, any restrictive criteria or guidelines for use can lead to exclusion from treatment for some patients who might ultimately benefit from therapy. Will the hospital or clinician incur additional liability for not using this therapy in all patients with sepsis? A recognized expert in the field believes that the current status of information and experimental data are inadequate to support a finding of negligence if these products are not used, especially in the absence of confirming gram-negative culture results.[4]

P&T committees must develop meaningful drug-use control mechanisms for monoclonal antibody treatment. These drug-use controls should be applied not only to restrict inappropriate use of this therapy but also to promote its appropriate use. The development of controls must be multidisciplinary, incorporating input not just from physicians but from pharmacists and health-care administrators as well. Criteria for drug-use control that have been developed at a major referral and teaching hospital appear in this issue of *Clinical Pharmacy*.[5] While these criteria may not be fully applicable to all settings, they do represent an example of what needs to be addressed as the drug-use control process is applied to antiendotoxin monoclonal antibody therapy. Monitoring of the use of such therapy must be prospective, and patterns of use should be reviewed regularly by the P&T committee and the medical staff to identify and address problems in a timely manner.

In addition to the need to develop guidelines for use, P&T committees will be faced with new questions about selecting products for formulary admission. Potential issues for selection of antibody drugs in general relate to the source of the antibody (mouse or human), whether it is polyclonal or monoclonal, and the specific isotype (i.e., IgG or IgM). From a clinical perspective, drugs produced by advanced technologies are not intrinsically superior to traditional agents. In evaluations of drug products derived from advanced technologies, the factors of primary importance—efficacy and safety—should take precedence over specific technical details.

Many clinicians are eagerly awaiting the opportunity to use this new therapy for patients with known or suspected gram-negative sepsis. Nevertheless, until better data are available to clarify and confirm the actual benefit of antiendotoxin monoclonal antibody therapy, many questions will remain unanswered. In the face of limited financial resources, monoclonal antibodies directed against endotoxin cannot be indiscriminately prescribed. Clinicians must attempt to ensure that use is limited only to those patients with the greatest potential to benefit.

1. Barriere SL, Guglielmo BJ. Gram-negative sepsis, the sepsis syndrome, and the role of antiendotoxin monoclonal antibodies. *Clin Pharm*. 1992; 11:223-35.
2. Ziegler EJ, Fisher CJ, Sprung CL et al. Treatment of gram-negative bacteremia and septic shock with HA-1A human monoclonal antibody against endotoxin. *N Engl J Med*. 1991; 324:429-36.
3. Greenman RL, Schein RM, Martin MA et al. A controlled clinical trial of E5 murine monoclonal IgM antibody to endotoxin in the treatment of gram-negative sepsis. *JAMA*. 1991; 266:1097-102.
4. Bone RC. Monoclonal antibodies to endotoxin—new allies against sepsis? *JAMA*. 1991; 266:1125-6. Editorial.
5. Shepherd MF. Criteria for use of antiendotoxin monoclonal antibodies (HA-1A and E5) in adult and pediatric inpatients. *Clin Pharm*. 1992; 11:257-60.

Thomas C. Hardin, Pharm.D., FCCP
Clinical Coordinator, Pharmacy
Audie L. Murphy Memorial Veterans Hospital
San Antonio, TX 78284

Joseph T. DiPiro, Pharm.D., FCCP
Professor of Pharmacy
The University of Georgia
Augusta, GA 30912

Future Management of Septic Shock

Although monoclonal antibodies to endotoxin provide important insights regarding septic shock pathogenesis and have important evolving clinical applications, this technology only represents the initial stages of our ability to inhibit mediators in the treatment of this serious disease. Pharmacologic inhibitors of the lipid A portion of endotoxin have been shown to inhibit several of endotoxin's effects and may prove therapeutic in the near future. Monoclonal antibodies to other important sepsis mediators, such as tumor necrosis factor and interleukin-1, may prove to have a therapeutic role in gram-positive and gram-negative septic shock. Other innovative methods of mediator inhibition include administration of an interleukin-1 receptor antagonist or soluble (inactivating) receptors for tumor necrosis factor.

In the near future, we hope to be able to inhibit the septic shock pathogenetic sequence at multiple key steps and thereby reduce the high mortality that is presently associated with this very serious disease.

—Parrillo JE. Management of septic shock: present and future. *Ann Intern Med*. 1991; 115:491-2. Editorial.

DUE Criteria

The DUE Criteria *section of* Clinical Pharmacy *features model drug-use evaluation criteria that may be employed as a component of a comprehensive quality assurance program. The criteria sets are presented in the format used in the ASHP book* Criteria for Drug Use Evaluation. *Some of the criteria sets will have been originally published in that book; others will be presented here for the first time and published in future volumes of the ASHP book. The practitioners who developed a criteria set are acknowledged.*

In selecting drug products for coverage in DUE Criteria, *priority is given to products that have been recently marketed, those that are frequently prescribed, those that have high potential risk associated with their use, and those that are expensive. When feasible, a criteria set will be linked with a* Drug Review *that appears in the same issue.*

These criteria sets are a starting point for the development of DUE Criteria for a specific practice setting. Readers are encouraged to modify the model criteria to fit their own circumstances.

Criteria for use of antiendotoxin monoclonal antibodies (HA-1A and E5) in adult and pediatric inpatients[a]

Element	Standard 100%	Standard 0%	Exception[b] or Critical Preventive/ Responsive Measure[c]	Sources of Information
Justification for Use				
1. For HA-1A, management of suspected or confirmed gram-negative infection in patient with all of the following signs of sepsis (sepsis syndrome)[1-3]: a. Fever (temperature >38.3 °C) or unexplained hypothermia (temperature <35.6 °C) b. Tachycardia (heart rate [HR] >90 beats/min if >15 yr old, ≥110 beats/min if 6–15 yr old, ≥125 beats/min if 3 mo–5 yr old) c. Tachypnea (respiratory rate [RR] >20 breaths/min if >15 yr old, ≥20 breaths/min if 6–15 yr old, ≥25 breaths/min if 3 mo–5 yr old) or requirement for mechanical ventilation d. Hypotension (supine, cuff systolic blood pressure [BP] ≤90 mm Hg if >15 yr old, <85 mm Hg if 6–15 yr old, <80 mm Hg if 3 mo–5 yr old or, for adult, sustained systolic BP drop of ≥40 mm Hg after adequate fluid challenge or after use of vasopressors) or signs and symptoms of peripheral hypoperfusion, as manifested	X		1A. Patient receiving β-adrenergic antagonists or antihypertensive medication 1B. Patient receiving β-adrenergic agents, corticosteroids, antipyretic agents, sedative agents, anticoagulants, or antiarrhythmic agents[2] 1C. Patient receiving long-term hemodialysis	1. History and physical (H&P), physician orders, progress notes, intensive-care unit (ICU) flow sheets, laboratory reports 1A,B. Physician orders, progress notes, medication administration record (MAR) 1C. Physician orders, progress notes

Prepared by Michele F. Shepherd, Pharm.D., Clinical Specialist, Department of Pharmacy, Abbott Northwestern Hospital, Minneapolis, MN, and Clinical Assistant Professor, College of Pharmacy, University of Minnesota, Minneapolis.

 0278-2677/92/0301-0257$01.00.

Element	Standard 100%	Standard 0%	Exception[b] or Critical Preventive/Responsive Measure[c]	Sources of Information
by presence of at least two of the following: (1) Unexplained metabolic acidosis (pH ≤7.3, base deficit >5 meq/L, or elevated plasma lactate concentration) (2) Arterial hypoxemia (arterial P_{O_2} ≤75 mm Hg or arterial P_{O_2}: F_{IO_2} ratio <250) (3) Acute renal failure (urine output <30 mL/hr for ≥1 hr despite adequate fluid volume, increasing serum creatinine concentration, or need for dialysis) (4) Recent (within 24 hr) unexplained coagulation abnormalities (elevated prothrombin time [PT] or partial thromboplastin time [PTT]) or recent (within 24 hr) unexplained thrombocytopenia (<100,000 platelets/cu mm) or decrease in platelet count to ≤50% of previous value (5) Sudden deterioration of mental status (6) Elevated cardiac index (>4 L/min/sq m) with low systemic vascular resistance (<800 dyne · sec/cm^5)				
2. For E5, management of suspected or confirmed gram-negative infection in patient with at least two of the following (a–d): a. Core temperature >38 °C or <35 °C b. Peripheral white blood cell count (WBC) >12,000/cu mm, <3000/cu mm, or ≥20% immature forms c. Gram-negative pathogens growing in blood culture from sample drawn within the preceding 48 hr d. Documented or suspected site of gram-negative infection and e. Signs of systemic septic response, as manifested by presence of at least one of the following: (1) Arterial hypotension (systolic BP <90 mm Hg or acute drop in systolic BP of ≥30 mm Hg) (2) Metabolic acidosis (base deficit >5 meq/L) (3) Decreased systemic vascular resistance (<800 dyne · sec/cm^5)	X		2A. Patient receiving β-adrenergic antagonists, antihypertensive medication, or cancer chemotherapy 2B. Patient receiving β-adrenergic agents, corticosteroids, antipyretic agents, sedative agents, anticoagulants, or antiarrhythmic agents[2] 2C. Patient receiving long-term hemodialysis	2. H&P, physician orders, progress notes, ICU flow sheets, laboratory reports 2A,B. Physician orders, progress notes, MAR 2C. Physician orders, progress notes

Element	Standard 100%	Standard 0%	Exception[b] or Critical Preventive/Responsive Measure[c]	Sources of Information
(4) Tachypnea (RR >20 breaths/min) or, if mechanically ventilated, ventilation >10 L/min				
(5) Unexplained dysfunction of kidneys (urine output <30 mL/hr), lungs (arterial P_{O_2} <75 mm Hg on room air, or arterial P_{O_2}:F_{IO_2} ratio <280), central nervous system, or coagulation (thrombocytopenia, 25% decrease in platelet count, or elevated PT or PTT)				
Critical (Process) Indicators				
3. For HA-1A and E5, appropriate intensive-care therapies and monitoring in place	X		3A. None	3. Physician orders, progress notes, nursing notes, ICU flow sheets
4. For HA-1A and E5, appropriate samples obtained for Gram's stains, cultures, and susceptibility testing	X		4A. None	4. H&P, physician orders, progress notes, infectious diseases consultation report
5. For HA-1A and E5, appropriate empirical or therapeutic antimicrobial therapy administered	X		5A. None	5. Physician orders, progress notes, MAR
6. For HA-1A and E5, sepsis not suspected to be caused by infectious agents other than gram-negative bacteria[1,2]	X		6A. None	6. H&P, progress notes, laboratory reports
7. For HA-1A and E5, cardiogenic or hemorrhagic shock without gram-negative sepsis not suspected[1-3]	X		7A. None	7. H&P, progress notes, ICU flow sheets, nursing notes
8. HA-1A or E5 not used in pregnant or breast-feeding patient[1-4,d]	X		8A. Benefit outweighs risk to fetus or baby	8. H&P, progress notes 8A. Progress notes
9. HA-1A or E5 not used in patient whose clinical course is rapidly fatal or whose condition is considered irreversible[1,2,4]	X		9A. None	9. H&P, progress notes, nursing notes
10. E5 not used in patient with prior therapy with or known allergy to murine products[4]	X		10A. Benefit outweighs risk	10. H&P, physician orders, progress notes, MAR 10A. Progress notes
11. E5 not used in children[4]	X		11A. Benefit outweighs risk to child	11. H&P, progress notes, nursing notes 11A. Progress notes
12. HA-1A adult dose: 100 mg i.v. infused over 15–30 min[2]	X		12A. Patient may receive up to two additional 100-mg doses (300 mg total) with 24 hours between each dose	12,12A. Physician orders, progress notes, MAR
13. HA-1A pediatric dose: 3 mg/kg (maximum 100 mg) i.v. infused over 15–30 min[2]	X		13A. Age is <3 months 13B. In presumed fulminant meningococcemia, one dose of 6 mg/kg (maximum 100 mg) infused over 15–30 min[2]	13. Physician orders, progress notes, MAR 13A. H&P 13B. Physician orders, progress notes, MAR, laboratory reports
14. HA-1A infusion diluted with 0.9% sodium chloride injection 50 mL[2]	X		14A. None	14. Physician orders, progress notes, MAR
15. HA-1A administered in a separate i.v. line and not mixed with other medications[d]	X		15A. Limited number of i.v. sites available	15. Physician orders, MAR, nursing notes, i.v. administration flow sheets 15A. Progress notes, nursing notes
16. E5 adult dose: 2 mg/kg i.v. infused over 60 min. Dose	X		16A. Second dose not administered if patient	16,16A. Physician orders, progress notes, MAR, nursing notes

Element	Standard 100%	Standard 0%	Exception[b] or Critical Preventive/Responsive Measure[c]		Sources of Information	
repeated 24 hr after the first dose[4]				experienced severe reaction to first dose		
17. E5 infusion diluted with 5% dextrose and 0.9% sodium chloride injection 200 mL[4]	X		17A.	None	17.	Physician orders, progress notes, MAR
Complications						
18. For HA-1A[2,d] or E5,[4] allergic or anaphylactic reaction (bronchospasm, urticaria, hypotension, flushing, edema, erythema)		X	18A.	Identify other drug and nondrug causes	18.	Progress notes, physician orders, MAR, nursing notes
			18B.	Provide symptomatic care and supportive therapy	18A.	Progress notes, MAR
			18C.	If severe reaction, discontinue HA-1A or E5	18B,C.	Physician orders, progress notes, MAR
19. For E5, seizures[4]		X	19A.	Identify other drug and nondrug causes	19.	Progress notes, physician orders, MAR, nursing notes
			19B.	Provide symptomatic care and supportive therapy	19A.	Progress notes, MAR
			19C.	If severe reaction, discontinue E5	19B,C.	Physician orders, progress notes, MAR
Outcome Measures						
20. Improvement in or resolution of clinical signs and symptoms of sepsis	X		20A.	Patient died	20,20A.	Progress notes, nursing notes
21. Patient survived septic episode	X		21A.	Patient died	21,21A.	Progress notes, nursing notes

[a] Criteria address justification for use (indications), critical (process) indicators, complications of therapy, and patient outcome. Each criterion consists of an element, a standard, exceptions to the standard, and sources of information. The element is the minimum level of evidence needed to show that patient care was optimal. The standard defines the deviation from an element that is acceptable. If no deviation is acceptable, the standard is 100%. Exceptions are circumstances in which deviation is allowable. Sources of information listed are the most reliable sources. Sources pertaining to an element or exception are identified by the number assigned to the element or exception (e.g., 1, 1A).

[b] For justification for use and critical (process) indicators.

[c] For complications and outcome measures.

[d] Tynan K, Centocor Inc. Personal communication. 1991 July 23.

References

1. Ziegler EJ, Fisher CJ, Sprung CL et al. Treatment of gram-negative bacteremia and septic shock with HA-1A human monoclonal antibody against endotoxin. *N Engl J Med.* 1991;324:429-36.
2. Centocor, Inc. Open label trial of Centoxin (HA-1A) treatment of presumed gram-negative sepsis: protocol number COO41T07. Malvern, PA; 1991 July 11.
3. Fisher CJ, Zimmerman J, Khazaeli MB et al. Initial evaluation of human monoclonal anti-lipid A antibody (HA-1A) in patients with sepsis syndrome. *Crit Care Med.* 1990; 18:1311-5.
4. Greenman RL, Schein RMH, Martin MA et al. A controlled clinical trial of E5 murine monoclonal IgM antibody to endotoxin in the treatment of gram-negative sepsis. *JAMA.* 1991; 266:1097-102.

Current Literature

Drug Reaction Alerts 273

Book Reviews

Guide to Clinical Trials 277
By Bert Spilker
Reviewed by James E. Tisdale

Pharmacokinetics and Pharmacodynamics, Volume 3: Peptides, Peptoids, and Proteins 277
Edited by Pamela D. Garzone, Wayne A. Colburn, and Michael Mokotoff
Reviewed by C. Lindsay DeVane

Drug Reaction Alerts

Drug Reaction Alerts focuses primarily on serious, unlabeled reactions to new chemical entities. The citations are compiled monthly from International Pharmaceutical Abstracts, which covers over 800 pharmacy and health-related journals worldwide. An address for reprints (when available) follows the name of the corresponding author in each citation.

Pharmacists may use the FDA Adverse Reaction Report form that appears in the January and July issues of Clinical Pharmacy for submitting reports of adverse drug reactions directly to FDA.

Antithyroid Drugs

Pasquier E, Genereau T, Baudrimont M et al. (Imbert JC, Service of Internal Medicine, Service of Anatomical Pathology, and Regional Center for Pharmacovigilance, Hôpital St. Antoine, 75571 Paris, France). Biopsy-proven myositis with microvasculitis in association with **carbimazole**. *Lancet.* 1991; 338:1082-3. Case. (36-year-old woman with Graves' disease; received carbimazole 60 mg/day tapered to 45 mg/day within two months, and became euthyroid; developed intermittent muscle pain approximately three months after starting carbimazole therapy; muscle pain progressed to severe pain with weakness within one month of onset; muscle tissue biopsy revealed microvasculitis; withdrawal of carbimazole and therapy with propylthiouracil led to rapid clinical and biological improvement over two weeks and no muscle pain or weakness after two months)

Antivirals

Eck P, Silver SM, Clark EC (Rochester General Hospital, Rochester, NY 14621). Acute renal failure and coma after a high dose of oral **acyclovir**. *N Engl J Med.* 1991; 325:1178. Case. (70-year-old woman with herpes zoster; received oral acyclovir 800 mg five times daily and propoxyphene napsylate 100 mg every six hours for seven days; developed weakness, intermittent confusion, and vague pain in lower left abdominal quadrant; white blood cell count, 21,000/cu mm; diagnosed presumptively with diverticulosis at hospital admission; withdrawal of acyclovir and propoxyphene napsylate and therapy with i.v. hydration, cimetidine, and cefoxitin did not lead to improvement, and woman became unresponsive within 36 hours; withdrawal of all drugs and therapy with i.v. naloxone did not lead to improved mental status; blood urea nitrogen and serum creatinine concentrations increased from 25 to 44 mg/dL and from 1.8 to 5.0 mg/dL, respectively; plasma acyclovir concentration 60 hours after last dose, 3.0 μg/mL [normal range of trough concentration, 0.14–1.2 μg/mL]; renal function and neurological condition improved without specific therapy over three days; discharged from hospital on hospital day 7)

Continued on page 277

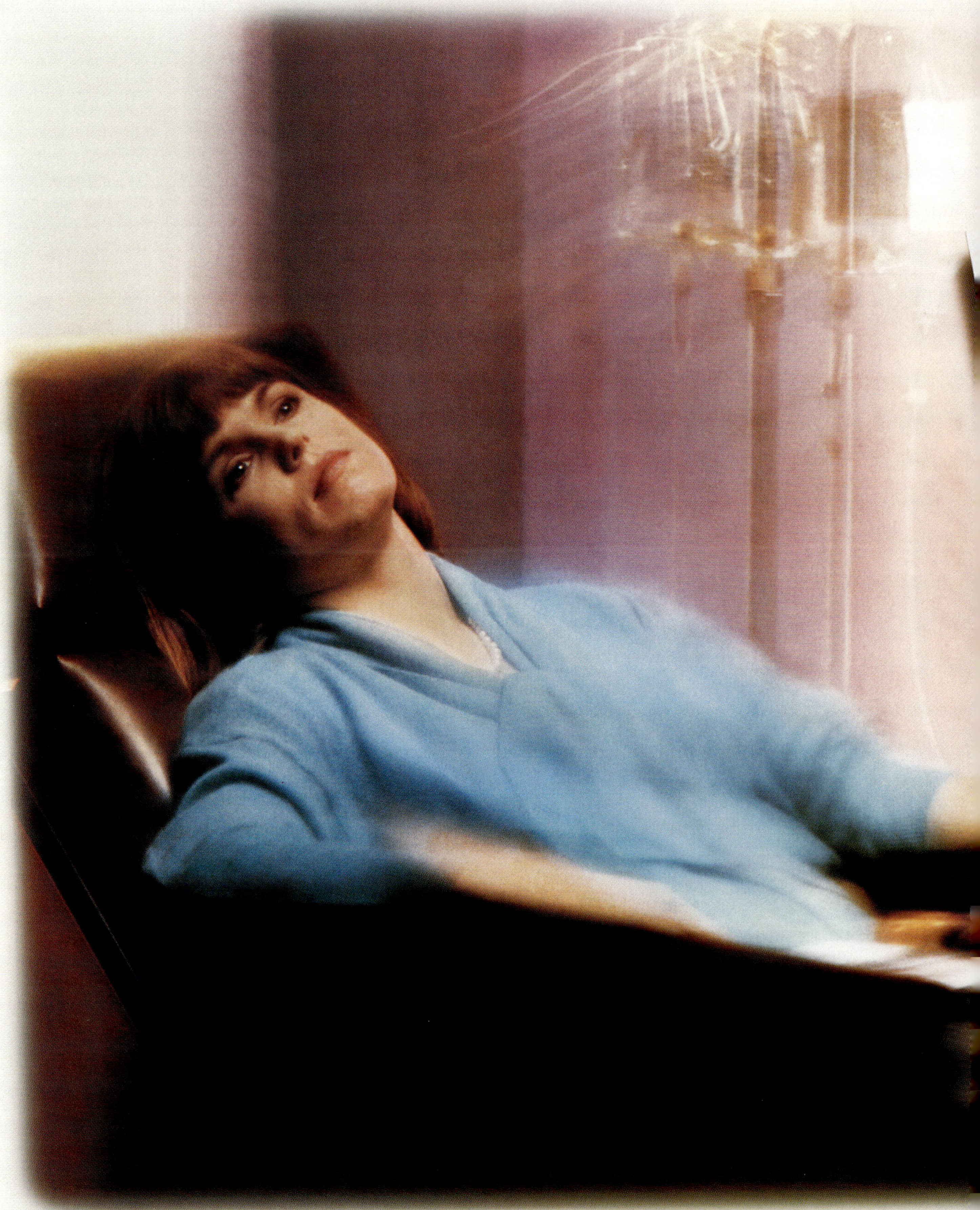

Continued from page 273

Drug Abuse

Hudson MM, Edmonds M, Watkins PJ (Dulwich Hospital, London SE22 8PT, England). Misuse of **temazepam**. *Br Med J.* 1991; 303:993. Case. (28-year-old woman; extracted temazepam 80 mg from liquid-filled capsules, and injected drug intra-arterially; developed macular rash, edema, and tenderness of right leg; serum creatine kinase concentration increased from 5,900 IU/L four hours after temazepam injection to 25,000 IU/L five days after injection; therapy with i.v. fluids to maintain diuresis led to complete recovery)

Drugs, Adverse Reactions

McCormack K, Rustin GJ, Smith DB et al. (Newlands ES, Department of Medical Oncology, Charing Cross Hospital, London W6 8RF, England). *Pneumocystis carinii* pneumonia and high-dose **dexamethasone** to prevent emesis of chemotherapy. *Lancet.* 1991; 338:946-7. Cases. (two women with cancer, aged 26 and 41 years; received dexamethasone 8 mg three times daily for two days for prevention of antineoplastic-induced emesis; developed life-threatening *Pneumocystis carinii* pneumonia-like infection; therapy with high-dose sulfamethoxazole combined with trimethoprim and ventilatory support with continuous positive airway pressure led to recovery)

Fertility Agents

Kobayashi N, Matsui I, Tanimura M et al. (Nagahara N, Japan Children's Cancer Registry, Department of Child Ecology, National Children's Medical Research Center, Setagaya-ku, Tokyo 154, Japan). Childhood neuroectodermal tumors and malignant lymphoma after maternal ovulation induction. *Lancet.* 1991; 338:955. Study. (retrospective; mothers of 6236 children with malignant diseases diagnosed from 1985 to 1989; reviewed preconception drug therapies; children born to mothers who underwent ovulation induction developed more cases of childhood malignant disease than children born to mothers who did not undergo ovulation induction; **clomiphene** was widely used as first choice for infertility therapy)

Gastrointestinal Drugs

Dutertre JP, Soutif D, Jonville AP et al. (Autret E, Department of Clinical Pharmacology and Rheumatology, CHU Hôpital Bretonneau, 37044 Tours, France). Sexual disturbances during **omeprazole** therapy. *Lancet.* 1991; 338:1022. Case. (77-year-old man with esophagitis; received omeprazole 20 mg/day for at least six weeks; developed painful nocturnal erections; withdrawal of omepazole led to disappearance of nocturnal erections; positive rechallenge)

Book Reviews

Guide to Clinical Trials

By Bert Spilker.
Published by Raven Press, 1185 Avenue of the Americas, New York, NY 10036, 1991. xxv + 1156 p. Price $130.

Guide to Clinical Trials provides general information and guidelines for planning and conducting clinical research projects. Spilker, a widely published author in the area of clinical trial methodology, compiled material from three of his previously published books and wrote more than 40 new chapters specifically for this book.

The book contains much useful information for pharmacists who are interested in or actively conducting clinical research. A glossary of terms appears at the beginning of the book. The author has liberally used tables and figures and provided numerous checklists and sample forms. There are well-written discussions on topics such as the advantages and disadvantages of various types of study design, bias in clinical research, types of study controls, randomization procedures, and patient recruitment strategies. In addition, guidelines for developing and writing protocols are provided including discussions of ethical issues, informed consent and institutional review processes, and preparation of data collection forms.

Sections about the interpretation of clinical data are valuable, particularly the general 10-step approach to interpreting clinical data, as well as nonspecific advice to interpreting efficacy and adverse effect data. Pharmacists who are involved in preparing, packaging, or dispensing drugs for clinical trials will be especially interested in the chapter that addresses these issues. The guidelines for preparing a clinical research article for publication are also very useful.

The book provides a substantial amount of information on clinical research in the pharmaceutical industry. Included are discussions of Phase I–IV trials; bioequivalence studies; regulatory, patent, and legal considerations; evaluation of orphan drugs; marketing-oriented studies; interactions of academic investigators with pharmaceutical companies; drug development processes; data required for drug approval; and postmarketing surveillance studies.

Guide to Clinical Trials is aimed at a diverse audience that includes university students in pharmacy, pharmacology, or medical programs; persons with little research experience as well as experienced researchers; and nonscientists such as marketing and sales personnel in the pharmaceutical industry. As a result, much of the information provided is general. Pharmacists may find the discussions of pharmacokinetic principles, dosage forms and formulations, design of pharmacokinetics trials, and interpretation of pharmacokinetics data to be very basic. Discussions of trial methodologies for specific therapeutic and disease areas are not provided; however, the author includes references that interested readers may consult. Overall, the information contained in this volume is of great interest and practical value to pharmacists and anyone else involved in clinical research.

Guide to Clinical Trials is a comprehensive reference that provides valuable guidelines, suggestions, and information on clinical trials from conception to publication. This book is essential and well worth the cost to any individual who wants to become or is already involved in clinical research, participates in a clinical research training program such as a post-Pharm.D. fellowship, or teaches courses in research design.

Reviewed by James E. Tisdale, Pharm.D., College of Pharmacy and Allied Health Professions, Wayne State University, 105 Shapero Hall, Detroit, MI 48202-3489.

Pharmacokinetics and Pharmacodynamics, Volume 3: Peptides, Peptoids, and Proteins

Edited by Pamela D. Garzone, Wayne A. Colburn, and Michael Mokotoff.
Published by Harvey Whitney Books Company, P.O. Box 42696, Cincinnati, OH 45242, 1991. viii + 200 p. Price $35.

Continued on page 280

AWARDS PROGRAM

The ASHP Research and Education Foundation conducts annually an Awards Program recognizing important contributions to the literature of hospital pharmacy. The Awards Program has been administered by the Foundation since 1971.

The Awards Program is made possible by grants to the Foundation from Bristol-Myers Squibb U.S. Pharmaceutical Division and the American Society of Hospital Pharmacists.

Award recipients are chosen by selection panels appointed by the Foundation's Board of Directors.

The Awards Program of the Foundation is based on the concept that recognition through awards stimulates research and fosters improvement in the quality of published professional articles. The program provides annual awards, if a recipient is chosen, in the following areas:

A **RESEARCH AWARD** is offered for an important contribution to the scientific pharmaceutical literature of research in hospital pharmacy during the calendar year preceding the year in which the award is granted. (For this award, "research" refers not only to the formalized testing of hypotheses using the scientific approach, but also includes methods improvement studies, product development, demonstration projects with built-in evaluation, problem-solving using research methods, and controlled clinical studies involving drugs.)

An **AWARD FOR ACHIEVEMENT FOR SUSTAINED CONTRIBUTIONS TO THE LITERATURE OF HOSPITAL PHARMACY** is offered to an individual for publishing in the pharmaceutical literature, over several years, papers of consistently high quality and importance.

An **AWARD FOR ACHIEVEMENT IN THE PROFESSIONAL PRACTICE OF HOSPITAL PHARMACY** is offered for the most noteworthy contribution to the literature in the professional practice of hospital pharmacy in the calendar year preceding the year in which the award is granted. (For this award, "professional practice of hospital pharmacy" refers to all aspects of professional practice, including management, drug use control, technological services, clinical services, and information processing.)

A **STUDENT AWARD** is offered to an undergraduate or graduate pharmacy student for an unpublished paper on a subject relevant to hospital pharmacy prepared during the academic year preceding the Midyear Clinical Meeting at which the award is presented. Students in B.S., M.S., and Pharm.D. programs are eligible.

The Research and Achievement awards each consist of a $4,000 honorarium, a $700 expense allowance to attend the ASHP Midyear Clinical Meeting for the award presentation, and a plaque.

The Student Award consists of a $1000 honorarium, $700 expense allowance to attend the ASHP Midyear Clinical Meeting, and a plaque.

Nominations
Criteria and procedures for submitting nominations for the Awards may be obtained by completing and mailing the attached form or by writing to the ASHP Research and Education Foundation.

Deadlines

May 15
Nominations must be mailed (postmarked) no later than this date.

August 1
Date after which Award recipients will be announced.

Request Form

To:
ASHP Research and Education Foundation
4630 Montgomery Avenue
Bethesda, Maryland 20814

Please send me the criteria and procedures for submitting nominations for the ASHP Foundation Awards.

Submit this request form, together with a self-addressed label, to:

ASHP Foundation
4630 Montgomery Avenue, Bethesda, MD 20814
(301) 657-3000

Continued from page 277

This book is the third in a series of published proceedings from symposia held at the University of Pittsburgh. The first, held in 1985, dealt with traditional aspects of pharmacokinetic drug studies and was appropriately titled *Research Design and Analysis*. The second, held in 1987 and published as *Current Problems/Potential Solutions*, focused on the interface between pharmacokinetic data and measures of pharmacodynamic response. These volumes still serve as excellent references for design and analysis of pharmacokinetic studies. The latest book in this series, *Peptides, Peptoids, and Proteins*, presents in-depth discussions on many aspects of drug pharmacokinetics and dynamics that were covered in the first two volumes but are now applied to drugs developed by modern biotechnological techniques. Some examples familiar to clinical pharmacists include tissue plasminogen activator, granulocyte–macrophage colony-stimulating factor, and growth hormone. Publication of this set of proceedings results in a much-needed, comprehensive reference.

The text is divided into three major sections that cover design and synthesis of peptides, analytic and pharmacokinetic perspectives, and safety and regulatory aspects. Most chapters discuss highly specialized topics. For example, chapters 1–3 present medicinal chemistry surveys and would be of greatest interest to scientists involved in drug synthesis; chapter 4 provides some insight into the problems inherent in choosing between luteinizing hormone-releasing hormone (luliberin) agonists and antagonists, major new classes of therapeutic drugs.

The eight chapters in the middle section constitute most of the book and discuss assay, delivery, and pharmacokinetics of peptides and proteins. I highly recommend that anyone who reads this book should start with chapter 9 in this section, which discusses the pharmacokinetics and pharmacodynamics of growth hormone-releasing hormone (somatoliberin). It provides an overview for the entire book and its theme: new biotechnology results in the development of many potentially useful therapeutic agents, but understanding the pharmacokinetics and pharmacodynamics of these drugs requires solutions to problems that did not exist with older drugs. Chapter 9 provides definitions for all the terms in the book except for "peptoid," which is never defined in spite of its use in the book's title and major subsections. With the background provided by this chapter, the earlier chapters on drug synthesis and the later ones on bioassays, derivative approaches to analysis and quantitation, problems of drug delivery and administration, and complexities of quantitating biological actions assume more relevance.

Although this book is a valuable and up-to-date survey of an important topic, I have reservations about its current suitability for many pharmacists, particularly those who practice clinically. The delivery of pharmaceutical care will not immediately improve after a pharmacist reads this book; however, the book presents a broad yet detailed and well-referenced survey of a rapidly evolving pharmaceutical field that will eventually affect the practice of all pharmacists. Pharmacists involved in oncology, immunology, or endocrinology practice may find the coverage of cyclosporine and insulin to be useful. As for my practice in clinical psychopharmacology, the peptide and protein drugs have yet to make a major impact in therapeutics; however, I expect this situation to change in the near future. When the topic becomes more germane to my practice, this book is probably the first one I'll reach for when seeking information and direction before heading off to the library. Like the first two volumes in this series, this book should serve as a useful reference for many years.

Reviewed by C. Lindsay DeVane, Pharm.D., Department of Pharmacy Practice, College of Pharmacy, J. Hillis Miller Health Center (Box J-486), University of Florida, Gainesville, FL 32610-0486.

Advertising Index

American Society of Hospital Pharmacists
Clinical Pharmacy, 221
Concepts in Oncology Therapeutics, 279
Amgen Inc.
Epogen, 207
Neupogen, 265-272
ASHP Research and Education Foundation
Awards Program, 278
Burroughs Wellcome Company
Exosurf Neonatal, 213-217
Eisenhower Medical Center
Position Available, 219
Eli Lilly and Company
Hospital Division, 209
PLAN International USA
Childreach Sponsorship, 264
SmithKline Beecham
Timentin, inside back cover, outside back cover
UMI Article Clearinghouse
Microform Reproductions, 221
The Upjohn Company
Zefazone, 210-212
Virginia Mason Hospital
Positions Available, 219
Wyeth-Ayerst Laboratories, Inc.
Ativan Injection, 274-276
Tubex, inside front cover

News

Benzodiazepine antagonist approved by FDA 287

Acellular pertussis vaccine approved by FDA 290

Third HMG-CoA reductase inhibitor marketed for cholesterol reduction 290

Cefprozil enters oral antibiotic market 295

FDA seeks changes in benzodiazepine packaging and labeling 295

EPA seeks information on efficacy of sterilants and disinfectants 295

Expert panel issues guidelines on asthma management 295

Guidelines address systemic glucocorticosteroid use for infection management 295

News Briefs 296

Upcoming Specialty Meetings 296

Benzodiazepine antagonist approved by FDA

A benzodiazepine-receptor antagonist, flumazenil (Mazicon, Hoffmann-La Roche), has been approved by FDA for the management of benzodiazepine overdoses and for complete or partial reversal of sedation when benzodiazepines are used to induce or maintain general anesthesia or to produce conscious sedation for diagnostic or therapeutic procedures.

After intravenous administration, flumazenil has an initial distribution half-life of 7–15 minutes and a terminal half-life of 40–80 minutes. Flumazenil has an apparent distribution volume of 0.5 L/kg. Clearance, primarily by hepatic metabolism, is dependent on hepatic blood flow. The major metabolites are the demethylated free acid and its glucuronide conjugate.

Intravenous flumazenil has been shown to antagonize benzodiazepine-induced sedation, impairment of recall, and psychomotor impairment. Reversal of amnesia can be incomplete.

The dosage should be individualized. When used after general anesthesia or conscious sedation, the recommended dosage is 0.2 mg administered intravenously over 15 seconds at one-minute intervals until the desired level of consciousness is obtained (maximum dose, 1 mg). If sedation recurs, additional doses may be given. A maximum of 1 mg (administered in 0.2-mg increments) should be given at any one time, and no more than 3 mg should be given within one hour.

For the initial management of suspected benzodiazepine overdoses, 0.2 mg should be given intravenously over 30 seconds. After 30 seconds has elapsed, a 0.3-mg dose can be given if the desired level of consciousness has not been obtained. Additional doses of 0.5 mg can be given at one-minute intervals (maximum dose, 3 mg). If sedation recurs, doses may be repeated.

Using more than the minimum effective dose of flumazenil can complicate the management of patients who are physically dependent on benzodiazepines or patients who are taking benzodiazepines for a therapeutic effect (e.g., seizure control).

Use of flumazenil has been associated with seizures, most commonly in patients who have received long-term therapy for sedation or when patients have taken overdoses involving cyclic antidepressants. Flumazenil should not be given to patients who show signs of serious cyclic antidepressant poisoning. Seizures associated with

Continued on page 290

News *Continued from page 287*

flumazenil administration generally require treatment with phenytoin, barbiturates, or higher than usual doses of benzodiazepines.

Flumazenil is not a substitute for adequate post-procedural monitoring. When flumazenil is used after conscious sedation or general anesthesia, patients should be monitored for recurrent sedation, respiratory depression, or other residual benzodiazepine effects for a period appropriate for the benzodiazepine used. Flumazenil may not fully reverse ventilatory insufficiency. If flumazenil is initially effective, hypoventilation may recur because the effects of flumazenil may be more short-lived than those of the benzodiazepine.

Nausea and vomiting are the most common adverse effects of flumazenil. Other adverse effects include dizziness, agitation, pain at the injection site, headache, and emotional lability.

Mazicon is supplied as a 0.1-mg/mL solution in 5- and 10-mL vials.

Acellular pertussis vaccine approved by FDA

A diphtheria and tetanus toxoids and pertussis (DTP) vaccine that includes an acellular pertussis vaccine component (Acel-Imune, Lederle–Praxis) was approved by FDA at the end of 1991. The vaccine is indicated for use as the fourth and fifth doses (given at 18 months and at four to six years of age) in the immunization series. Use of Acel-Imune may be considered for children as young as 15 months if it is expected that they will not return at 18 months for vaccination; however, studies in this age group have not been completed.

Other DTP vaccine formulations licensed in the United States contain inactivated whole-cell pertussis vaccine. The acellular vaccine contains four inactivated antigenic components of the pertussis cell: filamentous hemagglutinin, lymphocytosis promoting factor, a 69-kilodalton outer membrane protein, and type 2 fimbriae.

Compared with a whole-cell DTP vaccine produced by Lederle, Acel-Imune caused fewer reactions at the injection site and less drowsiness, fretfulness, and fever.

The recommended dose is 0.5 mL injected intramuscularly.

Acel-Imune is supplied in a 5-mL vial.

Third HMG-CoA reductase inhibitor marketed for cholesterol reduction

Marketing of simvastatin (Zocor, Merck Sharp & Dohme) was approved by FDA in late 1991. It is labeled for use as an adjunct to diet for the reduction of elevated total and low-density lipoprotein (LDL) cholesterol levels in patients with primary hypercholesterolemia (types IIa and IIb) when the response to dietary restriction of cholesterol and saturated fat is inadequate. Simvastatin is an inhibitor of 3-hydroxy-3-methylglutaryl-coenzyme A (HMG-CoA) reductase.

Simvastatin undergoes extensive first-pass extraction

Continued on page 295

Continued from page 290

in the liver. About 13% of a radiolabeled oral dose is excreted in urine and 60% is recovered in feces.

Simvastatin reduces total cholesterol and LDL-cholesterol levels in patients with heterozygous familial or nonfamilial forms of primary hypercholesterolemia or patients with mixed hyperlipidemia. Maximum response usually occurs in four to six weeks.

Use of simvastatin has been associated with elevated serum aminotransferase levels and, rarely, with rhabdomyolysis. In clinical trials involving 2423 patients, 1.4% of patients discontinued therapy because of adverse reactions attributed to simvastatin.

The recommended starting dosage of simvastatin is 5–10 mg daily in the evening; elderly persons and individuals with an LDL-cholesterol concentration of ≤190 mg/dL should receive a starting dose of 5 mg. The recommended dosage range is 5–40 mg/day, with the daily dosage given as a single evening dose.

Zocor is supplied as 5-mg tablets in unit-of-use bottles of 60 and 90, 10-mg tablets in unit-of-use bottles of 60 and 90 and unit dose packages of 100, and 20- and 40-mg tablets in unit-of-use bottles of 60.

Cefprozil enters oral antibiotic market

The oral cephalosporin cefprozil (Cefzil, Bristol–Myers Squibb) was among the drugs approved by FDA at the end of 1991. Cefprozil is indicated for the treatment of pharyngitis or tonsillitis caused by susceptible strains of *Streptococcus pyogenes*; otitis media caused by *Streptococcus pneumoniae, Haemophilus influenzae,* and *Moraxella catarrhalis;* secondary bacterial infection of acute bronchitis or acute bacterial exacerbation of chronic bronchitis caused by *Strep. pneumoniae, H. influenzae,* and *M. catarrhalis;* uncomplicated skin and skin-structuce infections caused by *Staphylococcus aureus* (including penicillinase-producing strains) and *Strep. pyogenes.*

Cefprozil is 95% absorbed after oral administration. Peak concentrations occur within 1.5 hours after administration. Urinary recovery accounts for about 60% of a dose. The average plasma half-life is 1.3 hours in healthy subjects but may be prolonged to 6 hours in patients with severe renal dysfunction. The average area under the serum concentration–time curve (AUC) is 35–60% larger in elderly persons than in young adults and is 15–20% larger in women than in men. These differences in AUC are not large enough to require dosage adjustments.

About 2% of clinical trial participants discontinued cefprozil therapy because of adverse effects. Adverse effects reported in more than 2% of patients treated with cefprozil include diarrhea (2.9%), nausea (3.5%), and eosinophilia (2.3%).

The recommended adult dosage for most indications is 500 mg once or twice daily. Patients with severe renal impairment should receive lower dosages. A dosage of 15 mg/kg twice daily is recommended for children less than 13 years of age.

Cefzil is supplied as 250- and 500-mg tablets in bottles and unit dose packages of 100 and as a powder for oral suspension (125 mg/5 mL or 250 mg/5 mL) in 50- and 100-mL bottles.

FDA seeks changes in benzodiazepine packaging and labeling

As part of FDA's ongoing review of the safety of triazolam, the agency has asked manufacturers of benzodiazepine sleep aid products to make several changes in product packaging and labeling. Manufacturers are being asked to develop unit-of-use packages intended for outpatient use and to attach to the packages a patient package insert that describes the risks and benefits of the drug. The new packages will provide no more than a 10-day supply of medication. FDA is also seeking revisions in the professional product labeling that will be classwide and will strengthen current warnings and emphasize appropriate use for the short-term treatment of insomnia.

EPA seeks information on efficacy of sterilants and disinfectants

Prompted by concerns that some chemical sterilants and disinfectants are ineffective when used as directed, the Environmental Protection Agency (EPA) is funding a one-year pilot project for gathering information about problems associated with use of these products for infection control. The Department of Preventive Medicine at Texas Tech University Health Sciences Center will run the program, entitled Antimicrobial Complaint System. A toll-free telephone number has been established (800-447-6349); calls can be received daily between 0700 and 1900 (central time).

Expert panel issues guidelines on asthma management

"Guidelines for the Diagnosis and Management of Asthma," an expert panel report from the National Asthma Education Program of the National Heart, Lung, and Blood Institute, was published as a supplement to the September 1991 issue of the *Journal of Allergy and Clinical Immunology*. The 109-page document emphasizes the importance of inflammation to the pathogenesis and treatment of asthma, the use of a peak flow meter to assess the severity of asthma and the response to therapy, and the importance of patient education. Flow charts provide a stepped-care approach to the treatment of asthma of various severities.

Guidelines address systemic glucocorticosteroid use for infection management

General guidelines for the use of systemic glucocorticosteroids in the treatment of selected infections have been issued by a working group of the Antimicrobial Agents Committee of the Infectious Diseases Society of America. For each infection or condition considered, the recommendation for or against glucocortico-

Continued on page 296

News *Continued from page 295*

steroid use is classified according to the strength of the recommendation and the quality of the supporting evidence. The guidelines were published in the January 1992 issue of the *Journal of Infectious Diseases*.[1]

1. McGowan JE Jr, Chesney PJ, Crossley KB et al. Guidelines for the use of systemic glucocorticosteroids in the management of selected infections. *J Infect Dis*. 1992; 165:1-13.

News Briefs

• FDA has asked all manufacturers of **oral, injectable, or inhaled corticosteroids** to include in the product labeling a warning that high-dose or long-term treatment with corticosteroids may place children who have been exposed to chicken pox or measles at risk for serious or fatal disease.

• As part of an ongoing review of nonprescription drugs, FDA has identified five active ingredients as being safe and effective for treatment of **dandruff, seborrheic dermatitis, or psoriasis.** Dandruff-control products may contain coal tar preparations, pyrithione zinc, salicylic acid, selenium sulfide, sulfur, or combinations of sulfur and salicylic acid. Coal tar and salicylic acid were judged safe and effective for the treatment of psoriasis. Products marketed for seborrheic dermatitis may contain coal tar preparations, pyrithione zinc, salicylic acid, or selenium sulfide.

• Extended-release **metoprolol** succinate tablets (Toprol XL) have been marketed by Astra for once-daily use in the treatment of hypertension and angina.

Upcoming Specialty Meetings

Maternal Nutrition and Pregnancy Outcome. San Diego, CA, May 17–20; contact G. Busacco, New York Academy of Sciences, 2 East 63rd Street, New York, NY 10021; 212-838-0230.

International Conference of Lyme Borreliosis (5th). Arlington, VA, May 31–June 2; contact Secretary, 5th International Conference of Lyme Borreliosis, Federation of American Societies for Experimental Biology, 9650 Rockville Pike, Bethesda, MD 20814; 301-530-7010.

Conference on Drug Research in Immunologic and Infectious Disease (3rd). Washington, DC, June 27–July 1; contact G. Busacco, New York Academy of Sciences, 2 East 63rd Street, New York, NY 10021; 212-838-0230.

Medinfo '92 Satellite Conference on Estimation and Control of Patient Variability in Clinical Pharmacokinetics of Antibiotics. Lyon, France, September 21–23; contact Pascal Maire, Pharm.D., Hopital A. Charial, Hospices Civils de Lyon, 40, Avenue de la Table de Pierre, 69 340 Francheville, France; 33 72 32 34 39, (fax) 33 72 32 34 38.

PRAVACHOL® (Pravastatin Sodium Tablets)

CONTRAINDICATIONS

Hypersensitivity to any component of this medication.

Active liver disease or unexplained, persistent elevations in liver function tests (see WARNINGS).

Pregnancy and lactation. Atherosclerosis is a chronic process and discontinuation of lipid-lowering drugs during pregnancy should have little impact on the outcome of long-term therapy of primary hypercholesterolemia. Cholesterol and other products of cholesterol biosynthesis are essential components for fetal development (including synthesis of steroids and cell membranes). Since HMG-CoA reductase inhibitors decrease cholesterol synthesis and possibly the synthesis of other biologically active substances derived from cholesterol, they may cause fetal harm when administered to pregnant women. Therefore, HMG-CoA reductase inhibitors are contraindicated during pregnancy and in nursing mothers. **Pravastatin should be administered to women of childbearing age only when such patients are highly unlikely to conceive and have been informed of the potential hazards.** If the patient becomes pregnant while taking this class of drug, therapy should be discontinued and the patient apprised of the potential hazard to the fetus.

WARNINGS

Liver Enzymes: HMG-CoA reductase inhibitors, like some other lipid-lowering therapies, have been associated with biochemical abnormalities of liver function. Increases of serum transaminase (ALT, AST) values to more than 3 times the upper limit of normal occurring on 2 or more (not necessarily sequential) occasions have been reported in 1.3% of patients treated with pravastatin in the U.S. over an average period of 18 months. These abnormalities were not associated with cholestasis and did not appear to be related to treatment duration. In those patients in whom these abnormalities were believed to be related to pravastatin and who were discontinued from therapy, the transaminase levels usually fell slowly to pretreatment levels. These biochemical findings are usually asymptomatic although worldwide experience indicates that anorexia, weakness, and/or abdominal pain may also be present in rare patients.

As with other lipid-lowering agents, liver function tests should be performed during therapy with pravastatin. Serum aminotransferases, including ALT (SGPT), should be monitored before treatment begins, every six weeks for the first three months, every eight weeks during the remainder of the first year, and periodically thereafter (e.g., at about six-month intervals). Special attention should be given to patients who develop increased transaminase levels. Liver function tests should be repeated to confirm an elevation and subsequently monitored at more frequent intervals. If increases in AST and ALT equal or exceed three times the upper limit of normal and persist, then therapy should be discontinued. Persistence of significant aminotransferase elevations following discontinuation of therapy may warrant consideration of liver biopsy.

Active liver disease or unexplained transaminase elevations are contraindications to the use of pravastatin (see CONTRAINDICATIONS). Caution should be exercised when pravastatin is administered to patients with a history of liver disease or heavy alcohol ingestion (see CLINICAL PHARMACOLOGY: Pharmacokinetics/Metabolism). Such patients should be closely monitored, started at the lower end of the recommended dosing range, and titrated to the desired therapeutic effect.

Skeletal Muscle: Rhabdomyolysis with renal dysfunction secondary to myoglobinuria has been reported with pravastatin and other drugs in this class. Uncomplicated myalgia has also been reported in pravastatin-treated patients (see ADVERSE REACTIONS). Myopathy, defined as muscle aching or muscle weakness in conjunction with increases in creatine phosphokinase (CPK) values to greater than 10 times the upper limit of normal was reported to be possibly due to pravastatin in only one patient in clinical trials (< 0.1%). Myopathy should be considered in any patient with diffuse myalgias, muscle tenderness or weakness, and/or marked elevation of CPK. Patients should be advised to report promptly unexplained muscle pain, tenderness or weakness, particularly if accompanied by malaise or fever. **Pravastatin therapy should be discontinued if markedly elevated CPK levels occur or myopathy is diagnosed or suspected. Pravastatin therapy should also be temporarily withheld in any patient experiencing an acute or serious condition predisposing to the development of renal failure secondary to rhabdomyolysis, e.g., sepsis; hypotension; major surgery; trauma; severe metabolic, endocrine, or electrolyte disorders; or uncontrolled epilepsy.**

The risk of myopathy during treatment with lovastatin is increased if therapy with either cyclosporine, gemfibrozil, erythromycin, or niacin is administered concurrently. There is no experience with the use of pravastatin together with cyclosporine. Myopathy has not been observed in clinical trials involving small numbers of patients who were treated with pravastatin together with niacin. One trial of limited size involving combined therapy with pravastatin and gemfibrozil showed a trend toward more frequent CPK elevations and patient withdrawals due to musculoskeletal symptoms in the group receiving combined treatment as compared with the groups receiving placebo, gemfibrozil, or pravastatin monotherapy. Myopathy was not reported in this trial (see PRECAUTIONS: Drug Interactions). One patient developed myopathy when clofibrate was added to a previously well tolerated regimen of pravastatin; the myopathy resolved when clofibrate therapy was stopped and pravastatin treatment continued. **The use of fibrates alone may occasionally be associated with myopathy. The combined use of pravastatin and fibrates should generally be avoided.**

PRECAUTIONS

General: Pravastatin may elevate creatine phosphokinase and transaminase levels (see ADVERSE REACTIONS). This should be considered in the differential diagnosis of chest pain in a patient on therapy with pravastatin.

Homozygous Familial Hypercholesterolemia. Pravastatin has not been evaluated in patients with rare homozygous familial hypercholesterolemia. In this group of patients, it has been reported that HMG-CoA reductase inhibitors are less effective because the patients lack functional LDL receptors.

Renal Insufficiency. A single 20 mg oral dose of pravastatin was administered to 24 patients with varying degrees of renal impairment (as determined by creatinine clearance). No effect was observed on the pharmacokinetics of pravastatin or its 3α-hydroxy isomeric metabolite (SQ 31,906). A small increase was seen in mean AUC values and half-life ($t_{1/2}$) for the inactive enzymatic ring hydroxylation metabolite (SQ 31,945). Given this small sample size, the dosage administered, and the degree of individual variability, patients with renal impairment who are receiving pravastatin should be closely monitored.

Information for Patients: Patients should be advised to report promptly unexplained muscle pain, tenderness or weakness, particularly if accompanied by malaise or fever.

Drug Interactions: *Immunosuppressive Drugs, Gemfibrozil, Niacin (Nicotinic Acid), Erythromycin:* See WARNINGS: Skeletal Muscle.

Antipyrine: Clearance by the cytochrome P450 system was unaltered by concomitant administration of pravastatin. Since pravastatin does not appear to induce hepatic drug-metabolizing enzymes, it is not expected that any significant interaction of pravastatin with other drugs (e.g., phenytoin, quinidine) metabolized by the cytochrome P450 system will occur.

Cholestyramine/Colestipol: Concomitant administration resulted in an approximately 40 to 50% decrease in the mean AUC of pravastatin. However, when pravastatin was administered 1 hour before or 4 hours after cholestyramine or 1 hour before colestipol and a standard meal, there was no clinically significant decrease in bioavailability or therapeutic effect. (See DOSAGE AND ADMINISTRATION: Concomitant Therapy.)

Warfarin: In a study involving 10 healthy male subjects given pravastatin and warfarin concomitantly for 6 days, bioavailability parameters at steady state for pravastatin (parent compound) were not altered. Pravastatin did not alter the plasma protein-binding of warfarin. Concomitant dosing did increase the AUC and Cmax of warfarin but did not produce any changes in its anticoagulant action (i.e., no increase was seen in mean prothrombin time after 6 days of concomitant therapy). However, bleeding and extreme prolongation of prothrombin time has been reported with another drug in this class. Patients receiving warfarin-type anticoagulants should have their prothrombin times closely monitored when pravastatin is initiated or the dosage of pravastatin is changed.

Cimetidine: The $AUC_{0\text{-}12hr}$ for pravastatin when given with cimetidine was not significantly different from the AUC for pravastatin when given alone. A significant difference was observed between the AUC's for pravastatin when given with cimetidine compared to when administered with antacid.

Digoxin: In a crossover trial involving 18 healthy male subjects given pravastatin and digoxin concurrently for 9 days, the bioavailability parameters of digoxin were not affected. The AUC of pravastatin tended to increase, but the overall bioavailability of pravastatin plus its metabolites SQ 31,906 and SQ 31,945 was not altered.

Gemfibrozil: In a crossover study in 20 healthy male volunteers given concomitant single doses of pravastatin and gemfibrozil, there was a significant decrease in urinary excretion and protein binding of pravastatin. In addition, there was a significant increase in AUC, Cmax, and Tmax for the pravastatin metabolite SQ 31,906. Combination therapy with pravastatin and gemfibrozil is generally not recommended.

In interaction studies with *aspirin, antacids* (1 hour prior to PRAVACHOL), *cimetidine, nicotinic acid,* or *probucol*, no statistically significant differences in bioavailability were seen when PRAVACHOL (pravastatin sodium) was administered.

Other Drugs: During clinical trials, no noticeable drug interactions were reported when PRAVACHOL was added to: diuretics, antihypertensives, digitalis, converting-enzyme inhibitors, calcium channel blockers, beta-blockers, or nitroglycerin.

Endocrine Function: HMG-CoA reductase inhibitors interfere with cholesterol synthesis and lower circulating cholesterol levels and, as such, might theoretically blunt adrenal or gonadal steroid hormone production. Results of clinical trials with pravastatin in males and post-menopausal females were inconsistent with regard to possible effects of the drug on basal steroid hormone levels. In a study of 21 males, the mean testosterone response to human chorionic gonadotropin was significantly reduced ($p < 0.004$) after 16 weeks of treatment with 40 mg of pravastatin. However, the percentage of patients showing a $\geq$ 50% rise in plasma testosterone after human chorionic gonadotropin stimulation did not change significantly after therapy in these patients. The effects of HMG-CoA reductase inhibitors on spermatogenesis and fertility have not been studied in adequate numbers of patients. The effects, if any, of pravastatin on the pituitary-gonadal axis in pre-menopausal females are unknown. Patients treated with pravastatin who display clinical evidence of endocrine dysfunction should be evaluated appropriately. Caution should also be exercised if an HMG-CoA reductase inhibitor or other agent used to lower cholesterol levels is administered to patients also receiving other drugs (e.g., ketoconazole, spironolactone, cimetidine) that may diminish the levels or activity of steroid hormones.

CNS Toxicity: CNS vascular lesions, characterized by perivascular hemorrhage and edema and mononuclear cell infiltration of perivascular spaces, were seen in dogs treated with pravastatin at a dose of 25 mg/kg/day, a dose that produced a plasma drug level about 50 times higher than the mean drug level in humans taking 40 mg/day. Similar CNS vascular lesions have been observed with several other drugs in this class.

A chemically similar drug in this class produced optic nerve degeneration (Wallerian degeneration of retinogeniculate fibers) in clinically normal dogs in a dose-dependent fashion starting at 60 mg/kg/day, a dose that produced mean plasma drug levels about 30 times higher than the mean drug level in humans taking the highest recommended dose (as measured by total enzyme inhibitory activity). This same drug also produced vestibulocochlear Wallerian-like degeneration and retinal ganglion cell chromatolysis in dogs treated for 14 weeks at 180 mg/kg/day, a dose which resulted in a mean plasma drug level similar to that seen with the 60 mg/kg dose.

Carcinogenesis, Mutagenesis, Impairment of Fertility: In a 2-year study in rats fed pravastatin at doses of 10, 30, or 100 mg/kg body weight, there was an increased incidence of hepatocellular carcinomas in males at the highest dose ($p < 0.01$). Although rats were given up to 125 times the human dose (HD) on a mg/kg body weight basis, their serum drug levels were only 6 to 10 times higher than those measured in humans given 40 mg pravastatin as measured by AUC.

The oral administration of 10, 30, or 100 mg/kg (producing plasma drug levels approximately 0.5 to 5.0 times human drug levels at 40 mg) of pravastatin to mice for 22 months resulted in a statistically significant increase in the incidence of malignant lymphomas in treated females when all treatment groups were pooled and compared to controls ($p < 0.05$). The incidence was not dose-related and male mice were not affected.

A chemically similar drug in this class was administered to mice for 72 weeks at 25, 100, and 400 mg/kg body weight, which resulted in mean serum drug levels approximately 3, 15, and 33 times higher than the mean human serum drug concentration (as total inhibitory activity) after a 40 mg oral dose. Liver carcinomas were significantly increased in high-dose females and mid- and high-dose males, with a maximum incidence of 90 percent in males. The incidence of adenomas of the liver was significantly increased in mid- and high-dose females. Drug treatment also significantly increased the incidence of lung adenomas in mid- and high-dose males and females. Adenomas of the eye Harderian gland (a gland of the eye of rodents) were significantly higher in high-dose mice than in controls.

No evidence of mutagenicity was observed *in vitro*, with or without rat-liver metabolic activation, in the following studies: microbial mutagen tests, using mutant strains of *Salmonella typhimurium* or *Escherichia coli*; a forward mutation assay in L5178Y TK +/− mouse lymphoma cells; a chromosomal aberration test in hamster cells; and a gene conversion assay using *Saccharomyces cerevisiae*. In addition, there was no evidence of mutagenicity in either a dominant lethal test in mice or a micronucleus test in mice.

In a study in rats, with daily doses up to 500 mg/kg, pravastatin did not produce any adverse effects on fertility or general reproductive performance. However, in a study with another HMG-CoA reductase inhibitor, there was decreased fertility in male rats treated for 34 weeks at 25 mg/kg body weight, although this effect was not observed in a subsequent fertility study when this same dose was administered for 11 weeks (the entire cycle of spermatogenesis, including epididymal maturation). In rats treated with this same reductase inhibitor at 180 mg/kg/day, seminiferous tubule degeneration (necrosis and loss of spermatogenic epithelium) was observed. Although not seen with pravastatin, two similar drugs in this class caused drug-related testicular atrophy, decreased spermatogenesis, spermatocytic degeneration, and giant cell formation in dogs. The clinical significance of these findings is unclear.

Pregnancy: Pregnancy Category X: See CONTRAINDICATIONS.

Safety in pregnant women has not been established. Pravastatin was not teratogenic in rats at doses up to 1000 mg/kg daily or in rabbits at doses of up to 50 mg/kg daily. These doses resulted in 20x (rabbit) or 240x (rat) the human exposure based on surface area (mg/meter^2). However, in studies with another HMG-CoA reductase inhibitor, skeletal malformations were observed in rats and mice. PRAVACHOL (pravastatin sodium) should be administered to women of child-bearing potential only when such patients are highly unlikely to conceive and have been informed of the potential hazards. If the woman becomes pregnant while taking PRAVACHOL (pravastatin sodium), it should be discontinued and the patient advised again as to the potential hazards to the fetus.

Nursing Mothers: A small amount of pravastatin is excreted in human breast milk. Because of the potential for serious adverse reactions in nursing infants, women taking PRAVACHOL should not nurse (see CONTRAINDICATIONS).

Pediatric Use: Safety and effectiveness in individuals less than 18 years old have not been established. Hence, treatment in patients less than 18 years old is not recommended at this time. (See also PRECAUTIONS: **General.**)

ADVERSE REACTIONS

Pravastatin is generally well tolerated; adverse reactions have usually been mild and transient. In 4-month long placebo-controlled trials, 1.7% of pravastatin-treated patients and 1.2% of placebo-treated patients were discontinued from treatment because of adverse experiences attributed to study drug therapy; this difference was not statistically significant. In long-term studies, the most common reasons for discontinuation were asymptomatic serum transaminase increases and mild, non-specific gastrointestinal complaints. During clinical trials the overall incidence of adverse events in the elderly was not different from the incidence observed in younger patients.

Adverse Clinical Events: All adverse clinical events (regardless of attribution) reported in more than 2% of pravastatin-treated patients in the placebo-controlled trials are identified in the table below; also shown are the percentages of patients in whom these medical events were believed to be related or possibly related to the drug:

	All Events %		Events Attributed to Study Drug %	
Body System/Event	Pravastatin (N=900)	Placebo (N=411)	Pravastatin (N=900)	Placebo (N=411)
Cardiovascular				
Cardiac Chest Pain	4.0	3.4	0.1	0.0
Dermatologic				
Rash	4.0*	1.1	1.3	0.9
Gastrointestinal				
Nausea/Vomiting	7.3	7.1	2.9	3.4
Diarrhea	6.2	5.6	2.0	1.9
Abdominal Pain	5.4	6.9	2.0	3.9
Constipation	4.0	7.1	2.4	5.1
Flatulence	3.3	3.6	2.7	3.4
Heartburn	2.9	1.9	2.0	0.7
General				
Fatigue	3.8	3.4	1.9	1.0
Chest Pain	3.7	1.9	0.3	0.2
Influenza	2.4*	0.7	0.0	0.0
Musculoskeletal				
Localized Pain	10.0	9.0	1.4	1.5
Myalgia	2.7	1.0	0.6	0.0
Nervous System				
Headache	6.2	3.9	1.7*	0.2
Dizziness	3.3	3.2	1.0	0.5
Renal/Genitourinary				
Urinary Abnormality	2.4	2.9	0.7	1.2
Respiratory				
Common Cold	7.0	6.3	0.0	0.0
Rhinitis	4.0	4.1	0.1	0.0
Cough	2.6	1.7	0.1	0.0

*Statistically significantly different from placebo.

The following effects have been reported with drugs in this class:

Skeletal: myopathy, rhabdomyolysis.

Neurological: dysfunction of certain cranial nerves (including alteration of taste, impairment of extra-ocular movement, facial paresis), tremor, vertigo, memory loss, paresthesia, peripheral neuropathy, peripheral nerve palsy.

Hypersensitivity Reactions: An apparent hypersensitivity syndrome has been reported rarely which has included one or more of the following features: anaphylaxis, angioedema, lupus erythematous-like syndrome, polymyalgia rheumatica, vasculitis, purpura, thrombocytopenia, leukopenia, hemolytic anemia, positive ANA, ESR increase, arthritis, arthralgia, urticaria, asthenia, photosensitivity, fever, chills, flushing, malaise, dyspnea, toxic epidermal necrolysis, erythema multiforme, including Stevens-Johnson syndrome.

Gastrointestinal: pancreatitis, hepatitis, including chronic active hepatitis, cholestatic jaundice, fatty change in liver, and, rarely, cirrhosis, fulminant hepatic necrosis, and hepatoma; anorexia, vomiting.

Reproductive: gynecomastia, loss of libido, erectile dysfunction.

Eye: progression of cataracts (lens opacities), ophthalmoplegia.

Laboratory Test Abnormalities: Increases in serum transaminase (ALT, AST) values and CPK have been observed (see WARNINGS).

Transient, asymptomatic eosinophilia has been reported. Eosinophil counts usually returned to normal despite continued therapy. Anemia, thrombocytopenia, and leukopenia have been reported with other HMG-CoA reductase inhibitors.

Concomitant Therapy: Pravastatin has been administered concurrently with cholestyramine, colestipol, nicotinic acid, probucol and gemfibrozil. Preliminary data suggest that the addition of either probucol or gemfibrozil to therapy with lovastatin or pravastatin is **not** associated with greater reduction in LDL-cholesterol than that achieved with lovastatin or pravastatin alone. No adverse reactions unique to the combination or in addition to those previously reported for each drug alone have been reported. Myopathy and rhabdomyolysis (with or without acute renal failure) have been reported when another HMG-CoA reductase inhibitor was used in combination with immunosuppressive drugs, gemfibrozil, erythromycin, or lipid-lowering doses of nicotinic acid. Concomitant therapy with HMG-CoA reductase inhibitors and these agents is generally not recommended. (See WARNINGS: **Skeletal Muscle** and PRECAUTIONS: **Drug Interactions.**)

OVERDOSAGE

There have been no reports of overdoses with pravastatin.

Should an accidental overdose occur, treat symptomatically and institute supportive measures as required.

(J4-422A)

Issued: January 1992

Letters

The Letters *column is a forum for rapid exchange of ideas among readers of* Clinical Pharmacy. *Liberal criteria are applied in the review of submissions to encourage contributions to this column.*

Letters need not be submitted with the journal's manuscript checklist. The following conditions, however, must be adhered to: (1) the body of the letter must be no longer than two typewritten pages, (2) the use of references, tables, and illustrations should be minimized, (3) the authors' names, affiliations, and mailing addresses must be typed at the end of the letter in the format used by Clinical Pharmacy, *and (4) the entire letter (including references, tables, and authors' names) must be typed double-spaced on plain white paper (not letterhead). Following acceptance of a letter, the authors are required to sign an exclusive publication statement and a copyright transferal form.*

Topical capsaicin for osteoarthritis

We would like to supplement the comments by Miller[1] that appeared in the Therapy Consultation section of October's issue of *Clinical Pharmacy*. Miller discussed the treatment of osteoarthritis in a patient with a history of duodenal ulcers.

One therapeutic option that Miller did not mention is capsaicin topical cream. Capsaicin 0.025% and 0.075% creams (Zostrix and Zostrix HP, respectively; GenDerm) are indicated for the relief of pain associated with osteoarthritis or rheumatoid arthritis. In animal and human studies, purified capsaicin has depleted substance P, the neurotransmitter implicated in the pathogenesis of pain and inflammation associated with rheumatoid arthritis and osteoarthritis.[2-6]

Two double-blind, randomized clinical studies have demonstrated capsaicin's superiority over cream vehicle in attenuating the pain associated with osteoarthritis and rheumatoid arthritis. In one trial ($n = 101$), four weeks of treatment with capsaicin 0.025% reduced pain by a mean of 57% and 33% in patients with rheumatoid arthritis and osteoarthritis, respectively, as rated on a visual analog scale ($p \le 0.05$).[7] Among patients with rheumatoid arthritis, 79% reported improvement in arthritis condition on the physician's global evaluation after four weeks of capsaicin treatment; 60% of those who were treated with vehicle reported improvement ($p = 0.027$). Among patients with osteoarthritis, 70% reported improvement after capsaicin treatment, and 49% reported improvement after treatment with the vehicle ($p = 0.023$).

In the other trial ($n = 21$), patients with osteoarthritis who were treated with capsaicin 0.075% had a 42% reduction in articular tenderness, as assessed by dolorimeter scores, and a 40% reduction in pain, as rated on a visual analog scale, after four weeks of therapy.[8] The reductions were greater than those that occurred in vehicle-treated patients ($p \le 0.05$).

As Miller stated, because osteoarthritis is not a systemic disease, systemic therapy may not constitute optimal treatment. Use of topical capsaicin localizes therapy to the desired site of action. Unlike therapy with nonsteroidal anti-inflammatory agents, topical capsaicin has no known systemic adverse effects. A local, transient, and usually mild burning sensation may occur after application of capsaicin. In considering a treatment regimen for elderly patients with osteoarthritis and concomitant illnesses, the possibility of drug interactions must be considered; capsaicin has not been shown to interact with any systemic therapies to produce untoward adverse effects.

Zostrix and Zostrix HP contain purified capsaicin, the chemical shown to deplete substance P. Other products for which capsaicin or a related substance is listed as an active ingredient contain either capsaicin oleoresin or capsicum oleoresin. Because of its route of administration, efficacy in reducing arthritic pain, and safety, topical capsaicin is a reasonable alternative to conventional systemic therapy for arthritis.

1. Miller DR. Treatment options for a patient with osteoarthritis and a history of ulcer disease. *Clin Pharm.* 1991; 10:740-1.
2. Lam FY, Ferrell WR. Capsaicin suppresses substance P-induced joint inflammation in the rat. *Neuroscience.* 1989; 105:155-8.
3. Jessell TM, Iversen LL, Cuello AC. Capsaicin-induced depletion of substance P from primary sensory neurones. *Brain Res.* 1978; 152:183-8.
4. Inman RD, Chiu B, Rabinovich S et al. Neuromodulation of synovitis: capsaicin effect on severity of experimental arthritis. *J Neuroimmunol.* 1989; 24:17-22.
5. Carpenter SE, Lynn B. Vascular and sensory responses of human skin to mild injury after topical treatment with capsaicin. *Br J Pharmacol.* 1981; 73:755-8.
6. Anand P, Bloom SR, McGregor GP. Topical capsaicin pretreatment inhibits axon reflex vasodilatation caused by somatostatin and vasoactive intestinal polypeptide in human skin. *Br J Pharmacol.* 1983; 78:665-9.
7. Deal CL, Schnitzer TJ, Lipstein E et al. Treatment of arthritis with topical capsaicin: a double-blind trial. *Clin Ther.* 1991; 13:383-93.
8. McCarthy GM, Bernstein JE, McCarty DJ. Topical capsaicin reduces pain and tenderness in osteo-arthritic finger joints. *J Rheumatol.* 1992; (in press).

Patrice L. Flynn, Associate Director of Clinical Research
Dennis West, M.S., FCCP, Vice President for Scientific Affairs

GenDerm Corporation
600 Knightsbridge Parkway
Lincolnshire, IL 60069

Correction

Clarithromycin and azithromycin: New macrolide antibiotics (February 1992, Drug Review). On page 144, the last sentence of the fourth full paragraph should read as follows: In one of these trials, failure of clarithromycin to eradicate *Haemophilus* spp. was seen in 5 of 17 cultured strains.[88]

Special Feature

Acute pain management: Operative or medical procedures and trauma, part 1

Agency for Health Care Policy and Research

Foreword

Approximately 23.3 million operations were performed in 1989 in the United States, and most of these involved some form of pain management. Unfortunately, clinical surveys continue to indicate that routine orders for intramuscular injections of opioid "as needed"—the standard practice in many clinical settings—fail to relieve pain in about half of postoperative patients. Postoperative pain contributes to patient discomfort, longer recovery periods, and greater use of scarce health care resources and may compromise patient outcomes.

There is wide variation in the methods used to manage postoperative and other acute pain, ranging from no set strategy to a comprehensive team ap-

Acute pain management guideline panel members included Daniel B. Carr, M.D., Panel Co-Chair, Director, Division of Pain Management, Department of Anesthesia, Massachusetts General Hospital; Ada K. Jacox, R.N., Ph.D., Panel Co-Chair, Independence Foundation Chair in Health Policy, School of Nursing, The Johns Hopkins University; C. Richard Chapman, Ph.D., Professor of Anesthesiology, School of Medicine, University of Washington; Betty R. Ferrell, R.N., Ph.D., Research Scientist, Nursing Research, City of Hope Medical Center; Howard L. Fields, M.D., Ph.D., Departments of Neurology and Physiology, University of California, San Francisco; George Heidrich III, R.N., M.A., Instructor, Department of Neurology, University of Wisconsin Medical School; Nancy K. Hester, R.N., Ph.D., Assistant Director, Center for Nursing Research, and Associate Professor, School of Nursing, Health Sciences Center, University of Colorado; C. Stratton Hill, Jr., M.D., Professor of Medicine, M.D. Anderson Cancer Hospital, University of Texas; Arthur G. Lipman, Pharm.D., Professor of Clinical Pharmacy, College of Pharmacy, University of Utah; Charles L. McGarvey, M.S., Chief, Physical Therapy Service, Department of Rehabilitation Medicine, National Institutes of Health; Christine A. Miaskowski, R.N., Ph.D., Associate Professor, Department of Physiological Nursing, University of California, San Francisco; David Stevenson Mulder, M.D., Professor of Surgery, McGill University, and Surgeon-in-Chief, Montreal General Hospital; Richard Payne, M.D., Associate Professor of Neurology, University of Cincinnati Medical Center; Neil Schecter, M.D., Associate Professor of Pediatrics, Head, Division of Developmental and Behavioral Pediatrics, University of Connecticut School of Medicine, and Co-Director, Children's Pain Service, University of Connecticut Health Center; Barbara S. Shapiro, M.D., Associate Director, Multidisciplinary Pain Management Program, Division of General Pediatrics, Children's Hospital of Philadelphia; Robert S. Smith, Ph.L., Director, Institute for Medicine in Contemporary Society, State University Medical Center at Stony Brook; Carole V. Tsou, M.D., Division of Family Medicine, UCLA Center for Health Sciences; and Loretta Vecchiarelli, Rehabilitation Counselor and Burn Survivor, Rehabilitation Hospital of Western New England. Panel staff members were Jane Ballantyne, M.B., B.S., Technology Assessment Group, Harvard School of Public Health; Donna Mahrenholz, R.N., Ph.D., School of Nursing, The Johns Hopkins University; and Janice Ulmer, R.N., Ph.D., School of Nursing, The Johns Hopkins University. The consultants were Thomas C. Chalmers, M.D., Technology Assessment Group, Harvard School of Public Health; Frederick Mosteller, Ph.D., Department of Health Policy and Management, Harvard School of Public Health; and Barker Bausell, Ph.D., Center for Research, School of Nursing, University of Maryland.

The Acute Pain Management Guideline Panel expresses profound appreciation to the patients who helped us in the development of the consumer version of the guideline and to our numerous colleagues in many disciplines who made valuable contributions during the development of the guideline. We are especially grateful to Dr. Mitchell Max of the American Pain Society for his continuous and enthusiastic support and advice. Dr. Ada Jacox thanks her colleagues at The Johns Hopkins University for their thoughtful contributions and encouragement.

Numerous colleagues in the Departments of Surgery, Anesthesia, and Nursing at Massachusetts General Hospital provided informal yet valuable input as portions of the guideline were being written at that site. Dr. Daniel Carr's clinical colleagues in the Division of Pain Management of the Department of Anesthesia willingly increased their clinical load when the guideline development process became particularly time consuming. This extra workload fell particularly upon the shoulders of the Postoperative Pain Service, directed by Dr. Buckman McPeek, and the Diagnostic and Therapeutic Nerve Blocking Unit, directed by Dr. Donald P. Todd. Dr. Richard J. Kitz, the Henry Isaiah Dorr Professor and Chairman of Anesthesiology, and Dr. George E. Battit, Vice-Chairman, provided constant encouragement for this project and facilitated it in many practical ways. Miss Evelyn Hall provided expert and dedicated administrative and secretarial assistance.

Reprinted with permission of the Agency for Health Care Policy Research.

This article is being published in two parts; the final part will appear in the May issue.

The Agency for Health Care Policy and Research (AHCPR) was established in December 1989 under Public Law 101-239 (Omnibus Budget Reconciliation Act of 1989) to enhance the quality, appropriateness, and effectiveness of health care services and access to these services. AHCPR carries out its mission through conduct and support of general health services research, including medical effectiveness research, facilitating development of clinical practice guidelines, and dissemination of research findings and guidelines to health care providers, policymakers, and the public.

The legislation also established within AHCPR the Office of the Forum for Quality and Effectiveness in Health Care (the Forum). The Forum has primary responsibility for facilitating the development, periodic review, and updating of clinical practice guidelines. The guidelines will assist practitioners in the prevention, diagnosis, treatment, and management of clinical conditions.

Other components of AHCPR include the Center for Medical Effectiveness Research, which has principal responsibility for patient outcomes research and studies of variations in clinical practice; the Center for General Health Services Extramural Research, which supports research on primary care, the cost and financing of health care, and access to care for underserved and rural populations; the Center for General Health Services Intramural Research, which uses large data sets for policy research on national health care expenditures and utilization, hospital studies, and long-term care; the Center for Research Dissemination and Liaison, which produces and disseminates findings from AHCPR-supported research, including guidelines, and conducts research on dissemination methods; the Office of Health Technology Assessment, which responds to requests from federal health programs for assessment of health care technologies; and the Office of Science and Data Development, which develops specialized databases and enhances techniques for using existing databases for patient outcomes research.

Guidelines are available in formats suitable for health care practitioners, the scientific community, educators, and consumers. The AHCPR invites comments and suggestions from users for consideration in development and updating of future guidelines. Please send written comments to Director, Office of the Forum, Executive Office Center, Suite 401, 2101 East Jefferson Street, Rockville, MD 20852.

proach as advocated in this clinical practice guideline. This guideline sets forth procedures to minimize the incidence and severity of acute pain after surgical and medical procedures and pain associated with trauma in adults and children. It offers clinicians a coherent yet flexible approach to pain assessment and management for use in daily practice.

Although it is not practical or desirable to eliminate all postoperative and other acute pain, an aggressive approach to pain assessment and management can reduce such pain, increase patient comfort and satisfaction, and in some cases, contribute to improved patient outcomes and shorter hospital stays.

This clinical practice guideline was developed under the sponsorship of the Agency for Health Care Policy and Research (AHCPR), Public Health Service, U.S. Department of Health and Human Services. To develop the guideline, AHCPR convened an interdisciplinary expert panel made up of physicians, nurses, a pharmacist, a psychologist, a physical therapist, a patient/consumer, and an ethicist. The panel first undertook an extensive and interdisciplinary clinical review of current needs, therapeutic practices and principles, and emerging technologies for pain assessment and management. Second, the panel conducted a comprehensive review of the field to define the existing knowledge base and critically evaluate the assumptions and common wisdom in the field. Third, the panel initiated peer review of guideline drafts and field review with intended users in clinical sites. Comments from these reviews were assessed and used in developing the guideline.

This is the first edition of the *Clinical Practice Guideline for Acute Pain Management: Operative or Medical Procedures and Trauma*. Further editions will be produced as needed to reflect new research findings and experience with emerging technologies for pain assessment and relief.

Introduction. This guideline addresses the care of patients with acute pain after operation, medical procedures, or trauma. (Methods used to develop the guideline are in Appendix A.) It outlines the physiological basis for pain and cites clinical studies linking effective postoperative pain management with improved patient outcomes. The guideline also describes practices that can minimize or eliminate acute pain. Rigid prescriptions for postoperative pain control are inappropriate because patients vary greatly in the severity of their pre-existing pain, medical conditions, and pain experiences; the extensiveness of pathology and associated operations; responses to interventions; personal preferences; and the settings in which they receive care. Instead, this guideline offers clinicians a coherent yet flexible approach to pain assessment and management in daily practice. This guideline has four major goals:

1. Reduce the incidence and severity of patients' postoperative or posttraumatic pain.
2. Educate patients about the need to communicate unrelieved pain so they can receive prompt evaluation and effective treatment.
3. Enhance patient comfort and satisfaction.
4. Contribute to fewer postoperative complications and, in some cases, shorter stays after surgical procedures.

Organization of the Guideline. To derive maximum benefit, clinicians should read the entire guideline. However, the guideline is organized so that users can go easily to those sections of immediate interest. Following a discussion of why clinicians should take an aggressive approach to prevention and control of postoperative pain, methods of pain assessment are described. Pharmacologic and nonpharmacologic methods of pain control are then presented for general control of postoperative pain, followed by discussion of pain control for specific operative sites and for specific types of patients. The final section discusses institutional responsibility for effective pain management.

This guideline reflects the state of knowledge, current at the time of publication, on effective and appropriate acute pain management following surgery, medical procedures, and trauma. The recommendations are primarily based on published scientific literature. (For a complete list of the literature surveyed, see the bibliography of the *Guideline Report for Acute Pain Management: Operative or Medical Procedures and Trauma* (in press). Rockville, MD: Agency for Health Care Policy and Research.) When the scientific literature was incomplete or inconsistent in a particular area, the recommendations reflect the professional judgment of the panel members, in consultation with expert peer reviewers and practitioners. Decisions to adopt any particular recommendation must be made by the practitioner in light of available resources and circumstances presented by individual patients.

Need for Aggressive Postoperative Pain Control

Pain is an unpleasant sensory and emotional experience arising from actual or potential tissue damage or described in terms of such damage.[1,2] No matter how successful or how deftly conducted, operations produce tissue trauma and release potent mediators of inflammation and pain.[3]

Pain is just one response to the trauma of surgery, however. In addition to the major stress of surgical trauma and pain, the substances released from injured tissue evoke "stress hormone" responses in the patient. Such responses promote breakdown of body tissue; increase metabolic rate, blood clotting, and water retention; impair immune function; and trigger a "fight or flight" alarm reaction with autonomic features (e.g., rapid pulse) and negative emotions.[4-7] Pain itself may lead to shallow breathing and cough suppression in an attempt to "splint" the injured site, followed by retained pulmonary secretions and pneumonia.[8-12] Unrelieved pain also may delay the return of normal gastric and bowel function in the postoperative patient.[13]

The physiological and psychosocial risks associated with untreated pain are greatest in frail patients with other illnesses such as heart or lung disease, those undergoing major surgical procedures such as aortic surgery, and the very young or very old. Because of advances in surgical and anesthetic techniques, it is now common for such patients to undergo operations once dismissed as prohibitively risky.

Unfortunately, clinical surveys continue to show that routine orders for intramuscular injections of opioid as needed will leave more than half of postoperative patients with unrelieved pain due to undermedication.[14-17] In the past, postoperative pain was thought to be inevitable, a harmless though intense discomfort that the patient had to tolerate. Unrelieved pain after surgery or trauma is often unhealthy; fortunately, it is preventable or controllable in an overwhelming majority of cases. Patients have a right to treatment that includes prevention or adequate relief of pain.

Recognition of the widespread inadequacy of pain management has prompted recent corrective efforts within multiple health care disciplines, including surgery,[18,19] anesthesiology,[20,21] nursing,[22,23] and pain management groups.[24-26] Although it is not practical or desirable to entirely eliminate all postoperative pain, this clinical practice guideline sets forth procedures to minimize the incidence and severity of acute pain after surgical or medical procedures and trauma. The guideline is designed to help clinicians, patients, and patients' families understand the assessment and treatment of postoperative and other acute pain in both adults and children.

Health care is both a technical and an ethical enterprise. The ethical obligation to manage pain and relieve the patient's suffering is at the core of a health care professional's commitment. While medical treatments often involve risks and burdens, anything harmful to the patient, including postoperative pain, should be minimized or prevented if possible. The ethical importance of pain management is further increased when additional benefits for the patient are realized—earlier mobilization, shortened hospital stay, and reduced costs. If inadequate pain management results from a clinician's conflict between reducing pain and avoiding potential side effects and/or legal liability, achieving greater technical competence and knowledge of risks and benefits can help to reduce such conflicts.

Prevention Is Better than Treatment. Pain is dynamic. Without treatment, sensory input from injured tissue reaches spinal cord neurons and causes subsequent responses to be enhanced. Pain receptors in the periphery also become more sensitive after injury. Recent studies demonstrate long-lasting changes in cells within spinal cord pain pathways after a brief painful stimulus.[27-31] Such physiological studies confirm longstanding clinical impressions that established pain is more difficult to suppress.[32-34] The health care team should encourage patients to request pain medication before the pain becomes severe and difficult to control. Furthermore, the team should teach patients simple relaxation exercises to help decrease postoperative pain.[35]

Aggressive pain prevention and control that occur before, during, and after surgery can yield both short-term and long-term benefits. In the very short term, for example, a patient's first request for analgesia after orthopedic surgery occurs later after operations performed with opioid premedication and intraoperative nerve blocks than after general anesthesia alone.[36] In the short term, patients who undergo cesarean section under epidural anesthesia request less postoperative pain medication in the next three days than patients who have general anesthesia.[37] Also in the short term, postoperative patients able to self-medicate with small intravenous doses of opioids such as morphine metered out by a programmable infusion pump—patient-controlled analgesia or PCA[38]—have less pain and are more satisfied with their pain relief. These patients tend to be discharged earlier from the hospital compared with those given the same drug on an as-needed basis.[39-43]

In the long term, after elective limb amputation for vascular insufficiency, patients who receive epidural analgesia before an operation are less likely to have chronic phantom limb pain, in contrast to those conventionally treated.[44] Pilot studies such as these that show diverse benefits of aggressive pain treatment complement controlled clinical trials that indicate that postoperative morbidity and mortality decrease in high-risk populations such as the very young[45] or very old[46] when postoperative care includes aggressive pain relief.

Much of the clinical research cited here is preliminary and needs to be confirmed by properly designed clinical trials. Yet, when considered with laboratory reports and well-documented undertreatment of pain in hospitalized patients, it is likely that routine provision of proactive, aggressive pain treatment will benefit large numbers of postoperative patients. To ensure these benefits, institutions must develop and use formal procedures to assess pain and employ patient-based feedback to gauge the effectiveness of pain control.[47,48] The flow charts shown in Figures 1 and 2 indicate the points at which caregivers must make decisions about assessing and controlling patient pain.

Process of Pain Assessment and Reassessment

Pain is a complex, subjective response with several quantifiable features, including intensity, time course, quality, impact, and personal meaning. The reporting of pain is a social transaction between caregiver and patient. Therefore, successful assessment and control of postoperative pain depends in part on establishing a positive relationship between health care providers, patients, and (when appropriate) their families. Studies have shown that patients provided with information related to physiological coping (instruction in coughing, deep breathing, turning, and ambulation) reported less pain,[49] were given fewer analgesics postoperatively,[50,51] and had shorter lengths of stay.[51] Egbert et al.[52] found that providing patients sensory information preoperatively (i.e., detailed descriptions of discomforts to be expected postoperatively) decreased pain, analgesic use, and length of stay. Still other researchers found that patients provided with procedural and sensory information as well as instructions related to physiological coping tended to receive fewer analgesics[53,54] and had shorter lengths of stay than patients who were given less complete information.[54]

As noted in Figures 1 and 2, the subject of postoperative pain and its control is a critical part of the initial review of all relevant aspects of the planned procedure. The surgeon should discuss this with the patient and the family. In addition, pain assessment and management issues should be a part of the preoperative workups of the anesthesia and nursing staffs. Patients and their families should be informed that pain reports are valuable and important information and also that pain may herald surgical complications that demand prompt diagnosis and therapy. To aid in planning and discussing pain control strategies

Figure 1. Pain treatment flow chart: preoperative and intraoperative phases.

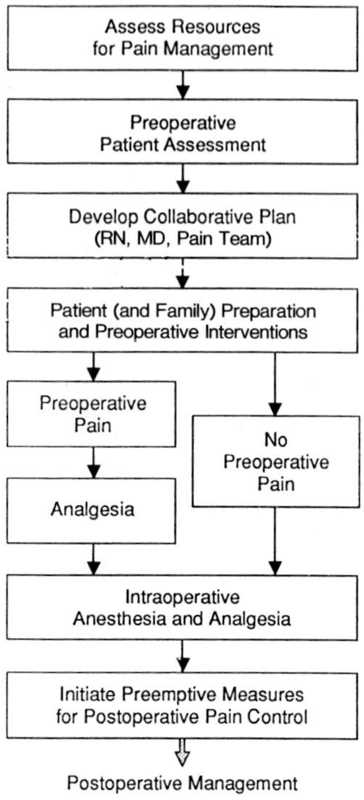

Figure 2. Pain treatment flow chart: postoperative phase.

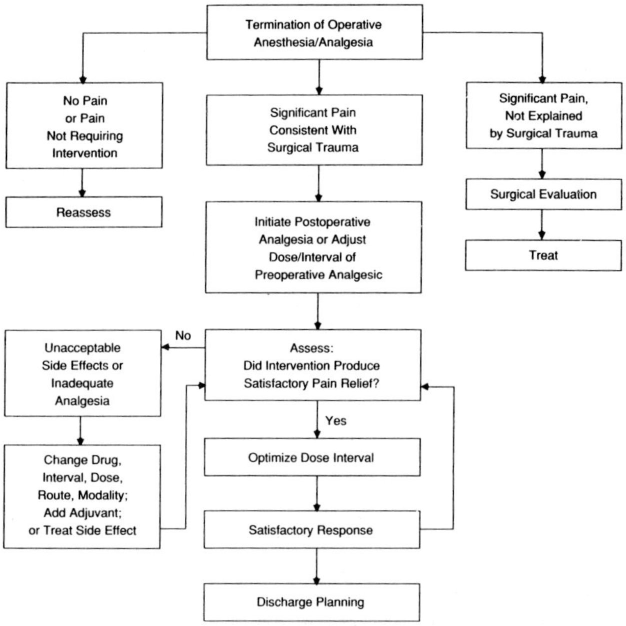

with the patient, a member of the anesthesiology department should obtain a pain history during the preoperative visit. The pain history should include:

- Significant previous and/or ongoing instances of pain and its effect on the patient;
- Previously used methods for pain control that the patient has found either helpful or unhelpful;
- The patient's attitude toward and use of opioid, anxiolytic, or other medications, including any history of substance abuse;
- The patient's typical coping response for stress or pain, including more broadly, the presence or absence of psychiatric disorders such as depression, anxiety, or psychosis;
- Family expectations and beliefs concerning pain, stress, and postoperative course;
- Ways the patient describes or shows pain; and
- The patient's knowledge of, expectations about, and preferences for pain management methods and for receiving information about pain management.

Some patients fear overmedication (e.g., "They will medicate me into oblivion so that I won't be any trouble"). Others know from previous experience that they are prone to side effects of certain drugs (e.g., dysphoria or nausea). Patients who express fears or concerns related to previous analgesic effects may require a cautious approach to medication. Preoperative anxiety may indicate a concurrent medical condition such as substance abuse or withdrawal, hyperthyroidism, anxiety disorder, affective disorder, psychosis, or a medication side effect. Excessive preoperative anxiety should be assessed and a psychiatric or psychologic consultation considered to assist with perioperative management. When the preoperative assessment is complete (as noted in Figure 1), the health care team should develop a pain management plan in collaboration with the patient. When developing the pain management plan, clinicians must consider the relative risks, benefits, and costs of available pain control options. They also should attempt to correct patient misconceptions about the use of pharmacologic or nonpharmacologic strategies.

Once a pain management plan is in place, preoperative preparation of the patient and family is extremely important. Preoperative preparation of patients (and families, when appropriate) assists patients in understanding their responsibilities in pain management. To ensure that postoperative pain measurement is both valid and reliable, the staff should review the selected pain measurement tool—for example, a simple descriptive scale or a visual analogue scale—with the patient before surgery. Pain assessment instruments are discussed below and samples are provided in Figures 3–7 and Tables 1–3. The patient should be told how frequently pain will be assessed and asked to select a measurement tool. A member of the health care team should advise the patient that a score above some predetermined criterion of the patient's choosing (e.g., a score of 3–4 on a 10-point scale) will result in a dose increment or other intervention. The patient's negotiation of this criterion is particularly important if the patient fears overmedication or intends to cope psychologically with the pain. Patient preferences should be supported.

Figure 3. Examples of pain intensity scales. If the simple descriptive pain intensity scale or the 0–10 numeric pain intensity scale is used as a graphic rating scale, a 10-cm baseline is recommended. A 10-cm baseline is also recommended for the visual analogue scale.

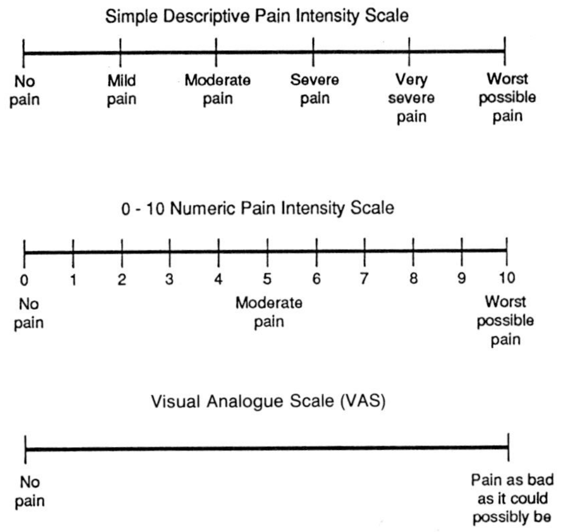

Figure 4. Examples of pain distress scales. If the simple descriptive pain distress scale or the 0–10 numeric pain distress scale is used as a graphic rating scale, a 10-cm baseline is recommended. A 10-cm baseline is also recommended for the visual analogue scale.

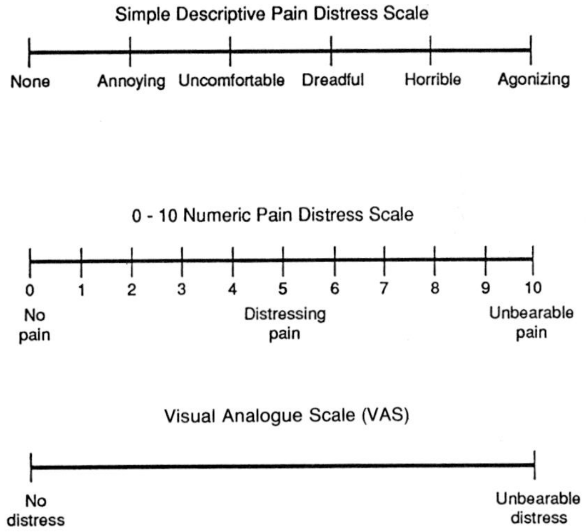

Assessment of pain after surgery should be frequent and simple. Many different measurement tools are available, and several factors help determine the best choices.[55] First, consider the patient's age; developmental status; physical, emotional, or cognitive condition; and preference. Second, consider the expertise, time, and effort available from the individual performing the assessment. Third, examine the

Figure 5. Initial pain assessment tool. May be duplicated for use in clinical practice. (McCaffrey M, Beebe A. Pain: clinical manual for nursing practice. St. Louis: C.V. Mosby; 1989.)

Date ____________

Patient's Name ____________ Age ______ Room ______

Diagnosis ____________ Physician ____________

Nurse ____________

I. Location: Patient or nurse mark drawing.

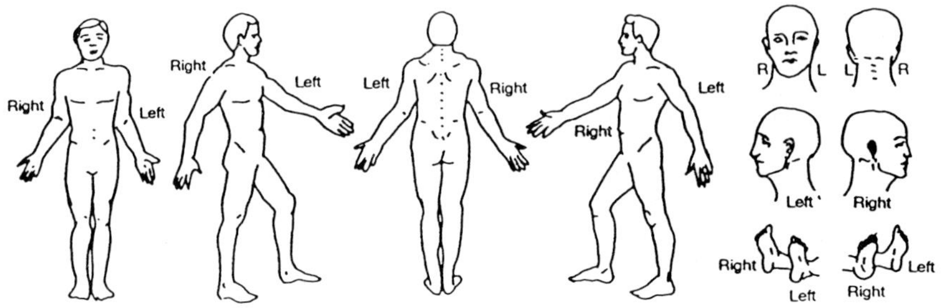

II. Intensity: Patient rates the pain. Scale used ____________
Present: ____________
Worst pain gets: ____________
Best pain gets: ____________
Acceptable level of pain: ____________

III. Quality: (Use patient's own words, e.g. prick, ache, burn, throb, pull, sharp) ____________

IV. Onset, duration variations, rhythms: ____________

V. Manner of expressing pain: ____________

VI. What relieves the pain? ____________

VII. What causes or increases the pain? ____________

VIII. Effects of pain: (Note decreased function, decreased quality of life.)
Accompanying symptoms (e.g. nausea) ____________
Sleep ____________
Appetite ____________
Physical activity ____________
Relationship with others (e.g. irritability) ____________
Emotions (e.g. anger, suicidal, crying) ____________
Concentration ____________
Other ____________

IX. Other comments: ____________

X. Plan: ____________

institution's requirements for monitoring and documentation for quality assurance purposes. Based on these factors, each health care institution should educate staff in the proper and consistent use of a valid assessment tool(s) and establish its own quality assurance program for evaluation of postoperative pain assessment and management.[47,48,56] For example, recording pain intensity on the bedside vital sign chart may be considered necessary to make the assessment easily accessible to members of the health care team. In addition, each institution should identify individuals responsible for postoperative pain assessment and control.

A comprehensive approach to postoperative pain assessment requires evaluation of (1) patient perceptions, (2) physiological responses, (3) behavioral responses, and (4) cognitive attempts by the patient to manage pain. Physiological responses such as heart rate, blood pressure, and respiratory rate provide critical information in the immediate postoperative period. Once the patient has recovered from anesthesia, the mainstay of pain assessment should be the patient's self-report to assess pain perceptions (including description, location, intensity/severity, and aggravating and relieving factors) and cognitive response. Patient self-report is the single most reliable indicator of the existence and intensity of pain and any concomitant affective discomfort or distress.[56] Neither behavior nor vital signs can substitute for a self-report.[57] Patients may be experiencing excruciat-

Figure 6. Flow sheet for pain assessment. May be duplicated for use in clinical practice. (McCaffrey M, Beebe A. Pain: clinical manual for nursing practice. St. Louis: C.V. Mosby; 1989.)

Patient ______________________ Date ____________

* Pain rating scale used ______________________

Purpose: to evaluate the safety and effectiveness of the analgesic(s).

Analgesic(s) prescribed: ______________________

Time	Pain rating	Analgesic	R	P	BP	Level of arousal	Other†	Plan & comments

* *Pain rating*: A number of different scales may be used. Indicate which scale is used and use the same one each time. For example, 0-10 (0= no pain, 10 = worst pain).

† *Possibilities for other columns:* bowel function, activities, nausea and vomiting, other pain relief measures. Identify the side effects of greatest concern to patient, family, physician, and nurses.

ing pain even while smiling and using laughter as coping mechanisms.[58]

Samples of commonly used pain assessment tools are in Figures 3–7 and Tables 1–3. Three common self-report measurement tools useful for assessment of pain intensity and affective distress in adults and many children are (1) a numerical rating scale (NRS), (2) a visual analogue scale (VAS), and (3) an adjective rating scale (ARS). While many researchers prefer visual analogue measures,[59,60] each of these tools can be a valid and reliable instrument as long as endpoints and adjective descriptors are carefully selected.[61-63]

In practical use, the visual analogue scale is always presented graphically, usually with a 10-cm baseline and endpoint adjective descriptors. Patients are asked to place a mark on the line at a point that best represents their pain. The visual analogue scale is scored by measuring the distance of a patient's mark from the zero. The numerical and adjective rating scales may be presented graphically (see Figures 3 and 4) or in other formats. For example, numerical rating scales are sometimes presented verbally, and adjective rating scales are presented as a list of pain descriptors. In a graphic format, scoring of the numerical and adjective rating scales may be the same as that described above for the visual analogue scale, or they can be scored as numeric integers.

For each of these scales, the clinician should request the patient's self-report, not only with the patient at rest but also during routine activity such as coughing, deep breathing, or moving (e.g., turning in bed). Complaints of pain must be heeded. The patient should be observed for behaviors that often indicate pain, such as splinting the operative site, distorted posture, impaired mobility, insomnia, anxiety, attention seeking, and depression. Patient awareness of pain and the ability to control pain are important components of pain assessment. If pain behavior is observed or if the patient expresses feelings of inadequate control, a member of the health care team should discuss these with the patient and share this information with other members of the team. The management plan should then be revised as needed.

The clinician should document the patient's preferred tool for pain assessment and the goal for postoperative pain control as expressed by a score on a pain scale in the patient's chart as part of the pain history. Simply to record patient responses to the question "How is your pain?" invites misunderstanding or denial and hinders quantification. Pain should be assessed and documented (1) preoperatively; (2) routinely at regular intervals postoperatively, as determined by the operation and severity of the pain (e.g., every two hours while awake for one day after surgery); (3) with each new report of pain; and (4) at a suitable interval after each analgesic intervention (e.g., 30 minutes after parenteral drug therapy and one hour after oral analgesics). Most important, the team should evaluate immediately each instance of unexpected intense pain, particularly if sudden or associated with oliguria or altered vital signs such as hypotension, tachycardia, or fever and consider new diagnoses such as wound dehiscence, infection, or deep venous thrombosis.

Occasionally, apparent discrepancies between behaviors and a patient's self-report of pain may occur. For example, patients may describe pain as an 8 out of 10 on a pain scale while smiling and walking freely or as 2 out of 10 while tachycardic, splinting, and sweating. Discrepancies between behavior and a patient's self-report may result from excellent coping skills. The patient who uses distraction and relaxation techniques may engage in diversionary activities while still experiencing severe pain. Patients may deny severe pain for a variety of reasons, including fear of inadequate pain control or a perception that stoicism is expected or rewarded. Similarly, patients managed with as-needed analgesia may perceive that medication will be given only if the pain score is very high. Patients who perceive staff as inattentive to their concerns may use pain as a way to get help for other reasons.

When discussing pain assessment and control with patients, members of the health care team should emphasize the importance of a factual report, thereby avoiding both stoicism and exaggeration. Patients with anxiety or other concerns should rate their mood and emotional distress separately from their pain by using similar scales (Figure 4). When discrepancies between behaviors and self-reports of pain occur, clinicians should address these differences with the patient. The pain team and the patient should then renegotiate the pain management plan.

Patients unable to communicate effectively with staff require special consideration for pain assessment, e.g., neonates and children, developmentally

Figure 7. Word-graphic rating scale. *Instructions:"This is a line with words to describe how much pain you may have. This side of the line means no pain and over here the line means worst possible pain."* (Point with your finger where "no pain" is, and run your finger along the line to "worst possible pain," as you say it.) *"If you have no pain, you would mark like this."* (Show example.) *"If you have some pain, you would mark somewhere along the line, depending on how much pain you have."* (Show example.) *"The more pain you have, the closer to worst pain you would mark. The worst pain possible is marked like this."* (Show example.) *"Show me how much pain you have right now by marking with a straight, up and down line anywhere along the line to show how much pain you have right now."* (Used with permission. This word-graphic rating scale is from the Adolescent Pediatric Pain Tool in: Savedra MC, Tesler MD, Holzemer WL et al. Adolescent pediatric pain tool (APPT) preliminary user's manual. San Francisco: University of California; 1989.)

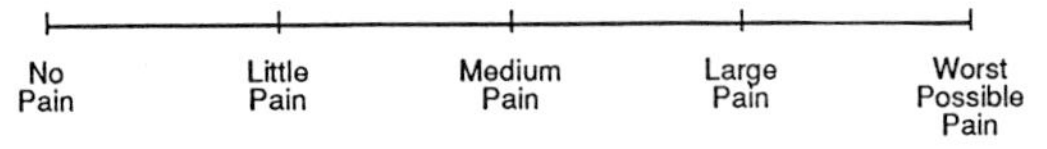

Table 1.
Pain Experience History for Pediatric Patients[a]

Child Form	Parent Form
Tell me what pain is.	What word(s) does your child use in regard to pain?
Tell me about the hurt you have had before.	Describe the pain experiences your child has had before.
Do you tell others when you hurt? If yes, who?	Does your child tell you or others when he/she is hurting?
What do you do for yourself when you are hurting?	How do you know when your child is in pain?
What do you want others to do for you when you hurt?	How does your child usually react to pain?
What don't you want others to do for you when you hurt?	What do you do for your child when he/she is hurting?
What helps the most to take your hurt away?	What does your child do for him/herself when he/she is hurting?
Is there anything special that you want me to know about you when you hurt? (If yes, have child describe.)	What works best to decrease or take away your child's pain?
	Is there anything special that you would like me to know about your child and pain? (If yes, describe)

[a]Adapted with permission from Hester NO, Barcus CS. Assessment and management of pain in children. *Pediatr Nurs Update.* 1986;1(14):2-8.

Table 2.
Self-Report Measures—Poker Chip Tool Instructions[a]

English Instructions
1. Use four red poker chips.
2. Align the chips horizontally in front of the child on the bedside table, a clipboard, or other firm surface.
3. Tell the child, *"These are pieces of hurt."* Beginning at the chip nearest the child's left side and ending at the one nearest the right side, point to the chips and say. *"This* (the first chip) *is a little bit of hurt and this* (the fourth chip) *is the most hurt you could ever have."* For a young child or for any child who does not comprehend the instructions, clarify by saying, *"That means this* (the first chip) *is just a little hurt; this* (the second chip) *is a little more hurt; this* (the third chip) *is more hurt; and this* (the fourth chip) *is the most hurt you could ever have."*
4. Ask the child, *"How many pieces of hurt do you have right now?"* Children without pain will say they don't have any.
5. Clarify the child's answer by words such as "Oh, you have a little hurt? Tell me about the hurt." (Use the pain interview.)
6. Record the number of chips selected on the bedside flowsheet.

Spanish Instructions[b]
1. Follow the English instructions, substituting the following words.
2. Tell the parent, if present: *"Estas fichas son una manera de medir dolor. Usamos cuatro fichas."*
3. Say to the child: *"Estas son pedazos de dolor: una es un poquito de dolor y cuatro son el dolor maximo que tu puedes sentir. Cuantos pedazos de dolor tienes?"*

[a]Hester NO, Foster RL, Kristensen K. Measurement of pain in children: generalizability and validity of the pain ladder and poker chip tool. In: Tyler DC, Krane EJ, eds. Advances in pain research and therapy, Vol. 15: pediatric pain. New York: Raven Press; 1990:79-84. Reprinted with permission.
[b]Spanish instructions used with permission from Jordan-Marsh M, Hall D, Yoder L et al. The Harbor-UCLA Medical Center Humor Project for Children. Los Angeles, Harbor-UCLA Medical Center: 1990.

delayed persons, psychotic patients, patients with dementia, and non-English-speaking patients. Children and cognitively impaired patients require simpler or modified pain measurement scales and assessment approaches (see section on pain in children). The staff should work with both the patient and parent or guardian preoperatively and postoperatively. Staff should endeavor to find a translator for the non-English-speaking patient, at least once, to determine a convenient way to assess pain. Members of the health care team should attend to the preferences and needs of patients whose education or cultural tradition may impede effective communication. Certain cultures have strong beliefs about pain and its management, and these patients may hesitate to complain about unrelieved pain. Such beliefs and preferences should be determined and respected, if at all possible.

In summary, health care providers should view good pain control as a source of pride and a major responsibility in quality care. Support personnel not trained in pain assessment should be encouraged to be "pain vigilant" and report to the health care team any patient discomfort, such as during transport or transfer to an x-ray table. At the institutional level, periodic evaluation studies should be conducted to monitor the effectiveness of pain assessment and management procedures. Without institutional support for an organized process by which pain is recognized, documented, assessed, and reassessed on a regular basis, staff efforts to treat pain may become sporadic and ineffectual. A pain care process relying on patients' or families' demands for analgesia as needed will produce intervals of inadequate pain control and worsen burdens of anxiety, loss of personal control, sleeplessness, and fatigue after surgery. Patients and their families should understand that pain relief is an important part of their health care, that information about options to control pain is available, and that they are welcome to discuss their preferences with the health care team. Patients should recognize that health professionals will elicit and respond quickly to their pain reports. Before a patient's discharge, those taking care of the patient should describe the interventions used to manage pain and assess their effectiveness. This review, while good practice for each patient, is especially important when initial management was unsuccessful and/or when side effects or other complications occurred.

Table 3.
Pain Interview for Pediatric Patients[a]

Child Form	Parent Form
Tell me about the hurt you're having now.	Tell me about the pain your child is having now.
Elicit descriptors, location, and cause.	Elicit descriptors, location, and cause.
What would you like me to do for you?	What would you like me to do for your child?

[a]Adapted with permission from Hester NO, Barcus CS. Assessment and management of pain in children. *Pediatr Nurs Update.* 1986;1(14):2-8.

Options to Prevent and Control Postoperative Pain

Patient education and reduction of any pre-existing pain should occur before the operation. Because the goal of the treatment plan is to prevent significant postoperative pain from the outset, treatment alternatives, potential risks, dosage adjustments, or adjunctive therapies should be described to the patient and family. Teaching emphasizes what the patient is likely to experience postoperatively, including the specific method(s) of pain assessment, intervention(s) the staff will employ, and the level of patient participation required. Staff also should inform patients that it is easier to prevent pain than to "chase" or treat it once it has become established and that communication of unrelieved pain is essential to its relief.

Pain control options include:

- Cognitive-behavioral interventions such as relaxation, distraction, and imagery; these can be taught preoperatively and can reduce pain, anxiety, and the amount of drugs needed for pain control;

- Systemic administration of nonsteroidal anti-inflammatory drugs (NSAIDs) or opioids using the traditional as-needed schedule or around-the-clock administration[25];
- Patient-controlled analgesia (PCA), usually meaning self-medication with intravenous doses of an opioid; this can include other classes of drugs administered orally or by other routes;
- Spinal analgesia, usually by means of an epidural opioid and/or local anesthetic injected intermittently or infused continuously;
- Intermittent or continuous local neural blockade (examples of the former include intercostal nerve blockade with local anesthetic or cryoprobe; the latter includes infusion of local anesthetic through an interpleural catheter);
- Physical agents such as massage or application of heat or cold; and
- Electroanalgesia such as transcutaneous electrical nerve stimulation (TENS).

A postoperative pain management plan might include several of these options. A pamphlet, or "menu" of alternative strategies, can help focus discussion of these options between caregivers and the patient. The postoperative pain management plan should reflect co-existing and/or ongoing problems such as cancer-related pain or opioid tolerance. The plan should be consistent with the overall surgical and anesthetic plans. For example, an elixir form of analgesic is preferable to a tablet when painful or difficult swallowing is anticipated. Also, if the patient is to have an epidural catheter placed during surgery that could make postoperative pain control simpler or more effective, it should not be removed in the postanesthesia care unit (PACU). Staff should note their plans for preoperative, intraoperative, and postoperative pain management in the patient's chart so that other members of the care team can respond to patient questions and coordinate plans for rehabilitation and discharge.

Intraoperative management is often key to the success of postoperative pain control. If pain prevention and control are to be achieved through an epidural catheter, the catheter should be placed and its function verified preoperatively to assure its effective intraoperative and postoperative use. This is particularly true in patients whose position, body casts, or subsequent anticoagulation make postoperative catheter insertion problematic. The planned preoperative and intraoperative use of opioids and timing of the first postoperative opioid dose by the anesthesiologist, nurse anesthetist, surgeon, or PACU nurse are important in the postoperative care plan. Equally important are decisions during surgery on the concurrent use of local anesthetics (e.g., for intraoperative nerve blocks) and the nature of the surgical incision and placement of drains or tubes (e.g., chest and nasogastric). If TENS is to be used for postoperative pain management, the electrodes may need to be placed intraoperatively. Finally, intraoperative placement of casts and splints to provide support and restrict postoperative movement may enhance other pain management efforts.

Pharmacologic Management. Pharmacologic management of mild to moderate postoperative pain should begin, unless there is a contraindication, with an NSAID. Moderately severe to severe pain normally should be treated initially with an opioid analgesic. After many relatively noninvasive surgical procedures, NSAIDs alone can achieve excellent pain control.[64,65] NSAIDs decrease levels of inflammatory mediators generated at the site of tissue injury. Even when insufficient alone to control pain, NSAIDs have a significant opioid dose-sparing effect upon postoperative pain and can be useful in reducing opioid side effects.[39,66,67] The concurrent use of opioids and NSAIDs often provides more effective analgesia than either of the drug classes alone. Although it is likely that NSAIDs also act within the central nervous system, in contrast to opioids, they do not cause sedation or respiratory depression, nor do they interfere with bowel or bladder function. Acetaminophen does not affect platelet aggregation, nor does it provide peripheral anti-inflammatory activity. Some evidence exists that two salicylates do not affect platelet aggregation profoundly; these are salsalate[68] and choline magnesium trisalicylate.[69] All other NSAIDs appear to produce a risk of platelet dysfunction that may impair blood clotting and carry a small risk of gastrointestinal bleeding. At present, one NSAID (ketorolac) is approved by the Food and Drug Administration (FDA) for parenteral use. Tables 4–6 include information on NSAIDs, opioids, and other analgesic drugs.

Opioid analgesics are the cornerstone of pharmacological postoperative pain management, especially for more extensive surgical procedures that cause moderate to severe pain. Other agents such as NSAIDs or single injections of local anesthetics may control mild to moderate pain after relatively minor procedures or reduce opioid dose requirements after more extensive operations when this is a goal.[39,70-76] Even in the absence of pre-emptive efforts targeted at postoperative analgesia, adequate postoperative pain control can usually be achieved with opioid analgesics. When increasing doses of opioids are ineffective in controlling postoperative pain, a prompt search for residual pathology is indicated, and other diagnoses such as neuropathic pain should be considered.

Opioid tolerance or physiological dependence is unusual in short-term postoperative use in opioid-naive patients. Likewise, psychologic dependence and addiction are extremely unlikely to develop after patients without prior drug abuse histories use opioids for acute pain.[77] Proper use of opioids involves selecting a particular drug and route of administration and judging (1) suitable initial dose; (2) frequency of administration; (3) optimal doses of non-opioid analgesics, if these are also to be given; (4) incidence and severity of side effects; and (5) whether the analgesic will be given in an inpatient or ambulatory setting. Titration to achieve the desired therapeutic effect in

Table 4.
Summary Evidence Table for Pharmacologic Interventions[a]

Intervention[b]	Route[c]	Type of Evidence[d]	Comments
NSAIDs	Oral (alone)	Ib, IV	Effective for mild to moderate pain. Begin preoperatively. Relatively contraindicated in patients with renal disease and risk of or actual coagulopathy. May mask fever.
	Oral (adjunct to opioid)	Ia, IV	Potentiating effect resulting in opioid sparing. Begin preoperatively. Cautions as above.
	Parenteral (ketorolac)	Ib, IV	Effective for moderate to severe pain. Expensive. Useful where opioids contraindicated, especially to avoid respiratory depression and sedation. Advance to opioid.
Opioids	Oral	IV	As effective as parenteral in appropriate doses. Use as soon as oral medication tolerated. Route of choice.
	I.M.	Ib, IV	Has been the standard parenteral route, but injections painful and absorption unreliable. Hence, avoid this route when possible.
	S.C.	Ib, IV	Preferable to i.m. when a low-volume continuous infusion is needed and i.v. access is difficult to maintain. Injections painful and absorption unreliable. Avoid this route for long-term repetitive dosing.
	I.V.	Ib, IV	Parenteral route of choice after major surgery. Suitable for titrated bolus or continuous administration (including PCA), but requires monitoring. Significant risk of respiratory depression with inappropriate dosing.
	PCA (systemic)	Ia, IV	I.V. or S.C. routes recommended. Good steady level of analgesia. Popular with patients but requires special infusion pumps and staff education. See cautions about opioids above.
	Epidural and intrathecal	Ib, IV	When suitable, provides good analgesia. Significant risk of respiratory depression, sometimes delayed in onset. Requires careful monitoring. Use of infusion pumps requires additional equipment and staff education. Expensive if infusion pumps employed.
Local anesthetics	Epidural and intrathecal	Ia, IV	Limited indications. Effective regional analgesia. Opioid sparing. Addition of opioid to local anesthetic may improve analgesia. Risks of hypotension, weakness, numbness. Requires careful monitoring. Use of infusion pump requires additional equipment and staff education.
	Peripheral nerve block	Ia, IV	Limited indications and duration of action. Effective regional analgesia. Opioid sparing.

[a]Selected references are included in this clinical guideline. More complete references are available in the *Guideline Report. Acute Pain Management: Operative or Medical Procedures and Trauma* (AHCPR Pub. No. 92-0022) (in press). Rockville, MD: Agency for Health Care Policy and Research.
[b]NSAIDs = Nonsteroidal anti-inflammatory drugs.
[c]PCA = patient-controlled analgesia.
[d]Ia = evidence obtained from meta-analysis of randomized controlled trials. Ib = evidence obtained from at least one randomized controlled trial. IV = evidence obtained from expert committee reports or opinions and/or clinical experiences of respected authorities.

the immediate postoperative period and to maintain that effect over time should be emphasized.

Opioids produce analgesia by binding to opioid receptors both within and outside the central nervous system. Opioid analgesics are classified as full agonists, partial agonists, or mixed agonist-antagonists, depending on the manner in which they interact with opioid receptors. Full agonists produce a maximal response within the cells to which they bind; partial agonists produce a lesser response, regardless of their concentration; and mixed agonist-antagonists activate one type of opioid receptor while simultaneously blocking another type. Several types and subtypes of such receptors exist. The most important receptor type for clinical analgesia is named mu because of its affinity for morphine. Other commonly used mu opioid agonists include hydromorphone, codeine, oxycodone and hydrocodone, methadone, levorphanol, and fentanyl. All mu opioid agonists have the potential to cause constipation, urinary retention, sedation, and respiratory depression and frequently also produce nausea or confusion. Mixed agonist-antagonists in clinical use include pentazocine (Talwin), butorphanol tartrate (Stadol), and nalbuphine hydrochloride (Nubain); each of these blocks or is neutral at the mu opioid receptor while simultaneously activating a different type of opioid receptor termed kappa. Patients receiving mu opioid agonists should not be given a mixed agonist-antagonist because doing so may precipitate a withdrawal syndrome and increase pain. Mixed agonist-antagonists and partial agonists may exhibit a ceiling effect not only with respect to

Table 5.
Dosing Data for Nonsteroidal Anti-inflammatory Drugs (NSAIDs)[a]

Drug	Usual Adult Dosage	Usual Pediatric Dosage[b]	Comments
Oral NSAIDs			
Aspirin	650–975 mg q 4 hr	10–15 mg/kg q 4 hr[c]	The standard against which other NSAIDs are compared. Inhibits platelet aggregation; may cause postoperative bleeding.
Acetaminophen	650–975 mg q 4 hr	10–15 mg/kg q 4 hr	Acetaminophen lacks the peripheral anti-inflammatory activity of the other NSAIDs.
Ibuprofen (Motrin, others)	400 mg q 4–6 hr	10 mg/kg q 6–8 hr	Available as several brand names and as generic; also available as an oral suspension.
Choline magnesium trisalicylate (Trilisate)	1000–1500 mg b.i.d.	25 mg/kg b.i.d.	May have minimal antiplatelet activity; also available as oral liquid.
Diflunisal (Dolobid)	1000-mg initial dose followed by 500 mg q 12 hr		
Etodolac (Lodine)	200–400 mg q 6–8 hr		
Fenoprofen calcium (Nalfon)	200 mg q 4–6 hr		
Ketoprofen (Orudis)	25–75 mg q 6–8 hr		
Magnesium salicylate	650 mg q 4 hr		Many brands and generic forms are available.
Meclofenamate sodium (Meclomen)[c]	50 mg q 4–6 hr		
Mefenamic acid (Ponstel)	250 mg q 6 hr		
Naproxen (Naprosyn)	500-mg initial dose followed by 250 mg q 6–8 hr	5 mg/kg q 12 hr	Also available as oral liquid.
Naproxen sodium (Anaprox)	550-mg initial dose followed by 275 mg q 6–8 hr		
Salsalate (Disalcid, others)	500 mg q 4 hr		May have minimal antiplatelet activity.
Sodium salicylate	325–650 mg q 3–4 hr		Available in generic form from several distributors.
Parenteral NSAID			
Ketorolac tromethamine (Toradol)	30 or 60 mg i.m. initially, then 15 or 30 mg q 6 hr; oral dose following i.m. dose: 10 mg q 6–8 hr		I.M. dose not to exceed 5 days.

[a]These NSAIDs have FDA approval for use as simple analgesics, but clinical experience has been gained with other drugs as well.
[b]Drug recommendations are limited to NSAIDs for which pediatric dosing experience is available.
[c]Contraindicated in presence of fever or other evidence of viral illness.

respiratory depression[78,79] but also in regard to their analgesic activity. In the awake patient, there is a clinical ceiling analgesic effect even with morphine because side effects such as respiratory depression limit the dose that may be safely given. However, this does not limit the ability of clinicians to effectively increase the drug dose when the painful stimulus increases and respiratory status is monitored.

Meperidine (Demerol), a mu opioid analgesic, is commonly used for postoperative pain control. Meperidine is commonly underdosed and administered too infrequently even by physicians aware of its pharmacokinetics.[14] The common postoperative meperidine order of 75 mg parenterally every four hours as needed often is inadequate for several reasons. Meperidine produces clinical analgesia for only 2.5–3.5 hours, and a dose of 75 mg every four hours is equivalent to only 5–7.5 mg of morphine. Therefore, to obtain postoperative analgesia equal to that from 10 mg of morphine sulfate every four hours, a clinician would have to use 100–150 mg of meperidine every three hours. Because of its unique toxicity, meperidine is often contraindicated in patients with impaired renal function and those receiving antidepressants of the monoamine oxidase inhibitor class.[80] Normeperidine (6-*N*-desmethylmeperidine) is a toxic meperidine metabolite excreted through the kidney. In patients with normal renal function, normeperidine has a half-life of 15–20 hours; this time is extended greatly in elderly individuals and patients with impaired renal function. Normeperidine is a cerebral irritant that can cause effects ranging from dysphoria and irritable mood to convulsions.[81,82] These effects have been observed even in young, otherwise healthy patients given sufficiently high doses of normeperidine postoperatively. Therefore, meperidine should be reserved for very brief courses in otherwise healthy patients who have demonstrated an unusual reaction (e.g., local histamine release at the infusion site) or allergic response during treatment with other opioids such as morphine or hydromorphone.

Titration of opioids should be based on the patient's analgesic response and side effects. Remember that patients vary greatly in their analgesic dose requirements and responses to opioid analgesics. Relative potency estimates provide a rational basis for selecting the appropriate starting dose to initiate analgesic therapy, changing the route of administration (e.g., from parenteral to oral), or when switching to another opioid. Dosage conversion factors based on relative potency estimates may differ somewhat between individual patients. When estimating the initial postoperative dose of an opioid analgesic, a clinician should consider whether patients have been receiving opioid analgesics preoperatively. In such patients, supplemental postoperative doses should be adjusted above the preoperative baseline requirement unless the operation itself is likely to remove the painful stimulus.

An as-needed order for opioid administration can result in prolonged delays while the nurse unlocks the controlled substances cabinet and prepares the drug for administration and until the drug takes effect. These delays can be eliminated by administering analgesics on a regular time schedule initially. For example, if the patient is likely to have pain requiring opioid analgesics for 48 hours following surgery, morphine could be ordered every four hours by the clock (not as needed) for 36 hours. Once the duration of analgesic action is determined for a patient, the dosage frequency should be adjusted to prevent pain from recurring. Depending on patient preferences, the orders may be written so that the patient can refuse an analgesic if not in pain or forego it if asleep. However, as in dosing with other drugs that require a steady blood level to remain effective, interruption of an around-the-clock dosage schedule during the hours of sleep may cause the patient to be suddenly awakened by intense pain as blood analgesic levels decline.

It may be acceptable late in the postoperative course to give the same drug every four hours as requested. Switching from an around-the-clock to an as-needed dosage schedule later in the patient's course is one way to provide pain relief while minimizing the risk of adverse effects as the patient's analgesic dose requirement diminishes. As part of this schedule, a patient's pain should be assessed at regular intervals to determine the efficacy of the drug intervention, the presence of side effects, or the need for dosage adjustment or supplemental doses for breakthrough pain. Effective use of opioid analgesics should facilitate routine postoperative activities—e.g., coughing and deep breathing exercises, ambulation, and physical therapy.[43,83,84] The opioid should be withheld if the patient is sedated when awake or whenever there is respiratory depression (usually fewer than 10 breaths per minute).

Opioids may be administered by a variety of routes; oral dosing is usually the most convenient and least expensive route of administration. It is appropriate as soon as the patient can tolerate oral intake and is the mainstay of pain management in the ambulatory surgical population.

Preoperative intravenous or epidural access may be appropriate for postoperative management of severe pain, even when the oral route is available. Relatively few side effects will occur ordinarily, provided that these modalities are carefully managed by clinicians with appropriate expertise. Using potent analgesics or invasive techniques postoperatively, at a time when a patient's level of consciousness and physical function are returning to normal, requires careful titration and patient assessment.

Drug dosage, frequency, side effects, and risks differ even more noticeably between the intravenous and epidural routes than between the oral and intravenous routes. Clinicians not familiar with epidural opioid doses and pharmacokinetics must review the literature carefully before using that route. In addition, side effects (e.g., confusion, respiratory depression, hypotension, urinary retention, or pruritus) associated with opioids can be greater with intravenous and epidural administration and require ongoing assessment and monitoring. Other potential problems that dictate expert vigilance and follow-up during epidural analgesia include abscess development or anesthesia of a nerve root at the site of catheter tip. These routes of administration are best limited to specially trained staff who are knowledgeable and skilled in the management of patients receiving intravenous or epidural opioids, typically under the direction of an acute or postoperative pain treatment service.

Patient-controlled analgesia (PCA) is a safe method for postoperative pain management that many patients prefer to intermittent injections. Systemic PCA usually connotes intravenous drug administration, but it also can be subcutaneous or intramuscular. Few studies of the use of PCA drug delivery to the epidural space exist. A typical intravenous PCA prescription applicable to many contexts relies on a series of loading doses; for example, 3 to 5 mg of morphine, repeated every five minutes until the initial postoperative pain (if present) diminishes. A low-dose basal infusion (0.5–1 mg per hour) at night allows uninterrupted sleep. On-demand doses typically add 1 mg of morphine every six minutes, with a total hourly limit of 10 mg. Once the patient is able to take oral medications, an around-the-clock schedule of an oral opioid such as a codeine–acetaminophen combination is provided, and the basal infusion rate is discontinued. By observing the number of on-demand doses self-administered by the patient, the clinician can assess the adequacy of the oral medication and titrate it further, change to a stronger compound such as oxycodone with acetaminophen, or discontinue the PCA pump.

Intravenous administration is the preferred route for postoperative opioid therapy when the patient cannot take oral medications. When intravenous access is problematic, sublingual and rectal routes

Table 6.
Dosing Data for Opioid Analgesics[a-c] *(table spreads across two pages)*

Dosages	Morphine	Codeine	Hydromorphone (Dilaudid)	Hydrocodone (in Lorcet, Lortab, Vicodin, others)	Levorphanol (Levo-Dromoran)	Meperidine (Demerol)
Approximate equianalgesic oral dose	30 mg q 3–4 hr (around-the-clock dosing); 60 mg q 3–4 hr (single dose or intermittent dosing)	130 mg q 3–4 hr[d]	7.5 mg q 3–4 hr	30 mg q 3–4 hr	4 mg q 6–8 hr	300 mg q 2–3 hr
Approximate equianalgesic parenteral dose	10 mg q 3–4 hr	75 mg q 3–4 hr	1.5 mg q 3–4 hr	Not available	2 mg q 6–8 hr	100 mg q 3 hr
Recommended oral starting dose (adults > 50 kg body weight)	30 mg q 3–4 hr	60 mg q 3–4 hr	6 mg q 3–4 hr	10 mg q 3–4 hr	4 mg q 6–8 hr	Not recommended
Recommended parenteral starting dose (adults > 50 kg body weight)	10 mg q 3–4 hr	60 mg q 2 hr (i.m./s.c.)	1.5 mg q 3–4 hr	Not available	2 mg q 6–8 hr	100 mg q 3 hr
Recommended oral starting dose (children and adults < 50 kg body weight)[e]	0.3 mg/kg q 3-4 hr	1 mg/kg q 3–4 hr[f]	0.06 mg/kg q 3–4 hr	0.2 mg/kg q 3–4 hr[f]	0.04 mg/kg q 6–8 hr	Not recommended
Recommended parenteral starting dose (children and adults < 50 kg body weight)[e]	0.1 mg/kg q 3–4 hr	Not recommended	0.015 mg/kg q 3–4 hr	Not available	0.02 mg/kg q 6–8 hr	0.75 mg/kg q 2–3 hr

[a]Published tables vary in the suggested doses that are equianalgesic to morphine. Clinical response is the criterion that must be applied for each patient; titration to clinical response is necessary. Because there is not complete cross-tolerance among these drugs, it is usually necessary to use a lower than equianalgesic dose when changing drugs and to retitrate to response.

[b]For morphine, hydromorphone, and oxymorphone, rectal administration is an alternate route for patients unable to take oral medications, but equianalgesic doses may differ from oral and parenteral doses because of pharmacokinetic differences.

should be considered as alternatives to traditional intramuscular or subcutaneous injections. All routes other than intravenous require a lag time for absorption of the drug into the circulation. In addition, repeated injections with associated pain and trauma may deter some patients, especially children, from requesting pain medication. Continuous administration of low doses of opioids intravenously or transdermally and intermittent delivery across the buccal mucosa are relatively new but apparently effective methods to administer opioids postoperatively. Further experience is needed to define the clinical roles of these innovative methods in relation to more well-established methods.

Opioids and local anesthetic agents interact favorably. Continuous administration into the epidural space of low concentrations of opioids in dilute solutions of local anesthetic provides excellent analgesia, while reducing the potential risks (e.g., respiratory depression or motor block) associated with equianalgesic concentrations of either agent administered singly. In a less technologically demanding approach, systemically administered opioids given preoperatively, intraoperatively, or postoperatively augment the duration and effectiveness of local anesthetics given spinally or epidurally. Local anesthetics alone may be applied intermittently to specific nerves to interrupt pain pathways. For example, injecting local anesthetics around the intercostal nerves after thoracotomy significantly improves pulmonary function.[39,72,73,76] Catheters for continuous or repeated intermittent dosing of local anesthetic also have been employed postoperatively in the pleural space or adjacent to nerves such as the brachial plexus or cervical sympathetic ganglia. However, a clinical role for interpleural or perineural local anesthetics in the postoperative setting has not yet been defined.

Nonpharmacologic Management. Nonpharmacologic interventions can be classified as either cognitive-behavioral interventions or physical agents. Cog-

Methadone (Dolophine)	Oxycodone (Roxicodone, also in Percocet, Percodan, Tylox, others)	Oxymorphone (Numorphan)	Buprenorphine (Buprenex)	Butorphanol (Stadol)	Nalbuphine (Nubain)	Pentazocine (Talwin)
20 mg q 6–8 hr	30 mg q 3–4 hr	Not available	Not available	Not available	Not available	150 mg q 3–4 hr
10 mg q 6–8 hr	Not available	1 mg q 3–4 hr	0.3–0.4 mg q 6–8 hr	2 mg q 3–4 hr	10 mg q 3–4 hr	60 mg q 3–4 hr
20 mg q 6–8 hr	10 mg q 3–4 hr	Not available	Not available	Not available	Not available	50 mg q 4–6 hr
10 mg q 6–8 hr	Not available	1 mg q 3–4 hr	0.4 mg q 6–8 hr	2 mg q 3–4 hr	10 mg q 3–4 hr	Not recommended
0.2 mg/kg q 6–8 hr	0.2 mg/kg q 3–4 hr[f]	Not recommended	Not available	Not available	Not available	Not recommended
0.1 mg/kg q 6–8 hr	Not available	Not recommended	0.004 mg/kg q 6–8 hr	Not recommended	0.1 mg/kg q 3–4 hr	Not recommended

[c]Recommended doses do not apply to patients with renal or hepatic insufficiency or other conditions affecting drug metabolism and kinetics.
[d]Codeine doses above 65 mg often are not appropriate because of diminishing incremental analgesia with increasing doses but continually increasing constipation and other side effects. Consult the section on management of pain in neonates for recommendations.
[e]Doses listed for patients with body weight less than 50 kg cannot be used as initial starting doses in babies less than six months of age.
[f]Doses of aspirin and acetaminophen in combination opioid/NSAID preparations must also be adjusted to the patient's body weight.

nitive and behaviorally based approaches include several ways to help patients understand more about their pain and take an active part in its assessment and control. The goals of interventions classified as cognitive-behavioral therapies are to change patients' perceptions of pain, alter pain behavior, and provide patients with a greater sense of control over pain. The goals of interventions classified as physical agents or modalities are to provide comfort, correct physical dysfunction, alter physiological responses, and reduce fears associated with pain-related immobility or activity restriction. Nonpharmacologic approaches are intended to supplement, not substitute for, the pharmacologic or invasive techniques described above.

Nonpharmacologic interventions are appropriate for the patient who (1) is interested; (2) is experiencing anxiety or fear, as long as the anxiety is not incapacitating or due to a medical or psychiatric condition that has a more specific treatment; (3) may benefit from avoiding or reducing drug therapy (e.g., history of adverse reactions, fear of or physiological reason to avoid oversedation); (4) is likely to experience and need to cope with a prolonged interval of postoperative pain, particularly if punctuated by recurrent episodes of intense treatment- or procedure-related pain; or (5) has incomplete pain relief following appropriate pharmacologic interventions. Cognitive-behavioral approaches include preparatory information, simple relaxation, imagery, hypnosis, and biofeedback. Physical therapeutic agents and modalities include application of superficial heat or cold, massage, exercise, immobility, and electroanalgesia such as TENS therapy.

Giving a patient a detailed description of all medical procedures, expected postoperative discomfort, and instruction aimed at decreasing treatment- and mobility-related pain can decrease self-reported pain, analgesic use, and postoperative length of stay.[39,49,50,52,54] Patients should receive sufficient procedural and sensory information to satisfy their interest and enable them to assess, evaluate, and communicate postoperative pain. In addition, all preoperative patients should receive instruction emphasizing the importance of coughing, deep breathing, turning, and walking, along with suggestions on how to decrease physical discomforts from such activities. When fear or anxiety occur, it is important to assess psychological coping skills and provide practical suggestions for managing pain and maintaining a positive outlook. Patients who appear anxious or fearful before surgery, and others who express an interest in cognitive-behavioral strategies, should be assisted in selecting an intervention (e.g., simple relaxation or imagery) and taught how to use it. In some patients, particularly those with high levels of anxiety, too much information or too many demanding decisions can exacerbate fear and pain.[85,86] Psychiatric evaluation is appropriate for patients who manifest disabling or disruptive anxiety symptoms such as emotional instability, restlessness, inability to sleep, and dulled thinking.

Relaxation is the most widely evaluated cognitive-behavioral approach to postoperative pain management. (Examples of relaxation exercises are in Table 7.) Relaxation strategies, including simple relaxation,[87-90] imagery,[90,91] hypnosis,[92] biofeedback,[93] and music-assisted relaxation[94,95] have all shown some degree of effectiveness in reducing pain. Relaxation strategies and imagery techniques need not be complex to be effective. Relatively simple approaches such as the brief jaw relaxation procedure described in Table 8 have been successful in decreasing self-reported pain and analgesic use.[96,97] These strategies take only a few minutes to teach but must be reinforced periodically by encouraging and coaching their use. They are simple and can be reinforced by using audiotapes or supportive family members. (Sample relaxation and imagery exercises are included in Table 9, and printed resource materials or manuals are available elsewhere.[98,99]) A relaxation strategy that can be used informally is music distraction. Both patients' personally preferred music[94] and "easy listening" music[95] have significantly decreased postoperative pain in clinical studies. Patients who need repeated coaching may benefit from the use of a commercially prepared relaxation or music-assisted relaxation audiotape.

Other cognitive-behavioral strategies require greater professional involvement; these include complex imagery, hypnosis, biofeedback, and combined therapies. Such strategies are commonly applied when patients have chronic pain even before surgery.

Although some data suggest that the use of complex imagery may reduce pain,[90,91] that biofeedback may lessen pain and operative site muscle tension,[93,100] and that interventions that combine imagery and relaxation may decrease pain,[101-103] each requires specialized training and, for biofeedback, the use of special equipment. Findings from studies of hypnosis for control of postoperative pain are inconsistent.[92,104-106] Lack of research sufficient to demonstrate effectiveness in reducing postoperative pain, and the need for special training or equipment, preclude the recommendation of complex imagery, biofeedback, or hypnosis for routine postoperative pain control. This is not to say that patients who have a high level of preoperative anxiety, whose pain is severe and enduring, or who suffer recurrent episodes of procedure-related pain will not benefit from these strategies. However, for such patients a more comprehensive pain management program must include active involvement of professionals skilled in cognitive-behavioral therapy and psychological assessment.

In addition to cognitive-behavioral interventions, several physical therapeutic methods can be used to manage pain.[107] Commonly used physical agents include applications of heat and cold, massage, exercise, and rest or immobilization. Applications of heat or cold are used to alter pain threshold, reduce muscle spasm, and decrease congestion in an injured area. Applications of cold are used initially to decrease tissue injury response. Later, heat is used to facilitate clearance of tissue toxins and accumulated fluids. Massage and exercise are used to stretch and regain muscle and tendon length. Immobilization is used following many musculoskeletal procedures to provide rest and maintain the alignment necessary for proper healing. With the exception of applications of cold and immobilization, these interventions typically are not used following surgery unless complications occur or an extended postoperative course is expected. When physical modalities are used, it is often for a physiological goal other than pain relief. Of these modalities only cryotherapy (application of cold) has been evaluated in the literature.[108-110] Lanham and colleagues[109] and Rooney and colleagues[110] used cryotherapy in association with TENS therapy. There is insufficient evidence to suggest that cryotherapy alone is effective in reducing postoperative pain. Cryotherapy is different from cryoanalgesia (application of a cryoprobe to specific peripheral nerves), which has proven effective for post-thoracotomy pain.[39]

TENS therapy is one physical modality for which there is considerable support. TENS therapy has been effective in reducing self-reported pain and analgesic use following abdominal surgery,[111,112] orthopedic surgery,[113,114] thoracic surgery,[110,115] mixed surgical procedures,[116-118] and cesarean section.[119,120] TENS therapy also has improved physical mobility following thoracic[115,121] and orthopedic[113,114] surgery. Both TENS therapy and sham TENS therapy (that is, application of electrodes without transmission of electric current) significantly reduced analgesic use and subjective reports of pain.[39] No significant differences were found between TENS therapy and sham TENS.[112,122,123] Even though these findings suggest a placebo effect underlies the reduction of perceived pain and analgesic use during TENS therapy, beneficial effects do, in fact, result.[39] The physical modalities

Table 7.
Summary Evidence Table for Nonpharmacologic Interventions[a,b]

Intervention[c]	Technique	Type of Evidence[d]	Comments
Simple relaxation (begin preoperatively)	Jaw relaxation, progressive muscle relaxation, or simple imagery	Ia, IIa, IIb, IV	Effective in reducing mild to moderate pain and as an adjunct to analgesic drugs for severe pain. Use when patients express an interest in relaxation. Requires 3–5 minutes of staff time for instructions.
	Music	Ib, IIa, IV	Both patient-preferred and "easy listening" music are effective in reducing mild to moderate pain.
Complex relaxation (begin preoperatively)	Biofeedback	Ib, IIa, IV	Effective in reducing mild to moderate pain and operative site muscle tension. Requires skilled personnel and special equipment.
	Imagery	Ib, IIa, IIb, IV	Effective for reduction of mild to moderate pain. Requires skilled personnel.
Education/instruction (begin preoperatively)		Ia, IIa, IIb, IV	Effective for reduction of pain. Should include sensory and procedural information and instruction aimed at reducing activity-related pain. Requires 5–15 minutes of staff time.
TENS		Ia, IIa, III, IV	Effective in reducing pain and improving physical function. Requires skilled personnel and special equipment. May be useful as an adjunct to drug therapy.

[a]Selected references are included in this clinical guideline. More complete references are available in the *Guideline Report. Acute Pain Management: Operative or Medical Procedures and Trauma* (AHCPR Pub. No. 92-0022) (in press). Rockville, MD: Agency for Health Care Policy and Research.
[b]Insufficient scientific evidence is available to provide specific recommendations regarding the use of hypnosis, acupuncture, and other physical modalities for relief of postoperative pain.
[c]TENS = transcutaneous electrical nerve stimulation.
[d]Ia = evidence obtained from meta-analysis of randomized controlled trials. Ib = evidence obtained from at least one randomized controlled trial. IIa = evidence obtained from at least one well-designed controlled study without randomization. IIb = evidence obtained from at least one other type of well-designed quasi-experimental study. III = evidence obtained from well-designed nonexperimental studies, such as comparative studies, correlational studies, and case studies. IV = evidence obtained from expert committee reports or opinions and/or clinical experiences of respected authorities.

Table 8.
Jaw Relaxation Instructions[a]

1. Let your lower jaw drop slightly, as though you were starting a small yawn.
2. Keep your tongue quiet and resting on the bottom of your mouth.
3. Let your lips get soft.
4. Breathe slowly, evenly, and rhythmically: inhale, exhale, and rest.
5. Allow yourself to stop forming words with your lips and stop thinking in words.

[a]McCaffery M, Beebe A. Pain: Clinical manual for nursing practice. St. Louis: C.V. Mosby; 1989. Reprinted with permission.

of acupuncture and electroacupuncture also have been clinically evaluated in postoperative patients, with conflicting findings; no clear analgesic effect has been demonstrated.[124-127]

How each patient's postoperative pain management program is designed and implemented will vary according to the type of medical facility and services available to support a pain management program. At the least, clinicians should be introduced to these methods so they recognize the benefits of cognitive-behavioral and physical interventions, know the indications for their use, and are able to provide information and counseling to patients. In addition, patients should have access to written information about available therapies, why and when to use them, and sources for self-management materials or professional consultations.

Catastrophic postoperative events are rarely, if ever, masked by any of the approaches to postoperative pain control previously described. Any sudden or unexplained change in pain intensity requires immediate evaluation by the surgeon. Likewise, a sudden increase in anxiety may signal cardiac or pulmonary decompensation and requires prompt medical or surgical assessment.

Process of Effective Pain Management. *Postoperative Pain Management.* As illustrated in Figure 2, the process of postoperative pain management is ongoing. Following intraoperative anesthesia and analgesia, postoperative pain assessment and management begins. Based on the preoperative plan, postoperative drug and nondrug interventions are initiated. Pa-

Table 9.
Relaxation Exercises[a]

Example 1: Deep breath/tense, exhale/relax, yawn for quick relaxation

1. Clench your fists; breathe in deeply and hold it a moment.
2. Breathe out slowly and go limp as a rag doll.
3. Start yawning.

Additional points: Yawning becomes spontaneous. It is also contagious, so others may begin yawning and relaxing, too.

Example 2: Slow rhythmic breathing for relaxation

1. Breathe in slowly and deeply.
2. As you breathe out slowly, feel yourself beginning to relax; feel the tension leaving your body.
3. Now breathe in and out slowly and regularly, at whatever rate is comfortable for you. You may wish to try abdominal breathing.
4. To help you focus on your breathing and breathe slowly and rhythmically: Breathe in as you say silently to yourself, "in, two, three." Breathe out as you say silently to yourself, "out, two, three," *or* each time you breathe out, say silently to yourself a word such as peace or relax.
5. You may imagine that you are doing this in a place you have found very calming and relaxing for you, such as lying in the sun at the beach.
6. Do steps 1 through 4 only once or repeat steps 3 and 4 for up to 20 minutes.
7. End with a slow deep breath. As you breathe out say to yourself "I feel alert and relaxed."

Additional points: If you intend to do this for more than a few seconds, try to get in a comfortable position in a quiet environment, you may close your eyes or focus on an object. If you do not know how to do abdominal breathing, ask your nurse for help. This technique has the advantage of being very adaptable in that it may be used for only a few seconds or for up to 20 minutes.

Example 3: Peaceful past

Something may have happened to you a while ago that brought you peace and comfort. You may be able to draw on that past experience to bring you peace or comfort now. Think about these questions:

1. Can you remember any situation, even when you were a child, when you felt calm, peaceful, secure, hopeful, comfortable?
2. Have you ever daydreamed about something peaceful? What were you thinking of?
3. Do you get a dreamy feeling when you listen to music? Do you have any favorite music?
4. Do you have any favorite poetry that you find uplifting or reassuring?
5. Have you ever been religiously active? Do you have favorite readings, hymns, or prayers? Even if you haven't heard or thought of them for many years, childhood religious experiences may still be very soothing.

Additional points: Very likely some of the things you think of in answer to these questions can be recorded for you, such as your favorite music or a prayer. Then you can listen to the tape whenever you wish. Or, if your memory is strong, you may simply close your eyes and recall the events or words.

[a]Adapted with permission from McCaffery M, Beebe A. Pain: Clinical manual for nursing practice. St. Louis: C.V. Mosby, 1989.

tients should be reassessed at frequent intervals (not less than every two to four hours for the first 24 hours) to determine the efficacy of the intervention in reducing pain. If the intervention is ineffective, additional causes of pain should be considered, the plan should then be re-evaluated, and appropriate modifications should be made. Pharmacologic interventions should be titrated to achieve optimal pain control with minimal adverse effects. Ongoing reassessment ensures satisfactory pain relief with the most appropriate balance of drug and nondrug strategies.

Discharge Planning. Inpatients, as well as ambulatory surgical patients, should be given a written pain management plan at discharge. Pertinent discharge instructions related to pain management include specific drugs to be taken, frequency of drug administration, potential side effects of the medication, potential drug interactions, specific precautions to follow when taking the medication (e.g., physical activity limitations, dietary restrictions), and name of the person to notify about pain problems and other postoperative concerns.

References

1. International Association for the Study of Pain. Pain terms: a list with definitions and notes on usage. *Pain*. 1979; 6:249.
2. Merskey H. An investigation of pain in psychological illness. Oxford: Oxford University; 1964. Thesis.
3. Hargreaves KM, Dionne RA. Evaluating endogenous mediators of pain and analagesia in clinical studies. In: Max M, Portenoy R, Laska, E, eds. Advances in pain research and therapy: the design of analgesic clinical trials. Vol. 18. New York: Raven Press; 1991:579-98.
4. Dinarello C. Interleukin-1. *Rev Infect Dis*. 1984; 6:51-95.
5. Egdahl G. Pituitary-adrenal response following trauma to the isolated leg. *Surgery*. 1959; 46:9-21.
6. Kehlet H. The endocrine-metabolic response to postoperative pain. *Acta Anaesthesiol Scand*. 1982; 74(Suppl):173-5.
7. Kehlet H, Brandt MR, Rem J. Role of neurogenic stimuli in mediating the endocrine-metabolic response to surgery. *J Parenter Enter Nutr*. 1980; 4:152-6.
8. Anscombe AR, Buxton RJ. Effect of abdominal operations on total lung capacity and its subdivisions. *Br Med J*. 1958; 2:84-7.
9. Hewlett AM, Branthwaite MA. Postoperative pulmonary function. *Br J Anaesth*. 1975; 47:102-7.
10. Latimer RG, Dickman M, Day WC et al. Ventilatory patterns and pulmonary complications after upper abdominal surgery determined by preoperative and postoperative computerized spirometry and blood gas analysis. *Am J Surg*. 1971; 122:622-32.
11. Marshall BE, Wyche MQ Jr. Hypoxemia during and after anesthesia. *Anesthesiology*. 1972; 37:178-209.
12. Sydow FW. The influence of anesthesia and postoperative analgesic management on lung function. *Acta Chir Scand*. 1989; 550(Suppl):159-65.
13. Wattwil M. Postoperative pain relief and gastrointestinal motility. *Acta Chir Scand*. 1989; 550(Suppl):140-5.

14. Marks RM, Sachar EJ. Undertreatment of medical inpatients with narcotic analgesics. *Ann Intern Med.* 1973; 78:173-81.
15. Sriwatanakul K, Weis OF, Alloza JL et al. Analysis of narcotic usage in the treatment of postoperative pain. *JAMA.* 1983; 250:926-9.
16. Donovan M, Dillon P, McGuire L. Incidence and characteristics of pain in a sample of medical-surgical inpatients. *Pain.* 1987; 30:69-78.
17. Oden R. Acute postoperative pain: incidence, severity, and the etiology of inadequate treatment. *Anesthesiol Clin North Am.* 1989; 7:1-15.
18. Kehlet H. Postoperative pain. In: Committee on Pre- and Postoperative Care, American College of Surgeons. Care of the surgical patient. Vol. 1. New York: Scientific American Medicine; 1989:3-12.
19. Royal College of Surgeons of England, the College of Anesthetists. Report of the Working Party on Pain After Surgery. London: Royal College of Surgeons; 1990.
20. Phillips GD, Cousins MJ. Practical decision making. In: Cousins JM, Phillips GD, eds. Acute pain management. New York: Churchill Livingstone; 1986:275-90.
21. Ready LB, Oden R, Chadwick HS et al. Development of an anesthesiology-based postoperative pain service. *Anesthesiology.* 1988; 68:100-6.
22. Jacox AK, ed. Pain: a sourcebook for nurses and other health professionals. Boston: Little, Brown; 1977.
23. American Nurses Association. Position statement on the registered nurse's (RN) role in the management of patients receiving i.v. conscious sedation for short-term therapeutic, diagnostic, or surgical procedures. Kansas City: American Nurses Association; 1991.
24. National Health and Medical Research Council [Australia]. Management of severe pain. Canberra, Australia: National Health and Medical Research Council; 1988.
25. American Pain Society. Principles of analgesic use in the treatment of acute pain and chronic cancer pain: a concise guide to medical practice. 2nd ed. Skokie, IL: American Pain Society; 1989.
26. International Association for the Study of Pain. Report of the task force on acute pain management. (in press).
27. Bullit E. Induction of c-fos-like protein within the lumbar spinal cord and thalamus of the rat following peripheral stimulation. *Brain Res.* 1989; 493:391-7.
28. Fitzgerald M. C-fos and changing the face of pain. *Trends Neurosci.* 1990; 13:439-40.
29. Hanley MR. Proto-oncogenes in the nervous system. *Neuron.* 1988; 1:175-82.
30. Hunt SP, Pini A, Evan G. Induction of c-fos-like protein in spinal cord neurons following sensory stimulation. *Nature.* 1987; 328:632-4.
31. Przewlocki R, Haarmann I, Nikolarakis K et al. Prodynorphin gene expression in spinal cord is enhanced after traumatic injury in the rat. *Brain Res.* 1988; 464:37-41.
32. McQuay H. Opioids in chronic pain. *Br J Anaesth.* 1989; 63:213-26.
33. Wall PD. The prevention of postoperative pain. *Pain.* 1988; 24,33:289-90.
34. Woolf CJ, Wall PD. Morphine-sensitive and morphine-insensitive actions of C-fibre input on the rat spinal cord. *Neurosci Lett.* 1986; 64:221-5.
35. Ceccio CM. Postoperative pain relief through relaxation in elderly patients with fractured hips. *Orthop Nurs.* 1984; 3(3):11-9.
36. McQuay HJ, Carroll D, Moore RA. Postoperative orthopaedic pain: the effect of opiate premedication and local anaesthetic blocks. *Pain.* 1988; 33:291-5.
37. Hanson AL, Hanson B, Matousek M. Epidural anesthesia for cesarean section. The effect of morphine-bupivacaine administered epidurally for intra- and postoperative pain relief. *Acta Obstet Gynecol Scand.* 1984; 63:135-40.
38. Ferrante FM, Ostheimer GW, Covino BG, eds. Patient-controlled analgesia. Chicago: Blackwell; 1990.
39. Acute pain management: operative or medical procedures and trauma. Guideline report. Rockville, MD: Agency for Health Care Policy and Research, Public Health Service, U.S. Department of Health and Human Services; (AHCPR publication no. 92-0022). (in press).
40. Bollish SJ, Collins CL, Kirking DM et al. Efficacy of patient-controlled versus conventional analgesia for postoperative pain. *Clin Pharm.* 1985; 4:48-52.
41. Eisenach JC, Grice SC, Dewan DM. Patient-controlled analgesia following cesarean section: a comparison with epidural and intramuscular narcotics. *Anesthesiology.* 1988; 68:444-8.
42. Jackson D. A study of pain management: patient controlled analgesia versus intramuscular analgesia. *J Intraven Nurs.* 1989; 12(1):42-51.
43. Wasylak TJ, Abbott FV, English MJ et al. Reduction of postoperative morbidity following patient-controlled morphine. *Can J Anaesth.* 1990; 37:726-31.
44. Bach S, Noreng MF, Tjellden NU. Phantom limb pain in amputees during the first 12 months following limb amputation, after preoperative lumbar epidural blockade. *Pain.* 1988; 33:297-301.
45. Anand KJ, Sippell WG, Aynsley-Green A. Randomized trial of fentanyl anaesthesia in preterm babies undergoing surgery: effects on the stress response. *Lancet.* 1987; 1:62-6. [Published erratum appears in *Lancet.* 1987; 1:234.]
46. Egbert AM, Parks LH, Short LM et al. Randomized trial of postoperative patient controlled analgesia vs intramuscular narcotics in frail elderly men. *Arch Intern Med.* 1990; 150:1897-903.
47. American Pain Society, Committee on Quality Assurance Standards. Standards for monitoring quality of analgesic treatment of acute pain and cancer pain. *Oncol Nurs Forum.* 1990; 17:952-4.
48. American Pain Society quality assurance standards for relief of acute pain and cancer pain. In: Bond MR, Charlton JE, Woolf CJ, eds. Proceedings of the 6th World Congress on Pain. Amsterdam: Elsevier; 1991.
49. Fortin F, Kirouac S. A randomized controlled trial of preoperative patient education. *Int J Nurs Stud.* 1976; 13:11-24.
50. Voshall B. The effects of preoperative teaching on postoperative pain. *Top Clin Nurs.* 1980; 2(1):39-43.
51. Van Aernam B, Lindeman C. Nursing intervention with the presurgical patient: the effects of structured and unstructured preoperative teaching. *Nurs Res.* 1971; 20:319-32.
52. Egbert LD, Battit GE, Welch CE et al. Reduction of postoperative pain by encouragement and instruction of patients. *N Engl J Med.* 1964; 270:825-7.
53. Reading AE. The effects of psychological preparation on pain and recovery after minor gynecological surgery: a preliminary report. *J Clin Psychol.* 1982; 38:504-12.
54. Schmitt F, Wooldridge PJ. Psychological preparation of surgical patients. *Nurs Res.* 1973; 22:108-16.
55. Chapman CR, Syrjala KL. Measurement of pain. In: Bonica JJ, ed. The management of pain. 2nd ed. Vol. 1. Philadelphia: Lea & Febiger; 1990:580-94.
56. National Institutes of Health. The integrated approach to the management of pain. *J Pain Symptom Manage.* 1987; 2:35-44.
57. Beyer JE, McGrath PJ, Berde CV. Discordance between self-report and behavioral pain measures in children age 3-7 years after surgery. *J Pain Symptom Manage.* 1990; 5:350-6.
58. Fritz DJ. Noninvasive pain control methods used by cancer outpatients. *Oncol Nurs Forum.* 1988; Suppl 108: Abstract.
59. Scott J, Huskisson EC. Graphic representation of pain. *Pain.* 1976; 2:175-84.
60. Sriwatanakul K, Kelvie W, Lasagna L et al. Studies with different types of visual analog scales for measurement of pain. *Clin Pharmacol Ther.* 1983; 34:234-9.
61. Gracely RH, Wolskee PJ. Semantic functional measurement of pain: integrating perception and language. *Pain.*

1983; 15:389-98.
62. Houde RW. Methods for measuring clinical pain in humans. *Acta Anesthesiol Scand.* 1982; 74(Suppl):25-9.
63. Sriwatanakul K, Kelvie W, Lasagna L. The quantification of pain: an analysis of words used to describe pain and analgesia in clinical trials. *Clin Pharmacol Ther.* 1982; 32:143-8.
64. Davie IT, Slawson KB, Burt RA. A double-blind comparison of parenteral morphine, placebo, and oral fenoprofen in management of postoperative pain. *Anesth Analg.* 1982; 61:1002-5.
65. Rosen H, Absi EG, Webster JA. Suprofen compared to dextropropoxyphene hydrochloride and paracetamol (Cosalgesic) after extraction of wisdom teeth under general anesthesia. *Anaesthesia.* 1985; 40:639-41.
66. Hodsman NB, Burns J, Blyth A et al. The morphine sparing effects of diclofenac sodium following abdominal surgery. *Anaesthesia.* 1987; 42:1005-8.
67. Martens M. A significant decrease of narcotic drug dosage after orthopaedic surgery. A double-blind study with naproxen. *Acta Orthop Belg.* 1982; 48:900-6.
68. Estes D, Kaplan K. Lack of platelet effect with the aspirin analog, salsalate. *Arthritis Rheum.* 1980; 23:1301-7.
69. Danesh BJ, Saniabadi AR, Russell RI et al. Therapeutic potential of choline magnesium trisalicylate as an alternative to aspirin for patients with bleeding tendencies. *Scot Med J.* 1987; 32:167-8.
70. Egan TM, Herman SJ, Doucette EJ et al. A randomized, controlled trial to determine the effectiveness of fascial infiltration of bupivacaine in preventing respiratory complications after elective abdominal surgery. *Surgery.* 1988; 104:734-40.
71. Engberg G. Factors influencing the respiratory capacity after upper abdominal surgery. *Acta Anaesthesiol Scand.* 1985; 29:434-45.
72. Engberg G. Respiratory performance after upper abdominal surgery: a comparison of pain relief with intercostal blocks and centrally acting analgesics. *Acta Anaesthesiol Scand.* 1985; 29:427-33.
73. Kaplan JA, Miller ED Jr, Gallagher EG Jr. Postoperative analgesia for thoracotomy patients. *Anesth Analg.* 1975; 54:773-7.
74. Patel JM, Lanzafame RJ, Williams JS et al. The effect of incisional infiltration of bupivacaine hydrochloride upon pulmonary functions, atelectasis, and narcotic need following elective cholecystectomy. *Surg Gynecol Obstet.* 1983; 157:338-40.
75. Sabanathan S, Mearns AJ, Bickford Smith PJ et al. Efficacy of continuous extrapleural intercostal nerve block on post-thoracotomy pain and pulmonary mechanics. *Br J Surg.* 1990; 77:221-5.
76. Toledo-Pereyra LH, DeMeester TR. Prospective randomized evaluation of intrathoracic intercostal nerve block with bupivacaine on postoperative ventilatory function. *Ann Thorac Surg.* 1979; 27:203-5.
77. Porter J, Jick H. Addiction rare in patients treated with narcotics. *N Engl J Med.* 1980; 302:123. Letter.
78. Nagashima H, Karamanian A, Malovany R et al. Respiratory and circulatory effects of intravenous butorphanol and morphine. *Clin Pharmacol Ther.* 1976; 19:738-45.
79. Kallos T, Caruso FS. Respiratory effects of butorphanol and pethidine. *Anaesthesia.* 1979; 34:633-7.
80. Wood MM, Cousins MJ. Iatrogenic neurotoxicity in cancer patients. *Pain.* 1989; 39:1-3.
81. Kaiko RF, Foley KM, Grabinski PY et al. Central nervous system excitatory effects of meperidine in cancer patients. *Ann Neurol.* 1983; 13:180-5.
82. Szeto H, Inturrisi C, Houde R et al. Accumulation of normeperidine, an active metabolite of meperidine, in patients with renal failure of cancer. *Ann Intern Med.* 1977; 86:738-41.
83. Alexander JI, Parikh RK, Spence AA. Postoperative analgesia and lung function: a comparison of narcotic analgesic regimens. *Br J Anaesth.* 1973; 45:346-52.
84. Rawal N, Sjostrand UH. Clinical application of epidural and intrathecal opioids for pain management. *Int Anesthesiol Clin.* 1986; 24:43-57.
85. Johnson J, Fuller S, Endress P et al. Altering patients' responses to surgery: an extension and replication. *Res Nurs Health.* 1978; 1(3):111-21.
86. Johnson J, Rice V, Fuller S et al. Sensory information, instruction in a coping strategy, and recovery from surgery. *Res Nurs Health.* 1978; 1(1):4-17.
87. Horowitz BF, Fitzpatrick JJ, Flaherty GG. Relaxation techniques for pain relief after open heart surgery. *Dimens Crit Care Nurs.* 1984; 3(6):364-71.
88. Lawlis GF, Selby D, Hinnant D et al. Reduction of postoperative pain parameters by presurgical relaxation instructions for spinal pain patients. *Spine.* 1985; 10:649-51.
89. Levin RF, Malloy GB, Hyman RB. Nursing management of postoperative pain: use of relaxation techniques with female cholecystectomy patients. *J Adv Nurs.* 1987; 12:463-72.
90. Daake DR, Gueldner SH. Imagery instruction and the control of postsurgical pain. *Appl Nurs Res.* 1989; 2(3):114-20.
91. Horan JJ, Laying FC, Pursell CH. Preliminary study of effects of "in vivo" emotive imagery on dental discomfort. *Percept Mot Skills.* 1976; 42:105-6.
92. Kiefer RC, Hospodarsky J. The use of hypnotic technique in anesthesia to decrease postoperative meperidine requirements. *J Am Osteopath Assoc.* 1980; 79:693-5.
93. Madden C, Singer G, Peck C et al. The effect of EMG biofeedback on postoperative pain following abdominal surgery. *Anaesth Intensive Care.* 1978; 6:333-6.
94. Locsin RG. The effect of music on the pain of selected postoperative patients. *J Adv Nurs.* 1981; 6:19-25.
95. Mullooly VM, Levin RF, Feldman HR. Music for postoperative pain and anxiety. *J NY State Nurs Assoc.* 1988; 19(3):4-7.
96. Flaherty GG, Fitzpatrick JJ. Relaxation technique to increase comfort level of postoperative patients: a preliminary study. *Nurs Res.* 1978; 27:352-5.
97. Wells N. The effect of relaxation on postoperative muscle tension and pain. *Nurs Res.* 1982; 31:236-8.
98. McCaffery M, Beebe A. Pain: clinical manual for nursing practice. St. Louis: C.V. Mosby; 1989.
99. Syrjala KL. Relaxation techniques. In: Bonica JJ, ed. The management of pain. Vol. 2. Philadelphia: Lea & Febiger; 1990:1742-50.
100. Moon MH, Gibbs JM. The control of postoperative pain by EMG biofeedback in patients undergoing hysterectomy. *N Z Med J.* 1984; 97:643-6.
101. Mogan J, Wells N, Robertson E. Effects of preoperative teaching on postoperative pain: a replication and expansion. *Int J Nurs Stud.* 1985; 22:267-80.
102. Pickett C, Clum GA. Comparative treatment strategies and their interaction with locus of control in the reduction of postsurgical pain and anxiety. *J Consult Clin Psychol.* 1982; 50:439-41.
103. Swinford P. Relaxation and positive imagery for the surgical patient: a research study. *Perioper Nurs Q.* 1987; 3(3):9-16.
104. Daniels LK. The treatment of acute anxiety and postoperative gingival pain by hypnosis and covert conditioning: a case report. *Am J Clin Hypn.* 1976; 19:116-9.
105. John ME Jr, Parrino JP. Practical hypnotic suggestion in ophthalmic surgery. *Am J Ophthalmol.* 1983; 96:540-2.
106. Snow BR. The use of hypnosis in the management of preoperative anxiety and postoperative pain in a patient undergoing laminectomy. *Bull Hosp Jt Dis Orthop Inst.* 1985; 45:143-9.
107. Lee M, Itoh M, Yang GW et al. Physical therapy and rehabilitation medicine. In: Bonica JJ, ed. The management of pain. 2nd ed. Vol. 2. Philadelphia: Lea & Febiger; 1990:1769-88.
108. Cohn BT, Draeger RI, Jackson DW. The effects of cold therapy in the postoperative management of pain in patients undergoing anterior cruciate ligament reconstruc-

tion. *Am J Sports Med.* 1989; 17:344-9.
109. Lanham RH Jr, Powell S, Hendrix BE. Efficacy of hypothermia and transcutaneous electrical nerve stimulation in podiatric surgery. *J Foot Surg.* 1984; 23:152-8.
110. Rooney SM, Jain S, McCormack P et al. A comparison of pulmonary function tests for postthoracotomy pain using cryoanalgesia and transcutaneous nerve stimulation. *Ann Thorac Surg.* 1986; 41:204-7.
111. Cooperman AM, Hall B, Mikalacki K et al. Use of transcutaneous electrical stimulation in the control of postoperative pain. *Am J Surg.* 1977; 133:185-7.
112. Hargreaves A, Lander J. Use of transcutaneous electrical nerve stimulation for postoperative pain. *Nurs Res.* 1989; 38(3):159-61.
113. Jensen JE, Conn RR, Hazelrigg G et al. The use of transcutaneous neural stimulation and isokinetic testing in arthroscopic knee surgery. *Am J Sports Med.* 1985; 13:27-33.
114. Smith MJ, Hutchins RC, Hehenberger D. Transcutaneous neural stimulation use in postoperative knee rehabilitation. *Am J Sports Med.* 1983; 11:75-82.
115. Liu YC, Liao WS, Lien IN. Effect of transcutaneous electrical nerve stimulation for post-thoracotomic pain. *J Formosan Med Assoc.* 1985; 84:801-9.
116. Neary J. Transcutaneous electrical nerve stimulation for the relief of post-incisional surgical pain. *J Am Assoc Nurse Anesth.* 1981; 149(2):151-5.
117. Solomon R, Viernstein M, Long D. Reduction of postoperative pain and narcotic use by transcutaneous electrical nerve stimulation. *Surgery.* 1980; 87:142-6.
118. VanderArk G, McGrath K. Transcutaneous electrical stimulation in treatment of postoperative pain. *Am J Surg.* 1975; 130:338-40.
119. Davies JR. Ineffective transcutaneous nerve stimulation following epidural anaesthesia. *Anaesthesia.* 1982; 37:453-7.
120. Smith CM, Guralnick MS, Gelfand MM et al. The effects of transcutaneous electrical nerve stimulation on post-cesarean pain. *Pain.* 1986; 27:181-93.
121. Warfield C, Stein J, Frank H. The effect of transcutaneous electrical nerve stimulation on pain after thoracotomy. *Ann Thorac Surg.* 1985; 39:462-5.
122. Conn IG, Marshall AH, Yadav SN et al. Transcutaneous electrical nerve stimulation following appendicectomy: the placebo effect. *Ann R Coll Surg Engl.* 1986; 68:191-2.
123. Taylor AG, West BA, Simon B et al. How effective is TENS for acute pain? *Am J Nurs.* 1983; 83:1171-4.
124. Evron S, Schenker JG, Olshwang D et al. Postoperative analgesia by percutaneous electrical stimulation in gynecology and obstetrics. *Eur J Obstet Gynecol Reprod Biol.* 1981; 12:305-13.
125. Facco E, Manani G, Angel A et al. Comparison study between acupuncture and pentazocine analgesic and respiratory post-operative effects. *Am J Chin Med.* 1981; 9:225-35.
126. Hansson P, Ekblom A. Influence of stimulus frequency and probe size on vibration-induced alleviation of acute orofacial pain. *Appl Neurophysiol.* 1986; 49(3):155-65.
127. Wigram JR, Lewith GT, Machin D et al. Electroacupuncture for postoperative pain. *Physiother Pract.* 1986; 2(2):83-8.

Appendix A—Methods Used To Develop Clinical Practice Guideline

Three processes were used for the development of the guideline. First was an extensive interdisciplinary clinical review of current needs, therapeutic practices and principles, and emerging technologies for postoperative pain control. This process included review of all pertinent guidelines and standards, receipt of information and opinion from external consultants, a commissioned paper on the ethical aspects of postoperative pain management, an open forum to receive input from concerned parties, and extensive discussion among the panel members.

The second process was a comprehensive review of published research on management of acute postoperative pain and, to a lesser extent, pain associated with trauma and procedure-induced pain. The panel determined that the review should include research related to pain assessment and both pharmacologic and nonpharmacologic treatments. The panel was particularly interested in the effects of the interventions on pain, complications, patient satisfaction, length of stay, and treatment costs.

Articles selected for review were (1) published empirical studies of pain in adults and children after elective and nonelective surgery, pain associated with diagnostic and treatment procedures, and pain associated with posttraumatic injuries and burns; (2) research-based articles on measurement and assessment of pain; (3) pain management guidelines; and (4) review articles.

Articles excluded from review included reports of animal studies and surgical interventions outside the scope of interventions accessible to specialized pain treatment teams or primary caregivers, studies of chronic benign or malignant pain except when also relevant to postoperative or procedural pain, studies comparing within-class analgesic potencies, descriptions of basic pain mechanisms except where specific clinical interventions were tested, editorials and commentaries, discussions of the etiology of pain, studies written in non-English languages, discussions of psychological characteristics, and pure dose-efficacy studies.

The literature review was done at sites in Boston (Harvard University and Massachusetts General Hospital), Baltimore (University of Maryland and The Johns Hopkins University), and Denver (University of Colorado). A group at the School of Public Health, Harvard University, performed meta-analyses of drug and TENS studies. Nondrug studies were reviewed at the Baltimore and Denver sites.

The search strategy was developed in conjunction with the National Library of Medicine (NLM). Twelve databases were searched, producing a list of approximately 2400 drug citations and 2750 nondrug citations; additional citations were retrieved through other sources; for example, another 4314 nondrug and pain assessment citations and 42 drug citations were obtained from bibliographies of review articles, annotated bibliographies, and the like. From these, approximately 600 drug studies and 500 nondrug articles were reviewed and coded for analysis. Using a best-evidence synthesis, the research relevant to particular aspects of pain management was summarized and analyzed. Best-evidence synthesis is based on the best-evidence principle as used in law, in which the same evidence that would be essential in one case might be disregarded in another because better evidence is available.[1] When possible, meta-analyses were performed on the randomized controlled trials. The evidence used for recommendations regarding various interventions in adults is summarized in Tables 4 and 7. The tables include the intervention, the type of evidence, and comments regarding use of the intervention.

The third process was peer review of drafts of the guideline and pilot review with intended users. Thirty-three experts in various aspects of pain management reviewed and commented on an early draft of the guideline, using as a framework for their evaluation the attributes of clinical practice guidelines developed by the Institute of Medicine (IOM) of the National Academy of Sciences.[2] Nine experts in pain management or practice guideline development reviewed a later draft, using the IOM attributes of guidelines and methods suggested by the Agency for Health Care Policy and Research (AHCPR). Nine additional experts in pain management in children reviewed the section of the guideline on neonates, infants, and children. Pilot review of a later draft was done with physicians, nurses, and others (n = 151) involved in pain management at 15 clinical sites. They reviewed and commented on the clarity, clinical applicability, flexibility, resources, or training needed to implement the guideline, and cost implications of the guideline if implemented. A consumer version was developed and tested in clinical sites with 54 patients and 62 nurses and physicians, who reviewed it for clarity and accuracy.

Health policy issues related to ethical, economic, and legal aspects of postoperative pain management were addressed by the panel in several ways. A paper was commissioned on the ethical aspects of postoperative pain management, and the legal implications of pain management were addressed through the limited information available in the literature.

The entire process was anchored by an interdisciplinary panel of experts who used an integrated approach to synthesize the scientific evidence with the knowledge of experts to develop the guideline. Prior to printing of this guidance, drug dosage tables were reviewed by the U.S. Food and Drug Administration. The panel recommends that the guideline be updated two years after its publication.

1. Slavin RE. Best-evidence synthesis: an alternative to meta-analytic and traditional reviews. *Educational Researcher*. 1986; 15(9):5-11.
2. Field MD, Lohr KN, eds. Clinical practice guidelines: directions for a new program. Committee to Advise the Public Health Service on Clinical Practice Guidelines, Institute of Medicine. Washington: National Academy Press; 1990.

Appendix B—Glossary

General Terms

AHCPR: Agency for Health Care Policy and Research; federal agency established in 1989.

Best-evidence synthesis: Evidence based on the best-evidence principle as used in law, in which the same evidence that would be essential in one case might be disregarded in a second case because better evidence becomes available.

Case study design: A nonexperimental study that extensively explores a single unit (a unit may be a person, family, or group) or a very small number of units.

Descriptive study: A nonexperimental study in which variables or subject characteristics are examined as they naturally occur for the purpose of describing or comparing samples or examining relationships among a set of variables.

Experimental study (Randomized controlled trial or randomized clinical trial): An experiment that uses random assignment to create treatment and control groups so that changes can be inferred or attributed to the experimental treatment.

Meta-analysis: The process of combining the results of several related studies to obtain more reliable conclusions.

Peer review: Evaluation of the present guideline document by an interdisciplinary panel of experts using the Institute of Medicine attributes of clinical practice guidelines as evaluation criteria.

Pilot review: Review and testing of the present guideline by clinicians to evaluate aspects of the guideline such as clarity, clinical applicability, flexibility, resource utilization, training needs, and cost of guideline implementation. Review of a consumer version of the present guideline by consumers and clinicians to evaluate its clarity, usefulness, flexibility, and accuracy.

Quasi-experimental study (Includes nonrandomized controlled trial or nonrandomized clinical trial): A design that does not use random assignment to create treatment and control groups but uses other methods to control validity threats so that changes can be inferred or attributed to the experimental treatment.

Scientific review: An exhaustive literature search to define and critically evaluate the knowledge base for pain assessment and interventions.

Pain Physiology

Anxiolysis: Sedation or hypnosis used to reduce anxiety, agitation, or tension.

Neuropathic pain: Pain that arises from a damaged nerve.

Nociception: The process of pain transmission; usually relating to a receptive neuron for painful sensations.

Pain: An unpleasant sensory and emotional experience associated with actual or potential tissue damage or described in terms of such damage.

Pain threshold level: The level of intensity at which pain becomes appreciable or perceptible.

Nonpharmacologic Management

Acupuncture: The piercing of specific body sites with needles to produce pain relief.

Counterirritant: An agent that is applied to produce irritation at one site so as to decrease perception of pain at the same or a distant site.

Cryoanalgesia: The destruction of peripheral nerves by extreme cold to achieve prolonged pain relief.

Cryotherapy: The therapeutic use of cold to reduce discomfort, limit progression of tissue edema, or break a cycle of muscle spasm.

Patient education: Providing the patient with an explanation of perioperative procedures, expected postoperative sensations, and instruction to help decrease mobility-related discomfort.

Relaxation methods: A variety of techniques to help decrease anxiety and muscle tension; these may include imagery, distraction, and progressive muscle relaxation.

Tactile strategies: Strategies that provide comfort through the sense of touch, such as stroking or massage.

TENS (transcutaneous electrical nerve stimulation): A method of producing electroanalgesia through electrodes applied to the skin.

Pain Assessment

Conscious sedation: "Light sedation" during which the patient retains airway reflexes and responses to verbal stimuli.

Oximetry: Determination of the oxygen saturation of arterial blood, typically by means of an external probe applied around a finger or toe.

Paradoxical reaction: A response (e.g., to a drug) that is the opposite of the usual response, such as agitation produced in an individual patient by a drug normally considered to be a sedative.

Pharmacologic Management

EMLA (eutectic mixture of local anesthetic): An ointment that contains local anesthetics so that topical application causes local anesthesia without the need for injection.

Epidural: Situated within the spinal canal, on or outside the dura mater (tough membrane surrounding the spinal cord); synonyms are "extradural" and "peridural."

Equianalgesic: Having equal pain-killing effect; for example, morphine sulfate 10 mg i.m. is generally used for opioid analgesic comparisons.

Interpleural: Situated between the membrane surrounding the lungs and the membrane lining the thoracic cavity.

Intrathecal: Within a sheath (e.g., cerebrospinal fluid that is contained within the dura mater).

Local nerve block: Infiltration of a local anesthetic around a peripheral nerve so as to produce anesthesia in the area supplied by the nerve.

Mixed opioid agonist-antagonist: A compound that has an affinity for two or more types of opioid receptors and blocks opioid effects on one receptor type while producing opioid effects on a second receptor type.

NSAID (nonsteroidal anti-inflammatory drug): Aspirin-like drug that reduces pain and inflammation arising from injured tissue.

Opioid agonist: Any morphine-like compound that produces bodily effects including pain relief, sedation, constipation, and respiratory depression.

Opioid partial agonist: A compound that has an affinity for and stimulates physiological activity at the same cell receptors as opioid agonists but that produces only a partial (i.e., submaximal) bodily response.

PCA (patient-controlled analgesia): Self-administration of an analgesic by a patient instructed in doing so; usually refers to self-dosing with intravenous opioid (e.g., morphine) administered by means of a programmable pump.

Peridural: Synonym for "epidural" and "extradural."
Perineural: Surrounding a nerve.

1. Cook TD, Campbell DT. Quasi-experimentation: design and analysis issues for field settings. Chicago: Rand McNally College Publishing Co; 1979.
2. International Association for the Study of Pain. Pain terms: a list with definitions and notes on usage. *Pain*. 1979; 6:249.
3. Field MD, Lohr KN. Clinical practice guidelines: directions for a new program. Committee to Advise the Public Health Service on Clinical Practice Guidelines, Institute of Medicine. Washington, DC: National Academy Press; 1990.

Therapy Updates

New considerations for *Haemophilus influenzae* type b vaccination

Julianne B. Pinson and C. Wayne Weart

Abstract: The immunogenicity, efficacy, adverse effects, dosage recommendations, and cost of the three commercially available *Haemophilus influenzae* type b (Hib) conjugate vaccines are discussed.

Three Hib conjugate vaccines are licensed for use in children 15 months of age or older: ProHIBiT (Connaught), HibTITER (Praxis), and PedvaxHIB (Merck). HibTITER and PedvaxHIB were recently approved for use in infants as young as two months of age; both have demonstrated efficacy in preventing Hib disease in this age group, whereas ProHIBIT has not been shown to afford adequate protection in young infants. Because the three vaccines induce markedly different immunologic responses, they cannot be considered interchangeable and the recommended dosage schedules differ. The Centers for Disease Control Immunization Practices Advisory Committee (ACIP) and the American Academy of Pediatrics (AAP) both recommend that all infants be immunized with a complete series of either HibTITER or PedvaxHIB beginning routinely at two months or as soon as possible thereafter. The cost of a single dose is similar for the three Hib conjugate vaccines; full immunization with HibTITER is more expensive than with ProHIBiT or PedvaxHIB because four doses are required for completion of the series.

Selection of the appropriate Hib vaccine for infants should be based on availability, cost, and the clinician's interpretation of existing data.

Index terms: Complexes; Costs; Dosage; Equivalency; *Haemophilus* b oligosaccharide conjugate vaccines; *Haemophilus* b polysaccharide conjugate vaccines; *Haemophilus influenzae*; Immunization; Immunogenicity; Pediatrics; Toxicity; Vaccines
Clin Pharm. 1992; 11:332-6

Infections caused by *Haemophilus influenzae* type b (Hib) pose a serious health threat to infants and children in the United States. This organism is the leading cause of bacterial meningitis in children three months to five years of age, accounting for approximately 12,000 cases annually.[1] The mortality rate for Hib meningitis is 5%, and 20–30% of survivors suffer serious morbidity in the form of neurologic sequelae.[1,2] Other invasive diseases in children that may be attributable to Hib include septicemia, pneumonia, epiglottitis, cellulitis, arthritis, osteomyelitis, and pericarditis. Approximately 79% of all Hib cases occur in infants younger than 15 months, with a peak incidence between 6 and 12 months.[2,3]

In 1985, *Haemophilus* b polysaccharide vaccine was licensed in the United States.[4] The vaccine was designed to induce antibodies against polyribosylribitol phosphate (PRP), the capsular polysaccharide and major virulence factor for Hib. Despite proven efficacy in a large Finnish trial,[5] use of the vaccine in the United States was associated with a large number of failures and a postlicensure efficacy ranging from 41% to 88%.[2] Moreover, the vaccine was clearly ineffective in infants and was approved only for use in children 24 months or older, a group that is not at highest risk for Hib infection.

To obtain infant protection and improve immunogenicity, conjugate vaccines were developed in which the PRP capsule of the polysaccharide vaccine was linked to a protein carrier.[4] Three conjugate vaccines have been licensed for use in children 15 months of age or older: ProHIBiT (Connaught Laboratories,

Julianne B. Pinson, Pharm.D., is Family Medicine Fellow, Department of Community Pharmacy Practice and Administration, Medical University of South Carolina (MUSC), Charleston. C. Wayne Weart, Pharm.D., is Professor, Department of Community Pharmacy Practice and Administration, and Associate Professor, Department of Family Medicine, MUSC, Charleston.

Address reprint requests to Dr. Pinson at the Family Medicine Center, Medical University of South Carolina, 171 Ashley Avenue, Charleston, SC 29425.

Swiftwater, PA), HibTITER (Praxis Biologics, Rochester, NY), and PedvaxHIB (Merck Sharp & Dohme, West Point, PA). Two of these vaccines, HibTITER and PedvaxHIB, have recently been approved for use in infants as young as two months.[6,7] A PRP–tetanus toxoid conjugate vaccine has also been developed and is being tested for efficacy and immunogenicity in infants. Each of the conjugate vaccines differs in protein carrier, polysaccharide size, and method of chemical conjugation (Table 1).[2,8] Although each of the vaccines is intended to induce the production of antibodies protective against Hib, these immunogenic and biochemical differences make each vaccine unique.

The availability of three different vaccines for the same purpose has generated considerable confusion among immunization advisory panels and pediatric practitioners. Because the three conjugate vaccines induce markedly different immunologic responses, they cannot be considered interchangeable and the recommended dosage schedules differ. Both the Immunization Practices Advisory Committee (ACIP) of the Centers for Disease Control and the American Academy of Pediatrics (AAP) have issued recent statements regarding use of the vaccines in infants and children.[2,8] However, differences between these recommendations and those issued previously,[6,7] as well as inherent differences in the vaccines, can make practitioners uncertain of which vaccine to use and how to use these vaccines appropriately.

Immunogenicity

Increasing levels of antibody to PRP (anti-PRP) are associated with decreasing risk of invasive Hib disease. Although these levels have not been precisely defined, existing data suggest that serum anti-PRP concentrations ranging from 0.15 to 1.0 μg/mL are protective against Hib infection.[4,9] Each of the three available conjugate vaccines has been demonstrated to induce protective concentrations of antibody; however, the magnitude of the concentrations, the number and scheduling of the doses necessary to achieve them, and the duration of protective concentrations vary among the vaccines.

Preliminary results from a study conducted in Alaskan infants suggested that PedvaxHIB was most immunogenic after two doses, but the anti-PRP concentrations achieved with two doses of Pedvax HIB were lower than those achieved after three doses of HibTITER.[10] Antibody concentrations at 12 to 15 months (pre-booster age) were markedly lower for PedvaxHIB than for HibTITER. Although this finding suggests a shorter duration of protection with PedvaxHIB, the clinical significance of this difference is unknown. ProHIBiT was the least immunogenic vaccine after three doses and at pre-booster age. Results of this study are depicted in Figure 1. Another trial conducted in infants in California demonstrated similar trends in immunogenicity among the vaccines.[11]

When the conjugate vaccines are used in children older than 15 months, there appears to be no clear immunologic advantage of one over another. Turner et al.[9] found that HibTITER produced protective antibody response in 96% of 47 patients 17–22 months of age as compared with 72% of 46 patients of the same age vaccinated with ProHIBiT. In another study conducted in 319 children 17–19 months of age, all three conjugate vaccines induced large antibody responses, although significant differences in the anti-PRP concentration were achieved by the vaccines.[12] The clinical implication of these findings is that, although there may be differences in the magnitude of antibody response, each vaccine is immunogenic in this age group.

Efficacy

Because serum antibody concentrations after vaccination do not always correlate with protection,[4] the efficacy of the Hib vaccines is expressed as the percentage of patients who do not contract Hib disease after vaccination. Two trials have investigated the efficacy of ProHIBiT in infants.[13,14] The first study was a large-scale trial in Finnish infants that demonstrated a protective efficacy of 89% despite a relatively poor immunogenicity (<40% of patients attained anti-PRP

Table 1.
***H. influenzae* Type b Conjugate Vaccines**[8]

Trade Name	Manufacturer	Abbreviation	Carrier Protein	Licensed Indication	Cost ($) Single Dose[a]	Cost ($) Full Series[a]
ProHIBiT	Connaught Laboratories	PRP-D	Diphtheria toxoid	Children (≥15 mo)	16.00	16.00
HibTITER	Praxis Biologics (distributed by Lederle)	HbOC	CRM197 (nontoxic mutant diphtheria toxin)	Infants and children (≥2 mo)	16.13	64.52
PedvaxHIB	Merck Sharp & Dohme	PRP-OMP	OMP (outer membrane protein complex of *Neisseria meningitidis*)	Infants and children (≥2 mo)	16.00	48.00

[a]Prices calculated from Cardinale VA, ed. Drug topics red book 1991. Oradell, NJ: Medical Economics Company; 1991:327, 492, 537.

Figure 1. Comparative immunogenicity of conjugate Hib vaccines.[10] ProHIBiT and HibTITER given as a total of three doses at two, four, and six months of age. PedvaxHIB given as a total of two doses at two and four months of age. Pre = anti-PRP concentration before any vaccine is administered, post-1 = anti-PRP concentration after one dose of vaccine, post-2 = anti-PRP concentration after two doses of vaccine, post-3 = anti-PRP concentration after three doses of vaccine, and pre-booster = age at which booster dose is required (after two or three doses of vaccine).

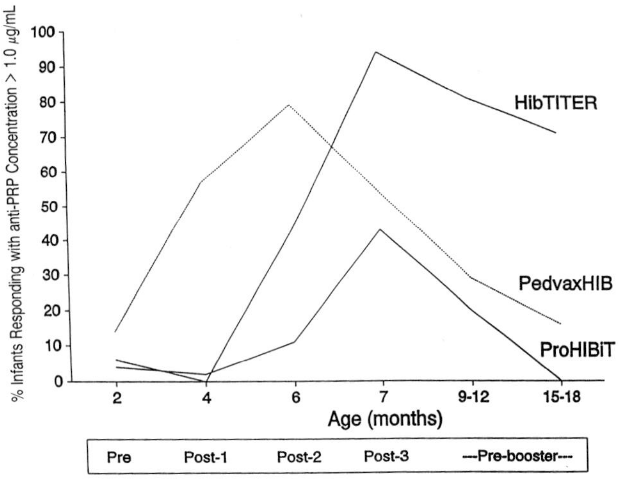

concentrations greater than 1.0 μg/mL). In contrast, a study conducted in Alaskan natives demonstrated poor immunogenicity in infants and an estimated efficacy of only 35%.[14] Confounding factors that may have influenced these results include the following facts: A higher proportion of Hib invasive disease occurs in Alaskan infants than in Finnish infants, the Alaskan infants were vaccinated at an earlier age (two months versus three months) than the Finnish infants, and the Alaskan study used a smaller sample size than did the Finnish study.[4] Regardless of these differences, the poor efficacy demonstrated in the Alaskan study, coupled with the poor immunogenicity reported in both studies, led the FDA to refuse to license ProHIBiT for use in infants younger than 15 months.

The data on the efficacy of HibTITER are derived primarily from a clinical trial involving approximately 60,000 infants enrolled in the Northern California Kaiser Permanente Health Plan.[15] Of the 30,000 infants who received three doses of the vaccine, none contracted Hib disease, indicating a protective efficacy of 100%. However, only a 26% efficacy was noted in those infants receiving one dose, and the possibility that one dose of vaccine had no efficacy could not be excluded. PedvaxHIB has been demonstrated to be 93% effective in 2,588 Navajo infants who received two doses of the vaccine at two and four months of age.[16] None of these infants contracted Hib disease in the interval between the first and second doses of the vaccine. However, the occurrence of one case of Hib disease in a patient receiving only two doses of PedvaxHIB and several documented cases in those receiving only one dose of HibTITER underscore the importance of completing the entire regimen to ensure immunity.[8]

Although all three vaccines are approved for use in children older than 15 months, few published studies demonstrate their efficacy in this age group. Licensure of ProHIBiT was based on demonstrated safety and immunogenicity superior to that of the plain (nonconjugated) polysaccharide vaccine, which had previously been proven effective in a 1974 Finnish trial.[4,5] The efficacy of ProHIBiT has since been confirmed by Greenberg et al.,[17] who demonstrated a protective efficacy of 88% in 79 children 18–59 months of age. Both HibTITER and PedvaxHIB were licensed for use in children older than 15 months on the basis of their safety and immunogenicity, although no data on their protective efficacy in this age group exist. Ongoing case-control studies will evaluate the efficacy of these vaccines in this age group.

Adverse Effects

Each of the conjugate vaccines seems to be extremely safe when administered to infants and children.[18-20] Minor adverse effects that have been reported include temperature greater than 38.3 °C and local reactions such as erythema, swelling, induration, and tenderness. The incidence of these reactions is low, ranging from less than 1% to 4.6%.[18-20] These reactions occurred more frequently after the third dose of HibTITER than after the first two doses.[2] Similarly, adverse events were more frequent after the second dose of PedvaxHIB than after the first dose. Most of the reactions reported with all three vaccines appear more frequently at 24 hours after the dose than at 48 hours.[18]

Dosage Recommendations

On the basis of the recent trials conducted in infants, both ACIP and AAP recommend that all infants be immunized with either HibTITER or PedvaxHIB beginning routinely at two months of age or as soon as possible thereafter.[2,8] The vaccine series may be initiated as early as six weeks of age. Recent statements from ACIP and AAP regarding the scheduling of the vaccine series are virtually identical (Table 2).[2,8]

There are no data on the interchangeability of the conjugate vaccines. Consequently, both the ACIP and the AAP agree that the same conjugate vaccine should be used throughout the entire vaccination series.[2,8] However, this recommendation may be difficult to follow when patients move before completing the series or receive doses at different clinics. Parents may be aware that the child has received a "meningitis shot" without knowing or having records of which vaccine was given. Although there are no specific guidelines to manage such situations, it is prudent to ensure that infants two to six months old receive a primary series of at least three doses of the same con-

Table 2.
Recommended Vaccination Schedules for *H. influenzae* Type b Conjugate Vaccines[2,8]

Age Immunization Initiated (mo)	Vaccine Product Used at Initiation	Primary Series	Booster[a,b]	Total No. Doses
2–6	HibTITER	3 doses, 2 mo apart	15 mo	4
	PedvaxHIB	2 doses, 2 mo apart	12 mo	3
7–11	HibTITER or PedvaxHIB	2 doses, 2 mo apart	15 mo	3
12–14	HibTITER or PedvaxHIB	1 dose	15 mo	2
15–59	HibTITER, PedvaxHIB, or ProHIBIT	1 dose	...	1
≥60[c]	HibTITER, PedvaxHIB, or ProHiBiT	1 dose	...	1

[a]American Academy of Pediatrics considers that safety and efficacy are likely to be equivalent for ProHIBiT, HibTITER, and PedvaxHIB for use in children 15 months of age or older.[8]
[b]Booster should be administered at least two months after previous dose. In special circumstances requiring "catch-up" immunizations, the minimal acceptable interval between doses is one month.[2,8]
[c]Only for children with chronic illness known to be associated with an increased risk for *Haemophilus influenzae* type b disease.[8]

jugate vaccine.[2]

All of the conjugate vaccines can be administered simultaneously with diphtheria and tetanus toxoids and pertussis vaccine adsorbed (DTP); combined measles, mumps, and rubella virus vaccine (MMR); oral live attenuated poliovirus vaccine (OPV); or inactivated poliovirus vaccine (IPV).[2] Additionally, there are no known contraindications to simultaneous administration of the Hib vaccines with either pneumococcal or meningococcal vaccine.[2,8] However, the Hib vaccines should be administered in a separate syringe from other vaccines because it is not known what effect combining agents would have on the immunogenicity and tolerability of the vaccines.[8,a] Similarly, Hib conjugate vaccines should be administered at a separate site when given concurrently with other vaccines.[2] Merck Sharp & Dohme is developing a combination PedvaxHIB/MMR-II vaccine and a combination PedvaxHIB and DPT vaccine, but it is not known when, if ever, these formulations may be available.[a] A combination HibTITER and DPT vaccine is also under development at Lederle Laboratories.

Cost

The comparative costs of the conjugate vaccines are depicted in Table 1. Although the costs of a single dose are similar among the vaccines, full immunization with HibTITER is more expensive than with ProHIBiT or PedvaxHIB because it requires four doses for completion. When considering these costs, parents and practitioners alike should realize that the vaccines do not protect against noninvasive (nontypable) *H. influenzae* diseases such as otitis media, sinusitis, and bronchitis. Parents who believe the cost of the Hib vaccines will be justified by avoiding these more common, noninvasive illnesses are likely to be disappointed.

Conclusion

Based on experience to date, the three commercially available Hib conjugate vaccines elicit different immune responses and efficacy rates in infants. The immunogenicity of ProHIBiT in infants is clearly inferior to that of HibTITER and PedvaxHIB, although studies of its efficacy have produced conflicting results. Until more data are made available, ProHIBiT should not be given to infants younger than 15 months.

The comparative immunogenicity and efficacy in infants of HibTITER and PedvaxHIB are difficult to evaluate. The lack of standardization of laboratory tests for anti-PRP, differences in study design, and epidemiologic differences in study populations make interpretation of available data difficult. PedvaxHIB elicits a greater antibody response after two doses than does HibTITER; however, this response does not persist as long as the response elicited by three doses of HibTITER. The clinical implication of these trends is unclear because the efficacy rates of the two vaccines are similar. The AAP considers the safety and efficacy of the two vaccines, when initiated in infants younger than seven months, likely to be equivalent. The ACIP has made no such statement. Both committees agree, however, that for children older than 15 months, any of the three vaccines are acceptable. This position has been supported by immunogenicity trials but has not yet been confirmed in efficacy trials.

Until data on the interchangeability of the vaccines are available, ProHIBiT, HibTITER, and PedvaxHIB must be considered different vaccines and should be used according to their approved recommendations only. Based on existing efficacy data, it is not possible to define a clear advantage of PedvaxHIB over HibTITER, or vice versa. Some factors to consider when choosing a Hib conjugate vaccine include daycare status and presence of school-aged children or young infants in the home, which place a child at increased risk for contracting and spreading Hib infection. These factors may become very important in choosing between PedvaxHIB and HibTITER if differences in immunogenicity trends between the two vaccines are shown to correlate with differences in onset or duration of protection. The only certain differences to date, however, are the number of required doses and cost; HibTITER is more expensive than PedvaxHIB because of its four-dose schedule. Selection of the appropriate Hib vaccine for infants should therefore be based on availability, cost, and the clinician's interpretation of existing data.

---

[a]Robert W. Shackleford, M.D., Merck Sharp & Dohme. Written communication. 1991 Mar 11.

References

1. Wilfert CM. Epidemiology of *Haemophilus influenzae* type b infections. *Pediatrics*. 1990; 85(4 Part 2):676-81.
2. Centers for Disease Control. Haemophilus b conjugate vaccines for prevention of *Haemophilus influenzae* type b disease among infants and children two months of age and older: recommendations of the Immunization Practices Advisory Committee (ACIP). *MMWR*. 1991; 40:1-7.
3. Anon. *H. influenzae* vaccine for infants. *Med Lett Drugs Ther*. 1991; 33:5-7.
4. Shapiro ED. New vaccines against *Haemophilus influenzae* type b. *Pediatr Clin North Am*. 1990; 37:567-83.
5. Peltola H, Kayhty H, Virtamen M et al. Prevention of *Haemophilus influenzae* type b bacteremic infection with the capsular polysaccharide vaccine. *N Engl J Med*. 1984; 310:1561-5.
6. Centers for Disease Control. FDA approval for use of *Haemophilus* b conjugate vaccine for infants. *MMWR*. 1990; 39:698-9.
7. Centers for Disease Control. FDA approval for use of *Haemophilus* b conjugate vaccine for infants. *MMWR*. 1990; 39:925-6.
8. Committee on Infectious Diseases. *Haemophilus influenzae* type b conjugate vaccines: recommendations for immunization of infants and children two months of age and older: update. *AAP News*. 1991; Mar.
9. Turner RB, Cimino CO, Sullivan BJ. Prospective comparison of the immune response of infants to three *Haemophilus influenzae* type b vaccines. *Pediatr Infect Dis J*. 1991; 10:108-12.
10. Wainwright JI, Letson GW, Chiu CY et al. Immunogenicity of three *Haemophilus influenzae* type b Hib conjugate vaccines in Alaska USA native infants. Paper presented at Joint Meeting of the American Pediatric Society and the Society for Pediatric Research. Anaheim, CA, May 7–10, 1990.
11. Ward JI, Berkowitz C, Burkart K et al. Comparative immunogenicity of *Haemophilus influenzae* type b (Hib) conjugate vaccines (PRP-D/PRP-OMP) in infants less than 6 months of age. Paper presented at 28th Interscience Conference of Antimicrobial Agents and Chemotherapy, Los Angeles, CA, October 26, 1988.
12. Holmess SJ, Murphy TV, Anderson RS et al. Immunogenicity of four *Haemophilus influenzae* type b conjugate vaccines in 17- to 19-month-old children. *J Pediatr*. 1991; 118:364-71.
13. Eskola J, Peltola H, Takala AK et al. Efficacy of *Haemophilus influenzae* type b polysaccharide–diphtheria toxoid conjugate vaccine in infancy. *N Engl J Med*. 1987; 317:717-21.
14. Ward J, Brenneman G, Letson GW et al. Limited efficacy of a *Haemophilus influenzae* type b conjugate vaccine in Alaska Native infants. *N Engl J Med*. 1990; 323:1393-401.
15. Black SB, Shinefield HR, Fireman B et al. Efficacy in infancy of oligosaccharide conjugate *Haemophilus influenzae* type b (HbOC) vaccine in a United States population of 61 080 children. *Pediatr Infect Dis J*. 1991; 10:97-104.
16. Santosham M, Wolff M, Reid R et al. The efficacy in Navajo infants of a conjugate vaccine consisting of *Haemophilus influenzae* type b polysaccharide and *Neisseria meningitidis* outer-membrane protein complex. *N Engl J Med*. 1991; 324:1767-72.
17. Greenberg DP, Vadheim CM, Bordenave N et al. Protective efficacy of *Haemophilus influenzae* type b polysaccharide and conjugate vaccines in children 18 months of age and older. *JAMA*. 1991; 265:987-92.
18. Connaught Laboratories. ProHIBiT package insert. Swiftwater, PA; 1987 Dec.
19. Praxis Biologics. HibTITER package insert. Rochester, NY; 1990 Oct.
20. Merck Sharp & Dohme. PedvaxHIB package insert. West Point, PA; 1990 Dec.

When Immunization Programs Falter

"Among children in developed nations, death and discomfort from contagious diseases have declined markedly during the past half century, in large measure due to widespread immunization. In the United States, for example, reported cases of measles decreased by 95% within 5 years of vaccine licensure; and the incidence of whooping cough (pertussis), a disease which showed little or no decline before immunization, decreased to one hundredth of prevaccination levels just 10 years after routine immunization began. Case rates of paralytic poliomyelitis in this country dropped even more precipitously; by 1965, reported incidence was less than 0.5% of a decade earlier, when the first vaccine became available. All these diseases remain important causes of childhood mortality in the developing world.

Experience confirms that when immunization programs falter, dramatic increases in preventable diseases ensue. . . .

Indisputably effective, routine immunization is also relatively inexpensive; careful analysis has confirmed its cost-effectiveness. Immunization programs in developed nations have few opponents on other grounds. It is therefore perplexing that rates of routine immunization among U.S. preschool children appear to be falling steadily. Recent outbreaks of measles, mumps, and a surge in reported pertussis cases have all occurred among unvaccinated populations. The U.S. Immunization Survey was discontinued after 1985 figures were tabulated; current, reliable rates of immunization prior to school entry in the U.S. are not available.

—Williams BC. Immunization coverage among preschool children: the United States and selected European countries. *Pediatrics*. 1990; 86(Suppl):1052-6."

β-Adrenergic antagonists for primary prevention of gastrointestinal hemorrhage in patients with cirrhosis and esophageal varices

CHERYL A. ELDER AND MARYANN S. REYNOLDS RESTINO

Abstract: The use of β-adrenergic antagonists for primary prevention of gastrointestinal hemorrhage in patients with cirrhosis and esophageal varices is discussed.

In five controlled trials, patients with cirrhosis and endoscopically proven esophageal varices were treated with either propranolol or nadolol in doses to reduce heart rate by 20–25% or in doses to decrease hepatic vein pressure by 25% of basal levels or to a level of less than 12 mm Hg.

In two of three studies, investigators found that propranolol significantly reduced frequency of initial bleeding in patients with esophageal varices. In one of two studies, nadolol significantly decreased the risk of variceal bleeding in patients with cirrhosis; in the other study, a significant difference in the frequency of initial bleeding was found only among patients who were compliant with therapy. Only one of the five studies showed a significant difference in survival between the treatment group and the placebo group. Adverse effects of therapy included dizziness, fatigue, cardiac insufficiency, Raynaud's phenomenon, and risk of bleeding associated with propranolol withdrawal.

Therapy with a nonselective β-adrenergic antagonist should be considered for primary prevention of gastrointestinal hemorrhage in patients with cirrhosis and suspected or documented large varices; however, abrupt discontinuation of the medication is associated with risk of bleeding.

Index terms: Esophageal and gastric varices; Gastrointestinal hemorrhage; Liver cirrhosis; Nadolol; Propranolol; Sympatholytic agents; Toxicity
Clin Pharm. 1992; 11:337-41

Portal hypertension is often caused by hepatic cirrhosis. Elevated portal venous pressure is believed to result from two mechanisms: increased portal vascular resistance and increased splanchnic blood flow.[1] Increased portal vascular resistance appears to be the primary mechanism of portal hypertension. Retrograde flow of blood from the high-pressure portal venous circulation to the lower-pressure systemic venous circulation occurs through portosystemic collateral channels. Blood vessels that may form collateral channels include veins around the rectum, the gastroesophageal junction, the retroperitoneal space, and the falciform ligament of the liver.[2] Increased vascular resistance within these collaterals maintains the elevated portal pressure.

A second mechanism thought to contribute to portal hypertension is the development of a hyperdynamic circulation. Increased levels of circulating vasodilators in conjunction with decreased vascular sensitivity to vasoconstrictors result in increased blood flow secondary to peripheral and splanchnic vasodilatation.[1]

Hemorrhage from a portosystemic venous collateral is a common clinical manifestation of portal hypertension. Hemorrhage most commonly occurs in collaterals at the gastroesophageal junction, which are known as esophageal varices. Factors contributing to variceal rupture have not been fully elucidated but are believed to include portal and intravariceal pressure, varix size, wall tension,[1] and local irritation from ethanol consumption. Variceal bleeding often occurs spontaneously and usually presents as painless but massive hematemesis. Depending on the extent of blood loss and degree of subsequent hypovolemia, associated signs may range from mild postural tachycardia to severe shock.[2]

Hemorrhage from esophageal varices is associated with a high mortality rate and an increased risk of recurrent bleeding. Initial episodes of variceal bleeding have been shown to have a 40–70% mortality rate.[3] Treatment strategies focus on preventing the first episode of variceal bleeding in patients with cirrhosis, thus improving survival.

A variety of pharmacologic agents have been found to possess portal antihypertensive effects, including the following: the central α-agonist clonidine; the long-acting organic nitrates, such as isosorbide dinitrate; and the nonselective β-adrenergic antagonists, such as propranolol.[4] Clonidine has been found to normalize cardiac output and to decrease portal pressure.[5] Isosorbide dinitrate has also been found to

CHERYL A. ELDER is a Pharm.D. degree candidate, Philadelphia College of Pharmacy and Science, Philadelphia, PA. MARYANN S. REYNOLDS RESTINO, PHARM.D., is Pharmacy Education Coordinator, North Carolina Baptist Hospital, Winston-Salem, NC; at the time of this report, she was Director, Drug Information Center, Department of Pharmacy Practice and Pharmacy Administration, Philadelphia College of Pharmacy and Science.

Address reprint requests to Dr. Restino at the Pharmacy Department, North Carolina Baptist Hospital, Medical Center Boulevard, Winston-Salem, NC 27157.

Table 1.
Summary of Study Characteristics and Results from Primary Prevention Trials[a]

Source	Study Design	Treatment	No. Patients in Group	Child-Pugh Classification (% Study population)	Duration of Follow-up[b] (mo)	Patients Not Bleeding[c] (Cum. %) Treatment	Patients Not Bleeding[c] (Cum. %) Control	Patients Surviving[c] (Cum. %) Treatment	Patients Surviving[c] (Cum. %) Control	Withdrawal because of Adverse Effects (%)
Pascal et al.[11]	R MC SB	Propranolol Placebo	118 112	A, 17 B, 37 C, 46	24	74[d]	39	72[d]	51	11
Italian Multicenter Project[12]	R MC SB	Propranolol Vitamin K	85 89	A, 59 B, 34 C, 7	42	74	59	51	59	27
Bosch et al.[13]	R MC DB	Propranolol Placebo	51 51	N/A	60	N/A[e]	N/A	N/A[e]	N/A	8
Lebrec et al.[14]	R MC SB	Nadolol Placebo	53 53	A, 58 B, 42 C, 0	12	83	80	78	80	10
Ideo et al.[15]	R SB	Nadolol Placebo or ranitidine	30 49	A or B, 76 C, 24	24	94[f]	70	94	78	1.3

[a]R = randomized, MC = multicenter, SB = single-blind, DB = double-blind, N/A = not available, Cum. = cumulative.
[b]Patients followed until end of study or study end point.
[c]Based on Kaplan-Meier analysis assessed by log-rank test.
[d]Treatment and control values were significantly different ($p < 0.05$).
[e]Kaplan-Meier analysis not reported.
[f]Treatment and control values were significantly different ($p < 0.02$).

decrease portal pressure without markedly affecting hepatic perfusion.[6,7] However, controlled trials evaluating the long-term effect of these agents on portal hypertension and variceal bleeding are not available.

The only pharmacologic modality for the prevention of variceal bleeding that has been sufficiently evaluated is the nonselective β-adrenergic antagonists. Propranolol has been shown to decrease portal venous pressure,[8] decrease blood flow in the splanchnic region,[9] and decrease blood flow in the superior portosystemic collateral circulation.[10] Both primary prevention trials (the drug was used to prevent hemorrhage in patients who had never bled) and secondary prevention trials (the drug was used to prevent recurrent bleeding) have been conducted. This article focuses on the use of β-adrenergic antagonists for primary prevention of gastrointestinal hemorrhage in patients with cirrhosis and esophageal varices.

Primary Prevention Trials of β-Adrenergic Antagonists

Five controlled trials evaluating primary prophylaxis with β-adrenergic antagonists have been performed—three with propranolol[11-13] and two with nadolol.[14,15] Study characteristics and results are presented in Table 1. All patients in the five trials had cirrhosis and endoscopically proven esophageal varices. The patients were treated with either propranolol or nadolol in doses intended to reduce the heart rate by 20–25%[11,12,14,15] or in doses to decrease the hepatic vein pressure gradient by 25% of basal levels or to a level of less than 12 mm Hg.[13]

Table 2.
Child-Pugh Criteria for Assigning Points in a System for Grading Severity of Liver Disease[16]

Variable	Point Value[a] 1	2	3
Ascites	None	Slight	Moderate
Encephalopathy (grade)	None	1 or 2	3 or 4
Bilirubin (μmol/L)	<25	25–40	>40
Albumin (g/L)	>35	28–35	<28
Prothrombin time (seconds greater than control)	1–4	4–6	>6

[a]Increasing point value corresponds to increasing severity of disease.

All patients were reported as having large varices, the definition of which varied among the studies. Pascal et al.[11] enrolled patients with grade II and grade III varices; that is, the varices are not flattened by insufflation but are (grade II) or are not (grade III) separated by areas of normal tissue. Two trials defined large varices as occupying greater than one third of the esophageal lumen.[12,15] In the study by Lebrec et al.,[14] varices ranged in size from 4 to 6 mm.

The severity of cirrhosis also varied among the trials. Patients were graded on the severity of liver disease according to the Child-Pugh classification (Table 2).[16] In this weighted system, one, two, or three points are scored for increasing abnormality of each of the five variables assessed. Patients who score 5 or 6 points are classified as grade A; patients with 7–9 points, grade B; and patients with 10–15 points, grade C. Most patients were grade A or grade B, although there was a significant percentage of patients classified as grade C in two trials.[11,15] Bosch et al.[13] did not report information on variceal size or severity of disease.

The percentages of patients not bleeding and the survival rates were dissimilar in each of the studies. In the trial by Pascal et al.,[11] propranolol significantly reduced the incidence of first bleeding and death from all causes during a two-year follow-up period. The incidence of each of these events among patients receiving propranolol was approximately two thirds lower than that of the placebo group. Significant beneficial effects of treatment, however, were apparent only in patients with grade C disease, not in patients with grade A or B disease.

The investigators suggest that the lack of an apparent effect of propranolol on the incidence of bleeding in patients with grade A or B disease may be due to the small size of these groups (44 patients in both the propranolol and placebo groups) and to the low number of events in these groups (six and nine for the propranolol and placebo groups, respectively). Deaths from hemorrhage occurred less frequently in the group of patients receiving propranolol, but the difference did not achieve statistical significance. No difference among the classes of severity of disease was found for this variable. This trial has been criticized because only 42% of the patients who bled were evaluated by endoscopy at the time of hemorrhage to determine the source of bleeding.[1]

In contrast to the results of Pascal et al.,[11] the Italian Multicenter Project[12] found propranolol to have no significant overall effect on bleeding or survival. However, upon retrospective analysis it was found that, in the subset of patients without ascites at the time of randomization, the proportion of patients free of bleeding was significantly higher in the propranolol group than in the placebo group (83% versus 61%, $p = 0.028$). This difference was more pronounced during ascites-free intervals and may be related to the proposed decrease in responsiveness to β-blockade in decompensated patients.[17] The investigators thus concluded that propranolol can prevent initial bleeding in patients without ascites but has no effect on survival.

This conclusion raises several issues. First, the rate of deterioration in liver function or clinical status before the occurrence of hemorrhage would seem to be a more useful index of risk of bleeding than the clinical status at entry into the study, particularly in a study of this duration (up to 42 months).[1] Second, the lack of a significant effect of treatment on survival may be attributed to the low number of deaths from bleeding (10 in the propranolol group and 12 in the control group). In addition, nine patients in the control group received propranolol after their first episode of bleeding and subsequently did not bleed again during the trial. This form of secondary prophylaxis may have reduced the incidence of bleeding and death, thereby minimizing the possibility of showing a different survival rate. Furthermore, the investigators admit that the trial was designed to test the effect of treatment on the incidence of bleeding and not on the improvement of survival, which would have required more patients or a longer follow-up period.

In the trial by Bosch et al.,[13] only patients with a hepatic vein pressure gradient greater than or equal to 12 mm Hg (normal, <5 mm Hg) were included. Daily propranolol doses were determined by progressively increasing the dose until the hepatic vein pressure gradient was reduced by 25% of baseline or measured less than 12 mm Hg or until the dose was limited by a heart rate less than 55 beats per minute. Although survival was not influenced, the frequency of bleeding was significantly reduced ($p < 0.01$) in the propranolol group (22%) compared with the placebo group (4%). This trial has been cited as evidence for a threshold pressure for variceal development and bleeding.[1] Hepatic vein pressure gradients at the time of hemorrhage were not reported.

Lebrec and colleagues[14] evaluated the prophylactic effect of nadolol, another nonselective β-adrenergic antagonist, in patients with grade A and grade B cirrhosis. This study failed to demonstrate an overall beneficial effect of treatment. The investigators point out, however, that therapy was interrupted or discontinued in several noncompliant patients, defined as those who admitted to not taking their medication for at least two consecutive days. If only compliant patients were considered, a statistically significant difference ($p < 0.02$) in percentages of patients free of bleeding was observed for the nadolol group (97%) compared with the placebo group (77%). Compliance, or the lack thereof, had no significant effect on survival. The results of this trial are thus limited in application to those patients with grade A or grade B cirrhosis who are compliant with therapy, a behavior which is often difficult to assess.

Favorable results with nadolol were also reported by Ideo and colleagues.[15] In this trial, which consisted of patients with all grades of disease severity, nadolol significantly decreased the risk of bleeding and improved the endoscopic appearance of the varices. Although the death rate tended to be lower in the nadolol group, the difference was not significant.

Three main weaknesses are common to the trials reported thus far. First, the trials generally lack an adequate sample size to demonstrate a beneficial effect of treatment on bleeding and mortality. Second, with the exception of the trial by Bosch et al.,[13] the protocols were not double-blind. This study design would be ideal but is often difficult to maintain with this type of drug. Third, there was often no standardization of emergency treatment for bleeding. There are many types of therapeutic interventions, including vasopressin, balloon tamponade, sclerotherapy, and surgery, that are used to treat variceal bleeding and may account, at least in part, for the differences in mortality rates.

The dissimilar results reported in these trials have been a source of considerable debate. When evaluated separately, none of the trials is able to define without question the role of β-adrenergic antagonists in the primary prevention of variceal bleeding. In an attempt to clarify discrepant findings and thus better determine the effect of this drug therapy, several groups have performed a meta-analysis of the data from various trials.[18-20] This type of analysis compares each treated group with the controls from the same study and combines the treatment effect across all studies in an attempt to provide any information about the presence and size of any significant effects.

Poynard et al.[20] analyzed data on individual patients from four randomized clinical trials.[11,12,14,15] Of the 589 patients studied, 286 received a nonselective β-adrenergic antagonist (propranolol, 203; nadolol, 83) and 303 received placebo. Endpoints for comparison after two years of follow-up were the percentage of patients who had no bleeding; the percentage who did not have fatal bleeding, which was defined as occurring when a patient died within six weeks of a bleeding episode; the percentage who survived; and the percentage who survived without any bleeding. There were significant differences between the treatment group and the control group in the mean percentages of patients who had no upper gastrointestinal bleeding (78% in the treatment group versus 65% in the control group, $p = 0.002$) and who had no fatal bleeding (90% in the treatment group versus 82% in the control group, $p = 0.01$). However, there was no overall difference in the percentage of patients surviving after two years (71% in the treatment group versus 68% in the control group, $p = 0.34$).

These data suggest that β-adrenergic antagonists significantly reduce the mortality from bleeding but that patients then die from other causes. The percentage of surviving patients who had no bleeding after two years was 62% in the treatment group and 53% in the control group ($p = 0.04$). Meta-analysis[18-20] has revealed an overall positive effect of β-adrenergic antagonists in the primary prevention of bleeding in patients with cirrhosis and large varices. The greatest efficacy was in patients with good compliance who did not have ascites and in patients with less severe disease. No significant difference in efficacy was found between propranolol and nadolol.[20]

Adverse Effects of Therapy

A final issue in the use of β-adrenergic antagonists for primary prophylaxis is whether patients are likely to tolerate this therapy. A wide range of incidences of withdrawal because of adverse effects was reported in each of the trials (Table 1). Adverse effects generally consisted of dizziness, fatigue, cardiac insufficiency, and Raynaud's phenomenon.

Hayes and colleagues[21] conducted a double-blind, placebo-controlled trial to investigate the safety of propranolol in an outpatient population of patients with mild to moderate liver disease. Although the overall incidence of adverse effects and study withdrawal was high, no significant difference was observed between the propranolol and the placebo groups. The investigators suggest that these high incidences of adverse effects and withdrawal may reflect on the study population, of which approximately one half had alcohol-related liver disease. Because this population is often the target for treatment, their tolerance to long-term propranolol therapy may limit its usefulness as a prophylactic agent.

It has been theorized that the high incidence of adverse effects occurring with propranolol in patients with cirrhosis may be related to higher serum concentrations of the drug secondary to decreased liver metabolism.[15] Because nadolol is not metabolized by the liver, its metabolism would not be influenced by decreased liver function and drug accumulation would not occur. This potential for decreased incidence of adverse effects with nadolol may be a consideration for some patients.

Other concerns associated with the use of β-adrenergic antagonist therapy are related to its effect on renal and portal blood flow, particularly in patients with more severe disease who are prone to hepatorenal syndrome and hepatic encephalopathy. Although it has been reported that renal blood flow and sodium excretion remain unchanged in patients with cirrhosis and ascites following long-term propranolol therapy,[22] the potential for the induction or exacerbation of hepatorenal syndrome in patients with severe disease makes this a valid concern. However, no deleterious effects on renal function were reported in any of the reviewed trials. The risk of inducing hepatic encephalopathy is somewhat less of a concern. Although serum ammonia concentrations may increase,[23] clinically evident hepatic encephalopathy generally does not develop.[24,25] However, β-adrenergic antagonist therapy may worsen pre-existing encephalopathy.[25]

Bleeding associated with propranolol withdrawal has been reported[26] and was noted in two patients in the Italian Multicenter Project.[12] In this study, two patients who abruptly discontinued their medications bled on the first day after propranolol withdrawal; one of these patients died. Because of this risk, alcoholic patients who continue to drink are not good candidates for prophylactic therapy with β-adrenergic antagonists. Additionally, it is recommended that therapy be tapered over a period of four to seven days before discontinuation.[26]

Conclusion

The primary goal of prophylactic therapy for esophageal varices is to improve survival by preventing the first episode of bleeding. One trial has shown the survival rate to be significantly higher in patients who received a nonselective β-adrenergic antagonist.[11] Three studies have demonstrated treatment to be more effective than placebo in preventing the initial episode of bleeding,[11,13,15] while two studies found treatment to be effective only in the subset of patients who either were compliant with therapy[14] or were without ascites at the time of enrollment into the study.[12] In view of the distressing nature of variceal hemorrhage and the high medical costs associated with its emergency treatment, a secondary goal of prophylactic therapy to reduce bleeding, even if overall mortality is not influenced, is justified.[3]

Based on the available data, therapy with a nonselective β-adrenergic antagonist should be considered for primary prevention of gastrointestinal hemorrhage in patients with cirrhosis and suspected or documented large varices. Because of the risk of bleeding associated with abrupt discontinuation of the medication, however, therapy should be limited to those patients who will be compliant. More studies are needed to further identify the target population in which therapy will be most beneficial.

References

1. MacMathuna P, Westaby D, Williams R. Taking tension out of the portal system: an approach to the management of portal hypertension in the 1990s. *Scand J Gastroenterol*. 1990; 25(Suppl 175):131-45 .
2. Podolsky DK, Isselbacher KJ. Cirrhosis of the liver. In: Braunwald E, Isselbacher KJ, Petersdorf RG et al., eds. Harrison's principles of internal medicine. New York: MacMillan; 1991:1340-50.
3. Burroughs AK, D'Heygere F, McIntyre N. Pitfalls in studies of prophylactic therapy for variceal bleeding in cirrhotics. *Hepatology*. 1986; 6:1407-13.
4. Reichen J. Liver function and pharmacological considerations in pathogenesis and treatment of portal hypertension. *Hepatology*. 1990; 11:1066-78.
5. Moreau R, Lee SS, Hadengue A et al. Hemodynamic effects of a clonidine-induced decrease in sympathetic tone in patients with cirrhosis. *Hepatology*. 1987; 7:149-54.
6. Freeman JG, Baron JR, Record CO. Effect of isosorbide dinitrate, verapamil and labetalol on portal pressure in cirrhosis. *Br Med J*. 1985; 291:561-2.
7. Merkel C, Finucci G, Zuin R et al. Effects of isosorbide dinitrate on portal hypertension in alcoholic cirrhosis. *J Hepatol*. 1987; 4:174-80.
8. Lebrec D, Hillon P, Munoz C et al. The effect of propranolol on portal hypertension in patients with cirrhosis: a hemodynamic study. *Hepatology*. 1982; 2:523-7.
9. Cales P, Braillon A, Girad C et al. Acute effect of propranolol on splanchnic circulation in normal and portal hypertensive rats. *J Hepatol*. 1985; 1:349-57.
10. Cales P, Braillon A, Jiron MI et al. Superior portosystemic collateral circulation estimated by azygos blood flow in patients with cirrhosis: lack of correlation with oesophageal varices and gastrointestinal bleeding: effect of propranolol. *J Hepatol*. 1985; 1:37-46.
11. Pascal JP, Cales P, Multicenter Study Group. Propranolol in the prevention of first upper gastrointestinal tract hemorrhage in patients with cirrhosis of the liver and esophageal varices. *N Engl J Med*. 1987; 317:856-61.
12. The Italian Multicenter Project for Propranolol in Prevention of Bleeding. Propranolol prevents first gastrointestinal bleeding in non-ascitic cirrhotic patients: final report of a multicenter randomized trial. *J Hepatol*. 1989; 9:75-83.
13. Bosch J, Groszmann RJ, Grace N et al. Propranolol in the prevention of the first hemorrhage from esophageal varices: results of a randomized, double-blind, cooperative clinical trial. *J Hepatol*. 1988; 7(Suppl):S12. Abstract.
14. Lebrec D, Poynard T, Capron JP et al. Nadolol for prophylaxis of gastro-intestinal bleeding in patients with cirrhosis: a randomized trial. *J Hepatol*. 1988; 7:118-25.
15. Ideo G, Bellati G, Fesce E et al. Nadolol can prevent the first gastrointestinal bleeding in cirrhotics: a prospective, randomized study. *Hepatology*. 1988; 8:6-9.
16. Pugh RNH, Murray-Lyon IM, Dawson JL et al. Tran-section of the oesophagus for bleeding oesophageal varices. *Br J Surg*. 1973; 60:646-9.
17. Gerbes AL, Remien J, Jungst D et al. Evidence for down-regulation of beta-2-adrenoreceptors in cirrhotic patients with severe ascites. *Lancet*. 1986; 1:1409-11.
18. Pagliaro L, Burroughs AK, Sorenson TIA et al. Therapeutic controversies and randomised controlled trials: prevention of bleeding and rebleeding in cirrhosis. *Gastroenterol Int*. 1989; 2:71-84.
19. Hayes PC, Davis JM, Lewis JA et al. Meta-analysis of the value of propranolol in prevention of variceal hemorrhage. *Lancet*. 1990; 336:153-6.
20. Poynard T, Cales P, Pasta L et al. Beta-adrenergic-antagonist drugs in the prevention of gastrointestinal bleeding in patients with cirrhosis and esophageal varices: an analysis of data and prognostic factors in 589 patients from four randomized clinical trials. *N Engl J Med*. 1991; 324:1532-8.
21. Hayes PC, Crichton S, Shepherd AN et al. Propranolol in chronic liver disease: a controlled trial of its effect and safety over twelve months. *Q J Med*. 1987; 65:828-34.
22. Wilkinson SP, Bernardi M, Smith IK et al. Effect of beta adrenergic blocking drugs on the renin–aldosterone system, sodium excretion and renal haemodynamics in cirrhosis with ascites. *Gastroenterology*. 1977; 73:659-63.
23. van Buuren HR, van der Velden PC, Koorevaar G et al. Propranolol increases arterial ammonia in liver cirrhosis. *Lancet*. 1982; 2:951-2.
24. Cales P, Nicolas MP, Guell A et al. Propranolol does not alter cerebral flow and functions in cirrhotic patients without previous hepatic encephalopathy. *Hepatology*. 1989; 9:439-42.
25. Reding P. Risk of hepatic encephalopathy in patients taking propranolol for portal hypertension. *Lancet*. 1982; 2:550. Letter.
26. Lebrec D, Bernuau J, Rueff B et al. Gastrointestinal bleeding after abrupt cessation of propranolol administration in cirrhosis. *N Engl J Med*. 1982; 307:560. Letter.

Research Notes

Multicenter evaluation of a patient-controlled analgesia device for the treatment of postoperative pain

DANIEL P. WERMELING, STAN A. GREENE, BRADLEY A. BOUCHER, MARK E. LEHMAN, GERALD G. BRIGGS, EDWARD R. BEZARRO, AND THOMAS S. FOSTER

Clin Pharm. 1992; 11:342-6

Patient-controlled analgesia (PCA) delivery systems were first tested in the 1960s and 1970s.[1-4] Commercial devices became available in the United States in the early 1980s, and PCA was accepted by the medical community.[5-8] Although PCA technology was relatively expensive, many university teaching hospitals and private hospitals offered PCA as a marketed service throughout the 1980s. At least nine manufacturers offer PCA devices, including large bedside devices, small portable pumps, and disposable systems.[9]

Further evaluation of PCA infusion devices is needed. Several manufacturers have sponsored extensive preclinical and clinical studies by independent contract or academic researchers. Less evaluative information of device performance is available for some devices.[10] Comparisons of the clinical performance of PCA devices are difficult because of differences in the designs of initial studies.

The Baxter infusor and patient control module (Baxter Laboratories, Deerfield, IL) is a disposable, nonelectronic, lightweight device that consists of two components. The 5-mL/hour infusor is a continuous-infusion drug delivery device that uses a balloon reservoir to store medication and to produce an energy source for the system. Microbore tubing from the infusor is attached to a wristband activation device, the patient control module. A needle attached to exit tubing of the module is inserted into the Y-site injection port of the patient's primary intravenous line. The patient depresses a button on the face of the control module to self-administer a 0.5-mL dose of analgesic medication. The infusor flow rate limits patients to a full dose every six minutes. The patient can receive a proportion of the dose should the device be activated before six minutes elapse.

The initial clinical evaluation of this device was a single-center evaluation of 50 patients.[11] The protocol was conducted under highly supervised conditions because this was the first time the device was used in humans for analgesic purposes. The purpose of this study was to perform a pharmacy-coordinated, national, multicenter clinical trial to evaluate the use of the PCA system for postoperative pain relief in 150 patients.

Methods. The College of Pharmacy, University of Kentucky, Lexington, served as the research coordination center. Five medical centers representing a broad geographical distribution were chosen to evaluate the PCA device: Beth Israel Hospital, Boston,

DANIEL P. WERMELING, PHARM.D., is Assistant Research Professor and Director, Drug Product Evaluation Unit, College of Pharmacy, University of Kentucky, Lexington. STAN A. GREENE, PHARM.D., is Clinical Pharmacy Coordinator, Drug Information and Clinical Research Services, Department of Pharmacy, St. John's Regional Health Center, Springfield, MO. BRADLEY A. BOUCHER, PHARM.D., is Associate Professor, Department of Clinical Pharmacy, University of Tennessee, Memphis, and Regional Medical Center at Memphis. MARK E. LEHMAN, PHARM.D., is Medical Services Manager, Squibb U.S. Pharmaceutical Group, Bristol-Myers Squibb, Cincinnati, OH; at the time of this study, he was Associate Director of Pharmacy Services, Medical College of Virginia Hospitals, and Associate Professor, Department of Pharmacy and Pharmaceutics, Medical College of Virginia, Virginia Commonwealth University, Richmond. GERALD G. BRIGGS is Clinical Pharmacist, Department of Pharmacy, Women's Hospital, Long Beach Memorial Medical Center, Long Beach, CA. EDWARD R. BEZARRO is Clinical Pharmacist, Department of Pharmacy, Beth Israel Hospital, Boston, MA. THOMAS S. FOSTER, PHARM.D., is Professor and Director, Center for Pharmaceutical Science and Technology, College of Pharmacy, University of Kentucky.

Address reprint requests to Dr. Wermeling at the Drug Product Evaluation Unit, College of Pharmacy, University of Kentucky, Room 319, Rose Street, Lexington, KY 40536-0082.

Baxter Laboratories, Deerfield, IL, supplied infusors and patient control modules.

The following individuals and institutions are acknowledged as key participants in this trial: Stephen Christiansen, M.D., Department of Surgery, St. John's Regional Health Center, Springfield, MO; Anne Marie Bombassaro, Pharm.D., Department of Clinical Pharmacy, University of Tennessee and the Regional Medical Center at Memphis; C. Richard Patterson, M.D., Department of Surgery, University of Tennessee and the Regional Medical Center at Memphis; Molly Collier, R.N., M.S.N., Department of Nursing, Beth Israel Hospital, Boston, MA; Medical College of Virginia, Richmond, VA; and Women's Hospital, Long Beach Memorial Medical Center, Long Beach, CA.

MA; Medical College of Virginia Hospitals, Richmond, VA; Long Beach Memorial Medical Center, Long Beach, CA; The Regional Medical Center at Memphis, Memphis, TN; and St. John's Regional Health Center, Springfield, MO. These hospitals represent university teaching or private hospitals and had experience with PCA devices ranging from none to established pain management programs. Factors evaluated across and within sites included narcotic use, pain and sedation scores, adverse effects, patient satisfaction, and whether the number of devices used was related to institutional policies regarding frequency of set change.

Investigators and hospitals agreed to follow a common protocol previously developed at the University of Kentucky.[11] Each investigator received a sample informed consent document and data collection forms. Modifications of the protocol were allowed to accommodate hospital service programs for providing analgesic medication to postoperative patients. Investigators submitted a study proposal based on these documents to their respective institutional review boards for approval. Each of the investigators organized a study team consisting of pharmacists, nurses, and physicians to oversee conduct of the investigation. Each site agreed to provide evaluable data on 30 patients who were expected to require morphine sulfate for postoperative pain management.

We expected that most patients enrolled would be undergoing general surgery or gynecologic or orthopedic surgical procedures. Male and female patients 18 to 65 years of age with American Society of Anesthesiology (ASA) class I to II physiologic status were eligible. Patients whose surgical procedure was of a nature that generally required postoperative pain management with injectable narcotics for at least 36 hours were identified consecutively and asked to participate. Patients with serious debilitating disorders, sepsis, allergy to narcotics, or history of drug or alcohol abuse and patients receiving narcotics for pain management before this surgical procedure were excluded from study participation.

Potential patient candidates were interviewed before surgery and asked questions concerning their medical history, including the use of prescription drugs, alcoholic beverage consumption, and possible abuse of prescription or illicit drugs. During the interview, patients were given an orientation to PCA therapy and the use of the PCA device. Informed consent was obtained from every patient after he or she had reviewed the purpose of the study and operation of the PCA device.

Upon emergence of the patient from anesthesia, an intravenous loading dose of morphine could be administered by an anesthesiologist for pain relief if deemed necessary. Patients were permitted to use the device in the postoperative recovery room after emergence from anesthesia and in their rooms after surgery. Standing orders for intramuscular morphine administration were written at some hospitals in case the PCA device was not immediately available after surgery or in case analgesia was not maintained with the device. Methods for compounding morphine solutions were those commonly employed at each hospital. Morphine solutions for the infusor were prepared in the pharmacy and placed in the device by study personnel or hospital pharmacy staff. Distribution of the PCA device to recovery rooms or wards followed hospital policies for transfer of controlled substances.

The dose of morphine delivered to the patient upon each activation of the device is dependent on the concentration of morphine filling the infusor. Most patients were prescribed a morphine sulfate concentration of 2 mg/mL, which delivers 1 mg of morphine sulfate per activation of the control module. The initial choice of morphine concentration was left to the investigators.

Adjustment of the bolus dose to optimize analgesic therapy was permitted. This was accomplished by exchanging the infusor in use with an infusor containing morphine at the desired concentration. Morphine sulfate concentrations of 3 or 4 mg/mL were permitted for dosage adjustment.

Infusor and control modules were exchanged at intervals consistent with the medical centers' policies for intravenous set change (24–72 hours). Therapy with the PCA device proceeded until intravenous fluid therapy was discontinued or until PCA treatment was deemed unnecessary. PCA therapy was discontinued at any time upon patient request or if therapy was judged by the investigators to be producing significant adverse effects.

Study charting by the nursing staff was performed every four hours for the duration of the trial with measurement of vital signs and overall degree of sedation on a five-point scale (wide-awake, drowsy, dozing intermittently, mostly sleeping, awakes only when aroused). Medication use was determined every four hours from a volume indicator tape attached to the infusor. Patients were asked to provide a ranking of their level of pain relief (comfortable, mild discomfort, in pain, bad pain, very bad pain) every four hours during waking hours. After the study, a questionnaire to determine overall satisfaction was given to each patient (appendix).

At the conclusion of the clinical trial phase of the investigation, each investigator encoded data on a computer diskette using a preset reporting format. From this database, each hospital compiled an individual study report. The research coordination center used data from diskettes and final reports to develop a composite profile of PCA therapy for all patients studied at the five hospitals. Data on demographics, morphine use, and PCA device use were compiled and analyzed within and across all hospitals using descriptive statistics.

Results. A total of 155 patients participated in the study. Demographic data for these patients are summarized in Table 1. Patients were comparable in height and weight with the exception of patients at

Medical College of Virginia Hospitals, where more gastric bypass operations were performed on obese patients. The study was not balanced by gender because of the high number of gynecologic surgeries performed at some hospitals; 21% of the patients were men. Table 1 provides a breakdown of surgical procedures performed at each investigative site.

A total of 17 patients (10.9%) withdrew or were withdrawn by the investigators from the study (Table 1). Seven of the 17 patients were unevaluable because of cancellation of surgery (1), operative complications (3), or allergic reaction to morphine (3). Of the remaining 148 evaluable patients, 10 were withdrawn from the study while using the device. Six of the 10 patients were withdrawn because of adverse effects of morphine including nausea (4), rash (1), and respiratory depression (1). The patient suffering from respiratory depression had received intramuscular injections of morphine in addition to morphine self-administered by PCA. This patient had a history of alcohol abuse. Two other patients were withdrawn because of poor pain relief. One of these patients had a history of chronic back pain; the second patient had a history of alcohol abuse. One patient was withdrawn from the study because of phlebitis at the intravenous catheter site. One patient failed to respond to morphine and was given hydromorphone instead.

A summary of morphine sulfate use during PCA therapy is described in Table 2. The mean morphine sulfate dose ranged from 0.46 mg/sq m to 0.56 mg/sq m (mean, 0.53 mg/sq m). One site had a lower standardized dose because of a subject population mostly composed of morbidly obese patients. On average, each patient consumed 99 mg of morphine sulfate (0–434 mg) over a 67-hour period (8–144 hours). The average hourly morphine sulfate dosing rate was 1.5 mg/hour. Figure 1 demonstrates graphically the average daily dosing rates for all sites. A pattern described in other studies was seen with higher morphine use during postoperative days 1 and 2.[5-7,11] The

Table 1.
Demographic Data by Site

Variable	MA	VA	CA	TN	MO	Total
Patients						
No. enrolled	30	30	33	30	32	155
Gender (M/F)	8/22	4/26	0/33	5/25	16/16	33/122
Height in cm (mean ± S.D.)	170 ± 8.6	169 ± 7.9	163 ± 8.9	162 ± 30	170 ± 9.6	
Weight in kg (mean ± S.D.)	73 ± 18	110 ± 34	72 ± 22	78 ± 22	78 ± 15	
Operation						
Cholecystectomy	11	4	0	14	14	43
Colon resection	4	6	1	3	5	19
Hysterectomy	12	0	27	0	1	40
Gastric bypass	0	19	0	0	0	19
Hip repair	0	0	0	0	5	5
Mastectomy	0	1	0	5	0	6
Other	3	0	5	8	7	23
Total	30	30	33	30	32	155
Patient Dropouts						
Nausea	3	0	0	0	1	4
Rash	1	0	0	2	1	4
Operative complications	1	0	1	0	1	3
Poor pain relief	1	0	1	0	0	2
Respiratory depression	0	0	0	1	0	1
Other	0	0	2	1	0	3
Total	6	0	4	4	3	17

Table 2.
Morphine Use[a] by Site

Variable	MA	VA	CA	TN	MO	Mean
Morphine sulfate dose per PCA[b] injection (mg/sq m)	0.54 ± 0.10	0.46 ± 0.14	0.56 ± 0.12	0.55 ± 0.12	0.53 ± 0.10	0.53 ± 0.03
Total dosage of PCA morphine sulfate (mg)	85 ± 60	150 ± 96	107 ± 78	72 ± 92	80 ± 49	99 ± 82
Total PCA hours	50 ± 21	84 ± 26	91 ± 28	53 ± 18	60 ± 24	67 ± 29
Avg. dosing rate (mg/hr)	1.7 ± 1.0	1.8 ± 1.0	1.2 ± 0.6	1.4 ± 1.1	1.3 ± 0.7	1.5 ± 1.1

[a]Expressed as mean ± S.D.
[b]PCA = patient-controlled analgesia.

rate declined substantially over the next two to three days. Figure 2 provides a similar scenario for average morphine use by each investigative site.

A total of 221 control modules and 283 infusors were dispensed to 149 patients (Table 3). Only seven patients (4.7%) had a dosage increase requiring a new infusor with higher morphine concentration. One patient had a dosage decrease requiring a new infusor with lower morphine concentration. Patients required additional PCA sets for the following reasons: (1) replacement of the set if PCA therapy extended beyond the time interval for intravenous set change dictated by institutional policy, or (2) requirement of additional morphine beyond what was provided with the initial infusor.

According to pain scores taken every four hours, patients had mild or no pain for approximately 79% of the responses. Summary of sedation scores revealed that patients were alert or drowsy for approximately 83% of the responses.

Responses to the poststudy questionnaire indicated that more than 80% of the patients experienced no worse than moderate pain after the operative procedure; 70% experienced only mild to moderate drowsiness. Forty-two percent of the patients reported not sleeping well. However, when questioned about the nature of the insomnia, only 14% stated that the main cause of their inability to sleep was pain. Sixty percent of the patients reported that they were awakened by pain. Almost all patients (93%) thought that it was not inconvenient to administer medications during sleeping hours and that no design modifications were necessary to prevent interruption of sleep for self-administration of medication. Ninety percent of the patients reported that they would rather have PCA than intramuscular injections for future postoperative pain management.

Discussion. The results of this multicenter study demonstrate the utility of the Baxter infusor and patient control module as a PCA device and support the findings of the initial clinical trial.[11] This study employed the same morphine doses and lockout intervals reported in previous trials. Although we used no comparison group, our data are consistent with those reported in other clinical evaluations of PCA therapy.[5-7,11]

There were no serious adverse effects caused by device defects or operator error as described in earlier reports.[12,13] Reasons for patient withdrawal from the clinical trial were not associated with use of the system.

The responses to the poststudy questionnaire reveal that patients were quite satisfied with the device. Additional comments made about the device by patients or nurses were as follows: (1) lengthen the wristband to accommodate larger wrist circumferences, (2) increase length of tubing from the infusor to the patient control module, and (3) develop a better volume indicator for the infusor.

Independent in vitro evaluation of this and other

Figure 1. Average daily morphine use by all patients.

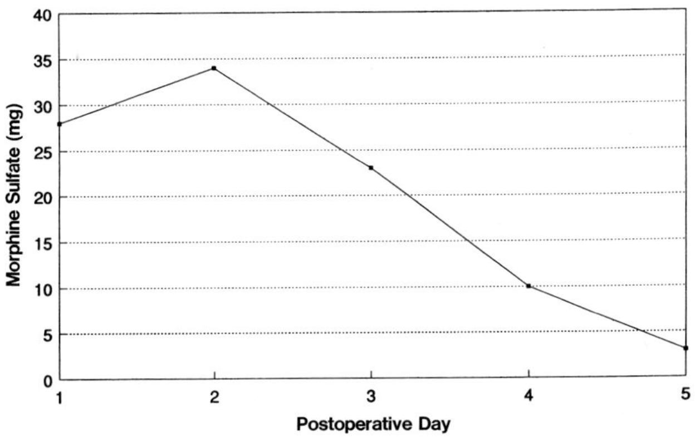

Figure 2. Average daily morphine use, by center.

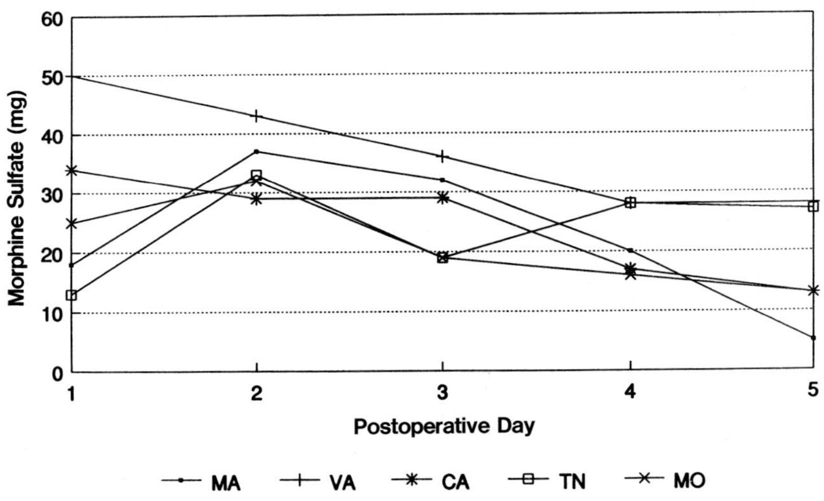

PCA devices was published by a nonprofit agency.[10] The agency rated the Baxter device as acceptable for patient use and gave it good marks for ease of setup and operation. Many of the stated disadvantages of the device (difficult dose adjustment, poor security, infusor rate variation, patient dexterity) were not observed in this study.

The ultimate evaluation and success of this device rests with the product selection and evaluation committees of medical institutions. Pharmacists, physicians, nurses, and biomedical engineers play an integral role in evaluating the performance of medical equipment. Moreover, as experts in drug delivery systems, pharmacists provide leadership regarding the evaluation and selection of vitally important equipment, such as infusion devices. This study of the Baxter device provides selection committees with a starting point for their own evaluations.

The development and evaluation of the Baxter PCA device could serve as a model for the development of new infusion equipment. Pharmacy and industry collaborated in the design and modification of the new device during rigorous in vitro testing, a preliminary clinical trial, and a multicenter clinical trial. Pharmacy should continually strive to create partnerships with industry to codevelop infusion devices.

Conclusion. The Baxter infusor and patient control module was studied at five medical centers in the United States. Use of the device was consistent with previous evaluations of PCA therapy for postoperative pain.

References

1. Sechzer PH. Studies in pain with analgesic delivery system. *Anesth Analg*. 1971; 50:1-10.
2. Scott JS. Obstetric analgesia. *Am J Obstet Gynecol*. 1970; 106:959-78.
3. Forrest WH Jr, Smethurst PWR, Kienitz ME. Self-administration of intravenous analgesics. *Anesthesiology*. 1970; 33:363-5.
4. Keeri-Szanto M. Apparatus for demand analgesia. *Can Anaesth Soc J*. 1971; 18:581-2.
5. Bennett RL, Baumann TJ, Batenhorst RL et al. Morphine titration in postoperative laparotomy patients using patient-controlled analgesia. *Curr Ther Res*. 1982; 32:45-52.
6. Tamsen A, Hartvig P, Dahlstrom B et al. Patient-controlled analgesic therapy in the early postoperative period. *Acta Anaesthesiol Scand*. 1979; 23:462-70.
7. Bollish SJ, Collins CL, Kirking DM et al. Efficacy of patient-controlled analgesia versus conventional analgesia for postoperative pain. *Clin Pharm*. 1985; 4:48-52.
8. Vinik HR, Anton KE, Barbarash RA et al. Patient-controlled analgesia in hospitalized patients: a multicenter evaluation. *Postgrad Med Spec Rep*. 1986; Aug 28:41-5.
9. Rapp RP, Bivins BA, Littrell RA et al. Patient-controlled analgesia: a review of effectiveness of therapy and an evaluation of currently available devices. *DICP*. 1989; 23:899-904.
10. Anon. Patient-controlled analgesic infusion pumps. *Health Devices*. 1988; 17:136-67.
11. Wermeling DP, Foster TS, Rapp RP et al. Evaluation of a disposable, nonelectronic, patient-controlled analgesia device for postoperative pain. *Clin Pharm*. 1987; 6:307-14.
12. White PF. Mishaps with patient-controlled analgesia. *Anesthesiology*. 1987; 66:81-3.
13. Grey TC, Sweeney ES. Patient-controlled analgesia. *JAMA*. 1988; 259:2240.

Table 3.
Patient Control Module and Infusor Use by Site

Variable	MA	VA	CA	TN	MO	Total
No. PCMs[a] used	30	58	62	36	35	221
No. infusors used	63	67	65	42	46	283
No. patients with dose increase	2	1	0	1	3	7
No. patients with dose decrease	0	0	1	0	0	1
Set change interval (hr)	. . .[b]	48	48	72	72	

[a]PCM = patient control module.
[b]72 hours for PCM, 24 hours for infusor.

Appendix—Poststudy Questionnaire

1. On the whole, how much pain have you had since the operation?
   a. No pain
   b. Mild pain
   c. Moderate pain
   d. Bad pain
   e. Very bad pain
2. Except on the day of the operation, which of the following describes how sleepy you felt since the time of the operation?
   a. Wide-awake
   b. Slightly drowsy
   c. Moderately drowsy
   d. Very drowsy
3. Have you slept well since the operation?
   a. Yes
   b. No
4. What was the main cause of any trouble you may have had sleeping?
   a. Pain
   b. Activity in the room
   c. Restlessness
   d. Other
5. Do you remember awakening from sleep at night just because you were in pain and needed an additional dose of pain medication?
   a. Yes
   b. No
6. Did giving pain medication during sleeping hours cause you any significant inconvenience?
   a. Yes
   b. No
7. Should we redesign the device so that you would not have to give yourself medication while trying to sleep?
   a. Yes
   b. No
8. As opposed to having intramuscular shots for pain relief, do you feel you would
   a. Rather have PCA therapy as pain treatment for future surgery
   b. Rather have intramuscular shots for future surgery
   c. Not care which type of pain treatment you received

Effect of lidocaine–prilocaine cream on pain from subcutaneous injection

ANNA TADDIO, ISABELLE ROBIEUX, AND GIDEON KOREN

Clin Pharm. 1992; 11:347-9

EMLA 5% cream (Astra Pharma Inc.) is a eutectic mixture of equal parts of lidocaine and prilocaine that is applied topically to induce skin anesthesia. It is currently marketed as a nonprescription medication in Canada but is not available in the United States.

The anesthesia produced by EMLA may be apparent at a depth of up to 5 mm, and the effect persists after the cream's removal.[1] EMLA has been used effectively as an anesthetic for needle puncture,[2-6] superficial skin surgery,[7] and removal of molluscum contagiosum lesions.[8,9] However, its effectiveness in reducing the pain associated with subcutaneous injection has not been tested.

The objective of this study was to evaluate EMLA's ability to make subcutaneous injection less painful.

Methods. Healthy adult volunteers participated in a randomized, double-blind, prospective trial. Exclusion criteria for the study were a history of sensitivity or allergy to amide-type anesthetics and receipt of any anesthetic or sedative within two hours of the study. The study was approved by the human subject review committee of our hospital, and all subjects gave written informed consent. All participants were given an information sheet that described EMLA and its uses, as well as the purpose of the study and its blinded and placebo-controlled design. The sheet indicated how EMLA was to be applied, that it would take one hour to become effective, that 1 mL of sterile 0.9% sodium chloride solution would be injected into each arm, and that subjects would be asked to record the amount of pain they experienced for each injection. The sheet noted that redness or itching could occur.

Subjects received one 2.5-g application of either EMLA or placebo cream to the left arm over the middle of the deltoid muscle, and an occlusive dressing was applied immediately. The other cream was applied in a similar fashion to the right arm and covered. The order of cream application was random for each subject. Both placebo and EMLA creams contained the same ingredients, except that the active ingredients in EMLA were replaced with coconut oil (Miglyol 812, Dynamit Nobel, Sweden) in the placebo cream. Both formulations were visually and cosmetically identical. The creams were applied in a circular pattern, with a radius of approximately 1.5 cm. After 60–75 minutes, the dressings were removed and the creams were wiped off with a tissue. Within five minutes of cream removal, investigators rated local skin reactions (i.e., pallor, edema, or redness) as being not present, mild, moderate, or severe. The investigators were blinded to site of drug and placebo. After the area was wiped with an alcohol swab, each subject received one subcutaneous injection of 1.0 mL of room-temperature 0.9% sodium chloride injection (Astra Pharma Inc.) in each site, starting with the left arm. A 25-gauge, 5/8-inch needle was used. For each injection, the needle was inserted in the middle of the deltoid area at a 90° angle to the skin. The solution was injected over five seconds, as counted by the investigator. All injections were performed by one investigator. The area on the skin where the cream was applied was not identified with a marker because the application area was consistent and also because the dressing left markings on the skin.

The pain associated with the procedure was scored by each subject by using an ungraded 100-mm visual analog scale (VAS) with zero denoting "no pain" and 100 mm denoting "worst possible pain." All subjects were pretested for understanding of the VAS. In this comprehension test, subjects scored the pain they would feel in the following situations: receiving a mosquito bite, falling in the snow, falling on the pavement, and slamming a door on their fingers. For each injection, subjects used one VAS to score the pain felt from the needle insertion and another to score the pain felt from the actual injection of solution. The pretest and pain evaluations were administered by the same investigator, who did not give the injections. All subjects filled out a short questionnaire about EMLA cream after receiving both injections.

The differences between the pain scores were evaluated using the Wilcoxon signed-rank test. The effect of the side of injection and the location of EMLA cream was studied using the Mann-Whitney *U* test. The a priori level of significance was ≤ 0.05.

Results. Twenty subjects participated in the study. The mean age was 30 years (range, 19–46 years). Sixteen subjects (80%) were women. Eighteen subjects (90%) were white, one was Asian and one was black. Fifteen subjects (75%) reported no history of skin allergies. Five others (25%) reported allergies to skin cleaners, perfumes, mosquito bites, animals, or plants. Eleven subjects (55%) received EMLA on the left arm, and the remainder received it on the right arm.

Table 1 shows the pain scores from the VAS comprehension test and injections. Needle insertion caused significantly less pain in EMLA-treated arms than in placebo-treated arms ($p < 0.01$). There was also a significant difference between the pain associated with

---

ANNA TADDIO is Motherisk Counsellor and graduate student in the Faculty of Pharmacy; ISABELLE ROBIEUX, M.D., is Pediatrician; and GIDEON KOREN, M.D., is Pediatrician, Division of Clinical Pharmacology, The Hospital for Sick Children, Toronto.

Address reprint requests to Dr. Koren at The Hospital for Sick Children, 555 University Avenue, Toronto, Ontario M5G 1X8, Canada.

Supported by a grant from Astra Pharma Inc., Canada.

Anna Taddio received support from the Motherisk Research Fund, the Norman Aronson Award (Syntex Inc.), and the University of Toronto Open Fellowship.

needle entry and the pain of actual injection in EMLA-treated arms ($p < 0.01$). There was no significant difference between these variables in the placebo group. Pain caused by the injection was not significantly different between EMLA- and placebo-treated arms. When other variables were held constant, there was no difference in pain between left and right arms or between left and right EMLA-treated arms.

All subjects reported that they believed they would be able to properly apply EMLA at home one hour before having their next injection. Eighty percent reported that they thought the one-hour application time was not difficult to fit into their schedule, and 50% stated that they would be willing to purchase EMLA for their next injection. (The wholesale price of a 5-g tube is approximately $6 Canadian, but subjects were not given this information.)

Table 2 lists the frequency of adverse effects. No serious adverse effects were noted. EMLA and placebo were associated with adverse effects in 85% and 35% of subjects, respectively. Skin pallor was the most frequent reaction, occurring in 13 subjects (65%) on the EMLA-treated arm, compared with three subjects (15%) on the placebo-treated arm.

Discussion. Our study showed that needle insertion causes less pain if the injection site has been pretreated with EMLA. However, the pain of solution injection was not lessened by EMLA pretreatment. Since subcutaneous injection is commonly used in children for administration of routine vaccinations, it seems reasonable to test EMLA in children during vaccination. Because needles are perceived as painful by children and parents, administration of EMLA cream may alleviate anxiety by decreasing pain.

Bjerring and Arendt-Nielson[1] used an 18-gauge needle in their study to determine that the depth of analgesia after topical application of EMLA cream was 5 mm during the 30 minutes after a 90-minute application time and during the 60 minutes after a 120-minute application time. Our study, which employed a 25-gauge needle inserted to a depth of 5/8 inch (16 mm), suggests that the depth of analgesia provided by EMLA may extend into the subcutaneous tissue. This is supported by the fact that EMLA provides analgesia for venous cannulation.[6]

In our study, subjects scored pain intensity on a VAS. This method has been used successfully in evaluating EMLA's efficacy in other trials as well. Halperin et al.[6] found that children reported significantly less pain from venipuncture, subcutaneous drug reservoir puncture, and lumbar puncture after treatment with EMLA. Manner et al.[4] also used the VAS in their evaluation of pain associated with venous cannulation in children. DeWaard-van der Spek et al.[9] found that children, evaluating their own pain by using a VAS, reported less pain from curettage of molluscum contagiosum after treatment with EMLA cream, compared with placebo.

Our study did not address differences in pain perception resulting from the properties of the injected substance, such as pH, temperature, and osmolality. Therefore, the perception of pain in this study may not reflect the perception of pain caused by routine vaccinations. Nevertheless, this does not mean that EMLA is not useful under other conditions. In fact, it may have a greater impact on pain perception when less physiologic substances are injected. Also, the quality of pain associated with insertion of the needle versus that of solution injection may be different, and we are uncertain of the contribution of each to the pain from the entire procedure.

EMLA cream was associated with more adverse reactions than placebo, but the reactions were mild and

Table 1.
Ratings of Pain from Imagined Sources and from Subcutaneous Injection ($n = 20$)

Pain Source	Scores on Visual Analog Scale (mm)[a]		
	Mean ± S.D.	Median	Range
Imagined pain			
Mosquito bite	7.9 ± 10.0	2.5	0–35
Falling in snow	10.9 ± 10.0	8.8	0–38
Falling on pavement	31.3 ± 13.9	33.0	4–55
Slamming door on finger	74.6 ± 18.9	74.5	27–99
Needle insertion			
EMLA-treated arm	3.9 ± 8.5[b]	1.0	0–32
Placebo-treated arm	9.1 ± 11.2	4.5	1–44
Injection of 0.9% sodium chloride			
EMLA-treated arm	13.9 ± 15.8	7.0	0–48
Placebo-treated arm	18.3 ± 21.2	4.5	1–60

[a]100-mm scale, where 0 mm = no pain and 100 mm = worst possible pain.
[b]Significantly different from scores for needle insertion into the placebo-treated arm and for injection of 0.9% sodium chloride solution into the EMLA-treated arm ($p < 0.01$, Wilcoxon signed-rank test).

Table 2.
Adverse Effects Associated with EMLA and Placebo Administration ($n = 20$)

Effect and Severity[a]	No. (%) Subjects with Effect	
	EMLA	Placebo
Pallor		
Mild	12 (60)	3 (15)
Moderate	1 (5)	0
Redness, mild	2 (10)	2 (10)
Other[b]		
Mild	6 (30)	2 (10)
Moderate	1 (5)	1 (5)
Total[c]	17 (85)	7 (35)

[a]Adverse effects were rated by investigators as nonexistent, mild, moderate, or severe.
[b]Includes heat sensation, itching, soreness, aching sensation, blotchiness or variation in skin color, redness where adhesive tape was applied, numbness, or heaviness.
[c]Three subjects had two adverse effects each when treated with EMLA, one subject had three adverse effects when treated with EMLA, and one subject had two adverse effects when treated with placebo.

consisted mainly of skin pallor. Pallor is a recognized effect of EMLA cream.[10]

Conclusion. Subcutaneous needle insertion in adult volunteers was less painful after EMLA, rather than placebo, was used to pretreat the injection site.

References

1. Bjerring P, Arendt-Nielson L. Depth and duration of skin analgesia to needle insertion after topical application of EMLA cream. *Br J Anaesth.* 1990; 64:173-7.
2. Hallen B, Uppfeldt A. Does lidocaine–prilocaine cream permit painfree insertion of iv catheters in children? *Anaesthesiology.* 1982; 57:340-2.
3. Maunuksela EL, Korpela R. Double-blind evaluation of a lignocaine–prilocaine cream (EMLA) in children: effect on the pain associated with venous cannulation. *Br J Anaesth.* 1986; 58:1242-5.
4. Manner T, Kanto J, Iisalo E et al. Reduction of pain at venous cannulation in children with a eutectic mixture of lidocaine and prilocaine (EMLA cream): comparison with placebo cream and no local premedication. *Acta Anaesthesiol Scand.* 1987; 31:735-9.
5. Hopkins CS, Buckley CJ, Bush GH. Pain-free injection in infants: use of a lignocaine–prilocaine cream to prevent pain at intravenous induction of general anaesthesia in 1–5-year-old children. *Anaesthesia.* 1988; 43:198-201.
6. Halperin DL, Koren G, Attias D et al. Topical skin anesthesia for venous, subcutaneous drug reservoir and lumbar punctures in children. *Pediatrics.* 1989; 84:281-4.
7. Juhlin L, Evers H, Broberg F. A lidocaine–prilocaine cream for superficial skin surgery and painful lesions. *Acta Derm Venereol.* 1980; 60:544-6.
8. Rosdahl I, Edmar B, Gisslen H et al. Curettage of molluscum contagiosum in children: analgesia by topical application of a lidocaine/prilocaine cream (EMLA). *Acta Derm Venereol.* 1988; 68:149-53.
9. DeWaard-van der Spek FB, Oranje AP, Lillieborg S et al. Treatment of molluscum contagiosum using a lidocaine/prilocaine cream (EMLA) for analgesia. *J Am Acad Dermatol.* 1990; 23:685-8.
10. Astra Pharma Inc. EMLA cream product monograph. Mississauga, Ontario, Canada: 1990 Dec 7.

Commentary

Treating ischemic stroke: Is nimodipine the answer?

EDZARD ERNST

Clin Pharm. 1992; 11:350-1

Ischemic stroke makes a sad and sizable contribution to mortality and disability in most countries, although insights into the risk factors are beginning to aid in prevention.[1] Many unsolved problems surround stroke rehabilitation,[2] and effective treatment of acute ischemic stroke is still highly controversial. Hemodilution, anticoagulants, corticosteroids, and metabolic activators and inhibitors have all failed to be demonstrably and indisputably effective.[3]

Recently, nimodipine, a calcium-channel blocker with alleged preferential cerebrovascular action,[4] has been claimed to be effective in the treatment of ischemic stroke, possibly by increasing cerebral blood flow[5] and preventing brain cell necrosis by limiting transcellular calcium flux.[6] The drug improves the outcome of cerebral ischemia in primates, dogs, and rats.[7-9] Yet these findings might, for a number of reasons, not be applicable to the clinical situation of acute ischemic stroke in humans. The ultimate test for nimodipine is therefore the controlled clinical trial.

Clinical Trials. Gelmers[10] was the first to report that nimodipine benefits ischemic stroke patients. He randomly assigned patients to a nimodipine group (120 mg/day) and a control group. After four weeks of treatment, the Mathew score indicated significantly greater improvement in the nimodipine-treated group. Although this study had obvious limitations—a single-blind design, a short observation period—it stimulated the performance of more rigorous trials.

Gelmers and coworkers[11] conducted a second study, this time double-blind. They gave 186 patients with ischemic stroke oral nimodipine (30 mg every six hours) or placebo. Treatment began within 24 hours after the onset of symptoms and again was continued for four weeks. The mortality rate was much lower in the nimodipine group than among the controls (8 versus 19 fatalities during the first four weeks and 16 versus 27 deaths during the first six months). The Mathew score at six months indicated a significantly better outcome in treated patients. The drug was most beneficial in men and in patients with moderate to severe cases. It is unclear whether patients who were treated relatively early after the onset of symptoms profited more than those treated less promptly.

In a multicenter trial with a similar design, patients were enrolled up to 48 hours after the onset of symptoms.[12] Neither mortality rates nor neurological scores differed between patients given nimodipine (120 mg/day for four weeks) and those given placebo. However, when patients with moderate to severe cases were analyzed separately, the outcome was found to be significantly better in those who received nimodipine. This study was limited by its relatively short observation period of only 28 days.

A Swiss group conducted a double-blind, randomized, placebo-controlled trial admitting only moderately affected patients with a Mathew score of 50 to 75.[13] The dosage of nimodipine was 30 mg q.i.d., and follow-up lasted four months. There was no difference between the groups in the Mathew score at four months. The drawbacks of this study were its small sample size ($n = 60$) and the entry of patients up to 48 hours after symptoms began.

In a large ($n = 1215$), randomized, double-blind, placebo-controlled multicenter study, the same nimodipine dosage (30 mg q.i.d.) was used, patients were enrolled up to 48 hours after the onset of symptoms, patients with severe and mild cases were excluded, and the Barthel index was used at six months as the primary endpoint.[14] Neither survival nor neurological outcome differed between the groups. Patients admitted within 24 hours of symptom onset also showed no greater benefit.

In another trial, oral nimodipine 120 mg or placebo was given daily for three weeks to patients who had suffered supratentorial infarction within 48 hours.[15] At the end of the three weeks, mortality rates were not significantly different (5.9% for nimodipine and 8.6% for placebo). Neurological function, however, differed in favor of nimodipine in a subgroup of severely affected patients.

Bridgers et al.[16] reported studies in which patients with moderate to severe deficits were enrolled within 24 hours of symptom onset and given intravenous nimodipine (1 or 2 mg/hr for five days) followed by

---

EDZARD ERNST, PH.D., M.D., is Professor and Head, Department of Physical Medicine and Rehabilitation, University of Vienna, Währinger Gürtel 18-20, A-1097 Vienna, Austria.

oral nimodipine (120 mg/day). An interim analysis (28% of the sample) revealed a worse outcome for patients on the high-dose regimen (compared with placebo), while patients with moderate deficits who received low-dose nimodipine seemed to benefit (compared with placebo).

A recent U.S. multicenter study showed no significant advantage of nimodipine for the sample analyzed as a whole.[17] In 1064 patients, three dosages (60, 120, and 240 mg/day) were compared with placebo. Only patients whose treatment started within 18 hours of stroke with 120 mg/day had a significantly better outcome than did placebo-treated patients. These somewhat disappointing results could again have been due to the relatively long time (48 hours) allowed between the acute event and the beginning of treatment.

Possible Explanations of Inconsistent Findings. How can the discrepancies among studies be explained? Perhaps there is a subgroup of nimodipine responders that has not been identified. Most of the data imply that patients are more likely to be helped by nimodipine if they are affected only moderately by the stroke. Since the aim of the therapy is to salvage tissue in the ischemic penumbra, it makes sense that patients with an appreciable amount of salvageable tissue would be the most likely to benefit.[18] The dosage, route of administration, and use of concomitant therapy should also be considered.

The time window during which treatment has a chance to work may be much smaller than has been believed. Animal experiments indicate that this window may consist not of days but of hours or even minutes.[6,19] The clinical data available to date strongly suggest that the delay between the onset of symptoms and the initiation of treatment should be as short as possible. Thus, study designs allowing 48 hours seem unreasonable.

One study[11] suggests that men are more likely to benefit than women. This possibility requires further investigation.

Other problems complicate interpretation of the clinical trial results. For instance, studies using both mortality rate and neurological outcome as endpoints can be burdened with a severe systematic error. A nimodipine-induced reduction in mortality would lead to worsening of the average neurological score (because survivors, who are likely to have relatively low scores, would be included). In contrast, the most severely afflicted control patients might die, leading to a false-positive result in terms of the average neurological score for surviving controls.

The Swiss group[13] used a follow-up period of four months, while others[11] used longer periods. Some investigators used the Barthel index and others the Mathew scale; neither has been truly validated.[11] The Mathew scale correlates well with the patient's condition,[20] while the Barthel index parallels motor status.[21]

Conclusion. Nimodipine may help in the treatment of ischemic stroke, but it is unlikely to be a complete treatment. The age of therapeutic nihilism in stroke therapy[22] continues to change to one of cautious optimism.

References

1. Harmsen P, Rosengren A, Tsipogianni A et al. Risk factors for stroke in middle-aged men in Göteberg, Sweden. *Stroke*. 1990; 21:223-9.
2. Ernst E. A review of stroke rehabilitation and physiotherapy. *Stroke*. 1990; 21:1081-5.
3. Byer JA, Easton JD. Therapy of ischemic cerebrovascular disease. *Ann Intern Med*. 1980; 93:742-56.
4. Kazda S, Towart R. Nimodipine: a new calcium antagonist drug with a preferential cerebrovascular action. *Acta Neurochir (Wien)*. 1982; 63:259-65.
5. White RP, Cunningham MP, Robertson JT. Effect of the calcium antagonist nimodipine on contractile responses of isolated canine basilar arteries induced by serotonin, prostaglandin $F_{2\text{-}\alpha}$, thrombin, and whole blood. *Neurosurgery*. 1982; 10:344-8.
6. Uematsu D, Greenberg JH, Hickey WF et al. Nimodipine attenuates both increase in cytotoxic free calcium and histologic damage following focal cerebral ischemia and reperfusion in cats. *Stroke*. 1989; 20:1531-7.
7. Steen PA, Gisvold SE, Milde JH et al. Nimodipine improves outcome when given after complete cerebral ischemia in primates. *Anesthesiology*. 1985; 62:406-14.
8. Steen PA, Newberg LA, Milde JH et al. Nimodipine improves cerebral blood flow and neurologic recovery after complete ischemia in the dog. *J Cereb Blood Flow Metab*. 1983; 3:38-43.
9. Bederson JB, Bartkowski HM, Obana W et al. Nimodipine in rat MCA occlusion (MCAO). *Stroke*. 1985; 16:142. Abstract.
10. Gelmers HJ. The effects of nimodipine on the clinical course of patients with acute ischemic stroke. *Acta Neurol Scand*. 1984; 69:232-9.
11. Gelmers HJ, Gorter K, de Weerdt CJ et al. A controlled trial of nimodipine in acute ischemic stroke. *N Engl J Med*. 1988; 318:203-7.
12. Martinez-Vila E, Guillen F, Villanueva A et al. Placebo-controlled trial of nimodipine in the treatment of acute ischemic cerebral ischemia. *Stroke*. 1990; 21:1023-8.
13. Bogousslavsky J, Regli F, Zumstein V et al. Double-blind study of nimodipine in non-severe stroke. *Eur Neurol*. 1990; 30:23-6.
14. Trust Study Group. Randomised, double blind, placebo-controlled trial of nimodipine in acute stroke. *Lancet*. 1990; 336:1205-9.
15. Hornig CR, Kaps M, Hacke W et al. Nimodipine in acute stroke: results of the Nimodipine German–Austrian Stroke Trial. *Stroke*. 1991; 22:153. Abstract.
16. Bridgers SL, Koch G, Munera C et al. Intravenous nimodipine in acute stroke: interim analysis of randomized trials. *Stroke*. 1991; 22:153. Abstract.
17. American Nimodipine Group. Clinical trial of nimodipine in acute ischemic stroke. *Stroke*. 1992; (in press).
18. Heiss WD. Flow thresholds of functional and morphological damage of brain tissue. *Stroke*. 1983; 14:329-31.
19. Barsan WG, Brott TG, Olinger CP et al. Early treatment for acute ischemic stroke. *Ann Intern Med*. 1989; 111:449-51. Editorial.
20. Mathew NT, Meyer JS, Rivera VM et al. Double-blind evaluation of glycerol treatment in acute cerebral infarction. *Lancet*. 1972; 2:1327-9.
21. Loewen SC, Anderson BA. Predictors of stroke outcome using objective measurement scales. *Stroke*. 1990; 21:78-81.
22. Biller J, Love BB. Nihilism and stroke therapy. *Stroke*. 1991; 22:1105-7. Editorial.

Drug Experience

Straightforward reports of unusual drug experiences are included in this section. These may be confirmations of previously reported drug experiences or brief apparent first reports. While selected references may be cited, the purpose of a Drug Experience *report is not to present an extensive review of the literature.*

A related section, Grand Rounds, *includes papers that are well-documented patient case reports with a thorough review of the important literature to help put the case in perspective.*

Simultaneous concentrations of ciprofloxacin in breast milk and in serum in mother and breast-fed infant

DEBRA K. GARDNER, STEVEN G. GABBE, AND CHRIS HARTER

Clin Pharm. 1992; 11:352-4

Ciprofloxacin is a new fluoroquinone with a broad spectrum of aerobic gram-positive and gram-negative activity. Its pharmacokinetic properties contribute to its ability to achieve high tissue concentrations after oral dosing. Because ciprofloxacin produced permanent lesions of the cartilage in immature dogs, the manufacturer has warned against its use in children and pregnant women.[1] Ciprofloxacin-induced arthropathies have also been reported in three children with cystic fibrosis who received high doses of ciprofloxacin for three weeks to three months for pulmonary infections.[2,3] In all cases, the arthropathies resolved after the drug was discontinued. It is not known whether subtherapeutic doses ingested from breast milk would adversely affect an infant, but ciprofloxacin is currently not recommended during breast-feeding if another effective antimicrobial is available.[4]

To date there are two published reports of ciprofloxacin concentrations in breast milk.[5,6] However, in neither of these studies had infants consumed the breast milk. Therefore, to our knowledge, there is no published information on serum concentrations of ciprofloxacin in infants fed breast milk from mothers taking the drug. We report a case in which a woman receiving ciprofloxacin for an episiotomy infection continued to breast-feed her infant, enabling us to determine the concentrations of ciprofloxacin in the breast milk and in the mother's and the infant's serum.

Case Report. A 32-year-old gravida 1, para 0 white woman with insulin-dependent diabetes mellitus of one year's duration was admitted to the hospital at 36 weeks' gestational age with ruptured membranes and contractions every two to three minutes. Her diabetes had been well controlled by three insulin injections per day, as evidenced by a hemoglobin A_{Ic} of 6.3% (normal, 4.4–8%). At delivery, the patient experienced a third-degree laceration with a 4-cm lateral extension, which was repaired with a layered closure. The infant was a 3570-g female, large for her gestational age, with Apgar scores of 8 at one minute and 9 at five minutes. Examination of the patient's perineum on the first postpartum day revealed edematous hemorrhoids, but otherwise the episiotomy appeared to be healing normally. By the second postpartum day, the patient was breast-feeding successfully and was discharged from the hospital.

At a two-week follow-up appointment, the patient was doing well and her episiotomy appeared to be healing satisfactorily. Three weeks later, however, she complained of a yellowish-green discharge from the episiotomy site. Upon examination the area was tender, erythematous, and warm to the touch. The patient was afebrile, and sitz baths four times a day were prescribed.

One week later, an unhealed area of the episiotomy continued to drain purulent fluid, which was sent for culture. Rectal examination revealed hemorrhoids, but no detectable fistula. Sitz baths and perineal irrigations with hydrogen peroxide were prescribed. Cultures grew *Escherichia coli* and α-streptococci; therefore, cephalexin 500 mg p.o. q.i.d. for one week was prescribed, and hydrogen peroxide and saline irrigations were continued. Treatment with irrigation

DEBRA K. GARDNER, PHARM.D., is Clinical Pharmacist, Neonatal Intensive-Care Unit and Obstetrics Unit, Department of Pharmacy, The Ohio State University Hospitals, and Clinical Assistant Professor, College of Pharmacy, The Ohio State University, Columbus. STEVEN G. GABBE, M.D., is Professor and Chairman, Department of Obstetrics and Gynecology, and CHRIS HARTER, R.N., is Nursing Staff Development Coordinator and Lactation Nurse Coordinator, The Ohio State University Hospitals.

Address reprint requests to Dr. Gardner at the Department of Pharmacy, The Ohio State University Hospitals, 410 West 10th Avenue, Columbus, OH 43210.

and warm compresses was continued after antimicrobial therapy was completed.

Because the perineum had not healed at three months postpartum, a small fistula from the sinus tract to the rectum was suspected. Surgical intervention was considered, but it was decided to try a second course of antimicrobials. A culture of the drainage grew *E. coli* sensitive to all standard antimicrobials tested. Because of its ability to achieve high concentrations in gynecologic tissues with oral dosing[7] and its spectrum of gram-negative enteric activity, ciprofloxacin 500 mg (as the hydrochloride salt) p.o. once daily was initiated.

Since there is little information on ciprofloxacin excretion into breast milk and none on the absorption and resulting serum concentrations of ciprofloxacin in the breast-fed infant, we obtained consent from the mother to determine simultaneous milk concentration and maternal and infant serum concentrations of ciprofloxacin during her follow-up appointment. The mother had completed 10 days of ciprofloxacin therapy by taking 500 mg orally at midnight each night after the infant's last breast-feeding. The mother's last dose was at 0001 on the day of the study. The infant was being exclusively breast-fed six times a day; however, she was sleeping through the night at this time. Therefore, on the day of the study the infant's first and only breast-feeding was at 0800, eight hours after the last maternal dose.

Five milliliters of the mother's blood was drawn and 20 mL of breast milk was expressed at approximately 1040. Approximately 1 mL of the infant's blood was also drawn at this time. Both blood samples were immediately spun and the serum was separated. The serum samples and the breast milk were frozen at −20 °C and were shipped on dry ice by overnight delivery to Miles Pharmaceutical Division, Miles Inc., West Haven, Connecticut.

At Miles Inc., a microbiological assay using *Klebsiella pneumoniae* was conducted to determine ciprofloxacin concentrations in the samples. Miles Inc. assured us that the samples were received frozen and the amounts sent were adequate for the assay. The assay's limit of detection is 0.03 μg/mL. The correlation coefficient was 0.995 for the assay of the serum samples and 0.999 for the assay of the breast milk sample. The mother's serum concentration was 0.21 μg/mL and the breast milk concentration was 0.98 μg/mL. The infant's serum concentration was undetectable, or <0.03 μg/mL.

The patient improved during her course of ciprofloxacin. Erythema decreased, and the discharge ceased.

On the day the serum and milk samples were obtained for ciprofloxacin assay, the mother expressed concern about continuing to expose the infant to the antimicrobial. Therefore, the patient was prescribed amoxicillin 500 mg (as the trihydrate) with clavulanic acid 125 mg (as clavulanate potassium) t.i.d. for three weeks. The patient has continued to do well.

Discussion. Giamarellou et al.[5] published the first study on ciprofloxacin in breast milk. In their study, 10 lactating women were given ciprofloxacin 750 mg every 12 hours for three doses and six simultaneous serum and breast milk concentrations were obtained 2–24 hours after the third dose. Peak serum and milk concentrations occurred simultaneously at two hours and were 2.06 μg/mL and 3.79 μg/mL, respectively. Concentrations in both milk and serum declined with a similar curve, with the milk:plasma concentration ratio being highest (2.13) at four hours and averaging 1.7 at most other points. Whether these women continued breast-feeding during the study was not stated, and no data were obtained for their infants.

Cover and Mueller[6] reported the case of a 27-year-old white woman, 17 days postpartum, who was recovering from acute renal failure that required hemodialysis. The patient received one 500-mg dose of ciprofloxacin concomitantly with ferrous sulfate 325 mg. Breast milk concentrations were obtained every four hours for 16 hours after the dose. No maternal serum concentrations were obtained and the patient was not allowed to breast-feed her infant. The ciprofloxacin concentration in her breast milk was 9.1 μmol/L (3.0 μg/mL) at 4, 8, and 12 hours after the dose, and it decreased to 6.0 μmol/L (1.98 μg/mL) by 16 hours. The authors calculated that the infant would have received a cumulative dose of 0.44 mg of ciprofloxacin in that 16-hour period. The breast milk concentration may have remained high in this patient because of her renal impairment.

In our study, serum and breast milk concentrations were lower than those previously published. This is probably because the dosage prescribed was low, 500 mg p.o. daily, and because the breast milk sample was drawn more than 10 hours after the last dose was taken.

The infant in our case was a healthy, exclusively breast-fed four-month-old who weighed 6.1 kg. Infants of this size and age consume an average of 150 mL/kg/day of milk. The ciprofloxacin concentration in our patient's breast milk was obtained at approximately the midpoint of the dosage interval. To estimate the daily dose received by the infant, the milk concentration of approximately 1 μg/mL at the midpoint of the dosage interval was assumed to be the average milk concentration throughout the day. Therefore, the infant would have ingested approximately 0.92 mg per day, or 0.15 mg/kg/day, a very low dose. However, since the maternal dose was taken after the last nursing of the day and the morning breast-feeding occurred eight hours after the dose, the infant may have been exposed to peak rather than average milk concentrations. This issue cannot be resolved, since the concentration of ciprofloxacin in the milk consumed at 0800 is not known, but it does tend to emphasize the importance of timing the dose with respect to breast-feeding.

Conclusion. Although ciprofloxacin was undetectable in the serum sample obtained from this infant, this should not be interpreted as proof that ciprofloxacin can safely be administered during lactation, especially if maternal doses are higher than 500 mg per day and the infant is a small neonate with immature renal function. More information is needed on the excretion of ciprofloxacin in breast milk and the safety of low doses in the infant.

References

1. Gough AW, Barsoum NJ, Renlund RC et al. Fine structural changes during reparative phase of canine drug-induced arthropathy. *Vet Pathol.* 1985; 22:82-4.
2. Jawad ASM. Cystic fibrosis and drug-induced arthropathy. *Br J Rheumatol.* 1989; 28:179-80.
3. Alfaham M, Holt ME, Goodchild MC. Arthropathy in a patient with cystic fibrosis taking ciprofloxacin. *Br Med J.* 1987; 295:699.
4. Briggs GG, Freeman RK, Yaffe SJ. Drugs in pregnancy and lactation. 3rd ed. Baltimore: Williams & Wilkins; 1990; 3(4):19-20.
5. Giamarellou H, Kolokythas E, Petrikkos G et al. Pharmacokinetics of three newer quinolones in pregnant and lactating women. *Am J Med.* 1989; 87(Suppl 5A):49S-51S.
6. Cover DL, Mueller BA. Ciprofloxacin penetration into human breast milk: a case report. *DICP.* 1990; 24:703-4.
7. Dalhoff A, Weuta H. Penetration of ciprofloxacin into gynecologic tissues. *Am J Med.* 1987; 82:133-8.

DUE Criteria

The DUE Criteria *section of* Clinical Pharmacy *features model drug-use evaluation criteria that may be employed as a component of a comprehensive quality assurance program. The criteria sets are presented in the format used in the ASHP book* Criteria for Drug Use Evaluation. *Some of the criteria sets will have been originally published in that book; others will be presented here for the first time and published in future volumes of the ASHP book. The practitioners who developed a criteria set are acknowledged.*

In selecting drug products for coverage in DUE Criteria, *priority is given to products that have been recently marketed, those that are frequently prescribed, those that have high potential risk associated with their use, and those that are expensive. When feasible, a criteria set will be linked with a* Drug Review *that appears in the same issue.*

These criteria sets are a starting point for the development of DUE Criteria for a specific practice setting. Readers are encouraged to modify the model criteria to fit their own circumstances.

Criteria for use of colfosceril (Exosurf Neonatal) in neonates[a]

Element	Standard 100%	Standard 0%	Exception[b] or Critical Preventive/ Responsive Measure[c]	Sources of Information
Justification for Use				
1. Treatment of established respiratory distress syndrome (RDS) in patient requiring mechanical ventilation[1-3] or	X		1A. None	1. History and physical examination (H&P), laboratory reports, radiology reports, physician orders
2. Prophylaxis in infant at risk for developing RDS[4-6] who meets one or more of the following criteria: a. Estimated gestational age (EGA) <28 wk b. Birth weight (BW) <1250 g c. Absence of fetal lung maturity documented by amniotic fluid analysis or	X		2A. None	2. Maternal medical record, laboratory reports, H&P, progress notes, physician orders
3. Treatment of respiratory distress (RD) that requires mechanical ventilation and is due to sepsis, adult respiratory distress syndrome (ARDS), or meconium aspiration syndrome (MAS)[7,8]	X		3A. None	3. H&P, progress notes, laboratory reports, radiology reports, physician orders
Critical (Process) Indicators				
4. Treatment of RDS or RD: mechanical ventilation required and diagnosis of RDS or RD confirmed by chest roentgenogram and arterial blood gas determination	X		4A. None	4. H&P, laboratory reports, radiology reports, respiratory therapy flow sheets, progress notes, maternal medical record
5. Prophylactic use for preterm infant: BW and EGA or amniotic fluid studies support use	X		5A. None	5. H&P, prenatal and birth history, maternal medical record, laboratory reports of amniotic fluid analysis
6. Appropriate dosage for treatment of RDS due to	X		6A. Assisted ventilation terminated before completion of two	6. Physician orders, medication administration record (MAR),

Prepared by Varsha Bhatt-Mehta, Pharm.D., Clinical Pharmacist, Newborn Intensive Care Unit, University of Michigan Medical Center, Ann Arbor, and Clinical Assistant Professor of Pharmacy, College of Pharmacy, University of Michigan, and Robert E. Schumacher, M.D., Assistant Professor of Pediatrics, Department of Pediatrics and Communicable Diseases, University of Michigan Medical Center.

Element	Standard 100%	Standard 0%	Exception[b] or Critical Preventive/ Responsive Measure[c]		Sources of Information
surfactant deficiency or RD due to sepsis, ARDS, or MAS: 5 mL/kg every 12 hr for two doses[9]			doses 6B. Up to 4–6 doses needed for patient with persistent requirement for mechanical ventilation due to RDS 6C. Dosage interval shortened on basis of clinical response	 6A. 6B,C.	respiratory therapy notes Physician orders, MAR, respiratory therapy notes Physician orders, MAR, laboratory reports, radiology reports, respiratory therapy notes
7. Appropriate dosage for prophylactic use: 5 mL/kg every 12 hr for three doses with first dose administered as soon as possible after birth[9]	X		7A. Assisted ventilation terminated before completion of three doses 7B. Up to 4–6 doses needed for patient with persistent requirement for mechanical ventilation	7. 7A. 7B.	Physician orders, MAR Physician orders, MAR, respiratory therapy notes Physician orders, MAR, laboratory reports, respiratory therapy notes
8. All doses administered via endotracheal tube without disturbing mechanical ventilator in accordance with product labeling[9]	X		8A. None	8.	Product labeling, MAR, respiratory therapy notes
9. Endotracheal tube suctioned before dose given[9]	X		9A. None	9.	Respiratory therapy notes
Complications					
10. Pulmonary hemorrhage		X	10A. Provide supportive care 10B. Investigate for presence of significant patent ductus arteriosus[4,9]	10. 10A. 10B.	Progress notes, radiology reports, nursing notes, respiratory therapy notes Physician orders, progress notes Physician orders, progress notes
11. Mucus plugs in the endotracheal tube		X	11A. Suction if mucus plug suspected[9] 11B. Replace endotracheal tube if suctioning unsuccessful[9]	11,11A,B.	Progress notes, nursing notes, respiratory therapy notes
12. Apnea		X	12A. Provide supportive care (e.g., methylxanthines)	12. 12A.	Progress notes, nursing notes Physician orders, MAR
13. Reflux of drug in endotracheal tube during dosing		X	13A. Stop drug administration until endotracheal tube clears (may need to increase peak inspiratory pressure to clear tube)[9]	13,13A.	Progress notes, respiratory therapy notes, nursing notes
14. Decrease in transcutaneous oxygen saturation		X	14A. Stop drug administration[9] 14B. Temporarily increase inspired oxygen fraction (Fio_2) and peak inspiratory pressure[9]	14,14A,B.	Progress notes, respiratory therapy notes, laboratory reports, nursing notes
Outcome Measures					
15. Treatment of established RDS: decreased severity of RDS (decrease in Fio_2 needs, decrease in ventilator rate and pressures, increase in arterial blood oxygen tension)	X		15A. Patient died 15B. Patient did not tolerate treatment	15. 15A. 15B.	Progress notes, respiratory therapy notes, radiology reports Progress notes Progress notes, respiratory therapy notes, nursing notes
16. RDS prophylaxis: patient did not develop RDS	X		16A. Patient died 16B. Patient did not tolerate treatment	16. 16A. 16B.	Progress notes, laboratory reports, radiology reports Progress notes Progress notes, respiratory therapy notes, nursing notes
17. Treatment of RD due to sepsis, ARDS, or MAS: decreased severity of RD (i.e., decrease in Fio_2 needs)	X		17A. Patient died 17B. Patient did not tolerate treatment	17. 17A. 17B.	Progress notes, laboratory reports, radiology reports Progress notes Progress notes, respiratory therapy notes, nursing notes

[a] Criteria address justification for use (indications), critical (process) indicators, complications of therapy, and patient outcome. Each criterion consists of an element, a standard, exceptions to the standard, and sources of information. The element is the minimum level of evidence needed to show that patient care was optimal. The standard defines the deviation from an element that is acceptable. If no deviation is acceptable, the standard is 100%. Exceptions are circumstances in which deviation is allowable. Sources of information listed are the most reliable sources. Sources pertaining to an element or exception are identified by the number assigned to the element or exception (e.g., 6, 6A).

[b] For justification for use and critical (process) indicators.

[c] For complications and outcome measures.

References

1. Long W, Thompson T, Sundell H et al. Effects of two rescue doses of a synthetic surfactant on mortality rate and survival without bronchopulmonary dysplasia in 700- to 1350-gram infants with respiratory distress syndrome. *J Pediatr.* 1991; 118:595-605.
2. Canadian Exosurf Pediatric Study Group. Effects of two rescue doses of Exosurf Pediatric in 342 750–1249 gram infants. *Pediatr Res.* 1990; 27:200A.
3. U.S. and Canadian Exosurf Pediatric Study Group. Effects of two rescue doses of Exosurf Pediatric in 1232 infants ≥1250 grams. *Pediatr Res.* 1990; 27:320A.
4. Corbet A, Bucciarelli R, Goldman S et al. Decreased mortality rate among small premature infants treated at birth with a single dose of synthetic surfactant: a multicenter controlled trial. *J Pediatr.* 1991; 118:277-84.
5. Corbet A, Bose C, Long W et al. Effects of a single prophylactic dose of Exosurf Pediatric at birth in 700–1350 gram infants. *Pediatr Res.* 1990; 27:298A.
6. Kendig JW, Notter RH, Cox C et al. A comparison of surfactant as immediate prophylaxis and as rescue therapy in newborns of less than 30 weeks' gestation. *N Engl J Med.* 1991; 324:865-71.
7. U.S. Exosurf Pediatric Study Group. Effects of Exosurf Pediatric on infants with occult congenital pneumonia. *Pediatr Res.* 1990; 27:228A.
8. Auten RL, Notter RH, Kendig JW et al. Surfactant treatment of full-term newborns with respiratory failure. *Pediatrics.* 1991; 87:101-7.
9. Burroughs Wellcome. Exosurf Neonatal package insert. Research Triangle Park, NC; 1990 Aug.

Criteria for use of beractant (Survanta) in neonates[a]

Element	Standard 100%	Standard 0%	Exception[b] or Critical Preventive/Responsive Measure[c]	Sources of Information
Justification for Use				
1. Prevention of respiratory distress syndrome (RDS) in patient with one or both of the following risk factors: a. Estimated gestational age ≤30 weeks[1] b. Estimated birth weight <1250 g[2] or	X		1A. Lecithin : sphingomyelin (L:S) ratio >2[3] 1B. No clinical signs of RDS on examination in operating room (OR)	1. Maternal progress notes, fetal ultrasound report 1A. Report of amniocentesis with L:S ratio 1B. OR notes
2. Treatment of RDS in patient who meets all of the following criteria: a. Age ≤8 hr[2,4] b. Radiographic evidence of RDS[2] c. Mechanical ventilation with inspired oxygen fraction (FIO_2) ≥0.3 required to maintain arterial PO_2 >50 mm Hg[2]	X		2A. Therapy delayed because of patient transfer 2B. Therapy delayed because of patient instability (e.g., pneumothorax, hypotension)	2. Progress notes, nursing flow sheets, radiology reports, laboratory reports 2A, B. Progress notes, physician orders
Critical (Process) Indicators				
For Prophylactic Use				
3. First dose given within 15 min after birth[2]	X		3A. Resuscitation necessary or patient unstable	3, 3A. Physician orders, progress notes, anesthesia records, medication administration record (MAR)
4. Need for additional doses supported by radiographic evidence of RDS[2]	X		4A. None	4. Radiology reports
For Prophylactic Use or Treatment of RDS				
5. FIO_2 >0.3 required to maintain arterial PO_2 >50 mm Hg at time of additional doses[2]	X		5A. None	5. Nursing flow sheets, laboratory reports, MAR
6. Beractant administered using technique described in the package insert[2]	X		6A. None	6. Nursing notes, package insert

Prepared by Rebecca Rogers Prevost, Pharm.D., Clinical Pharmacist for Obstetrics–Gynecology–Neonatology, Regional Medical Center, Memphis, TN; Robert Mirro, M.D, Neonatologist and Associate Professor, Departments of Pediatrics, Obstetrics and Gynecology, and Physiology, University of Tennessee, Memphis; and Sheldon B. Korones, M.D., Medical Director of the Newborn Center and Professor, Departments of Pediatrics and Obstetrics and Gynecology, University of Tennessee.

Element	Standard 100%	Standard 0%	Exception[b] or Critical Preventive/ Responsive Measure[c]	Sources of Information	
7. Appropriate dose administered: 4 mL/kg[2]	X		7A. None	7.	Physician orders, MAR
8. Additional doses administered at intervals no less than six hours apart[2]	X		8A. None	8.	Physician orders, MAR
9. Endotracheal tube not suctioned within one hour after dose administration[2]	X		9A. Endotracheal tube plugged 9B. Pulmonary hemorrhage	9, 9A, B.	Nursing flow sheets, progress notes, physician orders
10. Infant closely monitored (e.g., oxygen saturation, heart rate, blood pressure, arterial blood gases) for 30 min after dose administration for changes that require adjustments in ventilator settings[5,6]	X		10A. None	10.	Nursing flow sheets, laboratory reports
11. No more than four doses given	X		11A. None	11.	Physician orders, MAR
Complications					
12. Endotracheal tube blockage[2]		X	12A. Suction endotracheal tube 12B. Replace endotracheal tube if suctioning is unsuccessful	12, 12A, B.	Nursing notes, progress notes
13. Reflux of drug in endotracheal tube during administration		X	13A. Stop drug administration until infant is stable 13B. Increase peak inspiratory pressure (PIP)	13, 13A, B.	Nursing notes, progress notes
14. Decrease in oxygen saturation with dosing[2]		X	14A. Stop drug administration until infant is stable 14B. Increase PIP, FiO_2	14, 14A, B.	Nursing flow sheets, laboratory reports
15. Pulmonary air leak[2]		X	15A. Insert chest tube	15,15A.	Nursing notes, progress notes
16. Bradycardia[2]		X	16A. Support heart rate, check for blocked endotracheal tube, check endotracheal tube placement, check for air leaks	16, 16A.	Nursing flow sheets, progress notes
17. Pallor[2]		X	17A. Provide supportive care, check for blocked endotracheal tube, check endotracheal tube placement, check for air leaks	17, 17A.	Nursing notes, progress notes
18. Hypertension or hypotension[2]		X	18A. Provide supportive care	18, 18A.	Nursing flow sheets
19. Cyanosis		X	19A. Adjust ventilator settings as needed, check for blocked endotracheal tube, check endotracheal tube placement, check for air leaks	19, 19A.	Nursing notes, progress notes
Outcome Measures					
20. RDS prophylaxis: RDS prevented or course attenuated[7]	X		20A. Patient died 20B. Patient did not tolerate therapy	20. 20A. 20B.	Progress notes, nursing notes, radiology reports, laboratory reports Progress notes Progress notes, nursing notes
21. Treatment of established RDS: RDS less severe (mean airway pressure <5 cm H_2O within 7 days, infant weaned from oxygen therapy within 28 days, FiO_2 reduced by 20% after dose administration, no progression to bronchopulmonary dysplasia)	X		21A. Patient died 21B. Patient did not tolerate therapy	21. 21A. 21B.	Progress notes, nursing notes, radiology reports, laboratory reports Progress notes Progress notes, nursing notes
22. RDS prophylaxis or treatment: death due to RDS prevented[8]	X		22A. Patient died 22B Patient did not tolerate therapy	22, 22A. 22B.	Progress notes Progress notes, nursing notes

[a] Criteria address justification for use (indications), critical (process) indicators, complications of therapy, and patient outcome. Each criterion consists of an element, a standard, exceptions to the standard, and sources of information. The element is the minimum level of evidence needed to show that patient care was optimal. The standard defines the deviation from an element that is acceptable. If no deviation is acceptable, the standard is 100%. Exceptions are circumstances in which deviation is allowable. Sources of information listed are the most reliable sources. Sources pertaining to an element or exception are identified by the number assigned to the element or exception (e.g., 1, 1A).

[b] For justification for use and critical (process) indicators.

[c] For complications and outcome measures.

References

1. Kendig JW, Notter RH, Cox C et al. A comparison of surfactant as immediate prophylaxis and as rescue in newborns of less than thirty weeks' gestation. *N Engl J Med.* 1991; 324:865-71.
2. Ross Laboratories. Survanta package insert. Columbus, OH; 1991 Aug.
3. Gluck L. Evaluation of fetal lung maturation by analysis of phospholipid indicators in amniotic fluid. In: Lung maturation and the prevention of hyaline membrane disease. Proceedings of the 70th Ross conference on pediatric research. Columbus, OH: Ross Laboratories; 1976:47-9.
4. Rosenburg AA. Surfactant replacement therapy and the respiratory distress syndrome. *Pediatr Update.* 1991; 2:2-6.
5. Horbar JD, Soll RF, Sutherland JM et al. A multicenter randomized, placebo-controlled trial of surfactant therapy for respiratory distress syndrome. *N Engl J Med.* 1989; 320:959-65.
6. Bhat R, Dziedzic K, Bhutani VK. Effect of single dose surfactant on pulmonary function. *Crit Care Med.* 1990; 18:590-5.
7. Hoekstra RE, Jackson JC, Myers TF et al. Improved neonatal survival following multiple doses of bovine surfactant in very premature neonates at risk for respiratory distress syndrome. *Pediatrics.* 1991; 88:10-8.
8. Liechty EA, Donovan E, Purohit D et al. Reduction of neonatal mortality after multiple doses of bovine surfactant in low birth weight neonates with respiratory distress syndrome. *Pediatrics.* 1991; 88:19-28.

A change to Zefazone is no small change

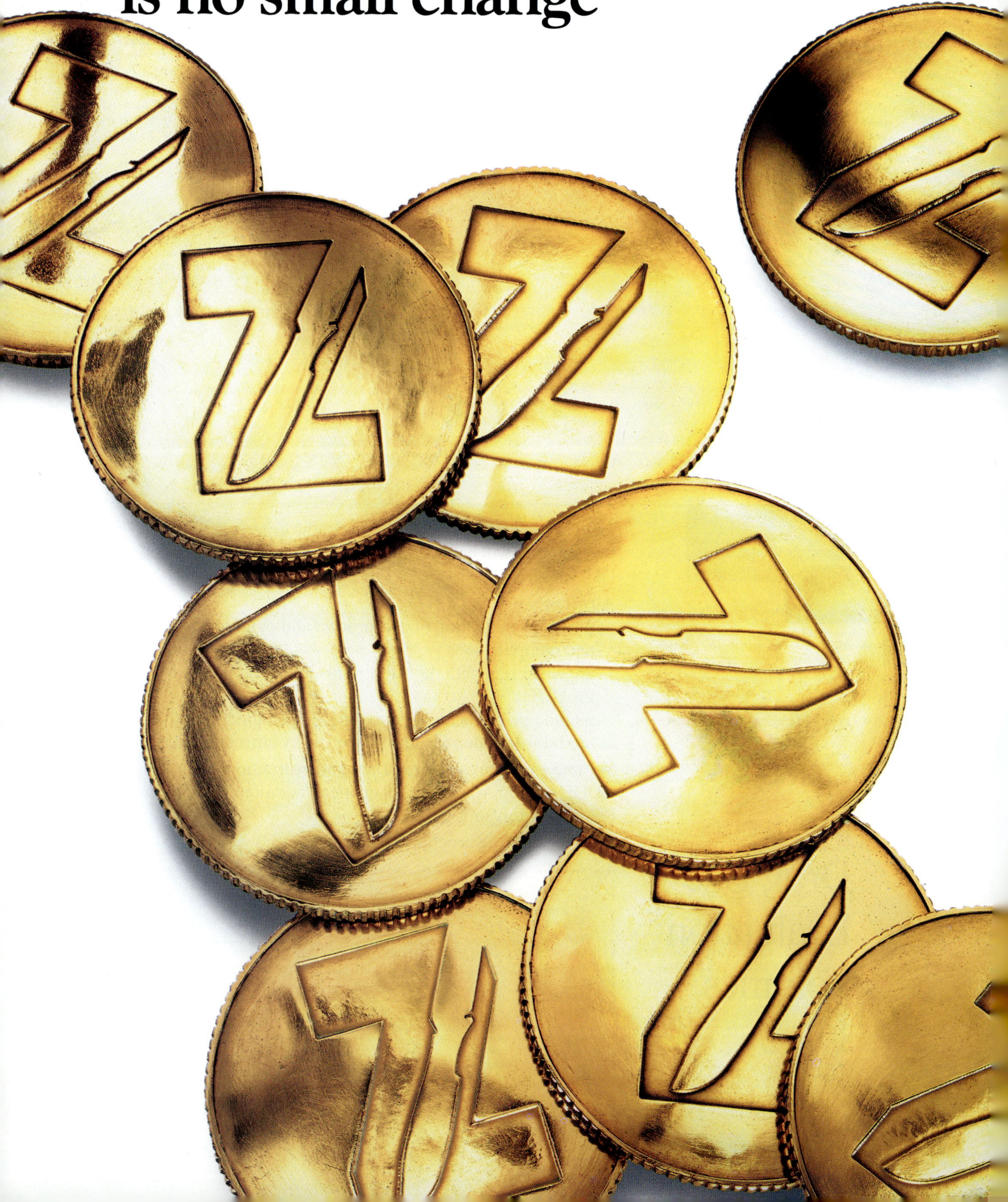

EXOSURF® Neonatal™

(COLFOSCERIL PALMITATE, CETYL ALCOHOL, TYLOXAPOL) For Intratracheal Suspension / 10 mL vials

PLEASE CONSULT FULL PRODUCT INFORMATION BEFORE PRESCRIBING.

INDICATIONS AND USAGE: Exosurf Neonatal is indicated for:

1. **Prophylactic** treatment of infants with birth weights of less than 1350 grams who are at risk of developing RDS (see PRECAUTIONS),
2. **Prophylactic** treatment of infants with birth weights greater than 1350 grams who have evidence of pulmonary immaturity, and
3. **Rescue** treatment of infants who have developed RDS.

CONTRAINDICATIONS: There are no known contraindications to treatment with Exosurf Neonatal.

WARNINGS: Intratracheal Administration Only: Exosurf Neonatal should be administered only by instillation into the trachea. **General:** The use of Exosurf Neonatal requires expert clinical care by experienced neonatologists and other clinicians who are accomplished at neonatal intubation and ventilatory management. Adequate personnel, facilities, equipment, and medications are required to optimize perinatal outcome in premature infants. Instillation of Exosurf Neonatal should be performed **only** by trained medical personnel experienced in airway and clinical management of unstable premature infants. Vigilant clinical attention should be given to all infants prior to, during, and after administration of Exosurf Neonatal. **Acute Effects:** Exosurf Neonatal can rapidly affect oxygenation and lung compliance. **Lung Compliance:** If chest expansion improves substantially after dosing, peak ventilator inspiratory pressures should be reduced immediately, without waiting for confirmation of respiratory improvement by blood gas assessment. Failure to reduce inspiratory ventilator pressures rapidly in such instances can result in lung overdistention and fatal pulmonary air leak. **Hyperoxia:** If the infant becomes pink and transcutaneous oxygen saturation is in excess of 95%, FiO_2 should be reduced in small but repeated steps (until saturation is 90 to 95%) without waiting for confirmation of elevated arterial pO_2 by blood gas assessment. Failure to reduce FiO_2 in such instances can result in hyperoxia. **Hypocarbia:** If arterial or transcutaneous CO_2 measurements are <30 torr, the ventilator rate should be reduced at once. Failure to reduce ventilator rates in such instances can result in marked hypocarbia, which is known to reduce brain blood flow. **Pulmonary Hemorrhage:** In the single study conducted in infants weighing <700 grams at birth, the incidence of pulmonary hemorrhage (10% vs 2% in the placebo group) was significantly increased in the Exosurf Neonatal group. None of the five studies involving infants with birth weights >700 grams showed a significant increase in pulmonary hemorrhage in the Exosurf Neonatal group. In a cross-study analysis of these five studies, pulmonary hemorrhage was reported for 1% (14/1420) of infants in the placebo group and 2% (27/1411) of infants in the Exosurf Neonatal group. Fatal pulmonary hemorrhage occurred in three infants; two in the Exosurf Neonatal group and one in the placebo group. Mortality from all causes among infants who developed pulmonary hemorrhage was 43% in the placebo group and 37% in the Exosurf Neonatal group. Pulmonary hemorrhage in both Exosurf Neonatal and placebo infants was more frequent in infants who were younger, smaller, male, or who had a patent ductus arteriosus. Pulmonary hemorrhage typically occurred in the first 2 days of life in both treatment groups. In more than 7700 infants in the open, uncontrolled study, pulmonary hemorrhage was reported in 4%, but fatal pulmonary hemorrhage was reported rarely (0.4%). In the controlled clinical studies, Exosurf Neonatal treated infants who received steroids more than 24 hours prior to delivery or indomethacin postnatally had a lower rate of pulmonary hemorrhage than other Exosurf Neonatal treated infants. Attention should be paid to early and aggressive diagnosis and treatment (unless contraindicated) of patent ductus arteriosus during the first 2 days of life (while the ductus arteriosus is often clinically silent). Other potentially protective measures include attempting to decrease FiO_2 preferentially over ventilator pressures during the first 24 to 48 hours after dosing, and attempting to decrease PEEP minimally for at least 48 hours after dosing. **Mucous Plugs:** Infants whose ventilation becomes markedly impaired during or shortly after dosing may have mucous plugging of the endotracheal tube, particularly if pulmonary secretions were prominent prior to drug administration. Suctioning of all infants prior to dosing may lessen the chance of mucous plugs obstructing the endotracheal tube. If endotracheal tube obstruction from such plugs is suspected, and suctioning is unsuccessful in removing the obstruction, the blocked endotracheal tube should be replaced immediately.

PRECAUTIONS:

General: In the controlled clinical studies, infants known prenatally or postnatally to have major congenital anomalies, or who were suspected of having congenital infection, were excluded from entry. However, these disorders cannot be recognized early in life in all cases, and a few infants with these conditions were entered. The benefits of Exosurf Neonatal in the affected infants who received drug appeared to be similar to the benefits observed in infants without anomalies or occult infection. **Prophylactic Treatment-Infants <700 Grams:** In infants weighing 500 to 700 grams, a single prophylactic dose of Exosurf Neonatal significantly: improved FiO_2 and ventilator settings, reduced pneumothorax, and reduced death from RDS, but increased pulmonary hemorrhage (see WARNINGS). Overall mortality did not differ significantly between the placebo and Exosurf Neonatal groups (see Table 1 in full product information). Data on multiple doses in infants in this weight class are not yet available. Accordingly, clinicians should carefully evaluate the potential risks and benefits of Exosurf Neonatal administration in these infants. **Rescue Treatment-Number of Doses:** A small number of infants with RDS have received more than two doses of Exosurf Neonatal as rescue treatment. Definitive data on the safety and efficacy of these additional doses are not available. **Carcinogenesis, Mutagenesis, Impairment of Fertility:** Exosurf Neonatal at concentrations up to 10,000 μg/plate was not mutagenic in the Ames Salmonella assay. Long-term studies have not been performed in animals to evaluate the carcinogenic potential of Exosurf Neonatal. The effects of Exosurf Neonatal on fertility have not been studied.

ADVERSE REACTIONS:

General: Premature birth is associated with a high incidence of morbidity and mortality. Despite significant reductions in overall mortality associated with Exosurf Neonatal, some infants who received Exosurf Neonatal developed severe complications and either survived with permanent handicaps or died.

In controlled clinical studies evaluating the safety and efficacy of Exosurf Neonatal, numerous safety assessments were made. In infants receiving Exosurf Neonatal, pulmonary hemorrhage, apnea and use of methylxanthines were increased. A number of other adverse events were significantly reduced in the Exosurf Neonatal group, particularly various forms of pulmonary air leak and use of pancuronium. Tables 3 and 4 summarize the results of the major safety evaluations from the controlled clinical studies.

Table 3: Safety Assessments[a]—Prophylactic Treatment

Number of Doses:	Single Dose		Single Dose		Single Dose		1 vs 3 Doses	
Birth Weight Range:	500 to 700 grams		700 to 1350 grams		700 to 1100 grams		700 to 1100 grams	
Treatment Group:	Placebo (Air)	EXOSURF	Placebo (Air)	EXOSURF	Placebo (Air)	EXOSURF	EXOSURF 1 Dose	EXOSURF 3 Doses
Number of Infants:	N=108	N=107	N=193	N=192	N=222	N=224	N=356	N=360
	% of Infants		% of Infants		% of Infants		% of Infants	
Intraventricular Hemorrhage (IVH)								
Overall	51	57	31	27	36	36	38	35
Severe IVH	26	25	10	8	13	14	9	9
Pulmonary Air Leak (PAL)								
Overall	52	48	16	11	32	25	29	27
Pneumothorax	23	10*	5	6	19	11*	14	12
Pneumopericardium	1	4	2	0	<1	1	1	1
Pneumomediastinum	2	1	2	3	7	1**	3	2
Pulmonary Interstitial Emphysema	43	44	13	7*	26	20	23	22
Death from PAL	4	6	<1	<1	2	1	2	1
Patent Ductus Arteriosus	49	53	66	70	50	55	59	57
Necrotizing Enterocolitis	2	4	11	13	3	4	6	2*
Pulmonary Hemorrhage	2	10**	2	4	1	4	4	6
Congenital Pneumonia	4	4	2	4	2	2	1	1
Nosocomial Pneumonia	10	10	2	4	4	7	14	15
Non-Pulmonary Infections	33	35	34	39	28	29	35	34
Sepsis	30	34	30	34	23	24	30	27
Death From Sepsis	4	4	3	3	1	2	3	2
Meningitis	4	6	3	1	2	3	1	2
Other Infections	7	4	5	3	6	10	10	11
Major Anomalies	3	1	2	4	7	4	4	4

Table 3: Safety Assessments[a]—Prophylactic Treatment (Cont.)

Number of Doses:	Single Dose		Single Dose		Single Dose		1 vs 3 Doses	
Birth Weight Range:	500 to 700 grams		700 to 1350 grams		700 to 1100 grams		700 to 1100 grams	
Treatment Group:	Placebo (Air)	EXOSURF	Placebo (Air)	EXOSURF	Placebo (Air)	EXOSURF	EXOSURF 1 Dose	EXOSURF 3 Doses
Number of Infants:	N=108	N=107	N=193	N=192	N=222	N=224	N=356	N=360
	% of Infants		% of Infants		% of Infants		% of Infants	
Hypotension	70	77	52	47	59	62	54	50
Hyperbilirubinemia	22	21	63	61	27	31	20	21
Exchange Transfusion	4	3	1	2	2	2	3	1
Thrombocytopenia[b]	21	25	not available		9	8	12	10
Persistent Fetal Circulation	0	1	1	1	0	2*	1	<1
Seizures	11	8	2	2	11	9	6	5
Apnea	34	33	76	73	55	65*	62	68
Drug Therapy								
Antibiotics	96	99	98	96	98	99	>99	99
Diuretics	55	60	39	37	59	63	64	65
Anticonvulsants	14	18	23	24	20	16	9	8
Inotropes	46	40	20	20	26	20	28	27
Sedatives	62	71	65	64	63	57	52	52
Pancuronium	19	11	22	14*	19	13*	15	11
Methylxanthines	38	43	77	77	61	72*	75	82*

[a] All parameters were examined with "as-treated" analyses. * $p<0.05$
[b] Thrombocytopenia requiring platelet transfusion. ** $p<0.01$

Table 4: Safety Assessments[a]—Rescue Treatment

Number of Doses:	Two Doses		Two Doses	
Birth Weight Range:	700 to 1350 grams		1250 grams and above	
Treatment Group:	Placebo (Air)	EXOSURF	Placebo (Air)	EXOSURF
Number of Infants:	N=213	N=206	N=622	N=615
	% of Infants		% of Infants	
Intraventricular Hemorrhage (IVH)				
Overall	48	52	23	18*
Severe IVH	13	9	5	4
Pulmonary Air Leak (PAL)				
Overall	54	34***	30	18***
Pneumothorax	29	20*	20	10***
Pneumopericardium	4	1	1	2
Pneumomediastinum	8	4	5	2**
Pulmonary Interstitial Emphysema	48	25***	24	13***
Death from PAL	7	3	<1	1
Patent Ductus Arteriosus	66	57	54	45*
Necrotizing Enterocolitis	3	3	1	2
Pulmonary Hemorrhage	3	1	<1	1
Congenital Pneumonia	2	3	2	2
Nosocomial Pneumonia	5	7	2	2
Non-Pulmonary Infections	19	22	13	13
Sepsis	15	17	8	8
Death From Sepsis	<1	<1	1	<1
Meningitis	1	<1	1	<1*
Other Infections	5	8	5	6
Major Anomalies	3	3	4	4
Hypotension	62	57	50	39**
Hyperbilirubinemia	17	19	12	10
Exchange Transfusion	3	4	1	2
Thrombocytopenia[b]	10	11	4	<1**
Persistent Fetal Circulation	1	1	6	2**
Seizures	10	10	6	3*
Apnea	48	65**	37	44*
Drug Therapy				
Antibiotics	100	99	98	98
Diuretics	60	65	45	34***
Anticonvulsants	17	17	10	5**
Inotropes	36	31	27	16***
Sedatives	72	68	76	64***
Pancuronium	34	17**	33	15***
Methylxanthines	62	74**	49	53

[a] All parameters were examined with "as-treated" analyses. * $p<0.05$ *** $p<0.001$
[b] Thrombocytopenia requiring platelet transfusion. ** $p<0.01$

Pulmonary Hemorrhage: See WARNINGS. **Abnormal Laboratory Values:** Abnormal laboratory values are common in critically ill, mechanically ventilated, premature infants. A higher incidence of abnormal laboratory values in the Exosurf Neonatal group was not reported. **Events During Dosing:** Data on events during dosing are available from more than 8800 infants in the open, uncontrolled clinical study (Table 5).

Table 5: Events During Dosing in the Open, Uncontrolled Study[a]

Treatment Type:	Prophylactic Treatment	Rescue Treatment
Number of Infants:	N=1127	N=7711
	% of Infants	% of Infants
Reflux of Exosurf	20	31
Drop in O_2 saturation ($\geq$20%)	6	22
Rise in O_2 saturation ($\geq$10%)	5	6
Drop in transcutaneous pO_2 ($\geq$20 mm Hg)	1	8
Rise in transcutaneous pO_2 ($\geq$20 mm Hg)	2	5
Drop in transcutaneous pCO_2 ($\geq$20 mm Hg)	<1	1
Rise in transcutaneous pCO_2 ($\geq$20 mm Hg)	1	3
Bradycardia (<60 beats/min)	1	3
Tachycardia (>200 beats/min)	<1	<1
Gagging	1	5
Mucous Plugs	<1	<1

[a] Infants may have experienced more than one event.
Investigators were prohibited from adjusting FiO_2 and/or ventilator settings during dosing unless significant clinical deterioration occurred.

Reflux: Reflux of Exosurf Neonatal into the endotracheal tube during dosing has been observed and may be associated with rapid drug administration. If reflux occurs, drug administration should be halted and, if necessary, peak inspiratory pressure on the ventilator should be increased by 4 to 5 cm H_2O until the endotracheal tube clears. ***>20% Drop in Transcutaneous Oxygen Saturation:*** If transcutaneous oxygen saturation declines during dosing, drug administration should be halted and, if necessary, peak inspiratory pressure on the ventilator should be increased by 4 to 5 cm H_2O for 1 to 2 minutes. In addition, increases of FiO_2 may be required for 1 to 2 minutes. ***Mucous Plugs:*** See WARNINGS.

DOSAGE AND ADMINISTRATION: See full product information.

Wellcome
BURROUGHS WELLCOME CO., Research Triangle Park, NC 27709

Printed in U.S.A. EX-Y01228

Current Literature

Drug Reaction Alerts 368

Book Review

Data Collection Forms in Clinical Trials 373
By Bert Spilker and John Schoenfelder
Reviewed by Karen J. Schoenbrun

Books Received 374

Drug Reaction Alerts

Drug Reaction Alerts focuses primarily on serious, unlabeled reactions to new chemical entities. The citations are compiled monthly from International Pharmaceutical Abstracts, which covers over 800 pharmacy and health-related journals worldwide. An address for reprints (when available) follows the name of the corresponding author in each citation.

Pharmacists may use the FDA Adverse Reaction Report form that appears in the January and July issues of Clinical Pharmacy for submitting reports of adverse drug reactions directly to FDA.

Anticoagulants

De Keyser J, Herroelen L (Department of Neurology, Academisch, Ziekenhuis, Free University of Brussels, B 1090 Brussels, Belgium). Strokes soon after oral anticoagulant therapy in patients with atrial fibrillation. *Lancet*. 1991; 338:1158. Cases. (63-year-old woman and 71-year-old man with atrial fibrillation; woman received **acenocoumarol** 4 mg on day 1 and 3 mg on day 2; man received acenocoumarol 8 mg on day 1 and 4 mg on day 2; developed hemiplegia within 48 hours after first dose of acenocoumarol; computed tomography scan five days later revealed nonhemorrhagic infarction in territory of a cerebral artery; woman slowly improved, but man died from bronchopneumonia 20 days after hemiplegic event)

Antifungals

Persons DA, Laughlin M, Tanner D et al. (Hathorn JW, Duke University Medical Center, Durham, NC 27710). **Fluconazole** and *Candida krusei* fungemia. *N Engl J Med*. 1991; 325:1315. Cases. (four immunocompromised patients with cancer; received fluconazole 100–200 mg daily as i.v. infusion as primary therapy or chemoprophylaxis for oropharyngeal candidiasis; developed *Candida krusei* infections; three patients developed episodes of fever and received therapy with broad-spectrum antimicrobials; blood cultures grew *C. krusei*; therapy with amphotericin B led to improvement in two patients but other two patients deteriorated and died)

Wingard JR (Bone Marrow Transplant Program, Division of Hematology/Oncology, Department of Medicine, Emory University School of Medicine, Atlanta, GA 30322), Merz WG, Rinaldi MG et al. Increase in *Candida krusei* infection among patients with bone marrow transplantation and neutropenia treated prophylactically with **fluconazole**. *N Engl J Med*. 1991; 325:1274-7. Study. (retrospective; 439 adult inpatients who had undergone bone marrow transplantation or who had leukemia during 1989–90; 84 patients received fluconazole 400 mg daily as chemoprophylaxis for disseminated candidal infection, and 355 patients did not receive fluconazole; 8.3% of fluconazole-treated patients developed *C. krusei* infections compared with 1.2% of untreated patients [$p = 0.002$]; colonization by *C. krusei* occurred in 40.5% of fluconazole-treated patients versus 16.7% of untreated patients [$p < 0.0001$])

Anti-inflammatory Agents

Ahmed M (128 Knight's Manor Way, Dartford, Kent DA1 5SP, England), Davison OW. Severe cystitis associated with

tiaprofenic acid. *Br Med J*. 1991; 303:1376. Cases. (three women, aged 69–82 years; received tiaprofenic acid 300–600 mg/day for a few weeks to eight months; developed severe cystitis; withdrawal of tiaprofenic acid led to resolution of symptoms)

Antimalarial Agents

Shlim DR (The CIWEC Clinic, Kathmandu, Nepal). Severe facial rash associated with **mefloquine**. *JAMA*. 1991; 266:2560. Case. (23-year-old female tourist to central Asia; received mefloquine 250 mg twice in two weeks; developed burning sensation on face three days after first dose; symptom progressed to raised, bullous lesions in symmetrical pattern on day of second dose; concomitant oral contraceptive tablets; therapy with cephalexin and topical hydrocortisone for presumed bedbug bites did not lead to resolution of rash; therapy with tapered six-day course of prednisone led to improvement of patient's rash and complete resolution of rash four months later)

Antineoplastic Agents

Durand JM (Department of Internal Medicine, Hôpital Sainte-Marguerite, 13009 Marseilles, France), Kaplanski G, Portal I et al. Liver failure due to recombinant alpha interferon. *Lancet*. 1991; 338:1268-9. Case. (60-year-old man with hairy cell leukemia; received **interferon alfa-2b** 3 million units three times weekly as s.c. injections for nine months; developed liver failure; liver tissue biopsy revealed widespread periportal fibrosis, cholestatis of liver canaliculi, centrilobular zonal necrosis, and mild portal and periportal inflammation without hairy cell infiltration; developed *Staphylococcus aureus* infection and died from septic shock)

Miles DW, Longhurst SJ, Harper PG et al. (Balkwill FR, Biological Therapies Laboratory, Imperial Cancer Research Fund, London WC2, England). Toxicity and reconstitution of recombinant interleukin 2 with albumin. *Lancet*. 1991; 338:1464. Case. (47-year-old woman with metastatic malignant melanoma; received **aldesleukin** 18 million IU/sq m/day for five days as continuous infusion; for first course, dextrose injection without albumin was used to reconstitute aldesleukin; for second course, dextrose injection and albumin were used to reconstitute drug; blood pressure fell by 20 mm Hg during first infusion compared with 50 mm Hg during second infusion; withdrawal of aldesleukin infusion during second course and therapy with plasma expanders led to recovery of blood pressure; reinstitution of aldesleukin infusion at 9 million IU/sq m/day led to substantial hypotension, and aldesleukin was withdrawn; blood concentrations of tumor necrosis factor, interferon gamma, and neopterin were increased after addition of albumin)

Antithyroid Drugs

Shiran A, Shechner C, Dickstein G (Haifa Medical Center, Haifa, Israel). **Propylthiouracil**-induced agranulocytosis in four patients previously treated with the drug. *JAMA*. 1991; 266:3129-30. Study. (case series; 178 patients who received propylthiouracil for hyperthyroidism during 1985–90; 178 patients received propylthiouracil 300–900 mg/day for 12–18 months, and 55 patients who relapsed received second course; four patients, aged 46–65, developed agranulocytosis [neutrophil count $<0.2 \times 10^9/L$] after three to six weeks of receiving second course of therapy at 300 mg/day; agranulocytosis manifested as one case of peritonsillar cellulitis and two cases of tonsillitis; 10 patients received methimazole instead of propylthiouracil because of minor adverse effects)

Cardiac Drugs

Packer M (Center for Heart Failure Research, Mount Sinai School of Medicine, 1 Gustave Levy Place, New York, NY 10029), Carver JR, Rodeheffer RJ et al. Effect of oral **milrinone** on mortality in severe chronic heart failure. *N Engl J Med*. 1991; 325:1468-75. Study. (double-blind randomized controlled; 1088 patients with severe chronic heart failure and advanced left ventricular dysfunction at 119 medical centers; 561 patients received oral milrinone 40 mg/day, and 527 received placebo; all patients received digoxin, a diuretic, and an angiotensin-converting-enzyme inhibitor for at least four weeks before study and during study; milrinone therapy associated with 28% increase in mortality from all causes [95% confidence interval, 1–6%] and 34% increase in cardiovascular mortality [95% confidence interval, 6–69%] compared with placebo; no beneficial effect on survival observed for any milrinone-treated subgroup; study ended five months prematurely because of adverse effect of milrinone on patients' survival)

Drug Interactions

DiPadova C, Roine R, Frezza M et al. (Lieber CS, Alcohol Research and Treatment Center, Veterans Affairs Medical Center, 130 W. Kingsbridge Road, Bronx, NY 10468). Effects of **ranitidine** on blood alcohol levels after ethanol ingestion: comparison with other H_2-receptor antagonists. *JAMA*. 1992; 267:83-6. Study. (nonrandomized, controlled; eight men received ranitidine 300 mg/day, six men received **cimetidine** 1000 mg/day, and six men received **famotidine** 40 mg/day for eight days; all men received ethanol 0.3 g/kg as oral solution or i.v. injection before start of drug therapy and after last dose; ranitidine increased mean peak ethanol concentration by 34% [$p < 0.05$] and mean area under concentration–time curve by 41% [$p < 0.01$], compared with baseline; ranitidine decreased mean first-pass metabolism of ethanol from 70 to 31 mg/kg [$p < 0.05$] and increased ethanol bioavailability from 79.6% to 92.6% [$p < 0.05$]; cimetidine had greater effect than ranitidine on blood ethanol concentration, while famotidine had no significant effect)

Gastrointestinal Drugs

Convens C, Verhelst J, Mahler C (Department of Internal Medicine and Endocrinology, Middelheim Hospital, Antwerp 2020, Belgium). Painful gynaecomastia during **omeprazole** therapy. *Lancet*. 1991; 338:1153. Case. (68-year-old man with reflux esophagitis; received omeprazole 20 mg/day for three months; developed painful gynecomastia on left side; concomitant methylprednisolone, indomethacin, indapamide, and allopurinol; physical examination and mammography showed bilateral gynecomastia that was more pronounced on left side; serum testosterone, dihydrotestosterone, estradiol, follicle-stimulating hormone, luteinizing hormone, prolactin, and human chorionic gonadotropin concentrations within normal ranges; withdrawal of omeprazole led to regression of gynecomastia within about three weeks; rechallenge refused)

Hemostatics

Hadley T, Djulbegovic B (Division of Medical Oncology/Hematology, Department of Medicine, University of Louisville, James Graham Brown Cancer Center, 529 S. Jackson Street, Louisville, KY 40292). Disseminated intravascular coagulation after **factor IX complex** resolved using purified factor IX concentrate. *Arch Intern Med*. 1991; 115:621-2. Case. (41-year-old man with hemophilia B and cerebral hemorrhage; received nonpurified factor IX complex; developed disseminated intravascular coagulation; substitution of nonpurified factor IX complex with monoclonal antibody-purified factor IX led to resolution of coagulation disorder; computed tomography scan of head showed resolution of hemorrhage)

Hormones

Leclerq F, Fille A, Albat B et al. (Jaffiol C, Cardiology and Endocrinology Service, Centre Hospitalier Régional Universitaire, 34059 Montpellier, France). Congestive heart failure worsening with **octreotide** in acromegalic patient. *Lancet*. 1991; 338:1272-3. Case. (44-year-old acromegalic man with conges-

Continued on page 373

Continued from page 369

tive heart failure; received octreotide 300 μg/day increased to 600 μg/day by continuous s.c. infusion; condition deteriorated, requiring inotropic drugs for therapy of congestive heart failure; tumor volume shrank, and plasma growth hormone concentration decreased from 40.4 to 2.2 ng/mL during octreotide therapy; withdrawal of octreotide and reinstitution at 100 μg/day by continuous s.c. infusion led to reduction of left ventricular ejection fraction from 15% to 6%; discontinuation of octreotide led to no further acute events)

Hypotensive Agents

Sever PS (Hypertension Clinic, St. Mary's Hospital, London W2 1NY, England). Hypertrichosis and **verapamil**. *Lancet*. 1991; 338:1215-6. Case. (50-year-old hypertensive man with coexisting hyperlipidemia and history of bronchial asthma; received extended-release verapamil 240 mg/day for three to four weeks; man noticed thickening of his head hair, hair growth over bald patch on head, first-time hair growth on chest and abdomen, and new hair growth on arms and legs; therapy with verapamil led to satisfactory control of blood pressure)

Pediatrics

Bergman I (Children's Hospital, 3705 Fifth Avenue, Pittsburgh, PA 15213), Steeves M, Burckart G et al. Reversible neurologic abnormalities associated with prolonged intravenous **midazolam** and **fentanyl** administration. *J Pediatr*. 1991; 119:644-9. Cases. (three baby girls, aged 3–15 months, with endotracheal tubes; received i.v. midazolam and fentanyl for 4–11 days as sedation; developed encephalopathy; complete clearance of symptoms in five days to four weeks; retrospective review of 45 children who received continuous midazolam infusion for >12 hours, concomitant fentanyl therapy, and neurological assessment on withdrawal of sedation revealed that three children had definite and two had possible neurological sequelae)

Lane JC, Tennison MB (CB No. 7025, UNC-CH, Chapel Hill, NC 27599-7025), Lawless ST et al. Movement disorder after withdrawal of **fentanyl** infusion. *J Pediatr*. 1991; 119:649-51. Cases. (five children, aged 0.5–3.5 years, on mechanical ventilation in pediatric intensive-care unit; received fentanyl as continuous infusion [mean ± S.D. infusion rate, 3.0 μg/kg/hr] for three days at most then tapered over one or two days; developed withdrawal symptoms characterized by movement disorder and extreme irritability)

Wood EG (Division of Pediatric Nephrology, Cardinal Glennon Children's Hospital, St. Louis University, 1465 S. Grand Boulevard, St. Louis, MO 63104), Bunchman TE, Lynch RE. **Captopril**-induced reversible acute renal failure in an infant with coarctation of the aorta. *Pediatrics*. 1991; 88:816-8. Case. (1.73-kg baby girl with hypertension due to coarctation of aorta; received captopril 0.5 mg/kg/dose increased to 1.1 mg/kg/dose every six hours; developed acute renal insufficiency; withdrawal of captopril and therapy with other hypotensive agents led to control of blood pressure and improved serum creatinine concentration, but metabolic acidosis, gastric aspiration, and respiratory arrest developed two months later and patient died)

Toxicity

Tobin JR (Johns Hopkins Hospital, Department of Anesthesiology and Critical Care Medicine, Blalock 1508, 600 N. Wolfe Street, Baltimore, MD 21205), Doyle TP, Ackerman AD et al. **Astemizole**-induced cardiac conduction disturbances in a child. *JAMA*. 1991; 266:2737-40. Case. (12.5-kg three-year-old girl; accidentally ingested 10 10-mg astemizole tablets; developed multiple cardiac conduction abnormalities and became somnolent; therapy with gastric lavage, activated charcoal, and sorbitol led to normal electrocardiogram within seven hours)

Vaccines

Herroelen L (Department of Neurology, University Hospital, Free University of Brussels, Laarbeeklaan 101, B-1090 Brussels, Belgium), De Keyser J, Ebinger G. Central-nervous-system demyelination after immunisation with recombinant hepatitis B vaccine. *Lancet*. 1991; 338:1174-5. Cases. (two female health-care workers, aged 26 and 28 years; 26-year-old woman had multiple sclerosis, but 28-year-old woman had no previous neurological disease; received **hepatitis B virus vaccine inactivated** 20 μg as part of immunization plan; reported neurological adverse effects six weeks after inoculation; magnetic resonance imaging scans of brain showed hyperintense lesions; in 26-year-old woman, who became comatose after two weeks, therapy with dexamethasone and mannitol led to substantial improvement but persistence of hemiparesis on left side; in 28-year-old woman, therapy with methylprednisolone led to slight improvement but relapse occurred after one month)

Vasodilating Drugs

Moesch C (Department of Nephrology, CHRU Dupuytren, 87042 Limoges, France), Rince M, Daudon M et al. Renal intratubular crystallisation of calcium oxalate and naftidrofuryl oxalate. *Lancet*. 1991; 338:1219-20. Cases. (62-year-old man with arteritis, and 64-year-old man with arteritis and diabetes mellitus; received oral **nafronyl oxalate** 200 mg twice daily for 20 days; 62-year-old man also received nafronyl oxalate 400 mg in 5% dextrose injection by i.v. infusion three times daily for 20 days, and 64-year-old man also received nafronyl oxalate 400 mg by i.v. infusion two times daily for 10 days; developed acute renal failure; renal tissue biopsy showed calcium oxalate crystals in renal tubules; therapy with hemodialysis eventually led to partial recovery of renal function)

Book Review

Data Collection Forms in Clinical Trials

By Bert Spilker and John Schoenfelder.
Published by Raven Press, 1185 Avenue of the Americas, New York, NY 10036, 1990. xv + 672 p. Price $90.

Data Collection Forms in Clinical Trials is intended to aid researchers in developing high-quality data collection forms so that high-standard study protocols can be completed. The book is divided into two sections; the first thoroughly covers the process involved in creating data collection forms, and the second provides examples of data collection forms.

The process of form development is covered in a very organized and detailed manner. The idea of keeping a library of standardized forms is initially presented in the first chapter and then re-emphasized throughout the book. Other chapters focus on types of data collection forms, design of forms, preparation of the data collection form package, reproduction and assemblage of forms, design of data entry forms for use at remote clinical sites, data processing, and storage of completed forms. Many tables highlight the guidelines, considerations, and pitfalls to avoid when developing data collection forms. The authors offer insight on how to produce a form that will capture all the necessary data and provide consistency and clarity to the study.

Examples of data collection forms constitute most of the book. The authors chose to provide examples of well-

Continued on page 374

Continued from page 373

designed forms only, thereby focusing on the components of the well-designed form. The forms presented are divided into seven categories: background of a clinical trial, physical and other examinations, laboratory tests and evaluations, adverse events, medicines and assays of biological levels, efficacy, and patient termination and miscellaneous. To illustrate the ideas that were presented in the first section of the book, numerous sample forms are provided for each category. The wide variety of forms offered would aid any investigator in building or augmenting a forms library. The major problem with this section is that it is not self-explanatory. The authors needed to provide a set of instructions explaining the organization of the section. Another drawback is that the specific pointers and comments for individual forms are listed at the beginning of each chapter instead of alongside the form; much page turning is required to understand the comments.

This book would be an excellent resource for the researcher contemplating the design of a clinical investigation and the protocol team member wanting insight into how case study reports should be developed. The section on form development is well written and organized. Although the section with examples of forms was cumbersome to use, the variety of forms offered in *Data Collection Forms in Clinical Trials* should help anyone who needs to develop forms.

Reviewed by Karen J. Schoenbrun, Department of Pharmacy Services, University Hospital, Oregon Health Sciences University, 3181 S.W. Sam Jackson Park Road, OP16A, Portland, OR 97201-3098.

Books Received

Books are listed as soon as received; selected books may be reviewed in subsequent Book Reviews.

Cardiovascular Drugs and the Management of Heart Disease, Second Edition, edited by Gordon A. Ewy and Rubin Bressler. Published by Raven Press, 1185 Avenue of the Americas, New York, NY 10036, 1992. xvi + 496 p. Price $105.

Clinical Immunotoxicology, edited by David S. Newcombe, Noel R. Rose, and John C. Bloom. Published by Raven Press, 1185 Avenue of the Americas, New York, NY 10036, 1992. xii + 450 p. Price $95.

Manual of Antibiotics and Infectious Diseases, Seventh Edition, by John E. Conte, Jr., and Steven L. Barriere. Published by Lea & Febiger, 200 Chester Field Parkway, Malvern, PA 19355-9725, 1992. xvi + 419 p. Price $29.95.

USP DI, 12th Edition. Volume I (two books): Drug Information for the Health Care Professional. Volume II: Advice for the Patient—Drug Information in Lay Language. Volume III: Approved Drug Products and Legal Requirements. Published by The United States Pharmacopeial Convention, Inc., 12601 Twinbrook Parkway, Rockville, MD 20852, 1992. Volume IA and IB: 3146 p. total. Volume II: 1656 p. Volume III: 1141 p. Price (including monthly updates) $200, complete set; $140, Vol. I and II; $115, Vol. I only; $45, Vol. II only; $80, Vol. III only; plus shipping and handling.

Advertising Index

American Society of Hospital Pharmacists
Concepts in Oncology Therapeutics, 331
Criteria for Drug Use Evaluation, Volumes 1 and 2, 359
Medication Teaching Manual, 349
Pocket Guide to Injectable Drugs, 1991 Edition, 296
Rx Triage, 374
Amgen Inc.
Epogen, 283
Neupogen, 291-294
Bristol-Myers Squibb
Pravachol, 297-307
Burroughs Wellcome Company
Exosurf Neonatal, 363-367
Roche Laboratories, Division of Hoffmann-La Roche, Inc.
Rocephin, inside back cover, outside back cover
Roerig, A Division of Pfizer Pharmaceuticals
Diflucan, 370-372
Unasyn, 288-290
The Upjohn Company
Zefazone, 360-362
Wyeth-Ayerst Laboratories, Inc.
Ativan Injection, 284-286
Tubex, inside front cover

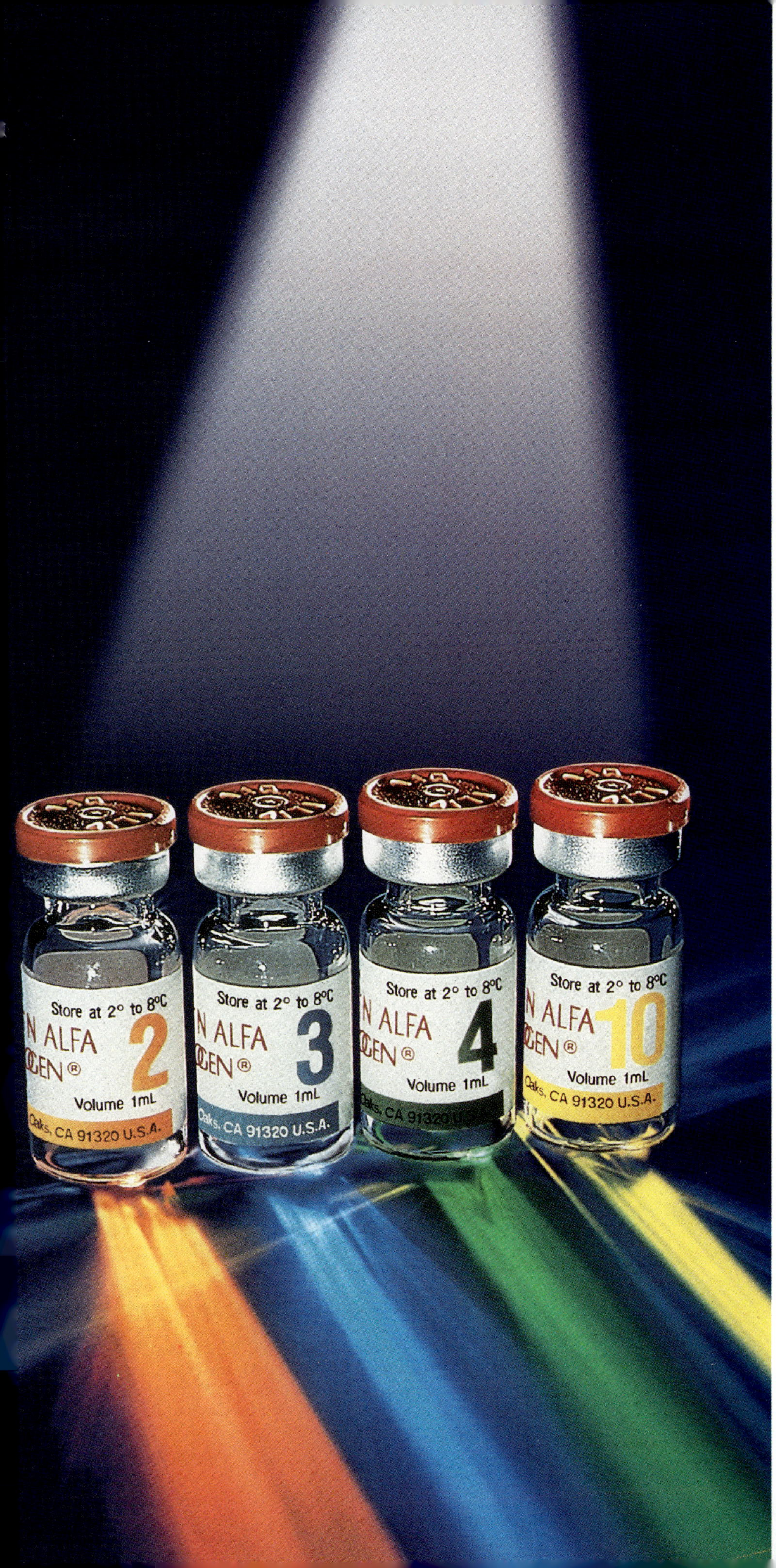

COLORS MAKE IT CONVENIENT.

SERVICES MAKE IT SHINE.

Every vial of EPOGEN® (Epoetin alfa) comes with a very important ingredient: a sophisticated and generous support system. Through seminars, symposia, in-service training, educational materials, direct consultation and many other services, we provide the kind of professional support that simply is not available anywhere else. We invite you to contact us for complete information about the total spectrum of services available to you. Do it soon. It will shed new light on the real significance of your source decision.

EPOGEN®
(EPOETIN ALFA)
RECOMBINANT

AMGEN®

Amgen Inc., Amgen Center
Thousand Oaks, CA 91320-1789
1-800-28-AMGEN
1-800-282-6436

News

HDL testing should be routine part of assessments of coronary heart disease risk, says consensus panel 378

Oral temafloxacin approved for U.S. market 381

Sertraline cleared for marketing as antidepressant 381

Nabumetone marketed for osteoarthritis, rheumatoid arthritis 381

FDA warns quality of underground zalcitabine is poor; Roche expands premarketing access programs 385

Tacrine made available under treatment IND protocol 385

News Briefs 385

Upcoming Specialty Meetings 385

HDL testing should be routine part of assessments of coronary heart disease risk, says consensus panel

Assessments of risk for coronary heart disease should routinely include measurements of high density lipoprotein (HDL) cholesterol in addition to total cholesterol, recommended the expert panel of the National Institutes of Health Consensus Development Conference on Triglyceride, High Density Lipoprotein, and Coronary Heart Disease, held in Bethesda, Maryland, February 26–28, 1992. At least two, and ideally three, measurements should be made at weekly intervals before final treatment decisions are made.

Risk Associated with Low HDL Cholesterol and High Triglycerides. The panel concluded that there is considerable evidence that a cause-and-effect relationship exists between low plasma HDL cholesterol and the development of coronary heart disease. Whether a comparable relationship exists between high plasma triglyceride concentrations and coronary heart disease has not been established. Limited data suggest that the risk of coronary heart disease increases as the triglyceride concentration increases in patients with high levels of total cholesterol or LDL cholesterol and low levels of HDL cholesterol. Elevated levels of triglycerides can increase several clotting factors and decrease fibrinolytic activity. Over time, these effects may contribute to atherosclerosis. Clinical trials do not establish whether lowering triglyceride concentrations will decrease the risk of coronary heart disease.

Indications for HDL-Cholesterol and Triglyceride Testing. When the risk of coronary heart disease in healthy individuals is being assessed, concentrations of both total cholesterol and HDL cholesterol should be determined. If the individual has a high total cholesterol concentration or at least two risk factors for coronary heart disease, testing should also include triglycerides. Triglyceride and HDL-cholesterol determinations are also indicated in patients with diabetes mellitus, central obesity, peripheral vascular disease, hypertension, or chronic renal disease or when familial hyperlipidemic disorders are suspected. If the patient has coronary heart disease, both HDL cholesterol and triglycerides should be measured. Concentrations of HDL cholesterol and triglycerides also need to be followed when hygienic or drug therapy is given with the intent of altering these components.

Treatment Recommendations. Regardless of the total cholesterol concentration, hygienic measures, such as dietary modifications, weight control, exercise, and smoking cessation, should always be used when the triglycer-

Continued on page 381

Continued from page 378

ide concentration is high or the HDL-cholesterol concentration is low. The panel recommended that drug therapy be used sparingly when these conditions exist in the absence of an elevated LDL-cholesterol concentration in a patient not known to have coronary heart disease: in these patients drug therapy should be limited to individuals who have multiple other risk factors that place them at high risk for coronary heart disease.

Oral temafloxacin approved for U.S. market

An oral formulation of temafloxacin hydrochloride (Omniflox, Abbott Laboratories) has received FDA approval for marketing. The new quinolone is labeled for use in the treatment of acute bacterial exacerbations of chronic bronchitis caused by *Haemophilus influenzae*, *Moraxella catarrhalis*, or *Streptococcus pneumoniae*; pneumonia caused by *H. influenzae* or *Strep. pneumoniae*; uncomplicated skin or skin-structure infections caused by *Acinetobacter calcoaceticus*, *Escherichia coli*, *Pseudomonas aeruginosa*, *Staphylococcus aureus*, or *Streptococcus pyogenes*; prostatitis caused by *Enterococcus faecalis*, *E. coli*, or *Proteus mirabilis*; uncomplicated urinary-tract infections caused by *E. coli*, *P. mirabilis*, or *Staphylococcus epidermidis*; or complicated urinary-tract infections caused by *E. coli* or *Klebsiella pneumoniae*.

About 80% of a single oral 600-mg dose is absorbed, with peak plasma concentrations occurring two to three hours after the dose. The elimination half-life in subjects with normal renal function is about eight hours. More than 60% of an administered dose is excreted unchanged in the urine within 48 hours after a dose. Fecal elimination accounts for 24% of a dose, and biliary excretion accounts for 3%.

The following adverse reactions were reported during premarketing clinical trials by more than 2% of patients treated with temafloxacin: nausea (5.6%), diarrhea (2.8%), dyspepsia (2.3%), headache (4.7%), and dizziness (4.2%). Concomitant administration of antacids or sucralfate may decrease the absorption of temafloxacin. Cimetidine has been reported to interfere with the elimination of temafloxacin.

Temafloxacin can be given every 24 hours for the treatment of uncomplicated urinary-tract infections. For other indications, a 12-hour dosage interval is recommended. The recommended dose is 400 or 600 mg, depending on the condition being treated. Patients with renal or hepatic dysfunction should receive reduced dosages. Use of temafloxacin in children is not recommended.

Omniflox is available as 400- and 600-mg tablets in bottles of 50 and unit dose packages of 100.

Sertraline cleared for marketing as antidepressant

Sertraline hydrochloride (Zoloft, Pfizer), a chemically distinct antidepressant, has been cleared for marketing in the United States. The mechanism of action is presumed to relate to the compound's ability to inhibit neuronal uptake of serotonin in the central nervous system.

After oral administration, sertraline undergoes extensive first-pass metabolism, primarily *N*-demethylation. *N*-desmethylsertraline is less active than sertraline and has a terminal elimination half-life of 62–104 hours. The terminal elimination half-life of sertraline is about 26 hours. Metabolic pathways for both sertraline and *N*-desmethylsertraline include oxidative deamination and subsequent reduction, hydroxylation, and glucuronide conjugation. Sertraline is highly bound to plasma proteins.

The most commonly reported adverse effects are gastrointestinal complaints (nausea, diarrhea, dyspepsia), tremors, dizziness, insomnia, somnolence, increased sweating, dry mouth, and male sexual dysfunction. Fifteen percent of patients treated with sertraline in premarketing clinical trials discontinued therapy because of adverse effects.

The recommended initial dosage of sertraline (as the hydrochloride salt) is 50 mg once daily, given in the morning or evening. A maximum dosage of 200 mg/day is recommended. At least one week should elapse between dosage changes.

Zoloft is available as 50- and 100-mg tablets in bottles of 50.

Nabumetone marketed for osteoarthritis, rheumatoid arthritis

A new nonsteroidal anti-inflammatory agent, nabumetone (Relafen, SmithKline Beecham), has been approved for the acute and long-term treatment of the signs and symptoms of osteoarthritis and rheumatoid arthritis. Nabumetone is being promoted as an agent that is comparable to other nonsteroidal anti-inflammatory agents in terms of efficacy but poses a lower risk of upper gastrointestinal ulcers.

Nabumetone, a naphthylalkanone, is at least 80% absorbed after oral administration. It is rapidly converted to an active metabolite, 6-methoxy-2-naphthylacetic acid, and to other unidentified metabolites. The active metabolite is highly protein bound and is transformed in the liver to inactive free metabolites and conjugates. The elimination half-life of 6-methoxy-2-naphthylacetic acid is about 24 hours.

The adverse effects reported most frequently by clinical trial participants were diarrhea (14%), dyspepsia (13%), and abdominal pain (12%). In controlled clinical trials, the cumulative incidence of peptic ulcers among patients taking nabumetone was 0.3% at three to six months of follow-up, 0.5% at one year, and 0.8% at two years; the studies involved 1677 patients treated with nabumetone for periods of one month to at least two years and included 1140 patients followed for one year and 927 followed for two years.

The recommended initial dosage of nabumetone is 1000 mg taken as a single dose with or without food. Some patients obtain greater relief with daily dosages of 1500 or 2000 mg. The drug may be given once or twice daily.

Relafen is supplied as 500- and 750-mg tablets in bottles of 100 and 500 and in unit dose packages of 100.

Continued on page 385

A change to Zefazone is no small change

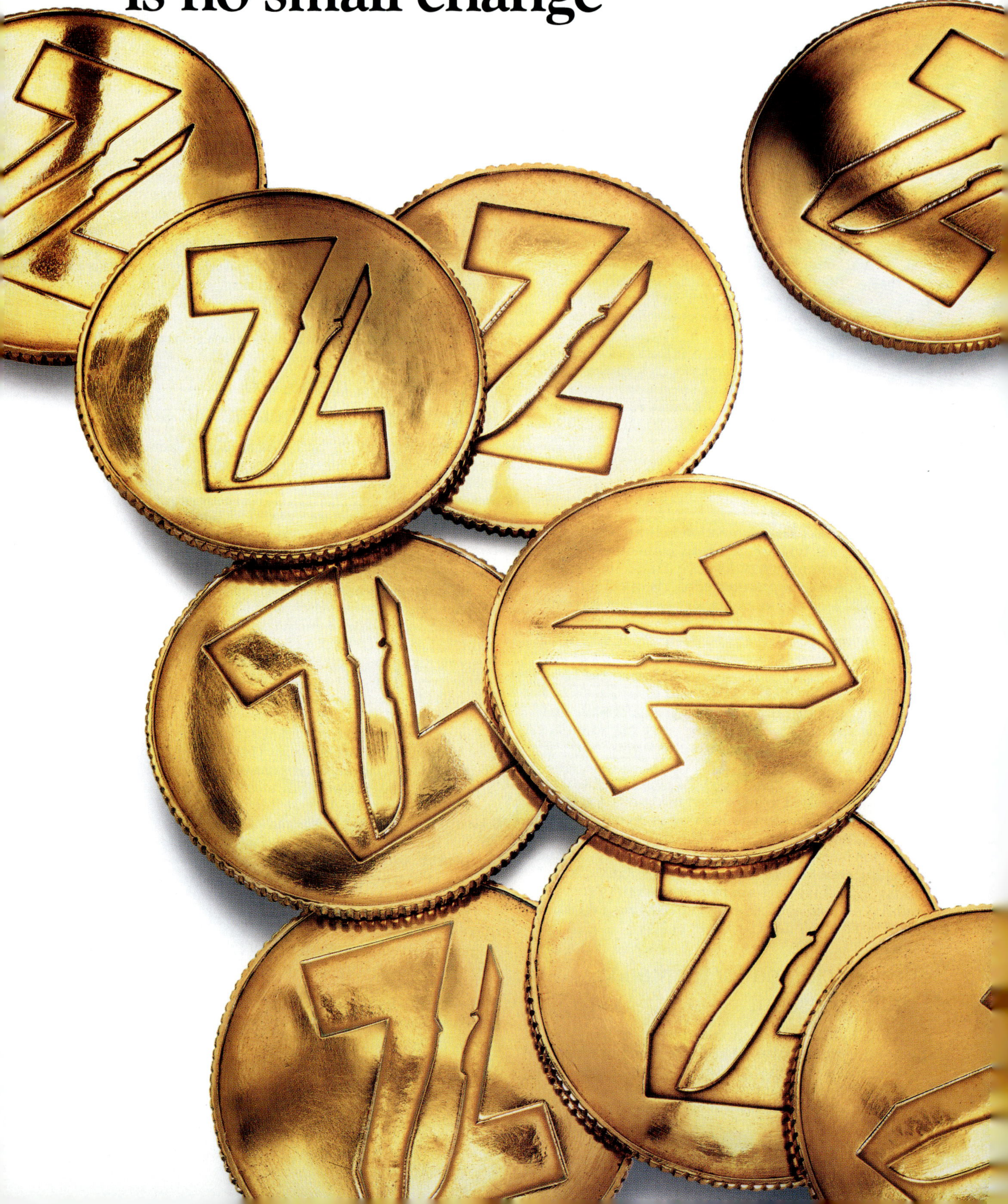

Continued from page 381

FDA warns quality of underground zalcitabine is poor; Roche expands premarketing access programs

FDA has urged AIDS buyers clubs to stop the sale and distribution of unauthorized versions of zalcitabine (dideoxycytidine, ddC). (Buyers clubs are groups that facilitate patient access to drugs purported to be useful for treatment of AIDS or associated conditions.) In January 1992, FDA received reports that the quantity of zalcitabine contained in some of the underground capsules varied substantially from the labeled amount. In response to these reports, FDA analyzed drug product samples obtained from various buyers clubs. According to FDA, these tests confirmed potentially serious variations in product potency and quality and reflect poor manufacturing practices. The amount of zalcitabine in assayed capsules ranged from no drug to twice the labeled amount.

FDA is currently reviewing a new drug application for zalcitabine, submitted in October 1991 by Hoffmann-La Roche. While the application is under review, Hoffmann-La Roche is expanding the programs that enable patients with human immunodeficiency virus (HIV) infection to gain access to the drug. The current program for patients who have not responded to or cannot tolerate zidovudine therapy will continue. Two new programs have been announced. One is an open-label protocol for symptomatic HIV-infected individuals with CD4 cell counts of <300/cu mm and asymptomatic persons with CD4 cell counts of <200/cu mm who cannot participate in controlled clinical trials. Complete patient enrollment information can be obtained from Hoffmann-La Roche by calling 800-332-2144. The second program will be designed to provide zalcitabine for use by individuals with CD4 cell counts of up to 500/cu mm.

Tacrine made available under treatment IND protocol

A treatment IND protocol approved for tacrine hydrochloride (Cognex, Warner-Lambert) will enable more patients with Alzheimer's disease to gain access to the drug. Patients will receive the drug at gradually increasing dosages, beginning at 40 mg daily for six weeks. Tacrine is known to cause hepatotoxicity in some patients. The dosage-escalation strategy was designed to identify and exclude patients who are sensitive to the drug's hepatotoxic effects. Additional information about the protocol and patient eligibility can be obtained by calling Warner-Lambert at 800-545-7627.

News Briefs

- Labeled indications for **acyclovir** (Zovirax, Burroughs Wellcome) have been expanded to include treatment of chickenpox.

- The American Academy of Pediatrics, in collaboration with the American Thoracic Society and the Division of Tuberculosis Control of the Centers for Disease Control, has issued recommendations for **treatment of tuberculosis in infants and children.** The statement was published in the January 1992 issue of *Pediatrics*.

- The examination for **board certification in pharmacotherapy** will be offered August 8, 1992, in Toronto, Ontario. To obtain information and an application, write to Board of Pharmaceutical Specialties, 2215 Constitution Avenue, N.W., Washington, DC 20037, or call 202-429-7591.

Upcoming Specialty Meetings

Clinical Issues in Nutrition Support. Dearborn, MI, May 28–29; contact American Society for Parenteral and Enteral Nutrition, 8630 Fenton Street, Suite 412, Silver Spring, MD 20910.

American Association for the Study of Headache. Toronto, Ontario, June 26–28; contact AASH, 875 Kings Highway, Suite 200, West Deptford, NJ 08096; 609-845-0322.

Fifth International Conference of Chronopharmacology and Chronotherapeutics. Amelia Island, FL, July 12–16; contact Michael Smolensky, Ph.D., Fifth International Conference of Chronopharmacology and Chronotherapeutics, School of Public Health, UTHSC–Houston, P.O. Box 20186, Houston, TX 77025.

International Congress: The Pain Clinic (5th). Jerusalem, Israel, September 14–18; contact Professor Y. Sharav, Scientific Committee, Hadassah School of Dentistry, P.O. Box 1172, 91 010 Jerusalem, Israel.

Letters

Asthma in children 386
Dennis M. Williams
Pamela A. Simon, Christine M. Murphy, and Shannon L. Coonce

Use of succimer 387
Steven M. Marcus, Bruce Ruck
Katherine V. Mann, John D. Travers
William Banner, Jr.

The Letters *column is a forum for rapid exchange of ideas among readers of* Clinical Pharmacy. *Liberal criteria are applied in the review of submissions to encourage contributions to this column.*

The Letters *column includes the following types of contributions: (1) comments, addenda, and minor updates on previously published work, (2) alerts on potential problems related to drug therapy or clinical research, (3) observations or comments on trends in drug therapy or clinical research, and (4) brief expressions of opinion about controversies in drug therapy or clinical research.*

Letters need not be submitted with the journal's manuscript checklist. The following conditions, however, must be adhered to: (1) the body of the letter must be no longer than two typewritten pages, (2) the use of references, tables, and illustrations should be minimized, (3) the authors' names, affiliations, and mailing addresses must be typed at the end of the letter in the format used by Clinical Pharmacy, *and (4) the entire letter (including references, tables, and authors' names) must be typed double-spaced on plain white paper (not letterhead). Following acceptance of a letter, the authors are required to sign an exclusive publication statement and a copyright transferal form.*

Asthma in children

I would like to comment on the review of childhood asthma that appeared in the September issue of *Clinical Pharmacy*.[1]

The authors commented that it is often difficult for children (and most adults) to use metered-dose inhalers (MDIs) correctly. Mastery of MDI technique is indeed difficult, but the primary shortcoming in this regard lies in the lack of understanding and sufficient instruction by health-care professionals, including pharmacists. If pharmacists would teach, observe, and periodically reinforce correct MDI technique, all asthma patients would benefit greatly.

The authors also noted an increasingly important role for inhaled corticosteroids in the management of asthma. In the future we are likely to see much higher dosages of currently available corticosteroids and the use of new, more potent corticosteroids. It is important for patients to understand the role of these drugs (i.e., suppression of inflammation) in their overall regimen. Improving MDI technique for these agents is important. Many clinicians now support the use of a spacer device to reduce oropharyngeal drug deposition for any patient receiving an inhaled corticosteroid.

Finally, the authors overlooked a crucial component in the management of asthma. Objective measures of lung function should be used to assess the severity of asthma and to monitor the course of therapy.[2] Routine monitoring of peak expiratory flow rates (peak flows) at home is an integral part of management for all patients with asthma except those with very mild disease. Home peak-flow monitoring involves the patient or family in management and can be used to optimize therapy or to detect changes that signal an asthmatic episode. Home peak-flow measurements should be used in asthma as home blood-glucose meters are used in diabetes. Peak-flow meters designed especially for children are available.

Pharmacists should recognize the value of patient education, especially that concerning the use of inhalation therapy and devices. Pharmacists should also be actively involved in providing peak-flow meters with proper instructions for patients with asthma.

1. Murphy CM, Coonce SL, Simon PA. Treatment of asthma in children. *Clin Pharm*. 1991; 10:685-703.
2. National Asthma Education Program. Executive summary: guidelines for the diagnosis and management of asthma. Bethesda, MD: National Institutes of Health, 1991; publication no. 91-3042A.

Dennis M. Williams, Pharm.D., Clinical Associate Professor
Division of Pharmacy Practice
School of Pharmacy
The University of North Carolina at Chapel Hill
Campus Box 7360, Beard Hall
Chapel Hill, NC 27599-7360

Home monitoring of peak expiratory flow rate (PEFR), at face value, provides a simple and relatively inexpensive method of objectively evaluating pulmonary function in all patients. However, peak-flow meter measurements must be interpreted carefully. The PEFR can be "normal" even when a patient has considerable symptoms.[1-3] Also, because the test is extremely effort-dependent,[4] the measured PEFR may be "abnormal" when the patient's disease is, in fact, controlled.

The insensitivity of the test requires that it be used in carefully selected situations. Home PEFR monitoring is particularly useful in the very stoic patient (e.g., a patient who consistently denies symptoms of asthma but consistently has poor spirometric measurements at follow-up).[5] In such a case, the clinician must determine the optimal PEFR for the patient by obtaining the measurement when the patient is optimally controlled (e.g., after prednisone burst therapy) and then using that value as the target PEFR. Routine home PEFR monitoring is also indicated for patients with severe asthma.

Long-term patient monitoring must include an assessment of the extent to which the disease interferes with the patient's life. Monitoring of an acute exacerbation in children must include assessment of the acute symptoms (e.g., coughing, dyspnea), some signs that the parents can easily assess at home (e.g., respiratory rate, presence of retractions, the patient's comfort level), and the response of these signs and symptoms to treatment. The response to treatment is critically important in determining the need for prednisone burst therapy, which should be instituted as soon as the indication is established.

Monitoring of patients with asthma includes involvement of the patient and parents in diligently following a number of signs and symptoms. Home PEFR monitoring may be part of the plan for selected patients. Educating the patient and parents about the appropriate response to clinical problems is an important role for pharmacists.

1. Johnston I, Anderson HR, Patel S. Variability of peak flow in wheezy children. *Thorax*. 1984; 39:583-7.
2. Sly PD, Hibbert ME, Landau LI. Diurnal variation of peak expiratory flow rate in asthmatic children. *Pediatr Pulmonol*. 1986; 2:141-6.
3. Mihatsch W, Geelhoed GC, Landau LI et al. Time course of change in oxygen saturation and peak expiratory flow in children admitted to hospital with acute asthma. *Thorax*. 1990; 45:438-41.
4. National Asthma Education Program. Guidelines for the diagnosis and management of asthma. Bethesda, MD: National Institutes of Health/National Heart, Lung and Blood Institute, 1991, publication no. 91-3042.
5. Weinberger M. Managing asthma. Baltimore: Williams & Wilkins; 1990.

Pamela A. Simon, Pharm.D., Clinical Assistant Professor
Christine M. Murphy, Pharm.D., Clinical Assistant Professor

Department of Pharmacy Practice
The University of Illinois at Chicago
833 South Wood Street, Room 244 (M/C 886)
Chicago, IL 60612

Shannon L. Coonce, Pharm.D., Clinical Pharmacist
University Medical Center of Southern Nevada
1800 West Charleston Boulevard
Las Vegas, NV 89102

Use of succimer

We would like to comment on the article[1] and editorial[2] about succimer in the December issue of *Clinical Pharmacy*.

McNeil Laboratories (a subsidiary of Johnson & Johnson) sought FDA approval for succimer as an orphan drug. Purely coincidental, perhaps, is the fact that the Agency for Toxic Substances and Disease Registry (ATSDR)[3] and the Centers for Disease Control (CDC)[4] estimated that there were approximately 200,000 children in the United States with a blood lead concentration (BLC) greater than 25 µg/dL. Consideration for orphan-drug status requires that the number of potential patients in the United States not exceed 200,000. More recent CDC guidelines, however, have stated that acceptable BLCs are <10 µg/dL; with this lower concentration, 2.4 million children in the United States might be candidates for succimer therapy.

Our understanding is that McNeil applied for orphan-drug status intentionally and that this action was not required by the FDA. Orphan-drug status gives some very specific advantages to the drug company. The drug is not patented because it is not, strictly speaking, a "new drug," and the company has an exclusive right to market the product. Further, the cost of evaluating an orphan drug becomes a tax write-off for the company. Finally, it is well known that a drug that becomes accepted in the treatment of one disease rapidly becomes usable in the treatment of other diseases. Because there is no restriction on how a physician uses a particular drug, succimer, which is effective in treating other metal poisonings, may be prescribed for indications not included in the package labeling.

To its credit, McNeil has taken the position that it will not advertise succimer or attempt to educate physicians about using the drug for any indication other than the treatment of lead poisoning.

The FDA approved succimer even though very few patients had been treated with the drug in the United States. Certainly, the FDA cannot be faulted for its action. The drug's orphan-drug status suggested that, since relatively few patients were thought to be eligible for treatment, it was unnecessary to subject a large number of patients to safety and efficacy studies.

We have had clinical experience using this drug since 1989. We recently reported that succimer-associated adverse effects occurred in a relatively high proportion of 68 patients.[5] Rash developed in 7–10% of adults and 5% of children. Small reductions in hemoglobin concentration occurred in 12% of the patients; we cannot relate this change to any clinical problems. One of our patients twice developed a potentially life-threatening hyperthermic reaction; one of these episodes occurred in a controlled clinical research setting. We have heard anecdotal accounts from other practitioners whose experience with succimer-associated adverse effects has paralleled ours. There are now reports of succimer-associated neutropenia and, in some animals, thrombocytopenia. The frequency of adverse effects may be so great that many physicians may be reluctant to use succimer for lead poisoning.

As to the editorial by Banner,[2] we believe the author missed the point of the succimer controversy. The FDA did not really establish a "cookbook" mandate for treatment. Unless we miss our guess, this drug will be used in large numbers of patients with a BLC below that specified in the package labeling.

1. Mann KV, Travers JD. Succimer, an oral lead chelator. *Clin*

Pharm. 1991; 10:914-22.
2. Banner W Jr. Succimer: controversial issues involving the release of a new product. *Clin Pharm*. 1991; 10:942. Editorial.
3. Agency for Toxic Substances and Disease Registry. The nature and extent of lead poisoning in children in the United States: a report to Congress. Atlanta, GA: Agency for Toxic Substances and Disease Registry; 1988.
4. Centers for Disease Control. Preventing lead poisoning in young children: a statement by the Centers for Disease Control, 1991. Atlanta, GA: Centers for Disease Control; 1991.
5. Marcus S, Okose P, Jennis T et al. Untoward effects of oral dimercaptosuccinic acid in the treatment of lead poisoning. Paper presented at the Annual Scientific Meeting of the American Academy of Clinical Toxicology, American Association of Poison Control Centers, American Board of Medical Toxicology, and Canadian Association of Poison Control Centers. Toronto, Ontario, Canada: 1991 Oct.

Steven M. Marcus, M.D., Medical Director
Bruce Ruck, Pharm.D., Coordinator of Drug Information

New Jersey Poison Information and Education System
210 Lyons Avenue
Newark, NJ 07112

Drs. Marcus and Ruck are in error regarding how the Orphan Drug Act was applied to the development and approval of succimer. The Orphan Drug Act, which amended the Federal Food, Drug and Cosmetic Act as of January 4, 1983, discussed rare diseases and conditions without specifying numerical prevalence thresholds. In March 1984 Johnson & Johnson Baby Products filed an orphan-drug designation request with the FDA's office of orphan products development, and in May 1984 the request was granted for the use of succimer in the treatment of lead poisoning in children. In October 1984 the Orphan Drug Act was amended to further define a rare disease or condition as one that (1) affects <200,000 persons in the United States or (2) affects >200,000 persons in the United States and for which there is no reasonable expectation that the cost of developing and making available in the United States a drug for the disease or condition will be recovered from United States sales of that drug. Among the relatively few incentives offered by the act are (1) tax credits for clinical research performed by the sponsor before approval and (2) a seven-year market exclusivity.

Neither the 1985 CDC guidelines[1] nor the 1988 ATSDR report to Congress[2] had been published when the orphan-designation request was made. The two documents most pertinent to the prevalence and management of lead poisoning in children were the 1978 CDC guidelines[3] and the report by Mahaffey et al.,[4] which described the data from the second National Health and Nutrition Examination Survey (NHANES II). The former defined lead poisoning in children (regardless of the presence of symptoms) as a BLC of ≥50 μg/dL with an erythrocyte protoporphyrin (EP) concentration of ≥250 μg/dL. The latter indicated that in 1978 approximately 30,000 children (six months to five years old) had a BLC of ≥50 μg/dL.

The 1985 CDC guidelines[1] redefined lead poisoning in children as a BLC of ≥25 μg/dL with an EP concentration of ≥35 μg/dL. Chelation therapy was recommended for children with either (1) a BLC of ≥55 μg/dL or (2) a BLC of ≥25 μg/dL in conjunction with an EP concentration of ≥35 μg/dL and a positive edetate (EDTA) provocative challenge. The 1988 ATSDR report[2] applied the data from NHANES II and projected them to the 1984 United States population; the estimate was that approximately 200,000 children had a BLC of >25 μg/dL. The 1985 CDC guidelines,[1] as mentioned above, indicated that only a fraction of these children were candidates for chelation therapy.

The 1991 CDC guidelines[5] still do not recommend chelation therapy for children with a BLC of <25 μg/dL. They do eliminate the recommendation that EP concentration be considered, but continue to recommend that, when possible, an EDTA provocative challenge be performed before a decision is made to start chelation therapy. Even with these revised guidelines, the ATSDR report would still estimate that <200,000 children in the United States would have been candidates for chelation therapy in 1984.

We mentioned in our paper that clinical experience with succimer has been limited. Mild to moderate neutropenia has been observed recently in some patients receiving the drug.[6] Although a causal relationship to succimer has not been definitely established, neutropenia has been reported with other drugs in the same chemical class. We have modified the product's package insert accordingly. Even so, oral succimer offers many advantages over previously available agents when it is used appropriately as part of a comprehensive therapeutic plan. Succimer can be used effectively to reduce the lead burden in children for whom the drug is indicated.

1. Centers for Disease Control. Preventing lead poisoning in young children: a statement by the Centers for Disease Control, 1985. Atlanta, GA: Centers for Disease Control, 1985; DHHS publication no. 99-2230.
2. Agency for Toxic Substances and Disease Registry. The nature and extent of lead poisoning in children in the United States: a report to Congress. Atlanta, GA: Agency for Toxic Substances and Disease Registry; 1988.
3. Centers for Disease Control. Preventing lead poisoning in young children: a statement by the Centers for Disease Control, April 1978. Atlanta, GA: Department of Health, Education, and Welfare; 1978.
4. Mahaffey KR, Annest JL, Roberts J et al. National estimates of blood lead levels: United States 1976–1980. Association with selected demographic and socioeconomic factors. *N Engl J Med*. 1982; 307:573-9.
5. Centers for Disease Control. Preventing lead poisoning in young children: a statement by the Centers for Disease Control, 1991. Atlanta, GA: Centers for Disease Control; 1991.
6. McNeil Consumer Products Company. Chemet package insert. Fort Washington, PA; 1991 November.

Katherine V. Mann, Pharm.D., Assistant Director
Medical Affairs

John D. Travers, M.D., M.P.H., Assistant Director
Clinical Research

McNeil Consumer Products Company
Camp Hill Road
Fort Washington, PA 19034

The primary issue raised in my editorial is generic: Should the FDA establish indications for drug use that are based solely on a single biochemical measure? This has not been the usual approach to prescribing drugs, and so to limit a drug's use to instances when this single indicator is present seems ill advised. The decision to treat an individual patient should be based on numerous factors, including age, exposure circumstances, other biochemical measures, and physical findings. It is easy to imagine circumstances in which reliance on the BLC alone could result in overtreatment or undertreatment of a specific child. Drs. Marcus and Ruck believe that children will be treated with succimer even if they have a BLC below that in the package labeling. Either the arbitrary labeling is then incorrect or these gentlemen have a rather cynical view of the community of practitioners.

The most recent CDC guidelines do not support the inappropriate prescribing of succimer, as Drs. Marcus and Ruck suggest, and would not alter the applicability of the Orphan Drug Act to this agent. If anything, the recent data in this country point to the diminishing size of the population with a BLC in the range suggested for treatment and reinforce the appropriateness of the Orphan Drug Act in helping to develop succimer.

The unimpressive and small series of adverse effects presented by Drs. Marcus and Ruck reinforces the need for adverse-effect monitoring but in no way diminishes the need for succimer. The frequency of adverse effects with the currently available chelators is well enough known that it does not bear repeating. All of the available data both here and abroad continue to support oral succimer as being safer than injectable chelation therapy.

It is surprising to read such a negative commentary on a drug that has been long awaited by the bulk of the toxicology community. Toxicologists should be taking an affirmative attitude by encouraging Phase IV data collection on succimer as it enters the market and by educating physicians on the drug's appropriate use.

William Banner, Jr., M.D., Ph.D., Associate Professor of Pediatrics
Department of Pediatrics
The University of Utah
Salt Lake City, UT 84113

Special Feature

Acute pain management: Operative or medical procedures and trauma, part 2

Agency for Health Care Policy and Research

Site-Specific Pain Control

Even for a single operation, there may be great variability in the approach to postoperative pain management based on patient factors such as age, weight, ability to understand and cooperate with plans for care, co-existing medical and psychological problems, and idiosyncratic sensitivity to analgesics; intraoperative course, such as size and location of incisions or drain placement or anesthetic management; and institutional resources available for treatment and monitoring in the particular setting.

Despite these variable factors, the clinician can still outline certain pain management options to present

Acute pain management guideline panel members included Daniel B. Carr, M.D., Panel Co-Chair, Director, Division of Pain Management, Department of Anesthesia, Massachusetts General Hospital; Ada K. Jacox, R.N., Ph.D., Panel Co-Chair, Independence Foundation Chair in Health Policy, School of Nursing, The Johns Hopkins University; C. Richard Chapman, Ph.D., Professor of Anesthesiology, School of Medicine, University of Washington; Betty R. Ferrell, R.N., Ph.D., Research Scientist, Nursing Research, City of Hope Medical Center; Howard L. Fields, M.D., Ph.D., Departments of Neurology and Physiology, University of California, San Francisco; George Heidrich III, R.N., M.A., Instructor, Department of Neurology, University of Wisconsin Medical School; Nancy K. Hester, R.N., Ph.D., Assistant Director, Center for Nursing Research, and Associate Professor, School of Nursing, Health Sciences Center, University of Colorado; C. Stratton Hill, Jr., M.D., Professor of Medicine, M.D. Anderson Cancer Hospital, University of Texas; Arthur G. Lipman, Pharm.D., Professor of Clinical Pharmacy, College of Pharmacy, University of Utah; Charles L. McGarvey, M.S., Chief, Physical Therapy Service, Department of Rehabilitation Medicine, National Institutes of Health; Christine A. Miaskowski, R.N., Ph.D., Associate Professor, Department of Physiological Nursing, University of California, San Francisco; David Stevenson Mulder, M.D., Professor of Surgery, McGill University, and Surgeon-in-Chief, Montreal General Hospital; Richard Payne, M.D., Associate Professor of Neurology, University of Cincinnati Medical Center; Neil Schecter, M.D., Associate Professor of Pediatrics, Head, Division of Developmental and Behavioral Pediatrics, University of Connecticut School of Medicine, and Co-Director, Children's Pain Service, University of Connecticut Health Center; Barbara S. Shapiro, M.D., Associate Director, Multidisciplinary Pain Management Program, Division of General Pediatrics, Children's Hospital of Philadelphia; Robert S. Smith, Ph.L., Director, Institute for Medicine in Contemporary Society, State University Medical Center at Stony Brook; Carole V. Tsou, M.D., Division of Family Medicine, UCLA Center for Health Sciences; and Loretta Vecchiarelli, Rehabilitation Counselor and Burn Survivor, Rehabilitation Hospital of Western New England. Panel staff members were Jane Ballantyne, M.B., B.S., Technology Assessment Group, Harvard School of Public Health; Donna Mahrenholz, R.N., Ph.D., School of Nursing, The Johns Hopkins University; and Janice Ulmer, R.N., Ph.D., School of Nursing, The Johns Hopkins University. The consultants were Thomas C. Chalmers, M.D., Technology Assessment Group, Harvard School of Public Health; Frederick Mosteller, Ph.D., Department of Health Policy and Management, Harvard School of Public Health; and Barker Bausell, Ph.D., Center for Research, School of Nursing, University of Maryland.

The Acute Pain Management Guideline Panel expresses profound appreciation to the patients who helped us in the development of the consumer version of the guideline and to our numerous colleagues in many disciplines who made valuable contributions during the development of the guideline. We are especially grateful to Dr. Mitchell Max of the American Pain Society for his continuous and enthusiastic support and advice. Dr. Ada Jacox thanks her colleagues at The Johns Hopkins University for their thoughtful contributions and encouragement.

Numerous colleagues in the Departments of Surgery, Anesthesia, and Nursing at Massachusetts General Hospital provided informal yet valuable input as portions of the guideline were being written at that site. Dr. Daniel Carr's clinical colleagues in the Division of Pain Management of the Department of Anesthesia willingly increased their clinical load when the guideline development process became particularly time consuming. This extra workload fell particularly upon the shoulders of the Postoperative Pain Service, directed by Dr. Buckman McPeek, and the Diagnostic and Therapeutic Nerve Blocking Unit, directed by Dr. Donald P. Todd. Dr. Richard J. Kitz, the Henry Isaiah Dorr Professor and Chairman of Anesthesiology, and Dr. George E. Battit, Vice-Chairman, provided constant encouragement for this project and facilitated it in many practical ways. Miss Evelyn Hall provided expert and dedicated administrative and secretarial assistance.

Reprinted with permission of the Agency for Health Care Policy and Research.

This article has been published in two parts; part 1 appeared in the April 1992 issue. The references cited in part 1 were published with that part.

to an otherwise uncomplicated adult patient. Many aspects of pain control are shared between operations on different parts of the body. For practical reference, pain management options for various surgical procedures are presented according to region of the body rather than by the pathophysiological mechanisms involved. In all cases, however, preoperative psychological preparation and medication should be considered, and ongoing postoperative assessment and reassessment of pain should be routine. In this way, pain can be controlled effectively. Vigilance for changes in postoperative pain will trigger prompt searches for diagnostically significant causes of new pain.

Head and Neck Surgery. *Dental Surgery.* The most common forms of dental surgery are brief and relatively noninvasive procedures often performed on an outpatient basis. A patient's anxiety is frequently disproportionate to the safety of the procedure; such a patient may benefit from behavioral or pharmacologic (anxiolytic) therapy. Mild pain associated with most forms of uncomplicated dental care such as simple tooth extractions, endodontic therapy, or scaling of the periodontal area or of a previously asymptomatic tooth is well managed by oral administration of an NSAID such as aspirin or ibuprofen. Preoperative administration of ibuprofen appears to delay the onset of postoperative pain and lessen its severity.[128] For patients unable to tolerate aspirin or ibuprofen, acetaminophen can provide an acceptable analgesic effect.

Dental procedures such as surgical removal of bony impactions and osseous periodontal surgery are more traumatic and typically produce intense and prolonged postoperative pain. The onset of such pain can be delayed by preoperative treatment with ibuprofen and/or application of a long-acting local anesthetic such as bupivacaine during the procedure.

Rarely, an intravascular or intraneural injection of local anesthetic in this context leads to bruising, bleeding, or systemic symptoms such as fainting, allergic reaction, or persistent pain due to direct nerve injury. When postoperative pain does emerge, it often requires the addition of an opioid to the nonsteroidal regimen. Codeine is frequently prescribed at a dosage of 30–60 mg every four to six hours. Increased analgesia but also an increased number of opioid side effects such as nausea, constipation, sedation, and respiratory depression follow dosage increases above this level. Alternative opioids include propoxyphene or oxycodone administered in doses that are equianalgesic to 30–60 mg of codeine.

Some operations on the oral cavity preclude the patient's taking oral medications postoperatively (e.g., wiring the mouth closed after an operation on a mandibular fracture). Alternative therapy should be based on the severity of the surgical procedure and expected pain associated with it, as well as the surroundings in which it will be managed. Formulations of NSAIDs such as rectal suppositories (indomethacin) or intramuscular injection (ketorolac) are now commonly available. Opioids may be administered by a variety of routes (intravenous, intramuscular, subcutaneous injection; transdermal; rectal) and schedules, including a patient-controlled schedule. Cost-efficacy analyses of parenteral opioid administration for oral surgery are not sufficient to permit any clear recommendations. Pain that does not respond to these measures should prompt a search for infection, osteitis, peripheral nerve injury, or the emergence of psychological and behavioral changes consistent with the development of chronic pain syndrome.

Radical Head and Neck Surgery. These operative procedures commonly interfere with oral intake for prolonged periods postoperatively and may be combined with a feeding gastrostomy or jejunostomy. Airway patency is always a consideration in these patients, and a tracheostomy frequently is an integral part of the operation. The use of flap coverage or skin grafts further increases the number of potentially painful sites. Prolonged preoperative pain, radiotherapy, and chemotherapy are important preoperative modifiers of pain therapy. Thus, the very nature of the operative procedure may dictate alternate routes for pain therapy in patients who have undergone major head and neck ablative procedures that may interfere with a patient's ability to describe pain and his or her response to analgesic intervention.

Intraoperative positioning of the head and neck are critical. Protective padding and avoidance of extreme flexion, extension, and rotation may help obviate or minimize muscle-spasm-induced pain after surgery. Foam cushion supports under the occiput can minimize decubitus-pressure-induced headache, palsies, and causalgia. Intraoperative traction on muscles and nerves should be started carefully and monitored during the operation to prevent reflex myalgias and causalgias. Painful swallowing after head and neck; ear, nose, and throat; and endocrine surgical procedures may require liquid forms of pain medicine, a modified diet, including liquid or soft foods, and occasional use of topical anesthetics such as viscous lidocaine.

Postoperative pain is often short term and of moderate intensity. Within one to three days, parenteral and oral opioids can be discontinued or replaced with nonopioid analgesics (which may have to be delivered via gastrostomy or jejunostomy). The use of most NSAIDs may be contraindicated for such procedures as thyroidectomy and parathyroidectomy where postoperative hemorrhage and risk of airway obstruction are significant. In such cases, acetaminophen or "platelet-sparing" NSAIDs may be ordered.

Neurosurgery. Patients undergoing an operation on the central nervous system frequently show abnormal neurologic signs and symptoms that must be closely followed in the postoperative period. In addition, these patients may receive drugs designed to reduce cerebral edema or prevent seizures. A major dilemma in this clinical setting is the need to carefully monitor critical neurologic signs such as pupillary reflexes and the level of consciousness that may be affected by conventional opioid analgesics used for the relief of postoperative pain.

Ideally, postoperative pain control should not interfere with the ability to assess a patient's neurologic status, particularly the level of consciousness, or with assessment of motor and sensory function following spinal cord surgery. Therefore, the administration of opioids, benzodiazepines, and anxiolytics, in particular, is relatively contraindicated. However, the clinician must balance the need for analgesia with the requirement for appropriate neurologic monitoring.

The uncomplicated postcraniotomy patient typically has mild to moderate pain and is readily managed by a short period of parenteral medications followed by oral analgesics. Laminectomy and other spinal procedures usually are more painful than craniotomies. Ketorolac, a parenteral NSAID, may be considered in this setting because it has no effect on the level of consciousness or pupillary reflexes. As mentioned previously, the use of nonsteroidal analgesics may be contraindicated in some postoperative settings when the risk of coagulopathy or hemorrhage is high, the need to assess fever is important, or the degree of pain is higher than the analgesic ceiling of the agent.

Epidural opioids and/or local anesthetics can minimize the need for systemic opioids and allow more accurate monitoring of brainstem and cerebral function. However, a single dose of epidural morphine may produce significant blood concentrations[129] that in turn cause effects within the central nervous system. A recent study could not demonstrate a difference in neuropsychiatric functioning between patients receiving oral and epidural morphine.[130] Furthermore, motor and sensory dysfunction associated with epidural local anesthetics (which are often coadministered with opioids) may obscure important neurologic signs. Again, remember to balance the need for adequate analgesia while minimizing the confounding central nervous system effects of analgesics and anesthetics.

Chest and Chest Wall Surgery. *Thoracic Surgery (Noncardiac).* Operative sites within the thorax include the heart, esophagus, and lungs and somatically innervated structures such as the ribs, superficial chest wall, and breast. Pre-existing disease of these organs (e.g., chronic obstructive pulmonary disease) or prior medical treatment (e.g., chemotherapy) are common. They contribute to postoperative morbidity through a variety of mechanisms, such as decreased pulmonary reserve. Drains and chest tubes can cause intense irritation and pain at entry sites or deeper. For this reason, NSAIDs such as indomethacin in suppository form are useful to reduce inflammation, although they are rarely enough for complete pain relief and indeed are not approved by the Food and Drug Administration as simple analgesics.

Good evidence exists that aggressive pain control in the form of epidural analgesia or neural blockade with local anesthetics after thoracic surgery improves pulmonary function; however, at present there is insufficient evidence from randomized controlled trials (RCTs) to conclude that after thoracic surgery these forms of aggressive pain control hasten walking or reduce morbidity and length of hospital stay.[38,72,74,131,132]

The greatest beneficial effects result from administration of opioids or a combination of opioid and local anesthetic in the thoracic epidural space. Reliance on a local anesthetic alone to secure postoperative epidural analgesia in the thoracic region carries possible side effects such as hypotension due to sympathetic blockade. Respiratory impairment because of somatic nerve block is another potential problem; therefore, intercostal nerve blocks are generally undesirable unless an opioid is contraindicated. Mixing a local anesthetic with an opioid produces better and more prolonged analgesia, but RCTs indicate that there is a tendency toward more side effects when an opioid is added to a local anesthetic, compared with the local anesthetic alone.[38,133,134] An example of a coordinated approach to postoperative analgesia is the placement of an epidural catheter prior to induction of anesthesia, which is used to deliver local anesthesia, either alone or mixed with an opioid for intraoperative analgesia and then is left in place postoperatively for infusion of a dilute analgesic. As previously emphasized, monitoring and care of patients with epidural catheters and assessment of the optimal time for switching to oral analgesia are best accomplished by a specially trained team.

Direct injection of local anesthetics alone to block intercostal nerves has been done for years as a means to provide postoperative analgesia and improved pulmonary function after thoracotomy. Unfortunately, such analgesia lasts only 6–12 hours, so that a single injection rarely suffices for the entire postoperative period. A clinician can overcome the brief duration of intercostal anesthesia by administering interpleural local anesthetics. To accomplish this, a catheter is placed between the parietal and visceral pleura, and anesthetic is injected at 4–6 hour intervals or infused continuously to produce continuous analgesia across several dermatomes.[135] As in all invasive techniques, this method requires skill in drug titration and vigilance for management of side effects such as pneumothorax.

The use of opioids to reduce postoperative pain after thoracotomy is well documented. Because of potential side effects, clinicians have tried to optimize delivery and closely match dose to need. In this context, PCA has resulted in incrementally improved analgesia, increased patient satisfaction, and tendencies toward improved pulmonary function and earlier recovery or discharge.[38,40-42,136] One strategy to manage pain after thoracotomy is to deliver epidural analgesia to prevent pain and then switch to patient-controlled intravenous analgesia if the epidural catheter ceases to function or is discontinued after several days on the ward.

A typical PCA prescription in this setting relies first on a series of loading doses; for example, 3–5 mg of morphine, repeated every five minutes until the initial postoperative pain diminishes. A low-dose basal infusion at night (e.g., 0.5–1.0 mg/hr) allows uninterrupted sleep for the patient. On-demand doses typically add 0.5–1.5 mg of morphine every 6 minutes. PCA doses of opioid are valuable to supplement analgesia during respiratory therapy or ambulation, even after the patient is taking oral analgesics and especially while chest tubes are in place. The transition from intravenous PCA to oral opioids is accomplished as described above. If adequate opioid analgesia yields undesired side effects, or if pain is not severe (e.g., when chest tubes are no longer in place), the patient can switch directly from epidural to oral analgesia using a combination of opioid and NSAID. Many opioid analgesics or mixtures are available in liquid form and are useful for patients unable to swallow tablets or capsules (e.g., after esophageal surgery).

Cardiac Surgery. Most cardiac operations involve a median sternotomy and anesthetic induction using high doses of opioids (morphine at 1 mg/kg or another opioid at an equivalent dose). Because somatic nerves are not divided by the surgical incision, postoperative pain is usually less than after conventional thoracotomy, even when lower doses of opioids are given during surgery. For procedures that use intercostal incisions, such as implantation of automatic defibrillatory devices, methods of pain control need not differ from those of other thoracic operations. Close observation is essential to distinguish postoperative pain originating in the chest wall and pleura from cardiac pain, which may signal myocardial ischemia due to a tachyrhythmia or threatened infarction from inadequate revascularization.

Abdominal and Perineal Surgery. *Upper Abdominal Surgery (Includes Cholecystectomy, Aortic Bypass).* Although outside the thorax, operations on the upper abdomen such as cholecystectomy compromise pulmonary function. Other associated morbidity (that may lead to mortality) includes immobility, hypercoagulability, venous thrombosis, and increased myocardial oxygen consumption when pain leads to an increase in blood pressure or rapid heart rate. Patients who undergo major vascular surgery frequently have co-existing myocardial disease, wide swings in blood pressure as their major vessels are clamped and unclamped, and significant fluid shifts associated with blood loss and replacement. These patients are particularly at risk for postoperative myocardial infarctions and arrhythmias. For operations on the abdominal aorta, intraoperative epidural anesthesia is widely used and simplifies the transition to postoperative epidural analgesia through the same catheter.

Hormonal indexes of stress are reduced postoperatively in patients given epidural analgesia using a local anesthetic (e.g., 0.25% bupivacaine) such as after cholecystectomy. Yet even when pain is completely eliminated by this technique, these hormonal stress responses do not vanish.[137] Normally, a minimum of three or four days will elapse postoperatively before oral analgesia is feasible following operations on the biliary system, stomach or intestine, or vasculature in the upper abdomen.

In preparing the patient for any upper abdominal operation, choices of pain management to be reviewed with the patient include intramuscular or subcutaneous injection of an opioid as needed, an around-the-clock schedule of injections (or continuous infusion of opioid) to be withheld in the event of side effects such as respiratory depression or nausea, intravenous PCA, or epidural analgesia in the manner described for postthoracotomy pain. Each of these approaches carries its own risks and benefits, which depend on the health care team's knowledge, expertise, and ability to recognize and treat side effects and correct inadequate pain relief. Other techniques have been used for postcholecystectomy pain, such as interpleural catheters or supplemental, long-acting local anesthetic blocks of the lower intercostal nerves and celiac plexus. These lie outside the range of most current clinical practice.

Lower Abdominal and Perineal Surgery (Abdominal Hysterectomy, Cesarean Section, Hernia Repair, Episiotomy, Urological and Gynecological Procedures, and Hemorrhoidectomy). The pain management plan for the patient undergoing lower abdominal or perineal surgery is based on the same principles as those for patients undergoing upper abdominal procedures. On the other hand, analgesia to control pain of active labor must be approached with special expertise and caution in light of side effects that may impair fetal well-being (e.g., fetal respiratory depression after maternal opioids or maternal hypotension after epidural local anesthetic). Suppression of pain and surgical stress responses is more complete with epidural local anesthesia after lower abdominal surgery than after upper abdominal operations.[138] Presumably this is because pathways such as phrenic or thoracic somatosensory afferents are less easily blocked by epidural anesthesia. Many obstetrical or urological procedures (e.g., cystoscopy) routinely are performed with spinal or epidural anesthesia, and the addition of low doses of opioid to a local spinal anesthetic appears to lengthen the duration of analgesia observed after the local anesthetic effect has subsided.[36,133,134,139,140] Pain after procedures on the anus is particularly severe and requires adjunctive measures such as stool softeners, dietary manipulation, and local anesthetic suppositories for control. Again, the precautions already outlined concerning spinal opioid use and the necessity for close monitoring apply. Goals of the postoperative pain management plan should include early ambulation. For obstetric procedures, opioid doses should be adjusted so as to produce minimum maternal and fetal sedation. Alternatively, if an epidural catheter has been placed for infusion of local anesthetic to control labor pain or to provide anesthesia for cesarean section, a dilute solution of local anesthetic may be infused through this catheter to control postoperative pain with little risk of sedating the nursing infant.

Musculoskeletal Surgery. *Back Surgery.* Operations on the spine at any level are frequently done in patients who have experienced chronic pain. Such patients may have the typical complications of chronic pain: depression, anxiety, irritability, and, if opioid analgesics were required preoperatively, a relative tolerance to opioid medications. All of these factors may complicate pain assessment and treatment in the postoperative period. In addition, the majority of procedures requiring a spinal operation are associated with paraspinal muscle spasm. In such cases, it is appropriate to add muscle relaxants to supplement conventional opioid therapy.

Operations on the spinal cord often involve laminectomy and bone grafting and may include opening the dura around the spinal cord. These procedures may limit the role of epidural and spinal delivery of pain medications. As with any neurologic procedure, postoperative patients require careful monitoring of neurologic functions, especially the assessment of sensory, motor, and autonomic functioning.

Surgery on Extremities (Orthopedic, Vascular). The most common operations performed on extremities are done electively and include total joint replacements. The high degree of morbidity related to venous thromboembolic complications must be considered. Pain control postoperatively should allow early ambulation and movement in the postoperative period. Supplementing conventional opioids with an epidural infusion of a local anesthetic may benefit these patients by decreasing the incidence of thromboembolism. Operations requiring a cast or other form of external fixation for stabilization demand frequent postoperative evaluation of circulation and neurologic functions. Pain therapy should not interfere with monitoring of the patient.

Orthopedic or vascular procedures on an extremity may result in a compartment syndrome; this is usually associated with a period of ischemia or perhaps injury to the muscles of the lower extremity. It is manifested by intracompartmental swelling with loss of function, the earliest manifestation being loss of dorsiflexion of the foot and pain. Once again, this requires continuous observation; pain control measures should not mask this process. If not treated promptly by decompression, a compartment syndrome may result in chronic postischemic neuropathy.

The traumatic amputation is often associated with phantom limb pain. Evidence now exists that infusion of epidural local anesthetic prior to elective amputation for inoperative vascular disease can minimize this symptom; the applicability of these pilot data to treatment of other conditions or trauma remains to be defined.[43]

The majority of operative procedures on extremities produce pain of moderate intensity usually controlled by early parenteral opioids supplemented by NSAIDs. Adding epidural analgesia is particularly attractive in terms of establishing early mobility and minimizing thromboembolic complications.[38,141-143]

Soft Tissue Surgery. Surgical procedures involving local soft tissue resections usually obtain pain control with oral opioids. Many of these procedures are done on an ambulatory basis and require careful patient education prior to and immediately after the procedure. Anxiety because of the potential results of a small surgical biopsy (e.g., feared results of a breast biopsy) may demand adjuvant drug or nondrug therapy. Preoperative and postoperative education and support by the surgeon and the health care team are supremely important.

Management of Postoperative and Procedural Pain in Infants, Children, and Adolescents

Much of the guideline thus far applies to both adults and children. The following section contains information specific to pain assessment and management in children. This section is not all-inclusive, and these recommendations should be used in conjunction with the entire guideline. This portion of the guideline, although based on a thorough review of the literature on procedure-induced and postoperative pain, is not a substitute for professional training and judgment. For further information, the clinician is referred to the bibliography and, when necessary, to experts for consultation.

Background. Children commonly experience postoperative pain. The incidence of moderate to severe pain in children in any health care setting is influenced by factors such as the child's medical condition, type of procedure performed, and attitudes of health care professionals toward pain management. In three studies on postoperative pain in children, the prevalence of moderate to severe pain varied from about 40% to 60%.[144-146]

Many children do not receive any opioid analgesics after surgical procedures, even though painful postoperative courses are expected.[144,147-151] Compared with adults undergoing similar procedures, less potent analgesic regimens usually are ordered for and given to children.[147,151] When used, opioid doses and intervals of administration are often inadequate; when a physician's order includes a selection of one or more analgesics, the tendency is to choose the least potent drugs.[146,147,149,152] In general, although children are less able than adults to articulate their treatment and medication needs, both opioid and nonopioid analgesics are commonly prescribed on an as-needed basis.[147,153] This type of prescription (1) requires the child or the family to describe the presence of pain and the need for analgesia and (2) focuses on the treatment of emerging pain rather than aggressive treatment to prevent pain.

Infants, even when premature, experience pain in response to aversive stimuli.[44,154-158] However, infants often do not receive opioid analgesia before or after major medical procedures.[159] Although the majority of ventilated infants receive postoperative opioid analgesia (but often in less than adequate doses), nonventilated infants often do not.[160-162] A survey of the beliefs and practices of anesthesiologists in the United Kingdom revealed that, although the majority believed neonates experience pain, few provided opioid analgesics for postoperative pain.[163] Discrepancies between beliefs and practices can occur for many reasons, but they have not been adequately explored.

Invasive and painful procedures are particularly distressing for children. Children often describe repeated invasive procedures as more distressing than any other aspect of illness or treatment.[148,164-166] Unlike adults, infants and young children may not understand the reason for procedures and may not participate actively in providing consent. Infants and young children also may not understand the time-limited nature of procedures. Although appropriate preparation and adequate analgesia for painful procedures are crucial for decreasing distress in children, these issues often are not addressed by health care providers, or they are approached haphazardly.[167]

Assessment. Pain is determined by many factors, including the medical condition, developmental level, emotional and cognitive state, personal concerns, meaning of pain, family issues and attitudes, culture, and environment. Caring for the child in pain requires frequent assessment and reassessment of the presence, amount, quality, and location of pain. It also means preventing or reducing anticipated pain and, when prevention is not possible, promptly alleviating pain. Because emotional distress accentuates the experience of pain, exploration of and intervention for possible sources of distress are necessary. For infants and children, the provider should recognize the potential for pain and pursue the possibility that a child is in pain. A knowledge of children, including their developmental level and their behavior, is necessary to adequately assess pain and distress.

Assessment includes a pain history, a search for diagnoses such as infection that could be increasing or causing pain, evaluation of the pain severity and location, and observation of the child and his or her responses to the environment. The inclusion of parents or guardians and other important family members is essential to pain assessment. Strategies for assessment should be tailored to the developmental level and personality of the child and to the context. Children who are developmentally delayed or retarded, learning disabled, emotionally disturbed, or non-English speaking require special assessment. Culturally determined beliefs about pain and medical care also should be considered. Getting to know the individual child is important for assessment and management of pain: obtaining a pain history and involving the parents in the child's care can optimize this process.

The pain history obtained prior to or at admission focuses on the language the child uses to describe pain (e.g., hurt, owie, boo-boo), previous pain experiences and coping strategies, how and to whom the child communicates pain, and the child's and the family's preferences to assess and treat pain.[168] The provider, child, and family can then decide together on their approach to pain assessment and treatment.

Routine assessment and documentation of pain are critical for effective pain control. The frequency of assessment is tailored to the severity of the pain. For example, after a major surgical procedure, assessment reasonably could occur at least every two hours on the day of surgery and the first postoperative day and at least every four hours on subsequent days. More frequent assessment is necessary if the pain is poorly controlled despite treatment. Pain intensity and its response to analgesics should be recorded on the bedside chart just as vital signs are recorded for easy review by health care providers. Structured documentation on a bedside flow sheet may increase the frequency of assessment and provision of analgesia.[169] Assessment methods should be easy to administer or perform, and documentation forms should be readily accessible to health care providers for use in recording pain. If the child is old enough to participate in assessment, his or her ease in response is important for accurate measurement. Young children may not understand the relationship between pain assessment and pain relief; therefore, they may not respond to questions if they are anxious or in severe pain.

Methods for Assessing Pain. No one method to assess pain offers a precise measure of the pediatric pain experience. Therefore, the use of more than one method of assessment may be helpful. Assessment tools should be appropriate for the child's age and cognitive development and for the context. A variety of assessment tools are available for all age groups; selection of appropriate tools depends on the psychometric adequacy of the tool as determined through estimates of reliability, validity, generalizability, and sensitivity. Several psychometrically sound and developmentally appropriate tools are available to assess pain for documentation on a bedside flow sheet. Representative tools are described in Figures 3–7 and Tables 1–3 in part 1.

As with adults, a self-report tool provides the most reliable and valid estimates of pain intensity, quality, and location. Self-reports can be used for developmentally normal children over the age of 4.[170] Self-report tools for children over the age of 4 include the Oucher,[171] the Poker Chip Tool,[172,173] and a faces scale.[174] Children over the age of 7 or 8 who understand the concept of order and number can use a numerical rating scale,[175] a horizontal word-graphic rating scale,[176] or a visual analogue scale.[177] In a recent study, 958 well children and adolescents and 175 hospitalized children and adolescents rated the visual analogue scale as the least preferred of five horizontal pain scales.[178] Reliability and validity for postoperative pain have been established for the Oucher, the Poker Chip Tool, and the horizontal word-graphic rating scale.

Children in pain or otherwise stressed may regress. For example, a child who before surgery uses a numerical scale appropriately may require a simpler scale after surgery. Similarly, children who are developmentally delayed or learning disabled may need assessment tools developed for younger children. If the child is unable or unwilling to respond, ratings can be obtained from the parents or health care providers. However, such ratings often underestimate moderate to severe pain and may overestimate lesser pain.[144] To increase accuracy and consistency, ratings from parents and health care providers are obtained using the same tool as the child uses.

Observation of behavior is the primary assessment method for the nonverbal child and may be an adjunct to assessment for the verbal child. Such observations focus on vocalizations, verbalizations, facial expressions, motor responses, and activity. To obtain meaningful observations, the health care professional watches for and documents behaviors associated with distress. Several aspects of behavior should be observed. For example, a child may move easily in bed, guard the surgical site when moving, or be completely immobilized and resist movement.

Various scales based on behavioral observations have been designed for clinical use in infants and preverbal children.[179-181] Although reliability and validity have not been well established, these scales offer a guide for observations of postoperative pain.

Use of behavioral observation to guide analgesia requires attention to the context of the child's behavior. For example, children cry not just in response to pain but also in response to fear, loneliness, and overstimulation or understimulation. Thus, additional assessment is necessary when the source of a behavior is not evident, so that all sources of distress can receive appropriate intervention. Sleeping, watching television, or joking may be misinterpreted as indicators of no pain while the child may, in fact, be attempting to control pain. Behavioral responses may be absent or attenuated in circumstances where vocalization or movement increases pain or where intubation, use of paralyzing agents or sedatives, extreme illness, weakness, or depression impedes vocalizations and movement. *If care providers are unsure whether a behavior indicates pain and if there is reason to suspect pain, an analgesic trial can be diagnostic as well as therapeutic.*

Unstructured observations of how a child looks and acts may provide additional information about the presence and amount of pain. Documenting observations over time may reveal specific changes in behavior that serve as important pain indicators. For example, a child may be alert and talkative and then appear sullen and withdrawn. Such a change warrants further investigation since it may indicate the onset of or an increase in pain.[182]

Scales for assessing procedure-related pain have been developed. Assessment of facial expressions and the quality of crying have been used with infants (e.g., Neonatal Facial Coding System[183]). The Procedure Behavior Rating Scale[184] and the Procedure Behavior Checklist[185] have been used with children. These tools are not applicable for routine postoperative use.

Physiologic indicators of pain and distress include heart rate, respiratory rate, blood pressure, and perspiration. However, these indicators are not specific for pain, and they vary among individual patients in pain. Therefore, the interpretation of physiological indicators should be done in the context of the clinical condition and in conjunction with other assessment methods.

Management. Pain is managed by the child, his or her parent(s), nurses, physicians, and other health care providers. Effective interaction is key to effective pain management. Although preferences of the child and the family deserve respect and careful consideration, the primary obligation of the health care provider is to ensure safe and competent care.

Children attempt to prevent or alleviate pain whether or not health care providers do so. When in pain, a child often prefers the use of medication and the presence of a parent.[186-188] However, children may not be in control of these strategies. Specific methods initiated by children that may be helpful include holding someone's hand, a stuffed toy, or favorite blanket; asking questions; using distraction; sleeping and resting; relaxing or using imagery; changing positions; and engaging in humor. Seemingly simple interventions such as holding someone's hand can have powerful effects. Facilitation of the child's usual strategies for decreasing pain is important.

Management of Pain Related to Procedures in Hospitalized Children. Diagnostic and therapeutic procedures are often associated with pain. A structured approach to pain management takes into consideration the type of procedure, anticipated range of pain, and individual factors such as age and condition.

Nonpainful procedures (e.g., computed tomographic scanning, magnetic resonance imaging, cast changes, and ultrasonic examination) often require a child to lie still. Preparatory education about the sensations and surroundings may decrease the child's distress and facilitate the procedure.[189] Nondrug approaches such as distraction and imagery may benefit the older child.[190] Sedation is appropriate in these situations, particularly if the child is under 6 years of age. Sedatives include oral chloral hydrate or pentobarbital. Pharmacologic sedation may result in the loss of the child's protective reflexes; therefore, children should be closely monitored even during "conscious sedation."

Painful procedures require a management plan that may include both drug and nondrug approaches. When planning the management of procedure-related pain and anxiety, a series of questions should be asked: (1) Why is the procedure being performed? (2) What is the expected intensity of pain? (3) What is the expected duration of pain? (4) What is the expected intensity of anxiety? (5) What is the expected duration of anxiety? (6) How often will the procedure be repeated? (7) How do the parents think the child will react? and (8) What are the child's and family's perceptions regarding the procedure? The following are general management principles for procedures:

- Treat anticipated procedure-related pain prophylactically.
- Ensure the competency of the person performing the procedure and the timeliness of the procedure.[190] Delays can escalate pain and anxiety. Children report that procedures are easier to tolerate if they know and trust the people doing them.
- Provide adequate and unhurried preparation of the child and family. Parental prediction of the child's response is highly correlated with the actual degree of distress.[191,192]
- Be attentive to environmental stimuli and the manner in which the child is handled. A room other than the child's room should be used whenever possible. Environmental factors, such as cold or crowded rooms or "beepers" on machines, can escalate distress.[164,187]
- Allow parents to be with the child during the procedure. The presence of a parent may be a source of great comfort for the child.[193,194] The parent's knowledge of the child can be invaluable. Parents should be educated, since they do not automatically know what to do, where to be, and what to say to help their child through the procedure.
- Tailor treatment options, both drug and nondrug, to the child's and the family's needs and preferences, to the procedure, and to the context. A child who undergoes a procedure as part of the treatment for a chronic or life-threatening disease has different needs from the child who has an occasional procedure as part of general well child care or for treatment of an acute but self-limited illness.
- If at all possible, administer pharmacologic agents by a route that is not painful (e.g., oral, transmucosal, or intravenous). If one or two doses of a parenteral agent are necessary and the child does not have intravenous access, a single injection may be preferable to multiple attempts at insertion of an intravenous catheter.
- Dovetail pharmacologic and nonpharmacologic options to complement one another.
- For repeated procedures, maximize treatment for the pain and anxiety of the first procedure to minimize anxiety before future procedures.
- Provide monitoring and resuscitative equipment if drugs are used for sedation. Facilities, equipment, and personnel to manage emergencies (e.g., vomiting and anaphylaxis) should be immediately available.
- Manage pre-existing pain optimally before beginning the procedure.
- After the procedure, review with the child and family their experiences and perceptions about the effectiveness of pain management strategies.

Pharmacologic Strategies for Procedural Pain. The needs of the individual child and the type of procedure to be performed shape the pharmacologic approach. As with assessment, the practitioner's expertise and experience with children are key to successful therapy. A pain-relieving agent, such as an opioid (see Table 7 for starting doses) or a local anesthetic, is needed to reduce the pain. Anxiolytics and sedatives are used specifically to reduce anxiety before and during the procedure; if used alone, they may blunt the behavioral response without relieving the pain. When anxiety is present, pharmacologic anxiolysis can complement analgesia to decrease overall distress. *The use of systemic analgesics and sedatives must be approached differently in the infant under 6 months of age* (see section on Managing Postoperative Pain in Neonates and Infants).

Agents that have a broad range of applicability include:

- *Local anesthetics*: These agents may be administered by local infiltration or topically. For topical use, a eutectic mixture of local anesthetics[195] is promising but not yet available in the United States.
- *Opioids*: These drugs can be given via the intravenous, oral, or transmucosal route. The intravenous route has the advantage of rapid effect and ease of titration. Intravenous opioids can be given in increments (e.g., 0.03–0.05 mg/kg of morphine every five minutes) and titrated to analgesic effect. Oral opioids can be used when close and rapid titration to effect is not required.
- *Benzodiazepines*: These agents can be given either orally or intravenously. Like opioids, intravenous benzodiazepines are given in increments and titrated to sedative effect.[190] Unlike diazepam, midazolam does not cause pain and local sclerosis when given intravenously.[190] Benzodiazepines provide sedation, not analgesia, and hence they often are used with opioids for painful procedures. If the combination of opioid plus benzodiazepine is used, the risk of respiratory depression is increased.
- *Barbiturates*: These drugs provide excellent sedation. They have no analgesic effects and are used with analgesics for painful procedures. For most patients, the sedation persists for many hours after the procedure is completed; rarely, some patients may have paradoxical reactions.[196] As with benzodiazepines, close observation for respiratory depression is essential, particularly when the intravenous route is employed or if an opioid is coadministered.

Exercise caution when using the mixture of meperidine (Demerol), promethazine (Phenergan), and chlorpromazine (Thorazine) (also known as DPT)—given intramuscularly—for painful procedures. The efficacy of this mixture is poor when compared with alternative approaches, and it has been associated with a high frequency of adverse effects.[197] It is not recommended for general use and should be used only in exceptional circumstances.

Agents such as nitrous oxide and ketamine can be used if trained personnel and appropriate monitoring procedures are available.[196] General anesthesia is appropriate in certain situations.[190]

Monitoring Conscious Sedation for Procedural Pain. Skilled supervision is necessary whenever systemic pharmacologic agents are used for conscious sedation (i.e., the patient maintains a response to verbal and physical stimuli). A health care provider not involved in performing the procedure or holding the child should monitor for conscious sedation including frequent assessment of heart rate, respiratory rate and effort, blood pressure, and level of consciousness. Continuous pulse oximetry to measure arterial oxygen saturation is strongly encouraged. Immediate accessibility of resuscitative drugs and equipment and the presence of at least one health professional trained in advanced life support are necessary. After completion of the procedure, monitoring should continue until the child is fully awake and has resumed the former level of function.

Deep sedation (i.e., the patient is not responsive to verbal or physical stimuli) is equivalent to general anesthesia and should be performed only under controlled circumstances by a professional trained in its use and skilled in pediatric airway management and pediatric basic life support. Reference to specific published guidelines is recommended.[198,199] To quote from the latter guideline, "The caveat that loss of consciousness should be unlikely is a particularly important aspect of the definition of conscious sedation, and the drugs and techniques used should carry a margin of safety wide enough to render unintended loss of consciousness highly unlikely. Since the patient who receives conscious sedation may progress into a state of deep sedation and obtundation, the practitioner should be prepared to increase the level of vigilance corresponding to that necessary for deep sedation."

Hospitalized children undergo procedures that include lumbar punctures, chest tube insertions, bone marrow aspirations and biopsies, cardiac catheterization, circumcisions, and burn dressing changes. General principles for the management of procedural pain and distress can be applied to all painful procedures:

- Most hospitalized children undergo minor invasive procedures, such as heel sticks and finger sticks, injections, venipunctures, and insertion of intravenous catheters. Such procedures, even though categorized as "minor," can be a major source of distress for sick or hospitalized children. The hospitalized child benefits from predictability as to time and frequency and "clustering" of procedures, with an identified block of time when no procedures are to be performed, barring emergencies. Intramuscular and subcutaneous routes should be avoided unless necessary for proper administration (e.g., immunizations).
- Nondrug strategies are effective for pain and anxiety associated with minor procedures. Providing emotional support, eliciting concerns, and providing information and age-appropriate choices are crucial. Infants can benefit from sensorimotor interventions (i.e., using a pacifier and using verbal or tactile strategies).[200-202] A variety of strategies have been studied in older children. The child and family can be prepared in several ways, such as provision of preparatory sensation information,[203,204] empathetic preparation,[205] and a multimodality approach using stories, art, and play.[206] Other potentially effective cognitive-behavioral strategies include distraction techniques such as music,[207,208] coping skills,[203,204] hypnosis,[209-211] play therapy,[212] and thought stopping.[213] Physical agents include TENS therapy[214] and counter-irritants such as ice.[190] One or more nonpharmacologic interventions in addition to preparation can be chosen by the health care team, family, and child. Choice should be based on the child's preference, personality, and coping style.

For lumbar punctures, local anesthetics are used for all age groups, although efficacy in infants is controversial. Systemic drugs that alter mental status cannot be used in acute medical illnesses, such as meningitis, where observation of the level of consciousness is crucial to treatment. In situations where such monitoring is not necessary, younger children and many older ones benefit from a benzodiazepine. Supplementation with opioids is helpful for some cases, especially when difficulty in performing the procedure is anticipated. Children over 5 years of age who have learned and can effectively use cognitive and behavioral coping skills may prefer not to use sedatives or opioids.[190]

Management strategies for bone marrow aspirations and biopsies include use of either general anesthesia or conscious sedation using benzodiazepines and opioids, along with local anesthesia. Adequate time is necessary for the local anesthetic agent to have full effect.

Nonpharmacologic methods with demonstrated efficacy for lumbar punctures and bone marrow aspirations and biopsies include hypnosis,[211] thought stopping,[213] and a multidimensional psychological intervention that includes a breathing exercise, reinforcement, imagery, behavioral rehearsal, and filmed modeling.[215] Additionally, the strategies described for minor invasive procedures can be used for lumbar punctures and bone marrow aspirations and biopsies.

The management of pain associated with circumcision is controversial. Circumcision often has a religious context, and the religious beliefs of the family should be respected. Pain associated with circumcision can be managed with a penile block.[216] However, recent evidence suggests that topical anesthesia may be a safe and effective option.[217,218]

Pain Related to Burn Dressing Changes. Burn dressing changes in the child with burns severe enough to require hospitalization are approached in a multidisciplinary fashion, using drug and nondrug strategies. Pain and anxiety co-exist in these situations and must be assessed and managed concurrently using opioids and benzodiazepines, respectively. Depending on the child and the level of anxiety, an opioid may be administered alone or used with a benzodiazepine. Since undertreatment of the pain can escalate anxiety, optimal pain control is necessary. Dressing changes occur repeatedly, and tolerance to opioids and benzodiazepines can develop, necessitating higher doses. For efficacy, doses should be increased as needed and titrated according to the response obtained during the previous procedure. The child also may have ongoing pain from the burns in addition to the pain and anxiety of the burn dressing changes. If the ongoing pain is not treated, the child's anxiety during the dressing changes may make it difficult to manage, even with significant doses of opioids and sedatives. Initial regimens for pain management may include a continuous infusion or around-the-clock intermittent doses of an opioid and additional bolus doses of an opioid and a benzodiazepine before the burn dressing changes. For extensive debridement procedures, conscious sedation may not be adequate; general anesthesia may be required.

A variety of nonpharmacologic approaches are effective adjuvants. These include hypnosis[219]; a multimodal approach involving distraction, relaxation, imagery, and positive reinforcement[220]; and cartoon viewing with positive reinforcement.[221] Children as young as 18 months do better during burn dressing changes if their participation and control are maximized.[222,223] For example, a child can help to remove his or her own dressings and call for a "time-out" if necessary. Dressing changes are performed in a treatment room or similar place, so that the child can consider his or her room as a safe place. The time and environment for the dressing change should be predictable to the child. The situation causing the burns may be one that produces emotional distress for the child (e.g., burns sustained as a result of the child playing with fire or disobeying rules), and the developing body image of the child may be threatened by the burns. Psychiatric and psychological intervention should be provided when necessary. Discharge planning initiated soon after admission can help relieve anxiety and increase compliance with the therapeutic regimen, particularly for children with burns on more than 30% of the body surface area.[224]

Management of Pain Associated with Surgical Procedures. Management of surgical pain involves three phases: preoperative, intraoperative, and postoperative.

Preoperative Management. Individual or group psychological preparation with or without home preparation[225-228] may decrease pain, anxiety, and distress before and after the operation. Parental presence during the induction of anesthesia decreases postoperative pain and reduces adverse psychological sequelae.[229-231] Preoperative medication should be given painlessly. For example, a child with intravenous access can receive medication by that route; alternative routes for the child without intravenous access include oral, rectal, and transmucosal administration.

Intraoperative Management. Adequate analgesia for preterm and fullterm infants significantly reduces surgical stress and postoperative morbidity.[232,233] This finding directly challenges the previous practice of providing minimal intraoperative anesthesia for infants based on concerns about the respiratory and hemodynamic side effects of opioids. High dose opioid anesthesia appears to be well tolerated, even in critically ill infants, provided it is used in a carefully monitored setting by skilled anesthesiologists.[234,235]

Other intraoperative techniques that may help to reduce, delay, or prevent postoperative pain include epidural blockade with opioids and/or local anesthetics and local anesthetic infiltrated into the wound or applied to block a peripheral nerve. These approaches should be limited to personnel qualified in these anesthetic techniques. Children who receive intraoperative epidural opioids require careful monitoring after the procedure; this method should be used only in settings where such monitoring is available.

Postoperative Management. Drug therapies are the most important aspect of pain management. Nondrug techniques to reduce postoperative pain are useful adjuncts; the approaches are similar to those described for procedural pain: relaxation, distraction, the presence of a parent or a special toy or blanket, and cognitive preparation for anticipated events.[187] Physical methods, such as positioning with blanket rolls for support and the use of heat or ice, also can be helpful. Pacifiers, swaddling, and a calming environment may be helpful for infants.[200,201]

Drug therapy for postoperative pain depends upon the child's age, medical condition, type of surgery, and expected postoperative course. Pain after minor surgery, such as herniorrhaphy or tonsillectomy, usually can be managed with acetaminophen with or without codeine when the oral route is available. Often children are sent home on the day of surgery after such procedures; thus, parental instruction in pain control is important.[236]

For major surgery, such as abdominal, thoracic, urologic, or orthopedic procedures, parenteral opioids are the mainstay of pain management. These drugs can be administered systemically or spinally, depending on individual needs. NSAIDs are useful in certain situations. Intravenous administration of NSAIDs is currently being studied in children; these and other agents may be used more widely in the future.

Some health care professionals are concerned about the potential for psychological dependence and addiction when using opioids for pain control in children. In adults, the risk of addiction after use of opioids for pain relief is small. Although studies of the risks in children are lacking, no known aspect of childhood development or physiology increases the risk of physiologic or psychological vulnerability to chemical dependence.

Several issues are pertinent to opioid administration:

- *Route*: In the immediate postoperative period, systemic opioids are delivered by either the intravenous or epidural routes. Intramuscular injections are painful and frightening to children; many children would rather have pain than a "shot."[148] Since an intravenous catheter is required for hydration after major surgery, this route is always available. After the child is able to take medication by mouth, an oral opioid can be given with a nonopioid analgesic.
- *Schedule*: Intermittent boluses of opioids can be provided on an around-the-clock basis, using a dose of about 0.1 mg/kg of morphine or its analgesic equivalent. Dosage intervals are the same as those recommended for adults. Continuous infusion of morphine (0.02–0.04 mg/kg/hr) for children over 6 months of age has been well studied.[237-239] Continuous infusion avoids the extreme variations that may occur with intermittent intravenous doses. "Rescue" doses for breakthrough or poorly controlled pain can be offered at regular intervals to patients receiving a continuous infusion. Because of wide variability in the opioid dose needed for adequate analgesia, no matter which route and schedule of administration is employed, pain and side effects (particularly respiratory depression) should be reassessed at frequent intervals and the dose and interval adjusted for the best pain relief.
- *Agent*: As in adults, morphine is the standard. Fentanyl may be preferable when cardiovascular stability is an issue and patients are closely monitored and/or intubated. Meperidine should be used only in exceptional circumstances.
- *Patient-controlled analgesia*: PCA provides safe and effective analgesia in children as young as 7 years of age.[240] This approach is appropriate for older children and adolescents, since it offers an element of developmentally appropriate control. The addition of a basal infusion may provide better analgesia without increasing the total dose of opioid.[240] Children and young adolescents may benefit from reminders to "push the button for pain" in the immediate postoperative period. Regular assessment and reassessment of pain and side effects, with adjustment of the PCA parameters as indicated, are necessary with PCA. Education of the patient and the family are key to the success of this approach. PCA must be supervised by professionals trained in its use.
- *Side effects*: The pharmacologic approach to managing side effects in children is similar to that in adults. However, young verbal children may have difficulty communicating subjective symptoms, like pruritus, nausea, and dysphoria; the preverbal child may show only generalized discomfort. Assessment of side effects occurs with assessment of pain relief. If an infant or preverbal child becomes increasingly restless or irritable despite an increased opioid dose, treatment of presumed side effects or a change to an alternative opioid can be considered.
- *Monitoring:* Regular assessment of vital signs and level of consciousness is necessary when parenteral opioids are used for managing postoperative pain. Because of wide interindividual and intraindividual variations in the response to opioids, an occasional child will have an adverse reaction despite even the most careful titration of doses and intervals. The use of cardiorespiratory monitors is controversial, and professional judgment is required. In any case, machines cannot substitute for skilled and frequent assessment and observation by the health care provider.

Regional Analgesia. Regional analgesia is now widely used for infants and children and may be particularly applicable for young infants as well. Hemodynamic and respiratory effects of major regional analgesia in infants appear minimal.[241] The proper use of infusions or intermittent doses of epidural opioids and/or local anesthetics requires expertise and close monitoring, at least equal to that needed for infants receiving systemic opioids. An acute or postoperative pain service is usually necessary to provide the expertise and vigilance required.

Continuous epidural analgesia is effective for thoracic, abdominal, urologic, and orthopedic procedures.[238] Epidural infusions can be administered caudally (especially in children under 6 months of age) or via lumbar or thoracic epidural catheters in older children. Solutions infused into the epidural space are similar to but often more dilute than those applied in adults. Other regional techniques available to children include interpleural continuous infusions, brachial plexus infusions, lumbar sympathetic catheter infusions, and peripheral nerve blockade such as penile blocks.

Managing Postoperative Pain in Neonates and Infants. Young infants, especially premature infants or those who have neurologic abnormalities or pulmonary disease, are susceptible to apnea and respiratory depression when systemic opioids are used.[163,242] Metabolism is altered so that the elimination half-life is prolonged, and the blood-brain barrier is more permeable.[234,243-245] Thus, the adequate management of pain in this age group requires special consideration and expertise.

Clearly, neonates and infants experience pain, and adequate analgesia after surgery is necessary for both physiologic and ethical reasons. Institutions in which major surgery on neonates and infants is performed should provide training for personnel in the effective and safe administration of analgesia for children in this age group, as well as the technologic capability to provide appropriate monitoring. Several aspects of care should be noted.

Age. Some evidence suggests that the clearance of opioids increases rapidly over the first few weeks of life, and approaches adult rates by one to two months of age.[244-246] Because the available data are based on small numbers of infants, most practitioners reduce the initial dose and use intensive monitoring for infants up to about six months of age; this age is arbitrary and based on a cautious interpretation of the literature. It is reasonable to continue intensive monitoring up to about one year of age, as extreme sedation and decreased effort of respiration may be more difficult to assess in this age group than in older children.

Dosing and Schedules. Although further investigation is necessary, apnea and respiratory depression appear to be dose related.[244] For nonventilated infants under six months of age, the initial opioid dose, calculated in milligrams per kilogram, should be about one fourth to one third of the dose recommended for older infants and children. For example, morphine could be used at a dose of 0.03 mg/kg, instead of the traditional 0.1 mg/kg. Careful assessment is necessary after any dose, so that the optimal dose and interval of administration can be determined from clinical parameters (e.g., when pain breaks through and whether the infant appears comfortable after the dose). Many infants have inadequate pain relief after the initial small dose and require upward titration, sometimes to doses used for older children. Continuous infusions can be used, but a reduced dose is again necessary.

Regional Analgesia. Regional analgesia for neonates and young infants is as previously described for older infants and children.

Monitoring. Close monitoring of heart and respiratory rates, respiratory effort, blood pressure, and responsiveness to stimuli is mandatory. Frequent or continuous assessment of arterial oxygen saturation using pulse oximetry is a valuable adjunct to close clinical observation. Serum levels of opioids may increase many hours after a one-time intramuscular or subcutaneous dose, presumably because of late release from tissue stores. Thus, monitoring is continued for 24 hours after an opioid dose.[243]

Nonopioid Analgesics. These analgesics (e.g., acetaminophen) can be safely administered to neonates and infants without concern for hepatotoxicity when given for short courses at the recommended doses.[247,248] Acetaminophen can be given rectally or orally to augment analgesia.

Responsibility for Effective Pain Relief in Children. A formal and structured institutional review of pain management is as necessary for children as for adults. It begins with affirming the rights of all children in any institution to receive the best level of pain relief that can be provided safely. The available methods of pain management should be appropriate for the medical conditions of the children and the surgical procedures that are performed. Recommendations in this guideline in the section entitled Responsibility for Effective Pain Relief apply to children as well as adults. Patient and family feedback is necessary to ascertain and ensure the adequacy of pain management in children of all ages.

An environment centered on the child is necessary for adequate communication and assessment and to decrease the emotional distress of hospitalization. In addition to a staff experienced in caring for children, a child-centered environment lets parents participate in child care and provides adequate toys and age-appropriate activities.

Critical Questions Regarding the Adequacy of Pain Management Strategies. Knowledge of children—developmentally, behaviorally, and physiologically—is necessary for optimal assessment and treatment. Children are likely to talk less about pain than adults. Thus, the burden of vigilance for pain rests with the health care provider. The following questions focus on decision points of pain management. These questions serve as a guide for the health care provider to optimize pain management. Some children, however, will present with pain that is difficult to manage. In these situations, consultation is recommended.

Critical questions to consider before and during pharmacologic management include

- Have the child and parent(s) been asked about their previous experiences with pain and their preferences for use of analgesics?
- Is the child being adequately assessed at appropriate intervals?
- Are analgesics ordered for prevention and relief of pain?
- Is the analgesic strong enough for the pain expected or the pain being experienced?
- Is the timing of drug administration appropriate for the pain expected or experienced?
- Is the route of administration appropriate (preferably oral or intravenous) for the child?
- Is the child adequately monitored for the occurrence of side effects?
- Are side effects appropriately managed?
- Has the analgesic regimen provided adequate comfort and satisfaction from the child's or parents' perspective?

Parallel questions regarding nonpharmacologic strategies include

- Have the child and parent(s) been asked about their experience with and preferences for a given strategy?
- Is the strategy appropriate for the child's developmental level, condition, and type of pain?
- Is the timing of the strategy sufficient to optimize its effects?
- Is the strategy adequately effective in preventing or alleviating the child's pain?
- Are the child and parent(s) satisfied with the strategy for prevention or relief of pain?
- Are the treatable sources of emotional distress for the child being addressed?

Elderly Patients

Elderly patients present several pain management problems. First, relatively little attention has been paid to the topic of geriatric pain control in medical or nursing texts.[249] This is ironic because elderly people often suffer acute and chronic painful diseases,[250] have multiple diseases, and take many medications. They may have more than one source of pain and an increased risk for drug-drug as well as drug-disease interactions.[251] It has been estimated from population studies that the prevalence of pain is twofold higher in those over age 60 (250 per thousand) compared with those under 60 (125 per thousand).[252] Among institutionalized elderly, the prevalence may be over 70%.[253] Indeed, more than 80% of elderly people suffer various forms of arthritis, and most will have acute pain at some time.[254] Many elective or emergent operations are performed in the elderly to correct orthopedic problems (e.g., fractures, degenerative joint disease). Acute and/or postoperative severe pain related to cancer and its treatment are also more common in the elderly.[255] Other acutely painful conditions that affect the elderly disproportionately include herpes zoster, temporal arteritis, polymyalgia rheumatica, and atherosclerotic peripheral vascular disease.[250]

Second, pain assessment may present unique problems in elderly patients. They often report pain very differently from younger patients because of physiologic as well as psychological and cultural changes associated with aging.[256] Institutionalized elderly are often stoic about pain.[255] Age-associated changes in acute pain perception have long been of interest. Elderly patients often demonstrate altered presentations of common illnesses including "silent" myocardial infarctions and "painless" intra-abdominal emergencies.[257,258] Whether these clinical observations are the result of age-associated changes in pain perception remains to be explained. The widespread belief among clinicians that aging results in increased pain thresholds may be a myth. A variety of experiments using heat, pressure, or electrical current have not disclosed a trend regarding age-associated changes in either pain threshold or tolerance. It should be noted that the clinical relevance of these studies remains questionable, since experimentally induced pain may not be analogous to clinically experienced pain.[259]

Cognitive impairment, delirium (common in acutely ill frail elderly), and dementia (occurring in as many as 50% of institutionalized elderly) represent serious barriers to pain assessment for which no solution exists in the literature. Whether behavioral observations (e.g., agitation, restlessness, groaning) are sensitive and specific for pain assessment among the demented elderly remains to be shown. Traditional approaches, including the use of visual analogue scales, verbal descriptor scales, and numerical scales, have not been psychometrically established in this population. Moreover, a high prevalence of visual, hearing, and motor impairments in the elderly may impede the universal use of such scales by clinicians. Preliminary reports from ongoing work in the nursing home population suggest that many patients with moderate to severe cognitive impairment are able to report acute pain reliably at the moment or when prompted, although pain recall and integration of pain experience over time may be less reliable. If these early observations prove correct, pain assessment in this population may require frequent monitoring. Monitoring may have major implications for quality assurance, quality of care, and quality of life in this large population of elderly people (Ferrell and Ferrell. Personal communication. Work in progress on the epidemiology of pain among community nursing homes. 1991 Jul).

Third, elderly people, especially the frail and old-old (those over 85) are at particular risk for both undertreatment and overtreatment. Unfortunately, few studies of analgesic dosage requirements are performed in the elderly, and most studies have systematically excluded all potential subjects over 65. Age-related observations are extremely variable among elderly people. Indeed, the variance in measurements of most physiologic and pharmacologic parameters increases with age in cross-sectional studies.[251] Age-related changes in pharmacokinetics and pharmacodynamics contribute to a variety of adverse drug effects that have been reported in the elderly.

Nonopioid analgesic drugs, including NSAIDs and acetaminophen, are effective and appropriate for a variety of pain complaints in the elderly. However, it is recognized that the risk for gastric and renal toxicity from NSAIDs is increased in elderly patients, and unusual drug reactions including cognitive impairment, constipation, and headaches are also more common in the elderly population.[260] If gastric ulceration is a particular concern, co-administration of misoprostol or use of "platelet-sparing" NSAIDs should be considered as a way to lessen the risk of gastrointestinal bleeding.

Opioid analgesic drugs are effective for the management of acute pain in most elderly patients. Cheyne-Stokes breathing patterns are not unusual during sleep in the elderly and need not prompt discontinuation of opioid analgesia unless such analgesia clearly is associated with unacceptable degrees of arterial oxygen desaturation (< 85%). PCA has been shown in at least one study to be safe and effective for postoperative pain relief in selected patients.[45] If PCA is used, careful titration of dosage is necessary to avoid undesirable effects due to drug accumulation or from a decrease in the arousal effect as painful stimuli subside later in the patient's course. Elderly people are more sensitive to the analgesic effects of opioid drugs as they experience a higher peak and longer duration of pain relief.[261-263] They are also more sensitive to sedation and respiratory depression, probably as a result of altered distribution and excretion of the drugs. This is especially true in opioid-naive patients. Caution is required in the use of longer acting drugs such as methadone for this reason.[249]

Elderly people, in general, have increased fat-to-lean body mass ratios and reduced glomerular filtration rates.[251] Opioids produce cognitive and neuropsychiatric dysfunction through poorly defined mechanisms that in part include the accumulation of biologically active metabolites such as morphine-6-glucuronide or normeperidine.[79] Opioid dosage titration should take account of not only analgesic effects but also side effects that extend beyond cognitive impairment. These side effects may include urinary retention that looms as a larger threat in elderly males with prostatic hypertrophy, constipation and intestinal obstruction, respiratory depression, or exacerbation of Parkinson's disease. The management of nausea using phenothiazines or antihistamines is fraught with problems, because elderly people are exquisitely sensitive to anticholinergic side effects including delirium, bladder and bowel dysfunction, and movement disorders.[249]

Local anesthetic infusions may result in cognitive impairment if significant blood levels are reached. Yet prior to that point, orthostatic hypotension may result from sympathetic blockade and clumsiness may ensue from partial motor or sensory anesthesia. Thus, appropriate precautions should be taken, such as help with ambulation or the use of side rails at night.

Finally, attitudes among health care professionals, the lay public, and patients themselves may impede appropriate care. Many members of all three groups consider acute and chronic pain a part of normal aging.[249,253]

Patients Who Are Known or Suspected Substance Abusers

Management of acute pain in the substance abuser is a difficult but increasingly common clinical problem. Substance abusers experience traumatic injuries (see section on Patients with Shock, Trauma, and Burns) and a variety of health problems more often than the general population. Often during their postoperative care, issues arise that prompt the staff to request consultation with specialized "pain teams." For example, the question of possible withdrawal from pre-existing opioid use may be raised because sympathetic nervous system stimulation (restlessness, tachycardia, sleeplessness) may be caused by either undertreated pain or relative opioid abstinence. The related issue of risk of development of substance abuse behaviors in opioid-naive patients given opioid analgesics postoperatively appears to be small based on survey data by Porter and Jick,[76] who found that only four such instances of iatrogenic drug abuse occurred in approximately 12,000 patients screened through the Boston Collaborative Drug Study.

A variety of reports, increasingly frequent in number, have addressed the difficult questions surrounding postoperative opioid use in substance abusers, and several recommendations have recently emerged from reviews of this literature.[264] First, every effort should be made to define the mechanism of the pain and to treat the primary problem. Infection, tissue ischemia, or a new surgical diagnosis in the postoperative period may require specific measures such as antibiotic therapy, fasciotomy, or reoperation rather than an increase in the opioid dose. Attention to the primary cause of pain symptoms may reduce greatly the requirement for and negotiations about opioid analgesics.

Second, clinicians should distinguish between the temporal characteristics of the abuse behavior. For example, a distant history of substance abuse might predispose to re-emergence of substance abuse behaviors with the stress of surgery and postoperative pain but may not require treatment approaches different from those appropriate for nonaddicted patients. The implications are different for patients with a recent history of active drug abuse, who may require higher than usual starting doses of opioids and who may not have acquired an ability to set limits on their drug use.

Third, one should follow relevant pharmacologic principles of opioid use. For example, treatment with an opioid agonist-antagonist should not be started in the patient who enters tolerant to opioid agonists such as methadone. Mixed agonist-antagonists may precipitate withdrawal if given in this setting. Loading doses of opioids will be required in normal patients as well as in substance abusers to reduce the intensity of postoperative pain to acceptable levels. PCA is being used with increasing frequency for many patients, including known substance abusers. This mode of opioid delivery can be utilized safely in substance abusers when appropriate lockout intervals and hourly dosage limits are programmed, and when the device is "tamper-resistant," so that the patient cannot reprogram the pump or remove any drug. If used for an opioid-tolerant patient, PCA doses must be increased to achieve the same analgesic effect as for opioid-naive or nonaddicted patients.

Fourth, just as for other patients, nonopioid therapies should be given concomitantly with or even to replace opioids. Such therapies include NSAIDs, local anesthetic solutions given via catheter into the epidural space or surrounding peripheral nerves, cryoanalgesia, TENS, and nondrug therapies. Appropriate use of nonopioid therapies frequently will reduce the dosage requirement for opioid analgesia.

Fifth, specific drug abuse behavior in the postoperative patient should be recognized and dealt with firmly. Such behavior includes tampering with PCA machines (or other drug delivery devices), hoarding of oral doses of opioid analgesics, or attempting to self-inject the melted contents of capsules or siphoned infusion solutions. At that point, limits of analgesic dosages and expected patient behavior should be made clear to the patient in a frank discussion that also considers the medical, ethical, and legal consequences to the patient and physician if drug abuse behaviors continue. For the most part, security measures already in place (locked closets and inventory checks each nursing shift, antitamper features on PCA machines) will frustrate such attempts. A toxicological screen may be ordered on an inpatient's urine or blood specimens to confirm or exclude a diagnosis of surreptitious drug use (e.g., cocaine administration).

In the outpatient setting, clear instructions (preferably written out and copied into the patient's record) should be offered regarding doses and frequency of medication and the number of days the prescription is expected to last. The addition of a random urine testing procedure to outpatient medication contracts should be considered in all outpatients with a known history of substance abuse who are given opioid analgesics for pain. Opioid medications should be prescribed by one physician only, and attempts to circumvent this restriction or to falsify prescriptions should not be tolerated. The claim of needing additional medication to make up for lost or stolen controlled substances should be accompanied by documentation that the patient has reported this to the police.

Sixth, caregivers should set limits to avoid excessive negotiation about drug selections or choices. For example, it is not appropriate to depart from an institutional policy for morphine use for postoperative analgesia just because of a substance abuser's request for meperidine, as long as the patient has no history of adverse reaction to morphine. Once every effort has been made by clinicians to adjust a patient's opioid regimen in light of the extent and site of the operation, the patient's prior tolerance to opioids, and clinical response to initial analgesic titration, it is not unreasonable to adhere to this regimen with few, if any, changes. When possible, the treatment plan should include clear criteria (e.g., number of days postoperatively, ability to ambulate) by which opioid doses will be tapered and stopped. Within such a treatment plan, requests for higher dosage by a patient who can walk easily or spends much of the time resting comfortably may appropriately be denied. Consultation should be obtained with appropriate services early in a difficult patient's course. Consultation should help develop a unified multidisciplinary plan that includes, usually, psychiatric, psychological, and substance abuse expertise. Medical input can be obtained beyond the scope of the immediate caretakers to evaluate these and other problematic behaviors. Medical and/or neurologic input can be valuable when neurologic symptoms such as seizures in patients who have recently discontinued alcohol or barbiturate use are assessed.

These guidelines will aid the clinician in distinguishing "drug seeking" behaviors from "pain avoidance" behaviors. Often patients who are undertreated for pain and who voice displeasure are labeled as "addicts." This phenomenon has been called "pseudo-addiction."[265] Careful and objective assessment and reassessment of the postoperative patient with an active or previous substance abuse history will minimize the chance of a clinician being "duped" into providing inappropriate opioids but still provide the patient with legitimate pain complaints the opportunity to obtain meaningful and safe pain relief with opioids.

Patients with Concurrent Medical Conditions

Postoperative pain frequently must be treated in patients who have concurrent medical conditions for which they are taking one or more medications. The medical condition per se or the medications taken for it may influence the choice of analgesic and its dosage. These medical conditions are frequently chronic, and it may not be possible to discontinue problematic medications because of surgery. The most common medications or classes of medications that produce clinically significant drug interactions with opioid analgesics include alcohol and any central nervous system depressants, phenytoin, rifampin, and monoamine oxidase inhibitors. Drugs whose primary site of action lies outside the central nervous system (e.g., antibiotics such as rifampin) also may interact with opioid analgesics.

Co-existing conditions themselves influence the type and doses of opioid analgesics and the relative risks of pain treatment in the postoperative period. For example, patients with chronic pain who have been treated recently with opioids (e.g., patients with cancer and sickle cell disease) will usually require higher than the recommended starting doses to overcome opioid tolerance. Coagulopathy, neutropenia, and sepsis may contraindicate the use of epidural catheters or other regional anesthetic techniques in which the risks of bleeding or "seeding" of infection are increased.

Drug pharmacokinetics may change following surgery because of changes in drug absorption and distribution caused by alterations in cardiac output, venous capacitance, extravascular fluid shifts ("third spacing"), and changes in protein binding. Fever and sepsis in the postoperative period may affect drug disposition, as do shock, trauma, and burns. In addition, patients may not attain clinically effective plasma concentrations of opioids following intramuscular and subcutaneous injections because of pharmacokinetic alterations.

The major factor to consider in selecting analgesics for patients with concurrent medical conditions is whether the disorder produces either hepatic or renal impairment. Most analgesics are metabolized by the liver or kidney, so that any impairment of function in these organs influences the pharmacokinetics of the analgesic. The net result can be drug accumulation. Therefore, caution is essential when using opioids in patients with altered hepatic or renal function. Morphine is metabolized in the liver, and the parent compound, along with the metabolites, is excreted through the kidney. Acute or chronic hepatic failure (e.g., viral hepatitis or cirrhosis) appears to lower plasma clearance of morphine, prolong the terminal elimination half-life, and increase oral bioavailability.[266] Even mild renal failure, such as that associated with a decline in glomerular filtration rate with aging, can impede excretion of the metabolites of many opioids, resulting in clinically significant narcosis and respiratory depression.[267] Physiological alterations during surgery (e.g., changes in regional blood flow to the liver or kidneys, hepatic enzyme activity, enterohepatic circulation, or hormonal responses) may also alter drug metabolism and excretion. Meperidine, pentazocine, and propoxyphene have increased bioavailability, prolonged half-lives, and decreased systemic clearance and thus accumulate in hepatic and renal dysfunction. Doses of these drugs must be decreased appropriately. In contrast, the disposition and elimination of methadone are not significantly altered in patients with chronic liver disease.

Renal excretion is a major route of elimination for pharmacologically active opioid metabolites: norpropoxyphene, normeperidine, morphine-6-glucuronide, and dihydrocodeine. Elimination is decreased in patients with renal failure, and doses must be lowered or given less frequently.

For individual patients, it is difficult to predict the degree of impairment of metabolism or excretion of the most commonly used analgesics from either the clinical condition or laboratory indicators of hepatic or renal function because many factors impinge on clinical response. A lowered initial dose, careful titration of the opioid to desired effect, and ongoing monitoring of clinical response, level of consciousness, and respiratory effort are indicated. Continuous infusions and opioid administration around-the-clock at conventional intervals can result in accumulation of the parent compound or clinically active metabolites. To avoid undertreatment of pain during as-needed dosage schedules, the patient can be assessed at regular intervals, and if stable, a dose of opioid can be offered. PCA does not necessarily protect against accumulation of opioids and respiratory depression.[268] In renal failure especially, a decreased dose and prolonged lockout interval may be required. Nonopioid analgesics are often contraindicated in patients with hepatic or renal dysfunction.

Other diseases that may influence the control of postoperative pain include psychiatric illnesses requiring tricyclic antidepressants and monoamine oxidase inhibitors for treatment, neurologic disorders, pulmonary diseases, and acute and chronic infections.

Patients with respiratory insufficiency and those with chronic obstructive pulmonary disease, cystic fibrosis, and neuromuscular disorders affecting respiratory effort (e.g., muscular dystrophy, myasthenia gravis) are vulnerable to the respiratory depressant effects of opioids. However, when a patient splints his or her respiratory effort because of uncontrolled pain, that also can impair gas exchange. Therefore, careful planning is required to provide effective and safe postoperative analgesia. Unless specific contraindications exist, the use of nonopioid analgesics can be optimized in this group of patients.

However, severe postoperative pain may not be adequately controlled with just these agents. Epidural opioids have a lesser effect on pulmonary function than do systemic opioids.[269] Other regional anesthetic techniques can also be applied in this setting as a way to lower the dosage of systemic opioids required for satisfactory postoperative analgesia. If epidural analgesia cannot be used, small doses of opioids given frequently, continuous infusion, or PCA may provide smoother control of pain with less impact on respiratory effort at the time of peak effect. Whichever method is used to administer systemic opioids, a low initial dose is recommended; later doses can then be titrated to the desired effect. Appropriate monitoring of respiratory rate and effort and adequacy of gas exchange is necessary. Oximetry may be useful in selected cases.

Neurologic disorders can influence postoperative pain management if they (1) produce weakness of the respiratory muscles (e.g., amyotrophic lateral sclerosis, poliomyelitis); (2) impair alertness and mental function so that the sedative effects of opioids are exaggerated, and pain cannot be assessed easily; and (3) cause seizures requiring use of chronic anticonvulsant medications that may interact with analgesics. The first two circumstances have been addressed in the discussion above and other sections of this guideline. Phenytoin, a very commonly used anticonvulsant, increases the biotransformation of meperidine, causing faster elimination and necessitating increased doses of this analgesic.[270]

Patients with psychiatric illnesses taking anxiolytics or other psychoactive drugs must be carefully evaluated for drug interactions between the psychotropic and pain medications they take. Because both opioids and psychotropic drugs generally have sedative effects, it is not uncommon for these effects to be additive when the drugs are combined. Further, the tricyclic antidepressants clomipramine and amitriptyline may increase morphine levels as measured by an increase in bioavailability and the half-life of morphine.[271] Of particular importance is avoiding meperidine in patients receiving monoamine oxidase inhibitors. Severe adverse reactions, including death through mechanisms that mimic malignant hyperthermia, have been reported when these drugs have been used together.[270,272]

Patients treated with drugs for cardiovascular and metabolic disease frequently must continue their drugs throughout the intraoperative and postoperative period. Fortunately, severe interactions between these drugs and opioids are unlikely.

Alcoholics who must have surgical procedures should be maintained on benzodiazepines or alcohol throughout the intraoperative and postoperative period to prevent a withdrawal reaction or delirium tremens.

Clinicians must remain aware that patients in the categories discussed in this section may not respond as expected to medications administered for symptom control following surgery. Careful assessment and reassessment of patients' responses to analgesics and dose titration to response are always necessary. The concomitant use of nonpharmacologic treatments as adjunctive therapy of postoperative pain is also strongly recommended.

Patients with Shock, Trauma, and Burns

Victims of injury frequently present in a state of cardiovascular or respiratory instability that mandates immediate life-saving procedures (e.g., endotracheal intubation, defibrillation, cut-down, and chest tube insertion) without analgesia. The trauma patient is usually young (58.4%), frequently male (72.8%), and commonly (51.2%) has used alcohol or drugs prior to injury.[273]

Beecher[274] was the first to point out the difficulties in providing analgesia via the intramuscular route following a significant burn or injury. He noted the variability in absorption from site to site and prolonged absorption times in soldiers with shock. He also provided the basis for modern day pain control after burns or injuries by suggesting the exclusive use of the intravenous route. Most authorities now recommend incremental small intravenous doses of an opioid analgesic (morphine) carefully titrated to cardiovascular and respiratory stability. Concern for cardiorespiratory instability is particularly important in the first hour after injury. Any analgesic therapy also must allow for continuous monitoring of neurologic status after a head injury and neurovascular status after limb injury.

Once the patient is resuscitated and requires definitive surgical procedures, analgesia should be provided as outlined in this guideline for the various operative sites. The use of NSAIDs in the trauma patient remains controversial. They are undoubtedly of value in the patient with minor trauma, but the risk of excessive bleeding and gastric stress ulcers may prohibit their use following closed head injury, burn injury, or other multisystem injuries. When not contraindicated by sepsis, coagulopathy, or cardiorespiratory instability, the use of regional anesthetic approaches may be beneficial as described earlier for particular operative sites. For example, discomfort and splinting due to flail chest injury may improve with epidural analgesia, and borderline perfusion of an injured limb can increase with a sympathetic blockade by an epidural local anesthetic. On the other hand, surgical evaluation must always take priority over analgesic titration in the face of sudden increases in pain (e.g., extremity swelling) or somnolence (e.g., from an expanding subdural hematoma).

The patient with serious burn injury will require very special pain control after the initial resuscitation. The myth that "third-degree burns don't hurt" unfortunately still serves as a basis for widespread institutional denial of pain assessment and treatment for burn patients.[275] Pain control is essentially absent from current reviews of burn management, scientific programs of national burn associations, or funding agendas of the federal government or major private burn treatment organizations, much as pediatric pain and cancer pain were a decade ago. In reality, after a brief (hours-long) period of endogenous analgesia evoked by the stress of immediate burn injury, pain is often severe and intermittently excruciating for months during burn dressing changes, skin grafts, reconstructive surgery, or other interventions related to needs for prolonged ventilation or intravascular access. Nonviable, insensate tissue is always surrounded by regenerating areas from which pain may arise, considering that viable perfused tissue typically forms the inner margin of an excision. Altered pharmacokinetics and pharmacodynamics in the burn patient, who may be intubated, splinted, and unable to articulate pain, further combine to render pain management an individualized challenge. The almost universal presence of hypotension and vasodilation with or without sepsis generally precludes the use of spinal or epidural routes for pain control until the burn wound is closed. While some authors have described analgesic regimens for burn dressing changes that call for nonnarcotic analgesics, such as ketamine or nitrous oxide, these approaches are best reserved for unusual or refractory instances because of side effects such as dysphoria[276] or bone marrow depression,[277] respectively. More typically, high doses of opioids are required to bring pain under control. Even then, there may be pain that is relatively refractory to opioid use, particularly if the burn site is deep or extensive. A morphine infusion alone is inadequate to produce anesthesia, such as for operative procedures or prolonged ventilation, since awareness often persists. Recent clinical studies suggest that damage to underlying nerves may account for the opioid-resistant quality of pain after severe burns,[273,276] and that the continuous infusion of low doses of lidocaine—known to lessen neuropathic pain in other settings—may be a useful analgesic option in patients with burns.[277] For these reasons, and also because fear and anxiety are an almost universal response to burn injury and trauma of any kind, sedatives such as benzodiazepines are useful to supplement opioid analgesics. In addition, cognitive-behavioral strategies such as relaxation, imagery, and hypnosis have been described by burn survivors as very helpful. The large full-thickness burn with its consequences of pain, separation from family and job, and (frequently) disfigurement is usually accompanied by depression that may require drugs and, in turn, influence analgesic effects.

Patients Who Undergo Procedures outside of the Operating Room

Thousands of patients undergo painful procedures each day outside of operating rooms in emergency departments, clinics, wards, and intensive-care units. Analgesia issues outside the operating room also broadly apply to patients who have ambulatory surgical procedures, after which same-day discharge is expected. In any of the above settings, many procedures can be safely performed under local infiltration or regional anesthesia or by adopting behavioral, nondrug strategies, but systemic analgesia is often required to provide optimal pain control.

Only when immediate treatment of cardiorespiratory instability is required, or if a competent patient declines treatment, should analgesia be withheld for a painful procedure. The presence of a condition that could eventually result in cardiovascular, hemodynamic, neurologic, or pulmonary instability (e.g., femur fracture, pneumothorax, skull fracture) is not an absolute contraindication to systemic analgesia, although careful titration and monitoring must be provided. Though pain control may not be needed for certain procedures (e.g., diagnostic computed tomography scan, intravenous pyelogram, or ultrasound examination), providing analgesia is likely to enhance the accuracy of these studies by reducing patient writhing or restlessness because of pain.

No anesthetic or analgesic agent should be used unless the clinician understands the proper technique of administration, dosage, contraindications, side effects, and treatment of overdose. As described earlier, the intravenous route is the preferred delivery mode because of its rapid onset and easy and reliable dosing. Using an intravenous route sidesteps the pain and the unpredictable absorption, onset, and duration of action associated with intramuscular or subcutaneous injections. An intravenous cannula may be placed painlessly following intradermal injection of 1 mL of 1–2% lidocaine through a 27–30 gauge needle. Most often, intravenous titration of an opioid like morphine, with observation for 5–10 minutes between doses, will provide safe and adequate analgesia. Intravenous morphine doses may range from 1 to 10 mg depending on the age, weight, pain intensity, opioid tolerance, and nature of the procedure to be done. Dose titration must be continued throughout the procedure, since pain may break through, for example, during reduction of a joint or vigorous probing of an abscess.

Contraindications to opioid analgesia include altered sensorium, lung disease, pregnancy near term, or an inability to monitor and manage side effects such as respiratory depression in the setting where care is given. Since respiratory depression is strongly correlated with the degree of sedation, stimulation of the patient as well as the administration of small doses of naloxone (e.g., 0.04 mg), may be adequate to reverse mild degrees of hypoventilation. Of course, assisted ventilation by bag and mask, or (ultimately) endotracheal intubation and repetitive naloxone dosing, may be required to reverse more severe degrees of respiratory depression. If such respiratory depression does occur, the patient should be observed until well after the naloxone effect has worn off (usually after one hour). Nausea, bradycardia, and hypotension are other side effects to watch for in the clinic, ward, or emergency department.

Other opioids may be used in place of morphine. Meperidine is suitable for brief, titrated dosing but not for prolonged use. Fentanyl may be used in small doses (25-μg increments in the above example) but carries a higher risk than morphine or meperidine of inducing chest wall rigidity that must be immediately managed by administering a quick-onset muscle relaxant and supporting ventilation. Apart from chest wall rigidity, any opioid may trigger an acute Parkinson's-like syndrome particularly in the elderly or in patients with Parkinson's disease under medical therapy. Some mixed agonist-antagonists have the advantage that they produce lesser degrees of biliary or ureteral smooth muscle spasm, but they also may precipitate a withdrawal syndrome in patients habituated to opioid agonists such as methadone or heroin (or in other patients taking opioids for chronic pain).

NSAIDs currently have a limited role in the management of pain during brief, painful procedures, but two other nonnarcotic agents have proven useful when administered in monitored settings by trained personnel. Intravenous ketamine has a rapid onset of action and produces a state of conscious sedation in which patients respond to verbal commands and maintain airway reflexes but experience analgesia. Possible side effects include dysphoria, tachycardia, increased salivary and tracheal secretions, and myocardial ischemia in patients with pre-existing cardiac disease. Inhalation of a nitrous oxide–oxygen mixture can provide prompt anxiolysis and moderate analgesia. As a precaution, the patient should breathe through a face mask that he or she is holding, so that the mask will drop away if the patient becomes somnolent. Appropriate precautions should be taken to prevent environmental contamination with nitrous oxide (i.e., scavenging system), to avoid the possible inhalation of pure nitrous oxide without oxygen, and to withhold nitrous oxide in cases of altered sensorium, entrapped air such as pneumothorax or pulmonary blebs, bowel obstruction, air embolism, chronic pulmonary disease, or suspected decompression sickness.

Benzodiazepines may be valuable adjuncts to opioids in this setting. Although they lack analgesic properties for treatment of pain due to acute tissue injury, benzodiazepines diminish skeletal muscle spasm (e.g., during orthopedic reduction), reduce anxiety, and in higher doses, provide amnesia. Coadministration of an opioid and a benzodiazepine carries a substantially higher risk of inducing respiratory depression than administration of either drug individually, so particular vigilance is necessary. Typically, in a 70 kg adult, midazolam is used in incremental doses of 1 mg intravenously. Other agents such as phenothiazines (as antiemetics) or antihistamines (because of their weak sedative and analgesic properties) are useful in individual cases.

Regardless of the analgesic or adjuvant given, patients should be monitored closely according to institutional standards. Such standards may include continuous observation of the electrocardiogram; frequent recording of heart rate, blood pressure, and respiratory rate; and pulse oximetry. Considering the risks associated with opioid, benzodiazepine, and other analgesic use, patients should not be left unattended between successive doses of these agents and should be watched for at least 30 minutes after the completion of outpatient procedures for which intravenous analgesia has been provided. In a transient care setting, patients should not be discharged until they are awake and can converse and ambulate. Once discharged they should be accompanied by an adult for at least two half-lives of the agents used (e.g., at least six hours for morphine) and should be advised not to drive an automobile or operate dangerous machinery until it is likely that all medication effects are resolved (usually 24–48 hours). Documentation of monitoring during the procedure, observation prior to discharge, and discharge instructions should be part of the patient's permanent record.

At any site where painful procedures may be performed, equipment should be available to treat promptly any untoward effects of the analgesics selected. Apart from monitoring devices, such equipment includes supplemental oxygen, devices to maintain airway patency (e.g., oral and nasal airways, face masks, endotracheal tubes, laryngoscopes, and a bag-valve device), suction, drugs for resuscitation (e.g., atropine, naloxone), and a defibrillator. Most important, there must be present on site a physician or other provider skilled in resuscitation, particularly airway management.

Responsibility for Effective Pain Relief

Optimal application of pain control methods depends on cooperation between different members of the health care team throughout the patient's course of treatment. To ensure that this process occurs effectively, formal means must be developed and used within each institution to assess pain and to obtain patient feedback to gauge the adequacy of its control.[46,47,55]

The institutional process of acute pain management begins with an affirmation that patients should have access to the best level of pain relief that may safely be provided. Each institution should develop the resources necessary to provide the best and most modern pain relief appropriate to its patients.

In any setting, the quality of pain control will be influenced by the availability of a pain management program and the training, expertise, and experience of its members. There is wide variation among institutions in size, complexity, volume of surgical procedures, and differing patient populations; therefore, different pain management programs are suitable. In all cases, responsibility for this care should be assigned to those most knowledgeable, experienced, interested, and available to deal with patients' needs in a timely fashion.

Risks associated with sophisticated options for effective pain relief, such as epidural analgesia or PCA, are minimized by encouraging their application in an organized, methodical fashion with frequent follow-up and titration. It is logical to assign responsibility for effective pain relief under such circumstances to experts working in dedicated groups. The sense of security present in many hospitals where such dedicated groups are active should not seduce other providers into offering sophisticated pain relief options beyond the institutional resources to manage them vigilantly. Patient-controlled or epidural analgesia, or even conventional analgesia given by injection, are all potentially lethal. Death can occur if dosages are not titrated, drug interactions are not watched for, and patients are not monitored for side effects like respiratory depression. In this sense, analgesics should be prescribed with no less care and expertise than other medications such as digitalis or insulin. In settings where pain management teams are not feasible (e.g., surgicenters, primary care clinics, or nursing homes), less sophisticated options may be appropriate, yet responsibility for effective pain control should still be assigned to interested individuals. Only if institutions recognize the importance of effective pain control and assign responsibility to designated, accountable individuals or groups can the quality of care in this area be at its best.

The key items to be considered when developing an institutional quality assurance program to monitor the provision of pain relief are:

- Patient comfort and satisfaction with pain management
- The range and appropriateness of options available within a particular institution
- How those options can best be applied
- Minimizing side effects and complications related to pain control

Implementation of this guideline requires more than quality assurance procedures: interdisciplinary, interprovider collaboration should occur. Three elements are essential for interdisciplinary collaboration: a common purpose, diverse professional skills and contributions, and effective coordinating and communicating processes. For nurses, physicians, and others treating acute pain, the common purpose is relief of patients' pain. The purpose should be *explicit*, and a *commitment* to this goal should be elicited from *every* provider who can influence the patient's pain. Each health professional's diverse and complementary skills and contributions should be recognized and used toward meeting the common goal of pain relief. Knowledgeable and talented providers with a common purpose may not achieve effective pain control without effective communication and coordination. The following elements will help ensure successful collaboration:

- Clarity among professionals about what they can and will contribute (such as, who will coordinate pain management—primary nurse and attending physician or specialized pain control team, and can consultants write prescriptions or orders?).
- Decision making that reflects input from the patient and family (when appropriate), such as providing, when feasible, a menu of pain control choices that includes pharmacologic and nonpharmacologic means.
- Contingency planning, such as orders to avert or treat possible drug side effects like constipation,

nausea, or urinary retention; a range of analgesic doses to deal with varying pain intensity; post-discharge follow-up of acute pain problems such as phantom pain; and clear coverage for off-shifts or weekends.
- Regular meetings (e.g., daily rounds) of *all* providers (as many and as interdisciplinary as possible) at *mutually* convenient times to maximize communication and information sharing.

In addition to the above clinical communications, interpersonal issues of power, leadership, and conflict can hamper efforts to relieve pain. An ability to analyze these situations, as well as interpersonal competence in leadership and conflict resolution, are vital for *building teams and keeping them focused on their shared purpose of relieving pain.*

Summary

Summary recommendations 1–5 and 7 should be implemented in every hospital where operations are performed on inpatients. The Acute Pain Management Guideline Panel recommends that any hospital in which abdominal or thoracic operations are routinely performed offer patients postoperative regional anesthetic, epidural or intrathecal opioids, PCA infusions, and other interventions requiring a similar level of expertise, under the supervision of an acute pain service as described in summary recommendation 6. For pain management to be effective, each hospital must designate who or which department will be responsible for all of the required activities.

There are a number of alternative approaches to preventing or relieving postoperative pain, many of which can give good results if attentively applied. The following elements, however, apply to most cases and might serve as a focus for assessing the results of these guidelines:

1. *Promise patients attentive analgesic care.* Patients should be informed before surgery, orally and in printed format, that effective pain relief is an important part of their treatment, that talking about unrelieved pain is essential, and that health professionals will respond quickly to their reports of pain. It should be made clear to patients and families, however, that the total absence of any postoperative discomfort is normally not a realistic or even a desirable goal.
2. *Chart and display assessment of pain and relief.* A simple assessment of pain intensity and pain relief should be recorded on the bedside vital sign chart or a similar record that encourages easy, regular review by members of the health care team and is incorporated in the patient's permanent record. The intensity of pain should be assessed and documented at regular intervals (depending on the severity of pain) and with each new report of pain. The degree of pain relief should be determined after each pain management intervention, once a sufficient time has elapsed for the treatment to reach peak effect. A simple, valid measure of intensity and relief should be selected by each clinical unit. For children, age-appropriate measures should be used.
3. *Define pain and relief levels to trigger a review.* Each institution should identify pain intensity and pain relief levels that will elicit a review of the current pain therapy, documentation of the proposed modifications in treatment, and subsequent review of its efficacy. This process of treatment review and follow-up should include participation by physicians and nurses involved in the patient's care.
4. *Survey patient satisfaction.* At regular intervals defined by the clinical unit and quality assurance committee, each clinical unit should assess a randomly selected sample of patients who have had surgery within 72 hours. Patients should be asked their current pain intensity, the worst pain intensity in the past 24 hours, the degree of relief obtained from pain management interventions, satisfaction with relief, and their satisfaction with the staff's responsiveness.
5. *Analgesic drug treatment should comply with several basic principles*:
   a. *Nonopioid "peripherally acting" analgesics.* Unless contraindicated, every patient should receive an around-the-clock postoperative regimen of an NSAID. For patients unable to take medications by mouth, it may be necessary to use the parenteral or rectal route.
   b. *Opioid analgesics.* Analgesic orders should allow for the great variation in individual opioid requirements, including a regularly scheduled dose and "rescue" doses for instances in which the usual regimen is insufficient.
6. *Specialized analgesic technologies.* Technologies including systemic or intraspinal continuous or intermittent opioid administration or patient-controlled dosing, local anesthetic infusion, and inhalational analgesia (e.g., nitrous oxide) should be governed by policies and standard procedures that define the acceptable level of patient monitoring and appropriate roles and limits of practice for all groups of health care providers involved. The policy should include definitions of physician and nurse accountability, physician and nurse responsibility to the patient, and the role of pharmacy.
7. *Nonpharmacologic interventions.* Cognitive and behaviorally based interventions include a number of methods to help patients understand more about their pain and to take an active part in its assessment and control. These interventions are intended to supplement, not replace, pharmacologic interventions. Staff should give patients information about these interventions and support patients in using them.
8. *Monitor the efficacy of pain treatment.* Periodically review pain treatment procedures as defined in summary recommendations 1–4 above, using the institution's quality assurance procedures.

References

128. Jackson DL, Moore PA, Hargreaves KM. Pre-operative nonsteroidal anti-inflammatory medication for the prevention of postoperative dental pain. *J Am Dent Assoc.* 1989; 119:641-7.

129. Max MB, Inturrisi CE, Kaiko RF et al. Epidural and intrathecal opiates: cerebrospinal fluid and plasma profiles in patients with chronic cancer pain. *Clin Pharmacol Ther.* 1985; 38:631-41.
130. Sjøgren P, Banning A. Pain, sedation, and reaction time during long-term treatment of cancer patients with oral and epidural opioids. *Pain.* 1989; 39:5-11.
131. Hasenbos M, van Egmond J, Gielen M et al. Post-operative analgesia by high thoracic epidural versus intramuscular nicomorphine after thoracotomy. Part III. The effects of pre- and post-operative analgesia on morbidity. *Acta Anaesthesiol Scand.* 1987; 31:608-15.
132. Shulman M, Sandler AN, Bradley JW et al. Postthoracotomy pain and pulmonary function following epidural and systemic morphine. *Anesthesiology.* 1984; 61:569-75.
133. Capogna G, Celleno D, Tagariello V et al. Intrathecal buprenorphine for postoperative analgesia in the elderly patient. *Anaesthesia.* 1988; 43:128-30.
134. Pybus DA, D'Bras BE, Goulding G et al. Postoperative analgesia for haemorrhoid surgery. *Anaesth Intensive Care.* 1983; 11:27-30.
135. Scott NB, Mogensen T, Bigler D et al. Comparison of the effects of continuous intrapleural vs epidural administration of 0.5% bupivacaine on pain, metabolic response and pulmonary function following cholecystectomy. *Acta Anaesthesiol Scand.* 1989; 33:535-9.
136. McGrath D, Thurston N, Wright D et al. Comparison of one technique of patient-controlled postoperative analgesia with intramuscular meperidine. *Pain.* 1989; 37:265-70.
137. Anon. Analgesia and the metabolic response to surgery. *Lancet.* 1985; 1:1018-9. Editorial.
138. Kehlet H. Surgical stress: the role of pain and analgesia. *Br J Anaesth.* 1989; 63:189-95.
139. Chawla R, Arora MK, Saksena R et al. Efficacy and dose-response of intrathecal pentazocine for post-operative pain relief. *Indian J Med Res.* 1989; 90:220-3.
140. Reay BA, Semple AJ, Macrae WA et al. Low-dose intrathecal diamorphine analgesia following major orthopaedic surgery. *Br J Anaesth.* 1989; 62:248-52.
141. Modig J, Borg T, Bagge L et al. Role of extradural and of general anaesthesia in fibrinolysis and coagulation after total hip replacement. *Br J Anaesth.* 1983; 55:625-9.
142. Modig J, Borg T, Karlstrom G et al. Thromboembolism after total hip replacement: role of epidural and general anesthesia. *Anesth Analg.* 1983; 62:174-80.
143. Pettine KA, Wedel DJ, Cabanela ME et al. The use of epidural bupivacaine following total knee arthroplasty. *Orthop Rev.* 1989; 18:894-901.
144. Hester NO, Foster R, Kristensen K et al. Measurement of children's pain by children, parents, and nurses: psychometric and clinical issues related to the poker chip tool and the pain ladder. Generalizability of procedures assessing pain in children: final report; 1989. Research funded by NIH, National Center for Nursing Research under Grant Number NR01382. [Available from N.O. Hester, Center for Nursing Research, School of Nursing, University of Colorado, Denver, CO 80262.]
145. Johnston CC, Jeans ME, Abbott FV et al. A survey of pain in hospitalized children: preliminary results. In: Tyler D, Krane E. Proceedings of the 1st International Symposium on Pediatric Pain. New York: Raven Press; 1988:80. Abstract.
146. Mather L, Mackie J. The incidence of postoperative pain in children. *Pain.* 1983; 15:271-82.
147. Beyer JE, DeGood DE, Ashley LC et al. Patterns of postoperative analgesic use with adults and children following cardiac surgery. *Pain.* 1983; 17:71-81.
148. Eland JM, Anderson JE. The experience of pain in children. In: Jacox AK, ed. Pain: a source book for nurses and other health professionals. Boston: Little, Brown; 1977:453-73.
149. Foster RL, Hester NO. Administration of analgesics for children's pain. *Pain.* 1990; Suppl 5:S27.
150. Foster RL, Hester NO. The relationship between pain ratings and pharmacologic interventions for children in pain. In: Tyler D, Krane E, eds. Advances in pain research and therapy: pediatric pain. Vol. 15. New York: Raven Press; 1990:31-6.
151. Schechter NL, Allen DA. Physician's attitudes toward pain in children. *J Dev Behav Pediatr.* 1986; 7:350-4.
152. Foster R, Hester N. The relationship between assessment and pharmacologic intervention for pain in children. In: Funk SG, Tornquist EM, Champagne, MT et al., eds. Key aspects of comfort: management of pain, fatigue, and nausea. New York: Springer; 1989:72-9.
153. Bush JP, Holmbeck GN, Cockrell JL. Patterns of PRN analgesic drug administration in children following elective surgery. *J Pediatr Psychol.* 1989; 14:433-48.
154. Anand, K. The biology of pain perception in newborn infants. In: Tyler D, Krane E, eds. Advances in pain research and therapy: pediatric pain. Vol. 15. New York: Raven Press; 1990:113-22.
155. Anand KJ, Aynsley-Green A. Measuring the severity of surgical stress in newborn infants. *J Pediatr Surg.* 1988; 23:297-305.
156. Fitzgerald M, Shaw A, MacIntosh N. Postnatal development of the cutaneous flexor reflex: comparative study of preterm infants and newborn rat pups. *Dev Med Child Neurol.* 1988; 30:520-6.
157. Fitzgerald M, Millard C, McIntosh N. Hyperalgesia in premature infants. *Lancet.* 1988; 1:292.
158. Fitzgerald M, Millard C, McIntosh N. Cutaneous hypersensitivity following peripheral tissue damage in newborn infants and its reversal with topical anesthesia. *Pain.* 1989; 39:31-6.
159. Franck LS. A national survey of the assessment and treatment of pain and agitation in the neonatal intensive care unit. *J Obstet Gynecol Neonatal Nurs.* 1987; 16:387-93.
160. Campbell NN, Reynolds GJ, Perkins G. Postoperative analgesia in neonates: an Australia-wide survey. *Anaesth Intensive Care.* 1989; 17:487-99.
161. Purcell-Jones G, Dormon F, Sumner E. Paediatric anaesthetists' perceptions of neonatal and infant pain. *Pain.* 1988; 33:181-7.
162. Schnurrer JA, Marvin JA, Heimbach DM. Evaluation of pediatric pain medications. *J Burn Care Rehabil.* 1985; 6:105-7.
163. Purcell-Jones G, Dormon F, Sumner E. The use of opioids in neonates. A retrospective study of 933 cases. *Anaesthesia.* 1987; 42:1316-20.
164. Fowler-Kerry S. Adolescent oncology survivors' recollection of pain. In: Tyler D, Krane E, eds. Advances in pain research and therapy: pediatric pain. Vol. 15. New York: Raven Press; 1990:365-71.
165. Jay SM, Ozolins M, Elliott CH et al. Assessment of children's distress during painful medical procedures. *Health Psychol.* 1983; 2:133-47.
166. Weekes D, Savedra M. Adolescent cancer: coping with treatment-related pain. *J Pediatr Nurs.* 1988; 3:318-28.
167. Schechter NL. The undertreatment of pain in children: an overview. *Pediatr Clin North Am.* 1989; 36:781-94.
168. Hester NO, Barcus CS. Assessment and management of pain in children. *Pediatr Nurs Update.* 1986; 1(14):1-8.
169. Stevens B. Development and testing of a pediatric pain management sheet. *Pediatr Nurs.* 1990; 16:543-8.
170. McGrath PA. Pain in children: nature, assessment, and treatment. New York: Guilford Press; 1990.
171. Beyer JE. The Oucher: a user's manual and technical report. 1984. [Available from Judith Beyer, University of Colorado, Denver, CO 80262.]
172. Hester NKO. The preoperational child's reaction to immunization. *Nurs Res.* 1979; 28:250-5.
173. Hester NO, Foster RL, Kristensen K. Measurement of pain in children: generalizability and validity of the pain ladder and the Poker Chip Tool. In: Tyler DC, Krane EJ, eds. Advances in pain research and therapy: pediatric pain.

Vol. 15. New York: Raven Press; 1990:79-84.
174. McGrath PA, de Veber LL, Hearn MT. Multidimensional pain assessment in children. In: Fields HL, Dubner R, Cervero F, eds. Proceedings of the Fourth World Conference on Pain. Advances in pain research and therapy. Vol. 9. New York: Raven Press; 1985:387-93.
175. McGrath PJ, Unruh AM. Pain in children and adolescents. Amsterdam: Elsevier; 1987.
176. Savedra MC, Tesler MD, Holzemer WL et al. Adolescent pediatric pain tool (APPT) preliminary user's manual. San Francisco: University of California; 1989. [Available from M.C. Savedra, UCSF School of Nursing, San Francisco, CA 94143-0606].
177. Aradine CR, Beyer JE, Tompkins JM. Children's pain perception before and after analgesia: a study of instrument construct validity and related issues. *J Pediatr Nurs*. 1988; 3(1):11-23.
178. Tesler MD, Savedra MC, Holzemer WL et al. The word-graphic rating scale as a measure of children's and adolescents' pain intensity. *Res Nurs Health*. 1991; 14:361-71.
179. Barrier G, Attia J, Mayer MN et al. Measurement of post-operative pain and narcotic administration in infants using a new clincal scoring system. *Intensive Care Med*. 1989; 15(Suppl 1):S37-S39.
180. Gauvain-Piquard A, Rodary C, Rezvani A et al. Pain in children aged 2-6 years: a new observational rating scale elaborated in a pediatric oncology unit; a preliminary report. *Pain*. 1987; 31:177-88.
181. McGrath PJ, Johnson G, Goodman JT et al. CHEOPS: a behavioral scale for rating postoperative pain in children. In: Fields HL, Dubner R, Cervero F, eds. Proceedings of the Fourth World Conference on Pain. Advances in pain research and therapy. Vol. 9. New York: Raven Press; 1985:395-402.
182. Hester NO, Foster RL. Cues nurses and parents use in making judgments about children's pain. *Pain*. 1990; Suppl 5:S31.
183. Grunau RVE, Craig KD. Pain expression in neonates: facial action and cry. *Pain*. 1987; 28:395-410.
184. Katz ER, Kellerman J, Siegel SE. Behavioral distress in children with cancer undergoing medical procedures: developmental considerations. *J Consult Clin Psychol*. 1980; 48:356-65.
185. LeBaron S, Zeltzer L. Assessment of acute pain and anxiety in children and adolescents by self-reports, observer reports, and a behavior checklist. *J Consult Clin Psychol*. 1984; 52:729-38.
186. Adams J. A methodological study of pain assessment in Anglo and Hispanic children with cancer. In: Tyler D, Krane E, eds. Advances in pain research and therapy: pediatric pain. Vol. 15. New York: Raven Press; 1990:43-52.
187. Hester NO. Comforting the child in pain. In: Funk SG, Tornquist EM, Champagne MT et al., eds. Key aspects of comfort: management of pain, fatigue, and nausea. New York: Springer; 1989:290-8.
188. Savedra M, Gibbons P, Tesler M et al. How do children describe pain? A tentative assessment. *Pain*. 1982; 14:95-104.
189. Johnson JE, Kirchoff K, Endress MP. Altering children's distress behavior during orthopedic cast removal. *Nurs Res*. 1975; 24:404-10.
190. Zeltzer LK, Altman A, Cohen D et al. American Academy of Pediatrics: report of the Subcommittee on Management of Pain Associated with Procedures in Children with Cancer. *Pediatrics*. 1990; 86(Suppl 5):826-31.
191. Fradet C, McGrath PJ, Kay J et al. A prospective survey of reactions to blood tests by children and adolescents. *Pain*. 1990; 40:53-60.
192. Schechter NL, Bernstein BA, Beck A et al. Individual differences in children's response to pain: role of temperament and parental characteristics. *Pediatrics*. 1991; 87:171-7.
193. Bauchner H, Waring C, Vinci R. Parental presence during procedures in an emergency room: results from 50 observations. *Pediatrics*. 1991; 87:544-8.
194. Shaw E, Routh D. Effect of mothers' presence on children's reaction to aversive procedures. *J Pediatr Psychol*. 1982; 7:33-42.
195. Maunuksela EL, Korpela R. Double-blind evaluation of a lignocaine-prilocaine cream (EMLA) in children. *Br J Anaesth*. 1986; 58:1242-5.
196. Zelzter LK, Jay SM, Fisher DM. The management of pain associated with pediatric procedures. *Pediatr Clin North Am*. 1989; 36:941-64.
197. Nahata M, Clotz M, Krogg E. Adverse effects of meperidine, promethazine, and chlorpromazine for sedation in pediatric patients. *Clin Pediatr*. 1985; 24:558-60.
198. American Academy of Pediatrics. Guidelines for the elective use of conscious sedation, deep sedation, and general anesthesia in pediatric patients. *Pediatrics*. 1985; 76:317-21.
199. American Academy of Pediatrics. Guidelines for monitoring and management of pediatric patients during and following sedation for diagnostic and therapeutic procedures. *Pediatrics*. (in press).
200. Campos RG. Soothing pain-elicited distress in infants with swaddling and pacifiers. *Child Dev*. 1989; 60:781-92.
201. Field T, Goldson E. Pacifying effects of nonnutritive sucking on term and preterm neonates during heelstick procedures. *Pediatrics*. 1984; 74:1012-5.
202. Triplett JL, Arneson SW. The use of verbal and tactile comfort to alleviate distress in young hospitalized children. *Res Nurs Health*. 1979; 2:17-23.
203. Siegel L, Peterson L. Stress reduction in young dental patients through coping skills and sensory information. *J Consult Clin Psychol*. 1980; 48:785-7.
204. Siegel L, Peterson L. Maintenance effects of coping skills and sensory information on young children's response to repeated dental procedures. *Behav Ther*. 1981; 12:530-5.
205. Fernald C, Corry J. Empathic versus directive preparation of children for needles. *Child Health Care*. 1981; 10:44-7.
206. Fassler D. The fear of needles in children. *Am J Orthopsychiatry*. 1985; 55:371-7.
207. Fowler-Kerry S, Lander JR. Management of injection pain in children. *Pain*. 1987; 30:169-75.
208. Ryan E. The effect of musical distraction on pain in hospitalized school-aged children. In: Funk W, Tournquist E, Champagne M et al., eds. Key aspects of comfort: management of pain, fatigue, and nausea. New York: Springer; 1989:101-4.
209. Andolsek K, Novik B. Use of hypnosis with children. *J Fam Pract*. 1980; 10:503-7.
210. Olness K. Imagery (self-hypnosis) as adjunct therapy in childhood cancer: clinical experience with 25 patients. *Am J Pediatr Hematol Oncol*. 1981; 3:313-21.
211. Zeltzer L, LeBaron S. Hypnosis and nonhypnotic techniques for reduction of pain and anxiety during painful procedures in children and adolescents with cancer. *J Pediatr*. 1982; 101:1032-5.
212. Ellerton M, Caty S, Ritchie J. Helping young children master intrusive procedures through play. *Child Health Care*. 1985; 13:167-73.
213. Ross DM. Thought-stopping: a coping strategy for impending feared events. *Issues Compr Pediatr Nurs*. 1984; 7:83-9.
214. Eland JM. The effectiveness of transcutaneous electrical nerve stimulation (TENS) with children experiencing cancer pain. In: Funk SG, Tornquist EM, Champagne MT et al., eds. Key aspects of comfort: management of pain, fatigue, and nausea. New York: Springer; 1989:87-100.
215. Jay SM, Elliot C, Ozolins M et al. Behavioral management of children's distress during painful medical procedures. *Behav Res Ther*. 1985; 23:513-20.
216. Maxwell L, Yaster M, Wetzel R et al. Penile nerve block for newborn circumcision. *Obstet Gynecol*. 1987; 70:415-9.
217. Andersen KH. A new method of analgesia for relief of circumcision pain. *Anaesthesia*. 1989; 44:118-20.
218. Tree-Trakarn T, Pirayavaraporn S, Lertakyamanee J. Topical analgesia for relief of post-circumcision pain. *Anesthesi-*

ology. 1987; 67:395-9.
219. Bernstein N. Management of burned children with the aid of hypnosis. *J Child Psychol Psychiatry*. 1963; 4:93-8.
220. Elliott CH, Olson RA. The management of children's distress in response to painful medical treatment for burn injuries. *Behav Res Ther*. 1983; 21:675-83.
221. Kelley ML, Jarvie GJ, Middlebrook JL et al. Decreasing burned children's pain behavior: impacting the trauma of hydrotherapy. *J Appl Behav Anal*. 1984; 17:147-58.
222. Kavanagh C. A new approach to dressing change in the severely burned child and its effects on burn-related psychopathology. *Heart Lung*. 1983; 12:612-9.
223. Kavanagh C. Psychological intervention with the severely burned child: report of an experimental comparison of two approaches and their effects on psychological sequelae. *J Am Acad Child Psychiatry*. 1983; 22:145-56.
224. Quay NB, Alexander LL. Preparation of burned children and their families for discharge. *J Burn Care Rehabil*. 1983; 4:288-90.
225. Ferguson BF. Preparing young children for hospitalization: a comparison of two methods. *Pediatrics*. 1979; 64:656-64.
226. McGrath MM. Group preparation of pediatric surgical patients. *Image*. 1979; 11:52-62.
227. Visintainer M, Wolfer J. Psychological preparation for surgical pediatric patients: the effects on children's and parents' stress responses and adjustment. *Pediatrics*. 1975; 56:187-202.
228. Wolfer J, Visintainer M. Prehospital psychological preparation for tonsillectomy patients: effects on children's and parents' adjustment. *Pediatrics*. 1979; 64:646-55.
229. Hannallah RS, Rosales JK. Experience with parents' presence during anaesthesia induction in children. *Can Anaesth Soc J*. 1983; 30:286-9.
230. Johnston CC, Bevan JC, Haig MJ et al. Parental presence during anesthesia induction. *Assoc Oper Room Nurs J*. 1988; 47:187-94.
231. Schofield N, White J. Interrelations among children, parents, premedication, and anaesthetists in paediatric day stay surgery. *Br Med J*. 1989; 299:1371-5.
232. Anand KJ, Brown MJ, Causon RC et al. Can the human neonate mount an endocrine and metabolic response to surgery? *J Pediatr Surg*. 1985; 20:41-8.
233. Anand KJ, Hickey P. Pain and its effects in the human neonate and fetus. *N Engl J Med*. 1987; 317:1321-9.
234. Collins C, Koren G, Crean P et al. Fentanyl pharmacokinetics and hemodynamic effects in preterm infants during ligation of patent ductus arteriosus. *Anesth Analg*. 1985; 64:1078-80.
235. Yaster M. The dose response of fentanyl in neonatal anesthesia. *Anesthesiology*. 1987; 66:433-5.
236. Gedaly-Duff V, Ziebarth D. Mothers' management of surgical pain in preschool children. *J Pain Symptom Manage*. 1991; 6:147. Abstract.
237. Bray RJ. Postoperative analgesia provided by morphine infusion in children. *Anaesthesia*. 1983; 38:1075-8.
238. Hendrickson M, Myre L, Johnson DG et al. Postoperative analgesia in children: a prospective study of intermittent intramuscular injections versus continuous intravenous infusion of morphine. *J Pediatr Surg*. 1990; 25:185-91.
239. Lynn AM, Opheim KE, Tyler DC. Morphine infusion after pediatric cardiac surgery. *Crit Care Med*. 1984; 12:863-6.
240. Berde CB, Lehn BM, Yee JD et al. Patient-controlled analgesia in children and adolescents: a randomized, prospective comparison with intramuscular administration of morphine for postoperative analgesia. *J Pediatr*. 1991; 118:460-6.
241. Meignier M, Souron R, LeNeel JC. Postoperative dorsal epidural analgesia in the child with respiratory disabilities. *Anesthesiology*. 1983; 59:473-5.
242. Way WL, Costley EC, Way EL. Respiratory sensitivity of the newborn infant to meperidine and morphine. *Clin Pharmacol Ther*. 1965; 6:454-61.
243. Koehntop D, Rodman J, Brundage D et al. Pharmacokinetics of fentanyl in neonates. *Anesth Analg*. 1986; 65:227-32.
244. Koren G, Butt W, Chinyanga H et al. Postoperative morphine infusion in newborn infants: assessment of disposition characteristics and safety. *J Pediatr*. 1985; 107:963-7.
245. Lynn AM, Slattery JT. Morphine pharmacokinetics in early infancy. *Anesthesiology*. 1987; 66:136-9.
246. Hertzka R, Gauntlett I, Fisher D et al. Fentanyl-induced ventilatory depression: effects of age. *Anesthesiology*. 1989; 70:213-8.
247. Berde CB. Pediatric postoperative pain management. *Pediatr Clin North Am*. 1989; 36:921-40.
248. Berde CB. Pediatric analgesic trials. In: Max MB, Portenoy RK, Laska EM, eds. Advances in pain research and therapy: the design of analgesic clinical trials. Vol. 18. New York: Raven Press; 1991:445-55.
249. Ferrell BA. Pain management in elderly people. *J Am Geriatr Soc*. 1991; 39:64-73.
250. Anon. Pain in the elderly: patterns change with age. *JAMA*. 1979; 241:2191-2.
251. Kane RL, Ouslander JG, Abrass IB, eds. Essentials of clinical geriatrics. 2nd ed. New York: McGraw-Hill; 1989.
252. Crook J, Rideout E, Browne G. The prevalence of pain complaints in a general population. *Pain*. 1984; 18:299-314.
253. Ferrell BA, Ferrell BR, Osterweil D. Pain in the nursing home. *J Am Geriatr Soc*. 1990; 38:409-14.
254. Davis MA. Epidemiology of osteoarthritis. *Clin Geriatr Med*. 1988; 4:241-55.
255. Foley KM. The treatment of cancer pain. *N Engl J Med*. 1985; 313:84-95.
256. Fordyce WE. Evaluating and managing chronic pain. *Geriatrics*. 1978; 33:59-62.
257. Bayer AJ, Chada JS, Farag RR et al. Changing presentations of myocardial infarctions with increasing old age. *J Am Geriatr Soc*. 1986; 34:263-6.
258. Bender JS. Approach to the acute abdomen. *Med Clin North Am*. 1989; 73:1413-22.
259. Harkins SW, Kwentus J, Price DD. Pain and the elderly. In: Benedetti C, Chapman C, Moricca G, eds. Advances in pain research and therapy. Recent advances in the management of pain. Vol. 7. New York: Raven Press; 1984:103-21.
260. Roth SH. Merits and liabilities of NSAID therapy. *Rheum Dis Clin North Am*. 1989; 15:479-98.
261. Bellville WJ, Forrest WH, Miller E et al. Influence of age on pain relief from analgesics. A study of postoperative patients. *JAMA*. 1971; 217:1835-41.
262. Kaiko RF. Age and morphine analgesia in cancer patients with post-operative pain. *Clin Pharmacol Ther*. 1980; 28:823-6.
263. Kaiko RF, Wallenstein SL, Rogers AG et al. Narcotics in the elderly. *Med Clin North Am*. 1982; 66:1079-89.
264. Portenoy RK, Payne R. Acute and chronic pain. In: Lowinson JH, Ruit P, Milman R et al., eds. Comprehensive textbook of substance abuse. Baltimore: Williams & Wilkins; (in press).
265. Weissman DE, Haddox JD. Opioid pseudoaddiction: an iatrogenic syndrome. *Pain*. 1989; 36:363-6.
266. Hasselstrom, Eriksson S, Persson A et al. The metabolism and bioavailability of morphine in patients with severe liver cirrhosis. *Br J Clin Pharmacol*. 1990; 29:289-97.
267. Sear JW, Hand CW, Moore RA et al. Studies on morphine disposition: influence of renal failure on the kinetics of morphine and its metabolites. *Br J Anaesth*. 1989; 62:28-32.
268. Covington EC, Gonsalves-Ebrahim L, Currie KO et al. Severe respiratory depression from patient-controlled analgesia in renal failure. *Psychosomatics*. 1988; 30:226-8.
269. Bromage PR, Campoersi E, Chestnut D. Epidural narcotics for postoperative analgesia. *Anesth Analg*. 1980; 59:473-80.
270. Foley KM, Inturrisi CE. Analgesic drug therapy in cancer pain: principles and practice. *Med Clin North Am*. 1987; 71:207-32.
271. Ventafridda V, Ripamonti C, DeConno F et al. Antidepres-

sants increase bioavailability of morphine in cancer patients. *Lancet*. 1987; 1:1204. Letter.
272. Armstrong PJ, Bersten A. Normeperidine toxicity. *Anesth Analg*. 1986; 65:536-8.
273. Soderstrom CA, Trifillis AL, Shankar BS et al. Marijuana and alcohol use among 1023 trauma patients. A prospective study. *Arch Surg*. 1988; 123:733-77.
274. Beecher HK. Measurement of subjective responses: quantitative effects of drugs. New York: Oxford University Press; 1959.
275. Atchison NE, Osgood PF, Carr DB et al. Pain during burn dressing change in children: relationship to burn area, depth, and analgesic regimens. *Pain*. 1991; 47:41-6.
276. Dripps RD, Eckenhoff JE, Vandam LD. Introduction to anesthesia: the principles of safe practice. Philadelphia: W.B. Saunders; 1982.
277. Skacel PO, Hewlett AM, Lewis JD et al. Studies on the haemopoetic toxicity of nitrous oxide in man. *Br J Haematol*. 1983; 53:189-200.
278. Choinière M, Melzack R, Papillon J. Pain and paresthesia in patients with healed burns: an exploratory study. *J Pain Symptom Manage*. 1991; 6:437-44.
279. Jönsson A, Cassuto J, Hanson B. Inhibition of burn pain by intravenous lignocaine infusion. *Lancet*. 1991; 338:151-2.

Drug Review

Doxazosin: A new α_1-adrenergic antagonist

Kenneth S. Babamoto and William T. Hirokawa

Abstract: The physicochemical properties, pharmacology, pharmacokinetics, cardiovascular and metabolic effects, adverse effects, dosage, and administration of doxazosin are described, and comparative clinical studies of doxazosin therapy in patients with mild to moderate hypertension are reviewed.

Doxazosin mesylate, an α_1-adrenoceptor antagonist, is rapidly absorbed after oral administration and undergoes extensive hepatic metabolism. The drug decreases blood pressure by reducing peripheral resistance. Maximum hypotensive effects occur four to eight hours after the dose. Doxazosin favorably affects serum lipids by increasing concentrations of high-density lipoprotein (HDL) cholesterol, increasing the HDL:total cholesterol ratio, and decreasing concentrations of low-density lipoprotein cholesterol, total cholesterol, and triglycerides. In comparative clinical trials, doxazosin lowered standing and supine systolic and diastolic blood pressures as effectively as other α-adrenoceptor antagonists, β-adrenoceptor antagonists, diuretics, angiotensin-converting-enzyme inhibitors, and calcium-channel-blocking agents. The most frequently reported adverse effects are dizziness, headache, nausea, lethargy, and fatigue. Doxazosin may be used either alone or in combination with a β-adrenoceptor inhibitor or a diuretic. Orthostatic hypotension after the first dose occurs infrequently and may be minimized by initiating therapy at a dosage of 1 mg/day. The dosage may be increased at two-week intervals as needed, and blood pressure should be closely monitored.

Doxazosin has blood-pressure-lowering effects comparable to those of other α_1-adrenoceptor inhibitors and to those of antihypertensives in other drug classes.

Index terms: Dosage; Doxazosin mesylate; Hypertension; Hypotensive agents; Pharmacokinetics; Toxicity

Clin Pharm. 1992; 11:415-27

An estimated 58 million people in the United States have high blood pressure or receive antihypertensive medications.[1,2] Defined as systolic blood pressure (SBP) of ≥140 mm Hg or diastolic blood pressure (DBP) of ≥90 mm Hg, hypertension is one of several major risk factors associated with the development of coronary heart disease (CHD), the leading cause of death in Western societies.[3-6] Approximately one of every two deaths in the United States is related to cardiovascular disease, representing an estimated annual expenditure of $127 billion.[2]

In the 1988 report by the Joint National Committee on the Detection, Evaluation, and Treatment of High Blood Pressure, the traditional stepped-care approach for the management of hypertension was expanded to include nonpharmacologic approaches such as alcohol restriction, dietary and weight control, and control of cardiovascular risk factors.[1] Diuretics and β-adrenergic-receptor antagonists were recommended as initial pharmacologic treatment, and calcium-channel blockers and angiotensin-converting-enzyme (ACE) inhibitors were included as alternative drug therapy. The current stepped-care approach does not advocate use of α_1-adrenergic receptor antagonists as primary therapy; however, many studies have demonstrated their safety and efficacy as first-line agents in the management of hypertension.[2,7-9]

Doxazosin mesylate is a new selective α_1-adrenergic-receptor antagonist approved by the FDA for the treatment of hypertension, either alone or in combination with diuretics or β-adrenergic-receptor antagonists. For the past 15 years, prazosin has been the only α_1-specific antagonist commercially available in the United States. Recently, doxazosin (Cardura; Roerig-

Kenneth S. Babamoto, Pharm.D., is Drug Information Pharmacist, and William T. Hirokawa, Pharm.D., is Coordinator, Investigational Drug Section, Department of Pharmaceutical Services, UCLA Medical Center, Los Angeles, CA.

Address reprint requests to Dr. Babamoto at the Drug Information Center, Department of Pharmaceutical Services, UCLA Medical Center, A4-190 CHS, 10833 LeConte Avenue, Los Angeles, CA 90024.

This is **article 680-204-9212** in the **ASHP Continuing Education System**; it qualifies for 1.0 hour of continuing-education credit. See page 442 for learning objectives and test questions.

Pfizer, New York, NY) and terazosin (Hytrin; Abbott, North Chicago, IL) were both approved for marketing and received an FDA rating of 1C, signifying a new molecular entity with little or no therapeutic advantage over existing drugs.

This article evaluates the clinical trials comparing doxazosin mesylate with other antihypertensive agents and reviews the chemistry, pharmacology, pharmacokinetics, metabolic and adverse drug effects, and economic impact of doxazosin therapy for the treatment of mild to moderate hypertension.

Physicochemical Properties

Doxazosin mesylate is a quinazoline derivative that is structurally related to prazosin and terazosin (Figure 1). The chemical name of doxazosin mesylate is 1-(4-amino-6,7-dimethoxy-2-quinazolinyl)-4-(1,4-benzodioxan-2-ylcarbonyl) piperazine monomethanesulfonate; the empiric formula is $C_{24}H_{29}N_5O_8S$, and the molecular weight is 547.6.[10]

The pK_a of doxazosin is 6.9, and the compound is fully soluble in dimethylsulfoxide; soluble in dimethylformamide; slightly soluble in water (0.8% at 25 °C), ethanol, and methanol; and very slightly soluble in methylene chloride and acetone.[10]

Doxazosin mesylate is available in oral tablets, containing 1, 2, 4, or 8 mg of doxazosin base, which should be stored at temperatures below 86 °F (30 °C).[10] In this review, doxazosin dosages are expressed as the free base.

Pharmacology

The initial classification of α-adrenergic receptors into subtypes α_1 and α_2 was based on receptor location relative to terminal adrenergic nerve endings and subsequently redesignated according to receptor-binding affinity of specific α-adrenergic-receptor agonists and antagonists, irrespective of function or location.[9,11-13]

Alpha$_1$-adrenoceptors are situated on effector cells, postjunctional from the terminal division of adrenergic nerve endings, and are under direct neuronal control in response to norepinephrine (NE) released by nerve stimulation.[11] NE activation of α_1-adrenergic receptors located on vascular smooth muscle results in contraction, increased resistance, and elevated blood pressure. Alpha$_1$-adrenoceptors are not located exclusively on vascular smooth muscle and may mediate other physiological effects, including proximal tubule sodium reabsorption, liver glycogenolysis, central nervous system locomotor activity, ejaculation, and contraction of sphincters, myocardium, and pregnant uterus.[11,12,14]

Alpha$_2$-adrenoceptors are located primarily on terminal adrenergic nerve endings and mediate NE release. The mechanism of receptor activity is unknown; however, observations from early studies suggest that nerve impulses stimulate release of NE, which binds to α_2-receptors, inhibiting further release by means of

Figure 1. Structures of doxazosin, prazosin, and terazosin.

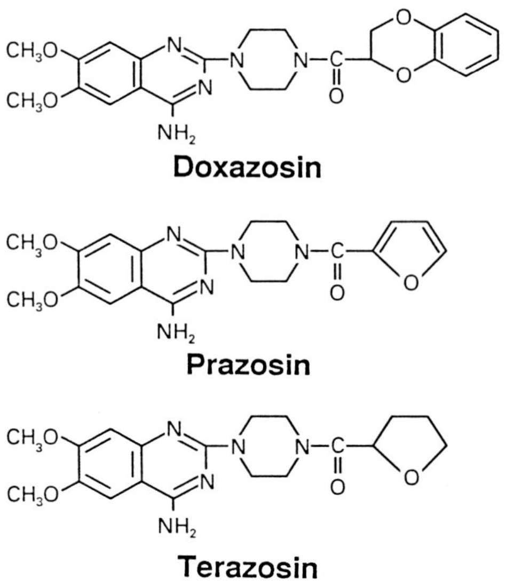

physiological feedback control.[12] Inhibition of α_2-receptors and loss of feedback control is associated with an increase in NE efflux to surrounding organs and tissues, including the densely innervated heart, resulting in tachycardia and arrhythmias.[11,15] Recent animal studies indicate the presence of postjunctional α_2-adrenoceptors that respond directly to circulating catecholamines; these receptors may play a role in maintaining peripheral vascular resistance.[11,12,14,16] However, other studies have not shown specific binding of either NE or epinephrine to postjunctional α_2-adrenergic receptors.[17,18]

Nonselective α-adrenergic receptor antagonists, such as phenoxybenzamine and phentolamine, lower blood pressure on a short-term basis.[11,19] Because these agents inhibit both α_1- and α_2-adrenoceptors, the loss of α_2-mediated feedback control increases circulating levels of NE and results in rapid development of tolerance, tachycardia, and tremors.[9,19]

Doxazosin is an α-adrenergic receptor antagonist that exhibits pharmacologic activity similar to that of prazosin; its selectivity and affinity for α_1-adrenoceptors have been demonstrated in both in vivo and in vitro studies.[20,21] In humans, doxazosin preferentially inhibits phenylephrine-induced SBP and DBP pressor responses and increases forearm blood flow in the presence of α_1-specific agonists.[18,22,23]

The mechanism of α-adrenoceptor stimulation, inhibition, and activity on effector organs and smooth muscle is not fully understood; however, evidence substantiates a relationship between increased intracellular calcium concentration and α-adrenergic receptor involvement.[14] Doxazosin does not act directly on smooth muscle; however, α_1-adrenoceptor inhibition may prevent influx of extracellular calcium and cause relaxation of vascular smooth muscle.[24]

Pharmacokinetics

Absorption. Single and multiple doses of doxazosin are rapidly absorbed; peak serum concentrations occur in 1.5 to 3 hours.[25-27] Oral bioavailability ranges from 65% to 70% after administration of doxazosin 2 mg with no observed difference between young (mean age, 29 years) and elderly (mean age, 71 years) normotensive volunteers.[28]

Mean peak and trough plasma concentrations increase in a linear dose-dependent manner.[29,30] In 18 elderly hypertensive patients (mean age, 71.4 years) who received oral doxazosin in daily dosages of 1, 2, 4, 8, and 16 mg for multiple days, mean ± S.D. peak plasma serum drug concentrations were 9.4 ± 1.5, 18.0 ± 3.2, 28.7 (no S.D. reported), 84.7 ± 10.6, and 168 ± 45.2 ng/mL, respectively, and trough concentrations ranged from 3.2 ± 1.0 to 57.8 ± 26.9 ng/mL.[29] Single-dose mean peak concentrations were similar to serum concentrations measured after one and six weeks of chronic therapy.[25,30]

The mean area under the curve (AUC) increases proportionally with increasing doses.[30] Doxazosin 2 to 8 mg was associated with an increase in mean ± S.D. $AUC_{0\text{-}24\,hr}$ from 208 ± 75 ng/hr/mL to 803 ± 264 ng/hr/mL at steady state; these values are approximately 1.3 to 1.7 times greater than those determined after administration of a 2-mg single dose.[25,30]

Distribution. Doxazosin is highly protein bound, with 98–99% complexed to human plasma proteins, independent of dose and duration of therapy.[30,31] The binding proteins have not been identified, although one study proposes that doxazosin may complex to α_1-acid glycoprotein, as demonstrated by displacement of ^{3}H-prazosin with concurrent doxazosin administration.[30] Human albumin may also bind with doxazosin.[30] Distribution in human tissue is unknown.

The apparent volume of distribution was significantly smaller in young normotensive subjects in comparison with elderly patients (1.0 L/kg and 1.7 L/kg, respectively) after a 2-mg oral and a 1-mg intravenous dose.[28] The disparity in volume of distribution may result from differences in body mass between age groups. In a dose-escalation study evaluating doxazosin 2, 4, and 8 mg at steady state, the volume of distribution was approximately 3.4 L/kg, irrespective of dose.[30] The increased volume of distribution may be a consequence of steady-state rather than single-dose administration.

Metabolism and Elimination. Doxazosin undergoes extensive hepatic metabolism following oral and intravenous administration. Less than 5% of the parent compound is excreted unchanged in feces, the major route of elimination.[31] The primary metabolic pathway is *O*-demethylation of the quinazoline nucleus to 6-*O*-desmethyl- and 7-*O*-desmethyl-doxazosin, accounting for 16% and 7% of an administered dose, respectively. Hydroxylation of the benzdioxan ring to 6'-hydroxy- and 7'-hydroxy-doxazosin accounts for 5% and 7% of the other major metabolites, respectively. Minor metabolites include 2-amino- and 2-piperazinyl-doxazosin. All metabolites reportedly have minimal, if any, pharmacologic activity.[30,32] In animal studies, isolated metabolites were similar to those identified in humans with the exception of a glucuronide conjugate that has not been found in humans.[31]

The major elimination pathway is through feces, with 63–65% of a 2-mg oral or 1-mg intravenous doxazosin dose recovered as radioactive metabolites and approximately 9% detected in urine.[31]

The mean elimination half-life ranges from 9 to 22 hours, independent of age, renal function, dose, or route of administration.[25-30,33,34] The wide range of half-life values may result from variances in sampling periods. In a bioequivalence study in which samples were collected for up to 96 hours after the dose was given, the mean elimination half-life was approximately 22 hours in patients receiving long-term therapy with doxazosin 8 mg/day.[33] Similarly, a study using a 54-hour sample period showed a mean half-life of 19 hours after single daily doses of 4 and 8 mg.[30] In this same study, blood sampling at 13–14 hours yielded half-life values of 9–12 hours; these values are similar to those observed in studies using 24-hour sampling periods.[35]

In a study of 18 elderly hypertensive patients (mean age, 71.4 years) receiving doxazosin 1–16 mg/day, a mean elimination half-life of 16.1 hours (range, 10.1–27.1 hours) was determined from samples collected up to 48 hours after the dose.[29]

Total body clearance was 1.2 and 2.1 mL/min/kg after a 1-mg intravenous dose was administered to young and elderly normotensive subjects, respectively.[28] Clearance values of 2.2 mL/min/kg were reported following oral doxazosin doses of 2, 4, and 8 mg at steady state.[30] Mean plasma clearance (88 mL/min) was substantially less than whole blood clearance (139 mL/min) in six healthy, normotensive male volunteers after intravenous administration of doxazosin 1 mg.[35]

Effect of Organ Dysfunction. The pharmacokinetic variables AUC, elimination half-life, peak serum concentration, and time to peak serum concentration are similar in individuals with renal insufficiency or renal failure and in healthy volunteers.[34,36] Mean half-life values were 12.6 hours and 15.5 hours in volunteers (glomerular filtration rate [GFR] range, 82–124 mL/min) and renal patients (GFR, 7–35 mL/min), respectively, with peak serum concentrations ranging from 7.6 to 9.4 ng/mL measured at 3.6 and 2.6 hours after administration of oral doxazosin 1 mg.[34]

In a study involving five patients with end-stage renal failure who required hemodialysis, serum doxazosin concentrations were measured four hours after a single 1-mg oral dose at the start of hemodialysis, and at one and two hours during hemodialysis.[34] Arterial and venous serum concentrations were unchanged from predialysis concentrations, signifying minimal drug removal.

Pharmacokinetic variables in patients with hepatic

dysfunction or failure have not been determined.

Cardiovascular Effects

Hemodynamics. Maximum hypotensive effects of oral and intravenous doxazosin occur within four to eight hours.[30,34,35] Peak serum concentrations, which occur 1.5 to 3 hours after an oral dose, do not correlate with observed blood pressure reduction. This delay in hypotensive activity may result from diffusion of doxazosin to peripheral α_1-receptor binding sites or into the "effect compartment" where hypotensive activity occurs.[30,35]

In a study involving 14 adult patients with essential hypertension, the acute hemodynamic effects of intravenous doxazosin 0.5–1.0 mg injected into the superior vena cava were determined in the supine and sitting positions at rest and during 100-watt ergometer bicycling exercise.[37] One hour after doxazosin administration, mean SBP was significantly reduced from pretreatment values by 16.9, 27.8, and 14.9 mm Hg, and DBP was significantly decreased by 8.4, 13.1, and 10.8 mm Hg in the supine and sitting positions, and during exercise, respectively. Similarly, mean arterial pressure (MAP) was significantly decreased from pretreatment values by 10.1 (supine), 11.7 (sitting), and 16.2 mm Hg (exercise).

After two days of oral therapy with doxazosin 1 mg to prevent potential first-dose-associated orthostatic hypotension, a single 2-mg oral dose was administered to 18 adult patients with mild to moderate essential hypertension. Supine SBP/DBP was reduced by 14.2/17.7 mm Hg and standing SBP/DBP was reduced by 20.8/15.1 mm Hg.[30] After dose escalations of 2, 4, and 8 mg for six weeks, steady-state standing SBP was significantly decreased by 21.2 mm Hg at an 8-mg daily dosage, compared with a reduction of 11.1 mm Hg at a 2-mg daily dosage. Standing DBP was decreased by 14.7, 18.7, and 21.5 mm Hg with the 2-, 4-, and 8-mg dose, respectively; however, reductions were statistically insignificant between dosage levels. In a double-blind, randomized placebo-controlled dose-titration study involving 135 patients with essential hypertension, the mean reduction in standing SBP and DBP was greater by 7.4 and 3.9 mm Hg, respectively, in patients receiving doxazosin than in patients receiving placebo.[38] Supine SBP and DBP decreased by 3.4 and 1.8 mm Hg more in the doxazosin-treated group than in the placebo group (p = 0.03 and 0.11, respectively). A dose–response effect was not observed in the 2-, 4- and 8-mg dose-escalation regimen.

After 10 weeks of therapy for 30 patients with elevated arterial pressure in a double-blind parallel-design protocol, standing SBP/DBP and supine SBP/DBP decreased by 14/14 mm Hg and 6/5 mm Hg, respectively, 24 hours after the last daily dose of doxazosin 1–16 mg.[39] Similar hypotensive effects were reported after nine weeks of doxazosin 1–16 mg/day (mean, 13.1 mg) administered to 20 patients who completed a placebo run-in and a four-week washout period.[40] Maximum standing DBP was reduced by 17.8 mm Hg four hours after the dose, and 24-hour standing and supine DBP were significantly reduced by 11.9 and 10.0 mm Hg, respectively, in comparison with results for patients receiving placebo.

In a study involving 14 adult patients, the total peripheral resistance index (TPRI) was reduced from pretreatment values by 5% at rest in the supine position (difference not significant), by 8.6% at rest in the sitting position ($p < 0.01$), and by 14% during 100-watt ergometer exercise ($p < 0.001$) one hour after an intravenous dose of doxazosin 0.5–1.0 mg.[37] The decrease in TPRI was associated with reductions in both SBP and DBP. After one year of oral therapy (2–16 mg/day), TPRI was reduced by 18.6% ($p < 0.01$), 19.7% ($p < 0.001$), and 18.3% ($p < 0.001$) in patients in the supine and sitting positions, and during exercise, respectively; this corresponds to MAP reduction of 12.9–16.8%.

Cardiac Effects. In this same patient population, stroke volume index was significantly decreased by 8.6% (supine) and 6.3% (sitting) one hour after intravenous doxazosin administration; a slight increase in stroke volume index (0.9%, not significant) was observed during exercise.[37] Cardiac index was increased by 4.1% ($p < 0.05$) during exercise, possibly because of a slight compensatory increase in heart rate; no significant changes were observed at rest. During long-term therapy, stroke volume index was not significantly changed from baseline values. Cardiac index was significantly increased from baseline measurements (8.1%) in the supine position only.

Maximum reductions in blood pressure were associated with peak heart rate elevations occurring at five to six hours after the dose, suggesting a reflex mechanism of activity.[30] However, measurements taken at steady state, 24 hours after the dose was given, showed that heart rate was unchanged from pretreatment values. Similar observations were reported in another study of 38 patients, in which standing and supine heart rate increased by 3.3 and 0.6 beats/min, ($p = 0.04$ and $p = 0.03$, respectively) in patients receiving doxazosin compared with patients receiving placebo, who had decreases in heart rate of 3.5 and 5.2 beats/min.[40]

Heart rate increased by 6.5% (supine), 4.7% (sitting), and 3.1% (exercise) one hour after intravenous injection of doxazosin.[37] The elevated heart rates were not significantly different from pretreatment values. After one year of doxazosin therapy, heart rate was insignificantly decreased by 0.3% (supine), 0.7% (sitting), and 0.9% (exercise).[37]

Renal Effects. In five hypertensive patients undergoing renal angiography, infusions of doxazosin 1.0 μg/kg/min into the renal artery for 10 minutes increased renal blood flow by approximately 10.6% with no measurable effects on systemic blood pressure.[41] At higher dosages, renal blood flow was further increased, but systemic hypotensive effects were observed. Renin secretion was essentially unchanged during the doxazosin infusion and concurrent isometric hand exercise.

After 12 weeks of oral doxazosin 1–8 mg/day (mean, 4.14 mg/day), 32 patients with mild to moderate essential hypertension were evaluated to assess the renal and adrenal hormonal effects of doxazosin in comparison with those of placebo.[42] In patients taking doxazosin, plasma renin activity, aldosterone concentration, body weight, urine volume, creatinine clearance, and urinary sodium and potassium excretion did not differ from pretreatment values or from values observed in patients receiving placebo. Kallikrein excretion was significantly increased over baseline and posttreatment placebo values by approximately 2.5-fold, which may be a direct effect of the drug or a physiological response to decreased intrarenal resistance.[42]

In 18 hypertensive patients with underlying renal failure receiving long-term treatment with doxazosin 1–16 mg/day, GFR (mean ± S.D.) significantly decreased from 68.7 ± 35.1 mL/min to 60.1 ± 30.9 mL/min and serum creatinine concentration (mean ± S.D.) significantly increased from 205 ± 219 µmol/L to 231 ± 256 µmol/L.[36] The mean effective renal plasma flow was unchanged in comparison with baseline values. However, other studies have reported insignificant changes in creatinine clearance, filtration fraction, para-aminohippurate clearance, and renal blood flow relative to baseline values in individuals with normal renal function and renal insufficiency.[43-45]

Metabolic Effects

Serum Lipids. Alpha$_1$-receptor antagonists, including doxazosin, have been reported to produce favorable effects on serum lipids, such as increasing high-density lipoprotein (HDL) cholesterol concentrations and the ratio of HDL to total cholesterol and decreasing low-density lipoprotein (LDL) cholesterol, total cholesterol, and triglyceride concentrations.[46,47] Although these factors may have an important role in the development of atherosclerosis and CHD, the relationship between the reported beneficial effects of doxazosin on serum lipids and the prevention of CHD and atherosclerosis remains unknown. The mechanism of doxazosin's positive effects on lipids has not been established, but several theories have been suggested, including the following: (1) increasing LDL receptor activity and thus reducing LDL and total cholesterol concentrations; (2) decreasing intracellular LDL cholesterol synthesis; (3) reducing the synthesis and secretion of very-low-density lipoprotein (VLDL) cholesterol; (4) stimulating lipoprotein lipase activity; (5) decreasing the rate of cholesterol absorption; and (6) inhibiting platelet aggregation.[3,48,49]

The serum lipoprotein effects of doxazosin and other antihypertensive agents reported in various clinical trials are summarized in Table 1. Pooled results from five studies, involving 142 patients receiving doxazosin and 155 patients receiving placebo, showed decreases in serum triglyceride and total cho-

Table 1.
Serum Lipid Effects Reported in Clinical Trials Involving Doxazosin and Various Antihypertensive Drugs[a]

Ref.	Final Drug Dosage (mg/day)	Duration (wk)	*n*	Posttreatment Serum Lipid Effects (% Change from Baseline) HDL	Trigly	Tot Chol	HDL:Chol
50	D, 4.6	24	32	−11.0	−12.3	−3.4	14.9
51	D, 11.6	9–24	142	7.6	−9.1	−1.2	8.9
	Pl	9–24	155	4.8	−3.0	0.6	4.1
52	D, 11.3	10–16	46	6.3	−12.6	−3.9	10.3
	Pl	10–16	49	8.5	−6.6	−1.6	10.6
	Pr, 13.8	10–16	49	2.0	−10.1	−6.4	8.8
53	D, 10.8	50	42	5.0	−11.7	−3.6	8.9
	Pr, 10.9	50	45	2.1	−10.3	−4.3	6.7
54	D, 1–16	10	38	2.1	−11.1	−2.9	5.2
	Pl	10	38	1.4	0.2	−0.2	1.1
	A, 50–100	10	40	6.2	10.4	−2.3	−4.1
55	D, 12.2	20-52	46	7.2	−5.9	−1.6	8.7
	A, 94.0	20-52	50	5.6	32.4	0.6	6.2
56	D, 5.2	156	83	3.7	−5.9	−2.1	5.9
	A, 66.4	156	81	−11.2	22.5	−10.3	−10.3
57	D, 4.4	11	25	5.0[b]	−6.8[b]	−4.5	9.8[b]
	E, 19.3	11	27	−5.0[b]	20.0[b]	−1.8	1.9[b]
58	D, 10.8	24	40	−0.7	−7.2	−3.9	3.1
	H, 89.1	24	39	−13.1	7.6	1.2	−14.1
59	D, 6.9	24	19	13.0	−17.4	−6.1	−19.7
	H, 84.6	24	16	8.4	26.3	9.8	19.4
60	D, 2.5	14	34	−16.3	6.1	−0.5	
	N, 13.2	14	33	3.0	16.7	3.4	

[a] HDL = high-density lipoprotein cholesterol, Trigly = triglycerides, Tot Chol = total cholesterol, D = doxazosin, Pl = placebo, Pr = prazosin, A = atenolol, E = enalapril, H = hydrochlorothiazide, N = nitrendipine.
[b] Approximate values derived from graphic representation.

lesterol concentrations of 9.1% and 1.2%, respectively.[51] HDL cholesterol concentration increased by 7.6% in the doxazosin group. These results were not significantly different from those found in the placebo group, which included a 3% reduction in the serum triglyceride concentration and 0.6% and 4.8% increases in serum total cholesterol and HDL cholesterol concentrations. The HDL:total cholesterol ratio was significantly increased (8.9%) in patients receiving doxazosin compared with those receiving placebo (4.1%).

Torvik and Madsbu[52] evaluated the serum lipid effects of doxazosin 1–16 mg/day (mean, 11.3 mg/day), prazosin 0.5–10 mg twice daily (mean, 13.8 mg/day), and placebo in a double-blind multicenter trial involving 144 patients (aged 26–71 years) with essential hypertension. Total cholesterol concentrations decreased from baseline values and HDL cholesterol concentrations increased with no statistical difference between the randomized groups. The HDL:total cholesterol ratio was significantly increased from pretreatment values with all three regimens. The triglyceride concentration was significantly reduced by 12.6% only in patients receiving doxazosin.

Although lipid changes were comparable among patients receiving doxazosin, prazosin, and placebo, patients receiving placebo reported a 1.2-kg decrease in weight, which may account for the favorable lipoprotein effects. Eighty-seven patients who successfully completed the 12-week trial were evaluated one year later.[53] Both doxazosin and prazosin demonstrated positive lipid effects, with total triglyceride concentration reduced by 11.7% and 10.3% and total cholesterol concentration decreased by 3.6% and 4.3% from pretreatment levels, respectively. HDL cholesterol concentration increased by 5.0% and 2.1% and the HDL:total cholesterol ratio increased by 8.9% and 6.7% with doxazosin and prazosin, respectively. Tests of statistical significance were not performed. The beneficial lipid effects observed at one year were similar to results observed at 12 weeks.

The serum lipid effects of doxazosin and atenolol have been compared in numerous clinical trials with similar results. In a double-blind study reported by Frick et al.,[55] doxazosin 1–16 mg/day (mean, 12.2 mg/day) and atenolol 50–100 mg/day (mean, 94.0 mg/day) were administered for 20–52 weeks to 96 patients with mild to moderate hypertension. Mean total triglyceride concentration was significantly decreased by 5.9% in patients receiving doxazosin and increased by 32.4% in patients on the atenolol-treatment regimen. Total cholesterol concentration was increased by 0.6% in atenolol-treated patients and reduced by 1.6% in doxazosin-treated patients; these findings were not statistically significant. Positive increases in HDL cholesterol concentration (7.2%, $p = 0.007$) were observed with doxazosin; the HDL:total cholesterol ratio increased by 8.7% ($p = 0.006$), compared with decreased HDL cholesterol concentrations (5.6%) and decreased HDL:total cholesterol ratios (6.2%) in patients receiving atenolol.

Talseth et al.,[56] reported serum lipid effects from a three-year follow-up study involving 83 patients receiving doxazosin and 81 patients receiving atenolol. In the doxazosin group, HDL cholesterol concentrations significantly increased by 3.7% and triglyceride concentrations significantly decreased by 5.9%; in atenolol-receiving patients, HDL concentrations decreased by 11.2% and triglyceride concentrations increased by 22.5%. The HDL:total cholesterol ratio increased by 5.9% ($p < 0.0001$) in patients receiving doxazosin and decreased by 10.3% in patients receiving atenolol. The 10-year risk of developing CHD, as determined by the Framingham Risk Equation, significantly decreased by 15.2% in patients receiving doxazosin and significantly increased by 25.4% in patients receiving atenolol. Values were significantly different between treatment regimens.

Changes in total and HDL cholesterol concentrations and HDL:total cholesterol ratio were not significantly different in 52 patients receiving doxazosin and enalapril.[57] However, total serum cholesterol concentrations significantly decreased by 4.5% during doxazosin therapy, compared with a 1.8% reduction during enalapril therapy. Calculated CHD risk was significantly reduced from pretreatment values in patients receiving either doxazosin (27.6%) or enalapril (18.5%).

In a 24-week trial involving 35 patients, Trost et al.[59] found significant reductions in total triglyceride (17.4%, $p = 0.002$) and cholesterol concentrations (6.1%, $p = 0.006$) in doxazosin-treated patients (mean dosage, 6.9 mg/day) compared with increases of 26.3% and 9.8%, respectively, in patients receiving hydrochlorothiazide (mean dosage, 84.6 mg/day). Favorable increases in HDL concentration (13.0%, $p = 0.075$) and HDL:total cholesterol ratio (19.7%, $p = 0.001$) were noted in patients receiving doxazosin therapy, and reductions of 8.4% and 19.4%, respectively, were observed in patients receiving hydrochlorothiazide.

Smoking Effects. Cigarette smoking is associated with stimulation of the adrenergic nervous system.[61] The proposed mechanism of activity is release of NE from terminal adrenergic nerve endings and release of adrenomedullary epinephrine, causing increases in SBP, DBP, and heart rate. In addition, smoking has been associated with changes in atherogenic lipoproteins.[62]

Westheim et al.[63] reported results from an open parallel trial involving 69 nonsmokers and 64 cigarette smokers receiving doxazosin antihypertensive therapy. Blood pressure was reduced in both study populations; rates of therapeutic success (defined as a reduction of ≥ 5 mm Hg in sitting DBP to a value of ≤ 90 mm Hg or a ≥10 mm Hg decrease from baseline) were 93.3% in smokers and 92.5% in nonsmokers. No changes in mean heart rate were reported at daily doses of 6.3 mg in smokers and 5.0 mg in nonsmokers.

Plasma lipid data were obtained for 53 smokers and 60 nonsmokers. In smokers, total cholesterol was reduced by 6.8%, total triglycerides decreased by 18.2%, and LDL cholesterol decreased by 12.8%. HDL cholesterol and HDL:total cholesterol ratio increased by 18.5% and 26.9%, respectively. All values were significantly different ($p < 0.001$) from baseline values in this group. In nonsmokers, total cholesterol decreased by 8.3% ($p < 0.001$), LDL cholesterol decreased by 11.0% ($p < 0.01$), HDL cholesterol increased by 8.2% ($p < 0.02$), and HDL:total cholesterol ratio increased by 17.6% ($p < 0.001$). The total triglyceride concentration decreased but was not significantly different from the baseline value. The only lipid changes that differed significantly between smokers and nonsmokers were elevation in HDL cholesterol and reduction in total triglycerides. Reductions in 10-year risk for CHD were significantly different between the smokers (39%) and nonsmokers (33%).

Similar findings were reported by Talseth et al.[64] in a retrospective subanalysis of 47 hypertensive smokers receiving either doxazosin or atenolol for 24 months. Both antihypertensive regimens produced comparable effects, with 73.5–75.0% of patients attaining blood pressure goals (defined as a reduction of ≥5 mm Hg in sitting DBP to a value of ≤90 mm Hg or a ≥10 mm Hg reduction from baseline values). Doxazosin was associated with a significant increase in HDL cholesterol (9.4%) and a nonsignificant reduction in total triglycerides (10.9%). Atenolol was associated with a nonsignificant reduction in HDL cholesterol (5.6%) and a significant increase in total triglycerides (20.7%) relative to baseline. The differences between drug regimens in lipid changes were significant ($p \leq 0.01$). Total cholesterol and LDL cholesterol concentrations were not significantly changed from baseline, and changes were not significantly different between treatment regimens.

Glucose Effects. Glucose intolerance and diabetes mellitus are risk factors associated with the development of CHD.[3] Non-insulin-dependent diabetes mellitus occurs in approximately 30–58% of patients with hypertension, primarily because of coincident obesity. The metabolic effects of doxazosin on blood glucose and insulin have been investigated in a small number of clinical trials involving normotensive and hypertensive patients with non-insulin-dependent diabetes mellitus. These studies showed minimal effects of doxazosin on blood glucose and insulin.[65,66]

In an open noncomparative trial evaluating the effects of doxazosin on glucose and serum insulin concentrations in 77 patients with mild essential hypertension, Lehtonen and the Finnish Multicenter Study Group[67] reported significantly reduced fasting blood glucose and insulin concentrations in patients after 26 weeks of doxazosin therapy (mean dosage, 6.4 mg/day).[67] At the end of the 26-week treatment period, fasting blood glucose concentrations and serum insulin concentrations had decreased significantly in comparison with values measured at the end of a four-week placebo period; fasting blood glucose concentration decreased from 81.7 mg/dL to 77.9 mg/dL (4.7%, $p < 0.05$) and serum insulin concentration decreased from 11.36 to 9.41 mU/L ($p < 0.001$).

Comparative Trials in Hypertension

Numerous comparative trials have examined the effectiveness of doxazosin in patients with mild to moderate hypertension, which is defined as diastolic blood pressure between 95 and 114 mm Hg on two separate occasions. The majority of trials were double-blind and involved three phases. The first phase typically was a placebo run-in period in which no concomitant antihypertensive treatment was permitted. This phase established the baseline blood pressure measurements without medication. Usually, this initial phase of four weeks was followed by a double-blind dosage titration period allowing the comparison of another antihypertensive medication. The typical goal of each study was to achieve target supine and standing DBP measurements of ≤90 mm Hg or to achieve a decrease of at least 5 mm Hg in supine DBP and a decrease of at least 10 mm Hg in standing DBP. The double-blind phase was generally followed by a maintenance period of at least four weeks.

Double-blind trials have been conducted that specifically examined the antihypertensive efficacy of doxazosin in comparison with placebo. Studies similar to the one conducted by Ames et al.[68] illustrate that there is a significant lowering of the standing arterial blood pressure with doxazosin as compared with placebo in patients with mild to moderate hypertension. Many trials have compared doxazosin with other commonly prescribed antihypertensive medications. Doxazosin has been compared with the α_1-adrenoceptor inhibitors terazosin and prazosin. Atenolol is the β_1-adrenoceptor antagonist that has been most often compared with doxazosin. Smaller studies have also compared metoprolol and nadolol with doxazosin. Other studies have examined drugs such as nitrendipine, enalapril, and hydrochlorothiazide in comparison with doxazosin.

Table 2 is a summary of therapeutic trials that compared doxazosin with other antihypertensive medications. Many of the studies were randomized, placebo-controlled, double-blind trials with a relatively large number of subjects. The studies confirm that doxazosin is as effective as any of the other antihypertensive drugs and may provide therapeutic attributes that make it preferable in certain clinical situations.

Comparison with α_1-Adrenoceptor Antagonists. In a study involving 172 patients with mild to moderate essential hypertension, Torvik and Madsbu[52] compared once-daily doses of doxazosin with prazosin given twice a day. Both antihypertensive agents produced reductions in standing and supine blood pressures that were statistically significant when compared with placebo. Of the 49 patients receiving prazosin, 29 (59%) were determined to be responders (using the previous definition), as compared with 25 (46%) of the 54 patients receiving doxazosin. Significant differences were not observed between the first-

Table 2.
Therapeutic Trials Comparing Various Antihypertensive Drugs with Doxazosin in Patients with Mild to Moderate Hypertension[a]

Ref.	Final Drug Dosage (mg/day)	Duration (wk)	*n*	% Responders	Mean Blood Pressure Changes (Systolic/Diastolic) Supine	Standing
51	D, 11.6	9–24	408	60	−10.2/−9.0	−14.5/−11.1
	Pr, 11.8	9–24	54	61	−12.3/−9.4	−8.7/−9.3
52	D, 11.3	12	54	46	−11.6/−9.1	−14.2/+10.0
	Pr, 13.8	12	49	59	−9.7/−8.6	−12.0/−10.4
69	D, 4.7	14	19	84.2	−20/−17	−20/−17[b]
	Pr, 6.7	14	23	56.5	−14/−10	−14/−10[b]
70	D, 2.4	14	26	73	−14.5/−15.3	−17.0/−16.0
	T, 5.6	14	28	64	−12.7/−13.4	−16.2/−15.8
51	D, 11.6	9–24	408	60	−10.2/−9.0	−14.5/−11.1
	A, 91	9–24	155	60	−15.4/−12.0	−13.4/−11.6
71	D, 3.3	8	20	80	−20/−18	−14/−10
	A, 100	8	20	70	−19/−16	−13/−11
72	D, 6.3	43	105	76	−13.1/−13.4[c]	−16.0/−13.8
	A, 66.5	43	117	82	−18.9/−15.0[c]	−18.1/−14.0
73	D, 4.6	8	20	65	−24.6/−17.0	−24.8/−17.0
	A, 100	8	20	60	−26.6/−14.8	−30.4/−15.4
74	D/A, 11/100	12	44	71	−13.2/−9.8	−17.0/−12.3
	A, 100	12	43	36	−9.2/−6.0	−6.2/−6.7
51	D, 11.6	9–24	408	60	−10.2/−9.0	−14.5/−11.1
	M, 187	9–24	33	70	−9.8/−8.9	−11.8/−10.6
51	D, 11.6	9–24	408	60	−10.2/−9.0	−14.5/−11.1
	Na, 100	9–24	26	54	−22.7/−16.2	−19.3/−15.3
75	D, 12	10	41	56	...	−9.3/+8.4
	Na, 124	10	43	51	...	−8.8/+8.3
57	D, 4.4	11	25	92	−32/−21	...
	E, 19.3	11	27	85	−26/−21	...
76	D, 5.6	14	31	74	−16/−14[c]	−17/−17
	E, 25.5	14	31	81	−30/−20[c]	−16/−14
51	D, 11.6	9–24	408	60	−10.2/−9.0	−14.5/−11.1
	H, 77	9–24	55	67	−21.7/−14.6	−23.9/−15.2
58	D, 10.8	24	45	60	−8.2/−8.8	−12.1/−11.3
	H, 89.1	24	39	51	−15.9/−9.0	−16.0/−8.4
59	D, 6.9	52	41	71	−14.0/−12.0	−17.8/−12.9
	H, 84.6	52	43	70	−14.4/+11.0	−16.9/−10.5
60	D, 2.3	101.0	34	94	−30/−19	−32/−19
	N, 13.2	101.7	33	91	−30/−21	−31/−21

[a] D = doxazosin, Pr = prazosin, T = terazosin, A = atenolol, M = metoprolol, Na = nadolol, E = enalapril, H = hydrochlorothiazide, N = nitrendipine.
[b] Approximate values obtained from graphic representation.
[c] Sitting position.

and second-generation α_1-adrenoceptor inhibitors. Reported adverse effects were similar in both the prazosin and doxazosin groups.

In a smaller study (54 patients) comparing doxazosin with terazosin, both drugs normalized blood pressure in similar numbers of patients.[70] Both drugs were administered once daily. Doxazosin (final mean daily dosage, 2.4 mg) and terazosin (final mean daily dosage, 5.6 mg) produced reductions in blood pressure that were not significantly different from each other. Both drugs were relatively well tolerated. Nausea was the most commonly reported adverse effect of terazosin, whereas vertigo was the most commonly reported adverse effect of doxazosin.

Comparison with β-Adrenoceptor Antagonists. Atenolol is one of the most frequently used cardioselective β-blockers, administered either alone or with other antihypertensive drugs, such as thiazides, to control mild to moderate hypertension. Doxazosin and atenolol have been compared by numerous investigators. In each of the studies, both doxazosin and atenolol produced the desired effect, reducing both the SBP and DBP in the supine and standing positions.[51,54,71-74,77,78]

Not surprisingly, atenolol therapy not only decreases blood pressure but also has an effect on heart rate. Heart rates typically were reduced by approximately 15 beats/min in patients receiving atenolol and 1–5 beats/min in patients receiving doxazosin. In most cases, these changes in heart rate were not clinically significant.[51,54,71-3]

Comparison with Enalapril. Taylor et al.[76] compared the antihypertensive effect of the ACE inhibitor enalapril with that of doxazosin.[76] This double-blind trial indicated that both drugs were comparable in their ability to reduce blood pressure in patients with mild or moderate hypertension. The final mean daily dosage was 5.6 mg for doxazosin and 25.5 mg for enalapril. Approximately 90% of patients in either drug group tolerated their medication well.

Comparison with Hydrochlorothiazide. In a double-blind comparison of doxazosin versus hydrochlorothiazide, Trost et al.[59] determined that both drugs significantly decreased supine and standing blood pressures. Differences between the two drugs were not significant. The mean daily dosage at the end of the treatment period was 6.9 mg for doxazosin and 84.6 mg for hydrochlorothiazide.

Responder rates were similar in a trial conducted by Cox et al.[51] Hydrochlorothiazide produced a greater decrease in both SBP and DBP. Sixty-seven percent of the hydrochlorothiazide-treated patients were deemed to be responders, compared with 60% of the doxazosin-treated patients. Similar results were reported by other investigators comparing the antihypertensive effects of doxazosin with those of hydrochlorothiazide.[58]

Summary of Comparative Trials. Doxazosin is as effective as other α_1-adrenoceptor antagonists, β-adrenoceptor antagonists, and antihypertensive agents from other drug classes in the treatment of mild to moderate hypertension. Studies examining the effectiveness of doxazosin therapy for severe hypertension still need to be conducted.

Other Clinical Uses

Alpha$_1$-adrenoceptor inhibitors have been shown to be useful in the treatment of benign prostatic hypertrophy.[79] Patients receiving prazosin at a dosage of 2 mg twice daily exhibited improvement in maximal urinary flow rate. This change in flow rate was not accompanied by a significant decrease in maximal micturition pressure. Despite the symptomatic benefit observed with prazosin, patients continued to have urinary obstruction. Additional studies are currently under way to determine the value of once-daily dosage regimens of doxazosin in the management of patients with prostatic obstruction.

Doxazosin administered concurrently with digoxin and diuretics may also be a useful adjunctive agent for the treatment of congestive heart failure (CHF). DiBianco et al.[80] evaluated once-daily administration of doxazosin in patients with CHF and observed a reduction in ventricular arrhythmias and a decrease in the episodes of worsening heart failure. More studies are required to determine the effectiveness and the role of doxazosin in symptomatic CHF patients.

Adverse Effects

As with most antihypertensive agents, the reported adverse effects of doxazosin can be attributed to the pharmacologic activity of the drug itself. The majority of studies reported mild to moderate adverse effects that seldom required the discontinuation of therapy; however, intolerable adverse effects resulted in discontinuation of doxazosin in approximately 2–7% of doxazosin-treated patients.[10,77] Headache (8%) and dizziness (7%) are the two most prevalent adverse effects reported in an overall summary involving 771 patients receiving doxazosin therapy.[81] In the manufacturer's placebo-controlled trials, 19% of patients (n = 339) receiving doxazosin complained of dizziness, as compared with 9% of patients receiving placebo (n = 336).[10] Headache was also commonly reported (14%); however, the placebo group had a similar frequency of complaints regarding headaches (16%). Nausea, lethargy, and fatigue are also commonly reported adverse events, which have been reported in 3–4% of patients. Other miscellaneous adverse effects, such as sexual dysfunction, anxiety, fluid retention, somnolence, and rhinitis, are similar to those reported for other antihypertensive agents.

Problems of first-dose hypotension, which were commonly observed in initial studies using high doses of prazosin, are generally not experienced by patients receiving doxazosin at starting doses of 1 mg/day.[7] The slower onset of doxazosin's hypotensive activity may be responsible for the lack of first-dose hypotension. Overall, postural syncope has been reported in less than 2% of patients receiving doxazosin.[7]

Contraindications and Precautions

No drug interactions involving doxazosin have been reported to date. The manufacturer has determined in an in vitro study that doxazosin does not affect the protein binding of digoxin, phenytoin, warfarin, and indomethacin.[10]

Doxazosin is classified as pregnancy category B, signifying that animal studies have not demonstrated adverse effects to the fetus, but no well-controlled or adequate trials in humans have been undertaken.[10] Doxazosin should be administered during pregnancy only when clinically warranted.

Dosage and Administration

Because of variability in hypotensive effects, doxazosin antihypertensive therapy must be individualized according to patient response. The initial starting dose for the treatment of hypertension is 1 mg administered once daily, which is generally not associated with first-dose hypotension. If required, dosage may be increased at two-week intervals according to blood-pressure-lowering effects. Mazzola et al.[82] reported the safety of a simplified dosage regimen in which the starting dose was given for two days and subsequent increases occurred over 12 to 14 days. Single daily doses up to 16 mg/day were administered in clinical trials, but doses greater than this are not recommended and are associated with an increase in postural hypotension.

The onset of hypotensive activity occurs between

two and six hours after doxazosin administration, and monitoring of blood pressure during this time interval is recommended. After dosage adjustments or addition of concomitant antihypertensive drug therapy, blood pressure should be closely monitored.

Availability and Cost

Doxazosin mesylate is indicated in FDA-approved labeling for the treatment of hypertension, either alone or in combination with β-adrenoceptor antagonists or diuretic therapy. Doxazosin is supplied as 1-, 2-, 4-, and 8-mg scored tablets in bottles of 100 tablets. The inactive ingredients for all strengths are microcrystalline cellulose, sodium starch glycoate, lactose, magnesium stearate, and sodium lauryl sulfate.[10] The 1-mg tablet is white; the 2-mg tablet is yellow, containing D & C Yellow No. 10 and FD & C Yellow No. 6; the 4-mg tablet is orange, containing FD & C Yellow No. 6; and the 8-mg tablet is green, containing FD & C Blue No. 10 and D & C Yellow No. 10.[10]

The average wholesale prices for a bottle of 100 tablets are as follows: 1 mg, $78.82; 2 mg, $78.82; 4 mg, $82.76; and 8 mg, $86.90.[83] Table 3 compares the costs of available α_1-adrenergic receptor antagonists and several antihypertensive agents evaluated in comparative clinical trials.

Table 3.
Representative Costs of Doxazosin and Various Antihypertensive Agents Evaluated in Clinical Studies

Product	Dose (mg)	Cost in Dollars[a] (per 100 tabs/caps)
Doxazosin tablets	1	78.82
(Cardura, Pfizer)	2	78.82
	4	82.76
	8	86.90
Prazosin capsules	1	32.11
(Minipress, Pfizer)	2	44.70
	5	76.20
Terazosin tablets	1	83.05
(Hytrin, Abbott)	2	83.05
	5	83.05
	10	83.05
Atenolol tablets	50	74.02
(Tenormin, ICI Pharma)	100	111.00
Enalapril tablets	2.5	58.85
(Vasotec, Merck Sharp & Dohme)	5	74.78
	10	78.53
	20	111.68
Hydrochlorothiazide tablets	25	11.05
(HydroDIURIL, Merck Sharp & Dohme)	50	17.51

[a] Average wholesale cost based on data from *Drug Topics Red Book*.[83]

Patient Instruction

Alpha$_1$-adrenergic receptor inhibitors, including doxazosin, are associated with hypotensive episodes, including orthostatic hypotension, syncope, dizziness, vertigo, or lightheadedness, primarily observed during initiation of therapy or after subsequent increases in dose. Patients should be advised to lie or sit down if they experience any of these symptoms and to exercise caution upon standing from the sitting or supine position.

Doxazosin has been reported to cause somnolence and drowsiness, and patients should be cautioned about performing hazardous tasks or tasks requiring mental alertness.

Formulary Considerations

The selection of antihypertensive drug therapy for the treatment of mild to moderate hypertension has evolved from the initial diuretic or β-adrenoceptor-antagonist stepped-care approach to a multifactorial, individualized treatment plan. No ideal antihypertensive agents are currently available, and selection of pharmacologic therapy should be based on efficacy, safety, patient compliance and acceptability, cost, and increasingly important, presence of underlying patient cardiovascular risk factors.

Prazosin has been available in the United States for approximately 15 years but represents only 4% of total antihypertensive prescriptions.[7] Various explanations have been suggested for this low use, including reduced efficacy, development of first-dose hypotension, tolerance, single-agent availability, and concomitant marketing of ACE inhibitors and calcium-channel-blocking agents. With the additional availability of doxazosin and terazosin, clinical experience with selective α_1-adrenoceptor antagonists may increase. Comparative trials have demonstrated similar blood-pressure-lowering effects between doxazosin and diuretics, β-adrenoceptor antagonists, enalapril, and nitrendipine, which is currently not available in the United States. Tolerance to the antihypertensive activity of doxazosin has not been observed, and first-dose hypotension may be minimized by initiating therapy with low doses. Because doxazosin has a long half-life, it may be administered in a single daily dose, which may possibly increase patient compliance. Doxazosin has also been associated with favorable serum lipid effects in hypertensive patients, including smokers and diabetic patients, without affecting blood glucose or insulin concentrations.

The availability of doxazosin does not constitute a major therapeutic advance in the treatment of mild to moderate hypertension; however, it does allow prescribers and pharmacists another blood-pressure-lowering therapeutic alternative that has been demonstrated to be safe, efficacious, convenient to administer, and competitively priced. Furthermore, doxazosin may provide positive CHD risk factor intervention with individualization of antihypertensive therapy.

In comparison with prazosin, both doxazosin and terazosin allow once-daily administration with similar antihypertensive efficacy. In addition, doxazosin is available in a scored-tablet dosage formulation that may be more cost-efficient than terazosin since tablets may be cut in half, decreasing patient drug costs by 50%. Because prazosin has been prescribed for over 15 years and is available in less costly generic formulations, it is doubtful that the introduction of doxazosin or terazosin will displace prazosin from drug formularies. However, in patients who require α_1-adrenoceptor antagonist therapy, doxazosin allows a once-daily, cost-effective alternative.

Conclusion

Doxazosin is a second-generation selective α_1-adrenoceptor antagonist with pharmacologic activity similar to that of its predecessor prazosin. The long elimination half-life of doxazosin allows once-daily administration, and its slow onset of hypotensive activity minimizes the first-dose hypotensive effect that is often reported with prazosin. Doxazosin's blood-pressure-lowering effects are comparable to those of other α_1-adrenoceptor antagonists and to those of antihypertensives in other drug classes.

References

1. 1988 Joint National Committee. The 1988 Report of the Joint National Committee on Detection, Evaluation, and Treatment of High Blood Pressure. *Arch Intern Med.* 1988; 148:1023-38.
2. Working Group on Management of Patients with Hypertension and High Blood Cholesterol. National Education Programs Working Group report on the management of patients with hypertension and high blood cholesterol. *Ann Intern Med.* 1991; 114:224-37.
3. Pool JL. Effects of doxazosin on serum lipids: a review of the clinical data and molecular basis for altered lipid metabolism. *Am Heart J.* 1991; 121:251-60.
4. MacMahon S, Peto R, Cutler J et al. Blood pressure, stroke, and coronary heart disease. Part 1: prolonged differences in blood pressure: prospective observational studies corrected for the regression dilution bias. *Lancet.* 1990; 335:765-74.
5. Dollery CT. Risk predictors, risk indicators, and benefit factors in hypertension. *Am J Med.* 1987; 82(Suppl 1A):2-8.
6. Taylor SH. Coronary artery disease risk factor management in the hypertensive patient. *Am J Cardiol.* 1987; 59:G2-8.
7. Khoury AF, Kaplan NM. Alpha-blocker therapy of hypertension: an unfulfilled promise. *JAMA.* 1991; 266:394-8.
8. Hayduk K. Efficacy and safety of doxazosin in hypertension therapy. *Am J Cardiol.* 1987; 59:G35-9.
9. Colucci WS. New developments in alpha-adrenergic receptor pharmacology: implications for the initial treatment of hypertension. *Am J Cardiol.* 1983; 51:639-43.
10. Pfizer-Roerig. Cardura package insert. New York, NY; 1990 Nov.
11. Davey MJ. Pharmacologic basis for the use of doxazosin in the treatment of essential hypertension. *Am J Med.* 1989; 87 (Suppl 2A):S36-44.
12. Davey M. Mechanism of alpha blockade for blood pressure control. *Am J Cardiol.* 1987; 59:G18-28.
13. Van Zwieten PA, Timmermans PBMWM, van Brummelen P. Role of alpha adrenoceptors in hypertension and in antihypertensive drug treatment. *Am J Med.* 1984; 77(Suppl 4A):17-25.
14. Cubeddu LX. New alpha$_1$-adrenergic receptor antagonists for the treatment of hypertension: role of vascular alpha receptors in the control of peripheral resistance. *Am Heart J.* 1988; 116(1 Part 1):133-62.
15. Corr PB, Heathers GP, Yamada KA. Mechanisms contributing to the arrhythmogenic influences of alpha$_1$-adrenergic stimulation in the ischemic heart. *Am J Med.* 1989; 87(Suppl 2A):S19-25.
16. Van Zwieten PA. Basic pharmacology of alpha-adrenoceptor antagonists and hybrid drugs. *J Hypertens.* 1988; 6(Suppl 2):S3-11.
17. Jie K, van Brummelen P, Timmermans PBMWM et al. Differences between exogenous and endogenous noradrenaline in the effects on vascular post-synaptic alpha$_1$- and alpha$_2$-adrenoceptors in man. *J Hypertens.* 1985; 3(Suppl 3):S145-7.
18. Van Brummelen PV, Jie K, Timmermans PBMWM et al. Postjunctional alpha-adrenoceptors and the regulation of arteriolar tone in humans. *J Cardiovasc Pharmacol.* 1985; 7 (Suppl 6):S149-52.
19. Nash DT. Alpha-adrenergic blockers: mechanism of action, blood pressure control, and effects on lipoprotein metabolism. *Clin Cardiol.* 1990; 13:764-72.
20. Timmermans PBMWM, Kwa HY, Karamat Ali F et al. Prazosin and its analogues UK-18,596 and UK-33,274: a comparative study on cardiovascular effects and alpha-adrenoceptor blocking activities. *Arch Int Pharmacodyn.* 1980; 245:218-35.
21. Alabaster VA, Davey MJ. The alpha$_1$-adrenoceptor antagonist profile of doxazosin: preclinical pharmacology. *Br J Clin Pharmacol.* 1986; 21:S9-17.
22. Singleton W, Saxton CAPD, Hernandez J et al. Postjunctional selectivity of alpha-blockade with prazosin, trimazosin, and UK-33,274 in man. *J Cardiovasc Pharmacol.* 1982; 4(Suppl 1):S145-51.
23. Jie K, van Brummelen P, Vermy P et al. Identification of vascular postsynaptic alpha$_1$- and alpha$_2$-adrenoceptors in man. *Circ Res.* 1984; 54:447-52.
24. Taylor SH. Clinical pharmacotherapeutics of doxazosin. *Am J Med.* 1989; 87 (Suppl 2A):S2-11.
25. Donnelly R, Elliott HL, Meredith PA et al. Concentration–effect relationships and individual responses to doxazosin in essential hypertension. *Br J Clin Pharmacol.* 1989; 28:517-26.
26. Conway EL, McNeil JJ, Meng L et al. Single-dose and steady-state pharmacokinetics of doxazosin given in combination with chlorothiazide to hypertensive subjects. *Clin Pharmacokinet.* 1989; 16:387-91.
27. Shionoiri H, Yasuda G, Yoshimura H et al. Antihypertensive effects and pharmacokinetics of single and consecutive administration of doxazosin in patients with mild to moderate essential hypertension. *J Cardiovasc Pharmacol.* 1987; 10:90-5.
28. Elliott HL, Meredith PA, Vincent J et al. Clinical pharmacological studies with doxazosin. *Br J Clin Pharmacol.* 1986; 21:S27-31.
29. Scott PJW, Hosie J, Scott MGB. A double-blind and crossover comparison of once daily doxazosin and placebo with steady-state pharmacokinetics in elderly hypertensive patients. *Eur J Clin Pharmacol.* 1988; 34:119-23.
30. Cubeddu LX, Fuenmayor N, Caplan N et al. Clinical pharmacology of doxazosin in patients with essential hypertension. *Clin Pharmacol Ther.* 1987; 41:439-49.
31. Kaye B, Cussans NJ, Faulkner JK et al. The metabolism and kinetics of doxazosin in man, mouse, rat, and dog. *Br J Clin Pharmacol.* 1986; 21:S19-25.
32. Elliott HL, Meredith PA, Reid JL. Pharmacokinetic overview of doxazosin. *Am J Cardiol.* 1987; 59:G78-81.
33. Conrad KA, Fagan TC, Mackie MJ et al. Doxazosin in patients with hypertension. *Eur J Clin Pharmacol.* 1988; 35:21-4.
34. Carlson RV, Bailey RR, Begg EJ et al. Pharmacokinetics and effect on blood pressure of doxazosin in normal subjects and patients with renal failure. *Clin Pharmacol Ther.* 1986; 40:561-6.
35. Vincent J, Elliott HL, Meredith PA et al. Doxazosin, an alpha$_1$-adrenoceptor antagonist: pharmacokinetics and concentration–effect relationships in man. *Br J Clin Pharmacol.* 1983; 15:719-25.
36. Oliver RM, Upward JW, Dewhurst AG et al. The pharmacokinetics of doxazosin in patients with hypertension and renal impairment. *Br J Clin Pharmacol.* 1990; 29:417-22.
37. Lund-Johansen P, Omvik P, Haugland H. Acute and chronic

hemodynamic effects of doxazosin in hypertension at rest and during exercise. *Br J Clin Pharmacol.* 1986; 21:S45-54.
38. Cubeddu LX, Pool JL, Bloomfield R et al. Effect of doxazosin monotherapy on blood pressure and plasma lipids in patients with essential hypertension. *Am J Hypertens.* 1988; 1:158-67.
39. Ames RP, Kiyasu JY. Alpha-1 adrenoceptor blockade with doxazosin in hypertension: effects on blood pressure and lipoproteins. *J Clin Pharmacol.* 1989; 29:123-7.
40. Smyth P, Pringle S, Jackson G et al. 24-Hour control of blood pressure by once daily doxazosin: a multicentre double-blind comparison with placebo. *Eur J Clin Pharmacol.* 1988; 34:613-8.
41. De Leeuw PW, Van Es PN, De Bos R et al. Acute renal effects of doxazosin in man. *Br J Clin Pharmacol.* 1986; 21:S41-3.
42. Oliveros-Palacios MC, Godoy-Godoy N, Colina-Chourio JA. Effects of doxazosin on blood pressure, renin–angiotensin–aldosterone and urinary kallikrein. *Am J Cardiol.* 1991; 67:157-61.
43. Bailey RR, Nairn PL, Walker RJ. Effect of doxazosin on blood pressure and renal hemodynamics of hypertensive patients with renal failure. *N Z Med J.* 1986; 99:942-5.
44. Wilner KD, Ziegler MG. Effects of $alpha_1$ inhibition on renal blood flow and sympathetic nervous activity in systemic hypertension. *Am J Cardiol.* 1987; 59:G82-6.
45. Bartels ACC, de Vries PMJM, Oe LP et al. Doxazosin in the treatment of patients with mild or moderate hypertension and mild or moderate renal insufficiency. *Am Heart J.* 1988; 116:1772-7.
46. Graham RM. Selective $alpha_1$-adrenergic blockade, lipids, and coronary heart disease risk. *Am J Med.* 1989; 87 (Suppl 2A):S53-6.
47. Lardinois CK, Neuman SL. The effects of antihypertensive agents on serum lipids and lipoproteins. *Arch Intern Med.* 1988; 148:1280-8.
48. Krone W, Nagele H. Effects of antihypertensives on plasma lipids and lipoprotein metabolism. *Am Heart J.* 1988; 116:1729-34.
49. Dzau VJ. Mechanism of the interaction of hypertension and hypercholesterolemia in atherogenesis: the effects of antihypertensive agents. *Am Heart J.* 1988; 116:1725-8.
50. Taylor SH. Efficacy and safety of doxazosin in the treatment of patients with mild or moderate hypertension and elevated levels of cholesterol. *Am Heart J.* 1991; 121:362-6
51. Cox DA, Leader JP, Milson JA et al. The antihypertensive effects of doxazosin: a clinical overview. *Br J Clin Pharmacol.* 1986; 21:S83-90.
52. Torvik D, Madsbu HP. Multicentre 12-week double-blind comparison of doxazosin, prazosin and placebo in patients with mild to moderate essential hypertension. *Br J Clin Pharmacol.* 1986; 21:S69-75.
53. Torvik D, Madsbu HP. An open one-year comparison of doxazosin and prazosin for mild to moderate essential hypertension. *Am J Cardiol.* 1987; 59:G68-72.
54. Nash DT, Schonfeld G, Reeves RL et al. A double-blind parallel trial to assess the efficacy of doxazosin, atenolol, and placebo in patients with mild to moderate systemic hypertension. *Am J Cardiol.* 1987; 59:G87-90.
55. Frick MH, Cox DA, Himanen P et al. Serum lipid changes in a one-year, multicenter, double-blind comparison of doxazosin and atenolol for mild to moderate essential hypertension. *Am J Cardiol.* 1987; 59:G61-7.
56. Talseth T, Westlie L, Daae L. Doxazosin and atenolol as monotherapy in mild and moderate hypertension: a randomized, parallel study with a three-year follow-up. *Am Heart J.* 1991; 121:280-5.
57. Wessels F. Double-blind comparison of doxazosin and enalapril in patients with mild or moderate essential hypertension. *Am Heart J.* 1991; 121:299-303.
58. Hjortdahl P, von Krogh H, Daae L et al. A 24-week multicenter double-blind study of doxazosin and hydrochlorothiazide in patients with mild to moderate essential hypertension. *Acta Med Scand.* 1987; 221:427-34.
59. Trost BN, Weidmann P, Riesen W et al. Comparative effects of doxazosin and hydrochlorothiazide on serum lipids and blood pressure in essential hypertension. *Am J Cardiol.* 1987; 59:G99-104.
60. Nechwatal W, Berger J, Blumrich W et al. A double-blind comparative study of doxazosin and nitrendipine in patients with mild-to-moderate essential hypertension. *Am Heart J.* 1988; 116:1806-14.
61. Cryer PE, Haymond MW, Santiago JV et al. Norepinephrine and epinephrine release and adrenergic mediation of smoking-associated hemodynamic and metabolic events. *N Engl J Med.* 1976; 295:573-7.
62. Craig WY, Palomaki GE, Haddow JE. Cigarette smoking and serum lipid and lipoprotein concentrations: an analysis of published data. *Br Med J.* 1989; 298:784-8.
63. Westheim A, Daae LNW, Kierulf P et al. Selective $alpha_1$ inhibition with doxazosin in hypertensive smokers and non-smokers: haemodynamic and metabolic effects. *J Hypertens.* 1990; 8(Suppl 5):S41-6.
64. Talseth T, Westlie L, Daae LNW. Long-term effects of doxazosin and atenolol on serum lipids and blood pressure in hypertensive smokers. *J Hypertens.* 1990; 8(Suppl 5):S47-51.
65. Castrignano R, D'Angelo A, Pati T et al. A single-blind study of doxazosin in the treatment of mild-to-moderate essential hypertensive patients with concomitant noninsulin-dependent diabetes mellitus. *Am Heart J.* 1988; 116:1778-84
66. Scheen AJ, Castillo M, Salvatore T et al. Lack of deleterious effects of the $alpha_1$-adrenoceptor blocking agent doxazosin on insulin secretion and insulin sensitivity in healthy men. *Curr Ther Res.* 1989; 46:200-9.
67. Lehtonen A, The Finnish Multicenter Study Group. Lowered levels of serum insulin, glucose, and cholesterol in hypertensive patients during treatment with doxazosin. *Curr Ther Res.* 1990; 47:278-84
68. Ames RP, Chrysant SG, Gonzalez F. Effectiveness of doxazosin in systemic hypertension. *Am J Cardiol.* 1989; 64:203-8.
69. De Planque BA. A double-blind comparative study of doxazosin and prazosin when administered with beta-blockers or diuretics. *Am Heart J.* 1991; 121:304-11.
70. Hayduk K, Schneider HT. Antihypertensive effects of doxazosin in systemic hypertension and comparison with terazosin. *Am J Cardiol.* 1987; 59:G95-8.
71. Giorgi G, Legramante JM, Fioravanti G et al. A comparative study of doxazosin versus atenolol in mild-to-moderate hypertension. *Am Heart J.* 1988; 116:1801-5.
72. Talseth T, Westlie L, Daae L et al. Comparison of the effects of doxazosin and atenolol on blood pressure and blood lipids: a one-year, double-blind study in 228 hypertensive patients. *Am Heart J.* 1988; 116:1790-6.
73. Mazzola C, Guerrasio E. Doxazosin versus atenolol: a randomized comparison of calculated coronary heart disease risk reduction. *Am Heart J.* 1988; 116:1797-801.
74. Searle M, Dathan R, Dean S et al. Doxazosin in combination with atenolol in essential hypertension: a double-blind placebo-controlled multicentre trial. *Eur J Clin Pharmacol.* 1990; 39:299-300.
75. Svetkey LP, Brobyn R, Deedwania P et al. Double-blind comparison of doxazosin, nadolol and placebo in patients with mild-to-moderate hypertension. *Curr Ther Res.* 1988; 43:969-78.
76. Taylor SH, Lee PS, Sharma SK. A comparison of doxazosin and enalapril in the treatment of mild and moderate essential hypertension. *Am Heart J.* 1988; 116:1820-5.
77. Lijnen P, Fagard R, Staessen J et al. Long-term double-blind comparison of doxazosin and atenolol in patients with mild to moderate hypertension. *J Cardiovasc Pharmacol.* 1989; 14:319-25.
78. Ott P, Storm TL, Krussell LR et al. Multicenter, double-blind comparison of doxazosin and atenolol in patients with mild to moderate hypertension. *Am J Cardiol.* 1987; 59:G73-7.
79. Kirby RS. Alpha-adrenoceptor inhibitors in the treatment of benign prostatic hyperplasia. *Am J Med.* 1989; 87 (Suppl

2A):S26-30.
80. DiBianco R, Parker JO, Chakko D et al. Doxazosin for the treatment of chronic congestive heart failure: results of a randomized double-blind and placebo controlled study. *Am Heart J*. 1991; 121:372-80.
81. Rosenthal J. Clinical experience with doxazosin in general medical practice. *Am Heart J*. 1988; 116:1748-57.
82. Mazzola C, Vaccarella A, Serra G et al. The efficacy and safety of doxazosin in the treatment of mild or moderate essential hypertension when dose adjustment is simplified. *Curr Ther Res*. 1990; 48:809-16.
83. Cardinale VA, Thurlow RM, eds. Drug Topics red book annual pharmacists' reference. Oradell, NJ: Medical Economics; 1991.

Research Notes

Absolute bioavailability of aminophylline liquid administered enterally in adults requiring mechanical ventilation

KAREN F. SHALANSKY, LEIGH M. VAUGHAN, CRISTINA USTAD, MARTIN G. TWEEDDALE, AND STEVEN A. SAHN

Clin Pharm. 1992; 11:428-32

Theophylline enhances bronchodilation and improves diaphragmatic contractility in the mechanically ventilated patient with severe obstructive lung disease.[1,2] Serum theophylline concentrations between 10 and 20 mg/L provide maximal benefit with minimal toxicity.[2,3] To achieve these levels, mechanically ventilated patients are initially treated with an intravenous theophylline infusion. When oral therapy can be prescribed, an equivalent liquid theophylline dose is typically administered intermittently by means of a nasogastric tube since endotracheal intubation prohibits the patient from swallowing.

Because the mechanically ventilated patient is often receiving enterally administered drugs and nutrition, the disposition of theophylline may be altered. Studies show decreased bioavailability of theophylline liquid when administered rectally or by way of colostomy rather than orally.[4,5] Continuous nasogastric feedings have also caused reduced absorption of oral theophylline, resulting in subtherapeutic serum theophylline concentrations and recurrent bronchospasm.[6] Other drugs exhibiting reduced bioavailability with nasogastric feedings include phenytoin and carbamazepine.[7,8]

Neither the bioavailability of theophylline when administered by way of nasogastric tube nor the disposition of this drug in the ventilator-dependent adult patient has been studied. The purpose of this study was to determine the bioavailability of an enterally administered liquid aminophylline formulation in adults requiring mechanical ventilation.

Methods. *Experimental Design.* This study was a prospective, multisite, nonrandomized, multiple-dose, crossover study, which was divided into two phases. During phase 1, aminophylline (equal to 80% theophylline) was administered intravenously by a continuous infusion. Loading and maintenance dosages were calculated to provide steady-state serum theophylline concentrations between 10 and 20 mg/L.[9] Steady-state conditions were confirmed by three consecutive theophylline concentrations within 20% of the mean measured in blood samples collected at least six hours apart.

In phase 2, i.v. aminophylline was discontinued and an equivalent daily dosage (to nearest 5 mg) of aminophylline liquid (Palaron, assayed as 20.90 mg of aminophylline per milliliter, equal to 86% theophylline, Fisons, Pickering, Ontario) was administered by way of nasogastric tube or gastrostomy tube in three equal doses given at 0800, 1600, and 2400. After a minimum of three half-lives, 2 mL blood specimens were drawn from established venous or arterial lines during one dosage interval at 0, 1, 2, 3, 4, 6, and 8 hours after an 0800 dose.

Blood specimens were drawn and placed in an evacuated blood collection tube without additives. All blood specimens were allowed to clot at room temperature and were centrifuged; the serum was frozen at –70 °C until assayed. Serum theophylline determinations were batched and measured using high-performance liquid chromatography[10] (patients 1–2) or fluorescence polarization immunoassay (TDx, Abbott Diagnostics, Irving, TX) (patients 3–8). All samples from a given patient were analyzed together using the same assay. The coefficients of variation were less than 5% for both assays

Subjects. Subjects had to meet the following criteria

KAREN F. SHALANSKY, PHARM.D., is Clinical Pharmacy Specialist, Critical Care, Vancouver General Hospital, Vancouver, British Columbia. LEIGH M. VAUGHAN, PHARM.D., is Assistant Professor and Clinical Pharmacist, Pulmonary and Critical Care, College of Pharmacy, Medical University of South Carolina, Charleston. CRISTINA USTAD is Clinical Pharmacist, Vancouver General Hospital. MARTIN G. TWEEDDALE, M.B., F.R.C.P.(C) is Director, Intensive Care Unit, Department of Medicine, Vancouver General Hospital. STEVEN A. SAHN, M.D., is Professor and Chairman, Division of Pulmonary and Critical Care, Department of Medicine, Medical University of South Carolina.

Address reprint requests to Dr. Vaughan at the College of Pharmacy, Medical University of South Carolina, 171 Ashley Avenue, Charleston, SC 29425-0810.

Supported in part by a grant from The Upjohn Company, Kalamazoo, MI.

Presented in part at the 25th Annual ASHP Midyear Clinical Meeting, Las Vegas, NV, December 10, 1990. Presented at the ACCP Annual Meeting, Minneapolis, MN, August 23, 1991.

to be admitted to the study: (1) 18–90 years old, (2) require mechanical ventilation, (3) reside in the intensive-care unit (ICU), and (4) require theophylline administration for treatment. Subjects were excluded if they (1) had known allergies to xanthines, (2) had medical contraindications (seizures or ventricular arrhythmias related to therapeutic concentrations of theophylline), (3) were receiving hemodialysis, plasmapheresis, or continuous arteriovenous hemofiltration, (4) had surgical removal of a section of the gastrointestinal tract, (5) were unable to ingest liquid medications enterally, or (6) displayed moderate to severe congestive heart failure as evidenced by echocardiographic ejection fraction less than 20%, presence of a third heart sound (S_3 gallop), or central venous pressure greater than 15 cm H_2O.

Patients who received medications that could potentially interact with theophylline were included in the study as long as steady-state conditions of all drugs were achieved.

This study was approved by the institution's review board for human research, and written informed consent was obtained from all subjects.

Pharmacokinetic Analysis. Serum theophylline concentrations were fitted to a one-compartment open model, assuming first-order absorption and elimination.

Theophylline clearance (CL) in phase 1 was calculated by dividing the dose (D) of theophylline infused each hour by the mean steady-state serum theophylline concentration (C_{ss}).[11] The C_{ss} value used was the average of the three consecutive concentrations.

Area under the concentration–time curve for phase 1 (AUC_{iv}) was calculated by multiplying C_{ss} by eight hours. AUC for phase 2 (AUC_{ng}) was calculated by using the trapezoidal method[12] and measuring the area under the curve for the eight-hour dosage interval. AUC_{ng} was normalized for differences in doses by dividing the eight-hour i.v. dose by the nasogastric dose, after converting both to the theophylline equivalent, then multiplying this by the AUC_{ng}.[13]

$$AUC_{ng}\text{ (adjusted)} = [(D_{iv} \times 8 \times 0.80)/(D_{ng} \times 0.86)] \times AUC_{ng}$$

The fraction of the oral dose absorbed ($F_{absolute}$) was calculated by dividing the adjusted AUC_{ng} by AUC_{iv}.

Percent fluctuation with liquid aminophylline in phase 2 was determined as follows:

$$\%\text{ Fluctuation} = [(\text{peak} - \text{trough})/\text{trough}] \times 100$$

Statistical Analysis. The two one-sided tests procedure was used to examine differences in AUCs.[14] The mean relative percent difference between AUCs (calculated as $[(AUC_{iv} - AUC_{ng})/AUC_{iv}] \times 100$) was described by a 90% confidence interval. The level of significance was set at $p < 0.05$.

A sample size of eight was required to detect a difference in AUC of 20% with a power of 0.81 and a level of significance of 0.05.

Results. Table 1 illustrates the demographics of the eight study subjects. Six patients had a smoking history before admission to hospital. All patients received continuous enteral feedings along with enterally administered aminophylline. Two patients had gastrostomy tube placements and received their oral medications, including aminophylline, and enteral feedings through the gastrostomy tube. Two patients received medications that could potentially interact with theophylline (patient 1 received ciprofloxacin, and patient 7 received phenytoin). Patient 2 had elevated liver function test results, which remained elevated throughout both phases of the study.

A summary of the pharmacokinetic values for both phases of the trial is shown in Table 2. Figure 1 illustrates the serum concentrations of theophylline during enteral administration. There were no significant differences in AUC for i.v. versus enteral aminophylline. The mean relative percent difference between the AUCs was –2.18% (90% confidence interval, –17.18 to 12.82). The absolute bioavailability of enterally administered aminophylline was 1.03 ± 0.22 (mean ± S.D.).

Discussion. When administered orally to asthmatic patients, liquid theophylline has a bioavailability that approaches 100%.[15] We observed complete absorption of a liquid aminophylline preparation administered by nasogastric tube or gastrostomy tube to critically ill patients requiring mechanical ventilation. Interpatient variability in absorption was similar to that reported in the literature[15,16] and can in part be attributed to assay error, dosing error, or fluctuation in clearance within a patient.

Studies evaluating the bioavailability of theophylline commonly employ healthy volunteers[4,17,18] or stable asthmatic patients.[15,19] Results from these populations are then extrapolated to more severely ill patients. Studies in critically ill patients[20] are difficult to undertake because of the severity of illness, the large number of prescribed medications, and difficulty in controlling external factors. Also, patients' conditions can change acutely, resulting in abrupt addition or discontinuation of medication.

Drug interactions are common in ICU patients receiving multiple medications. Two patients in our study concurrently received medications that are known to interact with theophylline. Patient 1 received ciprofloxacin, a drug that has been shown to reduce theophylline clearance by approximately 30%.[21-23] The maximal expression of this interaction occurs after three to five days of concomitant therapy.[21,22] Patient 1 entered the study after five days of concomitant therapy with ciprofloxacin. However, the mean serum theophylline concentration and AUC increased during phase 2, suggesting that ciprofloxacin's effect on theophylline clearance had not yet reached a plateau when the study began. This patient also had a history of cardiac dysfunction, which can reduce theophylline clearance[20]; however, there was no indication of cardiac problems during the study. Patient 7 had been stabilized on phenytoin for several years before the study. Although phenytoin can induce theophylline metabolism, the maximal effect of this interaction occurs within the first three to four weeks of therapy,[24] making

Table 1.
Demographic Characteristics of the Study Patients[a]

	Patient							
Characteristic[b]	1	2	3	4	5	6	7	8
Age (yr)	61	68	57	59	68	58	69	66
Sex	F	F	M	F	M	F	M	F
Weight (kg)	60	59	54	65	60	50	59	68
Disease state	Cardiomyopathy, AIDP, ARDS	Bronchitis, hypercapneic respiratory failure	COPD	Emphysema, pneumothorax	COPD, atrial fibrillation, intra-abdominal perforation and repair, GI bleed	COPD, lung cancer	Epilepsy, COPD, polycystic kidney disease	Asthma
Tube	GT	NG	NG	NG	GT	NG	NG	NG
Medication								
IV/SC	Furosemide	Heparin, ceftriaxone, ranitidine	Methylpred-nisolone, heparin, cefazolin	Methylpred-nisolone, dopamine, metoclopra-mide, piperacillin, tobramycin, albuterol	Furosemide, heparin, digoxin, dopamine, metoclopramide, amphotericin B, imipenem, tobramycin	Ranitidine, morphine, atropine, dexamethasone, cloxacillin, metoclopramide, lorazepam, dimenhydrinate	Metronidazole, ceftazidime, phenytoin, metoclopramide, fentanyl, diazepam	Methylprednisolone, cefamandole, diazepam, morphine
NG/GT	Ciprofloxacin, enalapril, digoxin, potassium chloride, ranitidine	. . .	Sucralfate	Sucralfate, multivitamins	Prednisone, diltiazem, metolazone, potassium chloride, ranitidine	. . .	Multivitamins, ranitidine	. . .
Smoker	Yes	Yes	Yes	Yes	Yes	Yes	No	No
Nutrition[c]	Isocal HCN	Isocal HCN	Osmolite HN	Osmolite HN	Magnacal HN	Osmolite HN	Magnacal HN	Osmolite HN

[a]AIDP = automatic implantable defibrillation placement, ARDS = adult respiratory distress syndrome, GT = gastrostomy tube, NG = nasogastric, COPD = chronic obstructive pulmonary disease, IV = intravenous, SC = subcutaneous, GI = gastrointestinal.
[b]All patients' liver function test results were normal, except for patient 2's aspartate aminotransferase (207-272 IU/L) and alkaline phosphatase (240–270 IU/L).
[c]Administered by continuous drip.

Table 2.
Pharmacokinetic Values for Theophylline[a]

Variable	Patient 1	2	3	4	5	6	7	8
Dosage[b]								
IV	5.2	6.5	14.2	13.3	9.6	16.1	11.7	6.8
NG	5.5	6.9	14.2	13.5	9.6	16.3	11.8	6.8
Mean serum theophylline concentration (mg/L)								
IV	8.4	9.2	11.5	11.7	14.7	11.8	8.5	11.5
NG	11.0	8.9	11.8	12.6	10.9	8.3	10.5	14.7
% Fluctuation								
NG	52	43	94	80	32	167	198	58.7
Clearance (L/hr)	1.52	1.30	2.78	3.07	1.63	2.85	3.39	1.67
$AUC_{0\text{-}8}$[c]								
IV	67.37	73.85	92.09	93.82	117.79	94.32	67.96	91.98
NG	81.75	66.86	94.75	103.89	87.70	67.48	84.95	120.15
$F_{absolute}$	1.19	0.91	1.03	1.11	0.74	0.72	1.25	1.31

[a]IV = intravenous, NG = nasogastric, $AUC_{0\text{-}8}$ = area under the concentration–time curve for the eight-hour dosage interval, $F_{absolute}$ = fraction of the oral dose absorbed.
[b]Dosage is expressed in terms of theophylline (mg/kg/day).
[c]Adjusted for differences in dosage.

Figure 1. Theophylline concentration versus time at steady-state conditions during enteral administration of aminophylline liquid.

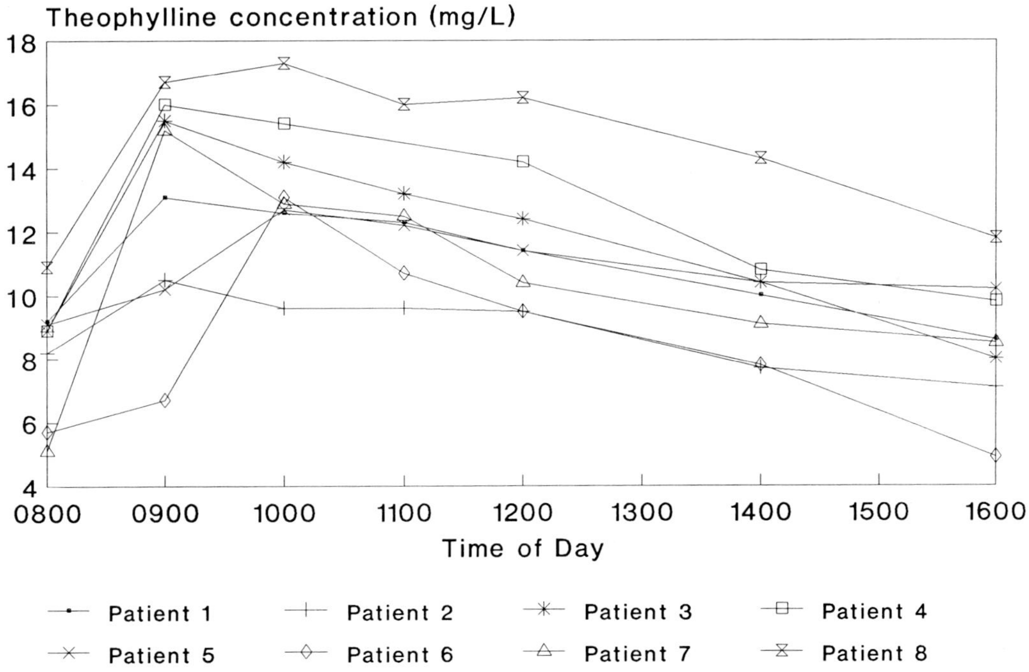

any additional effect of phenytoin on theophylline clearance during the course of this study unlikely.

The pharmacokinetics of theophylline are known to be affected by the administration of food.[25] Attributable factors include meal composition, alteration of gastric pH, and gut motility.[26] Enteral feedings have the potential to affect each of these factors and, thereby, theophylline pharmacokinetics. Our study demonstrates that continuous tube feedings of Isocal HCN (Mead Johnson Nutritionals, Evansville, IN), Osmolite HN (Ross, Columbus, OH), and Magnacal (Sherwood Medical, St. Louis, MO) do not affect the bioavailability of aminophylline. In several studies, theophylline has been shown to be visually compatible and pH stable when added to various enteral products.[27,28] Our results contrast with those of Gal and Layson,[6] who reported interference of oral theophylline absorption by continuous nasogastric feedings of Osmolite. In their study, theophylline extended-release tablets (Theo-Dur; Astra, Westboro, MA) were administered orally, as opposed to our study, in which aminophylline was administered enterally in a liquid formulation. It is not unusual for a food effect with theophylline to be formulation dependent.[25,26]

Conclusion. An aminophylline liquid was completely bioavailable when administered by way of nasogastric tube or gastrostomy tube to critically ill, mechanically ventilated patients.

References

1. Murciano D, Aubier M, Lecocguic Y et al. Effects of theophylline on diaphragmatic strength and fatigue in patients with chronic obstructive lung disease. *N Engl J Med*. 1984; 305:349-53.
2. Landsberg KF, Vaughan LM, Heffner JE. The effect of theophylline on respiratory muscle contractility and fatigue. *Pharmacotherapy*. 1990; 10:271-9.
3. Mitenko P, Ogilvie R. Rational intravenous doses of theophylline. *N Engl J Med*. 1973; 289:600-3.
4. Mason WD, Lanman RC, Amick EN et al. Bioavailability of theophylline following a rectally administered concentrated aminophylline solution. *J Allergy Clin Immunol*. 1980; 66:119-22.
5. Hooker KD, DiPiro JT, Stanfield JA et al. Absorption of theophylline administered via colostomy. *Clin Pharm*. 1989; 8:354-8.
6. Gal P, Layson R. Interference with oral theophylline absorption by continuous nasogastric feedings. *Ther Drug Monit*. 1986; 8:421-3.
7. Bauer LA. Interference of oral phenytoin absorption by continuous nasogastric feedings. *Neurology*. 1982; 32:570-2.
8. Bass H, Miles MV, Tennison MB et al. Effects of enteral tube feeding on the absorption and pharmacokinetic profile of carbamazepine suspension. *Epilepsia*. 1989; 30:364-9.
9. Ellis E, Hendeles L. Theophylline. In: Taylor WM, ed. A textbook for the clinical application of therapeutic drug monitoring. Irving, TX: Abbott Laboratories; 1986:185-201.
10. Orcutt JJ, Kozak PP, Gillman S et al. Micro-scale method for theophylline in body fluids by reversed-phase, high-pressure liquid chromatography. *Clin Chem*. 1977; 23:599-601.
11. Gibaldi M, Perrier D. Pharmacokinetics. 1st ed. New York: Marcel Dekker; 1975:16.
12. Gibaldi M. Biopharmaceutics and clinical pharmacokinetics. 3rd ed. Philadelphia: Lea & Febiger; 1984:315-6.
13. Hendeles L, Iafrate RP, Weinberger M. A clinical and pharmacokinetic basis for the selection and use of slow release theophylline products. *Clin Pharmacokinet*. 1984; 9:95-135.
14. Schuirmann DJ. A comparison of the two one-sided tests procedure and the power approach for assessing the equivalence of average bioavailability. *J Pharmacokinet Biopharm*. 1987; 15:657-80.
15. Hendeles L, Weinberger M, Bighley L. Absolute bioavailability of oral theophylline. *Am J Hosp Pharm*. 1977; 34:525-7.
16. Weinberger M, Hendeles L, Bighley L. The relation of product formulation to absorption of oral theophylline. *N Engl J Med*. 1978; 299:852-7.
17. Spangler DL, Kolof DD, Bloom FL et al. Theophylline bioavailability following oral administration of six sustained-release preparations. *Ann Allergy*. 1978; 40:6-11.
18. Welling PG, Lyons LL, Craig WA et al. Influence of diet and fluid on bioavailability of theophylline. *Clin Pharmacol Ther*. 1975; 17:475-80.
19. Guill M, Pruitt AW, Altman RE et al. Clinical and pharmacokinetic evaluation of a sustained-release liquid theophylline preparation. *J Allergy Clin Immunol*. 1988; 82:281-6.
20. Powell JR, Vozeh S, Hopewell P et al. Theophylline disposition in acutely ill hospitalized patients: the effect of smoking, heart failure, severe airway obstruction, and pneumonia. *Am Rev Respir Dis*. 1978; 118:229-38.
21. Wijnands WJA, Vree TB, van Herwaarden CLA. The influence of quinolone derivatives on theophylline clearance. *Br J Clin Pharmacol*. 1986; 22:677-83.
22. Schwartz J, Jaurequi L, Lettieri J et al. Impact of ciprofloxacin on theophylline clearance and steady-state concentrations in serum. *Antimicrob Agents Chemother*. 1988; 32:75-7.
23. Ryback MJ, Bowles SK, Prantharthi H et al. Increased theophylline concentrations secondary to ciprofloxacin. *Drug Intell Clin Pharm*. 1987; 21:879-81.
24. Landsberg KF, Shalansky S. Interaction between phenytoin and theophylline. *Can J Hosp Pharm*. 1988; 41:31-2.
25. Constance TD, Massey K. The effect of food on the absorption of sustained-release theophylline preparations in children. *Hosp Pharm*. 1988; 23:999-1002.
26. Plezia PM, Thornley SM, Kramer TH et al. The influence of enteral feedings on sustained-release theophylline absorption. *Pharmacotherapy*. 1990; 10:356-61.
27. Holtz L, Milton J, Sturek JK. Compatibility of medications with enteral feedings. *J Parenter Enter Nutr*. 1987; 11:183-6.
28. Cutie AJ, Altman E, Lenkel L. Compatibility of enteral products with commonly employed drug additives. *J Parenter Enter Nutr*. 1983; 7:186-91.

Possible ganciclovir-induced hepatotoxicity in patients with AIDS

Helen L. Figge, George R. Bailie,
Laurie L. Briceland, and Steven F. Kowalsky

Clin Pharm. 1992; 11:432-4

Cytomegalovirus (CMV) infection is a major cause of morbidity and mortality in patients with AIDS.[1,2] Ganciclovir has proved to be an effective anti-CMV agent, showing antiviral activity both in vitro and in vivo.[1] The major dose-limiting adverse effect of ganciclovir is neutropenia, which is reversible upon the discontinuation of therapy.[3] Ganciclovir has also been found to cause elevation in liver aminotransferases, thrombocytopenia, mental status changes, and phlebitis.[3,4]

Because there are few published data on the potential hepatotoxicity of ganciclovir, we undertook a retrospective review in an attempt to determine the frequency of ganciclovir-associated hepatotoxicity in patients with AIDS.

Methods. We reviewed the records of consecutive inpatients at Albany Medical Center Hospital who had

Helen L. Figge, Pharm.D., is Adjunct Assistant Professor; George R. Bailie, Pharm.D., FCCP, is Professor; and Laurie L. Briceland, Pharm.D., is Assistant Professor, Department of Pharmacy Practice, Albany College of Pharmacy (ACP), Albany, NY. Steven F. Kowalsky, Pharm.D., is Assistant Director, Anti-infectives, Miles Pharmaceuticals Inc., West Haven, CT; at the time of this study he was Professor, Department of Pharmacy Practice, ACP.

Address reprint requests to Dr. Bailie at the Department of Pharmacy Practice, Albany College of Pharmacy, 106 New Scotland Avenue, Albany, NY 12208.

Presented at the 12th Annual Meeting of the American College of Clinical Pharmacy, Minneapolis, MN, August 20, 1991.

AIDS and had been administered intravenous ganciclovir from January 1989 to December 1990. Institutional review board approval was not necessary as long as absolute confidentiality was maintained. Patients were identified from pharmacy computerized records. The criteria for inclusion in the study were confirmation of human immunodeficiency virus (HIV) positivity, satisfaction of the Centers for Disease Control (CDC) definition of AIDS, age greater than 16 years, administration of ganciclovir intravenously for at least three days for the treatment of a CMV infection, and availability of baseline and sequential liver function test (LFT) results. HIV positivity was confirmed by the Western blot assay. Renal transplant recipients were excluded. LFT results examined were serum aspartate aminotransferase (AST), alkaline phosphatase (ALP), and γ-glutamyltransferase (GGT) concentrations.

Hepatic damage was defined as either (1) an increase in AST to more than 50% above the patient's pretreatment baseline value or (2) a twofold elevation in both ALP and GGT over pretreatment baseline values. It was not necessary for the baseline values to be normal. Patients taking potentially hepatotoxic drugs other than ganciclovir were not excluded, but the drugs were documented.

Four independent reviewers analyzed the data for each patient and developed a consensus concerning the association between ganciclovir therapy and observed hepatic damage by considering the following criteria:

1. The hepatic damage is temporally related to the initiation of ganciclovir treatment (i.e., changes in liver function began within days of the start of treatment),
2. No infectious etiology is identifiable, and
3. No cause of hepatic damage other than drugs or infection is identifiable.

Improvements in LFT results after ganciclovir was discontinued in patients meeting the above criteria were taken as further evidence of a relationship between ganciclovir and a decline in liver function. The likelihood of ganciclovir causing hepatotoxicity was rated as follows:

1. *Highly probable:* All three of the criteria are met, and no potentially hepatotoxic drugs were coadministered with ganciclovir.
2. *Probable:* Two of the criteria are met, and no potentially hepatotoxic drugs were coadministered.
3. *Possible:* Three of the criteria are met, and potentially hepatotoxic drugs were coadministered.
4. *Remote:* Hepatic damage is believed to be due to some other cause.

Results. Sixteen courses of ganciclovir were administered to 12 men, but two courses in one patient were excluded from analysis because some necessary laboratory data were missing. The remaining 11 patients (14 courses) met the inclusion criteria; all were in group IV C-1 according to the system used by CDC to classify persons infected with HIV.[5,6] This category includes patients with at least one of the infectious diseases used in the CDC definition of AIDS. The mean ± S.D. patient age during the 14 courses was 38.2 ± 6.6 years (three patients are counted twice in this determination). The mean ± S.D. ganciclovir dosage for all 14 courses was 438 ± 149 mg/day (7.60 ± 2.38 mg/kg/day). The mean ± S.D. total dose was 5768 ± 3326 mg administered over 13.6 ± 4.8 days (range, 5–23 days).

Four patients had had five episodes of hepatic damage (Table 1); all five episodes were classified as possibly having been caused by ganciclovir. The mean ± S.D. total ganciclovir dose and number of days of therapy before the onset of hepatic damage for all five episodes were 2430 ± 1623 mg (range, 750–4800 mg) and 5.2 ± 1.9 days (range, 3–8 days), respectively. The four patients had been monitored for 5–12 days in the hospital after the onset of the hepatic damage.

In all five cases of possible ganciclovir-induced hepatotoxicity, other potentially hepatotoxic drugs had been administered (Table 1). Concomitant administration of such drugs precluded a more definitive association of ganciclovir with the hepatic damage. No countermeasures had been taken in four cases, but dosage reduction in the remaining case (patient 3) resulted in an improvement in LFT values, with ALP dropping from 360 IU/L to 268 IU/L and GGT from 175 IU/L to 134 IU/L. In the other four cases of possible ganciclovir-induced hepatotoxicity, the eventual outcome was unknown because of early patient discharge and inability to follow up. Patient 2 had had treatment courses that were nine months apart; Table 1 shows that liver function had improved by the time the second course was started (when the patient was 33 years old).

Of the nine courses of ganciclovir in eight patients that did not result in hepatic damage, potentially hepatotoxic drugs were concomitantly administered with five courses.

Discussion. Other reports of ganciclovir-induced toxicity mention only mild abnormalities in liver function.[3] The Collaborative DHPG Treatment Study Group[3] reported on 26 patients (22 of them patients with AIDS). Six patients were noted to have elevated LFT values that were believed to be drug related. However, the abnormal LFT values usually did not exceed twice the baseline values or twice the upper limit of normal. The true frequency of ganciclovir-induced hepatotoxicity in AIDS patients in the DHPG study cannot be determined, since some patients were excluded from analysis and it is not stated whether all six patients with LFT abnormalities had AIDS.

Shea et al.[4] reported a single case of ganciclovir-associated hepatotoxicity. The baseline LFT results were AST, 194 IU/L; ALP, 181 IU/L; and GGT, 542 IU/L, and after receiving ganciclovir 200 mg every eight hours (2.5 mg/kg/day), the patient's test values increased to AST, 900 IU/L; ALP, 250 IU/L; and GGT, 800 IU/L. AST declined when ganciclovir was stopped and increased to 1500 IU/L upon rechallenge with the drug (1.5 mg/kg/day). This is the only other

Table 1.
Characteristics of the Ganciclovir Treatment Courses[a]

Patient	Age (yr)	Ganciclovir Dosage (mg/kg/day)	Other Potentially Hepatotoxic Drugs Concurrently Administered	AST (IU/L)		ALP (IU/L)		GGT (IU/L)	
				Baseline	Peak	Baseline	Peak	Baseline	Peak
Courses with Hepatic Damage									
1	45	8.6	A, F, I	33	90	106	112	20	22
2	32	4.3	K	32	67	212	333	231	323
2	33	4.4	R	29	55	793	965	511	672
3	41	9.4, 4.3	Z	69	53	61	360	23	175
4	47	10.0	A	36	110	190	179	136	283
Mean ± S.D.	40 ± 7[b]	6.6 ± 2.6		40 ± 17	75 ± 24	272 ± 297	390 ± 338	184 ± 203	295 ± 241
Courses without Hepatic Damage									
4	47	4.9	K	95	135	166	167	127	108
5	34	8.8	A, I, K	32	42	136	160	20	30
6	27	8.9	None	52	49	265	232	100	105
7	31	8.9	None	43	50	112	141	61	100
8	44	7.8	K	39	45	96	115	50	47
8	44	10.0	None	49	32	250	216	279	252
9	33	5.1	N	94	108	126	138	278	288
10	38	9.0	M	33	41	146	119	N.A.	30
11	39	10.8	None	44	24	90	120	52	65
Mean ± S.D.	37 ± 8[b]	8.2 ± 2.0		53 ± 24	58 ± 37	154 ± 63	156 ± 42	129 ± 103	114 ± 94

[a]AST = serum aspartate aminotransferase concentration (normal, 15–25 IU/L), ALP = serum alkaline phosphatase concentration (normal, 30–115 IU/L), GGT = serum γ-glutamyltransferase concentration (normal, 0–65 IU/L), A = acyclovir, F = fluconazole, I = isoniazid, K = ketoconazole, R = rifampin, Z = zidovudine, N = nystatin, M = miconazole, N.A. = not available.
[b]Age of one patient counted twice.

well-documented case of ganciclovir-associated hepatotoxicity.

The magnitude of liver function abnormalities in our study ranged from mild (patient 1) to marked (patient 4). Most of the patients were taking other drugs with hepatotoxic potential, such as antituberculosis agents and acyclovir. This might have contributed to the hepatotoxicity observed. The hepatitis status of most of the patients was unknown; viral hepatitis could have contributed to the apparent hepatotoxicity. CMV-associated hepatitis is also a possible explanation. No other infections potentially involving the liver were documented.

Our report provides some additional evidence that hepatotoxicity can occur in patients with AIDS who are treated with ganciclovir. However, we cannot exclude the possibility that concurrently administered drugs or viral hepatitis or both contributed to the LFT abnormalities. Nevertheless, we recommend that all ganciclovir-treated AIDS patients undergo periodic LFTs, especially if they are receiving other potentially hepatotoxic drugs. Baseline LFTs should be performed in all patients and repeated every third day (based on the observed time of onset of possible hepatotoxicity in our sample). Substantial changes in LFTs may warrant a reduction in the ganciclovir dosage, but until larger studies are performed, such dosage reductions to counteract possible hepatotoxicity must be carefully weighed against the risk of exacerbating the patient's condition. Great caution should be exercised in extrapolating these findings to other patient groups with other characteristics.

Conclusion. Laboratory evidence of hepatic damage occurred in 5 of 14 courses of ganciclovir therapy in men with AIDS. The contribution of ganciclovir could not be separated from that of other drugs and infectious processes.

References

1. Fletcher CV, Balfour HH. Evaluation of ganciclovir for cytomegalovirus disease. *DICP*. 1989; 23:5-12.
2. Quinnan GV, Masur H, Rook AH et al. Herpes virus infections in the acquired immune deficiency syndrome. *JAMA*. 1984; 252:72-7.
3. Collaborative DHPG Treatment Study Group. Treatment of serious cytomegalovirus infections with 9-(1,3-di-hydroxy-2-propoxymethyl) guanine in patients with AIDS and other immunodeficiencies. *N Engl J Med*. 1986; 314:801-5.
4. Shea BF, Hoffman S, Sesin P et al. Ganciclovir hepatotoxicity. *Pharmacotherapy*. 1987; 7:223-6.
5. Centers for Disease Control. Classification system for human T-lymphotropic virus type III/lymphadenopathy-associated virus infections. *MMWR*. 1986; 35:334-9.
6. Centers for Disease Control. Revision of CDC surveillance case definition of acquired immunodeficiency syndrome. *MMWR*. 1987; 36(Suppl 1S):3S-14S.

DUE Criteria

The DUE Criteria *section of* Clinical Pharmacy *features model drug-use evaluation criteria that may be employed as a component of a comprehensive quality assurance program. The criteria sets are presented in the format used in the ASHP book* Criteria for Drug Use Evaluation. *Some of the criteria sets will have been originally published in that book; others will be presented here for the first time and published in future volumes of the ASHP book. The practitioners who developed a criteria set are acknowledged.*

In selecting drug products for coverage in DUE Criteria, *priority is given to products that have been recently marketed, those that are frequently prescribed, those that have high potential risk associated with their use, and those that are expensive. When feasible, a criteria set will be linked with a* Drug Review *that appears in the same issue.*

These criteria sets are a starting point for the development of DUE Criteria for a specific practice setting. Readers are encouraged to modify the model criteria to fit their own circumstances.

Criteria for use of pancuronium bromide, vecuronium bromide, atracurium besylate, tubocurarine chloride, metocurine iodide, pipecuronium bromide, and doxacurium chloride in adults[a]

Element	Standard 100%	Standard 0%	Exception[b] or Critical Preventive/ Responsive Measure[c]	Sources of Information
Justification for Use				
1. As an adjunct to general anesthesia, to facilitate endotracheal intubation[1-11] or	X		1A. None	1. Anesthesia records, preoperative notes, physician orders, nursing notes, progress notes, recovery room records
2. To provide muscle relaxation during surgery[1-11] or	X		2A. None	2. Anesthesia records, preoperative notes, physician orders, nursing notes, progress notes, recovery room records
3. To induce prolonged muscle paralysis in mechanically ventilated patient in intensive-care unit (ICU)[1-5,12]	X		3A. Doxacurium and pipecuronium use in ICU setting not studied	3. Physician orders, nursing notes, progress notes
Critical (Process) Indicators				
4. Administered by personnel trained in the use of neuromuscular blocking (NMB) agents, with facilities for intubation, artificial respiration, oxygen therapy, and NMB reversal agents readily available	X		4A. None	4. Anesthesia records, physician orders, nursing notes, progress notes, institutional policies and procedures, medication administration record (MAR)

Prepared by Andrew J. Donnelly, Pharm.D., M.B.A., Assistant Director, Clinical Services, and Clinical Pharmacist, Operating Room/Anesthesiology, Department of Pharmacy, Rush–Presbyterian–St. Luke's Medical Center, Chicago, IL; Julie A. Golembiewski, Pharmacist Practitioner, Operating Room, Department of Pharmacy, University of Illinois Hospital, Chicago, IL; Richard Skupski, M.D., Assistant Professor, Department of Anesthesiology, University of Illinois Hospital; and Jeffrey E. Wojtynek, Pharm.D., Pharmacist Practitioner, Investigational Drugs/Quality Assurance, Department of Pharmacy, University of Illinois Hospital.

Element	Standard 100%	Standard 0%	Exception[b] or Critical Preventive/ Responsive Measure[c]	Sources of Information
5. No history of hypersensitivity to NMB agent selected	X		5A. None	5. History and physical (H&P), allergies, anesthesia records, progress notes
6. Degree of neuromuscular blockade periodically monitored with peripheral nerve stimulator during surgery and as needed in ICU	X		6A. None	6. Anesthesia records, nursing notes, progress notes
7. Blood pressure, pulse, and respiration monitored continuously during surgery and periodically in ICU	X		7A. None	7. Anesthesia records, nursing notes, progress notes
8. Appropriate choice of agent[1-11] a. Pancuronium (1) Surgical case duration >90 minutes and (2) Patient without significant coronary artery disease (CAD) or significant renal impairment b. Vecuronium (1) Surgical case duration <120 minutes or for patient with significant CAD and (2) Patient has no significant hepatic or biliary disease c. Atracurium (1) Surgical case duration <90 minutes or patient with significant renal or hepatic impairment and (2) Patient has no significant CAD or history of asthma or anaphylactoid reaction d. Tubocurarine (1) Surgical case duration >90 minutes and (2) Patient has no significant renalimpairment or history of asthma or anaphylactoid reaction e. Metocurine (1) Surgical case duration >90 minutes and	X		8A. Vagolytic effect of pancuronium desired in patient with CAD to offset bradycardia caused by other agents (e.g., opioids) 8B. Unexpected prolongation of surgery when using vecuronium or atracurium 8C. Appropriate adjustment in dosage and dosing interval made for NMB agents eliminated renally	8. Anesthesia records, preoperative notes, physician orders, nursing notes, progress notes 8A. Anesthesia records 8B. Anesthesia records, preoperative notes, nursing notes 8C. Anesthesia records, preoperative notes, physician orders, nursing notes,

Element	Standard 100%	Standard 0%	Exception[b] or Critical Preventive/ Responsive Measure[c]	Sources of Information
(2) Patient has no significant renal impairment or history of asthma or anaphylactoid reaction f. Pipecuronium (1) Surgical case duration >90 minutes and (2) Patient has significant CAD and (3) Patient has no significant renal impairment g. Doxacurium (1) Surgical case duration >120 minutes and (2) Patient has significant CAD and (3) Patient has no significant renal impairment				
9. Appropriate i.v. dosage and dosing interval[1-12] a. Pancuronium bromide for anesthesia: (1) Priming dose: 0.015 mg/kg (2) Intubating dose: 0.08–0.20 mg/kg (3) Initial dose after succinylcholine: 0.04–0.10 mg/kg (4) Any additional doses of 0.01–0.06 mg/kg given 80–150 minutes after initial dose and then at 30- to 45-minute intervals or at twitch response ≥25% of control	X		9A. Doses reduced to lower end of dosage range and dosing intervals lengthened after maintenance doses of inhalational agents started[1-11] 9B. If patient obese, dose based on lean body weight (LBW)[6,7,9] 9C. Higher infusion rates required for mechanical ventilation in ICU setting because of tachyphylaxis[12] 9D. Doses reduced in patient with renal impairment (does not pertain to vecuronium or atracurium) and in geriatric patient (does not pertain to atracurium, pipecuronium, or doxacurium)[1-12]	9. Anesthesia records, preoperative notes, physician orders, nursing notes, progress notes, MAR 9A. Anesthesia records 9B. Anesthesia records, preoperative notes, nursing notes, progress notes 9C. Physician orders, nursing notes, progress notes 9D. Anesthesia records, preoperative notes, physician orders, nursing notes, progress notes
b. Pancuronium bromide for mechanical ventilation (ICU): (1) Loading dose: 0.03–0.10 mg/kg (2) Intermittent dosing: 0.1–0.2 mg/kg every 1–3 hours or (3) Continuous infusion: 1.0–1.7 μg/kg/min				
c. Vecuronium bromide for anesthesia:				

Element	Standard 100%	Standard 0%	Exception[b] or Critical Preventive/ Responsive Measure[c]	Sources of Information
(1) Priming dose: 0.01 mg/kg (2) Intubating dose: 0.08–0.30 mg/kg (3) Initial dose after succinylcholine: 0.04–0.06 mg/kg (4) Any additional doses of 0.01–0.05 mg/kg given 25–75 minutes after initial dose and then at 12- to 30-minute intervals or at twitch response ≥25% of control or (5) Continuous infusion: 0.7–1.3 μg/kg/min				
d. Vecuronium bromide for mechanical ventilation (ICU): (1) Loading dose: 0.1 mg/kg (2) Intermittent dosing: 0.1–0.2 mg/kg every hour or (3) Continuous infusion: 0.8–1.7 μg/kg/min				
e. Atracurium besylate for anesthesia: (1) Priming dose: 0.06–0.08 mg/kg (2) Intubating dose: 0.4–0.8 mg/kg (3) Initial dose after succinylcholine: 0.4–0.5 mg/kg (4) Any additional doses of 0.08–0.30 mg/kg given 20–60 minutes after initial dose and then at 15- to 30-minute intervals or at twitch response ≥25% of control or (5). Continuous infusion: 2–15 μg/kg/min				
f. Atracurium besylate for mechanical ventilation (ICU): (1) Loading dose: 0.4–0.5 mg/kg (2) Continuous infusion: 6–17 μg/kg/min				
g. Tubocurarine chloride for anesthesia: (1) Priming dose: 0.05 mg/kg (average dose = 3 mg) (2) Intubating dose: 0.5–0.6 mg/kg (3) Any additional doses of 0.3–0.4 mg/kg given 80–100 minutes after initial dose and then at 40-				

Element	Standard 100%	Standard 0%	Exception[b] or Critical Preventive/ Responsive Measure[c]	Sources of Information
to 60-minute intervals or at twitch response ≥25% of control h. Tubocurarine chloride for mechanical ventilation (ICU):(1) Loading dose: 0.5–0.6 mg/kg (2) Intermittent dosing: 0.25–0.50 mg/kg every 2–3 hours i. Metocurine iodide for anesthesia: (1) Priming dose: 0.05 mg/kg (2) Intubating dose: 0.2–0.5 mg/kg (3) Any additional doses of 0.10–0.25 mg/kg given approximately 25–150 minutes after initial dose and then at 30- to 45-minute intervals or at twitch response ≥25% of control j. Metocurine iodide for mechanical ventilation (ICU): (1) Loading dose: 0.2–0.5 mg/kg (2) Intermittent dosing: 0.25–0.50 mg/kg every three hours k. Pipecuronium bromide for anesthesia: (1) Intubating dose: 0.070–0.085 mg/kg (2) Initial dose after succinylcholine: 0.050–0.085 mg/kg (3) Any additional doses of 0.010–0.015 mg/kg given 30–200 minutes after initial dose and then at 17- to 175-minute intervals or at a twitch response ≥25% of control l. Doxacurium chloride for anesthesia: (1) Intubating dose: 0.05–0.08 mg/kg (2) Any additional doses of 0.005–0.025 mg/kg given 100–160 minutes after initial dose and then at 30- to 60-minute intervals or at twitch response ≥25% of control				
10. Appropriate reversal of neuromuscular blockade[8,10,13] a. Reversal at or near end of surgery b. Timing and dosing of i.v. reversal agents i. Neostigmine	X		10A. Train of four (TOF) ratio >0.7 or adequate clinical evidence of neuromuscular blockade reversal (e.g., five-second head lift)[8]	10. Anesthesia records, recovery room records 10A, C, D. Anesthesia records 10B. Anesthesia records, nursing notes 10E. Anesthesia records, preoperative notes, progress notes

Element	Standard 100%	Standard 0%	Exception[b] or Critical Preventive/ Responsive Measure[c]	Sources of Information
methylsulfate (0.025–0.075 mg/kg) and glycopyrrolate (5–15 μg/kg) 3–14 minutes before end of surgery or ii. Pyridostigmine bromide (0.1–0.3 mg/kg) and glycopyrrolate (5–15 μg/kg) 5–15 minutes before end of surgery or iii. Edrophonium chloride (0.5–1 mg/kg) and atropine sulfate (7–10 μg/kg) 0.5–9.0 minutes before end of surgery			10B. Surgeon miscalculated amount of time left for surgical procedure 10C. Doses reduced to lower end of dosage range for shallow neuromuscular blockade (TOF: four of four twitches visible with fade), higher end of range for deep neuromuscular blockade (TOF: zero to one twitches visible)[13] 10D. Edrophonium not used to reverse deep neuromuscular blockade[13] 10E. Planned postoperative intubation	
Complications				
11. Difficulty in reversal a. Patient transported to recovery room >20 minutes after end of surgery b. Patient transported to recovery room still intubated		X	11A. Identify other drug (e.g., amino-glycosides, magnesium) and nondrug causes (e.g., respiratory acidosis, hypothermia)[1-11,13] 11B. If maximum reversal dose given and other causes ruled out, control ventilation and allow neuromuscular blockade to terminate spontaneously[8]	11. Anesthesia records, nursing notes, recovery room records 11A. Anesthesia records, preoperative notes, physician orders, nursing notes, progress notes 11B. Anesthesia records, nursing notes, recovery room records
12. Cardiovascular effects[1-12] a. Hypotension b. Tachycardia c. Change in mean arterial pressure		X	12A. Identify other drug and nondrug causes (e.g., surgical stress or stimulation, "light" anesthesia, volume and metabolic status changes, limited cardiovascular reserve)[1-12] 12B. Provide supportive care	12. Anesthesia records, nursing notes, progress notes 12A. Anesthesia records, preoperative notes, physician orders, nursing notes, progress notes 12B. Anesthesia records, nursing notes, recovery room records
13. Histamine release[3-5,8] a. Bronchospasm b. Wheezing c. Erythema d. Flushing e. Anaphylactoid reaction		X	13A. Identify other drug and nondrug causes 13B. Pretreat with a histamine H_1 and H_2 antagonist[8] 13C. Administer doses slowly (e.g., atracurium, tubocurarine)[3-5,8] 13D. Provide supportive care	13. Anesthesia records, nursing notes, progress notes 13A. Anesthesia records, preoperative notes, physician orders, nursing notes, progress notes 13B. Anesthesia records, preoperative notes, nursing notes 13C. Anesthesia records, nursing notes 13D. Anesthesia records, nursing notes, progress notes, recovery room records

Element	Standard 100%	Standard 0%	Exception[b] or Critical Preventive/ Responsive Measure[c]		Sources of Information	
Outcome Measures						
14. Successful muscle relaxation[8]	X		14A.	None	14.	Anesthesia records, nursing notes, progress notes
15. Successful extubation[8]	X		15A.	Intubation required because of other drugs or	15, 15A.	Anesthesia records, nursing notes, progress notes, recovery room records
16. Extubation not delayed ≥10 minutes after surgery concluded	X		16A.	Extubation delayed because of other drugs or circumstances	16.	Anesthesia records, nursing notes
					16A.	Anesthesia records, nursing notes, recovery room records
			16B.	Postoperative intubation desired	16B.	Anesthesia records, preoperative notes

[a] Criteria address justifications for use (indications), critical (process) indicators, complications of therapy, and patient outcome. Each criterion consists of an element, a standard, exceptions to the standard, and sources of information. The element is the minimum level of evidence needed to show that patient care was optimal. The standard defines the deviation from an element that is acceptable. If no deviation is acceptable, the standard is 100%. Exceptions are circumstances in which deviation is allowable. Sources of information listed are the most reliable sources. Sources pertaining to an element or exception are identified by the number assigned to the element or exception (e.g., 8, 8A).

[b] For justification for use and critical (process) indicators.

[c] For complications and outcome measures.

References

1. Astra Pharmaceutical Products. Pancuronium bromide package insert. Westborough, MA; 1988 Dec.
2. Organon Pharmaceuticals. Norcuron package insert. West Orange, NJ; 1989 Mar.
3. Burroughs Wellcome. Tracrium package insert. Research Triangle Park, NC; 1989 Dec.
4. Quad Pharmaceuticals. Tubocurarine package insert. Indianapolis, IN; 1987 Oct.
5. Eli Lilly & Company. Metubine package insert. Indianapolis, IN; 1990 Mar.
6. Organon Pharmaceuticals. Arduan package insert. West Orange, NJ; 1990 Nov.
7. Burroughs Wellcome. Nuromax package insert. Research Triangle Park, NC; 1991 Mar.
8. Miller RD, Savarese JJ. Pharmacology of muscle relaxants and their antagonists. In: Miller RD, ed. Anesthesia. 3rd ed. New York: Churchill Livingstone; 1990:389-436.
9. Larijani GE, Gratz I, Silverberg M et al. Clinical pharmacology of the neuromuscular blocking agents. *DICP.* 1991; 25:54-64.
10. Bitetti J. Neuromuscular blockade. In: Firestone LL, Lebowitz PW, Cook CE, eds. Clinical Anesthesia Procedures of the Massachusetts General Hospital. 3rd ed. Boston: Little, Brown; 1988:167-84.
11. Basta SJ, Savarese JJ, Ali HH et al. Clinical pharmacology of doxacurium chloride. *Anesthesiology.* 1988; 69:478-86.
12. Buck ML, Reed MD. Use of nondepolarizing neuromuscular blocking agents in mechanically ventilated patients. *Clin Pharm.* 1991; 10:32-48.
13. Penn F. Neuromuscular blockade reversal agents. *Anesth Today.* 1989; 1(2):12-5.

CP Continuing Education

The ASHP Continuing-Education System gives readers a self-assessment mechanism for selected articles in Clinical Pharmacy *and* AJHP. *It allows readers to obtain continuing-education credit for these articles.*

For the purpose of CE-credit enrollment, a blank answer sheet is published at the end of each installment of the column for the CE articles in that issue. An enrollee accumulates these answer sheets until the enrollment is submitted, using the form that is published in the June and December issues of Clinical Pharmacy *and in the June and December issues of* AJHP. *Any combination of tests within an 18-month period, from both* Clinical Pharmacy *and* AJHP, *may be included in an enrollment. More complete details about enrollment in the system appear in the semiannual enrollment form.*

Article 680-204-9212 (see page 415)
Qualifies for 1.0 hour of CE credit

Doxazosin: A new α_1-adrenergic antagonist

Learning Objectives

After studying this article, the reader should be able to

1. Describe the pharmacology and pharmacokinetics of doxazosin.
2. Describe the effect of doxazosin on serum lipids.
3. List three adverse effects of doxazosin.
4. Recommend a doxazosin dosage regimen for the treatment of hypertension.
5. List two disorders other than hypertension for which doxazosin has been studied.

Self-assessment Questions

For each question there is only one best answer.

1. Inhibition of α_1-adrenergic receptors by doxazosin lowers blood pressure by

   a. Reducing cardiac contractility.
   b. Reducing heart rate.
   c. Reducing intravascular volume.
   d. Reducing vascular resistance.

2. When used in the treatment of hypertension, selective α_1-adrenergic antagonists, compared with nonselective α antagonists, should cause less

   a. Dizziness.
   b. Tachycardia.
   c. First-dose hypotension.
   d. Headache.

3. The disposition of orally administered doxazosin is characterized by

   a. Rapid absorption with extensive protein binding.
   b. Rapid absorption with little protein binding.
   c. Slow absorption with extensive protein binding.
   d. Slow absorption with little protein binding.

4. The elimination of doxazosin is characterized by

   a. Hepatic transformation to active metabolites, which are excreted primarily in the feces.
   b. Hepatic transformation to inactive metabolites, which are excreted primarily in the feces.
   c. Hepatic transformation to active metabolites, which are excreted primarily in the urine.
   d. Excretion of intact drug in the urine.

5. Maximum hypotensive effects generally occur well after peak serum doxazosin concentrations are achieved; one explanation of this phenomenon is that

   a. Doxazosin is a prodrug.
   b. Doxazosin activity depends on the slow process of altering protein synthesis.
   c. Diffusion of doxazosin to the active site may not occur immediately.
   d. All of the above alternatives are correct.

6. The effect of doxazosin on serum lipid concentrations is characterized by

   a. A decrease in total triglycerides and an increase in total cholesterol.
   b. A decrease in total cholesterol and an increase in high-density lipoprotein (HDL) cholesterol.
   c. Increases in the HDL:total cholesterol ratio and in total triglycerides.
   d. An increase in total cholesterol and a decrease in total triglycerides.

7. The most common adverse effect of doxazosin is

   a. Edema.
   b. Somnolence.
   c. Dizziness.
   d. Polyuria.

8. The recommended starting dosage of doxazosin (as

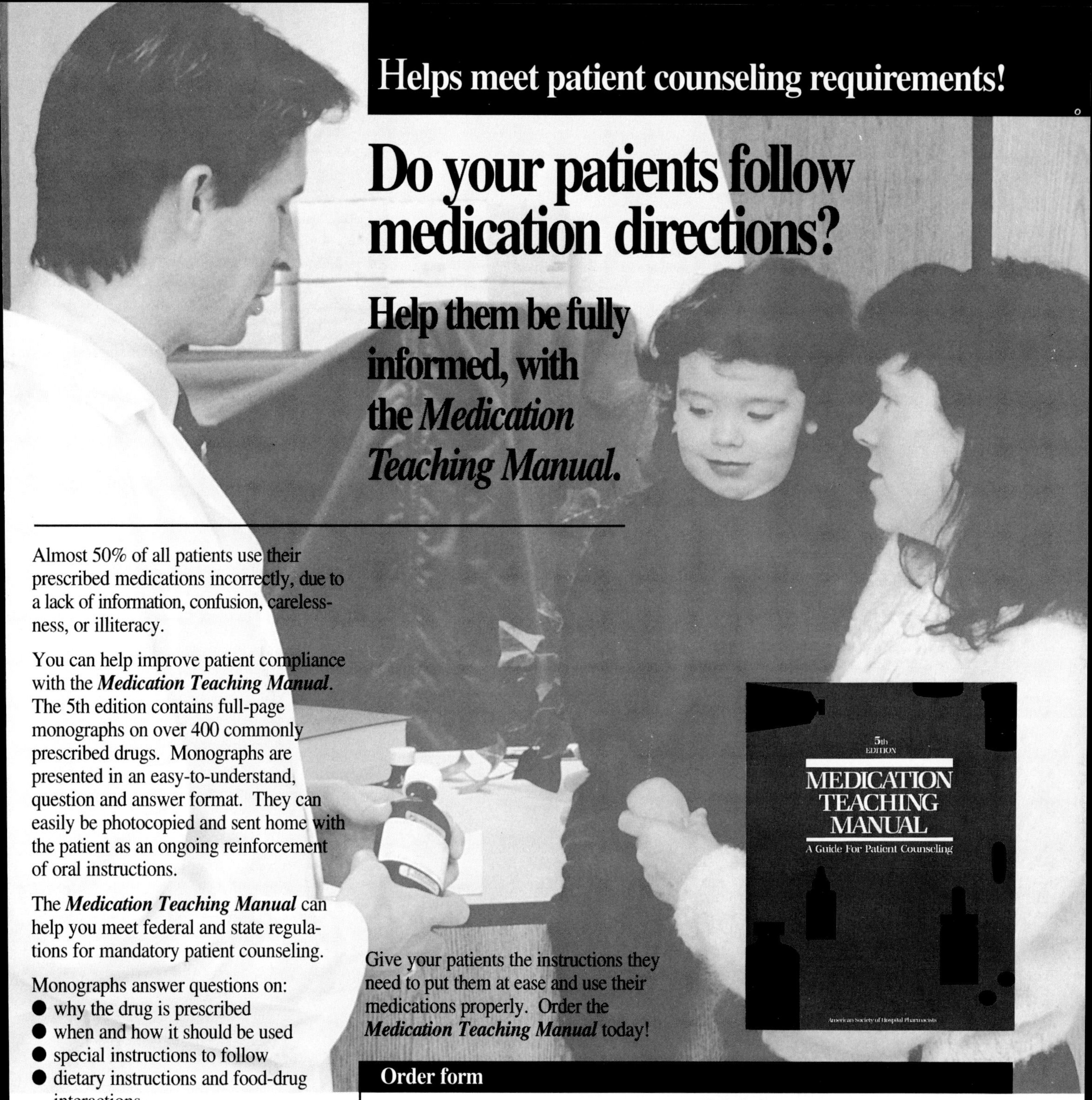
5th EDITION
MEDICATION TEACHING MANUAL
A Guide For Patient Counseling
American Society of Hospital Pharmacists

Current Literature

Drug Reaction Alerts

Drug Reaction Alerts focuses primarily on serious, unlabeled reactions to new chemical entities. The citations are compiled monthly from International Pharmaceutical Abstracts, which covers over 800 pharmacy and health-related journals worldwide. An address for reprints (when available) follows the name of the corresponding author in each citation.

Pharmacists may use the FDA Adverse Reaction Report form that appears in the January and July issues of Clinical Pharmacy for submitting reports of adverse drug reactions directly to FDA.

Antineoplastic Agents

Iveson TJ, Chan A (Department of Medicine, Royal Marsden Hospital, London SW3 6JJ, England). Pseudomembranous colitis complicating chemotherapy. *Lancet*. 1992; 339:192-3. Case. (43-year-old woman with breast cancer; received oral **cyclophosphamide** 100 mg/day on days 1–14 and **fluorouracil** 1 g and **methotrexate** 50 mg by i.v. injection on days 1 and 8 for four cycles as adjuvant therapy; developed diarrhea for 10 days, stabbing abdominal pains, and anorexia; *Clostridium difficile* toxin detected in stool specimen; therapy with oral vancomycin 125 mg four times daily and i.v. fluids led to end of diarrhea within 48 hours of starting vancomycin therapy)

Jones AL, Cropley I, O'Brien MER et al. (Gore ME, Biological Therapies Unit, Department of Medicine, Royal Marsden Hospital, London SW3 6JJ, England). Infectious complications of subcutaneous interleukin-2 and interferon-alpha. *Lancet*. 1992; 339:181-2. Study. (case series; four women and three men, aged 17–48 years, with metastatic cancer; received **aldesleukin** 4.8×10^6 units/sq m by s.c. injection three times daily on day 1 and twice daily on days 2–5, 8–12, and 15–19 and interferon alfa-2b 3×10^6 units/sq m by s.c. injection daily on days 3 and 5 and 6×10^6 units/sq m daily on days 8, 10, 12, 15, 17, and 19 for three-week cycles; blood and urine specimens were obtained weekly; two of two sets of blood cultures were positive for microbial growth in three patients, representing possible infections in 43% of patients and 13% of cycles)

Kemeny N (Memorial Sloan-Kettering Cancer Center, 1275 York Avenue, New York, NY 10021), Seiter K, Martin D et al. A new syndrome: ascites, hyperbilirubinemia, and hypoalbuminemia after biochemical modulation of fluorouracil with *N*-phosphonacetyl-L-aspartate (PALA). *Arch Intern Med*. 1991; 115:946-51. Study. (retrospective study; 44 patients with metastatic colorectal cancer; received **sparfosate sodium** 250 mg/sq m once weekly by 15-minute i.v. infusion followed 24 hours later by fluorouracil 600, 700, or 800 mg/sq m by i.v. bolus injection; 17 patients showed partial or complete responses to therapy; 15 responding patients developed ascites, hypoalbuminemia, hyperbilirubinemia, or elevated serum aspartate aminotransferase and alkaline phosphatase concentrations; significantly more responders to therapy developed at least one form of transient hepatic abnormality compared with nonresponders [88% versus 44%; $p = 0.004$])

Cardiac Drugs

Clarke KW, Brear SG, Hanley SP (Department of Medicine and Intensive Care Unit, North Manchester General Hospital, Manchester M8 6RB, England). Rise in intracranial pressure with intravenous **adenosine**. *Lancet*. 1992; 339:188-9. Case. (58-year-old man with paroxysmal supraventricular tachycardia after sustaining head injuries from a fall; received adenosine 50 µg/kg by i.v. injection and incremental 50-µg increases at two-minute intervals to a total dose of 250 µg/kg; developed decreased mean intra-arterial pressure and dose-related increased intracranial pressure without benefit from adenosine therapy; therapy with direct current countershock led to resolution of arrhythmia)

Cephalosporins

Lopez AJ, O'Keefe P (Section of Infectious Disease, Loyola University of Chicago, 2160 S. First Avenue, Maywood, IL 60153), Morrissey M et al. **Ceftriaxone**-induced cholelithiasis. *Arch Intern Med*. 1991; 115:712-14. Case. (42-year-old man with chronic active hepatitis and history of rheumatic heart disease; received ceftriaxone 2 g every 12 hours by i.v. injection for two months as chemoprophylaxis for endocarditis after placement of aortic homograft; developed acute pancreatitis; ultrasonography and computed tomography of gallbladder revealed gallstones; underwent cholecystectomy and operative cholangiography; infrared spectrophotometry of two of five gallstones showed stone composition of 80% ceftriaxone and 20% bilirubin)

Drug Interactions

Shah P (6 Presthope Road, Selly Oak, Birmingham B29 4LN, England), Dhurjon L, Metcalfe T et al. Acute angle closure glaucoma associated with nebulised **ipratropium bromide** and salbutamol. *Br Med J*. 1992; 304:40-1. Cases. (five patients, aged 67–78 years, with exacerbations of chronic obstructive pulmonary disease; received **albuterol** and ipratropium bromide by nebulization six times daily; developed symptoms of angle-closure glaucoma within nine days; withdrawal of albuterol and ipratropium bromide and therapy with pilocarpine, acetazolamide, and analgesics led to resolution of symptoms)

Hormones

James RA, Rhodes M, Rose P et al. (Kendall-Taylor P, Endocrine Unit, Royal Victoria Infirmary, Newcastle upon Tyne NE1 4LP, England). Biliary colic on abrupt withdrawal of **octreotide**. *Lancet*. 1991; 338:1527. Cases. (three women and one man, aged 37–65 years, with acromegaly; received octreotide acetate 150–600 µg/day for 28–46 months; abrupt withdrawal of octreotide acetate led to severe, short-term biliary colic within 12–16 hours; spontaneous recovery within 24 hours)

Immunotherapy

Nathan FE, Besa EC (Medical College of Pennsylvania, Philadelphia, PA 19129). GM-CSF and accelerated hemolysis. *N Engl J Med*. 1992; 326:417. Case. (42-year-old woman with non-Hodgkin's lymphoma; received full-dose chemotherapy followed by **regramostim** 250 mg/sq m/day for five days; hematocrit decreased from 18% on the previous day to 5%,

Continued on page 454

Continued from page 448

serum bilirubin concentration increased from 7 to 37 mg/dL, and serum lactate dehydrogenase concentration increased from 1200 to 1650 units/L; withdrawal of regramostim and therapy with packed red-blood-cell transfusions and vinblastine led to hematocrit of 25% on next day; negative rechallenge)

Wandl UB (Clinic of Internal Medicine and Polyclinic [Tumor Studies], University of Essen, 4300 Essen, Germany), Kloke O, Niederle N. Liver failure due to recombinant alpha interferon for chronic myelogenous leukemia. *Lancet*. 1992; 339:123-4. Case. (43-year-old woman with chronic myelogenous leukemia; received **interferon alfa-2b** 7×10^6 units by s.c. injection daily for six weeks then decreased to 4×10^6 units daily for two months; developed slight increases in serum hepatic enzyme concentrations; developed jaundice with greatly increased serum hepatic enzyme concentrations six months later; withdrawal of interferon alfa-2b did not lead to improvement; developed hepatic failure and hepatic coma and died)

Pediatrics

Veale KS (Department of Emergency Medicine, Texas Tech University, Regional Academic Health Center, 4800 Alberta Avenue, El Paso, TX 79905), Huff ES, Nelson BK et al. Pure red cell aplasia and hepatitis in a child receiving **isoniazid** therapy. *J Pediatr*. 1992; 120:146-8. Case. (seven-year-old boy; received isoniazid 12 mg/kg/day for approximately nine months after tuberculin skin test conversion; developed pure red-blood-cell aplasia and hepatitis; biopsy results of bone marrow sample were consistent with pure erythroid aplasia and eosinophilic hyperplasia; withdrawal of isoniazid and therapy with packed erythrocytes led to uneventful recovery)

Wales JK (University Department of Paediatrics, Sheffield Children's Hospital, Sheffield S10 2TH, England), Barnes ND, Swift PG. Growth retardation in children on steroids for asthma. *Lancet*. 1991; 338:1535. Cases. (six children, aged 2.5–9.5 years, with asthma; received **beclomethasone dipropionate** at a mean dose of 400–1000 μg/day by inhalation for a mean duration of 1.6–6.5 years; developed growth and adrenal suppression; withdrawal or reduction in dose of beclomethasone dipropionate led to increased growth of four children)

Vehicles

Bedichek E (Division of Nephrology, Medical College of Virginia, Box 160, Richmond, VA 23298-0160), Kirschbaum B. Case of **propylene glycol** toxic reaction associated with etomidate infusion. *Arch Intern Med*. 1991; 151:2297-8. Case. (70-year-old woman with increased intracranial pressure; received etomidate in propylene glycol at up to 0.9 mg of etomidate per hour for nearly 24 hours [total dose of propylene glycol as etomidate vehicle, 436 g]; developed lactic acidosis and hyperosmolality; withdrawal of etomidate led to complete resolution of acidosis and osmolar gap)

Books Received

Books are listed as soon as received; selected books may be reviewed in Book Reviews in subsequent issues.

Applied Therapeutics: The Clinical Use of Drugs, edited by Mary Anne Koda-Kimble and Lloyd Yee Young. Published by Applied Therapeutics, Inc., P.O. Box 5077, Vancouver, WA 98668-5077, 1992. xv + 1738 p. Price $85.

Drugs in Anaesthetic Practice, Seventh Edition, by M. D. Vickers, M. Morgan, and P.S.J. Spencer. Published by Butterworth-Heinemann Ltd., Halley Court, Jordan Hill, Oxford OX2 8EJ, England, 1991. Available from Butterworth, 80 Montvale Avenue, Stoneham, MA 02180-2422. xvi + 537 p. Price $95.

Effects of Drugs on Clinical Laboratory Tests, Third Edition, by Donald S. Young. Published by the American Association for Clinical Chemistry, Inc., 2029 K Street, N.W., Seventh Floor, Washington, DC 20006, 1990. ii + 937 p. Price $65 (AACC members), $100 (nonmembers).

Effects of Drugs on Clinical Laboratory Tests, 1991 Supplement, by Donald S. Young. Published by the American Association for Clinical Chemistry, Inc., 2029 K Street, N.W., Seventh Floor, Washington, DC 20006, 1991. ii + 360 p. Price $40 (AACC members), $60 (nonmembers).

Pharmacokinetic Self-Assessment Program: Module 1, Cardiovascular, Toni R. Host, Project Director and Assistant Editor. Published by the American College of Clinical Pharmacy, 3101 Broadway, Suite 380, Kansas City, MO 64111, 1991. Book A, Syllabus, Annotated References and Self-Assessment Questions, vii + 145 p. Book B, Answers, Rationale and References for Self-Assessment Questions, iii + 37 p. Price $95 (ACCP members), $150 (nonmembers). Subscription to complete program, consisting of six modules, $295 (ACCP members), $375 (nonmembers).

Physicians' Generix: The Official Drug Reference of FDA Prescribing Information and Therapeutic Equivalents, 1992 edition. Published by Data Pharmaceutica Inc., P.O. Box 1336, Smithtown, NY 11787, 1992. xxiii + 2679 p. Price $68 plus shipping and handling.

Neoplastic Diseases: Fundamentals of Clinical Oncology, C. Julian Rosenthal, editor. Published by Precept Press, Inc., 160 East Illinois Street, Chicago, IL 60611, 1991. xxvi + 891 p. Price $129.

Advertising Index

Alpha Therapeutic Corporation
Venoglobulin-I, 379-380
American Society of Hospital Pharmacists
AHFS Drug Information 92, 389
Concepts in Clinical Pharmacokinetics, 443
Concepts in Oncology Therapeutics, 453
Criteria for Drug Use Evaluation, Volumes 1 and 2, 441
Medication Teaching Manual, 447
MedTeach, 389
Safe Handling of Cytotoxic and Hazardous Drugs, 414
Amgen Inc.
Epogen, 377
Neupogen, 449-452
Critical Care America
Position Available, 385
Enzon, Inc.
Institutional, 390
SmithKline Beecham
Timentin, inside back cover, outside back cover
The Upjohn Company
Zefazone, 382-384
Wyeth-Ayerst Laboratories, Inc.
Ativan Injection, 444-446
Tubex, inside front cover

News

Heavy use of inhaled β agonists associated with increased risk of fatal or near-fatal asthma, study shows 458

Lomefloxacin reaches U.S. market 458

Warnings about use of angiotensin-converting-enzyme inhibitors in advanced pregnancy strengthened 467

New labeling and patient insert for triazolam approved by FDA 467

Cognitive enhancers illegal, says FDA 467

Call for applications to conduct research on patient outcomes associated with pharmaceutical therapy in ambulatory-care setting 467

News Briefs 467

Upcoming Specialty Meetings 470

Heavy use of inhaled β agonists associated with increased risk of fatal or near-fatal asthma, study shows

Regular use of β_2 agonists administered by metered-dose inhaler is associated with an increased risk of death or near death from asthma, according to a case–control study of subjects identified from a cohort who received prescriptions for asthma medications between 1978 and 1987.[1] Beta agonists may have been directly responsible for adverse effects, or heavy use of these agents may simply have been a marker for severe asthma. Patients who rely heavily on inhaled β agonists need to be re-evaluated medically.

From a cohort of 12,301 patients identified from computerized records of the Saskatchewan Prescription Drug Plan, 129 patients with fatal or near-fatal asthma were identified and matched with 655 controls. Use of β agonists was associated with an increased risk of fatal asthma (odds ratio, 2.6 per canister per month; 95% confidence interval, 1.7 to 3.9). The odds ratio for fatal or near-fatal asthma was 1.9 (95% confidence interval, 1.6 to 2.4). Fenoterol and albuterol were also analyzed separately. For fenoterol (200 μg/inhalation), the odds ratio for each additional canister dispensed per month was 5.4 for fatal asthma and 2.3 for fatal or near-fatal asthma; values for albuterol (100 μg/inhalation) were 2.4 and 1.9, respectively. When data for fenoterol and albuterol were analyzed on a microgram-for-microgram basis (100 μg of each drug), the odds ratios for fenoterol and albuterol were similar (2.3 and 2.4, respectively, for fatal asthma; 1.5 and 1.9, respectively, for fatal or near-fatal asthma).

1. Spitzer WO, Suissa S, Ernst P et al. The use of β-agonists and the risk of death and near death from asthma. *N Engl J Med.* 1992; 326:510-6.

Lomefloxacin reaches U.S. market

The oral quinolone lomefloxacin hydrochloride (Maxaquin, Searle) received marketing approval in February. It is indicated for the treatment of acute bacterial exacerbations of chronic bronchitis caused by *Haemophilus influenzae* or *Moraxella catarrhalis*; uncomplicated urinary-tract infections caused by *Escherichia coli*, *Klebsiella pneumoniae*, *Proteus mirabilis*, or *Staphylococcus saprophyticus*; or complicated urinary-tract infections caused by *E. coli*, *K. pneumoniae*, *Pr. mirabilis*, *Pseudomonas aeruginosa*, *Citrobacter diversus*, or *Enterobacter cloacae*. Lomefloxacin is also indicated for preoperative use to reduce the incidence of early postoperative urinary-

Continued on page 467

Continued from page 458

tract infections in patients undergoing transurethral surgical procedures.

The elimination half-life of lomefloxacin in subjects with normal renal function is approximately eight hours. About 65% of an oral dose is excreted unchanged in urine. Elimination is slower in elderly subjects, but no dosage adjustment is required if the estimated creatinine clearance is at least 40 mL/min/1.73 sq m.

Adverse events occurring in more than 1% of patients treated with lomefloxacin include nausea (3.7%), headache (3.2%), photosensitivity (2.4%), dizziness (2.3%), and diarrhea (1.4%). Sucralfate and antacids have been reported to decrease the bioavailability of lomefloxacin. Probenecid can slow renal elimination of lomefloxacin.

The recommended dosage of lomefloxacin (as the hydrochloride salt) is 400 mg once daily for 10 to 14 days. Patients with renal dysfunction should receive a reduced maintenance dosage. When lomefloxacin is used for prophylaxis, a single 400-mg dose should be given two to six hours before surgery.

Maxaquin is available as 400-mg tablets in bottles of 20 and unit dose packages of 100.

Warnings about use of angiotensin-converting-enzyme inhibitors in advanced pregnancy strengthened

The product labeling of all angiotensin-converting-enzyme (ACE) inhibitors is being revised to include stronger warnings about the risks associated with ACE-inhibitor use during the second and third trimesters of pregnancy. The new boxed warning will emphasize the risk of fetal harm, including kidney failure and deformities of the face or skull. Manufacturers of ACE inhibitors will also provide pharmacists with stickers to be placed on prescription bottles that read, "If you become pregnant, consult your doctor promptly about switching to a different drug."

New labeling and patient insert for triazolam approved by FDA

FDA has approved new labeling for triazolam (Halcion, Upjohn) and a patient insert to be attached to new 10-tablet unit-of-use packages.

The labeling now recommends that use of triazolam for treatment of insomnia be limited to 10 days and states that use for more than two or three weeks requires a complete re-evaluation of the patient. Expanded warnings place greater emphasis on the necessity of monitoring patients for underlying medical or psychiatric illnesses and adverse behavioral responses. The labeling describes bizarre behavioral events. It also emphasizes the facts that many adverse effects are dose related and that the elderly are more susceptible to adverse effects. Use of the smallest effective dosage is recommended, and maximum doses (intended for exceptional cases) are given: 0.5 mg for adults and 0.25 mg for elderly or debilitated patients.

The package insert for patients includes information on efficacy, adverse effects, and safe use of benzodiazepine sleep aids.

Cognitive enhancers illegal, says FDA

Any product being promoted as improving memory or intelligence is illegal, according to FDA officials responding to inquiries about the status of drugs that enhance cognitive function. The term "smart drugs" has been applied to various products that are touted as improving cognitive function in healthy individuals; the products include unapproved drugs, herbs, and nutrients such as amino acids, vitamins, or choline. Sources of these drugs include off-shore pharmacies, foreign mail-order firms, and health food outlets. According to FDA, claims regarding the cognitive effects of these products have not been subjected to scientific testing. Claims of efficacy are generally not placed on the product labeling; promotional efforts depend heavily on oral sales pitches and testimonials.

Call for applications to conduct research on patient outcomes associated with pharmaceutical therapy in ambulatory-care setting

The U.S. Public Health Service Agency for Health Care Policy and Research (AHCPR) Center for Medical Effectiveness Research is soliciting applications from nonprofit organizations to conduct research on patient outcomes associated with pharmaceutical therapy in the ambulatory-care setting. Three general areas of research are of particular interest: data and analytical methods, factors affecting the appropriateness of drug prescribing, and the role of the patient.

AHCPR expects to commit up to $3 million for 6 to 10 competitive awards under this request for applications. The deadline for applications is July 15, 1992. Details of this program announcement can be found in the *NIH Guide to Grants and Contracts* or can be obtained by contacting Lynn Bosco, M.D., or Eleanor M. Perfetto, Ph.D., at Center for Medical Effectiveness Research, 2101 East Jefferson Street, Suite 605, Rockville, MD 20852; 301-227-8485.

News Briefs

• FDA has approved a treatment IND protocol for **rifabutin** (Adria Laboratories). The drug will be made available to AIDS patients with CD4 cell counts of <200/cu mm to prevent or delay the onset of *Mycobacterium avium* complex infection. To obtain more information, call Adria Laboratories at 800-552-7228.

• To obtain a **cumulative list of drugs and biologics designated as orphan products** as of December 31, 1991, write to Dockets Management Branch (HFA-305), FDA, Room 1-23, 12420 Parklawn Drive, Rockville, MD 20857. Specify the docket number (84N-0102) in the request.

• **Pilocarpine hydrochloride** (Salagen, MGI Pharma) has been designated an orphan drug for the treatment of xerostomia and keratoconjunctivitis sicca in patients who have Sjögren's syndrome.

Continued on page 470

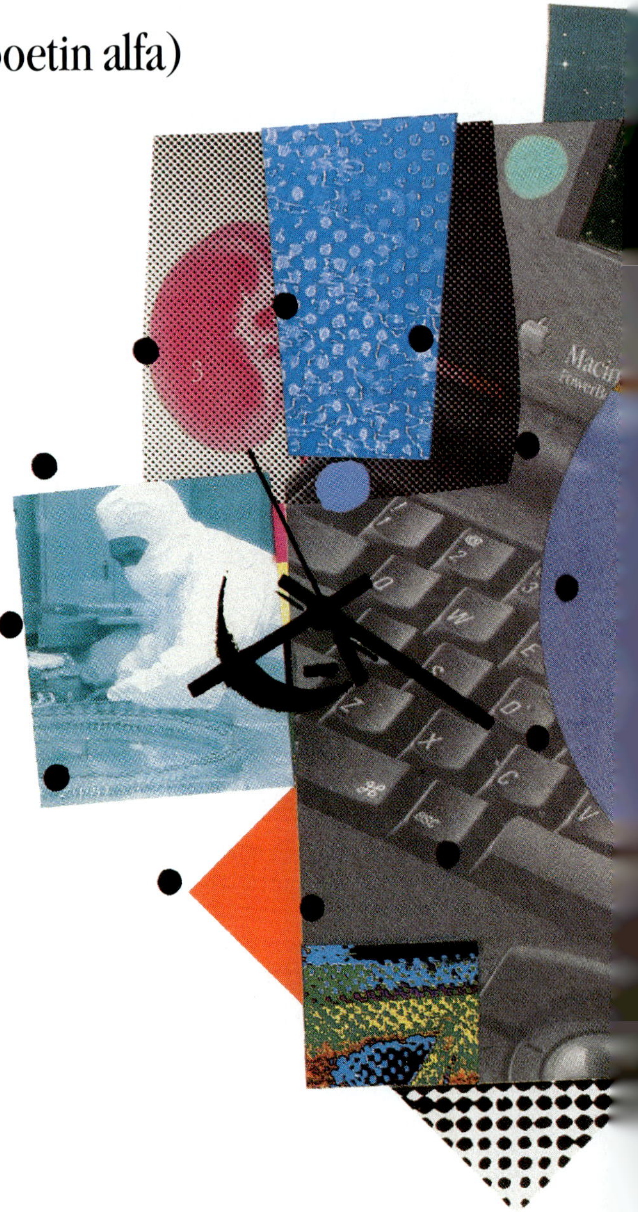

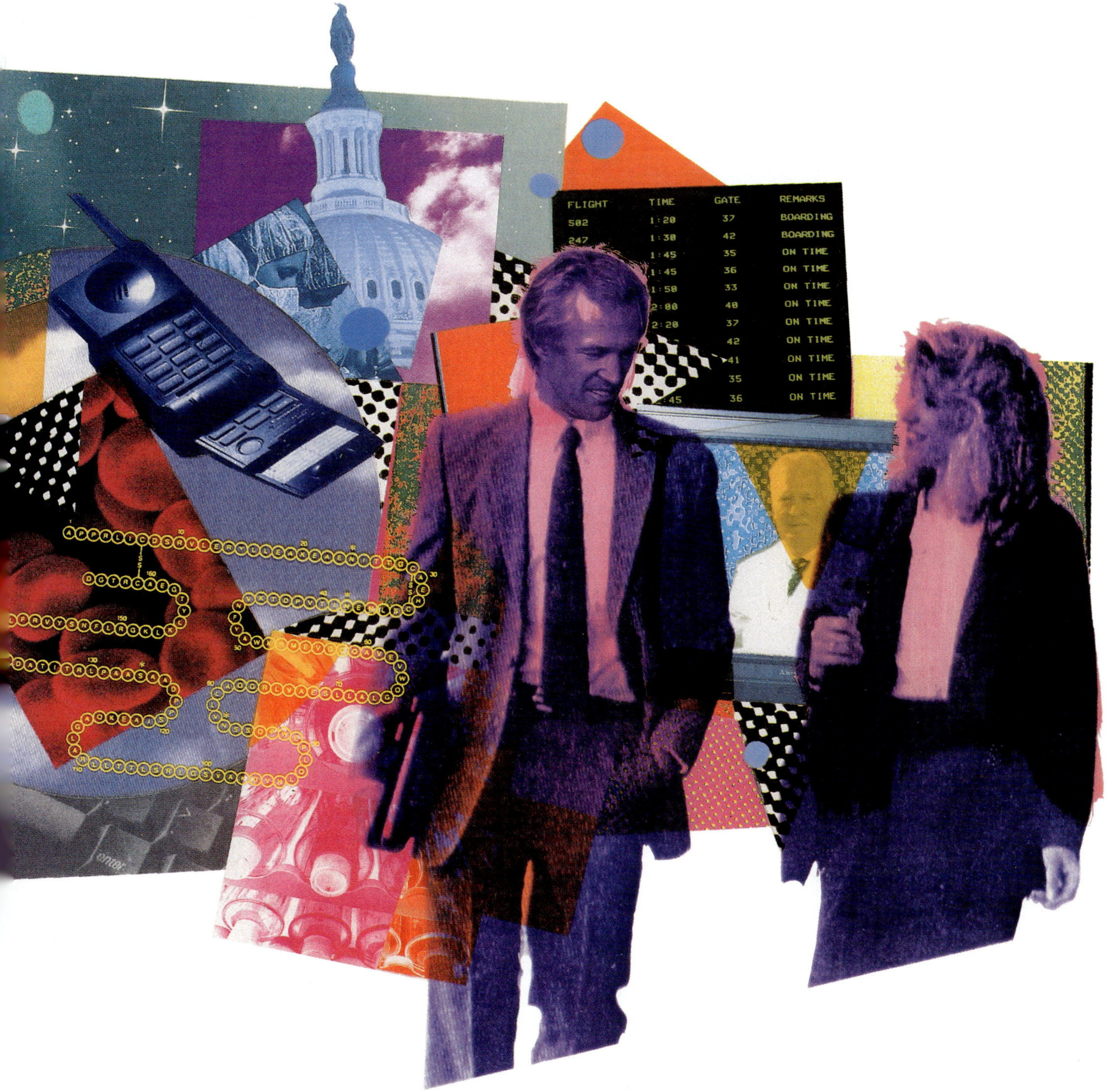
FLIGHT TIME GATE REMARKS
502 1:20 37 BOARDING
247 1:30 42 BOARDING
1:45 35 ON TIME
1:45 36 ON TIME
1:50 33 ON TIME
2:00 40 ON TIME
2:20 37 ON TIME
42 ON TIME
41 ON TIME
35 ON TIME
36 ON TIME
enter

News *Continued from page 467*

Upcoming Specialty Meetings

American College of Emergency Physicians. Seattle, WA, September 14–17; contact ACEP, P.O. Box 619911, Dallas, TX 75261-9911; 214-550-0911.

Current Concepts in the Treatment of Chronic Head Pain. Dayton, OH, September 19; contact Midwest Center for Head Pain Management, Upper Valley Medical Centers, 3130 North Dixie Highway, Miami County, OH 45373; 513-332-8544.

First National Conference on Asthma Management. Arlington, VA, October 11–13; contact National Asthma Conference/CHS, P.O. Box 30105, Bethesda, MD 20824-0105; 301-951-3275, (fax) 301-951-3269.

Special Feature

ASHP therapeutic guidelines on antimicrobial prophylaxis in surgery

ASHP Commission on Therapeutics

Clin Pharm. 1992; 11:483-513

The generally accepted principles of antimicrobial prophylaxis in surgery involve five considerations:

1. Surgical procedures for which prophylactic antimicrobials have been beneficial;
2. Timing of antimicrobial administration;
3. Duration of the antimicrobial regimen;
4. Route of antimicrobial administration; and
5. Selection of a particular antimicrobial agent.

Surgical Procedures

Antimicrobial prophylaxis is likely to be beneficial in surgical procedures associated with a high rate of infection (clean-contaminated or contaminated operations) and in any procedure in which postoperative infection, however unlikely, may be severe or fatal. Antimicrobial prophylaxis is justified for surgical procedures that enter the gastrointestinal tract (colorectal operations and high-risk gastroduodenal and biliary-tract operations) and pose the risk of bacterial contamination, as well as in head and neck operations. The value of antimicrobial prophylaxis for abdominal hysterectomies and neurosurgical procedures is controversial. Since most clean operations have a very low rate of postoperative infection, the prophylactic use of antimicrobials is usually not justified. However, recent data on procedures that entail placement of prosthetic materials (e.g., cardiopulmonary bypass, vascular procedures, total hip replacement, hip-fracture repair), in which the few infections that do occur can be quite serious, justify the prophylactic use of antimicrobials. A recently published study suggests that prophylactic antibiotics may be beneficial in other clean procedures, although this is controversial.[1] For some clean procedures (aortic resections, total hip replacements, hip-fracture repairs) the value of prophylactic antimicrobials has been demonstrated by placebo-controlled trials. Antimicrobial prophylaxis may be justified for any procedure if the patient is immunocompromised (e.g., malnourished, neutropenic, or receiving immunosuppressive agents).

Timing of Antimicrobial Administration

The timing of antimicrobial administration is important; antimicrobials given at inappropriate times can be ineffective for surgical prophylaxis. To be most effective in preventing postoperative infection, an antimicrobial must be present in the potentially contaminated tissues before bacteria enter the site (i.e., before the surgical incision) and must persist in tissues throughout the period of potential contamination.

Approved by the ASHP Commission on Therapeutics and the ASHP Board of Directors, April 22, 1992.

This document was written by the ASHP Commission on Therapeutics Task Force on Antimicrobial Prophylaxis in Surgery: Steven L. Barriere, Pharm.D., Specialist in Infectious Diseases, Department of Pharmaceutical Services, and Adjunct Professor of Medicine and Pharmacology, School of Medicine, University of California at Los Angeles Center for the Health Sciences, Los Angeles; John Connors, Pharm.D., Assistant Professor of Pharmacy Practice, Philadelphia College of Pharmacy and Science, Philadelphia, PA; Larry H. Danziger, Pharm.D., Assistant Professor of Pharmacy, College of Pharmacy, University of Illinois, Chicago; Joseph T. DiPiro, Pharm.D., Professor of Pharmacy and Surgery, Medical College of Georgia, Augusta; John F. Flaherty, Pharm.D., Associate Professor of Clinical Pharmacy, School of Pharmacy, University of California, San Francisco; B. Joseph Guglielmo, Pharm.D., Professor of Clinical Pharmacy, School of Pharmacy, University of California, San Francisco; Bruce Kreter, Pharm.D., Associate Director for Antiinfective Clinical Research, Bristol-Myers Squibb, Princeton, NJ; and Robert P. Rapp, Pharm.D., Professor and Chair, Division of Pharmacy Practice and Science, College of Pharmacy, University of Kentucky, Lexington.

The contributions of John M. Benson, Pharm.D., Douglas Fish, Pharm.D., and Paul O. Gubbins, Pharm.D., in the preparation of these guidelines are acknowledged.

The recommendations in this document do not indicate an exclusive course of treatment to be followed. Variations, taking into account individual circumstances, may be appropriate.

When antimicrobials are given after bacterial contamination, their ability to prevent infection is substantially reduced. Ideally, antimicrobials should be given immediately after the patient arrives in the operating room. During cesarean section, however, antimicrobial prophylaxis is administered after cross-clamping of the umbilical cord. Administering prophylaxis at this time is effective, and it minimizes neonatal exposure to antimicrobials. When antimicrobials are administered "on call" to the operating room, the time between administration and the start of the operation may be prolonged. This practice is not recommended. If short-acting agents are used, they should be readministered if the operation extends beyond three to four hours. If an operation is expected to last more than six to eight hours, it would be reasonable to administer an agent with a longer half-life and duration of action.

Duration of Antimicrobial Prophylaxis

The shortest duration of antimicrobial administration that is effective in preventing postoperative infection is not known; however, recent studies document that postoperative antimicrobial administration is not necessary for many operations.

Route of Antimicrobial Administration

Antimicrobials used for surgical prophylaxis may be administered intravenously, intramuscularly, orally, rectally, and topically (into the surgical wound). The preferred route of administration varies among surgeons; i.v. and i.m. routes are used most often. Oral antimicrobials are often used for gut decontamination in elective colorectal operations.

For most elective operations, i.m. and i.v. administration should be equivalent in terms of antimicrobial delivery to wound tissues. The antimicrobial agent should be given intravenously if the patient has an i.v. catheter in place. It is reasonable to wait to administer the agent until an i.v. line is placed in the operating room.

In situations where general anesthesia will interrupt bowel function or where nasogastric tubes may be placed, the absorption of orally administered antimicrobials may be unreliable. Orally administered antimicrobial agents are therefore not generally recommended for surgical prophylaxis.

Selection of Antimicrobial Agents

There is little evidence to suggest that the newer antimicrobials, which have broader in vitro antibacterial spectra, result in lower rates of postoperative wound infection than older drugs, whose spectra are narrower. The agent chosen should have antibacterial activity against the most common surgical wound pathogens. In clean operations, gram-positive cocci predominate. For clean-contaminated operations, the agent of choice should be effective against common pathogens found in the gastrointestinal or genitourinary tracts. For most operations, a first-generation cephalosporin such as cefazolin should be the agent of choice.

Specific recommendations for the selection of prophylactic antimicrobials for various surgical procedures are provided in Table 1. Recommendations for pediatric patients have been included where appropriate; however, it should be recognized that these recommendations are based on data derived primarily from adult patients and from clinical experience. Few data exist on the use of antimicrobial prophylaxis for surgery in the pediatric population. Cefazolin is most often recommended because of its relatively low cost and long duration of action and because it has activity against most of the pathogens commonly associated with clean and clean-contaminated operations. For clean operations where staphylococci are common pathogens, penicillinase-resistant penicillins (oxacillin, nafcillin) may be suitable alternatives. Vancomycin may sometimes be required in patients allergic to penicillins or cephalosporins or in cases involving a high number of methicillin-resistant staphylococci.

Numerous trials conducted in the 1970s and 1980s revealed no substantial differences in microbiological activity among the first-generation cephalosporins. In fact, the cephalothin disk has long served as the class disk for in vitro testing of all first-generation cephalosporins; individual agents have generally not been

Table 1.
Recommendations for Antimicrobial Surgical Prophylaxis[a]

Type of Surgery	Recommended Antimicrobial Regimen	Comments
Head and neck procedures (clean-contaminated)	Cefazolin 2 g i.v. at induction of anesthesia and repeated twice at 8-hr intervals or clindamycin 600 mg plus gentamicin 1.7 mg/kg given i.v. at induction of anesthesia and repeated twice at 8-hr intervals	Clindamycin alone appears to be effective, but more data are needed
Gastrointestinal procedures		
Cholecystectomy	Cefazolin 1 g i.v. at induction of anesthesia	Broad-spectrum agents and multiple doses have not been found to be more effective than narrow-spectrum agents administered in a single dose
Gastroduodenal	Cefazolin 1 g i.v. at induction of anesthesia	Indicated only for procedures entering stomach
Colonic	Oral neomycin sulfate 1 g plus erythromycin base 1 g (after mechanical bowel preparation is completed) at 1300, 1400, and 2300 on day before surgery If oral route is contraindicated: cefoxitin, cefotetan, cefmetazole, cefotaxime, or ceftizoxime 2 g i.v. at induction of anesthesia	Mechanical bowel preparation with polyethylene, glycol-electrolyte lavage solution should always be performed for nonobstructed patients undergoing elective operations Cefoxitin should be repeated if procedure exceeds three hours
Rectal or colostomy closure	Combination of oral and injectable antimicrobials	
Appendectomy	Uncomplicated: cefoxitin, cefotetan, cefmetazole, cefotaxime, or ceftizoxime 1-2 g i.v. at induction of anesthesia Complicated: continue antimicrobial for 3-5 days	
Obstetric/gynecologic procedures		
Cesarean section	Cefazolin 2 g i.v. as a single dose immediately after clamping of umbilical cord	Although controversial, recent data support prophylaxis in low-risk patients
Vaginal hysterectomy	Cefazolin 1 g i.v. at induction of anesthesia	Optional: 1-2 additional doses at 8-hr intervals
Abdominal hysterectomy	Cefazolin 1 g or cefotetan 1 g i.v. at induction of anesthesia	Probably most beneficial in risk patients
Neurosurgical procedures		
Elective craniotomy or laminectomy	Cefazolin or oxacillin or nafcillin 15 mg/kg up to 1 g i.v. at induction of anesthesia	Vancomycin 1 g i.v. should be substituted in hospitals with >10% prevalence of MRSA
CSF shunting	None	If prophylaxis is used, vancomycin 1 g i.v. at induction of anesthesia may be beneficial
Cardiothoracic procedures	Cefazolin 15 mg/kg (up to 1 g) q 8 hr or cefuroxime 50 mg/kg (up to 1.5 g) q 12 hr for 48-72 hr or until chest and mediastinal drainage tubes are removed	Cefamandole and cephalothin are effective alternatives
Orthopedic procedures		
Joint replacement	Cefazolin 15 mg/kg (up to 1 g) i.v. at induction of anesthesia and repeated twice at 8-hr intervals	Vancomycin is a suitable alternative
Hip-fracture repair	Cefazolin 1 g i.v. at induction of anesthesia and repeated q 8 hr for 48-72 hr	Vancomycin is a suitable alternative
Other clean orthopedic procedures	None	
Vascular procedures	Cefazolin 15 mg/kg (up to 1 g) i.v. at induction of anesthesia and repeated twice at 8-hr intervals	Vancomycin is a suitable alternative
Urologic procedures	Cefazolin 15 mg/kg (up to 1 g) i.v. at induction of anesthesia, trimethoprim 160 mg with sulfamethoxazole 800 mg p.o. 1-2 hr before surgery, or cephalexin or cephradine 500 mg p.o. 1-2 hr before surgery	Prophylaxis should be given to high-risk patients only (i.e., those with prolonged catheterization) or in hospitals where infection rates exceed 20%

[a]MRSA = methicillin-resistant *Staph. aureus*, CSF = cerebrospinal fluid.

tested. Most clinical microbiological laboratories assumed that susceptibility or resistance to cephalothin extended to all drugs in its class.

During the past several years, however, two important findings have emerged that might affect the selection of cefazolin as the prophylactic agent in clean surgical procedures. First, several investigators have demonstrated that there are marked differences in the rate and extent of hydrolysis that occurs when various cephalosporin antimicrobials are exposed to various staphylococcal β-lactamases.[2] Further, some strains of staphylococci produce β-lactamases capable of rapidly hydrolyzing cefazolin.[2] In several studies, cefazolin was found to be less effective than cefamandole or cefuroxime in preventing deep wound infection in patients who had undergone heart surgery.[3] Although the data are conflicting, microbiologic and clinical studies such as these have called into question the prominence of cefazolin as the first-generation cephalosporin of choice. New studies may be needed to reevaluate the use of agents such as cephalothin, cefamandole, and cefuroxime, which are more resistant to β-lactamase. A second factor influencing the selection of cefazolin is the recognition that methicillin- and oxacillin-resistant *Staphylococcus aureus* (MRSA) and methicillin-resistant, coagulase-negative staphylococci are resistant to all cephalosporins. These organisms are commonly associated with infection following cardiothoracic, orthopedic, vascular, and cerebrospinal-fluid shunting procedures. This new finding may influence drug selection in hospitals where the incidence of such isolates is high.

Although prophylactic antimicrobials play an important part in reducing the incidence of postoperative wound infection, it is important to recognize that a number of other factors, such as the surgeon's experience, length of the procedure, the hospital and operating-room environments, and the underlying medical condition of the patient, also have a strong impact on wound infection rates. These variables should be considered in evaluations of infection-control problems.

At the present time, cefazolin remains the preferred first-generation cephalosporin for surgical prophylaxis. Recent data notwithstanding, the demonstrated cost-effectiveness of cefazolin must be weighed against the increased cost and broader spectrum of newer antimicrobials. The use of other first-generation cephalosporins such as cephalothin or cephradine, which, although they have a shorter duration of action, are more resistant to staphylococcal β-lactamases, should be evaluated.

Head and Neck Surgery

Elective surgical procedures of the head and neck can be categorized according to their risk of postoperative infection as either clean or clean-contaminated procedures. Clean procedures include parotidectomy, thyroidectomy, and submandibular-gland excision. Clean-contaminated procedures include all those involving an incision through the oral or pharyngeal mucosa. They vary from a tonsillectomy to complicated tumor-debulking procedures requiring massive reconstruction. Patient-specific criteria that might influence postoperative wound infection rates include age, nutritional status, and the presence of concomitant medical conditions such as diabetes mellitus; if the patient has cancer, the stage of the malignancy before operation and preoperative radiation therapy must also be assessed.[4-6]

The normal flora of the mouth and oropharynx are responsible for most infections that follow head and neck procedures. The predominant oropharyngeal organisms include various streptococci (including aerobic and anaerobic species), *Staph. aureus*, peptococcus, peptostreptococcus, and numerous anaerobic gram-negative bacteria including *Bacteroides* species, *Neisseria*, and *Veillonella*. Nasal flora include staphylococci, *Streptococcus pyogenes*, *Strep. pneumoniae*, *Branhamella*, and *Haemophilus* species.

Anaerobic bacteria are approximately 10 times more prevalent than aerobic bacteria in the oropharynx. As a result, bacteria isolated from patients with postoperative wound infections are primarily polymicrobial. Both aerobic and anaerobic bacteria are routinely cultured from infected wounds in more than 90% of cases.[7-10] Johnson et al.[11] recently reviewed the need for gram-negative bacterial coverage in antimicrobial prophylaxis for clean-contaminated head and neck surgery. They concluded that clindamycin alone appears to be successful as a prophylactic agent and that broad-spectrum antimicrobials such as cefoxitin, while widely used for prophylaxis in this type of surgery, may be unnecessary. Since clindamycin does not offer any activity against aerobic gram-negative bacteria, the authors concluded that these bacteria are probably colonizers rather than pathogens in most patients.

The predominance of anaerobic bacteria in head and neck infection may explain why high-dose cefazolin (2 g) has been shown to be effective, whereas a 500-mg dose was not effective.[a] Cefazolin is known to inhibit many anaerobic bacteria at serum and tissue levels achieved with a 2-g dose.[12]

Clinical Trials. Systemic prophylactic antimicrobials have not proved effective in reducing wound infection rates among patients undergoing clean procedures of the head and neck. Johnson and Wagner[13] reviewed the records of 438 patients undergoing such procedures. Eighty percent of these patients had not received prophylactic antimicrobials, and the associated wound infection rate was 0.7%. The 20% of patients receiving antimicrobials had a similar rate of wound infection.

Patients undergoing clean-contaminated procedures of the head and neck or who received a placebo in double-blind clinical trials had wound infection rates between 24% and 87%. Patients in such studies who received antimicrobials had a dramatically lower incidence of postoperative wound infection. Brand et al.[14] enrolled 83 patients in a clinical trial; the treatment groups were as follows: cefazolin 500 mg every eight hours for one day; cefazolin 500 mg every eight hours for five days; gentamicin 1.7 mg/kg plus clindamycin 300 mg every eight hours for one day; and gentamicin plus clindamycin every eight hours for five days. The wound infection rate in the combined cefazolin groups was 27%, while that of the gentamicin/clindamycin combined group was 7%. Because the numbers of patients were small, no statistical analysis was performed. Mandell-Brown et al.[15] performed a double-blind trial with 101 patients who were divided into the following groups: placebo every eight hours for four doses; cefazolin 500 mg every eight hours for four doses; cefotaxime 2 g every eight hours for four doses; and cefoperazone 2 g every eight hours for four doses. Infection rates were 78% in the placebo group, 33% in the cefazolin group, 10% in the cefotaxime group, and 9% in the cefoperazone group. The difference between all antimicrobial groups and the placebo group was statistically significant. The hospital stay of infected patients was twice as long as that of noninfected patients. Johnson et al.[16] performed a similar trial with cefotaxime and cefoperazone and attained similar results. Other studies have produced similar results.[17-28]

Two additional trials deserve mention. In a randomized trial, Johnson et al.[17] compared cefazolin 2 g (as opposed to previous studies using 500 mg) with moxalactam 2 g. Each drug was given one hour before surgery and three more times, for a total of four doses. Infection rates were 8.5% in the cefazolin group and 3.4% in the moxalactam group. The difference did not reach statistical significance. Because of this study, the *Medical Letter on Drugs and Therapeutics* continues to recommend a 2-g dose of cefazolin for clean-contaminated head and neck surgery.[18] Gerard et al.[19] randomly assigned 113 patients to receive either amikacin plus clindamycin or ticarcillin/clavulanic acid. Infection rates were 10% in the amikacin/clindamycin group and 36% in the ticarcillin/clavulanic acid group. This difference was significant. Examination of the bacteria isolated from the ticarcillin/clavulanic acid group revealed a high prevalence of gram-negative and gram-positive anaerobic bacteria responsible for the wound infections. These results are difficult to reconcile, given the nearly complete in vitro coverage reported for ticarcillin/clavulanic acid against anaerobic bacteria.

Recommendations. *Clean Head and Neck Surgical Procedures.* Infection rates are generally less than 2%. Antimicrobial prophylaxis is not justified.

Clean-Contaminated Head and Neck Surgical Procedures. Systemic antimicrobial prophylaxis is mandatory. Wound infection rates are extraordinarily high (24–87%) when antimicrobials are not used. Rates below 10% may be expected when appropriate antimicrobial prophylaxis is given. Several regimens have been demonstrated to be effective in clinical trials. All agents should be given in regimens of one to four doses. In no case should prophylaxis exceed 24 hours. Single-dose regimens might be preferable, particularly when cost and the possibility of resistance are considered; however, this remains controversial.[4] Based on the marginal performance of ticarcillin/clavulanic acid in one clinical trial, the β-lactamase inhibitor combinations cannot be recommended at this time. The preferred regimens are clindamycin 600 mg (15 mg/kg for children) plus gentamicin 1.7 mg/kg given every 8 hours for 24 hours or cefazolin 2 g (20 mg/kg for children) every 8 hours for 24 hours.

Biliary-Tract Surgery

Operations involving the biliary tract are among the most commonly performed abdominal procedures. They include cholecystectomies, explorations of the common bile duct, and choledochoenterostomies (e.g., choledochoduodenostomy). Endoscopic sphincterotomy and liver transplantation, although related, will not be considered here. The postoperative wound infection rates after biliary-tract operations have been reported to be between 7% and 20%.[29-35] The incidence of postoperative wound infections is related to the microbial status of the biliary tract at the time of operation. In the majority of patients, the biliary tract is sterile, and the risk of infection is no higher than that of other clean operations (i.e., less than 5%). If bacteria colonize the biliary tract, the rate of infection may reach as high as 36%.[36] Appropriate use of antimicrobial prophylaxis in this setting therefore requires identification of patients likely to have bactibilia. High-risk groups include patients over 70 years of age and those with obstructed biliary tracts, acute cholecystitis, or common-bile-duct stones without jaundice.[37,38] Some studies have shown that patients 60 years of age and above are at increased risk of infection.[39,40] Moreover, some patients with bactibilia do not fit into any of the categories described above.

The organisms most likely to be associated with wound infection after biliary-tract surgery have been well characterized[33,36,39-46] and include *Escherichia coli*, *Klebsiella*, and enterococci. Other gram-negative bacilli, streptococci, and staphylococci are occasionally isolated. Anaerobes are infrequently isolated from the biliary tract; of these, species of clostridia are most common. Bacteria that are isolated from bile during surgery are those most likely to be associated with subsequent wound infections.

Clinical Trials. Controlled clinical trials of the use of preoperative antimicrobials for prevention of infection following biliary-tract operations have sought to answer three key questions: (1) Do antimicrobials prevent wound infections with biliary-tract operations? (2) Are certain agents more effective than others? and (3) What is the minimum duration of antimicrobial exposure necessary to prevent postoperative infection?

A recently published review and meta-analysis of 42 studies published between 1965 and 1988 has demonstrated that patients who receive prophylactic antimicrobials for biliary-tract surgery are less likely to develop infection than those who do not.[47] More than 4000 patients (both high-risk and low-risk) were included in this analysis. The overall incidence of postoperative infection was 15% in patients receiving no treatment and 9% less in those receiving antimicrobials (95% confidence interval, 7% to 11% reduction). Results for the control group were more favorable than those for the treatment group in only 4 of the 42 studies. A wide variety of antimicrobials, primarily cephalosporins, were used in these trials. The effectiveness of antimicrobial prophylaxis was demonstrated in both low-risk and high-risk patients.

Most recent antimicrobial prophylaxis trials involving biliary-tract operations have focused on the relative effectiveness of different antimicrobials, usually cephalosporins. Significant differences among agents have been demonstrated in only 2 of 16 comparative studies. Meta-analysis of these comparative trials has demonstrated no significant differences between first-, second-, and third-generation cephalosporins.[47] When first-generation cephalosporins were compared with second- or third-generation cephalosporins,[45,48-52] only one trial demonstrated a significant difference between regimens.[52] In that study, the wound infection rate was 0% with cefotetan and 14% with cefazolin. Second-generation cephalosporins have also been compared with second-generation agents or with third-generation agents.[39,40,53-57] In the latter group, only one trial reported a significant difference.[57] These investigators studied more than 1400 patients and found a wound infection rate of 3.3% with cefotaxime and 7.6% with cefoxitin. Other trials reported no significant differences between ampicillin and cefamandole,[44] cefonicid and mezlocillin,[58] and ceftriaxone and ciprofloxacin.[41]

The third major issue addressed by the clinical studies was the minimum duration of antimicrobial administration for prevention of postoperative wound infection. A number of different antimicrobials have been studied, including cefazolin,[33,58] cefonicid,[54,55,59] ceftriaxone,[48] cefotetan,[56] and cefotaxime.[57] Most of these studies compared a single preoperative antimicrobial dose with longer regimens. In all studies, the single-dose regimen was as effective as the multiple-dose regimen. Other trials have compared various single-dose regimens,[45,49,53] additionally demonstrating the effectiveness of single-dose cefotetan, cefazolin,[49] cefuroxime,[53] and moxalactam.[45]

Recommendations. The studies described above support the use of antimicrobial prophylaxis in all patients undergoing cholecystectomy. Although only patients with bactibilia are believed to be at increased risk of infection, it is difficult to identify these patients preoperatively, since they often do not fall into one of the recognized high-risk categories.

The recommended regimen is a single 1-g dose of cefazolin, given intravenously within 30 minutes of the start of the operation. Clinical trial data demonstrate that first-generation cephalosporins are as effective as second- or third-generation agents, and that a single preoperative dose is as effective as multiple doses.

Gastroduodenal Surgery

Common gastric operations for which antimicrobial prophylaxis may be considered include resection with or without vagotomy for gastric or duodenal ulcers, revision necessitated by development of strictures of the gastric outlet, resection for gastric carcinoma, and gastroplasty or gastric bypass for morbid obesity.

The risk of postoperative infection after gastroduodenal surgery varies markedly, depending on the type of operation performed and the patient's clinical status. Conditions with a relatively high risk of infection include gastric ulcer, gastric carcinoma, bleeding duodenal or gastric ulcers, and obstructing duodenal ulcers.[60] In one study, the wound infection rate was 4% after operations for duodenal ulcer, 29% for gastric ulcer, and 33% for gastric resection for cancer.[61] Infection rates in the placebo group in controlled studies have varied from 10% to 35%.[60,62,63] With gastric-bypass operations, a wound infection rate of 21% has been reported.[64] Another important factor associated with infection risk is the use of histamine H_2-receptor blockers or the presence of achlorhydria. Gastric bacterial counts are increased when H_2-receptor blockers are used; this may increase the risk of postoperative infection.[65,66]

In healthy individuals, the stomach is usually colonized by relatively few organisms (fewer than 10^4/mL). Among the most common are nasopharyngeal commensals (streptococci, lactobacilli, diphtheroids, and micrococci).[67,68] Increased pH from the use of H_2-receptor blockers, gastric obstruction, or bleeding can increase bacterial concentrations to 10^6/mL, and increased gastric bacterial concentrations are related to increased rate of infection.[63]

Wound infections after gastroduodenal surgery tend to be polymicrobial and usually involve coliforms, such as *E. coli*, and aerobic gram-positive cocci, such as enterococci.[61,69] In a study of patients undergoing gastric-bypass surgery, staphylococci were the most common organisms isolated from infected wounds, and gram-negative bacilli were isolated from two subphrenic abscesses.[64]

Clinical Trials. Relatively few studies have evaluated the effectiveness of antimicrobial prophylaxis for gastroduodenal operations. Of those published, most compared antimicrobials with placebo. Cephalosporins that have demonstrated efficacy over nonantimicrobial controls include cephaloridine,[63,70,71] cefazolin,[30,64] cefamandole,[61,72] and cefuroxime.[73,74] The latter two trials studied single doses of cefuroxime and involved relatively few patients. Pories et al.[64] demonstrated a reduction in wound infection rate from 21% to 4% with the use of antimicrobial prophylaxis for gastric-bypass surgery.

Few published studies have compared the effectiveness of the various antimicrobials used for gastroduodenal operations. Three studies reported no significant differences between cephalosporins and penicillins.[62,75,76] Another study, which included relatively few patients, demonstrated no significant difference between cefazolin and moxalactam.[50]

Recommendations. Prophylactic antimicrobials should be used when the stomach or duodenum is entered surgically, since such procedures place the patient at risk for postoperative infection. Antimicrobials are not needed when the lumen of the intestinal tract is not entered (e.g., selective vagotomy). Although some authors believe that antimicrobials are not necessary for patients undergoing gastric resection for nonobstructing ulcers, the widespread use of H_2-receptor blockers makes it likely that these patients will have high intraluminal bacterial concentrations, making antimicrobial prophylaxis advisable.

Most studies of antimicrobial prophylaxis with gastroduodenal operations have involved the cephalosporins. Although few comparative antimicrobial studies have been published, it appears that first-generation cephalosporins are as effective as second- or third-generation agents. Therefore, a first-generation agent such as cefazolin is preferred. Although the efficacy of single-dose prophylaxis in this setting has not been thoroughly studied, results of studies with cefuroxime suggest the effectiveness of a single, preoperative dose. Given the cumulative experience of single-dose prophylaxis for abdominal operations, it is justified to recommend single-dose prophylaxis for gastroduodenal operations as well.

Colorectal Surgery

Wound infections are the most common complication following elective colorectal surgery. This complication causes extensive morbidity and mortality and increases hospital costs. Factors associated with an increased risk for postoperative wound infections include impaired host defenses, age greater than 60 years, hypoalbuminemia, poor preoperative bowel preparation, and bacterial contamination of the surgical wound.[77]

Colonic aspirates obtained from patients undergoing colorectal surgery yield large numbers of aerobic and anaerobic microorganisms. More than 20 different aerobic and 50 anaerobic bacteria have been identified in the lumen of the bowel. These microorganisms make up to 20–30% of the fecal mass. *E. coli*, the most commonly isolated gram-negative aerobe, is found in concentrations of 10^6 to 10^8 organisms per gram of fecal contents. The concentration of anaerobes is 1,000 to 10,000 times greater. *Bacteroides fragilis* is the most frequently isolated of these organisms.

The goal of surgical prophylaxis for elective colorectal surgery is to reduce the risk of contamination of the operative wound by bacteria spilled from the colon and rectum at the time of surgery. Attaining this goal entails reduction in the concentration of the resident bacteria and eradication of any bacteria that may contaminate the surgical wound.

When no attempt is made to reduce the number of microorganisms present in the bowel, elective colorectal surgeries have been associated with infection rates as high as 40%.[78,79] Various methods of mechanical cleansing of the bowel have been devised to reduce these high concentrations of colorectal bacteria. Bartlett et al.[80] have shown that the use of a mechanical bowel preparation alone decreases the total number of bacteria but does not decrease the number of microorganisms per gram of stool in the colon at the time of operation. With conventional bowel-cleansing techniques alone, the wound infection rate is still 35–40%.[81,82] Until the mid-1980s, the conventional bowel-preparation technique required a minimum of 36–48 hours of enemas and oral cathartics in the immediate preoperative period. The goal was to reduce the concentration of bacteria, with the assumption that this was accomplished once the rectal effluent was clear. More recently, single-day (12 hours or less) orthograde lavage techniques using an isosmotic nonabsorbable electrolyte solution[83,84] or mannitol solution[85,86] have been used.

Since 1939, when Garlock and Seely[87] documented the value of preoperative administration of oral sulfonamides in reducing the incidence of wound infections after colonic surgery, investigators have searched for the most effective method to reduce postoperative infection. Antimicrobial agents, combined with mechanical cleansing of the colonic lumen, have significantly reduced postoperative wound infection rates, from 30–60% to less than 10% in clean-contaminated procedures.[88-97] Numerous studies have unequivocally shown this to be a safe and effective approach,[98,99] and it has become the standard approach for prophylaxis in elective colorectal surgery.

Although the method of bowel cleansing has been narrowed to one or two options, the choice of antimicrobial regimen is still vigorously debated. Given the nature of the microorganisms present in the colon and rectum, it seems reasonable that any prophylactic regimen should use an agent or combination of agents that is active against both aerobic and anaerobic bacteria. In the United States, three such antimicrobial regimens have been extensively studied. The first consists of the administration of one or more oral antimicrobials (erythromycin, neomycin) in doses high enough to decrease the resident colonic flora. The second involves the administration of injectable antimicrobials immediately before surgery and aims at attaining maximal tissue concentrations at the time the surgical wound is made. The third is a combination of the two previously mentioned techniques.

Various drug regimens have been studied and advocated for prophylaxis for colorectal surgery during the past two decades.[89] Many of these trials have presented inconsistent results. Problems in methodology have been well documented.[90-92]

Clinical Trials. With the exception of a few classic

studies, only reports published after 1980 were included in this analysis. The studies reviewed were predominantly prospective, randomized, controlled trials in which criteria for wound infection are clearly defined. Only half of the trials were blinded. Most experts agree that the rate for postoperative wound infection following clean-contaminated colorectal surgical procedures should be less than 10%, if an appropriate mechanical bowel-cleansing and antimicrobial regimen (active against aerobes and anaerobes) is used.[93-96] Therefore, studies that reported wound infection rates of greater than 15% when an antimicrobial regimen effective against both gram-negative aerobes and anaerobes was used were not evaluated for this review. Studies that did not discuss dosage and timing of antimicrobial administration and that had a placebo group were likewise excluded.

Preoperative Oral Antimicrobials. Washington et al.[97] were the first to document that the use of preoperative oral antimicrobials (neomycin and tetracycline) effective against both aerobes and anaerobes led to a dramatic reduction in the postoperative wound infection rate. Nichols et al.[98,99] and Clarke et al.[81] altered this approach, using neomycin and erythromycin in an attempt to increase effectiveness against anaerobic bacteria in the large bowel. Various agents, both singly and in combination, have been evaluated for prophylaxis for colorectal surgery.

Numerous studies using oral agents for prophylaxis have demonstrated that the combination of neomycin plus an effective anaerobic agent, generally either erythromycin[81,100-109] or metronidazole[86,105,110-116] (less commonly a tetracycline derivative[86,97,117] or clindamycin[111]), in conjunction with a bowel-cleansing technique reduced the incidence of postoperative wound infections to less than 10%. These results occurred in 19 (76%) of the 25 studies evaluated.[81,86,97,100,104-108] Forty-eight percent of these investigations documented a postoperative wound infection rate of less than 5%.[86,97,102-105,107-110,116]

The standard neomycin sulfate/erythromycin regimen (1 g of each drug orally at 1300, 1400, and 2300 one day preoperatively, with surgery performed at 0800 the next morning) used in the United States has resulted in postoperative infectious wound complications of less than 5% in half of the trials evaluated. In 90% of the studies evaluated, infectious wound complication rates were less than 10%.[86,97,102,104,108]

When metronidazole was combined with an agent active against gram-negative aerobes, only 44% of the treatment regimens reported a reduction of the postoperative wound infection rate to 5% or less.[86,105,107,112,114] Only 63% of the trials that evaluated metronidazole reported the wound infection rate to be less than 10%.[86,105,107,111,112,114] The difference in postoperative wound infections with a metronidazole combination versus the neomycin/erythromycin regimen may be a result of the different doses of metronidazole (2 g, 1 g, 750 mg, and 200 mg) used in these studies, as well as the fact that most of these studies were carried out in Europe.

Other combination regimens have been used as well. Neither tetracycline nor its derivatives have been shown to be more effective than neomycin/erythromycin in reducing postoperative wound infections.[86,97,117] With metronidazole alone, the postoperative wound infection rate is between 10% and 15%.[110,115,116]

Thus, available data demonstrate that the standard oral regimen of neomycin (nonabsorbable antibiotic) and erythromycin (which is absorbed and attains measurable tissue levels) provides the most effective means of preventing wound infection following elective colorectal surgery in adults. The safety and efficacy of this regimen in the pediatric population have not been documented; consequently, preoperative oral antimicrobials are not used in infants or young children.

Preoperative and Postoperative Regimens of Injectable Antimicrobials. In the late 1970s and early 1980s, debate about antimicrobial use in colorectal surgery centered on the issue of oral versus injectable antimicrobials. The oral, nonabsorbable antimicrobials were administered to reduce intraluminal concentrations of bacteria, whereas injectable antimicrobials were given to ensure high tissue concentrations at the time of surgery. All studies of wound infection rates following elective colorectal surgery have used oral absorbable antimicrobials (erythromycin, tetracycline, doxycycline, or metronidazole) as part of the standard bowel preparation.

One of the earliest studies evaluating the use of injectable agents alone was conducted by Polk and Lopez-Meyer,[78] who evaluated the use of i.m. cephaloridine. The wound infection rate in the treatment group was significantly lower than that of the control group.

In almost half of the studies that used only the i.v. route, a cephalosporin was among the treatment regimens evaluated.[85,100,104,118-130] Other antimicrobials evaluated, either singly or in combination, included aminoglycosides,[103,126,131-133]erythromycin,[132] ampicillin,[123,134] piperacillin, ticarcillin/clavulanic acid,[131,135] doxycycline,[127,136,137] lincosamides,[133] and metronidazole.[104,121,123,125-129,131-134,138]

When an injectable antimicrobial regimen (in conjunction with a mechanical bowel preparation) was used without any oral antimicrobial, only 26% of the studies evaluated reported postoperative infectious wound complication rates of 5% or less,[85,100,123,127-129,136,137] and only 65% of the treatment regimens studied reported infectious wound complication rates of less than 10%.[85,100,104,118,119,122,123,127-129,131-138] Those studies that evaluated injectable cephalosporins included first-,[116,117,128,129] second-,[85,100,118,120,121,123-125] and third-generation cephalosporins.[104,122,126] The first-generation cephalosporins have produced inconsistent results and do not appear to be of benefit in preventing postoperative wound infections.[107,116,117,128,129,139,140] The postoperative wound infection rate with these agents is generally greater than 20%. These results are not surprising, considering the relative inactivity of these agents against the anaerobic bacteria commonly associated with postoperative wound infections after elective colorectal surgery.

Cephalosporins with short half-lives, such as cefoxitin or cefotaxime, are associated with higher postoperative wound infections if the surgical procedures extend longer than four to five hours and the drugs are administered every six to eight hours.[130,141,142]

Evaluation of these studies seems to imply that the use of injectable antimicrobials, along with some mechanical bowel-cleansing procedure, is not as effective as an oral regimen in reducing postoperative wound infections. The use of an oral regimen effective against aerobes and anaerobes reduced postoperative wound infections to 5% or less in 48% of the treatment regimens evaluated. An injectable antimicrobial regimen produced a similar reduction in only 26% of the studies evaluated.

Combination of Oral and Injectable Antimicrobials. Attempting to further decrease the rate of postoperative wound infections, investigators have evaluated the combination of oral and i.v. antimicrobial agents for elective colorectal surgery. In theory, the goal is to reduce bacterial concentrations in the lumen and to attain sufficient tissue concentrations of antimicrobial to prevent postoperative infections.

Although some of these trials have documented significantly lower postoperative wound infection rates,[124,130,140,143,144] results are not consistent.[100,101,113,122]

Various i.v. antimicrobials have been added to oral antimicrobial regimens for prophylaxis for elective colorectal surgery.[100,101,112,113,122,124,131,139,143-146] Postoperative wound infection rates were 5% or less in 57% of the treatment regimens evaluated. All of the treatment regimens evaluated reported postoperative wound infection rates under 10% after elective colorectal surgery. These outcomes are similar to those achieved by oral regimens alone. The cephalosporins have been studied more than any other class of i.v. antimicrobials.[100,101,112,124,131,139,143,144]

It has recently been suggested that further stratification of the types of operative procedures may result in significantly different postoperative wound infection rates.[77,124,144,147] Coppa et al.[124,144] have presented data suggesting that operations involving the rectum are associated with a higher wound infection rate than operations involving the colon and that the use of a combination of oral and i.v. antimicrobials reduces the wound infection rate significantly more than does an oral regimen alone.

Other factors affecting postoperative wound infections after elective colorectal surgery include the length of the operative procedure[119,124,130,148] and the duration of antimicrobial administration after the surgical incision.[149-153] Unfortunately, the majority of studies do not report the duration of surgery. Kaiser et al.[130] reported a threefold increase in the incidence of postoperative wound infection when the operative procedure lasted for greater than four hours. If the procedure was less than four hours the infection rate was only 5%. In this study, cefoxitin, a short half-life cephalosporin, was given at six-hour intervals. Coppa et al.[124] reported an unacceptably high postoperative wound infection rate with cefoxitin alone when the surgical procedure lasted more than 3.5 hours. When cefoxitin was combined with an oral antimicrobial regimen the infection rate dropped to 6%, and if the procedure lasted less than 3.5 hours, the infection rate was 4% when cefoxitin was used alone. Jones et al.[141] and Shatney[142] reported that cefotaxime (also a short half-life cephalosporin) resulted in unacceptable postoperative wound infection rates when used for prophylaxis after prolonged colorectal surgery. These data imply that if the surgical procedure lasts longer than 3.5 to 4 hours, a cephalosporin with a relatively long half-life (i.e., cefotetan, ceftizoxime, cefmetazole) should be considered for prophylaxis. No published comparative trials have specifically addressed this issue.

Discussions of how many doses are needed to ensure adequate prophylaxis also merit careful review.[149-153] Stone et al.[154] was one of the first to document that prolonged administration of antimicrobials (five days) was no more beneficial than a shorter course of antimicrobials administered in the immediate operative period, as described by Polk and Lopez-Meyer.[78] This approach has now been confirmed by many other investigations. DiPiro et al.[149] recently reviewed 40 published clinical trials that evaluated single-dose systemic antimicrobial prophylaxis for several types of surgical procedures. Their review indicated that multiple-dose regimens were no more effective than single-dose prophylaxis. The authors stated that it was difficult to evaluate the literature on colorectal surgery because many studies combined a single i.v. dose of antimicrobial with an oral regimen.

In this review of the literature, five trials[85,104,118,119,136] evaluating colorectal surgery specifically were found to compare a single i.v. dose with multiple doses of an antimicrobial regimen. The postoperative wound infection rate for the single-dose studies was between 5% and 10% in three quarters of the reported regimens, and no significant differences in the postoperative wound infection rate after colorectal surgery were noted between the single- and multiple-dose regimens. While these studies indicate that the number of doses of antimicrobial prophylaxis is not of clinical importance, it is important to note that neither i.v. regimen is as effective as an oral regimen alone.

The review of evaluable studies of antimicrobial prophylaxis for elective colorectal surgery supports the use of an oral antimicrobial regimen (i.e., one that is active against aerobes and anaerobes and that attains adequate antianaerobic tissue concentrations immediately before surgical incision) and an adequate bowel-cleansing preparation. The use of i.v. antimicrobials alone does not reduce postoperative infectious wound complications to the same extent as do the oral regimens. The question of whether the combination of i.v. and oral antimicrobials is more efficacious than oral agents alone remains to be answered.

A recent survey of 352 board-certified colorectal surgeons concerning the use of bowel preparations and antimicrobials for prophylaxis revealed that all of the responding surgeons used some sort of bowel-cleansing procedure plus an antimicrobial regimen.[155] The preferred method of bowel cleansing, used by 58% of respondents, was oral polyethylene glycol– electrolyte lavage. The next-most-common approach, used by 36% of these surgeons, was a one- to three-day bowel preparation consisting of cathartics and enemas. The preferred regimen for the prevention of surgical infectious complications was a combined oral and injectable antimicrobial regimen plus bowel cleansing (88%). The most common oral regimen used by these surgeons consisted of an oral aminoglycoside (neomycin, kanamycin or gentamicin) plus erythromycin base (82%). The most common injectable antimicrobials used by these surgeons were the second-generation cephalosporins cefoxitin or cefotetan (74%).

Recommendations. *Mechanical Bowel Preparation.* Four liters of a polyethylene glycol–electrolyte lavage solution should be given over three hours starting the morning of the day before surgery; the lavage solution should always be used in conjunction with one of the following antimicrobial regimens.

Antimicrobial Regimen. Oral neomycin sulfate 1 g and erythromycin base 1 g should be given after the bowel preparation is complete at 19, 18, and 9 hours before surgery. If the oral route is contraindicated, a single 2-g i.v. dose of a cephalosporin that is effective against both aerobic and anaerobic bacteria and has a half-life of 60 minutes or longer (cefotetan, cefmetazole, cefotaxime, or ceftizoxime) should be administered at induction of anesthesia. If a cephalosporin with a half-life of 60 minutes or less is used (the half-life of cefoxitin is less than 60 minutes), and surgery lasts longer than three hours, a second dose of the i.v. antimicrobial should be given. The choice of cephalosporin should be based on cost to the institution. If the patient is to undergo a colostomy closure or rectal procedure, a combination of oral and i.v. agents should be given, following the dosage recommendations described above. Infants and young children should not receive oral antimicrobials. Ampicillin (50 mg/kg every six hours) and gentamicin (2.5 mg/kg every 8–12 hours) for three doses beginning at induction of anesthesia are recommended.

Appendectomy

The incidence of infectious complications following appendectomy is extremely variable and depends on the appearance of the appendix at the time of surgery. In uncomplicated appendectomy (appendix is normal or acutely inflamed), the postoperative infection rate is reported to range between 0% and 30%.[156-158] In the studies evaluated for this review, the rate of surgical wound infection in uncomplicated appendectomy without antimicrobial prophylaxis ranged from 8% to 27%.[159-169] However, if the appendix is gangrenous, perforated, or abscessed (complicated appendicitis), wound infection rates approach 80% without antimicrobial prophylaxis.[162] The goal of antimicrobial administration in patients with uncomplicated and complicated appendicitis is to reduce postoperative wound infection rates to less than 10% and between 10% and 25%, respectively.[158,164]

Appropriate antimicrobial prophylaxis has reduced surgical wound infection rates to as low as 1% in both uncomplicated and certain complicated appendectomies. The majority of studies have shown that even when appropriate antimicrobials are used, infectious complications will occur in 10–25% of patients with a gangrenous or perforated appendix.[162,170,171]

The most common microorganisms cultured from wound infections after appendectomy are anaerobic organisms (especially *B. fragilis*) and aerobic gram-negative enteric organisms (predominantly *E. coli*). Aerobic and anaerobic streptococci, *Staphylococcus* species, and *Enterococcus* species have also been cultured frequently, although not nearly as often as the aerobic and anaerobic gram-negative organisms. *Pseudomonas* species, reported by some researchers[172,173] to be a major pathogen in this setting, was not noted to be a problem in the studies reviewed for this discussion; in all, only 16 patients had a *Pseudomonas* species isolated in the studies reviewed.[166,167,172,173]

With the exception of certain classic articles, only studies published after 1979 were considered for this review. All studies evaluated were prospective, randomized, and blinded. Only those studies that reported specific criteria for postoperative infectious wound complications and presented a statistical analysis were considered for this review.

Time of administration was shown to be important in the studies reviewed. In two trials in which antimicrobials were administered after the abdomen had been opened and the appendix visualized, the rates of wound infection tended to be higher than in studies in which the antimicrobial was administered before the surgical incision was made.[161,174] To be most efficacious, drugs should be administered before incision. Therefore, in almost all studies evaluated for this review, the antimicrobial(s) were administered at induction of anesthesia.

Clinical Trials. *Uncomplicated Appendicitis.* In those studies involving patients with uncomplicated appendicitis, cefoxitin,[159,163,164,168] cefotaxime,[166,167] mezlocillin,[169] and clindamycin[162] were shown to be of approximately equal efficacy for prophylaxis; in all cases, the postoperative infectious wound complications were reduced to less than 10%. Overall, 80% of the treatment regimens evaluated noted a wound infection rate of 10% or less following appendectomy. Combination regimens including metronidazole[164-166] also resulted in a reduction in wound infections, but they were not shown to be more efficacious than single-drug therapy with cefoxitin or cefotaxime. Metronidazole as a single agent or the first-generation cephalosporins cefazolin[162] and cephalothin[168] were no more effective than placebo and resulted in more infectious complications than did other comparative regimens. These studies appear to indicate that first-generation cephalosporins are ineffective as prophylactic regimens for uncomplicated appendectomy.

Clindamycin,[162] while better than placebo, generally was associated with a higher rate of wound infection than cefoxitin (10% versus 0–7%, respectively).[159,163,164,168] Cefoxitin has been studied more extensively than the other cephalosporins. The use of a single 1-g i.v. dose was consistently shown to result in low rates of wound infection (less than 7%).[159,163,164,168] The studies were almost evenly split as to the duration of prophylaxis in the postoperative period. Five studies administered between 2 and 15 postoperative doses (> 60% used 2 or 3 doses)[159,160,163,165,168]; all reported infectious wound complication rates of less than 10%. The remaining six studies[161,162,164,166,167,169] administered a single preoperative dose; with one exception, wound complication rates were reduced to 10% or less.[161]

Evaluation of these studies indicates that the antimicrobial(s) used for prophylaxis in uncomplicated appendectomy should be active against aerobic bacteria. These data also support the use of a single preoperative dose.

Complicated Appendicitis. The studies evaluating antimicrobial prophylaxis in complicated appendicitis (gangrenous, perforated, or involving an abscess) report postoperative wound infection rates ranging from 0% to 80%.[162,164-169,172-176] The approach to management should comprise surgical and antimicrobial treatment of the contaminated area with the goal of preventing postoperative wound complications. The standard prophylaxis used for a clean or clean-contaminated surgical procedure is insufficient. Only 5 of 12 studies evaluated for this review studied patients diagnosed as having complicated appendicitis.[172-176]

Use of the first-generation cephalosporins cefazolin and cephalothin has resulted in an unacceptably high (27–80%) incidence of postoperative infectious wound complications.[162,168] While studies using a second-generation[164,166,168,173,174,176] or third-generation[166,167,173,176] cephalosporin report postoperative wound infection rates of 25% or less in more than three quarters of the clinical trials evaluated, only half of the treatment regimens that used either a second-generation[164,173,176] or third-generation[167,173,176] cephalosporin reported reductions to less than 10%.

Combination therapies including metronidazole[164-166,175] or clindamycin[164,172,173,175] plus an aminoglycoside have not been shown to be more efficacious than cefoxitin[164,168,174,177] in preventing wound infection, intra-abdominal infection, or both, following appendectomy. A single study comparing ceftizoxime with cefoxitin showed no difference in the rate of infection between the two agents; wound infection rates were 0% and 3%, respectively.[176]

In more than 71% of the antimicrobial regimens evaluated, patients treated with a single dose had postoperative wound infection rates of 25% or greater.[162,169,174,175] Postoperative wound infection rates of this magnitude were found in only 8% of the treatment regimens of three to five days' duration.[166,168,172,173,176] Treating for longer than five days has not proved to be of any additional benefit.[164,165]

Of all the evaluable studies of the cephalosporins, cefoxitin 1–2 g i.v. every six hours is considered by many to be the preferred regimen for antimicrobial prophylaxis before appendectomy and for treatment afterward. Based on their activity against aerobes and anaerobes, ceftizoxime, cefotaxime, cefmetazole, cefotetan, or combinations of an aminoglycoside plus metronidazole or clindamycin seem reasonable alternatives.

Recommendations. No single agent is clearly preferable to any other agent for prophylaxis in uncomplicated appendicitis or for the treatment of complicated appendicitis. Given the lack of data supporting a single-agent regimen for children, pediatric surgeons continue to prefer the combination of ampicillin, gentamicin, and clindamycin.

Uncomplicated Appendicitis. The recommended regimen is a cephalosporin having anaerobic and aerobic activity (cefoxitin, cefmetazole, ceftizoxime, cefotaxime, or cefotetan) given as a single 1- to 2-g i.v. dose at induction of anesthesia. If surgery lasts more than three hours, a second dose should be given. For pediatric patients, two doses of ampicillin, gentamicin, and clindamycin (5–15 mg/kg every eight hours) should be given.

Complicated Appendicitis. A cephalosporin having anaerobic and aerobic activity (cefoxitin, cefmetazole, ceftizoxime, cefotaxime, or cefotetan) should be given as a 1- to 2-g i.v. dose. The first dose should be administered at induction of anesthesia, and the regimen should be continued for three to five days. Alternatives include an aminoglycoside or aztreonam plus metronidazole or clindamycin. Additional options are imipenem or ticarcillin/clavulanate. For pediatric patients with complicated appendicitis, the regimen suggested for uncomplicated appendicitis should be continued for three to five days.

Cesarean Section

Approximately one million infants are born by cesarean section in the United States annually.[177] The rate of cesarean section has risen from 4.5 per 100 deliveries in 1965, to 16.5 in 1980, to 24.7 in 1988. Until 1986, repeat cesarean sections represented an increasingly large share of total cesareans, rising from approximately 25% of all cesareans in 1970 to more than 33% in 1986.[177] These increases now appear to have leveled off.

Postpartum infectious complications are common following cesarean section. Endometritis (infection of the uterine lining) has been reported to occur in high-risk populations at a rate as high as 85%.[178] High-risk patients are defined as women who have not received prenatal care, who are poorly nourished, who undergo multiple vaginal examinations, who have prolonged labor, and who have undergone frequent invasive monitoring. A majority of these women live in poverty. In contrast, patients in upper or middle socioeconomic populations, who tend to be better nourished and have received appropriate prenatal care, are at lower risk; the postpartum rate of endometritis in these patients ranges from 5% to 15%.

The factor most frequently associated with post-cesarean-section infectious morbidity is prolonged labor in the presence of ruptured membranes. Intact chorioamniotic membranes serve as a protective barrier against bacterial infection. Rupture of the membrane exposes the uterine surface to bacteria from the birth canal. The vaginal fluid with its bacterial flora is drawn up into the uterus when it relaxes between contractions during labor.[179] The flora include various aerobic and anaerobic streptococci, staphylococci, enteric gram-negative bacilli, and anaerobic gram-negative bacteria such as *Bacteroides bivius*, *B. fragilis*, and *Fusobacterium*.[180] In contrast, the organisms causing post-cesarean-section wound infections are *Staph. aureus* and other staphylococci, streptococci, and Enterobacteriaceae. Anaerobes are also present, but less commonly than in endometritis.[180] In addition to rupture of membranes, frequent vaginal examinations and invasive fetal monitoring also carry vaginal organisms into the uterine cavity. Other risk factors include systemic illness, poor hygiene, obesity, and anemia.[180]

Although febrile morbidity, or temperature elevation in an asymptomatic patient, is often considered in evaluations of antimicrobial prophylaxis, it appears that this temperature elevation is often not associated with an identifiable infection source or with symptoms specific for infection. It may occur in women with normal physical examination results and sometimes disappears without treatment. In controlled trials, it occurs with equal frequency in the placebo and treatment groups.[180,181] Moreover, women exhibiting febrile morbidity appear not to be those who later develop clinical infection. The presence or absence of febrile morbidity is probably not an appropriate indication of the efficacy of antimicrobial prophylaxis and therefore will not be considered.

Most of the investigations documenting the efficacy of prophylactic antimicrobials in cesarean section have been conducted in high-risk patients. Considerable controversy has existed regarding the necessity for prophylaxis in low-risk women undergoing cesarean section.

Two earlier investigations documented significant reductions in postcesarean endometritis following low-risk procedures with the use of prophylactic antimicrobials.[182,183] Some authorities have dismissed these benefits, arguing that limited morbidity, theoretical risks, and excess costs do not justify the use of prophylaxis in these patients.[184] From 1980 to 1982, Ehrenkranz et al.[185] undertook a large-scale prospective study of the efficacy of prophylaxis in more than 1800 low-risk women who underwent cesarean section.[185] Although the form of prophylaxis was not controlled and case controls were used, significant differences in endometritis and wound infection rates were found between women who did and did not receive prophylaxis. The investigators also found that primary cesarean section was associated with a fivefold higher rate of endometritis and that the odds of developing endometritis, wound infection, or both without timely antimicrobial prophylaxis were 3.7 to 1 in this cohort. Given their findings and assumptions regarding frequency of low-risk cesarean sections and efficacy and safety of the three 1-g doses of cefazolin used in the study, these authors concluded that more than $9 million could be saved annually by administration of prophylaxis to low-risk patients. The savings estimated from the lower limit of the odds ratio (1.4) is still $3.6 million annually. Thus, brief antimicrobial prophylaxis may be appropriate for all cesarean sections.

Clinical Trials. There have been more than 40 placebo-controlled, prospective trials evaluating the efficacy of antimicrobials in cesarean section, most of which have been carried out in high-risk populations. More than 50% of these trials have demonstrated benefit in terms of reduction of serious infection, and approximately 75% have revealed significant reductions in rates of postoperative endometritis.[186] The remaining 25% showed no statistical benefit in the prevention of serious infection or endometritis. Only approximately one in five of these trials demonstrated a statistically significant reduction in wound infection rates.[186]

A meta-analysis of these data by Enkin et al.[186] suggests a 75% reduction in serious infections and endometritis and a 65% reduction in wound infections for antimicrobial-treated patients compared with controls. These data are combined for high- and low-risk patients undergoing both emergency and elective procedures. When the data are cumulated via meta-analysis for the few trials of elective cesarean section, the summary odds ratios for endometritis (0.23, 95% confidence interval = 0.13–0.42) and wound infection (0.10, 95% confidence interval = 0.03–0.36) also support the use of prophylaxis in these procedures.

Timing of Prophylaxis. Unlike other surgical procedures, in which antimicrobials are ideally administered just before incision, administration of antimicrobials in cesarean section is usually delayed until after cord clamping. This is done principally to avoid suppression of the normal flora of the infant and minimize the risk of neonatal sepsis.

Although toxicity in the infant is of potential concern, the majority of drugs used for this procedure (primarily β lactams) have a documented record of safety in the treatment of infections in pregnancy, and many are used in the treatment of neonatal sepsis. The issue of timing has been addressed in two controlled trials. Cunningham et al.[187] and Gordon et al.[188] demonstrated no difference in infectious complications, regardless of whether the antimicrobials were given preoperatively or after cord clamping. In the study by Cunningham et al.[187] the infants who were not exposed to antimicrobial in utero underwent significantly fewer evaluations for neonatal sepsis. Thus, antimicrobials provide effective prophylaxis, even when given after clamping of the umbilical cord.

Duration of Prophylaxis. Most recent trials of antimicrobial prophylaxis have assessed the value of a single dose versus multiple doses (usually up to 24 hours). Earlier studies used regimens that lasted as long as five or six days. Studies by D'Angelo and Sokol[189] and Scarpignato et al.[190] found that a five-day course of cephalosporin prophylaxis is no more efficacious than a 24-hour course. Elliott et al.,[191] by contrast, found that three days of ampicillin was significantly more effective than three doses of ampicillin. The explanation for this difference is unclear. Faro et al.[192] assessed the efficacy of several types of β-lactam antimicrobials given in various regimens to nearly 1600 patients. One group of patients was given three doses of cefazolin and the two other groups received a single dose of cefazolin, either 1 g or 2 g. Results in patients receiving the single 2-g dose of cefazolin were statistically superior to those in patients receiving the other two cefazolin regimens.[192] Based on the data from the studies by D'Angelo and Scarpignato and more recent studies that demonstrated comparable efficacy of single doses, it does not seem necessary to extend prophylaxis beyond a single dose.

Route of Administration. Although the majority of studies have examined the effects of i.v. administration of antimicrobials, a few have evaluated the benefit of antimicrobial irrigations. Enkin et al.[186] summarized the data from six such trials. In one of these trials, Conover and Moore[193] found that intrauterine antimicrobial lavage was inferior to systemic administration of the same agents. None of the other trials demonstrated any difference in infectious morbidity. Therefore, given the adequate tissue penetration and demonstrated efficacy of injectable antimicrobials, irrigations of the uterine cavity are not warranted.

Selection of Antimicrobials. Guidelines for selection of antimicrobial prophylaxis established by Ledger et al.[194] more than 15 years ago are still applicable. The antimicrobial selected must (1) have a spectrum of activity effective against those bacteria likely to cause infection, (2) be present in tissue at the operative site in concentrations potentially effective against the infecting pathogen, (3) have been demonstrated to be clinically effective, (4) not be considered for first-line therapy of infection, (5) be nontoxic, (6) not promote the emergence of resistance, and (7) be cost-effective.

Although more than 20 different drugs have been used alone or in combination for prophylaxis, most obstetricians currently use either a penicillin or a cephalosporin.[195] A recent large-scale study by Faro et al.,[192] which involved more than 1500 high-risk patients, indicates that several single-dose regimens, including cefazolin 2 g, cefotetan 1 g, and piperacillin 4 g, are comparably effective. This provides three disparate choices, with drugs that offer differing spectra of activity with roughly equivalent efficacy. The earlier large-scale trials of Stiver et al.[196] and Rayburn et al.[197] offer a potential solution to this dilemma. Both studies involved hundreds of high-risk patients and compared cefazolin (poor *Bacteroides* coverage) with cefoxitin or moxalactam (good *Bacteroides* coverage). The Stiver study was placebo controlled. In both of these studies, cefoxitin and moxalactam were slightly less effective than cefazolin. In another study of nearly 350 high-risk women undergoing cesarean section, a 2-g dose of cefoxitin or piperacillin was given immediately after cord clamping and at four and eight hours after surgery.[198] Despite its superior in vitro activity against enterococci, *Pseudomonas aeruginosa*, and several enteric gram-negative bacillary species, piperacillin was found to be no more effective than cefoxitin.

Recommendations. Despite multiple clinical trials assessing the effectiveness of broad-spectrum antimicrobials or multiple doses of antimicrobials for prophylaxis in cesarean section, the data support the use of narrow-spectrum agents, such as first-generation cephalosporins, administered in a single dose immediately after clamping of the umbilical cord.[199,200] Given all of the above, it seems reasonable to use a single 2-g dose of cefazolin for all women undergoing cesarean section.

Hysterectomy

Hysterectomy is second only to cesarean section as the most frequently performed surgical procedure in the United States. Approximately 700,000 hysterectomies, or seven hysterectomies per 1000 women, are performed annually in this country. This rate has not changed substantially since the mid-1960s. The average hospital stay is now less than six days, a figure that has dropped by 50% in the past 25 years.[201]

Hysterectomy may be performed by a transvaginal or transabdominal approach. Uterine fibroid tumors account for 30% of all presurgical diagnoses leading to hysterectomy; the other most common diagnoses are endometriosis, uterine prolapse, cancer, and endometrial hyperplasia. The proportion of patients undergoing concurrent unilateral or bilateral oophorectomy increases with age; this procedure is done in approximately two thirds of women over the age of 60 years who undergo hysterectomy.[201] Radical hysterectomy, which entails removal of the uterus, fallopian tubes, and ovaries, as well as extensive stripping of the pelvic lymph nodes, is performed in patients with extension of cervical cancer.

Microbiology. The vagina is normally colonized with a wide variety of bacteria, including gram-positive and gram-negative aerobes and anaerobes. The normal flora of the vagina includes staphylococci, streptococci, enterococci, lactobacilli, diphtheroids, *E. coli*, anaerobic streptococci, *Bacteroides* species, and *Fusobacterium* species.[202-204] The vaginal flora changes during the menstrual cycle, which may affect the nature of postoperative infection.[202] Postoperative vaginal flora differs from preoperative flora; enterococci, gram-negative bacilli, and *Bacteroides* species increase postoperatively. Postoperative changes in flora may occur independently of prophylactic antimicrobial administration but are not by themselves predictive of postoperative infection.[203,205] Postoperative infections associated with vaginal hysterectomy are frequently polymicrobial, with enterococci, aerobic gram-negative bacilli, and *Bacteroides* species isolated most frequently. Postoperative wound infections following abdominal or radical hysterectomy are also polymicrobial; gram-positive cocci and enteric gram-negative bacilli predominate.[206,207]

Vaginal Hysterectomy. In a vaginal hysterectomy, the uterus and, occasionally, one or two fallopian tubes, the ovaries, or both, are removed through the vagina. No abdominal incision is made. Because the procedure is performed in an organ that is normally colonized with bacteria, it is associated with a higher risk of postoperative infection than is abdominal hysterectomy. The rate of postoperative infection (wound and pelvic sites) in women administered placebo or no prophylactic antimicrobials has generally fallen to between 17% and 40%, although it ranges from 12% to 78%.[208-261] A number of antimicrobial agents, including chloramphenicol, clindamycin, metronidazole, penicillin and tetracycline derivatives, streptomycin, and first-, second-, and third-generation cephalosporins, have been studied as perioperative prophylaxis for vaginal hysterectomy. Overall, the use of antimicrobials has markedly reduced the incidence of postoperative infection following vaginal hysterectomy to a generally acceptable rate of less than 10%.

The cephalosporins are used more frequently for prophylaxis in this procedure than any other class of drugs. Cefazolin has been associated with a postoperative infection rate ranging from 0% to 12%. Most recent studies have compared the efficacy of various second- and third-generation cephalosporins; postoperative infection rates have ranged between 0% and 16%. Studies directly comparing the newer second- or third-generation cephalosporins with cefazolin indicate that cefazolin is equivalent to the new agents in reducing the incidence of postoperative wound infections.[262-265]

The observation that *Bacteroides* species are commonly associated with infections following vaginal hysterectomy has prompted several investigators to study the efficacy of cephalosporins with enhanced anaerobic activity (cefmetazole, cefotetan, cefoxitin, ceftizoxime, and moxalactam) for perioperative prophylaxis. Postoperative infection rates associated with these agents have ranged from 0% to 15%.

The trend in recent years has been toward use of single-dose regimens of antimicrobials, administered immediately before surgery. Studies comparing single doses of one antimicrobial with multidose regimens of a different antimicrobial have shown the two regimens to be equally effective.

Abdominal Hysterectomy. Abdominal hysterectomy involves removal of the uterus and, in some cases, of one or both fallopian tubes, the ovaries, or both. Because bacterial contamination associated with this procedure is minimal, postoperative infection rates in women receiving no antimicrobial prophylaxis have generally been lower than those of women undergoing vaginal hysterectomy. The abdominal approach, however, takes more time, and this may predispose these patients to higher infection rates than patients undergoing vaginal hysterectomy with prophylaxis.[266] The need for antimicrobial prophylaxis in abdominal hysterectomy is controversial, although most obstetricians and gynecologists do currently employ prophylactic antimicrobials.

At least 25 placebo-controlled or no-antimicrobial-controlled studies have been performed in abdominal hysterectomy.[213,215,229,234-238,242,244,249,252,253,258,263,265,267-301] First- and second-generation cephalosporins and metronidazole have been studied more widely than any other agents. A meta-analysis recently demonstrated the general efficacy of antimicrobial prophylaxis for abdominal hysterectomy.[223] In this analysis, postoperative infection rates in the placebo group averaged 19.5%, whereas in women receiving prophylaxis the mean infection rate was 9.3%. A 24-hour regimen has been shown to be as effective as longer courses of prophylaxis, and many single-dose prophylaxis regimens have proved as effective as multiple-dose regimens.

The prophylactic efficacy of various cephalosporin regimens has recently been compared. Few comparisons have been made of second- and third-generation cephalosporins versus cefazolin; however, a number of second-generation cephalosporins have been compared. Single doses of cefotetan or cefotaxime appear to be as effective as multiple doses of cefoxitin.

Radical Hysterectomy. Many factors increase the risk of postoperative infection in women undergoing radical hysterectomy, including extended length of surgery, blood loss and replacement, presence of malignancy, prior radiation therapy, obesity, and presence of indwelling drainage catheters.[216,224] Nonetheless, because of the low degree of contamination associated with this procedure, the need for prophylaxis has not been definitively established. The use of prophylactic antimicrobials in radical hysterectomy has recently been reviewed by Hemsell.[217]

Six prospective, placebo-controlled trials have evaluated the impact of antimicrobial prophylaxis on wound infection following radical hysterectomy.[216,217,225-227,302,303] Rates of infection in the placebo groups ranged from 17% to 87%, whereas corresponding infection rates in antimicrobial-treated patients ranged from 0% to 15%. The incidence of postoperative infection was reduced in antimicrobial-treated patients in all of these trials. In one study, prophylaxis with cefamandole given by injection and by intraperitoneal irrigation reduced postoperative infection rates to less than 4%.[225] It should be noted, however, that other authors have noted similarly low infection rates in uncontrolled patient series and have been unable to recommend routine prophylaxis for radical hysterectomy.[226]

The optimal agent for and duration of antimicrobial prophylaxis for radical hysterectomy have not been determined; however, 24-hour regimens of mezlocillin or cefoperazone/sulbactam appear to be as effective as other antimicrobial regimens.[217,226] Antimicrobial prophylaxis is indicated for radical hysterectomy, and a 24-hour regimen is probably sufficient.

Recommendations. Infection is common in women who have undergone vaginal or abdominal hysterectomy without antimicrobial prophylaxis. Antimicrobial prophylaxis is indicated for all types of hysterectomy. Cefazolin is the drug of choice for surgical prophylaxis in vaginal hysterectomy. Although there have been few comparative trials involving single-dose cefazolin, clinical experience and the drug's relatively long serum half-life (1.8 hours) indicate that this regimen is effective for most women. A second dose of cefazolin may be administered if surgery lasts more than four hours. Single-dose regimens with cephalosporins such as cefazolin and cefotetan have been demonstrated to be as effective as multiple doses for abdominal hysterectomy. Extending antimicrobial prophylaxis beyond 24 hours for uncomplicated hysterectomy is unnecessary.

Neurosurgery

Clean neurosurgical procedures are those in which there is no break in surgical technique and no entry into the respiratory, gastrointestinal, or genitourinary tracts. Clean procedures usually carry a risk of postoperative wound infection of less than 5%, and in many hospitals the risk is 1–2%.[304] It is therefore understandable that the use of injectable antimicrobials in such procedures is quite controversial. In addition, it is difficult to design clinical trials that could distinguish between infection rates of 2% and 5%. A valid study would require placebo-controlled, randomized trials with at least 1000 patients in each study group.[305] Multicenter trials are usually required to accrue enough patients to avoid statistical errors.[306]

Among the clean neurosurgical procedures are elective craniotomies for the repair of aneurysms, correction of arteriovenous malformations, and removal of various types of brain tumors. There are major differences relating to such factors as immune status and nutrition between an individual who undergoes elective surgery for a nonmalignant condition and a patient with cancer; such variables make clinical trials difficult to assess. Some craniotomies for ruptured aneurysms must be done on an emergency basis, and meticulous preparation of the skin cannot be assured. Neurosurgical procedures following trauma occurring outside the hospital should never be included in comparative trials and would be considered contaminated surgery. Laminectomies (both with and without the use of the operating microscope) are performed by neurosurgeons, although in some centers this procedure is also performed by orthopedic surgeons. Many studies will include laminectomies as well as elective craniotomies in trials of clean neurosurgical procedures. The microscope introduces another variable (additional source of potential contamination) that should be taken into consideration. Ventricular-fluid shunting procedures (ventriculo-peritoneal shunts), performed to control increased intracranial pressure in patients with hydrocephalus, have also been included in some clinical trials of clean neurosurgical procedures. Since this procedure involves the placement of a foreign body (pressure-release valve and tubing) into the cranium, another variable is introduced. Most infectious-disease consultants believe that such shunting operations should be studied as a separate entity.[307] Ventricular-fluid shunting procedures are also performed following serious head trauma and in some elective craniotomy procedures to drain cerebrospinal fluid and lower intracranial pressure. The shunts are left in place for varying lengths of time, ranging from 48 hours to seven days. The rate of infection (usually ventriculitis) is generally reported to be between 5% and 20%.[308-310]

Data from most published clinical trials indicate that gram-positive bacteria are primarily associated with wound infections. *Staph. aureus* and coagulase-negative staphylococci are responsible for greater than 85% of such infections and are isolated in mixed cultures with other gram-positive bacteria in an additional 5–10% of cases. Gram-negative bacteria are isolated as the sole cause of postoperative neurosurgical wound infections in only 5–8% of cases.[311-317] Therefore most clinical trials of antimicrobial prophylaxis use a drug with primary activity against staphylococci. Drugs most frequently studied include clindamycin, erythromycin, penicillinase-stable penicillins (oxacillin, nafcillin, methicillin), first-generation cephalosporins, and vancomycin.

Clinical Trials. Before 1983, virtually all the published reports of antimicrobials used prophylactically in clean neurosurgery cases were based on uncontrolled, nonrandomized, retrospective studies.[311-313,318-322] These reports seem to favor some type of prophylactic regimen. In 1980, Haines[323] published an excellent review of these reports. He concluded that a final recommendation regarding antimicrobial prophylaxis in clean neurosurgical procedures must await the results of controlled clinical trials. In 1984, Geraghty and Feely[315] published the results of a randomized, nonblinded clinical trial reporting on 402 cases. The control group had a wound infection rate of 3.5%, versus 0% in the antimicrobial group. In 1986, Shapiro et al.[317] published a randomized, placebo-controlled, double-blind trial involving 148 neurosurgery cases. Operations included craniotomies, spinal surgery, and shunting procedures. The study was stopped prematurely because of an excess number of wound infections in the placebo group. The overall rate of infection was 2.8% in the antimicrobial group and 11.7% in the placebo group. Other publications involving retrospective chart reviews with large numbers of patients have also been published.[314,318,324,325] A neurosurgery group in the Netherlands performed a prospective, double-blind, placebo-controlled study of cloxacillin in craniotomy patients.[326] Postoperative infection rates in the cloxacillin group were 3.9% (6 of 156 patients) and in the placebo group 13% (20 of 154 patients). The difference was statistically significant ($p < 0.05$). Bullock et al.,[327] from South Africa, conducted a double-blind, placebo-controlled study in 417 patients undergoing clean elective neurosurgical procedures. Although the wound infection rate was significantly lower in the antimicrobial group than in the placebo group (2.0% versus 5.8%), the results of this study are questionable because the drug selected was piperacillin. This is an unusual choice for procedures where β-lactamase-producing staphylococci are the major bacteria causing wound infections. Piperacillin would not have stability against the β-lactamase produced by most staphylococci. Blomstedt and Kytta,[328] in a randomized study, used vancomycin in patients undergoing craniotomy with and without bone flaps. In comparison with groups of patients not receiving antimicrobials, only those patients with the bone-flap procedures demonstrated a reduction in postoperative infections after receiving vancomycin.

Postoperative central nervous system (CNS) shunt infections are a major complication associated with mortality and serious morbidity. Infections following surgery include meningitis, ventriculitis, and, less frequently, wound infections.[329] In most cases, antimicrobial therapy without shunt removal is not effective in eradicating the infecting organism.[330-335] Therefore, shunt removal or replacement, in addition to injectable antimicrobial therapy, is the preferred therapeutic modality. Staphylococci account for 75–80% of CNS and wound infections following shunting procedures. Gram-negative bacteria are responsible for only 10–20% of such infections.[336-344]

Because CNS infections following shunting procedures are responsible for substantial mortality and morbidity, especially in children, the possible role of prophylactic antimicrobials in such procedures has been the subject of numerous clinical trials.[345-353] Unfortunately, the majority of such trials have been neither randomized nor controlled, and many were retrospective. Reaching a conclusion about the effectiveness of prophylactic antimicrobials in shunting procedures is therefore difficult. Nonetheless, many neurosurgical services continue to use some type of prophylactic regimen. Further confusion exists because more than 50% of the time the isolated pathogen is a member of the coagulase-negative group of staphylococci. The majority of such isolates are methicillin resistant, which would make injectable vancomycin the only effective agent. Several trials using either intraventricular or i.v. vancomycin have failed to show a reduction in postoperative CNS infection rates.[328]

Recommendations. *Clean Neurosurgical Procedures: Elective Craniotomy and Laminectomy.* Although the effectiveness of antimicrobials in lowering postoperative wound infection rates following elective craniotomy and laminectomy has not been demonstrated in a single, large, pivotal clinical trial, there is enough evidence to suggest that a single dose of an antimicrobial, directed toward *Staph. aureus*, can be recommended. A single dose of cefazolin (1 g i.v. at the induction of anesthesia) appears to be the best choice. Alternatively, a single dose of one of the β-lactamase-stable penicillins might also be used (1 g of i.v. oxacillin or nafcillin). For elective procedures lasting longer than three hours, the dose of cefazolin should be repeated, and for procedures lasting more than two hours in which oxacillin or nafcillin has been used, the dose should likewise be repeated. In hospitals where methicillin-resistant *Staph. aureus* prevalence rates exceed 10%, the use of injectable vancomycin in a single-dose regimen is probably justified. Large-scale, randomized trials are needed to verify the need for prophylactic antimicrobials in clean neurosurgical procedures.

Cerebrospinal-Fluid Shunting Procedures. Meticulous surgical and aseptic technique and short operation time are important factors in lowering infection rates following shunt placement. The number of patients studied to date is small, and the results of trials do not lend support to the use of prophylactic antimicrobials. Therefore, antimicrobials cannot generally be recommended. However, clinicians must remember that the risk of Type II statistical errors in such studies is ever present.

Neurosurgeons who want to prescribe a single dose of an appropriate i.v. antimicrobial or to administer a dose of intraventricular antimicrobial through the shunt at the end of the procedure should be given the benefit of the doubt, provided that they understand the available research concerning such a practice. Unfortunately, because the majority of postoperative infections following shunting procedures are caused by methicillin-resistant, coagulase-negative staphylococci, the only reasonable drug at present is i.v. or intraventricular vancomycin.

Cardiothoracic Surgery

Approximately 600,000 cardiothoracic surgeries are performed annually in the United States.[354,355] Of these, 80% are coronary-artery bypass graft (CABG) procedures and 20% are heart-valve replacements. A relatively small number involve heart or heart–lung transplants and repair of congenital heart defects in children. Risk factors that predispose to infection following cardiothoracic surgery have been reviewed elsewhere.[355-358]

The selection, use, and efficacy of prophylactic antimicrobials for cardiothoracic surgery has been a source of controversy since the first study in this area was published in 1961 by Kittle and Reed,[359] who found no advantage to the administration of penicillin and streptomycin in a retrospective review of patients undergoing extracorporeal circulation for valve repair. At that time, antimicrobial prophylaxis was frequently not initiated until after surgery, and many surgeons believed it to be of no value.[359]

In 1963, Slonim[360] showed that patients undergoing open-heart surgery who had received penicillin and streptomycin had fewer infections than those who had received no antimicrobials. This evaluation was, however, performed retrospectively and was not randomized.

Two prospective, randomized, double-blind, placebo-controlled trials of cardiothoracic antimicrobial prophylaxis were published in the late 1960s.[361,362] These studies, which involved small numbers of patients who were primarily undergoing valve repair, found a modest benefit to the use of a semisynthetic penicillin or a combination of penicillin G and streptomycin in preventing postoperative wound infections.

The primary intent of early antimicrobial prophylaxis in open-heart surgery was to reduce the incidence of postoperative endocarditis following valve repair. Early studies showed that coagulase-positive and coagulase-negative staphylococci were the primary pathogens infecting prosthetic valves.[359-361] As a result, most early prophylactic regimens were directed against staphylococci, with semisynthetic penicillins and first-generation cephalosporins emerging as the drugs of choice.

With the advent of the CABG procedure and an expansion of the number of cardiothoracic procedures performed in the United States, the focus of prophylaxis has shifted to include a broader spectrum of gram-negative pathogens causing wound infections postoperatively, both at the sternal incision and the saphenous vein harvest sites.[361-364]

Clinical Trials. In 1979, a prospective, randomized, double-blind, placebo-controlled trial of antimicrobial prophylaxis for CABG confirmed the benefit of using a semisynthetic penicillin to prevent postoperative wound infection.[365] This study was terminated early because of a high incidence of postoperative wound infections in the placebo group, a finding that validated the ongoing practice of administering prophylactic antimicrobials for cardiothoracic surgery. Austin et al.[366] also terminated a double-blind, placebo-controlled study of cephalothin prophylaxis after 4 of the first 15 patients developed *Staph. aureus* sternal-wound infections. Penketh et al.[367] terminated a double-blind, placebo-controlled study evaluating cephradine after 12 of the first 22 placebo patients developed wound infections. Wound infection rates ranged from 9.1% to 54.5% in the placebo groups of these studies. Wound infection rates were reduced in all patient groups receiving antimicrobials; postoperative wound infection rates ranged from 0% to 6.7%. Postoperative wound infection rates since the routine administration of prophylactic antimicrobials for cardiothoracic surgeries have ranged from 0.8% to 25%.

The optimal duration of antimicrobial prophylaxis for cardiothoracic surgery has been addressed by four studies.[363,368-370] Cephalothin was the prophylactic cephalosporin in all four; in one study, it was combined with kanamycin. Doses and durations in the short groups ranged from a single 1-g-duration treatment dose of cephalothin to 2 g every six hours for two days. Long treatment regimens ranged from 2 g of cephalothin preoperatively followed by 1 g every six hours for three days to 2 g every six hours for six days. Two of the studies were performed before the development of the CABG procedure. Total wound infection rates were lower in the short-duration treatment groups in two of the four studies, although the differences were not statistically significant.

Cephalosporins were compared with antistaphylococcal penicillins as prophylactic agents in five studies. The antistaphylococcal penicillins were used in combination with another penicillin, an aminoglycoside, or both, in four of the five studies.[371-375] Four of the five studies revealed fewer total wound infections in the cephalosporin-treated patients; however, none of the results reached statistical significance.

Cephalothin was compared with the second-generation cephalosporins cefamandole or ceforanide in five studies, while cephradine was compared with cefamandole in one of these studies. Results from the six studies varied; no agent showed a significant advantage over the others.

Recently published trials comparing cefazolin, cefamandole, and cefuroxime as prophylactic antimicrobials for cardiothoracic surgery have shown a trend toward statistical significance in favor of the second-generation cephalosporins.[376-380] Total wound infection rates (sternal plus leg wound infection) ranged from 2.5% to 16.7% in cefazolin-treated patients and from 0% to 13.5% in cefamandole- or cefuroxime-treated patients. Total wound infection rates were lower in patients receiving the second-generation cephalosporin in seven of the eight comparison groups. Sternal wound infection rates were also reduced in seven of the eight treatment groups receiving either cefamandole or cefuroxime. Leg-wound infection rates were lower in five of the eight second-generation cephalosporin treatment groups. The study by Doebbeling et al.[380] demonstrated results that are contrary to those of the other studies, with cefuroxime-treated patients faring more poorly than cefazolin-treated patients with regard to sternal wound infections.

Two recent surveys by Woods[381,382] of antimicrobial prophylaxis practice in cardiothoracic surgery have shown that the choice of antimicrobials used for prophylaxis has changed in recent years to include the use of second-generation cephalosporins.

Cefamandole was compared directly with cefuroxime in two studies. Cefuroxime was associated with lower wound infection rates at sternal and leg sites in both studies, although the differences were not statistically significant. In both trials the total wound infection rate was less than 4%, and the study lacked sufficient power to distinguish a difference between treatment groups.[383]

Cefazolin was compared with ceftriaxone in two studies.[384,385] Cefazolin was associated with lower sternal and lower total wound infection rates in both studies, although the studies lacked statistical power to distinguish a significant difference between the two treatment groups.

Six other prospective, randomized, controlled studies of cardiothoracic prophylaxis have been performed. Kini et al.[386] compared cephalothin and cefazolin and found no differences in total wound infection rates. Pien et al.[387] compared cephalothin with clindamycin and found a nonstatistically significant reduction in both sternal and leg-wound infection rates in the clindamycin group. Geroulanos et al.[378] compared cefuroxime with ceftriaxone in 512 patients and found no differences in total wound infection rates. Kaiser et al.[377] compared cefazolin and cefamandole, both with the addition of gentamicin, and found a statistically significant reduction in sternal and total wound infection rates in the cefamandole/gentamicin group. Joyce and Szczepanski[388] compared penicillin G with vancomycin and found a significant reduction in total wound infections in the vancomycin group. Wilson et al.[389] evaluated 517 patients receiving teicoplanin, in two dosage regimens, or a combination of flucloxacillin and gentamicin. He found unacceptably high sternal-wound infection rates in the teicoplanin treatment group, although patients in the flucloxacillin/gentamicin groups also experienced high sternal-wound infection rates.

The postoperative infection rate in clean cardiothoracic surgeries is intrinsically low, and the degree of improvement of one regimen over another is relatively small. Antimicrobial prophylaxis in cardiothoracic surgery reduces the incidence of postoperative wound infection by fivefold when compared with placebo, to approximately 5%. On average, cefamandole and cefuroxime each reduced the incidence of wound infection by approximately 1.5-fold compared with cefazolin. Wound infections were not reduced in studies comparing cephalothin with either cefamandole or ceforanide, or when cefazolin was compared with ceftriaxone. Additionally, no differences in outcome were seen in studies comparing cefamandole with cefuroxime. No differences were found between short (single-dose to two-day) and long (three- to six-day) regimens. No differences were found between antistaphylococcal penicillin regimens (often used in combination with aminoglycosides or other penicillins) and single-agent first- or second-generation cephalosporin regimens.

The reduction in morbidity and mortality associated with postoperative wound infection is the most important result of antimicrobial prophylaxis in surgery. Financial constraints have led many individuals to reevaluate the use of antimicrobial prophylaxis. When the costs associated with the management of postoperative infection are factored into these calculations, the cost-effectiveness of prophylaxis becomes evident.[390,391]

Recommendations. Cephalosporins, as single agents, are at least as effective as combination regimens of antistaphylococcal penicillins and aminoglycosides, and are much easier to administer. Cephalothin and cefazolin have been the traditional cephalosporins of choice: however, cefamandole and cefuroxime have been shown to be slightly superior to cefazolin with regard to the overall incidence of postoperative wound infection. Further trials must be performed to confirm their superiority.

The frequency with which methicillin-resistant staphylococci have been recovered has increased steadily in recent years throughout the United States,[392,393] and one would predict that antistaphylococcal penicillins and cephalosporins might be ineffective in a patient colonized with this organism. Insufficient data exist regarding the prophylactic role of vancomycin in cardiothoracic surgery, either with or without an additional agent active against gram-negative pathogens.

It is recommended that cefazolin 1 g i.v. every 8 hours or cefuroxime 1.5 g i.v. every 12 hours be given for 48–72 hours, or until chest and mediastinal drainage tubes are removed. Cefamandole and cephalothin are suitable alternatives.

Insufficient data are available to document the appropriateness of cephalosporins in infants less than one month of age. Ampicillin (50 mg/kg every six hours for a total of four doses) and gentamicin (2.5 mg/kg every eight hours for a total of three doses) are generally used in this age group. Children older than one month should receive cefuroxime 50 mg/kg every eight hours for three doses.

Orthopedic Surgery

Postoperative wound infection is one of the more frequent complications of orthopedic surgery, and it often yields devastating results. Although early studies did not support the routine use of prophylactic antimicrobials,[394,395] these studies were flawed by an improper choice of agent(s), inappropriate dosage or route of administration, or failure to institute therapy until well beyond the time of the initial surgical incision. Later work has established that antimicrobial prophylaxis is indicated in some types of orthopedic procedures.[396-405] Antimicrobial prophylaxis will be discussed for total-joint-replacement surgery, repair of hip fractures, and clean orthopedic procedures. Open (compound) fractures are often associated with extensive wound contamination and are virtually always managed empirically with antimicrobial therapy as well as surgical debridement. This practice is viewed as treatment rather than prophylaxis.[406] The issue of whether patients with prosthetic joints who undergo dental, gastrointestinal, or genitourinary procedures should receive prophylaxis to reduce the likelihood of prosthesis infection has not been sufficiently studied, and no formal recommendations can be made at this time.

Organisms that make up the skin flora are the most frequent causes of postoperative infections in orthopedic surgery.[396-398,404] Gram-positive organisms such as *Staph. aureus*, *Staph. epidermidis*, and various streptococci, including enterococci, are responsible for more than two thirds of postoperative infections. Aerobic gram-negative bacilli (e.g., *E. coli*, *Proteus mirabilis*), anaerobes such as peptococci, and diphtheroids constitute the remainder of infecting organisms. The antimicrobials that have been studied most often for prophylaxis in orthopedic surgery include the antistaphylococcal penicillins and first-generation cephalosporins. First-generation cephalosporins (particularly cefazolin) are the most suitable agents for orthopedic prophylaxis, given their expanded spectrum, which includes gram-negative bacilli (such as *E. coli*), ease of administration, low cost, and safety. Second- and third-generation cephalosporins offer no major advantages over first-generation agents. Agents in the two former groups are more expensive; furthermore, indiscriminate use is likely to promote resistance, particularly to nosocomial gram-negative bacilli. Therefore, the use of second- and third-generation cephalosporins as surgical prophylaxis in orthopedic surgery should be avoided. In patients with serious β-lactam allergy, vancomycin is a suitable alternative agent for surgical prophylaxis.

Total Joint Replacement. The incidence of deep sepsis complicating joint replacements of the hip, knee, elbow, and shoulder is low, ranging from 0.6% to 11%.[396] With the introduction of prophylactic antimicrobials and the use of "ultraclean" operating rooms, the incidence of infection has declined substantially, generally to less than 1%.[396,399,400] The two main types of infectious complications of total joint arthroplasty are superficial wound infections and deep infections of the prosthesis. Deep sepsis of the joint prosthesis may occur as an early (less than one year after the procedure) or late (occurring after the first year) complication of joint-replacement surgery. Infection after joint arthroplasty can be disastrous, frequently requiring removal of the prosthesis and a prolonged course of antimicrobials for effective cure.

Clinical Trials. The majority of studies evaluating prophylactic antimicrobials in joint-replacement surgery have been conducted in patients undergoing total hip arthroplasty. Early double-blind, controlled trials demonstrated that 14 days of cloxacillin (given with probenecid) can significantly reduce the incidence of early and late infection.[397,398] Ericson et al.[397] reported 10 infections in 48 patients (17%) given placebo and none in those receiving cloxacillin, after a six-month period of follow-up. Carlsson et al.[398] found a 15% incidence of late, deep infection with no prophylaxis, compared with a 2% incidence with two weeks of cloxacillin prophylaxis in a total of 1065 hip-replacement procedures. Although these studies have been criticized because of the unusually high incidence of infection in the control group,[407] they demonstrate a clear-cut decrease in infectious complications with antistaphylococcal prophylaxis.

Hill et al.[399] evaluated the efficacy of prophylactic cefazolin in a double-blind, randomized, placebo-controlled trial involving 2137 hip replacements in 2097 patients. Cefazolin 1 g was given before surgery and continued every six hours for a total of five days. After a two-year follow-up period, "hip infection" was encountered in 3.3% of patients given placebo and in 0.9% of patients who received cefazolin ($p < 0.001$). When these results were further analyzed for the type of operating-room environment, a significant difference was observed only when surgery was carried out in a conventional operating room. Antimicrobial prophylaxis did not significantly reduce infection when hip-replacement surgery was performed in a "hypersterile" (laminar-airflow) operating room (1.3% with placebo versus 0.8% with cefazolin). This study was well designed in that sufficient numbers of patients were enrolled to avoid making either Type I or Type II errors in terms of the efficacy of prophylaxis.

The impact of ultraclean operating rooms on deep sepsis following joint-replacement surgery was further evaluated by Lidwell et al.,[400] in more than 8000 hip or knee operations. A significant decrease in deep infection was observed with the use of ultraclean operating rooms compared with conventional rooms (0.6% versus 1.5%, respectively). Although not strictly controlled in this study, the use of prophylactic antimicrobials (primarily flucloxacillin) was associated with a further reduction in the rate of deep infection of the prosthesis ($p < 0.01$).[400]

The issue of duration of prophylaxis was addressed by Pollard et al.,[401] who compared three 1-g i.m. doses of cephaloridine with a two-week course of flucloxacillin (500 mg i.m. for 24 hours, then orally thereafter) in a randomized trial of 297 patients. Wound infection developed in 1.7% of these patients; deep infections, 1.3%. Both occurred with equal frequency in the two treatment groups.

Taken together, the above studies suggest that a short course of antimicrobial prophylaxis can significantly reduce the incidence of postoperative infection in joint-replacement surgery, particularly of late, deep-seated infection. Although infectious complications are infrequent, the consequences of an infected joint prosthesis can be devastating. The use of ultraclean operating rooms has been shown to significantly reduce the incidence of deep sepsis after joint-replacement surgery, regardless of whether antimicrobials are also given.[399,400] Because such operating environments are not widely available, prophylactic administration of antimicrobials with activity directed primarily against *Staph. aureus* is indicated in patients undergoing joint-replacement surgery.

Recommendations. All patients undergoing total hip, elbow, knee, and shoulder arthroplasty should be given cefazolin 1 g i.v. immediately before surgery. Treatment should be continued every eight hours for a total of three doses. A longer prophylactic regimen does not further reduce the incidence of infection but may increase the likelihood of adverse effects. Patients with β-lactam allergy should be given vancomycin 15 mg/kg i.v. just before surgery. Therapy should be continued every 12 hours for two additional doses.

Repair of Hip Fractures. Because repair of hip fractures often involves internal fixation using foreign bodies such as nails, screws, plates, and wires, postoperative infection can produce extensive morbidity. Consequently, antimicrobial prophylaxis has become an accepted practice, even though the incidence of infection following hip fracture repairs is less than 5%.

Clinical Trials. The value of antimicrobial prophylaxis in hip-fracture repair has been studied in three double-blind, randomized, placebo-controlled trials. Boyd et al.[402] found postoperative wound infections in 7 of 145 patients (4.8%) receiving placebo and in 1 of 135 patients (0.8%) given nafcillin 0.5 g i.m. every six hours for two days ($p = 0.04$; one-tailed t test). The authors failed to detect a difference in the incidence of infected wound hematomas between the two groups.[402] It has been argued that had Boyd et al. used a two-tailed test, the p value would become 0.08, which is not statistically significant.[407] Given the authors' hypothesis that antimicrobial prophylaxis is likely to result only in a reduction in postoperative infection (as opposed to a possible increase in the incidence of infection), the use of a one-tailed test seems appropriate. In another study involving 307 patients, Burnett et al.[403] reported major postoperative wound infections in 4.7% of patients given placebo versus 0.7% of those given cephalothin 1 g i.v. on call to the operating room and every 4 hours for 72 hours thereafter ($p < 0.05$). Burnett et al. observed a trend toward colonization with cephalothin-resistant organisms in patients who received this drug as a prophylactic measure. Tengve et al.[404] compared no antimicrobial prophylaxis with cephalothin 2 g i.v. preoperatively and intraoperatively and continued every six hours for two days in 140 patients undergoing repair of trochanteric femur fractures. Patients receiving cephalothin were switched to cephalexin 1 g orally every six hours once they were able to take medication by mouth. Postoperative wound infections occurred in 12 of 71 patients (16.9%) given no prophylaxis and in 1 of 56 patients (1.8%) given cephalothin. Validity of this study may be questionable because of the small number of patients enrolled and the unusually high incidence of wound infections occurring in the control group. Nonetheless, results from the above three studies, taken together, support the efficacy of short-term prophylactic antimicrobials in reducing the incidence of postoperative wound infection in patients undergoing hip-fracture repair. The long-term benefits of prophylaxis have not been determined.

Recommendations. Patients undergoing repair of hip fractures, particularly those in whom nails, plates, or screws are to be used, should receive short-term prophylaxis using an agent with activity directed primarily against staphylococci. Intravenous cefazolin 1 g i.v. should be initiated before surgery and continued every eight hours for no more than 48 to 72 hours. Although cephalothin was used in two of the three studies cited above, cefazolin is preferred because it achieves better bone penetration[406] and higher and more sustained serum concentrations, causes less venous irritation, is more convenient to administer, and, in many cases, is more cost-effective. Second- and third-generation cephalosporins should not be used as prophylaxis in hip-fracture repairs. Patients with allergy to β-lactams should receive vancomycin at the dosages recommended for joint-replacement surgery.

Clean Orthopedic Procedures. The necessity for prophylactic antimicrobials for clean orthopedic procedures is not well established.[405,408] Included in this category are knee, hand, and foot surgery, and laminectomy, with and without fusion. These procedures are considered clean and do not normally involve the implantation of foreign materials. The risk of infection and long-term sequelae is therefore quite low. The risk of infection must be weighed against the cost and the potentially toxic effects of antimicrobial therapy before prophylaxis can be routinely recommended.

Clinical Trials. The most extensive investigation of the efficacy of antimicrobial prophylaxis in clean orthopedic procedures was performed in the early 1970s by Pavel et al.[405] In a randomized, double-blind, prospective study, these authors compared the efficacy of cephaloridine with that of placebo in reducing postoperative wound infection in more than 1500 patients. The incidence of infection was 5% with placebo and 2.8% with perioperative cephaloridine ($p = 0.025$). It was not until more than 1500 cases were assessed that a statistically significant difference between the treatment and control groups was seen.[405] Drug fever (loosely defined as fever occurring in any patient on the days he or she received the study drug) was noted in 34 antimicrobial-treated patients and in 14 patients in the placebo group ($p = 0.06$).

Given the small difference in infection rates between the groups and the lack of significant long-term sequelae associated with these procedures, many authorities have questioned the necessity for prophylactic antimicrobials. Attempts to correlate the incidence of infection with specific types of clean orthopedic procedures or with certain patient characteristics (e.g., age, disease state) have been unsuccessful. While one recent study has suggested that prophylaxis (with cefamandole) is more effective than placebo when procedures last longer than two hours,[408] these results were not supported by those observed by Pavel et al.,[405] whose series was much larger.

Recommendations. Antimicrobial prophylaxis is not

recommended for patients undergoing clean orthopedic procedures. The low incidence of infection, coupled with the absence of serious morbidity as a consequence of postoperative infection, does not justify the expense and potential for toxicity associated with routine use of antimicrobial prophylaxis in this setting.

Vascular Surgery

Infection following peripheral vascular surgery often is associated with extensive morbidity and mortality. Postoperative infection is particularly devastating if it involves the vascular-graft material. As a result, antimicrobial prophylaxis is widely used with surgical revascularization.[409]

Clinical Trials. In the first controlled study of antimicrobial prophylaxis in peripheral vascular surgery, Kaiser and colleagues[410] administered cefazolin intravenously on call and then every six hours for four doses. If the surgical procedure was longer than four hours, an additional 500-mg dose was administered. Only 2 of 225 patients (0.9%) who were given prophylaxis developed wound infection, compared with 16 of 237 (6.8%) in the control group. This difference was statistically significant. Four deep graft infections were observed in the control group; none occurred in the patients who received cefazolin. No infections were observed among 103 patients who underwent brachiocephalic procedures. Cefazolin-susceptible *Staph. aureus* was the predominant pathogen; however, gram-negative aerobic bacilli, coagulase-negative staphylococci, and enterococci were also isolated.

In a subsequent trial,[411] i.v. cephradine, topical cephradine, or both were compared with placebo in patients undergoing peripheral vascular surgery. Patients were randomly divided into four groups in the following manner: group 1, no antimicrobial; group 2, topical cephradine instilled in the incision before closure; group 3, a 24-hour perioperative course of i.v. cephradine; and group 4, topical and i.v. cephradine. Groups 2 through 4 had significantly fewer wound infections than did the control group. No infections were noted in patients receiving an i.v. or a topical drug; however, 3 of 51 patients in group 4 became infected. Thirteen of those patients receiving no antimicrobial (24.5%) developed wound infections. Ten of 16 infected patients grew *Staph. aureus*. *E. coli* and other gram-negative bacilli infrequently were associated with infection.

Patients undergoing vascular-access surgery for hemodialysis also benefit from the administration of antistaphylococcal antimicrobials. Perioperative cefamandole (1 g i.v. before surgery and every six hours for three doses) was compared with placebo in patients receiving placement of polytetrafluoroethylene vascular-access grafts.[412] Two of 19 cefamandole-treated patients became infected, compared with 8 of 19 placebo patients. This difference was statistically significant.

The duration of antimicrobial prophylaxis was investigated by Hasselgren et al.[413] Cefuroxime 1.5 g i.v. every eight hours was administered for either one or three days after surgery. The control group received placebo. The incidence of wound infection in control patients was 16.7%, versus 3.8% and 4.3% in the one- and three-day groups, respectively. The difference in the incidence of infection between the latter two groups was not significant, and the authors concluded that no benefit is derived from continuing prophylaxis for more than 24 hours in patients undergoing surgery of the lower abdominal vasculature. *Staph. aureus* was the dominant pathogen; however, *Staph. epidermidis* and occasional aerobic gram-negative bacilli were also isolated.

Recommendations. Prophylactic antimicrobials are efficacious in decreasing the rate of infection after vascular procedures involving the lower abdominal vasculature and procedures required for dialysis access. Patients undergoing brachiocephalic procedures do not appear to benefit from antimicrobial prophylaxis. Considering that second-generation cephalosporins (cefamandole, cefuroxime) have not been shown to be superior to first-generation agents (cefazolin, cephradine), the latter are recommended. Because of its long half-life, cefazolin is recommended over shorter-acting agents. Cefazolin 1 g (30 mg/kg for children) i.v. should be administered at the induction of anesthesia and every eight hours for 24 hours. Prolongation of prophylaxis for more than 24 postoperative hours is unnecessary. For patients with a history of an accelerated reaction to β-lactam agents, vancomycin is recommended.

Urological Surgery

The potential benefit of antimicrobial prophylaxis in urological surgery has been investigated in many clinical trials, particularly in patients undergoing transurethral resection of the prostate.[414-428] Many patients with resection of bladder tumors[429] have also been studied. A wide range of antimicrobial regimens, including cephalosporins,[415,417,419,421,423,425,426,429] aminoglycosides,[414,420,427,428] carbenicillin,[416,418] trimethoprim–sulfamethoxazole,[419,422] and nitrofurantoin,[424] has been used in these trials.

The most common infectious complication after urological procedures is bacteriuria, the incidence of which has varied from 0% to 54% in reported studies. More serious infection, including bacteremia, is rare after transurethral resection of the prostate. In general, *E. coli* is most commonly isolated in patients with postoperative bacteriuria; however, other gram-negative bacilli and enterococci also cause infection.

Considering that bacteriuria is the most common postoperative infection after urological surgery, it is important to emphasize certain points. First, in order to determine the effectiveness of antimicrobial prophylaxis, one must be certain that the urine was sterile before surgery. Patients with preoperative bacteriuria must be considered infected, and the use of antimicrobials becomes therapeutic rather than prophylactic. Second, since these patients are routinely catheterized, one must question whether postoperative bacteriuria has been caused by the catheter or the surgical procedure. Furthermore, the length of postoperative catheterization, mode of irrigation (closed versus open), and other factors must be incorporated into the analysis of the effectiveness of antimicrobial prophylaxis.

A review of the literature reveals that antimicrobials generally have not been found to decrease the incidence of postoperative bacteriuria when infection rates are less than 15%.[415-418] When the incidence of infection is greater than 20%, however, a marked antimicrobial effect has been observed.[420-422,424-428] Considering the low rate of serious postoperative infection, it is not surprising that prophylactic antimicrobials have not been shown to decrease the incidence of bacteremia.

The results of these studies suggest that no single antimicrobial regimen is superior to another. Broad-spectrum antimicrobials, such as aminoglycosides or second- and third-generation cephalosporins, are no more effective than first-generation cephalosporins or oral agents (trimethoprim–sulfamethoxazole, nitrofurantoin). Although a large number of the trials continued prophylaxis for up to three weeks postoperatively,[414,416,418,420-422,424,426] the most recent studies suggest that continuation of prophylaxis after the preoperative dose is unnecessary.[425,427,428]

Recommendations. Considering the low risk of serious infection after urological surgery, antimicrobial prophylaxis should be considered only in those patients considered to be at high risk of postoperative bacteriuria (e.g., those with prolonged postoperative catheterization) or in hospitals with infection rates of greater than 20%. Low-risk patients do not appear to benefit from the use of perioperative antimicrobials. If oral antimicrobials are used, a single dose of trimethoprim–sulfamethoxazole or cephalexin (or cephradine) 500 mg within two hours of surgery should be administered. If an injectable agent is recommended, cefazolin 1 g i.v. (30 mg/kg for pediatric patients), administered at the induction of anesthesia, is recommended. Continuation of antimicrobial prophylaxis postoperatively is not recommended.

---

[a]Dosages of ampicillin sodium, ampicillin trihydrate, cefamandole nafate, cefazolin sodium, cefmetazole sodium, cefoperazone sodium, cefotaxime sodium, cefotetan disodium, cefoxitin sodium, ceftizoxime sodium, cefuroxime sodium, cephalexin hydrochloride, cephalothin sodium, clindamycin phosphate, gentamicin sulfate, moxalactam disodium, nafcillin sodium, oxacillin sodium, piperacillin sodium, and vancomycin hydrochloride are expressed in terms of base. Salt forms are specified in the text and table only when dosage is expressed in terms of salt.

References

1. Platt R, Zaleznik DF, Hopkins CC et al. Perioperative antibiotic prophylaxis for herniorrhaphy and breast surgery. *N Engl J Med*. 1990; 322:153-60.
2. Kernodle DS, Classen DC, Burke JP et al. Failure of cephalosporins to prevent *Staphylococcus aureus* surgical wound infection. *JAMA*. 1990; 263:961-6.
3. Ariano RE, Zhanel GG. Antimicrobial prophylaxis in coronary bypass surgery: a critical appraisal. *DICP*. 1991; 25:478-84.
4. Robbins KT, Favrot S, Hanna D et al. Risk of wound infection in patients with head and neck cancer. *Head Neck*. 1990; (Mar/Apr):143-8.
5. Tabet JC, Johnson JT. Wound infection in head and neck surgery: prophylaxis, etiology and management. *J Otolaryngol*. 1990; 3:143-8.
6. Tramont EC. Host defense mechanisms. In: Mandell GL, Douglas RG, Bennett JE, eds. Principles and practice of infectious disease. 3rd ed. New York: Churchill; 1990:33-6.
7. Becker GD, Welch WD. Quantitative bacteriology of closed-suction wound drainage in contaminated surgery. *Laryngoscope*. 1990; 100:403-6.
8. Johnson JT, Yu VL. Role of aerobic gram-negative rods, anaerobes, and fungi in wound infection after head and neck surgery: implications for antibiotic prophylaxis. *Head Neck*. 1989; (Jan/Feb):27-9.
9. Rubin J, Johnson JT, Wagner RL et al. Bacteriologic analysis of wound infection following major head and neck surgery. *Arch Otolaryngol Head Neck Surg*. 1988; 114:969-72.
10. Brown BM, Johnson JT, Wagner RL. Etiologic factors in head and neck wound infections. *Laryngoscope*. 1987; 97:587-90.
11. Johnson JT, Yu VL, Myers EN et al. An assessment of the need for gram-negative bacterial coverage in antibiotic prophylaxis for oncological head and neck surgery. *J Infect Dis*. 1987; 155:331-3.
12. Atkinson BA. Species incidence, trends of susceptibility to antibiotics in the United States, and minimum inhibitory concentration. In: Lorian V, ed. Antibiotics in laboratory medicine. Baltimore: Williams & Wilkins; 1980:607-722.
13. Johnson JT, Wagner RL. Infection following uncontaminated head and neck surgery. *Arch Otolaryngol Head Neck Surg*. 1987; 113:368-9.
14. Brand B, Johnson JT, Myers EN et al. Prophylactic perioperative antibiotics in contaminated head and neck surgery. *Otolaryngol Head Neck Surg*. 1982; 90:315-8.
15. Mandell-Brown M, Johnson JT, Wagner RL. Cost-effectiveness of prophylactic antibiotics in head and neck surgery. *Otolaryngol Head Neck Surg*. 1984; 92:520-3.
16. Johnson JT, Yu VL, Myers EN et al. Efficacy of two third-generation cephalosporins in prophylaxis for head and neck surgery. *Arch Otolaryngol*. 1984; 110:224-7.
17. Johnson JT, Yu VL, Myers EN et al. Cefazolin vs moxalactam? A double blind randomized trial of cephalosporins in head and neck surgery. *Arch Otolaryngol Head Neck Surg*. 1986; 112:151-3.
18. Anon. Antimicrobial prophylaxis in surgery. *Med Lett Drugs Ther*. 1989; 31:105-8.
19. Gerard M, Meunier F, Dor P et al. Antimicrobial prophylaxis for major head and neck surgery in cancer patients. *Antimicrob Agents Chemother*. 1988; 32:1557-9.
20. Cuchural GJ, Tally FP, Macobus NV et al. Comparative activities of new beta-lactam agents against members of the *Bacteroides fragilis* group. *Antimicrob Agents Chemother*. 1990; 34:479-80.
21. Dor P, Klastersky J. Prophylactic antibiotics in oral pharyngeal and laryngeal surgery for cancer: a double-blind study. *Laryngoscope*. 1973; 83:1992-8.
22. Dor P, Klastersky J. Etude comparative de la ticarcillin et de la carbenicillin comme traitement prophylactique associé à la chirurgie carcinologique cervico-faciale. *Acta Chir*. 1976; 75:129-33.
23. Mombelli G, Coppens L, Dor P et al. Antibiotic prophylaxis in surgery for head and neck cancer. Comparative study of short and prolonged administration of carbenicillin. *J Antimicrob Chemother*. 1981; 7:665-7.

24. VanLaethem Y, Lagast H, Klastersky J. Anaerobic infections in cancer patients—comparison between therapy oriented strictly against anaerobes or both anaerobes and aerobes. *J Antimicrob Chemother*. 1982; 10:137-40.
25. Johnson JT, Meyers EN, Thearle PB et al. Antimicrobial prophylaxis for contaminated head and neck surgery. *Laryngoscope*. 1984; 94:46-51.
26. Saginur R, Odell PF, Poliquin JF. Antibiotic prophylaxis in head and neck cancer surgery. *J Otolaryngol*. 1988; 17:78-80.
27. Robbins KT, Byers RM, Fainstein V et al. Wound prophylaxis with metronidazole in head and neck surgical oncology. *Laryngoscope*. 1988; 98:803-6.
28. Gehanno P, Noisy N, Guedon C. Cefotaxime in the prophylaxis of otorhinolaryngological cancer surgery. *Drugs*. 1988; 35(Suppl 2):111-5.
29. Polk HC. Diminished surgical infection by systemic antibiotic administration in potentially contaminated operations. *Surgery*. 1974; 75:312-4.
30. Stone HH, Hooper CA, Kolb LD et al. Antibiotic prophylaxis in gastric, biliary and colonic surgery. *Ann Surg*. 1976; 184:443-52.
31. Renvall S, Nikoski J, Aho AJ. Wound infection in abdominal surgery. *Acta Chir Scand*. 1980; 146:25-30.
32. Cunha BA, Pyrtek LJ, Quintiliani R. Prophylactic antibiotic in cholecystectomy. *Lancet*. 1978; 2:207-8.
33. Strachan CJL, Black J, Powis SJA et al. Prophylactic use of cephazolin against wound sepsis after cholecystectomy. *Br Med J*. 1977; 1:1254-6.
34. McLeish AR, Keighley MRB, Bishop HM. Selecting patients requiring antibiotics in biliary surgery by immediate gram stains of bile at surgery. *Surgery*. 1977; 81:473-7.
35. Reiss R, Eliasive A, Deutsch A. Septic complication and bile culture in 800 consecutive cholecystectomies. *World J Surg*. 1982; 6:195-9.
36. Cainzos M, Potel J, Puente JL. Prospective randomized controlled study of prophylaxis with cefamandole in high risk patients undergoing operations upon the biliary tract. *Surg Gynecol Obstet*. 1985; 160:27-32.
37. Elliot DW. Biliary tract surgery. *South Med J*. 1977; 70(Suppl 1):31-4.
38. Chetlin SH, Elliot DW. Preoperative antibiotics in biliary surgery. *Arch Surg*. 1973; 107:319-23.
39. Berne TV, Yellin AE, Appleman MD et al. Controlled comparison of cefmetazole with cefoxitin for prophylaxis in elective cholecystectomy. *Surg Gynecol Obstet*. 1990; 170:137-40.
40. Wilson SE, Hopkins JA, Williams RA. A comparison of cefotaxime versus cefamandole in prophylaxis for surgical treatment of the biliary tract. *Surg Gynecol Obstet*. 1987; 164:207-12.
41. Kujath P. Brief report: Antibiotic prophylaxis in biliary tract surgery. *Am J Med*. 1989; 87(Suppl 5A):255-7.
42. Nanavati AL, Singer JA. Routine bile cultures during cholecystectomy. *Infect Surg*. 1977; 6:523-6.
43. Garibaldi RA, Skolnck D, Maglio S et al. Postcholecystectomy wound infection. *Ann Surg*. 1986; 204:650-4.
44. Levi JU, Martinez OV, Hutson DG et al. Ampicillin versus cefamandole in biliary tract surgery. *Am Surg*. 1984; 50:412-7.
45. Kellum JM, Duma RJ, Gorbach SL et al. Single-dose antibiotic prophylaxis for biliary surgery. *Arch Surg*. 1987; 122:918-22.
46. Muller EL, Pitt HA, Thompson JE et al. Antibiotics in infections of the biliary tract. *Surg Gynecol Obstet*. 1987; 165:285-92.
47. Meijer WS, Schmitz PIM, Jeeke J. Meta-analysis of randomized, controlled clinical trials of antibiotic prophylaxis in biliary tract surgery. *Br J Surg*. 1990; 77:282-90.
48. Kellum JM, Gargano S, Gorbach SL et al. Antibiotic prophylaxis in high-risk biliary operations: multicenter trial of single preoperative ceftriaxone versus multidose cefazolin. *Am J Surg*. 1984; 148:15-21.
49. Drumm J, Donovan IA, Wise R. A comparison of cefotetan and cephazolin for prophylaxis against wound infection after elective cholecystectomy. *J Hosp Infect*. 1985; 6:227-80.
50. Plouffe JF, Perkins RL, Fass RJ et al. Comparison of the effectiveness of moxalactam and cefazolin in the prevention of infection in patients undergoing abdominal operations. *Diagn Microbiol Infect Dis*. 1985; 3:25-31.
51. Crenshaw CA, Glanges E, Webber CE et al. A prospective randomized, double blind study of preventive cefamandole therapy in patients at high risk for undergoing cholecystectomy. *Surg Gynecol Obstet*. 1981; 153:546-52.
52. Leaper DJ, Cooper MJ, Turner A. A comparative trial between cefotetan and cephazolin for wound sepsis prophylaxis during elective upper gastrointestinal surgery with an investigation of cefotetan penetration into the obstructed biliary tree. *J Hosp Infect*. 1986; 7:269-76.
53. Hurlow RA, Strachan CJL, Wise R et al. A comparative study of the efficacy of cefuroxime for preventing wound sepsis after cholecystectomy. International Congress and Symposium series: Royal Society of Medicine. 1981: 1-8.
54. Maki DG, Lammers JL, Aughey DR. Comparative studies of multidose cefoxitin vs single dose cefonicid for surgical prophylaxis in patients undergoing biliary tract operations or hysterectomy. *Rev Infect Dis*. 1984; 6(Suppl):887-95.
55. Roufail WM. Comparison of cefonicid and cefoxitin for prophylaxis in biliary tract surgery. *Adv Ther*. 1985; 2:225-32.
56. Fabian TC, Zellner SR, Gazzaniga A et al. Multicenter open trial of cefotetan in elective biliary surgery. *Am J Surg*. 1988; 155:77-80.
57. Garcia-Rodriguez JA, Puig-LaCalle J, Arnau C et al. Antibiotic prophylaxis with cefotaxime in gastroduodenal and biliary surgery. *Am J Surg*. 1989; 158:428-32.
58. Lewis RT, Allan CM, Goodall RG et al. A single preoperative dose of cefazolin prevents postoperative sepsis in high-risk biliary surgery. *Dis Colon Rectum*. 1984; 27:44-7.
59. Targarona EM, Garau J, Munoz-Ramos C et al. Single-dose antibiotic prophylaxis in patients at high risk for infection in biliary surgery: a prospective and randomized study comparing cefonicid with mezlocillin. *Surgery*. 1990; 107:327-34.
60. Nichols RL, Webb WR, Jones JW et al. Efficacy of antibiotic prophylaxis in high risk gastroduodenal operations. *Am J Surg*. 1982; 143:94-8.
61. Stone HH. Gastric surgery. *South Med J*. 1977; 70(Suppl 1):35-7.
62. Morris DL, Yound D, Burdon DW et al. Prospective randomized trial of single dose cefuroxime against mezlocillin in elective gastric surgery. *J Hosp Infect*. 1984; 5:200-4.
63. Lewis RT, Allan CM, Goodall RG et al. Discriminate use of antibiotic prophylaxis in gastroduodenal surgery. *Am J Surg*. 1979; 138:640-3.
64. Pories WJ, Van Rij AM, Burlingham BT et al. Prophylactic cefazolin in gastric bypass surgery. *Surgery*. 1981; 90:426-32.
65. Ruddell WSJ, Axon ATR, Findlay JM et al. Effect of cimetidine on the gastric bacterial flora. *Lancet*. 1980; 1:672-4.
66. LoCiero J, Nichols RL. Sepsis after gastroduodenal operations; relationship to gastric acid, motility, and endogenous microflora. *South Med J*. 1980; 73:878-80.
67. Gorbach SL, Plaut AG, Nahas L et al. Studies of intestinal microflora: II. Microorganisms of the small intestine and their relations to oral fecal flora. *Gastroenterology*. 1967; 53:856-67.
68. Gorbach SL. Intestinal microflora. *Gastroenterology*. 1971; 60:1110-29.
69. Lewis RT, Allan CM, Goodall RG et al. Cefamandole in gastroduodenal surgery: a controlled prospective, randomized, double-blind study. *Can J Surg*. 1982; 25:561-3.
70. Polk HC, Lopez-Mayor JF. Postoperative wound infection: a prospective study of determinant factors and prevention. *Surgery*. 1969; 66:97-103.

71. Evans C, Pollock AV. The reduction of surgical wound infections by prophylactic parenteral cephaloridine. *Br J Surg*. 1973; 60:434-7.
72. Stone HH, Haney BB, Kolb LD et al. Prophylactic and preventive antibiotic therapy. *Ann Surg*. 1979; 189:691-9.
73. Mitchell NJ, Evans DS, Pollock D. Pre-operative, single-dose cefuroxime antimicrobial prophylaxis with and without metronidazole in elective gastrointestinal surgery. *J Antimicrob Chemother*. 1980; 6:393-9.
74. Hares MM, Hegarty MA, Warlow J et al. A controlled trial to compare systemic and intra-incisional cefuroxime prophylaxis in high risk gastric surgery. International Congress and Symposium series: Royal College of Medicine. 1981:9-15.
75. Brown JJ, Mutton TP, Wasilauskas BL et al. Prospective, randomized, controlled trial of ticarcillin and cephalothin as prophylactic antibiotics for gastrointestinal operations. *Am J Surg*. 1982; 143:343-8.
76. Polk HC, Trachtenberg L, George CD. A randomized, double-blind trial of single dose piperacillin versus multidose cefoxitin in alimentary tract operations. *Am J Surg*. 1986; 152:517-21.
77. Svensson LG. Prophylactic antibiotic administration. *S Afr J Surg*. 1985; 23:55-62.
78. Polk H, Lopez-Meyer J. Postoperative wound infection: a prospective study of determinant factors and prevention. *Surgery*. 1969; 66:97-103.
79. Burton RC. Postoperative wound infection in colon and rectal surgery. *Br J Surg*. 1973; 60:363-8.
80. Bartlett J, Condon R, Gorbach S et al. Veterans Administration Cooperative Study on bowel preparation for elective colorectal operations: impact of oral antibiotic regimen on colonic flora, wound irrigation cultures and bacteriology of septic complications. *Ann Surg*. 1978; 188:249-54.
81. Clarke J, Condon R, Bartlett J et al. Preoperative oral antibiotics reduce septic complications of colon operations: results of a prospective randomized, double-blind clinical study. *Ann Surg*. 1977; 186:251-9.
82. Nichols RL. Prophylaxis for elective bowel surgery. In: Wilson SE, Williams RA, Finegold S, eds. Intra-abdominal infections. New York: McGraw Hill; 1982:267-85.
83. Davis G. Santa Ana C, Morawiski S et al. Development of a lavage solution associated with minimal water and electrolyte absorption or secretion. *Gastroenterology*. 1980; 78:991-5.
84. Beck D, Harford F, DiPalma JA. Comparison of cleansing methods in preparation for colon surgery. *Dis Colon Rectum*. 1985; 28:491-5.
85. Jagelman D, Fazio V, Lavery I et al. Single dose piperacillin versus cefoxitin combined with 10 percent mannitol bowel preparation as prophylaxis in elective colorectal operations. *Am J Surg*. 1987; 154:478-81.
86. Wolff B, Beart R, Dozios R et al. A new bowel preparation for elective colon and rectal surgery: a prospective, randomized clinical trial. *Arch Surg*. 1988; 123:895-900.
87. Garlock JH, Seely GP. The use of sulfanilamide in surgery of the rectum and colon. *Surgery*. 1939; 5:787-90.
88. Baum M, Anish D, Chalmers T et al. A survey of clinical trials of antibiotic prophylaxis in colon surgery: evidence against further use of no treatment controls. *N Engl J Med*. 1981; 305:795-9.
89. Bartlett S, Burton R. Effects of prophylactic antibiotics on wound infection after elective colon and rectal surgery. *Am J Surg*. 1983; 145:300-9.
90. Chodak GW, Plaut ME. Use of systemic antibiotics for prophylaxis in surgery. *Arch Surg*. 1977; 112:326-34.
91. Berger SA, Nager H, Weitzman S. Prophylactic antibiotics in surgical procedures. *Surg Gynecol Obstet*. 1978; 146:469-75.
92. Evans M, Pollock AV. The inadequacy of published random control trials of antibacterial prophylaxis in colorectal surgery. *Dis Colon Rectum*. 1987; 30:743-6.
93. National Research Council, National Academy of Sciences. Postoperative wound infections: the influence of ultraviolet irradiation on the operating room and on various other factors. *Ann Surg*. 1965; 160(Suppl):1-192.
94. Cruse PJ, Foord R. The epidemiology of wound infection: a ten-year prospective study of 62,939 wounds. *Surg Clin North Am*. 1980; 60:27-40.
95. Nichols RL. Prophylaxis for intraabdominal surgery. *Rev Infect Dis*. 1984; 6(Suppl 1):276-82.
96. Condon RE. Preoperative antibiotic bowel preparation. *Drug Therapy*. 1983; (Jan):29-37.
97. Washington J, Dearing W, Judd E et al. Effect of preoperative antibiotic regimen on development of infection after intestinal surgery. *Ann Surg*. 1974; 180:567-72.
98. Nichols R, Condon R, Gorbach S et al. Efficacy of preoperative antimicrobial preparation of the bowel. *Ann Surg*. 1972; 176:227-32.
99. Nichols R, Broldo P, Condon R et al. Effect of preoperative neomycin–erythromycin intestinal preparation on the incidence of infectious complications following colon surgery. *Ann Surg*. 1973; 178:453-62.
100. Stellato T, Danziger L, Gordon N et al. Antibiotics in elective colon surgery: a randomized trial of oral, systemic, and oral/systemic antibiotics for prophylaxis. *Am Surg*. 1990; 56:251-4.
101. Maki D, Aughey D, Lammers J. Study of cefazolin, cefoxitin, and ceftizoxime for prophylaxis in colorectal surgery. Paper presented at 24th Interscience Conference on Antimicrobial Agents and Chemotherapy. Washington, DC: 1984 Oct 10.
102. Petrelli N, Contre C, Herrera L et al. A prospective randomized trial of perioperative prophylactic cefamandole in elective colorectal surgery for malignancy. *Dis Colon Rectum*. 1988; 31:427-9.
103. Felip JF, Bonet EB, Eisman FI et al. Oral is superior to systemic antibiotic prophylaxis in operations upon the colon and rectum. *Surg Gynecol Obstet*. 1984; 158:359-62.
104. Kling PA, Dahlgren S. Oral prophylaxis with neomycin and erythromycin in colorectal surgery; more proof for efficacy than failure. *Arch Surg*. 1989; 124:705-7.
105. Lewis RT, Goodall RG, Marien B et al. Is neomycin necessary for bowel preparation in surgery of the colon? Oral neomycin plus erythromycin versus erythromycin–metronidazole. *Dis Colon Rectum*. 1989; 32:265-70.
106. Keithly MR, Arabi Y, Alexander-Williams J et al. Comparison between systemic and oral antimicrobial prophylaxis in colorectal surgery. *Lancet*. 1979; 1:894-7.
107. Lewis RT, Allan CM, Goodall RG et al. Are first-generation cephalosporins effective for antibiotic prophylaxis in elective surgery of the colon? *Can J Surg*. 1983; 26:504-7.
108. Edmondson HT, Rissing JP. Prophylactic antibiotics in colon surgery: cephaloridine vs erythromycin and neomycin. *Arch Surg*. 1983; 118:227-1.
109. Wapnick S, Gunito R, Leveen HH et al. Reduction of postoperative infection in elective colorectal surgery with preoperative administration of kanamycin and erythromycin. *Surgery*. 1979; 85:317-21.
110. Hagen TB, Bergan T, Liavag I. Prophylactic metronidazole in elective colorectal surgery. *Acta Chir Scand*. 1980; 146:71-5.
111. Gahhos FN, Richards GK, Hinchey EJ et al. Elective colon surgery: clindamycin versus metronidazole prophylaxis. *Can J Surg*. 1982; 25:613-6.
112. Dion YM, Richards GK, Prentis JJ et al. The influence of oral metronidazole versus parenteral preoperative metronidazole on sepsis following colon surgery. *Ann Surg*. 1980; 192:221-6.
113. Beggs FD, Jobanputra RS, Holmes JT. A comparison of intravenous and oral metronidazole as prophylactic in colorectal surgery. *Br J Surg*. 1982; 69:226-7.
114. Goldring J, McNaught W, Scott A et al. Prophylactic oral antimicrobial agents in elective colonic surgery: a controlled trial. *Lancet*. 1975; 2:997-9.
115. Willis A, Fergunson I, Jones P et al. Metronidazole in prevention and treatment of *Bacteroides* infections in elective

colonic surgery. *Br Med J*. 1977; 1:607-10.
116. Bjerkesett T, Digranes A. Systemic prophylaxis with metronidazole (Flagyl) in elective surgery of the colon and rectum. *Surgery*. 1980; 87:560-6.
117. Hojer H, Wehherfors J. Systemic prophylaxis with doxycycline in surgery of the colon and rectum. *Ann Surg*. 1978; 187:362-8.
118. Periti P, Mazzei T, Tonelli F. Single dose cefotetan vs multiple dose cefoxitin-antimicrobial prophylaxis in colorectal surgery: results of a prospective, multicenter, randomized study. *Dis Colon Rectum*. 1989; 32:121-7.
119. Jagelman D, Fabian T, Nichols R et al. Single dose cefotetan versus multiple dose cefoxitin as prophylaxis in colorectal surgery. *Am J Surg*. 1988; 155:71-6.
120. Hoffman C, McDonald P, Watts J. Use of perioperative cefoxitin to prevent infection after colonic and rectal surgery. *Ann Surg*. 1981; 193:353-6.
121. Morton A, Taylor E, Wells G. A multicenter study to compare cefotetan alone with cefotetan and metronidazole as prophylaxis against infection in elective colorectal operations. *Surg Gynecol Obstet*. 1989; 169:4-45.
122. Hinchey E, Richards G, Lewis R et al. Moxalactam as single agent prophylaxis in the prevention of wound infection following colon surgery. *Surgery*. 1987; 101:15-9.
123. Madsen M, Toftgaard C, Graversen H et al. Cefoxitin for one day vs ampicillin and metronidazole for three days in elective colorectal surgery: a prospective, randomized, multicenter study. *Dis Colon Rectum*. 1988; 31:774-7.
124. Coppa G, Eng K. Factors involved in antibiotic selection in elective colon and rectal surgery. *Surgery*. 1988; 104:853-8.
125. Cunliffe WJ, Carr N, Schofield PF. Prophylactic metronidazole with and without cefuroxime in elective colorectal surgery. *J R Coll Surg Edinb*. 1985: 30:123-5.
126. McCulloch PG, Blamey SL, Finlay IG et al. A prospective comparison of gentamicin and metronidazole and moxalactam in the prevention of septic complications associated with elective operations of the colon and rectum. *Surg Gynecol Obstet*. 1986; 162:521-30.
127. Roland M. Prophylactic regimens in colorectal surgery: an open randomized consecutive trial of metronidazole used alone or in combination with ampicillin or doxycycline. *World J Surg*. 1986; 10:1003-8.
128. McDermott F, Polyglase A, Johnson W et al. Prevention of wound infection in colorectal resections by preoperative cephazolin with and without metronidazole. *Aust NZ J Surg*. 1981; 51:351-3.
129. Panichi G, Pantosto A, Giunchi G et al. Cephalothin, cefoxitin, or metronidazole in elective colorectal surgery? A single-blind randomized trial. *Am J Surg*. 1979; 137:68-74.
130. Kaiser A, Herrington J, Jacobs J et al. Cefoxitin vs erythromycin, neomycin and cefazolin in colorectal surgery: importance of the duration of the operative procedure. *Ann Surg*. 1983; 198:525-30.
131. Blair J, McLeod R, Cohen Z et al. Ticarcillin/clavulanic acid (Timentin) compared to metronidazole/netilmicin in preventing postoperative infection after elective colorectal surgery. *Can J Surg*. 1987; 30:120-2.
132. Bell GA, Smith JA, Murphy J. Prophylactic antibiotics in elective colon surgery. *Surgery*. 1983; 93:204-8.
133. Lozano F, Alonso AG, Almazan A et al. A comparison of three different prophylactic parenteral antibiotic regimens in colorectal surgery: a prospective study. *Int Surg*. 1985; 70:227-31.
134. Juul PZ. Klaaborg KE, Kronborg O. Single or multiple doses of metronidazole and ampicillin in elective colorectal surgery: a randomized trial. *Dis Colon Rectum*. 1987; 30:526-8.
135. University of Melbourne Colorectal Group. A comparison of single dose Timentin with mezlocillin for prophylaxis of wound infection in elective colorectal surgery. *Dis Colon Rectum*. 1989; 32:940-3.
136. Goransson G, Nilsson-Ehle I, Olsson S et al. Single versus multiple dose doxycycline prophylaxis in elective colorectal surgery. *Acta Chir Scand*. 1984; 150:245-9.
137. Bergman L, Solhaug JH. Single-dose chemoprophylaxis in elective colorectal surgery. *Ann Surg*. 1987; 205:77-81.
138. Olsen PR, Andersen HH, Hebjorn M et al. The prophylaxis of metronidazole in colorectal surgery. *Dan Med Bull*. 1983; 30:345-8.
139. Condon RE, Bartlett JG, Nichols RL et al. Preoperative prophylactic cephalothin fails to control septic complications of colorectal operations: results of a controlled clinical trial. *Am J Surg*. 1979; 137:68-74.
140. Stone HH, Hooper CA, Kolb LD et al. Antibiotic prophylaxis in gastric, biliary, and colonic surgery. *Ann Surg*. 1976; 184:443-50.
141. Jones RN, Wojeski W, Bakke J et al. Antibiotic prophylaxis to 1,036 patients undergoing elective surgical procedures. A prospective randomized comparative trial of cefazolin, cefoxitin, and cefotaxime in a prepaid medical practice. *Am J Surg*. 1987; 153:341-6.
142. Shatney CH. Antibiotic prophylaxis in elective gastrointestinal tract surgery: a comparison of single dose preoperative cefotaxime and multiple dose cefoxitin. *J Antimicrob Chemother*. 1984; 14(Suppl B):241-5.
143. Condon RE, Bartlett J, Greenlee H et al. Efficacy of oral and systemic antibiotic prophylaxis in colorectal operations. *Arch Surg*. 1983; 118:496-502.
144. Coppa G, Eng K, Gouge T et al. Parenteral and oral antibiotics in elective colorectal surgery: a prospective randomized trial. *Am J Surg*. 1983; 145:62-5.
145. Jagelman DG, Fazio VW, Lavery IC et al. A prospective, randomized double-blind study of 10% mannitol mechanical bowel preparation combined with oral neomycin and short-term, perioperative, intravenous Flagyl as prophylaxis in elective colorectal resections. *Surgery*. 1985; 98:861-5.
146. Barbar MS, Hirxberg BC, Rice C et al. Parenteral antibiotics in elective colon surgery? A prospective, controlled clinical study. *Surgery*. 1979; 86:23-9.
147. Galandiuk S, Polk HC, Jagelman DG et al. Reemphasis of priorities in surgical antibiotic prophylaxis. *Surg Gynecol Obstet*. 1989; 169:219-22.
148. Shapiro M, Munoz A, Tasger I et al. Risk factors for infection at the operative site after abdominal or vaginal hysterectomy. *N Engl J Med*. 1982; 307:1661-6.
149. DiPiro JT, Cheung RP, Bowden TA et al. Single dose systemic antibiotic prophylaxis of surgical wound infections. *Am J Surg*. 1986; 152:552-9.
150. Hall JC, Watts MK, O'Brien P et al. Single dose antibiotic prophylaxis in contaminated abdominal surgery. *Arch Surg*. 1989; 124:244-7.
151. Kasier AB. Antimicrobial prophylaxis in surgery. *N Engl J Med*. 1986; 315:1129-38.
152. Lambert WG, Mullinger BM. Single dose cefuroxime in the prophylaxis of abdominal wound sepsis. *Curr Med Res Opin*. 1980; 6:404-6.
153. DiPiro JT, Welage LS, Levine BA et al. Single dose cefmetazole versus multiple dose cefoxitin for prophylaxis in abdominal surgery. *J Antimicrob Chemother*. 1989; 23(Suppl D):71-7.
154. Stone H, Haney B, Kolb L et al. Prophylactic and preventative antibiotic therapy: timing, duration and economics. *Ann Surg*. 1979; 189:691-9.
155. Solla J, Rothenberger D. Preoperative bowel preparation: a survey of colon and rectal surgeons. *Dis Colon Rectum*. 1990; 33:154-9.
156. Gilmore OJ, Martin TD. Aetiology and prevention of wound infection in appendectomy. *Br J Surg*. 1974; 62:567-72.
157. Pinto DJ, Sanderson PJ. Rational use of antibiotic therapy after appendectomy. *Br Med J*. 1980; 280:275-7.
158. Keighley MR. Infection: prophylaxis. *Br Med Bull*. 1988; 44:374-402.
159. Winslow RE, Rem D, Harley JW. Acute nonperforating ap-

pendicitis: efficacy of brief antibiotic prophylaxis. *Arch Surg*. 1983; 118:651-5.
160. Keiser TA, Mackenzie RL, Feld LN. Prophylactic metronidazole in appendectomy: a double-blind controlled trial. *Surgery*. 1983; 93:201-3.
161. Ahmed ME, Ibrahim SZ, Arabi YE et al. Metronidazole prophylaxis in acute mural appendicitis: failure of a single intra-operative infusion to reduce wound infection. *J Hosp Infect*. 1987; 10:260-4.
162. Donovan IA, Ellis D, Gatehouse D et al. One-dose antibiotic prophylaxis against wound infection after appendectomy: a randomized trial of clindamycin, cefazolin sodium and a placebo. *Br J Surg*. 1979; 66:193-6.
163. O'Rourke MGE, Wynne MJ, Morahan RJ et al. Prophylactic antibiotics in appendectomy: a prospective double blind randomized study. *Aust NZ J Surg*. 1984; 54:535-41.
164. Lau WY, Fan ST, Chu KW et al. Cefoxitin versus gentamicin and metronidazole in prevention of post-appendectomy sepsis: a randomized, prospective trial. *J Antimicrob Chemother*. 1986; 18:613-9.
165. Lau WY, Fan ST, Yiu TF et al. Prophylaxis of postappendectomy sepsis by metronidazole and ampicillin; a randomized, prospective and double blind trial. *Br J Surg*. 1983; 70:155-7.
166. Lau WY, Fan ST, Yiu TF et al. Prophylaxis of post-appendectomy sepsis by metronidazole and cefotaxime; a randomized prospective and double blind trial. *Br J Surg*. 1983; 70:670-2.
167. Lau WY, Fan ST, Chu KW et al. Randomized, prospective, and double-blind trial of new beta-lactams in the treatment of appendicitis. *Antimicrob Agents Chemother*. 1985; 28:639-42.
168. Panichi G, Pantosti AL, Marsiglio F. Cephalothin or cefoxitin in appendectomy? *J Antimicrob Chemother*. 1980; 6:801-4. Letter.
169. McIntosh GS, Jacob G, Townell NH et al. Prevention of post-appendectomy sepsis by mezlocillin and metronidazole: a prospective randomized, double-blind trial. *J Antimicrob Chemother*. 1984; 14:537-42.
170. Jensen NG, Bach-Nilsen P, Damgaard B et al. A Danish multicenter study; cefoxitin versus ampicillin vs. metronidazole in perforated appendicitis. *Br J Surg*. 1984; 71:144-6.
171. Stone HH. Bacterial flora of appendicitis in children. *J Pediatr Surg*. 1976; 11:37-42.
172. Berne TV, Appleman MD, Chenella FC et al. Surgically treated gangrenous or perforated appendicitis: a comparison of aztreonam and clindamycin versus gentamicin and clindamycin. *Ann Surg*. 1987; 205:133-7.
173. Berne TV, Yellin AW, Appleman MD et al. Antibiotic management of surgically treated gangrenous or perforated appendicitis; comparison of gentamicin and clindamycin versus cefamandole versus cefoperazone. *Am J Surg*. 1982; 144:8-13.
174. Corder AP, Bates T, Prior JE et al. Metronidazole v. cefoxitin in severe appendicitis: a trial to compare a single intraoperative dose of two antibiotics given intravenously. *Postgrad Med J*. 1983; 59:720-3.
175. Flannigan GM, Clifford RP, Carver RA et al. Antibiotic prophylaxis in acute appendicitis. *Surg Gynecol Obstet*. 1983; 156:209-22.
176. Bennin RS, Thompson JE, Baron EJ et al. Gangrenous and perforated appendicitis with peritonitis: treatment and bacteriology. *Clin Ther*. 1990; 12(Suppl. B):I-XIV.
177. Taffel SM, Placek PJ, Meien M. 1988 U.S. C-section rate at 24.7 per 100 births—a plateau? *N Engl J Med*. 1990; 323:199-200.
178. Amstey MT, Sheldon GW, Blyth JF. Infectious morbidity after primary cesarean section in a private institution. *Am J Obstet Gynecol*. 1980; 136:205-10.
179. Faro S. Infectious disease relations to cesarean section. *Obstet Gynecol Clin North Am*. 1989; 16:363-71.
180. Faro S. Antibiotic prophylaxis. *Obstet Gynecol Clin North Am*. 1989; 16:279-89.
181. Hemsell DL. Infections after gynecologic surgery. *Obstet Gynecol Clin North Am*. 1989; 16:381-400.
182. Duff P, Smith PN, Keiser JF. Antibiotic prophylaxis in low-risk cesarean section. *J Reprod Med*. 1982; 27:133-8.
183. Apuzzio JJ, Reyelt C, Pelosi MA et al. Prophylactic antibiotics for cesarean section: comparison of high- and low-risk patients for endometritis. *Obstet Gynecol*. 1982; 59:693-8.
184. Duff P. Prophylactic antibiotics for cesarean delivery: a simple cost effective strategy for prevention of post-operative morbidity. *Am J Obstet Gynecol*. 1987; 157:794-8.
185. Ehrenkranz NJ, Blackwelder WC, Pfaff SJ et al. Infections complicating low-risk cesarean sections in community hospitals: efficacy of antimicrobial prophylaxis. *Am J Obstet Gynecol*. 1990; 162:337-43.
186. Enkin M, Enkin E, Chalmers I et al. Prophylactic antibiotics in association with cesarean section. In: Chalmers I, Enkin M, Keiser MJNC, eds. Effective care in pregnancy and childbirth. Vol 1. London: Oxford University; 1989:1246-69.
187. Cunningham FG, Leveno KJ, DePalma RT et al. Perioperative antimicrobials for cesarean delivery: before or after cord clamping. *Obstet Gynecol*. 1983; 62:151-4.
188. Gordon HP, Phelps D, Blanchard K. Prophylactic cesarean section antibiotics: maternal and neonatal morbidity before and after cord clamping. *Obstet Gynecol*. 1979; 53:151-6.
189. D'Angelo LJ, Sokol RJ. Short- versus long-course prophylactic antibiotic treatment in cesarean section patients. *Obstet Gynecol*. 1980; 55:583-6.
190. Scarpignato C, Caltabiano M, Condemi V et al. Short term vs long term cefuroxime prophylaxis in patients undergoing emergency cesarean-section. *Clin Ther*. 1982; 5:186-91.
191. Elliott JP, Freeman RK, Dorchester W. Short versus long course of prophylactic antibiotics in cesarean section. *Am J Obstet Gynecol*. 1982; 143:740-4.
192. Faro S, Martens MG, Hammill HA et al. Antibiotic prophylaxis: is there a difference? *Am J Obstet Gynecol*. 1990; 162:900-9.
193. Conover WB, Moore TR. Comparison of irrigation and intravenous antibiotic prophylaxis at cesarean section. *Obstet Gynecol*. 1984; 63:787-91.
194. Ledger WJ, Gee C, Lewis WP. Guidelines for antibiotic prophylaxis in gynecology. *Am J Obstet Gynecol*. 1975; 121:1038-45.
195. Galask R. Changing concepts in obstetric antibiotic prophylaxis. *Am J Obstet Gynecol*. 1987; 157:491-5.
196. Stiver HG, Forward KR, Livingstone RA et al. Multicenter comparison of cefoxitin vs cefazolin for prevention of infectious morbidity after nonelective cesarean section. *Am J Obstet Gynecol*. 1985; 145:158-63.
197. Rayburn W, Varner M, Galask R et al. Comparison of moxalactam and cefazolin as prophylactic antibiotics during cesarean section. *Antimicrob Agents Chemother*. 1985; 27:337-9.
198. Benigno BB, Ford LC, Lawrence WD et al. A double-blind, controlled comparison of piperacillin and cefoxitin in the prevention of post-operative infection in patients undergoing cesarean section. *Surg Gynecol Obstet*. 1986; 162:1-7.
199. Crombleholme WR. Use of prophylactic antibiotics in obstetrics and gynecology. *Clin Obstet Gynecol*. 1988; 31:466-72.
200. Jakobi P, Weissmann A, Zimmer EZ et al. Single dose cefazolin prophylaxis for cesarean section. *Am J Obstet Gynecol*. 1988; 158:1049-52.
201. Faro S. Antibiotic prophylaxis. *Obstet Gynecol Clin North Am*. 1989; 16:279-89.
202. Hemsell DL. Infections after gynecologic surgery. *Obstet Gynecol Clin North Am*. 1989; 16:381-400.
203. Crombleholme WR. Use of prophylactic antibiotics in obstetrics and gynecology. *Clin Obstet Gynecol*. 1988; 31:466-72.
204. Hirsch HA. Prophylactic antibiotics in obstetrics and gynecology. *Am J Med*. 1985; 78(Suppl 6B):170-6.
205. Gibbs RS. Obstetrics and gynecology. In: Conte JE, Jacob LS, Polk HC, eds. Antibiotic prophylaxis in surgery. Philadel-

phia: Lippincott; 1984:137-55.
206. Ohm MJ, Galask RP. The effect of antibiotic prophylaxis on patients undergoing total abdominal hysterectomy. II. Alterations of microbial flora. *Am J Obstet Gynecol*. 1976; 125:448-52.
207. Grossman JH, Adams RL. Vaginal flora in women undergoing hysterectomy with antibiotic prophylaxis. *Obstet Gynecol*. 1979; 53:23-9.
208. Hamod KA, Spence MR, Roshenshein NB et al. Single and multidose prophylaxis in vaginal hysterectomy: a comparison of sodium cephalothin and metronidazole. *Am J Obstet Gynecol*. 1980; 136:976-9.
209. Polk BF, Shapiro M, Goldstein P et al. Randomized clinical trial of perioperative cefazolin in preventing infection after hysterectomy. *Lancet*. 1980; 1:437-40.
210. Benigno BB, Evard J, Faro S et al. A comparison of piperacillin, cephalothin, and cefoxitin in the prevention of postoperative infections in patients undergoing vaginal hysterectomy. *Surg Gynecol Obstet*. 1986; 163:421-7.
211. Pokras R. Hysterectomy: past, present and future. *Stat Bull*. 1989; Oct-Dec:12-21.
212. Bartlett JG, Onderdonk AB, Durde E. Quantitative bacteriology of the vaginal flora. *J Infect Dis*. 1977; 136:271-5.
213. Grossman J, Greco T, Minkin MJ et al. Prophylactic antibiotics in gynecologic surgery. *Obstet Gynecol*. 1979; 53:537-44.
214. Levison ME, Corman LC, Carrington ER et al. Quantitative microflora of the vagina. *Am J Obstet Gynecol*. 1977; 127:80-5.
215. Ohm MJ, Galask RP. The effect of antibiotic prophylaxis on patients undergoing vaginal operations. II. Alterations of microbial flora. *Am J Obstet Gynecol*. 1975; 123:597-604.
216. Marsden DE, Cavanagh D, Wisniewski BJ et al. Factors affecting the incidence of infectious morbidity after radical hysterectomy. *Am J Obstet Gynecol*. 1985; 152:817-21.
217. Hemsell D, Bernstein S, Bawdon R et al. Preventing major operative site infection after radical hysterectomy and pelvic lymphadenectomy. *Gynecol Oncol*. 1989; 35:55-60.
218. Hemsell D, Menon M, Friedman A. Ceftriaxone or cefazolin prophylaxis for the prevention of infection after vaginal hysterectomy. *Am J Surg*. 1984; 148:22-6.
219. Hemsell D, Johnson E, Bawdon R et al. Ceftriaxone and cefazolin prophylaxis for hysterectomy. *Surg Gynecol Obstet*. 1985; 161:197-203.
220. Soper D, Yarwood R. Single-dose antibiotic prophylaxis in women undergoing vaginal hysterectomy. *Obstet Gynecol*. 1987; 53:879-82.
221. Hemsell D, Hemsell P, Nobles B et al. Moxalactam versus cefazolin prophylaxis for vaginal hysterectomy. *Am J Obstet Gynecol*. 1983; 147:379-85.
222. Shapiro M, Munoz A, Tager I et al. Risk factors for infection at the operative site after abdominal or vaginal hysterectomy. *N Engl J Med*. 1982; 107:1661-6.
223. Wtteewall-Evelaar E, Koreks M, Verbrugh H. The value of prophylaxis in abdominal hysterectomies: meta-analysis. Paper presented at the 29th Interscience Conference on Antimicrobial Agents and Chemotherapy. Houston, TX: 1989 Sep 18.
224. Mann W, Orr J, Shingleton H et al. Perioperative influences on infectious morbidity in radical hysterectomy. *Gynecol Oncol*. 1981; 11:207-12.
225. Miyazawa K, Hernandez E, Dillon MB. Prophylactic topical cefamandole in radical hysterectomy. *Int J Gynaecol Obstet*. 1987; 25:133-8.
226. Bendvold E, Kjorstad KE. Antibiotic prophylaxis for radical hysterectomy. *Gynecol Oncol*. 1987; 28:201-4.
227. Micha JP, Kucera PR, Birkett JP et al. Prophylactic mezlocillin in radical hysterectomy. *Obstet Gynecol*. 1987; 69:251-4.
228. Goosenberg J, Emich JP Jr, Schwarz RH. Prophylactic antibiotics in vaginal hysterectomy. *Am J Obstet Gynecol*. 1969; 105:503-6.
229. Allen J, Rampone J, Wheeless C. Use of a prophylactic antibiotic in elective major gynecologic operations. *Obstet Gynecol*. 1972; 39:218-24.
230. Ledger WJ, Sweet RL, Headington JT. Prophylactic cephaloridine in the prevention of postoperative pelvic infections in premenopausal women undergoing vaginal hysterectomy. *Am J Obstet Gynecol*. 1972; 115:766-74.
231. Breeden JT, Mayo JE. Low dose prophylactic antibiotics in vaginal hysterectomy. *Obstet Gynecol*. 1974; 43:379-85.
232. Ohm MJ, Galask RP. The effect of antibiotic prophylaxis on patients undergoing vaginal operations. I. The effect of morbidity. *Am J Obstet Gynecol*. 1975; 123:590-6.
233. Glover MW, Van Nagell JR Jr. The effect of prophylactic ampicillin on pelvic infection following vaginal hysterectomy. *Am J Obstet Gynecol*. 1976; 126:385-8 .
234. Swartz WH, Tenaree P. T-tube suction drainage and/or prophylactic antibiotics. A randomized study of 451 hysterectomies. *Obstet Gynecol*. 1976; 47:665-70.
235. Lett WJ, Ansbacher R, Davison BL et al. Prophylactic antibiotics for women undergoing vaginal hysterectomy. *J Reprod Med*. 1977; 19(Aug):51-4.
236. Jennings RH. Prophylactic antibiotics in vaginal and abdominal hysterectomy. *South Med J*. 1978; 71:251-4.
237. Homan J, McGowan J, Thompson J. Perioperative antibiotics in major elective gynecologic surgery. *South Med J*. 1978; 71:417-20.
238. Roberts JM, Homesley HD. Low-dose carbenicillin prophylaxis for vaginal and abdominal hysterectomy. *Obstet Gynecol*. 1978; 52:83-7.
239. Mendelson J, Portnoy J, De Saint Victor JR et al. Effect of single and multidose cephradine prophylaxis on infectious morbidity of vaginal hysterectomy. *Obstet Gynecol*. 1979; 53:31-5.
240. Mickal A, Curole D, Lewis C. Cefoxitin sodium: double-blind vaginal hysterectomy prophylaxis in premenopausal patients. *Obstet Gynecol*. 1980; 56:222-5.
241. Hemsell DL, Cunningham FG, Kappus S et al. Cefoxitin for prophylaxis in premenopausal women undergoing vaginal hysterectomy. *Obstet Gynecol*. 1980; 56:629-34.
242. Polk B, Tager I, Shapiro M et al. Randomized clinical trial of perioperative cefazolin in preventing infection after hysterectomy. *Lancet*. 1980; 1:437-40.
243. Ledger WJ, Child MA. The hospital care of patients undergoing hysterectomy: an analysis of 12,026 patients from the Professional Activity Study. *Am J Obstet Gynecol*. 1973; 117:423-30.
244. Agalle PC, Urban RB, Homesley HD et al. Single dose carbenicillin versus T-tube drainage in patients undergoing vaginal hysterectomy. *Surg Gynecol Obstet*. 1981; 153:351-2.
245. Karhunen M, Koskela O, Hannelin M. Single dose of tinidazole in prophylaxis of infections following hysterectomy. *Br J Obstet Gynaecol*. 1980; 87:70-2.
246. Rapp RP, Van Nagell JR, Donaldson ES et al. A double-blind randomized study of prophylactic antibiotics in vaginal hysterectomy. *Hosp Formul*. 1982; 1:524-9.
247. Jacobson JA, Hebertson R, Kasworm E. Comparison of ceforanide and cephalothin prophylaxis for vaginal hysterectomies. *Antimicrob Agents Chemother*. 1982; 22:643-7.
248. Stage AH, Glover DD, Vaughan JE. Low-dose cephradine prophylaxis in obstetric and gynecologic surgery. *J Reprod Med*. 1982; 27:113-9.
249. Vincelette J, Finkelstein F, Aoki FY et al. Double-blind trial of perioperative intravenous metronidazole prophylaxis for abdominal and vaginal hysterectomy. *Surgery*. 1983; 93:185-9.
250. Hemsell DL, Heard ML, Nobles BJ et al. Single-dose cefoxitin prophylaxis for premenopausal women undergoing vaginal hysterectomy. *Obstet Gynecol*. 1984; 63:285-90.
251. Roy S, Wilkins J. Single dose cefotaxime versus 3 to 5 dose cefoxitin for prophylaxis of vaginal or abdominal hysterectomy. *J Antimicrob Chemother*. 1984; 14(Suppl B):217-21.
252. Savage EW, Thadepalli H, Rambhatla K et al. Minocycline prophylaxis in elective hysterectomy. *J Reprod Med*. 1984; 29:81-7.
253. Maki DG, Lammers JL, Aughey DR. Comparative studies of multiple dose cefoxitin vs. single dose cefonicid for sur-

gical prophylaxis in patients undergoing biliary tract operations or hysterectomy. *Rev Infect Dis*. 1984; 6(Suppl 4):887-95.
254. Blanco JD, Lipscomb KA. Single-dose prophylaxis in vaginal hysterectomy: a double blind, randomized comparison of ceftazidime versus cefotaxime. *Curr Ther Res*. 1984; 36:389-93.
255. McDonald PJ, Sanders T, Higgins G et al. Antibiotic prophylaxis in hysterectomy: cefotaxime compared to ampicillin–tinidazole. *J Antimicrob Chemother*. 1985; 14(Suppl B):223-30.
256. Hemsell DI, Hemsell PG, Nobles BJ. Doxycycline and cefamandole prophylaxis for premenopausal women undergoing vaginal hysterectomy. *Surg Gynecol Obstet*. 1985; 161:462-4.
257. Benson WL, Brown RL, Schmidt PM. Comparison of short and long courses of ampicillin for vaginal hysterectomy. *J Reprod Med*. 1985; 30:874-6.
258. Hemsell DL, Johnson ER, Bawdon RE et al. Ceftriaxone and cefazolin prophylaxis for hysterectomy. *Surg Gynecol Obstet*. 1985; 161:197-203.
259. Forney JP, Morrow CP, Townsend DE et al. Impact of cephalosporin prophylaxis on colonization: vaginal hysterectomy morbidity. *Am J Obstet Gynecol*. 1976; 125:100-5.
260. Rapp RP, Connors JE, Hager WD et al. Comparison of single-dose moxalactam and a three-dose regimen of cefoxitin for prophylaxis in vaginal hysterectomy. *Clin Pharm*. 1986; 5:988-93.
261. Brautigam HH, Knothe H, Rangoonwala R. Impact of cefotaxime and ceftriaxone on the bowel and vaginal flora after single dose prophylaxis in vaginal hysterectomy. *Drugs*. 1988; 35(Suppl 2):163-8.
262. Faro S, Pastorek JG, Aldridge KE et al. Randomized double blind comparison of mezlocillin versus cefoxitin prophylaxis for vaginal hysterectomy. *Surg Gynecol Obstet*. 1988; 166:431-5.
263. Gordon SF. Results of a single center study of cefotetan prophylaxis in abdominal or vaginal hysterectomy *Am J Obstet Gynecol*. 1988; 158:710-4. (Erratum published in *Am J Obstet Gynecol*. 1989; 160:1025.)
264. Roy S, Wilkins J, Hemsell DL et al. Efficacy and safety of single dose ceftizoxime vs. multiple dose cefoxitin in preventing infection after vaginal hysterectomy. *J Reprod Med*. 1988; 33(1 Suppl):149-53.
265. Mercer LJ, Murphy HJ, Ismail MA et al. A comparison of cefonicid and cefoxitin for preventing infections after vaginal hysterectomy. *J Reprod Med*. 1988; 33:223-6.
266. Berkeley AS, Orr JW, Cavanagh D et al. Comparative effectiveness and safety of cefotetan and cefoxitin as prophylactic agents in patients undergoing abdominal or vaginal hysterectomy. *Am J Surg*. 1988; 155:81-5.
267. Davey PG, Duncan ID, Edward D et al. Cost–benefit analysis of cephradine and mezlocillin prophylaxis for abdominal and vaginal hysterectomy. *Br J Obstet Gynaecol*. 1988; 95:1170-7.
268. Mozzillo N, Dionigi R, Ventriglia L. Multicenter study of aztreonam in the prophylaxis of colorectal, gynecologic and urologic surgery. *Chemotherapy*. 1989; 35(Suppl 1):58-71.
269. The Multicenter Study Group. Single dose prophylaxis in patients undergoing vaginal hysterectomy: cefamandole versus cefotaxime. *Am J Obstet Gynecol*. 1989; 160:1198-201.
270. Roy S, Wilkins J, Galaif E et al. Comparative efficacy and safety of cefmetazole or cefoxitin in the prevention of postoperative infection following vaginal and abdominal hysterectomy. *J Antimicrob Chemother*. 1989; 23(Suppl D):109-17.
271. Friese S, Willems FTC, Loriaux SM et al. Prophylaxis in gynaecological surgery: a prospective randomized comparison between single-dose prophylaxis with amoxycillin/clavulanate and the combination of cefuroxime and metronidazole. *J Antimicrob Chemother*. 1989; 24(Suppl B):213-6.
272. Willis A, Bullen C, Ferguson I et al. Metronidazole in the prevention and treatment of *Bacteroides* infection in gynaecological patients. *Lancet*. 1974; 2:1540-3.
273. Mayer W, Gordon M, Rothbard MJ. Prophylactic antibiotics. Use in hysterectomy. *NY State J Med*. 1976; 76:2144-7.
274. Ohm MJ, Galask RP. The effect of antibiotic prophylaxis on patients undergoing total abdominal hysterectomy. II. Alterations of microbial flora. *Am J Obstet Gynecol*. 1976; 125:448-54.
275. Mathews D, Ross H. Randomized controlled trial of a short course of cephaloridine in the prevention of infection after abdominal hysterectomy. *Br J Obstet Gynecol*. 1978; 85:381-5.
276. Appelbaum P, Moodley J, Chatterton S et al. Metronidazole in the prophylaxis and treatment of anaerobic infection. *S Afr Med J*. 1978; 1:703-6.
277. Wheeless CR Jr, Dorsey JH, Wharton LR Jr. An evaluation of prophylactic doxycycline in hysterectomy patients. *J Reprod Med*. 1978; 21:146-50.
278. Duff P. Antibiotic prophylaxis for abdominal hysterectomy. *Obstet Gynecol*. 1982; 60:25-9.
279. Walker EM, Gordon AJ, Warren RE et al. Prophylactic single dose metronidazole before abdominal hysterectomy. *Br J Obstet Gynaecol*. 1982; 89:957-61.
280. Manthorpe T, Justesen T. Metronidazole prophylaxis in abdominal hysterectomy. A double blind controlled trial. *Acta Obstet Gynecol Scand*. 1982; 61:243-6.
281. Ohm MJ, Galask RP. The effect of antibiotic prophylaxis on patients undergoing total abdominal hysterectomy. I. Effect on morbidity. *Am J Obstet Gynecol*. 1976; 125:442-7.
282. Hemsell DL, Reisch J, Nobles B et al. Prevention of major infection after elective abdominal hysterectomy. Individual determination required. *Am J Obstet Gynecol*. 1983; 147:520-3.
283. Kvist-Poulsen H, Borel J. T-tube suction drainage and/or prophylactic two dose metronidazole in abdominal hysterectomy. *Acta Obstet Gynecol Scand*. 1984; 63:711-4.
284. Berkeley AS, Haywork SD, Hirsch JC et al. Controlled, comparative study of moxalactam and cefazolin for prophylaxis of abdominal hysterectomy. *Surg Gynecol Obstet*. 1985; 161:457-61.
285. Gonen R, Hakin M, Samberg I et al. Short term prophylactic antibiotic for elective abdominal hysterectomy: how short? *Eur J Obstet Gynecol Reprod Biol*. 1985; 20:229-34.
286. Senior C, Steirad J. Are preoperative antibiotics helpful in abdominal hysterectomy? *Am J Obstet Gynecol*. 1986; 154:1004-8.
287. Evaldson GR, Lindgren S, Malmborg AS et al. Single dose intravenous tinidazole prophylaxis in abdominal hysterectomy. *Acta Obstet Gynecol Scand*. 1986; 65:361-5.
288. Tuomala RE, Fischer SG, Munoz A et al. A comparative trial of cefazolin and moxalactam as prophylaxis for preventing infection after abdominal hysterectomy. *Obstet Gynecol*. 1985; 66:372-6.
289. Periti P, Mazzei T, Periti E. Prophylaxis in gynaecological and obstetric surgery: a comparative randomized multicentre study of single dose cefotetan versus two doses of cefazolin. *Chemioterapia*. 1988; 7:245-52.
290. Hemsell DL, Martin JN Jr, Pastorek JG II et al. Single dose antimicrobial prophylaxis at abdominal hysterectomy. Cefamandole vs cefotaxime. *J Reprod Med*. 1988; 33:939-44.
291. Scarpignato C, Labruna C, Condemi V et al. Comparative efficacy of two different regimens of antibiotic prophylaxis in total abdominal hysterectomy. *Pharmatherapeutica*. 1980; 2:450-5.
292. Wijma J, Kauer F, Van Saene H et al. Antibiotics and suction drainage as prophylaxis in vaginal and abdominal hysterectomy. *Obstet Gynecol*. 1987; 70:384-8.
293. Eron LJ, Gordon SF, Harvey LK et al. A trial using early preoperative administration of cefonicid for antimicrobial prophylaxis with hysterectomies. *DICP*. 1989; 23:655-8.
294. Hemsell DL, Johnson ER, Bawdon RE et al. Cefoperazone and cefoxitin prophylaxis for abdominal hysterectomy. *Obstet Gynecol*. 1984; 63:467-72.
295. Tchabo JG, Cutting ME, Butler C. Prophylactic antibiotics in patients undergoing total vaginal or abdominal hysterec-

tomy. *Int Surg*. 1985; 70:349-52.
296. Hemsell DL, Hemsell PG, Heard ML et al. Preoperative cefoxitin prophylaxis for elective abdominal hysterectomy. *Am J Obstet Gynecol*. 1985; 153:225-6.
297. Hemsell DL, Johnson ER, Heard. MC et al. Single dose piperacillin versus triple dose cefoxitin prophylaxis at vaginal and abdominal hysterectomy. *South Med J*. 1989; 82:438-42.
298. Orr JW Jr, Sisson PF, Barrett JM et al. Single center study results of cefotetan and cefoxitin prophylaxis for abdominal or vaginal hysterectomy. *Am J Obstet Gynecol*. 1988; 158:714-6.
299. Orr JW Jr, Varner RE, Kilgore LC et al. Cefotetan versus cefoxitin as prophylaxis in hysterectomy. *Am J Obstet Gynecol*. 1986; 154:960-3.
300. Berkeley AS, Freedman KS, Ledger WJ et al. Comparison of cefotetan and cefoxitin prophylaxis for abdominal and vaginal hysterectomy. *Am J Obstet Gynecol*. 1988; 158:706-9.
301. Periti P, Mazzei T, Lamanna S et al. Single dose ceftriaxone versus multi dose cefotaxime antimicrobial prophylaxis in gynecologic and obstetrical surgery. Preliminary results of a multicenter prospective randomized study. *Chemioterapia*. 1984; 3:299-304.
302. Sevin B, Ramos R, Lichtinger M et al. Antibiotic prevention of infection complicating radical abdominal hysterectomy. *Obstet Gynecol*. 1984; 64:539-45.
303. Rosenshein NB, Ruth JC, Villar J et al. A prospective randomized study of doxycycline as a prophylactic antibiotic in patients undergoing radical hysterectomy. *Gynecol Oncol*. 1983; 15:201-6.
304. Ehrenkranz NJ. Surgical wound infection occurrence in clean operations. Risk stratification for interhospital comparisons. *Am J Med*. 1981; 50:909-14.
305. Freiman JA, Chalmers TC, Smith H et al. The importance of beta, the type II error and sample size in the design and interpretation of the randomized control trial. *N Engl J Med*. 1978; 299:690-4.
306. Barza M. Guidelines for reports of clinical studies. *Antimicrob Agents Chemother*. 1989; 33:1829-30.
307. Fan-Havard P, Nahata MC. Treatment and prevention of infections of cerebrospinal fluid shunts. *Clin Pharm*. 1987; 6:866-80.
308. Keucher TR, Mealey J. Long term results after ventriculoatrial and ventriculoperitoneal shunting for infantile hydrocephalus. *J Neurosurg*. 1979; 50:179-86.
309. Yogev R, Davis T. Neurosurgical shunt infections—a review. *Childs Brain*. 1980; 6:74-80.
310. Renier D, Lacombe J, Pierre-Kahn A et al. Factors causing acute shunt infection—computer analysis of 1174 patients. *J Neurosurg*. 1984; 61:1072-8
311. Wright RL. Postoperative craniotomy infections. Springfield, IL: Charles C Thomas; 1966:26-31.
312. Horwitz NH, Curtin JA. Prophylactic antibiotics and wound infections following laminectomy for lumbar disc disease. A retrospective study. *J Neurosurg*. 1975; 43:727-31.
313. Savitz MH, Malis LI. Prophylactic clindamycin for neurosurgical patients. *NY State J Med*. 1976; 76:64-7.
314. Haines SJ, Goodman ML. Antibiotic prophylaxis of postoperative neurosurgical wound infection. *J Neurosurg*. 1982; 56:103-5.
315. Geraghty J, Feely M. Antibiotic prophylaxis in neurosurgery. A randomized controlled trial. *J Neurosurg*. 1984; 60:724-6.
316. Mollman HD, Haines SJ. Risk factors for postoperative neurosurgical wound infection. A case-control study. *J Neurosurg*. 1986; 64:902-6.
317. Shapiro M, Wald U, Simchen E et al. Randomized clinical trial of intra-operative antimicrobial prophylaxis of infection after neurosurgical procedures. *J Hosp Infect*. 1986; 8:283-95.
318. Wright RL. Postoperative craniotomy infections. Springfield, IL: Charles C Thomas; 1970:26-39.
319. Tenney JH, Vlahov D, Saleman M et al. Wide variation in risk of wound infection following clean neurosurgery. Implication for perioperative antibiotic prophylaxis. *J Meirpsirg*. 1986; 62:243-7.
320. Wright RL. Septic complication of neurosurgical spinal procedures. Springfield, IL: Charles C Thomas; 1970:26-39.
321. Savitz MH, Malis LI, Meyers BR. Prophylactic antibiotics in neurosurgery. *Surg Neurol*. 1974; 2:95-100.
322. Malis LI. Prevention of neurosurgical infection by intraoperative antibiotics. *Neurosurgery*. 1979; 5:339-43.
323. Haines SJ. Systemic antibiotic prophylaxis in neurological surgery. *Neurosurgery*. 1980; 6:355-61.
324. Quarterly GRC, Polyzoidis K. Intraoperative antibiotic prophylaxis in neurosurgery: a clinical study. *Neurosurgery*. 1981; 8:669-71.
325. Savitz MH, Katz SS. Prevention of primary wound infection in neurosurgical patients: a 10-year study. *Neurosurgery*. 1986; 18:685-8.
326. Van Ek B, Dijkmans BA, Van Dulken H et al. Antibiotic prophylaxis in craniotomy: a prospective, double-blind, placebo controlled study. *Scand J Infect Dis*. 1988; 20:633-9.
327. Bullock R, Van Dellen JR, Ketelbey W et al. A double-blind, placebo controlled trial of perioperative prophylactic antibiotics for elective neurosurgery. *J Neurosurgery*. 1988; 69:687-91.
328. Blomstedt GC, Kytta J. Results of a randomized trial of vancomycin prophylaxis in craniotomy. *J Neurosurgery*. 1988; 69:216-20.
329. Fan-Havard P, Nahata MC. Treatment and prevention of infections of cerebrospinal fluid shunts. *Clin Pharm*. 1987; 6:866-80.
330. O'Brien M. Parent A, Davis B. Management of ventricular shunt infections. *Childs Brain*. 1979; 5:304-9.
331. Schoenbaum SC, Gardner P, Shillito J. Infection of cerebrospinal fluid shunts: epidemiology, clinical manifestations and therapy. *J Infect Dis*. 1975; 131:534-52.
332. Walters BC, Hoffman HJ, Hendrick EB et al. Cerebrospinal fluid shunt infection. Influences on initial management and subsequent outcome. *J Neurosurg*. 1984; 60:1014-21.
333. Wilson HD, Bean JR, James HE et al. Cerebrospinal fluid antibiotic concentrations in ventricular shunt infections. *Childs Brain*. 1978; 4:74-82.
334. James HE, Walsh JW, Wilson HD et al. The management of cerebrospinal fluid shunt infections. A clinical experience. *Acta Neurochir*. 1981; 59:157-66.
335. Mates S, Glaser J, Shapiro K. Treatment of cerebrospinal fluid shunt infections with medical therapy alone. *Neurosurgery*. 1982; 11:781-3.
336. George R, Leibrock L, Epstein M. Long-term analysis of cerebrospinal fluid shunt infections—a 25-year experience. *J Neurosurg*. 1979; 51:804-11.
337. Bayston R. Hydrocephalus shunt infections and their treatment. *J Antimicrob Chemother*. 1985; 15:259-61.
338. Renier D, Lacombe J, Pierre-Kahn A et al. Factors causing acute shunt infection—computer analysis of 1174 patients. *J Neurosurg*. 1984; 61:1072-8.
339. Forrest DM, Cooper DG. Complications of ventriculoatrial shunts. A review of 455 cases. *J Neurosurg*. 1968; 29:506-2.
340. Odio C, McCracken JC, Nelson JD. CSF shunt infections in pediatrics—a seven-year experience. *Am J Dis Child*. 1984; 138:1103-8.
341. Petrak RM, Pottage JC, Harris AA et al. *Haemophilus influenzae* meningitis in the presence of a cerebrospinal fluid shunt. *Neurosurgery*. 1986; 18:79-81.
342. Sells CJ, Shurtleff DB, Coeser JD. Gram-negative cerebrospinal fluid shunt associated infections. *Pediatrics*. 1977; 59:614-8.
343. Shapiro S, Boaz J, Kleiman M et al. Origins of organisms infecting ventricular shunts. *Neurosurgery*. 1988; 22:868-72.
344. Gardner P, Leipzig TJ, Sadigh M. Infections of mechanical cerebrospinal fluid shunts. *Curr Clin Top Infect Dis*. 1988; 9:185-214.
345. Wang EL, Prober CG, Hendrick BE. Prophylactic sulfamethoxazole and trimethoprim in ventriculoperitoneal

shunt surgery. A double-blind, randomized, placebo-controlled trial. *JAMA*. 1984; 251:1174-7.
346. Blomstedt GC. Results in trimethoprim–sulfamethoxazole prophylaxis in ventriculostomy and shunting procedures. *J Neurosurg*. 1985; 62:694-7.
347. Djindjian M, Fevrier MJ, Ottervbein G et al. Oxacillin prophylaxis in cerebrospinal fluid shunt procedures: results of a randomized open study in 60 hydrocephalic patients. *Surg Neurol*. 1986; 25:178-80.
348. Blum J, Schwarz M, Voth D. Antibiotic single-dose prophylaxis of shunt infections. *Neurosurg Rev*. 1989; 12:239-44.
349. Shurtleff DB, Stuntz JT, Hayden PW. Experience with 1201 cerebrospinal fluid shunt procedures. *Pediatric Neurosci*. 1985-86; 12:49-57.
350. Shmidt K, Gjerris F, Osgaard O et al. Antibiotic prophylaxis in cerebrospinal fluid shunting: a prospective randomized trial in 152 hydrocephalic patients. *Neurosurgery*. 1985; 17:1-5.
351. Griebel R, Khan M, Tan L. CSF shunt complications: an analysis of contributory factors. *Childs Nerv Syst*. 1985; 1:77-80.
352. Lambert M, MacKinnon AE, Vaishnav A. Comparison of two methods of prophylaxis against CSF shunt infection. *Z Kinderchir*. 1984; 39(Suppl):109-10.
353. Odio C, Mohs E, Sklar FH et al. Adverse reactions to vancomycin used as prophylaxis for CSF shunt procedures. *Am J Dis Child*. 1984; 138:17-9.
354. Anon. Coronary bypass surgery charges. 1982-3 and 1986. *Stat Bull*. 1989; Jan–Mar:2-15.
355. National Heart Lung and Blood Advisory Council. Fifteenth report of the National Heart, Lung, and Blood Advisory Council: Progress and Challenge. Washington, DC: U.S. Department of Health and Human Services; 1988.
356. Beam T Jr. Perioperative prevention of infection in cardiac surgery. *Antibiot Chemother*. 1985; 33:114-39.
357. Bor D, Rose R, Modlin J et al. Mediastinitis after cardiovascular surgery. *Rev Infect Dis*. 1983; 5:885-97.
358. Nagachinta T, Stephens M, Reitz B et al. Risk factors for surgical-wound infection following cardiac surgery. *J Infect Dis*. 1987; 156:967-73.
359. Kittle C, Reed W. Antibiotics and extracorporeal circulation. *J Thorac Cardiovasc Surg*. 1961; 41:34-48.
360. Slonim R, Litwak R, Gadboys H et al. Antibiotic prophylaxis of infection complicating open-heart operations. *Antimicrob Agents Chemother*. 1963; 3:731-5.
361. Goodman J, Schaffner W, Collins H et al. Infection after cardiovascular surgery. *N Engl J Med*. 1968; 278:117-23.
362. Fekety F, Cluff L, Sabiston D et al. A study of antibiotic prophylaxis in cardiac surgery. *J Thorac Cardiovasc Surg*. 1969; 57:757-63.
363. Conte J, Cohen S, Roe B et al. Antibiotic prophylaxis and cardiac surgery: a prospective double-blind comparison of single-dose versus multi-dose regimens. *Ann Intern Med*. 1972; 76:943-9.
364. Firor W. Infection following open-heart surgery, with special reference to the role of prophylactic antibiotics. *J Thorac Cardiovasc Surg*. 1967; 53:371-8.
365. Fong I, Baker C, McKee D. The value of prophylactic antibiotics in aorta-coronary bypass operations. *J Thorac Cardiovasc Surg*. 1979; 78:908-13.
366. Austin T, Coles J, Burnett R et al. Aorta-coronary bypass procedures and sternotomy infections: a study of antistaphylococcal prophylaxis. *Can J Surg*. 1980; 23:483-5.
367. Penketh A, Wansbrough-Jones M, Wright E et al. Antibiotic prophylaxis for coronary artery bypass graft surgery. *Lancet*. 1985; 1:1500.
368. Goldman D, Hopkins C, Karchmer A et al. Cephalothin prophylaxis in cardiac valve surgery; a prospective, double-blind comparison of two-day and six-day regimens. *J Thorac Cardiovasc Surg*. 1977; 73:470-9.
369. Austin T, Coles J, McKechnie P et al. Cephalothin prophylaxis and valve replacement. *Ann Thorac Surg*. 1977; 23:333-6.
370. Hillis D, Rosenfeldt F, Spicer W et al. Antibiotic prophylaxis for coronary bypass grafting. *J Thorac Cardiovasc Surg*. 1983; 86:217-21.
371. Hill D, Yates A. Prophylactic antibiotics in open heart surgery. *Aust N Z J Med*. 1975; 81:414-7.
372. Myerowitz P, Caswell K, Lindsay W et al. Antibiotic prophylaxis for open-heart surgery. *J Thorac Cardiovasc Surg*. 1977; 73:625-9.
373. Cooper D, Norton R, Mobin M et al. A comparison of two prophylactic antibiotic regimes for open-heart surgery. *J Cardiovasc Surg (Torino)*. 1980; 21:279-86.
374. Bailey J, Perciva H. Cefamandole as a prophylactic in cardiac surgery. *Scand J Infect Dis*. 1980; (Suppl 25):112-7.
375. Ghoneim A, Tandon A, Ionescu M. Comparative study of cefamandole versus ampicillin plus cloxacillin: prophylactic antibiotics in cardiac surgery. *Ann Thorac Surg*. 1982; 33:152-8.
376. Slama T, Sklar S, Misinski J et al. Randomized comparison of cefamandole, cefazolin and cefuroxime prophylaxis in open-heart surgery. *Antimicrob Agents Chemother*. 1986; 29:744-7.
377. Kaiser A, Petracek M, Lea J et al. Efficacy of cefazolin, cefamandole, and gentamicin as prophylactic agents in cardiac surgery. *Ann Surg*. 1987; 206:791-7.
378. Geroulanos S, Oxelbark S, Donfried B et al. Antimicrobial prophylaxis in cardiovascular surgery. *Thorac Cardiovasc Surg*. 1987; 35:199-205.
379. Conklin C, Gray R, Neilson D et al. Determinants of wound infection incidence after isolated coronary artery bypass surgery in patients randomized to receive prophylactic cefuroxime or cefazolin. *Ann Thorac Surg*. 1988; 46:172-7.
380. Doebbeling B, Pfaller M, Kuhns K et al. Cardiovascular surgery prophylaxis: a randomized, controlled comparison of cefazolin and cefuroxime. *J Thorac Cardiovasc Surg*. 1990; 99:981-9.
381. Woods M, Rahija M. Survey of antimicrobial prophylaxis in cardiovascular surgery. Poster presented at the 43rd ASHP Annual Meeting. Denver, CO: 1986 Jun 5.
382. Woods M, LeBlanc K, Gersema L. Antibiotic prophylaxis in open heart surgery: results of a second survey. *Hosp. Pharm*. 1990; 25:641-3.
383. Gentry L, Zeluff B, Cooley D. Antibiotic prophylaxis in open-heart surgery: a comparison of cefamandole, cefuroxime and cefazolin. *Ann Thorac Surg*. 1988; 46:167-71.
384. Beam T, Raab T, Spooner J et al. Single-dose antimicrobial prophylaxis in open heart surgery. *Eur J Clin Microbiol*. 1984; 3:598-604.
385. Soteriou M, Recker F, Geroulanos S et al. Perioperative antibiotic prophylaxis in cardiovascular surgery: a prospective randomized comparative trial of cefazolin versus ceftriaxone. *World J Surg*. 1989; 13:798-802.
386. Kini P, Fernandez J, Causay R et al. Double-blind comparison of cefazolin and cephalothin in open-heart surgery. *J Thorac Cardiovasc Surg*. 1978; 76:506-9.
387. Pien F, Michael N, Mamiya R et al. Comparative study of prophylactic antibiotics in cardiac surgery: clindamycin versus cephalothin. *J Thorac Cardiovasc Surg*. 1979; 77:908-13.
388. Joyce F, Szczepanski K. A double-blind comparative study of prophylactic antibiotic therapy in open heart surgery: penicillin G versus vancomycin. *Thorac Cardiovasc Surg*. 1986; 34:100-3.
389. Wilson A, Treasure T, Gruneberg R et al. Antibiotic prophylaxis in cardiac surgery: a prospective comparison of two dosage regimens of teicoplanin with a combination of flucloxacillin and tobramycin. *J Antimicrob Chemother*. 1988; 21:213-23.
390. Boyce J, Potter-Bynoe G, Dziobek L. Hospital reimbursement patterns among patients with surgical wound infections following open heart surgery. *Infect Control Hosp Epidemiol*. 1990; 11:89-93.
391. Roach A, Kernodle D, Kaiser A. Selecting cost-effective antimicrobial prophylaxis in surgery: Are we getting what we pay for? *DICP*. 1990; 24:183-5.

392. Preheim L, Rimland D, Bittner M. Methicillin-resistant *Staphylococcus aureus* in Veterans Administration Medical Centers. *Infect Control*. 1987; 8:191-4.
393. Thornsberry C. Methicillin-resistant staphylococci. *Clin Lab Med*. 1989; 9:255-67.
394. Olix ML, Klug TJ, Coleman CR et al. Prophylactic penicillin and streptomycin in elective operations on bones, joints, and tendons. *Surg Forum*. 1960; 10:818-9.
395. Schonholtz GJ, Borgia CA, Blair JD. Wound sepsis in orthopedic surgery. *J Bone Joint Surg*. 1962; 44A:1548-52.
396. Fitzgerald RH. Infections of hip prostheses and artificial joints. *Infect Dis Clin North Am*. 1989; 3:329-38.
397. Ericson C, Lidgren L, Lindberg L. Cloxacillin in the prophylaxis of postoperative infections of the hip. *J Bone Joint Surg*. 1973; 55A:808-13.
398. Carlsson AS, Lidgren L, Lindberg L. Prophylactic antibiotics against early and late deep infections after total hip replacements. *Acta Orthop Scand*. 1977; 48:405-10.
399. Hill C, Mazas F, Flamant R et al. Prophylactic cefazolin versus placebo in total hip replacement. *Lancet*. 1981; 1:795-7.
400. Lidwell OM, Lowbury EJL, Whyte W et al. Effect of ultraclean air in operating rooms on deep sepsis in the joint after total hip or knee replacement: a randomized study. *Br Med J*. 1982; 285:10-4.
401. Pollard JP, Hughes SPF, Scott JE et al. Antibiotic prophylaxis in total hip replacement. *Br Med J*. 1979; 1:707-9.
402. Boyd RJ, Burke JF, Colton T. A double-blind clinical trial of prophylactic antibiotics in hip fractures. *J Bone Joint Surg*. 1973; 55A:1251-8.
403. Burnett JW, Gustilo RB, Williams DN et al. Prophylactic antibiotics in hip fractures. *J Bone Joint Surg*. 1980; 62A:457-62.
404. Tengve B, Kjellander J. Antibiotic prophylaxis in operations on trochanteric femoral fractures. *J Bone Joint Surg*. 1978; 60A:97-9.
405. Pavel A, Smith RL, Ballard A et al. Prophylactic antibiotics in clean orthopedic surgery. *J Bone Joint Surg*. 1974; 56A:777-82.
406. Eron LJ. Prevention of infection following orthopedic surgery. *Antibiot Chemother*. 1985; 33:140-64.
407. Norden CW. A critical review of antibiotic prophylaxis in orthopedic surgery. *Rev Infect Dis*. 1983; 5:928-32.
408. Henley MB, Jones RE, Wyatt RWB et al. Prophylaxis with cefamandole nafate in elective orthopedic surgery. *Clin Orthop*. 1986; 209:249-54.
409. Burnakis TG. Surgical antimicrobial prophylaxis: principles and guidelines. *Pharmacotherapy*. 1984: 4:248-71.
410. Kaiser AB, Clayson KR, Mulherin JL et al. Antibiotic prophylaxis in vascular surgery. *Ann Surg*. 1978; 188:283-9.
411. Pitt HA, Postier RG, Macgowan WA et al. Prophylactic antibiotics in vascular surgery. Topical, systemic, or both. *Ann Surg*. 1980; 192:356-64.
412. Bennion RS, Hiatt JR, Williams RA et al. A randomized, prospective study of perioperative antimicrobial prophylaxis for vascular access surgery. *J Cardiovasc Surg*. 1985; 26:270-4.
413. Hasselgren P-O, Ivarson L, Risberg B et al. Effects of prophylactic antibiotics in vascular surgery. A prospective, randomized double-blind study. *Ann Surg*. 1984; 200:86-92.
414. Gibbons RP, Stark RA, Gorrea RJ et al. The prophylactic use—or misuse—of antibiotics in transurethral prostatectomy. *J Urol*. 1978; 119:381-3.
415. Ferrie B, Scott R. Prophylactic cefuroxime in transurethral resection. *Urol Res*. 1984; 12:279-81.
416. Upton JD, Das S. Prophylactic antibiotics in transurethral resection of bladder tumors: are they necessary? *Urology*. 1986; 27:421-3.
417. Houle AM, Mokhless I, Sarto N et al. Perioperative antibiotic prophylaxis for transurethral resection of the prostate; is it justifiable? *J Urol*. 1989; 142:317-9.
418. Fair WR. Perioperative use of carbenicillin in transurethral resection of the prostate. *Urology*. 1986; 27(Suppl 2):15-8.
419. Shah P, Williams G, Chaudary M et al. Short-term antibiotic prophylaxis and prostatectomy. *Br J Urol*. 1981; 53:339-43.
420. Morris MJ, Golovsky D, Guinness MDG et al. The value of prophylactic antibiotics in transurethral prostatic resection: a controlled trial, with observations on the origin of postoperative infection. *Br J Urol*. 1976; 48:479-84.
421. Gonzalez R, Wright R, Blackard CE. Prophylactic antibiotics in transurethral prostatectomy. *J Urol*. 1976; 116:203-5.
422. Hills NH, Bultitude MI, Eykyn S. Co-trimoxazole in prevention of bacteriuria after prostatectomy. *Br Med J*. 1976; 2:498-9.
423. Dorflinger T, Madsen PO. Antibiotic prophylaxis in transurethral surgery. *Urology*. 1984; 24:643-6.
424. Matthew AD, Gonzales R, Jeffords D et al. Prevention of bacteriuria after transurethral prostatectomy with nitrofurantoin macrocrystals. *J Urol*. 1978; 120:442-3.
425. Childs SJ, Wells WG, Mirelman S. Antibiotic prophylaxis for genitourinary surgery in community hospitals. *J Urol*. 1983; 130:305-8.
426. Nielsen OS, Maigaard S, Frimødt-Møller N et al. Prophylactic antibiotics in transurethral prostatectomy. *J Urol*. 1981; 126:60-2.
427. Charton M, Vallancien G, Veillon B et al. Antibiotic prophylaxis or urinary tract infection after transurethral resection of the prostate: a randomized study. *J Urol*. 1987; 138:87-9.
428. Ramsey E, Sheth NK. Antibiotic prophylaxis in patients undergoing prostatectomy. *Urology*. 1983; 21:376-8.
429. DeBessonet DA, Merlin AS. Antibiotic prophylaxis in elective genitourinary tract surgery: a comparison of single-dose pre-operative cefotaxime and multiple-dose cefoxitin. *J Antimicrob Chemother*. 1984; 14(Suppl B):271-5.

Drug Review

Mesalamine and olsalazine: 5-Aminosalicylic acid agents for the treatment of inflammatory bowel disease

LARRY W. SEGARS AND BARRY J. GALES

Abstract: The history, pharmacology, pharmacokinetics, clinical uses and efficacy, adverse effects, drug interactions, and dosage and administration of rectal mesalamine and oral olsalazine in the treatment of inflammatory bowel disease (IBD) are reviewed.

The high incidence of toxicity associated with sulfasalazine led to the development of the nonsulfonamide 5-aminosalicylic acid products mesalamine and olsalazine. The exact mechanism of action of these agents in the treatment of IBD is unknown. In clinical trials, mesalamine was shown to be as effective as or more effective than sulfasalazine or corticosteroids in treating active ulcerative colitis, proctitis, and proctosigmoiditis. Mesalamine is effective in the maintenance of remission in patients with ulcerative colitis. Several studies have demonstrated the effectiveness of olsalazine in the treatment of active mild to moderate ulcerative colitis. Olsalazine is also effective in the maintenance of remission of ulcerative colitis.

The most common adverse effect associated with mesalamine enemas is perianal irritation or trauma secondary to insertion. The most common adverse effects associated with olsalazine are dose-dependent watery diarrhea and gastrointestinal upset. The recommended dosage of the mesalamine enema for the treatment of active mild to moderate ulcerative colitis is one 4-g (60-mL) retention enema daily for three to six weeks. The dosage of mesalamine suppositories for the treatment of active ulcerative proctitis is one 500-mg suppository inserted rectally twice daily for three to six weeks. The dosage of olsalazine is 1 g daily in divided doses for the maintenance of remission of ulcerative colitis.

Both rectal mesalamine and oral olsalazine provide clinicians with an effective therapeutic option for the treatment of ulcerative colitis, proctosigmoiditis, and proctitis in patients unresponsive to or intolerant of the effects of sulfasalazine or corticosteroids.

Index terms: Drug administration routes; Gastrointestinal drugs; Inflammatory bowel diseases; Mesalamine; Olsalazine sodium; Pharmacokinetics; Toxicity
Clin Pharm. 1992; 11:514-28

Treatment of inflammatory bowel disease (IBD) has focused primarily on reducing the severity of the symptoms and the number of relapses experienced by patients. Corticosteroids, first shown to be effective in 1955, have been administered orally, rectally, and intravenously for IBD.[1,2] The immunosuppressive agents azathioprine and mercaptopurine are effective in maintaining remission in patients with Crohn's disease. The antibiotic metronidazole has been shown to be effective in the treatment of Crohn's disease but not ulcerative colitis. Other agents including cromolyn sodium, clonidine, chloroquine, eicosapentaenoic acid, methotrexate, antitubercular agents, immune enhancers, and oxygen-derived free-radical scavengers are being examined for the treatment of IBD.[2] The drug sulfasalazine, which has been used for approximately 50 years, still remains a mainstay for the treatment of IBD.

This article reviews the history, pharmacology, pharmacokinetics, clinical efficacy, adverse effects, dosage, and administration of rectal mesalamine (5-aminosalicylic acid) and oral olsalazine (azodisal sodium), two related drugs recently introduced for the treatment of IBD.

LARRY W. SEGARS, PHARM.D., and BARRY J. GALES, PHARM.D., are Clinical Assistant Professors, College of Pharmacy, Southwestern Oklahoma State University (SWOSU), Weatherford, OK.

Address reprint requests to Dr. Segars at St. Anthony Hospital, 1000 North Lee Street, P.O. Box 205 (SWOSU), Oklahoma City, OK 73101.

This is **article 680-204-9213** in the **ASHP Continuing-Education System;** it qualifies for 1.0 hour of continuing-education credit. See page 559 for learning objectives and test questions.

Inflammatory Bowel Disease

Ulcerative colitis and Crohn's disease are categorized as types of IBD. While falling under the single heading of IBD, ulcerative colitis and Crohn's disease are two separate and distinct disorders, and only a small fraction of patients exhibit characteristics of both. Although ulcerative colitis and Crohn's disease are termed gastrointestinal tract disorders, systemic as well as local complications may occur.

Ulcerative colitis affects the rectum and extends proximally and continuously into the large bowel. In severe cases ulcerative colitis may affect the entire length of the colon. Prominent symptoms of ulcerative colitis include frequent, visibly bloody diarrhea accompanied by lower-left-quadrant abdominal pain, anorexia, weight loss, and fever. Pathologically, ulcerative colitis is characterized by the nontransmural infiltration of lymphocytes, plasma cells, eosinophils, and polymorphonuclear cells, which leads to ulceration and crypt abscess formation. These structural changes result in the intense, diffuse mucosal inflammation characteristic of ulcerative colitis.[3-6]

Crohn's disease most commonly occurs in the terminal ileum and proximal colon but may be present anywhere in the upper or lower gastrointestinal tract. Anal lesions are common, whereas the rectum is often spared. Prominent symptoms of Crohn's disease include fever, right-lower-quadrant abdominal pain, cramping, malabsorption, and intermittent diarrhea. The occurrence of strictures, obstructions, and perforations is more common in Crohn's disease than ulcerative colitis. Pathologically, Crohn's disease is characterized by localized transmural lesions with numerous epithelioid granulomas and substantial lymphangiectasia.[3-6]

The exact etiologies of ulcerative colitis and Crohn's disease are unknown. Studies have identified numerous abnormalities. However, it is unclear whether these findings are etiological or a result of the chronic inflammatory process. An infectious etiology hypothesis for IBD has been popular, with cytomegalovirus, *Pseudomonas* species, and atypical *Mycobacterium* species all being implicated. However, researchers searching for an infectious etiology have been unable to account for most episodes of IBD.[5] Findings that the incidence of IBD is higher in relatives of IBD patients suggest a genetic influence.[5,7,8]

Numerous immunological abnormalities have been identified in patients with IBD, including a reduction in neutrophil superoxide production,[9] increased IgG- and IgA-producing colonic mucosal B cells,[10] and increased T-suppressor-cell activity.[11] Crohn's disease has been postulated to be mediated by a continuous, poorly regulated immunological response to a mucosal antigen.[12]

Chemical mediators of inflammation are of great interest in the study of IBD. The production of prostaglandins through the cyclo-oxygenase pathway and the production of leukotrienes through the lipoxygenase pathway of arachidonic acid metabolism are both increased in IBD patients. The importance of the elevated levels of cyclo-oxygenase products, lipoxygenase products, C-reactive protein, and other inflammatory substances in patients with IBD is unknown.[13] These elevations may just be nonspecific markers of the ongoing inflammatory process.

Development of 5-Aminosalicylic Acid Compounds

Sulfasalazine was initially developed by a Scandinavian rheumatologist for the treatment of rheumatoid arthritis. Sulfasalazine utilizes a diazo bond to join a sulfonamide antibiotic, sulfapyridine, with an anti-inflammatory agent, mesalamine. (In this article, the name mesalamine refers to both the marketed drug product and the compound released by bacterial cleavage of sulfasalazine or olsalazine.) Case reports of the use of sulfasalazine in patients with ulcerative colitis first appeared in 1942,[14] and results of a large uncontrolled trial were published in 1948.[15] Subsequent controlled trials substantiated the effectiveness of sulfasalazine in treating[16,17] and maintaining remission[18,19] of IBD. Peppercorn and Goldman determined in 1972 that sulfasalazine was cleaved by intestinal bacteria at the diazo bond, liberating sulfapyridine and mesalamine.[20] Later studies showed mesalamine to be the active portion of sulfasalazine, with sulfapyridine acting as a carrier that releases mesalamine in the colon.[21-23]

Sulfasalazine is less than 10–20% absorbed in the upper gastrointestinal tract. Bacterial reduction of sulfasalazine's diazo bond occurs in the colon and is almost complete (<7% of a dose appears in the feces as sulfasalazine). Liberated sulfapyridine and mesalamine differ in their absorption profiles; mesalamine is poorly absorbed and sulfapyridine is well absorbed in the colon. Sulfapyridine is primarily metabolized by acetylation. This metabolism depends on the patient's acetylator phenotype. Toxicity occurs in 5–55% of patients during sulfasalazine therapy and is most common in slow acetylators. Adverse effects associated with sulfasalazine therapy include nausea, vomiting, diarrhea, headache, rash, blood dyscrasias, and oligospermia. Toxicity has been correlated with total serum sulfapyridine concentrations of >50 μg/mL. A similar positive correlation exists between sulfasalazine's efficacy and total sulfapyridine concentrations (20–40 μg/mL).[24,25]

The high incidence of toxicity associated with sulfasalazine led to the development of nonsulfonamide 5-aminosalicylic acid products, two of which are currently approved for use by the FDA. The first product is mesalamine (5-aminosalicylic acid, Rowasa, Reid-Rowell), available as a suspension for rectal administration and as rectal suppositories. The second 5-aminosalicylic acid product is olsalazine (Dipentum, Pharmacia, Inc.). Structurally, olsalazine is two mesalamine molecules joined by a diazo bond. Like sulfasalazine, olsalazine is poorly absorbed in the upper gastrointestinal tract, which allows most of the parent compound to reach the colon. Once the drug is in the colon, bacteria split olsalazine into two mesalamine molecules by reducing the diazo bond. Olsalazine releases only mesalamine when reduced, so adverse effects associated with carrier molecules like sulfapyridine are avoided.

Pharmacology of 5-Aminosalicylic Acid Compounds

The mechanism of action of 5-aminosalicylic acid compounds in the treatment of IBD is unknown. However, a number of potentially beneficial anti-inflammatory activities have been attributed to mesalamine. An area of early interest was the effect of mesalamine on prostaglandin production. Prostaglandins may alter mucosal water and electrolyte transport, mucus release, blood flow, and intestinal motility, thus contributing to diarrhea in patients with IBD. Prostaglandins may also contribute to the pain, fever, edema, free-radical formation, and lymphocyte activation seen in inflammatory reactions.[26,27] Studies have found prostaglandin levels to be elevated in the colonic mucosa of IBD patients.[28] Mesalamine has been shown to inhibit the enzyme cyclo-oxygenase in the arachidonic acid cascade, thus reducing inflammatory prostaglandin production. These findings led to the hypothesis that mesalamine activity depends on cyclo-oxygenase inhibition.[29] This hypothesis fell into disfavor when it was shown that indomethacin and flurbiprofen, both potent inhibitors of cyclo-oxygenase, were ineffective in treating IBD.[30,31] In fact, case reports have associated the use of cyclo-oxygenase inhibitors (nonsteroidal anti-inflammatory drugs) with relapses of IBD.[26,27,31]

The effects of mesalamine on the lipoxygenase pathway of arachidonic acid metabolism are currently under study. Leukotrienes stimulate chemotaxis, induce neutrophil aggregation and degranulation, and increase microvascular permeability.[26,27] Thus, leukotrienes and other lipoxygenase pathway products may contribute to the inflammatory process characteristic of IBD. Studies have shown that sulfasalazine, mesalamine, and *N*-acetylmesalamine, but not sulfapyridine, inhibit the production of soybean lipoxygenase in vitro at concentrations lower than those needed for cyclo-oxygenase inhibition.[32,33] Sulfasalazine and mesalamine, but not *N*-acetylmesalamine, have been shown to inhibit in vitro production of human neutrophil lipoxygenase.[34,35] Sulfidopeptide-leukotriene and leukotriene B_4 are lipoxygenase metabolites that are elevated in the colonic mucosal tissue of IBD patients. Sulfasalazine and mesalamine, but not indomethacin, inhibit the production of sulfidopeptide-leukotriene and leukotriene B_4 by colonic mucosal tissue.[36,37] This in vitro reduction in leukotriene production was confirmed by an in vivo experiment using topical mesalamine and rectal equilibrium dialysis.[38] Stenson[39] hypothesizes that mesalamine inhibits leukotriene B_4 production by attacking its unstable precursor, leukotriene A_4. The lack of a specific lipoxygenase inhibitor has made the detailed study of leukotrienes in patients with IBD difficult.[40,41]

Mesalamine exerts direct effects on the immune system. Macrophage and neutrophil chemotaxis is inhibited by sulfasalazine, mesalamine, and olsalazine.[42,43] Intestinal mononuclear cell production of both IgA and IgG antibodies is reduced by mesalamine.[44] Hypochlorous acid, which is released by activated neutrophils to induce cell lysis, is scavenged by mesalamine, possibly reducing cell damage and inflammation.[45] Production of oxygen-derived free radicals is increased in the intestinal mucosa of IBD patients. These reactive free radicals also are scavenged by mesalamine.[46,47]

Pharmacokinetics of Mesalamine and Olsalazine

The therapeutic activity of mesalamine depends on high intraluminal concentrations of the drug, making the importance of traditional systemic pharmacokinetic measurements unclear.

Orally administered mesalamine is rapidly and extensively absorbed in the upper gastrointestinal tract. Mesalamine absorption decreases from 75% in the small intestine to 19% in the colon. Most of the absorbed mesalamine is rapidly acetylated, independent of genetic phenotype, and renally excreted.[48-50] Colonic mucosa homogenates have been shown to presystemically acetylate mesalamine.[51] The elimination half-life of mesalamine varies with administration route and dosage form but usually is in the range of 0.7–2.4 hours.[48,52]

Mesalamine is 10–35% absorbed when administered as a rectal enema or suppository.[52-55] Absorption of mesalamine from enemas is pH dependent, with acidic solutions being less well absorbed than neutral solutions.[56] Absorption of mesalamine from enemas increases during remission of IBD and with increasing dose and enema volume.[55] Steady-state serum concentrations after rectal administration of 100-mL enemas containing 4 g of mesalamine were 0.92 μg/mL and 1.62 μg/mL for mesalamine and acetylmesalamine, respectively.[54] The spread of the enema is volume dependent; a 100-mL mesalamine enema reaches the splenic flexure, allowing for the effective treatment of left-sided colitis.[57] Retrograde spread of the 60-mL mesalamine enema available in the United States is less studied than that of the 100-mL enemas available elsewhere.

Orally administered olsalazine passes unabsorbed and uncleaved through the stomach and small intestines.[58] On reaching the colon, olsalazine undergoes almost complete (99.4%) diazo-bond reduction, resulting in the liberation of two mesalamine molecules.[59,60] Uncleaved olsalazine found in the feces accounts for only 3.6–5.9% of an oral maintenance dose.[61,62] Gastrointestinal tract intolerance has been associated with elevated concentrations of uncleaved olsalazine in fecal dialysates.[60] Oral olsalazine has a bioavailability of 2–5%, with high-fiber foods delaying and possibly diminishing absorption.[63] Peak olsalazine concentrations occur one to two hours after oral and rectal administration.[63,64] Serum olsalazine concentrations are low (2–4 μg/mL) and increase with dose.[60,63,65] Serum olsalazine concentrations are not significantly different in patients with active severe IBD and those with inactive IBD.[60] The clinical relevance of a small controlled trial reporting higher plasma olsalazine concentrations in responders than nonresponders is unknown.[66]

Urinary elimination of olsalazine is minimal; 0–1.1% of the drug appears in the urine after oral doses of up to 4 g or rectal doses of 2 g.[63,64] Small studies have reported extensive biliary elimination of absorbed olsalazine.[67] Systemically available olsalazine also may be hepatically converted to olsalazine-*O*-sulfate, which has a prolonged half-life. This metabolite is slowly converted back to olsalazine, resulting in an apparent olsalazine elimination half-life of 4–12.8 days after oral administration.[61-63,65,67] Steady-state serum olsalazine concentrations are reached within 5–19 days of maintenance therapy.[62,65,67]

The diazo-bond reduction product mesalamine and its metabolite acetylmesalamine account for most of the olsalazine administered. After oral 1- to 2-g/day maintenance doses of olsalazine, 6.3–18.2% of a dose may be recovered in the urine as mesalamine and acetylmesalamine. The majority of an oral olsalazine dose is found in the feces as mesalamine (13.4–30.2%) or acetylmesalamine (6.8–55.3%).[61,62]

Efficacy of Mesalamine Therapy for Ulcerative Colitis

Active Disease. In 1973, Peppercorn and Goldman described the metabolism of sulfasalazine.[68] Soon afterwards, researchers began to investigate which sulfasalazine component provided the drug's therapeutic activity. Several landmark studies were performed to determine the active moiety of sulfasalazine.[21-23] In the first trial, 62 patients with mild to moderate active ulcerative colitis were treated in a randomized fashion with sulfasalazine 2.0 g, oral sulfapyridine 1.3 g, or mesalamine 0.7 g administered nightly as retention enemas.[21] After two weeks of treatment, both the mesalamine and sulfasalazine groups had equal clinical, sigmoidoscopic, and histological improvement. No significant improvement was demonstrated in the sulfapyridine group. It was concluded that the mesalamine moiety provided the therapeutic activity of sulfasalazine. Two subsequent studies produced similar results.[22,23] In one of those studies 23 patients with ulcerative colitis and 9 patients with Crohn's disease were treated with mesalamine 0.5-g rectal suppositories, oral sulfasalazine 1.0 g, or oral sulfapyridine 0.5 g—each administered three times daily for six weeks.[22] Mesalamine and sulfasalazine provided substantial clinical improvement, whereas no improvement was demonstrated with sulfapyridine. The highest remission rates were seen in the mesalamine group (86% versus 64% with sulfasalazine).

Numerous other studies followed, demonstrating the effectiveness of mesalamine in the treatment of mild to moderate active ulcerative colitis.[69-85] Approximately half of the studies reviewed were randomized, double-blind comparisons.[23,70-72,74,77,84,80-83] A similar number of reviewed studies allowed patients to continue previous ulcerative-colitis drug therapy (oral sulfasalazine, oral corticosteroids, rectal corticosteroids) during the study period.[21,70-72,74,76,77,79,80,82-84] Many of the patients included in these trials were considered to be completely or partially unresponsive or intolerant to the effects of sulfasalazine or corticosteroids, or both. Two reviewed studies allowed previous medications to be continued for a few weeks into the study period, during which time these medications were tapered off.[73,79] In studies indicating no significant difference between treatments, adequate numbers of patients were enrolled in each group to prevent a Type II error.

Mesalamine Rectal Suppository. In a placebo-controlled trial by Williams et al.,[69] mesalamine 0.5 g or placebo suppositories were administered three times daily for six weeks to 27 patients with active distal proctitis involving less than 15 cm of the colon. Mesalamine provided patients with a significant improvement in their disease activity index (DAI) scores at three weeks ($p < 0.001$) and six weeks ($p < 0.01$). (A typical disease activity indexing system is shown in Table 1.) No significant improvement was demonstrated between week 3 and week 6. All but three patients receiving mesalamine achieved a DAI score of 0 (remission) by week 6. All three ultimately achieved a score of 0 with continued therapy. No significant

Table 1.
Disease Activity Index[a, b]

Stool Frequency
0 = Normal
1 = 1–2 Stools/day more than normal
2 = 3–4 Stools/day more than normal
3 = >4 Stools/day more than normal
Rectal Bleeding
0 = None
1 = Streaks of blood
2 = Obvious blood
3 = Mostly blood
Mucosal Appearance
0 = Normal
1 = Mild friability
2 = Moderate friability
3 = Exudation, spontaneous bleeding
Physician Rating of Disease Activity
0 = Normal
1 = Mild
2 = Moderate
3 = Severe

[a]Range of possible scores: 0–12.
[b]Reprinted with permission from reference 77.

improvement was demonstrated in the placebo group at three or six weeks.

In the largest study reviewed, 219 patients with ulcerative colitis involving less than 20 cm of the colon were treated with one of three dosages of mesalamine suppositories for four weeks.[70] Patients were randomized to receive 0.4 g three times daily, 0.25 g five times daily, or 1 g twice daily. All three groups had clinical and sigmoidoscopic improvements ranging from 82.5% to 89%. No significant differences were demonstrated among the three treatment groups.

Subsequently, Campieri et al.[71] compared two different dosages of mesalamine suppositories with placebo in 65 patients with proctitis and 29 patients with proctosigmoiditis involving less than 20 cm of the colon. Patients were randomized to one of the following groups to be treated for four weeks: 0.5-g twice daily, 0.5 g three times daily, or placebo three times daily. Both the mesalamine 1-g/day ($p < 0.05$) and mesalamine 1.5-g/day ($p < 0.01$) groups achieved clinical remission significantly more often than the placebo group after two weeks of therapy. Similar differences were demonstrated after four weeks ($p < 0.01$). Both mesalamine groups also had better response rates in endoscopic ($p < 0.02$) and histological ($p < 0.01$) evaluations compared with the placebo group. Once again, no significant difference was shown between the two mesalamine dosages. The authors concluded that 0.5-g mesalamine suppositories administered twice daily were both safe and effective for the treatment of mild to moderate active disease.

In a study to determine the spread of mesalamine suppositories, ^{99m}Tc-labeled suppositories were found to have retrograde spread to the rectum and sigmoid colon, thereby making them effective for the treatment of active distal proctitis.[69]

Mesalamine Enema. Several studies also have demonstrated the efficacy of the enema formulation of mesalamine for the treatment of active mild to moderate ulcerative colitis.[72-79] One early study found that 1- or 2-g mesalamine enemas administered nightly to 25 patients were equally effective in treating ulcerative colitis. The overall response rate was 62%.[72] A subsequent study was performed using mesalamine enemas in dosages that ranged from 1 to 4 g administered nightly.[73] During the open-label phase of the study, 74% of the patients developed clinical and proctosigmoidoscopic remission within three months, and an additional 13% achieved clinical but not proctosigmoidoscopic remission. During the placebo-controlled phase, 32 patients with ulcerative colitis, proctitis, or proctosigmoiditis were treated with 4-g mesalamine enemas nightly for 8–12 weeks or until remission developed. As soon as remission developed, the dosage was gradually reduced to 1 g nightly. Fifty-nine percent of the patients developed complete remission by 12 weeks. An additional 28% achieved complete remission with continued therapy (duration not provided). During or shortly after dosage reduction 40% of the patients experienced a relapse. Ninety-two percent of these patients developed remission again with the administration of nightly 4-g mesalamine enemas. The authors concluded that mesalamine enemas administered at a dosage of 4 g nightly were effective in inducing remission in patients with proctocolitis.

Similar results were produced in a study conducted by Biddle et al.[79] in which 90 patients with ulcerative colitis, proctitis, or proctosigmoiditis were treated with nightly 4-g mesalamine enemas for 12 weeks or until remission developed. Eighty-seven percent of the patients improved, and 54% achieved clinical remission after 12 weeks of therapy. An additional 26% of patients achieved remission after an additional 22 weeks of therapy. After the development of remission, the mesalamine dosage was tapered off. Of the 90 patients, 41 (45.6%) experienced a relapse. After retreatment with nightly 4-g mesalamine enemas, only one patient (2.5%) failed to again achieve remission.

Other studies also have demonstrated the safety and efficacy of mesalamine 4-g enemas administered nightly for the treatment of active mild to moderate ulcerative colitis.[72,74-78] The largest placebo-controlled trial reviewed included 153 patients with mild to moderate ulcerative colitis, proctitis, or proctosigmoiditis. Patients were randomized to be treated with 4-g mesalamine or placebo enemas nightly for six weeks. The physician assessment indicated that mesalamine produced clinical improvement more often than placebo ($p < 0.0001$), with DAI scores showing a greater decline with mesalamine than with placebo ($p < 0.0001$).[74]

Comparison of Suppository and Enema Formulations. Campieri et al.[86] compared the efficacy of the suppository and enema formulations of mesalamine for four weeks in 29 patients with mild to moderate distal proctitis (<20 cm). After four weeks both formulations produced 80–90% improvement in clinical, sigmoidoscopic, and histological evaluations. No significant difference in effectiveness was demonstrated between the two formulations of mesalamine. However, the suppositories were administered at 1 g twice daily, higher than the previously studied 0.5-g twice daily dosage. The enemas were given at a dosage of 2 g nightly, which was lower than the previously studied dosage of 4 g nightly. Patients were asked to rate both formulations according to practicality in self-administration and tolerability. All patients generally rated both formulations as "good" for both assessments. However, patients preferred the suppository over the enema ($p < 0.01$).

Comparison of Mesalamine with Corticosteroids. Mesalamine also has been shown to be more effective than corticosteroids in the treatment of mild to moderate active ulcerative colitis.[80-83] In one study conducted by Friedman et al.,[80] 16 patients with ulcerative colitis, proctitis, or proctosigmoiditis unresponsive to sulfasalazine were treated in a double-blind fashion with either 4-g mesalamine enemas or 0.1-g hydrocortisone enemas nightly for three weeks. Of the eight patients receiving mesalamine, seven (87.5%) had at least a 1-point improvement in their DAI scores, compared with only two of the eight patients (25%) receiving hydrocortisone. The histological and sigmoidoscopic scores improved in six patients receiving mesalamine (75%) and two patients receiving hydrocortisone (25%). The mean clinical and sigmoidoscopic scores significantly improved with the use of mesalamine ($p < 0.02$) compared with hydrocortisone. Histological scores were not significantly different between treatment groups.

A subsequent larger study ($n = 86$) with similar patients, medications, and dosages found that significantly more patients had clinical, sigmoidoscopic, and histological improvement with mesalamine than with hydrocortisone ($p < 0.0005$).[81] This study was also important because it demonstrated, with the use of ^{99m}Tc-labeled mesalamine enemas, the retrograde spread of the 100-mL enemas up to the splenic flexure, thereby indicating their usefulness in the treatment of left-sided colitis.

One other reviewed study found mesalamine only slightly more effective than prednisolone in providing ulcerative colitis patients with clinical, sigmoidoscopic, and histological improvement (60% versus 50%)[82] However, the 15 patients enrolled in the mesalamine group were treated with 3 g nightly, which is slightly lower than the previously studied 4-g dose.

Radiation-Induced Proctitis. Mesalamine was found to be of little benefit in the treatment of nine patients with radiation-induced proctitis.[84,85] Patients did not have any sustained improvement in their clinical symptoms or mucosal appearance. Only two patients treated with mesalamine had temporary improvement.[84,85] In contrast, mesalamine suppositories (1.2 g/day) and enemas (4 g/day) were found to be effective in treating three patients with inflammation of the ileal reservoir created by the ileoanal anastomosis after a colectomy.[87]

Summary. From the studies reviewed it can be concluded that the 4-g mesalamine retention enema administered nightly is effective for the treatment of active mild to moderate ulcerative colitis, especially when the patient is partially or completely unresponsive or intolerant to the effects of conventional IBD therapy.

Disease in Remission. Some patients may require continued therapy to lengthen the time until relapse or decrease the severity of the relapse. Several studies have demonstrated that both mesalamine formulations are effective in the maintenance of remission in patients with mild to moderate ulcerative colitis.[70,88-93] The studies reviewed ranged from three to seven weeks up to 24 months in duration.

Daily Therapy. In a study conducted by Campieri et al.,[70] 37 patients with ulcerative colitis in remission were randomized to be treated with either 0.4-g mesalamine suppositories twice daily for 6–12 months or 1-g mesalamine suppositories daily for 12 months. Three of 18 patients (16.6%) in the group receiving 0.4 g twice daily relapsed, compared with 9 of 19 patients (47.3%) in the group receiving 1 g daily.

Mesalamine also has been compared with placebo for the maintenance of remission.[88] Thirty patients with proctitis (n =17) or proctosigmoiditis (n =13) in remission were randomized to be treated with 0.4-g mesalamine suppositories twice daily or placebo for 12 months. Twelve of 13 mesalamine patients (92%) were still in remission compared with 3 of 14 placebo patients (21%) at the completion of the study. The time to relapse for the mesalamine group was 26 weeks, compared with 2–32 weeks for placebo ($p < 0.001$). The cumulative relapse rates were 8% in the mesalamine group and 79% in the placebo group ($p < 0.001$).

Various doses and dosage intervals of mesalamine enemas also have been shown to be effective for the maintenance of remission. In one study 1-g mesalamine enemas administered nightly were found to maintain remission over a 12-month period significantly better than placebo (75% versus 15.5%) ($p < 0.005$).[90] In a study conducted by Sutherland and Martin,[92] a dose of 2 g was found to maintain remission as well as a dose of 4 g when administered nightly for six months. No significant differences were observed between groups. The overall relapse rate was 15% after three months and 22% after six months.

Novel Dosage Strategies. Several investigators have studied unique dosage techniques for maintenance of remission. One investigator treated 20 patients with mild to moderate active ulcerative colitis with nightly 4-g mesalamine enemas.[91] Sixteen patients improved clinically; 15 achieved clinical remission and 14 achieved sigmoidoscopic remission. Once patients developed remission, they were entered into the dosage titration phase (n = 14) and were treated with 4-g enemas every other night. If remission was maintained for two weeks, the dosage was reduced to one 4-g enema every third night. Patients who relapsed were retreated with nightly 4-g mesalamine enemas until remission reoccurred; they then re-entered the dosage titration phase. Ultimately, eight patients maintained remission while receiving one 4-g enema every third night, three maintained remission while receiving one 4-g enema every other night, and three required nightly administration to maintain remission.

A second investigator compared the efficacy of 4-g mesalamine enemas administered nightly for the first seven days of each month with that of sulfasalazine 2 g administered orally each day of the month for the maintenance of remission.[93] Sixty patients with proctitis or proctosigmoiditis were randomized and treated for 24 months. The cumulative actuarial relapse rates were not significantly different at any time between groups ($p > 0.05$). Five patients receiving mesalamine relapsed during the first 12 months (20%), compared with eight patients receiving sulfasalazine (24%). Relapse rates during the subsequent 12 months likewise were similar in both groups. The actuarial relapse rates at 24 months were 37% in the mesalamine group and 43% in the sulfasalazine group. The mean time to relapse and the severity of relapse were similar in both groups.

Summary. From these studies it can be concluded that mesalamine is effective for the maintenance of remission in patients with mild to moderate ulcerative colitis. Dosages of 2 or 4 g nightly have been found to be equally effective, and some patients have been able to maintain remission while being treated with lower doses or extended frequencies.

Efficacy of Olsalazine Therapy for Ulcerative Colitis

Active Disease. Several studies have demonstrated the effectiveness of olsalazine in the treatment of active mild to moderate ulcerative colitis.[94-104] In one placebo-controlled trial olsalazine was found to be significantly more effective than placebo in providing patients with clinical and sigmoidoscopic improvement when given at a dosage of 0.5 g orally four times daily.[94] Similar results were reported in 105 patients with ulcerative colitis who were treated with 0.5 g twice daily.[96] After a four-week trial, olsalazine significantly improved rectal mucus discharge compared with placebo ($p = 0.0038$). Likewise, rectal bleeding decreased more with olsalazine than with placebo, although the difference was not significant ($p = 0.0536$). Rectoscopy findings improved in 62% of olsalazine patients and 46% of placebo patients ($p = 0.0127$). However, these results were not confirmed in a subsequent study that used a dosage of 1 g twice daily.[95] This dosage provided clinical improvement in only 6 of 15 patients receiving olsalazine, compared with 2 of 15 patients receiving placebo ($p = 0.11$). Sigmoidoscopy findings also were not significantly different between the olsalazine and placebo groups ($p = 0.19$).

Studies that followed began to use larger daily doses of olsalazine with better results. One study conducted by Meyers et al.[97] included 66 patients with active ulcerative colitis ($n = 26$) or proctosigmoiditis ($n = 40$) who were randomly assigned to treatment with olsalazine 0.75 g, 1.5 g, or 3 g or with placebo daily for three weeks. As was the case in previous olsalazine studies, the sigmoidoscopy scores for the combined olsalazine groups improved more than those for the placebo group ($p = 0.001$). The within-treatment group analysis demonstrated a significant improvement in the 1.5-g/day ($p = 0.01$) and 3-g/day ($p = 0.007$) groups only. The results for the group receiving 0.75 g/day were not provided. Subsequent studies that investigated the efficacy of olsalazine for the treatment of active mild to moderate ulcerative colitis found a response rate of 54.5% to 60% with dosages of 1 to 3 g daily.[98-104] Three reviewed studies demonstrated equal efficacy for olsalazine and sulfasalazine in treating patients with active ulcerative colitis.[102-104] Only one reviewed study included patients with severe ulcerative colitis ($n = 4$).[105] These four patients did not receive any clinical benefit despite the addition of other medicinal agents.

Although the FDA has not approved olsalazine for the treatment of active mild to moderate ulcerative colitis, these studies show that patients with mild to moderate active ulcerative colitis can be provided with clinical and sigmoidoscopic improvement when they receive dosages of up to 3 g/day. The one factor that may prevent the use of this agent at these doses for the treatment of active ulcerative colitis is its main adverse effect, which is dose-dependent watery diarrhea (see Adverse Effects of Mesalamine and Olsalazine). Because of this adverse effect, patients should be treated with olsalazine only for the maintenance of remission (see Disease in Remission, below).

Disease in Remission. Several studies demonstrated olsalazine's efficacy in the maintenance of remission of ulcerative colitis.[99,105-108] One study enrolled 102 patients with ulcerative colitis in remission and randomized them to be treated with either olsalazine 0.5 g or placebo twice daily for six months.[106] Twelve of 52 olsalazine patients (23%) relapsed compared with 24 of 49 placebo patients (49%) ($p < 0.01$). The histology exams did not differ significantly between the groups ($p = 0.10$). The largest study reviewed included 164 patients with ulcerative colitis in remission.[107] Patients were randomized to treatment with either olsalazine 1 g or sulfasalazine 2 g twice daily for six months. Sixteen olsalazine patients (19.5%) and 10 sulfasalazine patients (12.2%) relapsed ($p = 0.1632$). The time to relapse was not significantly different between the two treatment groups ($p = 0.1314$). Sandberg-Gertzen et al.[108] found that the relapse rates of patients in remission who received olsalazine 0.5 g twice daily were 19.2% after 6 months, an additional 21.4% during months 6–12, 11.9% during the subsequent 6 months, and 9.7% during months 18–24. Superior results were found in 12 patients treated with olsalazine 0.25 g four times daily for 36 weeks.[105] Ten of the 12 patients were still in remission one year later. Olsalazine 0.25 g four times daily or 0.5 g twice daily has been shown to be effective in maintaining remission and is associated with fewer adverse effects than the larger doses (up to 3 g/day).

Efficacy of Mesalamine and Olsalazine Therapy for Crohn's Disease

Mesalamine. Limited data are available describing the use of U.S.-approved mesalamine formulations in the treatment of Crohn's disease. Only one reviewed study included patients with Crohn's disease ($n = 9$).[22] The results in these 9 patients were less pronounced than those in the 23 patients with ulcerative colitis. Further investigation, performed in a larger population of patients with a full range of disease severities, must be conducted before a definitive recommendation can be made for the use of mesalamine in the treatment of or maintenance of remission of Crohn's disease.

Olsalazine. No reviewed studies used olsalazine in the treatment of Crohn's disease. Until supporting data are reported, olsalazine cannot be recommended for the treatment of or maintenance of remission of Crohn's disease.

Adverse Effects of Mesalamine and Olsalazine

Mesalamine. Sulfasalazine has been associated with a moderately high incidence of adverse effects (up to 55%).[16] Many investigators have attributed these adverse effects to the sulfapyridine component. Many of the patients who develop adverse reactions are found to have a slow acetylator phenotype.[109-112] Although adverse effects can occur with the use of mesalamine, in general the reviewed studies reported fewer adverse effects with mesalamine than previously reported with sulfasalazine. Many patients previously intolerant to the adverse effects of sulfasalazine have been safely and effectively treated with mesalamine.

The most frequently encountered adverse effects associated with the use of mesalamine enemas are perianal irritation or trauma secondary to enema insertion (19–42%),[73,90] rashes (2–13%),[71,75] headache (9%),[74] and fever (2–4%).[71,75,76] Fissures, fistulas, and abscesses also have been infrequently reported (2–4%),[73] although these can occur as a result of IBD. Other adverse effects include abdominal distention (5%),[83] dizziness (4%),[75] and buccal ulceration (2%).[76] Adverse effects that occurred in fewer than 1% of patients include fatigue and joint stiffness or arthralgia.[83] The majority of patients who experience adverse effects associated with the administration of mesalamine are able to continue therapy; only 2–14% require discontinuation of therapy.

One case report indicated the development of pancreatitis with the use of mesalamine.[113] Alterations in renal function were not reported in the human studies reviewed, and one investigator specifically reported that the use of mesalamine did not impair renal function.[114] A few case reports have described hair loss, and one reported the development of a Kawasaki-like syndrome.[74,76,115,116] Infrequent adverse effects induced by sulfasalazine, such as male infertility and pure red blood cell aplasia,[117-119] have not been demonstrated with mesalamine. The adverse effects experienced with the suppository formulation are similar to those seen with the enema, excluding the perianal irritation, trauma, and laceration. Other adverse effects reported with mesalamine products not available in the United States include watery diarrhea in an infant secondary to being breast-fed by a mother who was receiving rectal mesalamine[120] and myocardial hypersensitivity, of which one case was fatal.[121,122] Investigators using other mesalamine products not approved in the United States have reported cases of reversal of male infertility,[123-126] nephrotic syndrome,[127] pancreatitis,[128-130] pericardial effusion,[131] and acute interstitial nephritis.[132]

Although the incidence of adverse effects associated with mesalamine is less than that associated with sulfasalazine, allergic reactions such as rash, fever, and other systemic hypersensitivity reactions that are seen with sulfasalazine also may develop with the use of mesalamine and may require discontinuation of therapy.[133] Patients with previous hypersensitivity reactions to sulfasalazine, aspirin, or aspirin-containing compounds should be closely monitored and educated during initiation of mesalamine therapy.

Olsalazine. Adverse effects similar to those experienced with mesalamine also have been documented with olsalazine. Examples include rash (2–16%),[95,97,106,134-136] headache (2–13%),[94-96,102,104,106,135,136] and fever (2–4%).[106,136] Other adverse effects include lightheadedness and dizziness (2–5%),[94,99,105], hair loss (2%),[96] and arthralgia or weakness (0.5–3%).[96,105-107,134,136] Adverse effects that occurred in fewer than 1% of patients receiving olsalazine include lassitude, increased salivation, cough, irritability, pancreatitis, and hepatitis.[106,107,137,138] However, the two most frequently encountered adverse effects associated with olsalazine are dose-dependent watery diarrhea (3–50%)[94-99,101-107,139,140] and gastrointestinal upset (6–18%).[95,96,99-103,103,106,140] Patients describe the diarrhea induced by olsalazine as different from that associated with the disease. The diarrhea induced by olsalazine occurs more frequently, is watery, and does not contain blood. Olsalazine has been shown to accelerate gastric emptying and mouth-to-cecum transit time, as well as decreasing whole gut transit time after a solid meal. These effects are reportedly due to a direct effect on motility.[141] It has been reported that olsalazine induces anion secretion and decreased water and electrolyte absorption, resulting in a greater volume presented to an already diseased colon.[142,143] The diarrhea has been reported not to be mediated by PGE_2 or $PGE_{2\alpha}$.[141,142,144-146] It has been reported to occur more frequently in patients with more extensive, widespread disease, although the severity of disease did not correlate as well with the diarrhea.[106] However, the association between diarrhea and widespread disease was not demonstrated in a subsequent study.[135] The diarrhea returns to pretreatment levels after the dosage is lowered or therapy is discontinued. Up to 40–50% of patients who experience diarrhea require the discontinuation of olsalazine therapy. Olsalazine did not significantly increase bile acid loss compared with placebo in patients with permanent ileostomies, although olsalazine did increase ileostomy output.[145] Olsalazine has been shown to be safe in patients who have experienced sulfasalazine lung, defined as the development of fever, dyspnea, eosinophilia, and pulmonary infiltrates associated with the administration of sulfasalazine[147]; sulfasalazine-induced eosinophilic pneumonia[148]; and impotence induced by sulfasalazine.[136,149]

Drug Interactions and Contraindications to Use of Mesalamine and Olsalazine

Drug interactions have been infrequently reported with mesalamine and olsalazine. Concurrent use of nonsteroidal anti-inflammatory drugs may predispose patients to develop renal toxicity, although this has not been documented. Use of nonsteroidal anti-inflammatory drugs may also predispose patients to experience relapses of IBD. Relapses are postulated to be precipitated by increases in leukotriene production as a result of cyclo-oxygenase inhibition by nonsteroidal anti-inflammatory drugs.[150-152] Some researchers have reported an association between the use of oral contraceptives and an increased incidence of IBD.[5] Studies have not established a direct drug interaction between the aminosalicylates and either nonsteroidal anti-inflammatory drugs or oral contraceptives.

Contraindications to the use of these products include hypersensitivity to mesalamine, olsalazine, or salicylates. Mesalamine rectal suspension contains potassium metabisulfite, which may induce a severe hypersensitivity reaction in some patients. Use of mesalamine or olsalazine during pregnancy or in children less than 17 years of age has not been adequately studied and is not recommended.

Dosage and Administration of Mesalamine and Olsalazine

Mesalamine. The recommended dosage of the mesalamine enema for the treatment of active mild to moderate ulcerative colitis is one 4-g (60-mL) retention enema daily. The enema is usually administered at bedtime and should be retained for a minimum of eight hours. The recommended duration of therapy is three to six weeks. However, patients may require additional therapy to achieve remission. The safety and effectiveness of long-term therapy with mesalamine enemas have been demonstrated up to two years.[93] The frequency of administration may be extended to an every-other-night or every-third-night schedule to maintain remission in some patients. The dosage of mesalamine suppositories is one 500-mg suppository inserted rectally twice daily for the treatment of active mild to moderate distal proctitis. The suppository should be retained at least three hours. The duration of therapy for the suppositories is also three to six weeks. Patients may require a longer duration of therapy to develop remission. The safety and effectiveness of long-term therapy with mesalamine suppositories have been demonstrated up to one year.[88]

Olsalazine. The dosage of olsalazine is 1 g daily in divided doses (0.25 g four times daily or 0.5 g twice daily) for the maintenance of remission of ulcerative colitis. Olsalazine also has been shown to be effective for the induction of remission in patients with active mild to moderate ulcerative colitis; however, larger doses of 2–3 g/day may be necessary for patients to achieve remission.[94-98,101-104]

Patient Instructions

For best results the bowel should be emptied before administration of either mesalamine product. The suppository should be retained for at least three hours. The enema should be retained for a minimum of eight hours.

After removal of the enema from the box and protective foil package, the enema should be shaken well. The protective sheath should be removed from the applicator tip. For best positioning, the patient should lie on his or her left side with the left leg extended and the right leg flexed forward. The patient may also use the "knee–chest" position. After the applicator tip is lubricated, it should be gently inserted into the rectum with the tip pointed slightly toward the navel. After insertion, the patient should firmly grasp the bottle, tilt it toward the spine, and squeeze slowly. After complete administration of the contents, the bottle should be removed and discarded. The patient should remain in position for at least 30 minutes to allow for medication distribution. Patients should also be informed that the enemas may darken with time (one to two years) and should not be used if a dark brown color is observed. Administration instructions for patients, which include pictures, are located in each box of enemas. The olsalazine capsules should be taken orally as prescribed. The mesalamine suppository should be unwrapped and inserted rectally as prescribed.[153-155]

Cost and Availability of Mesalamine and Olsalazine

Mesalamine. Mesalamine is manufactured by Reid-Rowell under the trade name of Rowasa. The disposable retention enema is off-white to tan and contains 4 g of mesalamine in a 60-mL aqueous suspension. The enemas are supplied in boxed, foil-wrapped trays of seven at an average wholesale price of $52.40. The suppositories are individually foil wrapped, light tan, and bullet shaped; each contains 500 mg of mesalamine. They are supplied in boxes of 12 and 24 at an average wholesale price of $28.12 and $53.42, respectively.[153,154,156]

Olsalazine. Olsalazine is available from Pharmacia, Inc., marketed under the trade name Dipentum. It is supplied as the sodium salt in bottles of 100 capsules. Each capsule contains 250 mg of olsalazine and is beige. The capsules have an average wholesale price of $51.88 per 100. "DIPENTUM 250 mg" is imprinted on each capsule.[155,156]

Formulary Recommendation

Studies have found mesalamine enemas and suppositories to be safe and effective in the treatment of active mild to moderate ulcerative colitis, especially in patients previously unresponsive or intolerant to conventional therapy. Olsalazine also has been shown to be effective in the maintenance of remission. In a large portion of patients, mesalamine and olsalazine are associated with fewer adverse effects than sulfasalazine. Mesalamine and olsalazine will expand treatment options for patients with ulcerative colitis in relapse or remission and will most likely be a welcomed and clinically appropriate addition to an institution's formulary.

Investigational Aminosalicylate Agents

Numerous products designed to deliver locally high concentrations of aminosalicylates within the colon are under investigation. Oral products typically are either mesalamine tablets with a resin coating that is time or pH dependent, or both, or a mesalamine compound containing a diazo bond but no sulfonamide component.

Pentasa (Marion, United States, or Ferring, Denmark), commercially available in Europe as a 250-mg tablet, uses mesalamine microgranules coated with a semipermeable ethylcellulose membrane. This formulation exhibits both time-dependent and pH-dependent drug release characteristics. At a pH of 2 or 6, the drug is released linearly over 24 hours. When the pH is over 7.5, as it is in the terminal ileum and colon, the drug is released over eight hours. It is estimated that 35% of a dose is absorbed in the small intestine and 25% in the colon; 53% of a dose is eliminated in the urine.[157] The absorption of mesalamine from Pentasa is not significantly affected by concurrent famotidine administration.[158] Clinical trials show Pentasa to be equivalent to sulfasalazine for treating ulcerative colitis and effective in sulfasalazine-intolerant patients.[159,160] The efficacy of Pentasa in patients with Crohn's disease is less clear; one trial reported that 72% of the patients improved and another reported no significant difference between Pentasa and placebo.[161-163] It has been suggested that Pentasa may be less effective than other mesalamine agents for colonic disease because of its early release and subsequent absorption within the small intestine.[49]

Asacol (Norwich-Eaton, United States, or Tillotts, United Kingdom), available in the United Kingdom as a 400-mg mesalamine tablet, is coated with 80–130 μm of Eudragit S. Eudragit S is methacrylic acid copolymer B, which disintegrates at a pH greater than 7.[164-166] Approximately 20% of a dose can be recovered in the urine, suggesting that the product is minimally released in the small intestine and thus delivers more mesalamine to the colon.[49] Concurrent famotidine administration resulted in an unexpected and unexplained reduction in mesalamine absorption.[158] Asacol is more effective than placebo and similar to sulfasalazine in the treatment of ulcerative colitis.[167-169] High doses (2.7 g) of Asacol were no more effective than low doses (1.2 g) in the maintenance of remission of ulcerative colitis.[170] Sulfasalazine-intolerant patients with ulcerative colitis have responded to Asacol in several studies.[171-173] Use of Asacol in patients with Crohn's disease has not been extensively studied. Because mesalamine appears to be released in the colon, the effectiveness of Asacol in patients with Crohn's disease, which frequently involves the distal small intestine and proximal colon, is questioned.[49]

Mesalamine is also formulated as 250-mg and 500-mg tablets coated with Eudragit L (Rowasa, Reid-Rowell, United States; Salofalk, Falk, United Kingdom; Claversal, SmithKline Beecham, United States). Eudragit L disintegrates at a pH greater than 5.6, and complete dissolution occurs within two hours at a pH greater than 7.5.[4,174] These products are well absorbed; 55% of a dose is recovered in the urine.[163] Famotidine coadministration produces no significant increase in absorption.[158] Studies in patients with active ulcerative colitis have found these products to be as effective as sulfasalazine with fewer adverse effects.[163,174] In patients with active Crohn's disease, these products are equal to sulfasalazine in effectiveness and superior to placebo.[163] Because this formulation releases mesalamine in the distal ileum, it may be more effective for treatment of proximal than distal IBD.[49]

The other approach to delivering free mesalamine within the lower gastrointestinal tract is development of sulfasalazine analogues. These agents, like sulfasalazine and olsalazine, contain mesalamine that is liberated by bacterial reduction of the diazo bond within the colon. Compounds being studied include balsalazide, ipsalazide, and poly-ASA.[49,163,175,176] In general, diazo-bonded compounds release less mesalamine within the small bowel. This results in lower serum and urinary concentrations and higher luminal and fecal concentrations than are seen with the slow-release mesalamine products.[163,177,178]

Another salicylate compound being studied for the treatment of IBD is 4-aminosalicylic acid (*p*-aminosalicylic acid), an antitubercular agent. It appears that 4-aminosalicylic acid lacks mesalamine's ability to inhibit neutrophil-derived lipoxygenase and to scavenge oxygen-derived free radicals, which makes its possible mechanism of action even less clear.[179] A randomized, controlled trial of 1- and 2-g 4-aminosalicylic acid enemas found that the 1-g but not the 2-g 4-aminosalicylic acid enema was significantly more effective than placebo in reducing ulcerative-colitis symptoms.[180] A separate trial of longer duration showed that the nightly 2-g 4-aminosalicylic acid enemas were superior to placebo for treatment of active left-sided ulcerative colitis.[181] A study comparing 2-g mesalamine and 2-g 4-aminosalicylic acid enemas in patients with ulcerative colitis reported similar efficacies.[182] The activity of 4-aminosalicylic acid in patients with Crohn's disease has not been adequately studied to determine its effectiveness.

Conclusion

Sulfasalazine, with or without corticosteroids, has previously been the standard therapy for initial treatment of patients with newly diagnosed IBD or those whose disease has relapsed. Recently, studies have demonstrated the safety and effectiveness of mesalamine for the treatment of active mild to moderate ulcerative colitis and olsalazine for the maintenance of remission. Both agents are effective in inducing remission of ulcerative colitis, although olsalazine is not approved by the FDA for the treatment of active disease. Mesalamine and olsalazine also have been shown to be effective in the maintenance of remission for up to one to two years. Further study is needed before these agents can be routinely recommended for the treatment of active Crohn's disease or the maintenance of its remission. With fewer adverse effects associated with these newer agents and the acceptance of both dosage forms of mesalamine by patients, it is safe to say that mesalamine and olsalazine are to become viable and appropriate first-line therapeutic options for clinicians who want to treat patients with newly diagnosed or relapsed ulcerative colitis, especially those intolerant or unresponsive to previous conventional therapy.

References

1. Truelove SC, Witts LJ, Tunbridge RE et al. Cortisone in ulcerative colitis. Final report on a therapeutic trial. *Br Med J*. 1955; 2:1041-8.
2. Peppercorn MA. Advances in drug therapy for inflammatory bowel disease. *Ann Intern Med*. 1990; 112:50-60.
3. Malatjalian DA. Pathology of inflammatory bowel disease in colorectal mucosal biopsies. *Dig Dis Sci*. 1987; 32(Suppl 12):5S-15S.
4. Delgado JI, Cerda JJ. Medical treatment of inflammatory bowel disease. *Hosp Formul*. 1991; 26:466-73.
5. Calkins BM, Mendeloff AI. Epidemiology of inflammatory bowel disease. *Epidemiol Rev*. 1986; 8:60-91.
6. Sottile RF, Quandt CM, Present DH et al. Medical management of inflammatory bowel disease. *DICP*. 1989; 23:963-73.
7. Lashner BA, Evans AA, Kirsner JB et al. Prevalence and incidence of inflammatory bowel disease in family members. *Gastroenterology*. 1986; 91:1396-1400.
8. Bennett R, Rubin PH, Present DH. Inflammatory bowel disease (IBD) in husbands and wives. Frequency of IBD in 35 offspring of 19 couples. *Gastroenterology*. 1988; 94:A6111. Abstract.
9. Curran FT, Allan RN, Keighley MRB. Superoxide production by Crohn's disease neutrophils. *Gut*. 1991; 32:399-402.
10. Kett K, Brandtzaeg P. Local IgA subclass alterations in ulcerative colitis and Crohn's disease of the colon. *Gut*. 1987; 1013-21.
11. James SP, Neckers LM, Graeff AS et al. Suppression of immunoglobulin synthesis by lymphocyte subpopulations in patients with Crohn's disease. *Gastroenterology*. 1984; 86:1510-8.
12. James SP, Strober W, Quinn TC et al. Crohn's disease. New concepts of pathogenesis and current approaches to treatment. *Dig Dis Sci*. 1987; 32:1297-1310.
13. Boirvant M, Leoni M, Tariciotti D et al. The clinical significance of serum C reactive protein levels in Crohn's disease. Results of a prospective longitudinal study. *J Clin Gastroenterol*. 1988; 10:401-5.
14. Svartz N. Salazopyrin, a new sulfanilamide preparation. *Acta Med Scand*. 1942; 110:577-98.
15. Svartz N. The treatment of 124 cases of ulcerative colitis with salazopyrine and attempts of desensibilization in cases of hypersensitiveness to sulfa. *Acta Med Scand*. 1948; 130(Suppl 206):465-72.
16. Baron JH, Connell AM, Lennard-Jones JE et al. Sulphasalazine and salicylazosulphadimidine in ulcerative colitis. *Lancet*. 1962;1:1094-6.
17. Dick AP, Grayson MJ, Carpenter RG et al. Controlled trial of sulphasalazine in the treatment of ulcerative colitis. *Gut*. 1964; 5:437-42.
18. Misiewicz JJ, Lennard-Jones JE, Connell AM et al. Controlled trial of sulphasalazine in maintenance therapy for ulcerative colitis. *Lancet*. 1965; 1:185-8.
19. Dissanayake AS, Truelove SC. A controlled therapeutic trial of long-term maintenance treatment of ulcerative colitis with sulphasalazine (salazopyrin). *Gut*. 1973; 14:923-6.
20. Peppercorn MA, Goldman P. The role of intestinal bacteria in the metabolism of salicylazosulfapyridine. *J Pharmacol Exp Ther*. 1972; 181:555-62.
21. Azad Khan AK, Piris J, Truelove SC. An experiment to determine the active therapeutic moiety of sulphasalazine. *Lancet*. 1977; 2:892-5.
22. Klotz U, Maier K, Fischer C et al. Therapeutic efficacy of sulfasalazine and its metabolites in patients with ulcerative colitis and Crohn's disease. *N'Engl J Med*. 1980; 303:1499-1502.
23. Van Hees PAM, Bakker JH, Van Tongeren JHM. Effect of sulfapyridine, 5-aminosalicylic acid, and placebo in patients with idiopathic proctitis. A study to determine the active therapeutic moiety of sulphasalazine. *Gut*. 1980; 21:632-5.
24. Das KM, Dubin R. Clinical pharmacokinetics of sulphasalazine. *Clin Pharmacokinet*. 1976; 1:406-25.
25. Bondesen S, Nielsen OH, Schou JB et al. Steady-state kinetics of 5-aminosalicylic acid and sulfapyridine during sulfasalazine prophylaxis in ulcerative colitis. *Scand J Gastroenterol*. 1986; 21:693-700.
26. Rampton DS, Hawkey CJ. Prostaglandins and ulcerative colitis. *Gut*. 1984; 25:1399-1413.
27. Hawkey CJ, Rampton DS. Prostaglandins and the gastrointestinal mucosa. Are they important in its function, disease, or treatment? *Gastroenterology*. 1985; 89:1162-88.
28. Sharon P, Ligumsky M, Rachmilewitz D et al. Role of prostaglandins in ulcerative colitis. Enhanced production during active disease and inhibition by sulfasalazine. *Gastroenterology*. 1978; 75:638-40.
29. Ligumsky M, Karmeli F, Sharon P et al. Enhanced thromboxane A_2 and prostacyclin production by cultured rectal mucosa in ulcerative colitis and its inhibition by steroids and sulfasalazine. *Gastroenterology*. 1981; 81:444-9.
30. Hawkey CJ, Truelove SC. Inhibition of prostaglandin synthetase in human rectal mucosa. *Gut*. 1983; 24:213-7.
31. Rampton DS, Sladen GE. Prostaglandin synthesis inhibitors in ulcerative colitis. Flurbiprofen compared with conventional treatment. *Prostaglandins*. 1981; 21:417-25.
32. Sircar JC, Schwender CF, Carethers ME. Inhibition of soybean lipoxygenase by sulfasalazine and 5-aminosalicylic acid. A possible mode of action in ulcerative colitis. *Biochem Pharmacol*. 1983; 32:170-2.
33. Allgayer H, Eisenburg J, Paumgartner G. Soybean lipoxygenase inhibition. Studies with the sulphasalazine metabolites n-acetylaminosalicylic acid, 5-aminosalicylic acid and sulfapyridine. *Eur J Clin Pharmacol*. 1984; 26:449-51.
34. Stenson WF, Lobos E. Sulfasalazine inhibits the synthesis of chemotactic lipids by neutrophils. *J Clin Invest*. 1982; 69:494-7.
35. Nielsen OH, Bukhave K, Elmgreen J et al. Inhibition of 5-lipoxygenase pathway of arachidonic acid metabolism in human neutrophils by sulfasalazine and 5-aminosalicylic acid. *Dig Dis Sci*. 1987; 32:577-82.
36. Peskar BM, Dreyling KW, Peskar BA et al. Enhanced formation of sulfidopeptide-leukotrienes in ulcerative colitis and Crohn's disease. Inhibition by sulfasalazine and 5-aminosalicylic acid. *Agents Actions*. 1986; 18:381-3.
37. Peskar BM, Dreyling KW, May B et al. Possible mode of action of 5-aminosalicylic acid. *Dig Dis Sci*. 1987; 32(Suppl 12):51S-56S.
38. Lauritsen K, Laursen LS, Bukhave K et al. Effects of topical 5-aminosalicylic acid and prednisolone on prostaglandin E_2 and leukotriene B_4 levels determined by equilibrium in vivo dialysis of rectum in relapsing ulcerative colitis. *Gastroenterology*. 1986; 91:837-44.

39. Stenson WF. A molecular mechanism for the inhibition of the synthesis of leukotriene B_4 (LTB_4) by 5-aminosalicylate (5-ASA). *Gastroenterology*. 1986; 90:A1648. Abstract.
40. Sharon P, Stenson WF. Enhanced synthesis of leukotriene B_4 by colonic mucosa in inflammatory bowel disease. *Gastroenterology*. 1984; 86:453-60.
41. Lauritsen K, Laursen LS, Bukhave K et al. In vivo effects of orally administered prednisolone on prostaglandin and leucotriene production in ulcerative colitis. *Gut*. 1987; 28:1095-9.
42. Rhodes JM, Bartholomew TC, Jewell DP. Inhibition of leucocyte motility by drugs used in ulcerative colitis. *Gut*. 1981; 22:642-7.
43. Ireland A, Jewell DP. Mechanism of action of 5-aminosalicylic acid and its derivatives. *Clin Sci*. 1990; 78:119-25.
44. MacDermott RP, Schloemann SR, Bertovich MJ et al. Inhibition of antibody secretion by 5-aminosalicylic acid. *Gastroenterology*. 1989; 96:442-8.
45. Dallegri F, Ottonello L, Ballestrero A et al. Cytoprotection against neutrophil derived hypochlorous acid. A potential mechanism for the therapeutic action of 5-aminosalicylic acid in ulcerative colitis. *Gut*. 1990; 31:184-6.
46. Craven PA, Pfanstiel J, Saito R et al. Actions of sulfasalazine and 5-aminosalicylic acid as reactive oxygen scavengers in the suppression of bile acid-induced increases in colonic epithelial cell loss and proliferative activity. *Gastroenterology*. 1987; 92:1998-2008.
47. Ahnfelt-Ronne I, Nielsen OH, Christensen A et al. Clinical evidence supporting the radical scavenger mechanism of 5-aminosalicylic acid. *Gastroenterology*. 1990; 98:1162-9.
48. Myers B, Evans DNW, Rhodes J et al. Metabolism and urinary excretion of 5-amino salicylic acid in healthy volunteers when given intravenously or released for absorption at different sites in the gastrointestinal tract. *Gut*. 1987; 28:196-200.
49. Jarnerot G. Newer 5-aminosalicylic acid based drugs in chronic inflammatory bowel disease. *Drugs*. 1989; 37:73-86.
50. Brogden RN, Sorkin EM. Mesalazine. A review of its pharmacodynamic and pharmacokinetic properties, and therapeutic potential in chronic inflammatory bowel disease. *Drugs*. 1989; 38:500-23.
51. Allgayer H, Ahnfelt NO, Kruis W et al. Colonic n-acetylation of 5-aminosalicylic acid in inflammatory bowel disease. *Gastroenterology*. 1989; 97:38-41.
52. Klotz U, Maier KE. Pharmacology and pharmacokinetics of 5-aminosalicylic acid. *Dig Dis Sci*. 1987; 32(Suppl 12):46S-50S.
53. Jacobsen BA, Abildgaard K, Rasmussen HH et al. Availability of mesalazine (5-aminosalicylic acid) from enemas and suppositories during steady-state conditions. *Scand J Gastroenterol*. 1991; 26:374-8.
54. Almer S, Norlander B, Strom M et al. Steady-state pharmacokinetics of a new 4-gram 5-aminosalicylic acid retention enema in patients with ulcerative colitis in remission. *Scand J Gastroenterol*. 1991; 26:327-35.
55. Campieri M, Lanfranchi GA, Boschi S et al. Topical administration of 5-aminosalicylic acid enemas in patients with ulcerative colitis. Studies on rectal absorption and excretion. *Gut*. 1985; 26:400-5.
56. Bondesen S, Nielsen OH, Jacobsen O et al. 5-Aminosalicylic acid enemas in patients with active ulcerative colitis. Influence of acidity on the kinetic pattern. *Scand J Gastroenterol*. 1984; 19:677-82.
57. Campieri M, Lanfranchi GA, Brignola C et al. Retrograde spread of 5-aminosalicylic acid enemas in patients with active ulcerative colitis. *Dis Colon Rectum*. 1986; 29:108-10.
58. Sandberg-Gertzen H, Ryde M, Jarnerot G. Absorption and excretion of a single 1-g dose of azodisal sodium in subjects with ileostomy. *Scand J Gastroenterol*. 1983; 18:107-11.
59. Lauritsen K, Hansen J, Ryde M et al. Colonic azodisalicylate metabolism determined by in vivo dialysis in healthy volunteers and patients with ulcerative colitis. *Gastroenterology*. 1984; 86:1496-1500.
60. Lauritsen K, Laursen LS, Bukhave K et al. Long-term olsalazine treatment. Pharmacokinetics, tolerance and effects on local eicosanoid formation in ulcerative colitis and Crohn's colitis. *Gut*. 1988; 29:974-82.
61. Willoughby CP, Aronson JK, Agback H et al. Distribution and metabolism in healthy volunteers of disodium azodisalicylate, a potential therapeutic agent for ulcerative colitis. *Gut*. 1982; 23:1081-7.
62. Van Hogezand RA, Van Hees PAM, Zwanenburg B et al. Disposition of disodium azodisalicylate in healthy subjects. A possible new drug for inflammatory bowel disease. *Gastroenterology*. 1985; 88:717-22.
63. Ryde EM, Ahnfelt NO. The pharmacokinetics of olsalazine sodium in healthy volunteers after a single i.v. dose and after oral doses with and without food. *Eur J Clin Pharmacol*. 1988; 34:481-8.
64. Sandberg-Gertzen H, Ryde M, Jarnerot G. Absorption and excretion of azodisal sodium and its metabolites in man after rectal administration of a single 2-g dose. *Scand J Gastroenterol*. 1983; 18:571-5.
65. Campbell DES, Berglindh T. Pharmacology of olsalazine. *Scand J Gastroenterol*. 1988; 23(Suppl 148):7-12.
66. Hetzel DJ, Bochner F, Imhoff DM et al. Azodisalicylate (ADS) in the treatment of ulcerative colitis (UC). A controlled trial and assessment of drug disposition. *Gastroenterology*. 1985; 88:A1418. Abstract.
67. Van Hogezand RA. Pharmacokinetics of olsalazine and its metabolites. *Scand J Gastroenterol*. 1988; 23(Suppl 148):17-20.
68. Peppercorn MA, Goldman P. Distribution studies of salicylazosulfapyridine and its metabolites. *Gastroenterology*. 1973; 64:240-5.
69. Williams CN, Haber G, Aquino JA. Double-blind, placebo-controlled evaluation of 5-ASA suppositories in active distal proctitis and measurement of extent of spread using ^{99m}Tc-labeled 5-ASA suppositories. *Dig Dis Sci*. 1987; 32(Suppl 12):71S-75S.
70. Campieri M, Gionchetti P, Belluzzi A et al. 5-Aminosalicylic acid suppositories in the management of ulcerative colitis. *Dis Colon Rectum*. 1989; 32:398-9.
71. Campieri M, De Franchis R, Bianchi Porro G et al. Mesalazine (5-ASA) suppositories in the treatment of ulcerative proctitis or distal proctosigmoiditis. A randomized controlled trial. *Scand J Gastroenterol*. 1990; 25:663-8.
72. Powell-Tuck J, Parkins RA. Controlled comparison of enemas containing 1 g and 2 g 5-aminosalicylic acid in patients with ulcerative proctosigmoiditis. *Gut*. 1984; 25:A1143. Abstract.
73. McPhee MS, Swan JT, Biddle WL et al. Proctocolitis unresponsive to conventional therapy. Response to 5-aminosalicylic acid enemas. *Dig Dis Sci*. 1987; 32(Suppl 12):76S-81S.
74. Sutherland LR, Martin F, Greer S et al. 5-Aminosalicylic acid enema in the treatment of distal ulcerative colitis, proctosigmoiditis, and proctitis. *Gastroenterology*. 1987; 92:1894-8.
75. Campieri M, Lanfranchi GA, Brignola C et al. 5-Aminosalicylic acid as rectal enema in ulcerative colitis patients unable to take sulphasalazine. *Lancet*. 1984; 1:403. Letter.
76. Kandel G, Prokipchuk EJ. 5-ASA enemas for refractory distal ulcerative colitis. An open trial. *J Clin Gastroenterol*. 1987; 9:536-40.
77. Sutherland LR, Martin F. 5-Aminosalicylic acid enemas in treatment of distal ulcerative colitis and proctitis in Canada. *Dig Dis Sci*. 1987; 32(Suppl 12):64S-6S.
78. Barber GB, Lee DE, Antonioli DA et al. Refractory distal ulcerative colitis responsive to 5-aminosalicylate enemas. *Am J Gastroenterol*. 1985; 80:612-4.
79. Biddle WL, Miner PB. Long-term use of mesalamine enemas to induce remission in ulcerative colitis. *Gastroenterology*. 1990; 99:113-8.
80. Friedman LS, Richter JM, Kirkham SE et al. 5-Aminosalicylic acid enemas in refractory distal ulcerative colitis. A randomized, controlled trial. *Am J Gastroenterol*. 1986; 81:412-8.

81. Campieri M, Gionchetti P, Belluzzi A et al. Efficacy of 5-aminosalicylic acid enemas versus hydrocortisone enemas in ulcerative colitis. *Dig Dis Sci.* 1987; 32(Suppl 12):67S-70S.
82. Mulder CJJ, Tytgat GNJ, Wiltink EHH et al. Comparison of 5-aminosalicylic acid (3 g) and prednisolone phosphate sodium enemas (30 mg) in the treatment of distal ulcerative colitis. A prospective, randomized, double-blind trial. *Scand J Gastroenterol.* 1988; 23:1005-8.
83. Danish 5-ASA Group. Topical 5-aminosalicylic acid versus prednisolone in ulcerative proctosigmoiditis. A randomized, double-blind multicenter trial. *Dig Dis Sci.* 1987; 32:598-602.
84. Baum CA, Biddle WL, Miner PB. Failure of 5-aminosalicylic acid enemas to improve chronic radiation proctitis. *Dig Dis Sci.* 1989; 34:758-60.
85. Triantafillidis JK, Dadioti P, Nicolakis D et al. High doses of 5-aminosalicylic acid enemas in chronic radiation proctitis. Comparison with betamethasone enemas. *Am J Gastroenterol.* 1990; 85:1537-8. Letter.
86. Campieri M, Gionchetti P, Belluzzi A et al. 5-Aminosalicylic acid as enemas or suppositories in distal ulcerative colitis? *J Clin Gastroenterol.* 1988; 10:406-9.
87. Miglioli M, Barbara L, Di Febo G et al. Topical administration of 5-aminosalicylic acid. A therapeutic proposal for the treatment of pouchitis. *N Engl J Med.* 1989; 320:257. Letter.
88. DArienzo A, Panarese A, D'Armiento FP et al. 5-Aminosalicylic acid suppositories in the maintenance of remission in idiopathic proctitis or proctosigmoiditis. A double-blind placebo-controlled clinical trial. *Am J Gastroenterol.* 1990; 85:1079-82.
89. Mayberry JF, Balfour TW. Inflammation in the rectal stump. The role of 5-aminosalicylic acid suppositories. *J Clin Gastroenterol.* 1990; 12:119-20. Letter.
90. Biddle WL, Greenberger NJ, Swan JT et al. 5-Aminosalicylic acid enemas. Effective agent in maintaining remission in left-sided ulcerative colitis. *Gastroenterology.* 1988; 94:1075-9.
91. Guarino J, Chatzinoff M, Berk T et al. 5-Aminosalicylic acid enemas in refractory ulcerative colitis. Long-term results. *Am J Gastroenterol.* 1987; 82:732-7.
92. Sutherland LR, Martin F. 5-Aminosalicylic acid enemas in the maintenance of remission in distal ulcerative colitis and proctitis. *Can J Gastroenterol.* 1987; 1:3-6.
93. D'Albasio G, Trallori G, Ghetti A et al. Intermittent therapy with high-dose 5-aminosalicylic acid enemas for maintaining remission in ulcerative proctosigmoiditis. *Dis Colon Rectum.* 1990; 33:394-7.
94. Selby WS, Barr GD, Ireland A et al. Olsalazine in active ulcerative colitis. *Br Med J.* 1985; 291:1373-5.
95. Hetzel DJ, Shearman DJC, Labrooy J et al. Olsalazine in the treatment of active ulcerative colitis. A placebo controlled clinical trial and assessment of drug disposition. *Scand J Gastroenterol.* 1988: 23(Suppl 148):61-9.
96. Feurle GE, Theuer D, Velasco S et al. Olsalazine versus placebo in the treatment of mild to moderate ulcerative colitis. A randomized double blind trial. *Gut.* 1989; 30:1354-61.
97. Meyers S, Sachar DB, Present DH et al. Olsalazine sodium in the treatment of ulcerative colitis among patients intolerant to sulfasalazine. A prospective, randomized, placebo-controlled, double-blind, dose-ranging clinical trial. *Gastroenterology.* 1987; 93:1255-62.
98. Zinberg J, Molinas S, Das KM. Double-blind placebo-controlled study of olsalazine in the treatment of ulcerative colitis. *Am J Gastroenterol.* 1990; 85:562-6.
99. Smits BJ. Open study of olsalazine in ulcerative colitis. *Scand J Gastroenterol.* 1988; 23(Suppl 148):95.
100. Kildebo S. Open, uncontrolled trial of olsalazine. *Scand J Gastroenterol.* 1988; 23(Suppl 148):86.
101. Kondo M, Inoue M, Shiratori T et al. Olsalazine in active ulcerative colitis. Dose finding study in Japan. *Scand J Gastroenterol.* 1988; 23(Suppl 148):60.
102. Willoughby CP, Cowan RE, Gould SR et al. Double-blind comparison of olsalazine and sulphasalazine in active ulcerative colitis. *Scand J Gastroenterol.* 1988; 23(Suppl 148):40-4.
103. Ewe K, Eckardt V, Kanzler G. Treatment of ulcerative colitis with olsalazine and sulphasalazine. Efficacy and side-effects. *Scand J Gastroenterol.* 1988; 23(Suppl 148):70-5.
104. Rao SSC, Dundas SAC, Holdsworth CD et al. Olsalazine or sulphasalazine in first attacks of ulcerative colitis? A double blind study. *Gut.* 1989; 30:675-9.
105. Courtney MG, Weir DG. Olsalazine in the treatment of ulcerative colitis. *Scand J Gastroenterol.* 1988; 23(Suppl 148):83-5.
106. Sandberg-Gertzen H, Jarnerot G, Kraaz W. Azodisal sodium in the treatment of ulcerative colitis. A study of tolerance and relapse-prevention properties. *Gastroenterology.* 1986; 90:1024-30.
107. Ireland A, Mason CH, Jewell DP. Controlled trial comparing olsalazine and sulphasalazine for the maintenance treatment of ulcerative colitis. *Gut.* 1988; 29:835-7.
108. Sandberg-Gertzen H, Jarnerot G, Tysk C. Long-term treatment with olsalazine for ulcerative colitis. Safety and relapse prevention. A follow-up study. *Scand J Gastroenterol.* 1988; 23(Suppl 148):48-50.
109. Das KM, Eastwood MA, McManus JPA et al. Adverse reactions during salicylazosulfapyridine therapy and the relation with drug metabolism and acetylator phenotype. *N Engl J Med.* 1973; 289:491-5.
110. Schroder H, Evans DAP. Acetylator phenotype and adverse effects of sulphasalazine in healthy subjects. *Gut.* 1972; 13:278-84.
111. Taffet SL, Das KM. Sulfasalazine. Adverse effects and desensitization. *Dig Dis Sci.* 1983; 28:833-42.
112. Singleton JW, Law DH, Kelley ML et al. National cooperative Crohn's disease study. Adverse reactions to study drugs. *Gastroenterology.* 1979; 77:870-82.
113. Isaacs KL, Murphy D. Pancreatitis after rectal administration of 5-aminosalicylic acid. *J Clin Gastroenterol.* 1990; 12:198-9.
114. Diener U, Tuczek HV, Fischer C et al. Renal function was not impaired by treatment with 5-aminosalicylic acid in rats and man. *Naunyn-Schmiedeberg's Arch Pharmacol.* 1984; 326:278-82.
115. Kutty PK, Raman KRK, Hawken K et al. Hair loss and 5-aminosalicylic acid enemas. *Ann Intern Med.* 1982; 97:785-6. Letter.
116. Waanders H, Thompson J. Kawasaki-like syndrome after treatment with mesalamine. *Am J Gastroenterol.* 1991; 86:219-21.
117. Chatzinoff M, Guarino JM, Corson SL et al. Sulfasalazine-induced abnormal sperm penetration assay reversed on changing to 5-aminosalicylic acid enemas. *Dig Dis Sci.* 1988; 33:108-10.
118. Anttila PM, Valimaki M, Pentikainen PJ. Pure-red-cell aplasia associated with sulphasalazine but not 5-aminosalicylic acid. *Lancet.* 1985; 2:1006. Letter.
119. Zelissen PMJ, Van Hattum J, Poen H et al. Influence of salazosulphapyridine and 5-aminosalicylic acid on seminal qualities and male sex hormones. *Scand J Gastroenterol.* 1988; 23:1100-4.
120. Nelis GF. Diarrhoea due to 5-aminosalicylic acid in breast milk. *Lancet.* 1989; 1:383. Letter.
121. Agnholt J, Sorensen HT, Rasmussen SN et al. Cardiac hypersensitivity to 5-aminosalicylic acid. *Lancet.* 1989; 1:1135. Letter.
122. Kristensen KS, Hoegholm A, Bohr L et al. Fatal myocarditis associated with mesalazine. *Lancet.* 1990; 335:605. Letter.
123. Shaffer JL, Kershaw A, Berrisford MH. Sulphasalazine-induced infertility reversed on transfer to 5-aminosalicylic acid. *Lancet.* 1984; 1:1240. Letter.
124. Riley SA, LeCarpentier J, Mani V et al. Sulphasalazine induced seminal abnormalities in ulcerative colitis. Results of mesalazine substitution. *Gut.* 1987; 28:1008-12.
125. Cann PA, Holdsworth CD. Reversal of male infertility on changing treatment from sulphasalazine to 5-aminosali-

cylic acid. *Lancet*. 1984; 1:1119. Letter.
126. Kjaergaard N, Christensen LA, Lauritsen JG et al. Effects of mesalazine substitution on salicylazosulfapyridine-induced seminal abnormalities in men with ulcerative colitis. *Scand J Gastroenterol*. 1989; 24:891-6.
127. Novis BH, Korzets Z, Chen P et al. Nephrotic syndrome after treatment with 5-aminosalicylic acid. *Br Med J*. 1988; 296:1442.
128. Deprez P, Descamps C, Fiasse R. Pancreatitis induced by 5-aminosalicylic acid. *Lancet*. 1989; 2:445-6. Letter.
129. Sachedina B, Saibil F, Cohen LB et al. Acute pancreatitis due to 5-aminosalicylate. *Ann Intern Med*. 1989; 110:490-2.
130. Fiorentini MT, Fracchia M, Galatola G et al. Acute pancreatitis during oral 5-aminosalicylic acid therapy. *Dig Dis Sci*. 1990; 35:1180-2.
131. Jenss H, Becker EW, Weber P. Pericardial effusion during treatment with 5-aminosalicylic acid in a patient with Crohn's disease. *Am J Gastroenterol*. 1990; 85:332-3. Letter.
132. Mehta RP. Acute interstitial nephritis due to 5-aminosalicylic acid. *Can Med Assoc J*. 1990; 143:1031-2.
133. Turunen U, Elomaa I, Anttila VJ et al. Mesalazine tolerance in patients with inflammatory bowel disease and previous intolerance or allergy to sulphasalazine or sulphonamides. *Scand J Gastroenterol*. 1987; 22:798-802.
134. Rao SS, Cann PA, Holdsworth CD. Clinical experience of the tolerance of mesalazine and olsalazine in patients intolerant of sulphasalazine. *Scand J Gastroenterol*. 1987; 22:332-6.
135. Ireland A, Jewell DP. Olsalazine in patients intolerant to sulphasalazine. *Scand J Gastroenterol*. 1987; 22:1038-40.
136. Hetzel DJ, Hanrahan AN, Chapman PJ. Olsalazine treatment in patients intolerant of sulphasalazine. The Australian experience. *Scand J Gastroenterol*. 1988; 23(Suppl 148):89-94.
137. Poldermans D, Van Blankenstein M. Pancreatitis induced by disodium azodisalicylate. *Am J Gastroenterol*. 1988; 83:578-80.
138. Mulder H, Gratama S. Azodisalicylate (Dipentum)-induced hepatitis? *J Clin Gastroenterol*. 1989; 11:708-11.
139. Scherpenisse J, Van Hees PAM. Olsalazine in patients with serious side-effects or allergy due to sulphasalazine. *Scand J Gastroenterol*. 1988; 23(Suppl 148):108-9.
140. Jarnerot G. Clinical tolerance of olsalazine. *Scand J Gastroenterol*. 1988; 23(Suppl 148):21-3.
141. Rao SS, Holdsworth CD. Influence of olsalazine and sulphasalazine on gastrointestinal time. *Scand J Gastroenterol*. 1988; 23(Suppl 148):96-100.
142. Pamukcu R, Hanauer SB, Chang EB. Effect of disodium azodisalicylate on electrolyte transport in rabbit ileum and colon in vitro. *Gastroenterology*. 1988; 95:975-81.
143. Raimundo AH, Patil DH, Frost PG et al. Effects of olsalazine and sulphasalazine on jejunal and ileal water and electrolyte absorption in normal human subjects. *Gut*. 1991; 32:270-4.
144. Berglindh T, Landstrom E, Bergqvist E. Induction of and adaptation to olsalazine induced intestinal volume load. *Scand J Gastroenterol*. 1988; 23(Suppl 148):24-8.
145. Jarnerot G, Sandberg-Gertzen H, Tobiasson P et al. Olsalazine does not increase the bile acid losses in subjects with a permanent ileostomy. *Scand J Gastroenterol*. 1988; 23:489-92.
146. Sandberg-Gertzen H, Jarnerot G, Bukhave K et al. Effect of azodisal sodium and sulphasalazine on ileostomy output of fluid and PGE_2 and PGE_{2a} in subjects with a permanent ileostomy. *Gut*. 1986; 27:1306-11.
147. Sullivan S. Sulfasalazine lung. Desensitization to sulfasalazine and treatment with acrylic coated 5-ASA and azodisalicylate. *J Clin Gastroenterol*. 1987; 9:461-3.
148. Scherpenisse J, Van Der Valk PDLPM, Van Den Bosch JMM et al. Olsalazine as an alternative therapy in a patient with sulfasalazine-induced eosinophilic pneumonia. *J Clin Gastroenterol*. 1988; 10:218-20.
149. Ireland A, Jewell DP. Sulfasalazine-induced impotence. A beneficial resolution with olsalazine? *J Clin Gastroenterol*. 1989; 11:711. Letter.
150. Kaufmann HJ, Taubin HL. Nonsteroidal anti-inflammatory drugs activate quiescent inflammatory bowel disease. *Ann Intern Med*. 1987; 107:513-6.
151. Rampton DS, McNeil NI, Sarner M. Analgesic ingestion and other factors preceding relapse in ulcerative colitis. *Gut*. 1983; 24:187-9.
152. Rampton DS, Sladen GE. Relapse of ulcerative proctocolitis during treatment with non-steroidal anti-inflammatory drugs. *Postgrad Med J*. 1981; 57:297-9.
153. Reid-Rowell. Rowasa enema package insert. Marietta, GA: 1991 Aug.
154. Reid-Rowell. Rowasa suppository package insert. Marietta, GA: 1991 Aug.
155. Pharmacia, Inc. Dipentum package insert. Piscataway, NJ: 1991 Aug.
156. Drug Topics redbook annual pharmacists' reference. Sifton DW, ed. Montvale, NJ: Medical Economics; 1992.
157. Rasmussen SN, Bondesen S, Hvidberg EF et al. 5-Aminosalicylic acid in a slow-release preparation. Bioavailability, plasma level, and excretion in humans. *Gastroenterology*. 1982; 83:1062-70.
158. Wiltink EHH, Mulder CJJ, Stolk LML et al. Absorption of oral mesalazine-containing preparations and the influence of famotidine on the absorption. *Scand J Gastroenterol*. 1990; 25:579-84.
159. Mulder CJJ, Tytgat GNJ, Dekker W et al. Pentasa in lieu of sulfasalazine. *Ann Intern Med*. 1988; 106:911-2. Letter.
160. Mulder CJJ, Tytgat GNJ, Weterman IT et al. Double-blind comparison of slow-release 5-aminosalicylic acid and sulfasalazine in remission maintenance in ulcerative colitis. *Gastroenterology*. 1988; 95:1449-53.
161. Rasmussen SN, Binder V, Maier K et al. Treatment of Crohn's disease with peroral 5-aminosalicylic acid. *Gastroenterology*. 1983; 85:1350-3.
162. Rasmussen SN, Lauritsen K, Tage-Jensen U et al. 5-Aminosalicylic acid in the treatment of Crohn's disease. A 16-week double-blind, placebo-controlled, multicentre study with Pentasa. *Scand J Gastroenterol*. 1987; 22:877-83.
163. Martin F. Oral 5-aminosalicylic acid preparations in treatment of inflammatory bowel disease. An update. *Dig Dis Sci*. 1987; 32(Suppl 12):57S-63S.
164. Mardini HA, Lindsay DC, Deighton CM et al. Effects of polymer coating on faecal recovery of ingested 5-amino salicylic acid in patients with ulcerative colitis. *Gut*. 1987; 28:1084-9.
165. Dew MJ, Ryder REJ, Evans N et al. Colonic release of 5-amino salicylic acid from an oral preparation in active ulcerative colitis. *Br J Clin Pharmacol*. 1983; 16:185-7.
166. Dew MJ, Hughes PJ, Lee MG et al. An oral preparation to release drugs in the human colon. *Br J Clin Pharmacol*. 1982; 14:405-8.
167. Dew MJ, Hughes P, Harries AD et al. Maintenance of remission in ulcerative colitis with oral preparation of 5-aminosalicylic acid. *Br Med J*. 1982; 285:1012.
168. Riley SA, Mani V, Goodman MJ et al. Comparison of delayed-release 5-aminosalicylic acid (mesalazine) and sulfasalazine as maintenance treatment for patients with ulcerative colitis. *Gastroenterology*. 1988; 94:1383-9.
169. Schroeder KW, Tremaine WJ, Ilstrup DM. Coated oral 5-aminosalicylic acid therapy for mildly to moderately active ulcerative colitis. A randomized study. *N Engl J Med*. 1987; 317:1625-9.
170. Dew MJ, Harries AD, Evans N et al. Maintenance of remission in ulcerative colitis with 5-amino salicylic acid in high doses by mouth. *Br Med J*. 1983; 287:23-4.
171. Donald IP, Wilkinson SP. The value of 5-aminosalicylic acid in inflammatory bowel disease for patients intolerant or allergic to sulphasalazine. *Postgrad Med J*. 1985; 61:1047-8.
172. Dew MJ, Harries AD, Evans BK et al. Treatment of ulcerative colitis with oral 5-aminosalicylic acid in patients unable to take sulphasalazine. *Lancet*. 1983; 2:801. Letter.
173. Habal FM, Greenberg GR. Treatment of ulcerative colitis with oral 5-aminosalicylic acid including patients with ad-

verse reactions to sulfasalazine. *Am J Gastroenterol.* 1988; 83:15-9.

174. Rachmilewitz D. Coated mesalazine (5-aminosalicylic acid) versus sulphasalazine in the treatment of active ulcerative colitis. A randomized trial. *Br Med J.* 1989; 298:82-6.
175. Chan RP, Pope DJ, Gilbert AP et al. Studies of two novel sulfasalazine analogs, ipsalazide and balsalazide. *Dig Dis Sci.* 1983; 28:609-15.
176. Garretto M, Riddell RH, Winans CS. Treatment of chronic ulcerative colitis with poly-ASA. A new nonabsorbable carrier for release of 5-aminosalicylate in the colon. *Gastroenterology.* 1983; 84:A1162. Abstract.
177. Laursen LS, Stokholm M, Bukhave K et al. Disposition of 5-aminosalicylic acid by olsalazine and three mesalazine preparations in patients with ulcerative colitis. Comparison of intraluminal colonic concentrations, serum values, and urinary excretion. *Gut.* 1990; 31:1271-6.
178. Rijk MCM, Van Schaik A, Van Tongeren JHM. Disposition of 5-aminosalicylic acid by 5-aminosalicylic acid-delivering compounds. *Scand J Gastroenterol.* 1988; 23:107-12.
179. Nielsen OH, Ahnfelt-Ronne I. 4-Aminosalicylic acid, in contrast to 5-aminosalicylic acid, has no effect on arachidonic acid metabolism in human neutrophils, or on the free radical 1,1-diphenyl-2-picrylhydrazyl. *Pharmacol Toxicol.* 1988; 62:223-6.
180. Gandolfo J, Farthing M, Powers G et al. 4-Aminosalicylic acid retention enemas in treatment of distal colitis. *Dig Dis Sci.* 1987; 32:700-4.
181. Ginsberg AL, Beck LS, McIntosh TM et al. Treatment of left-sided ulcerative colitis with 4-aminosalicylic acid enemas. A double-blind, placebo-controlled trial. *Ann Intern Med.* 1988; 108:195-9.
182. Campieri M, Lanfranchi GA, Bertoni F et al. A double-blind clinical trial to compare the effects of 4-aminosalicylic acid to 5-aminosalicylic acid in topical treatment of ulcerative colitis. *Digestion.* 1984; 29:204-8.

Therapy Update

Methotrexate for treatment of unruptured ectopic pregnancy

REBECCA ROGERS PREVOST, THOMAS G. STOVALL, AND FRANK W. LING

Abstract: Clinical experience with and adverse effects of methotrexate for the treatment of unruptured ectopic pregnancy are described.

Ectopic pregnancy is suspected in the presence of the following: positive results on pregnancy test (e.g., test for β-human chorionic gonadotropin [β-hCG]), lower abdominal pain, a normal or slightly enlarged uterus, and a mass on either side of the midline. When laparoscopy is required for diagnosis, surgical correction is done at the same time. However, use of serial β-hCG titers, vaginal ultrasound examinations, serum progesterone concentrations, and dilation and curettage (when the pregnancy is confirmed to be nonviable) allows earlier detection of ectopic pregnancy without laparoscopy. If rupture has not occurred, i.v. or i.m. methotrexate is administered; usually, i.m. leucovorin is given, on alternate days, to prevent hematologic toxicity. Adverse effects of methotrexate include stomatitis, gastritis, and hepatic enzyme elevation. Use of a single-dose regimen of i.m. methotrexate without leucovorin has been associated with a lower frequency of toxicity. Selection criteria for patients are as follows: (1) an unruptured ectopic pregnancy less than or equal to 3.5 cm in greatest dimension on transvaginal ultrasound, (2) no active renal or hepatic disease, and (3) no evidence of leukopenia or thrombocytopenia.

Intramuscular methotrexate therapy is a safe and effective alternative to surgery for the treatment of unruptured ectopic pregnancy.

Index terms: Drug administration routes; Immunosuppressive agents; Methotrexate; Pregnancy; Toxicity
Clin Pharm. 1992; 11:529-32

An ectopic pregnancy results when a fertilized ovum becomes implanted outside the uterus. The most common site of extrauterine implantation is the fallopian tube, but other sites include the ovary, cervix, and abdominal cavity.[1] The incidence of ectopic pregnancy has increased fivefold since 1970 and is most closely correlated with an increase in pelvic inflammatory disease.[2] Other conditions associated with ectopic pregnancy include current use of an intrauterine device, history of infertility, prior tubal surgery, and any condition that prevents or retards migration of the fertilized ovum to the uterus. The risk of recurrence is estimated to be 20%. Of greatest concern is that rupture of ectopic pregnancy accounts for 12% of all maternal mortality and is the leading cause of maternal mortality in blacks.[2]

The most widely used treatment for ectopic pregnancy is surgical removal, and surgery is the only treatment for ruptured ectopic pregnancy. However, in an effort to improve subsequent fertility rates and to avoid the risks of surgical intervention, investigators have evaluated the use of methotrexate in resolving unruptured ectopic pregnancies. As an inhibitor of dihydrofolate reductase, methotrexate has the potential to prevent DNA replication in all cells. However, actively proliferating tissues, such as malignant cells, bone marrow, fetal and trophoblastic cells, dermal epithelium, buccal and intestinal mucosa, and the urinary bladder epithelium, are most susceptible. This article describes the role of methotrexate in the treatment of unruptured ectopic pregnancy and recent clinical experience with methotrexate, including its adverse effects.

Diagnosis of Ectopic Pregnancy

An ectopic pregnancy is usually suspected in the presence of a positive pregnancy test (i.e., positive test for urinary chorionic gonadotropin [UCG] or a positive serum quantitative test for the β-subunit of human

REBECCA ROGERS PREVOST, PHARM.D., is Clinical Pharmacist, Obstetrics/Gynecology and Neonatology, Regional Medical Center, Memphis, TN, and Assistant Professor, Department of Clinical Pharmacy, University of Tennessee, Memphis. THOMAS G. STOVALL, M.D., is Assistant Professor, and FRANK W. LING, M.D., is Associate Professor and Director, Division of Gynecology, Department of Obstetrics and Gynecology, University of Tennessee.

Address reprint requests to Dr. Prevost at the Regional Medical Center, 877 Jefferson Avenue, Memphis, TN 38103.

The Therapy Update *section provides concise analytical reviews of narrowly defined, important topics in pharmacotherapy. Priority is given to articles that focus on new or emerging standards in drug therapy. Articles are not intended to be comprehensive reviews of drugs or of disease states and their treatment.*

chorionic gonadotropin [β-hCG]), lower abdominal pain, a normal or slightly enlarged uterus, and a mass located to either side of the midline. Vaginal bleeding may or may not be present. After positive results are obtained for a pregnancy test, detection of an abnormal rise in the concentration of β-hCG and the serum concentration of progesterone further aids in the diagnosis of ectopic pregnancy.

Beta-hCG is produced by trophoblastic cells, which surround the embryo, and is responsible for maintaining the corpus luteum in early pregnancy. Beta-hCG is detectable as early as seven days after ovulation. Its amount doubles every 1.7 days in viable intrauterine pregnancies, achieving a peak concentration of approximately 60,000 mIU/mL by weeks 8–10 of pregnancy. Thereafter, β-hCG declines and remains at approximately 10,000 mIU/mL during weeks 18–40. Using radioimmunoassay technique, β-hCG is detectable at concentrations as low as 3 mIU/mL.[3]

Progesterone is secreted by the corpus luteum in early pregnancy, and then by the placenta after weeks 8–10. In 100% of viable intrauterine pregnancies, the serum concentration of progesterone is greater than 5 ng/mL. Therefore, values less than this are diagnostic of pregnancy nonviability.

Ectopic pregnancies are potentially life-threatening to the mother. If rupture has occurred, the patient may have hypotension or tachycardia, or may be in overt shock. However, if the ectopic pregnancy is unruptured, the patient may be asymptomatic. Therefore, all ectopic pregnancies should be considered as emergencies requiring definitive diagnosis and prompt treatment.

Laparoscopy is the mainstay of diagnosis. When laparoscopy is required for diagnosis, surgical treatment can be accomplished at the same time. However, Stovall et al.[4,5] have demonstrated that use of serial β-hCG titers, vaginal ultrasound, serum progesterone concentrations, and dilation and curettage when the pregnancy is confirmed to be nonviable allows for earlier detection of ectopic pregnancy without laparoscopy. Because laparoscopy is not performed immediately unless rupture is suspected, these diagnostic tests can shorten the length of time to diagnosis and treatment by one day. This approach may have a dramatic impact on the incidence of ruptured ectopic pregnancies. The use of serum progesterone concentration as a screening test for abnormal pregnancy has decreased the frequency of rupture in ectopic pregnancy from 79.2% to 38.8%.[5]

Clinical Experience with Methotrexate

Table 1 gives a comparison of parenteral methotrexate regimens, adverse effects, and efficacy rates. Methotrexate was first used to treat an ectopic pregnancy in 1965 in a patient with a nonviable abdominal pregnancy.[16] In this case, the fetus was removed surgically, but the placenta had implanted throughout the peritoneal cavity. The placenta could not be removed for concern of uncontrollable hemorrhage. Methotrexate 10 mg orally (as the sodium salt) was administered daily for four days to promote placental degeneration. This course of therapy was repeated twice during the following two weeks. The UCG titer declined after the first course of therapy and reached a nondetectable value by approximately 36 days. The patient experienced no adverse effects from the methotrexate therapy, and she remained asymptomatic during eight months of follow-up.

Ory et al.[8] employed methotrexate in six women with unruptured tubal pregnancies diagnosed by laparoscopy, ultrasound, and serum β-hCG concentrations. Patients received methotrexate 1 mg/kg (as the sodium salt) i.v. every other day during a seven-day period. Leucovorin 0.1 mg/kg (as the calcium salt) i.m. was administered on alternate days for prevention of hematologic toxicity. Blood chemistry, β-hCG concentrations, complete blood counts, and ultrasound examinations were monitored daily during therapy. Five of six patients had complete resolution of the ectopic pregnancy. One patient required surgery for arterial bleeding from the tubal implantation site; however, the fallopian tube did not rupture. Three patients had prompt declines in β-hCG concentrations, reaching nondetectable values within 5–20 days after therapy, while two patients had more prolonged courses, requiring 40–53 days for β-hCG values to fully decline. Stomatitis occurred in two patients, and serum aspartate aminotransferase (AST) concentrations increased in two patients. One patient experienced gastritis, and two patients required transfusion for a decreased hematocrit. No other morbidity was observed.

Rodi et al.[9] employed the same dosage (but used i.m. rather than i.v. methotrexate), diagnostic, and monitoring protocol in a study of seven women with unruptured ectopic pregnancy. Methotrexate treatment resulted in successful resolution in all cases. Posttherapy hysterosalpingograms were performed in five women: four demonstrated tubal patency on the side where the ectopic pregnancy had been, and one showed unilateral obstruction on the same side. One woman successfully achieved an intrauterine pregnancy before a hysterosalpingogram was performed. In all seven women, serum β-hCG concentrations fell to undetectable levels at a median of 31 days (range, 5–50 days). One patient experienced stomatitis, and two patients had increases in hepatic aminotransferase concentrations.

The authors extended their trial to 21 patients with ectopic pregnancies and showed successful resolution in 20 cases (95%) with medical therapy alone.[11] Methotrexate 1 mg/kg (as the sodium salt) was administered i.m. on days 1, 3, 5, and 7, and leucovorin 0.1 mg/kg (as the calcium salt) was administered i.m. on days 2, 4, 6, and 8. Five patients (24%) experienced methotrexate toxicity, including stomatitis, liver enzyme elevation, dermatitis, pleuritis, and mild nausea. All symptoms resolved within 96 hours of termination of therapy. Hysterosalpingograms performed at 12 weeks after methotrexate treatment revealed tubal patency in 75% of patients.

Stovall et al.[13] demonstrated a decrease in the incidence of adverse effects by using a protocol that adjusted the number of methotrexate and leucovorin doses according to the patient's β-hCG titer. Thirty-four patients with unruptured ectopic pregnancies were initially monitored with a baseline complete blood count and serum concentrations of AST, β-hCG, and progesterone. Methotrexate 1 mg/kg (as the sodium salt) was given i.m. followed by leucovorin 0.1 mg/kg (as the calcium salt) i.m. the next day. This regimen was continued until a 15% or greater decrease was noted in two consecutive daily β-hCG titers. Five patients (15%) required a single dose; 13 (38%) required two doses, 9 (26%) received three doses, and 7 (21%) received four doses. One patient required a second course of therapy 26 days after an initial two-dose course. Two patients (6%) developed a notable increase in serum AST concentration, which returned to baseline within 48 hours of drug discontinuation. The elevation in serum AST concentration was associated with a concurrent decline in β-hCG titer. One patient developed stomatitis, which spontaneously resolved within 24 hours of the fourth dose of methotrexate.

This individualized, multidose regimen was used by the same researchers to treat 100 patients.[14] Of 96 successfully treated patients, 17 (18%) had resolution of ectopic pregnancy with one methotrexate and leucovorin dose; 38 (40%), with two doses; 22 (23%), with three doses; and 19 (20%), with four doses. Among all 100 patients, one experienced a urinary tract infection (1%), two had increases in liver enzyme concentrations (2%), two experienced stomatitis (2%), and one experienced gastroenteritis (1%). Four (4%) of the 100 patients had ectopic rupture. Two of these patients received four methotrexate and leucovorin doses and two received doses before rupture occurred.

A simplified single-dose regimen has been used in our center and has resulted in an even lower frequency of methotrexate toxicity.[15] Thirty-one patients desiring future fertility who had an unruptured ectopic pregnancy less than 3.5 cm in greatest dimension on transvaginal ultrasound were treated as outpatients with a single i.m. injection of methotrexate 50 mg/sq

Table 1.
Trials of Methotrexate for Treatment of Unruptured Ectopic Pregnancy

Ref.	*n*	Methotrexate Dosage[a]	Leucovorin Dosage[b]	% Success	Complications[c] (*n*)
6	1	30 mg i.m. on day 1, then 15 mg i.m. on days 2–6, then 15 mg i.m. on days 8 and 9	None	100	Elevated LFT (1)
7	1	25 mg i.m. on days 1–3, then 20 mg i.m. on days 14–18	None	100	Gastritis (1), bone marrow suppression (1)
8	6	1 mg/kg i.v. on days 1, 3, 5, and 7	0.1 mg/kg i.m. on days 2, 4, 6, and 8	83	Stomatitis (2), elevated LFT (2), gastritis (1), decreased HCT (2)
9	7	1 mg/kg i.m. on days 1, 3, 5, and 7	0.1 mg/kg i.m. on days 2, 4, 6, and 8	100	Stomatitis (1), elevated LFT (2)
10	1	1 mg/kg i.m. on days 1, 3, and 5	0.1 mg/kg p.o. on days 2, 4, and 6	100	Stomatitis (1)
11	21	1 mg/kg i.m. on days 1, 3, 5, and 7	0.1 mg/kg i.m. on days 2, 4, 6, and 8	95	Stomatitis (2), elevated LFT (1), pleuritis (1), dermatitis (1), gastritis (1)
12	23	0.4 mg/kg i.m. on days 1–5	None	96	Elevated LFT (4), bone marrow suppression (1)
13	36	1 mg/kg i.m. on days 1, 3, 5, and 7 p.r.n.[d]	0.1 mg/kg i.m. on days 2, 4, 6, and 8 p.r.n.[d]	94	Stomatitis (1), elevated LFT (2)
14	100	1 mg/kg i.m. on days 1, 3, 5, and 7 p.r.n.[d]	0.1 mg/kg i.m. on days 2, 4, 6, and 8 p.r.n.[d]	96	Stomatitis (2), elevated AST (2), UTI (1), gastritis (1)
15	30	50 mg/sq m i.m. on day 1	None	97	None

[a]Given as the sodium salt.
[b]Given as the calcium salt.
[c]LFT = liver function test results, HCT = hematocrit, AST = serum aspartate aminotransferase concentration, UTI = urinary tract infection.
[d]Each methotrexate dose was followed by a dose of leucovorin. Methotrexate and leucovorin were given until there was a ≥15% reduction in two consecutive daily serum titers of human chorionic gonadotropin (β-subunit).

m (as the sodium salt) without leucovorin rescue. Ectopic pregnancy was diagnosed if the β-hCG titer was greater than 2000 mIU/mL without an associated intrauterine sac by transvaginal ultrasound, or if β-hCG titers rose persistently following endometrial curettage. After methotrexate administration, a β-hCG titer was obtained on days 1 (the day of methotrexate administration), 2, 4, and 7. A complete blood count and serum AST concentrations were obtained on days 1 and 7. Of 30 patients, 29 (97%) were successfully treated, as determined by a decline in serum β-hCG concentration to less than 10 mIU/mL. In the patient who did not respond to therapy, fetal cardiac activity had been noted on transvaginal ultrasound. No patient experienced any adverse effects of methotrexate during the initial treatment or the follow-up period.

We have treated 44 more patients by using this single-dose regimen and have continued to obtain similar results. This outpatient regimen is more attractive than previous treatment protocols because a lesser total dose of methotrexate is required, leucovorin rescue is not necessary, follow-up time is reduced, cost is reduced, and duration of hospitalization is minimized. Expansion of this protocol at our institution and at other centers is needed and anticipated.

Table 2.
Methotrexate Protocol Used at University of Tennessee, Memphis

Day	Methotrexate Dosage (mg/sq m)	Laboratory Tests and Procedures[a]
0		β-hCG, dilation and curettage, CBC, AST, BUN, SCr, blood type, Rh blood group
1	50 i.m.	β-hCG
2		β-hCG[b]
4		β-hCG
7	50 i.m.[c]	β-hCG,[d] CBC,[e] AST,[e] BUN,[e] SCr[e]

[a]β-hCG = serum concentration of β-subunit of human chorionic gonadotropin, CBC = complete blood count, AST = serum aspartate aminotransferase concentration, BUN = blood urea nitrogen, SCr = serum creatinine concentration.

[b]Probably unnecessary, but having patient appear for sample collection provides an opportunity to observe for clinical stability.

[c]Only given if decline in β-hCG is $<$15% between days 4 and 7.

[d]If decline is $\geq$15%, compared with day 4 value, then repeat β-hCG weekly until value is $<$10 mIU/mL.

[e]Probably unnecessary.

Recommendations

Patients receiving methotrexate for treatment of unruptured ectopic pregnancy should be chosen carefully. Patients eligible for methotrexate must meet the following criteria: (1) an unruptured ectopic pregnancy $\leq$ 3.5 cm in greatest dimension on transvaginal ultrasound, (2) no active renal or hepatic disease, and (3) no evidence of leukopenia or thrombocytopenia.

Although other methotrexate treatment regimens are effective, the single-dose regimen outlined in Table 2 is the most appropriate. Because of its simplicity, intramuscular administration of methotrexate seems most practical when compared with transvaginal or laparoscopy-directed injection. When laparoscopy is required for diagnostic confirmation, surgical treatment should be completed at that time.

After treatment is initiated, we instruct patients to refrain from alcohol, sexual intercourse, or the ingestion of folic acid, because these may exacerbate adverse effects of methotrexate or rupture of ectopic pregnancy. Patients are also instructed that they may have increased abdominal pain during treatment; this finding was observed during clinical trials.

Conclusion

Intramuscular methotrexate therapy is a safe and effective alternative to surgery for the treatment of unruptured ectopic pregnancy.

References

1. Wynn RM. Obstetrics and gynecology: the clinical core. Philadelphia: Lea & Febiger, 1983:114-7.
2. Nederlof KP, Lawson HW, Saftlas AF et al. Ectopic pregnancy surveillance, United States, 1970–1987. *MMWR*. 1990; 39(SS-4):9-17.
3. Cotton DB. Physiologic changes. In: Practical manual of obstetrical care. Zuspan FP, Quilligan EJ, eds. St Louis, MO: Mosby; 1982.
4. Stovall TG, Ling FW, Carsen SA et al. Non-surgical diagnosis and treatment of tubal pregnancy. *Fertil Steril*. 1991; 54:537-8.
5. Stovall TG, Ling FW, Cope BJ et al. Preventing ruptured ectopic pregnancy with a single serum progesterone. *Am J Obstet Gynecol*. 1989; 160:1425-31.
6. Tanaka T, Hayashi H, Kutsuzawa T et al. Treatment of interstitial ectopic pregnancy with methotrexate: report of a successful case. *Fertil Steril*. 1982; 37:851-2.
7. Chotiner HC. Nonsurgical management of ectopic pregnancy associated with severe hyperstimulation syndrome. *Obstet Gynecol*. 1985; 66:740-1.
8. Ory SJ, Villanueva AL, Sand PK et al. Conservative treatment of ectopic pregnancy with methotrexate. *Am J Obstet Gynecol*. 1986; 154:1299-306.
9. Rodi IA, Sauer MV, Gorrill MJ et al. The medical treatment of unruptured ectopic pregnancy with methotrexate and citrovorum rescue: preliminary experience. *Fertil Steril*. 1986; 46:811-3.
10. Cowan BD, McGehee RP, Bates GW. Treatment of persistent ectopic pregnancy with methotrexate and leukovorum rescue: a case report. *Obstet Gynecol*. 1986; 67(Suppl):S50-1.
11. Sauer MV, Gorrill MJ, Rodi IA. Non-surgical management of unruptured ectopic pregnancy: an extended clinical trial. *Fertil Steril*. 1987; 48:752-5.
12. Ichinoe K, Wake N, Shinkai N et al. Nonsurgical therapy to preserve oviduct function in patients with tubal pregnancies. *Am J Obstet Gynecol*. 1987; 156:484-7.
13. Stovall TG, Ling FW, Buster JE. Outpatient chemotherapy of unruptured ectopic pregnancy. *Fertil Steril*. 1989; 51:435-8.
14. Stovall TG, Ling FW, Gray LA et al. Methotrexate treatment of unruptured ectopic pregnancy: a report of 100 cases. *Obstet Gynecol*. 1991; 77:749-53.
15. Stovall TG, Ling FW, Gray LA. Single-dose methotrexate for treatment of ectopic pregnancy. *Obstet Gynecol*. 1991; 77:754-7.
16. Hreshchyshyn MM, Naples JD, Rondall CL. Amethopterin in abdominal pregnancy. *Am J Obstet Gynecol*. 1965; 93:286-7.

Research

Effect of a single dose of lactase on symptoms and expired hydrogen after lactose challenge in lactose-intolerant subjects

STEVEN W. SANDERS, KEITH G. TOLMAN, AND DONALD P. REITBERG

Abstract: The effect of a single dose of oral lactase on symptoms, breath hydrogen concentration, and glucose absorption in lactose-intolerant subjects challenged with lactose was studied

Volunteers underwent a lactose challenge test; those whose breath hydrogen concentrations increased 20 ppm or more and who met other criteria were admitted as subjects. After fasting, the subjects were given three chewable lactase tablets (total lactase dose, 9900 FCC units) or placebo tablets in a randomized, double-blind, crossover manner. The subjects also consumed 8 oz of whole milk in which 37.5 g of lactose powder was dissolved (total lactose content, 50 g). The washout period between lactose challenges was at least one week. Breath hydrogen and plasma glucose concentrations were measured before and at intervals after the challenges, and the subjects completed symptom-evaluation questionnaires every eight hours for four days.

Twenty-four subjects completed the study. The maximum mean breath hydrogen concentration was significantly lower after lactase treatment than after placebo treatment. In 21 subjects, the area under the hydrogen concentration–time curve (AUC) was lower after lactase than after placebo; three subjects had hydrogen AUCs more than 300 ppm · hr lower. There were no significant differences in plasma glucose levels. Subjective ratings of the severity of abdominal cramping, belching, flatulence, and diarrhea were lower during the first eight hours after challenge in lactase-treated subjects; ratings for bloating were lower during the next eight hours.

Single doses of a chewable lactase tablet reduced the concentration of expired hydrogen and symptoms of lactose intolerance after a lactose challenge.

Index terms: Dosage; Enzymes; Lactase; Lactose intolerance; Nutrition
Clin Pharm. 1992; 11:533-8

Lactase activity in the small bowel tends to diminish gradually with increasing age.[1,2] The propensity to develop frank intolerance of lactose-containing foods and beverages varies significantly among ethnic groups on the basis of their historical dependence on dairy cattle for survival.[2,3] A lactase deficiency rate of 2–30% is present even in ethnic populations with a relatively low incidence of lactose intolerance, such as nomadic Bedouins and Northern Europeans.[3] One of every four adults in the United States is estimated to be lactase deficient.[4]

Most persons with lactose intolerance adjust their diet by trial and error to minimize discomfort and the symptoms associated with lactose maldigestion. Symptoms of intolerance include flatulence, bloating, diarrhea, belching, and abdominal cramping, which vary in their severity. Loose stools and cramping result from osmotic redistribution of water into the bowel. Belching, bloating, and flatulence result from bacterial fermentation of lactose into free fatty acids, methane, carbon dioxide, and hydrogen. Noninvasive breath testing to measure the concentration of expired hydrogen provides an objective, rapid, and convenient method for evaluating patients with symptoms of lactose intolerance.[5,6]

Lactase harvested from *Aspergillus oryzae* has been

STEVEN W. SANDERS, PHARM.D., is Assistant Director of Clinical Research, TheraTech, Inc., Salt Lake City, UT; at the time of this study he was Clinical Director, Drug Research Center, Department of Internal Medicine, School of Medicine, University of Utah (UU), Salt Lake City. KEITH G. TOLMAN, M.D., is Chairman, Division of Gastroenterology and Professor of Medicine, Department of Medicine, School of Medicine, UU; at the time of this study he was also Director, Drug Research Center. DONALD P. REITBERG, PHARM.D., is Director of Clinical Research, Sterling Health, U.S.A., New York, NY.

Address reprint requests to Dr. Reitberg at Sterling Health U.S.A., 90 Park Avenue, New York, NY 10016.

Supported by a grant from Sterling Health, U.S.A.

Presented at the Annual Meeting of the American College of Gastroenterology, San Francisco, CA, October 31, 1990.

used extensively to supplement intestinal enzyme activity. The enzyme cleaves nonabsorbable lactose into the absorbable monosaccharides glucose and galactose.[3] The goal of this study was to evaluate the effect of a chewable, lactase-containing tablet, taken at the time of lactose ingestion, on lactose intolerance symptoms, breath hydrogen concentrations, and glucose absorption.

Methods

The study was approved by the University of Utah institutional review board. All subjects gave written informed consent before participating in the study.

Volunteers underwent a screening examination to determine their eligibility. All potential subjects underwent a lactose challenge test while fasting, a glucose tolerance test, and a physical examination. A medical history was taken, and clinical laboratory tests of blood and urine (serum chemistry, complete blood count, and macroscopic and microscopic urinalyses) were performed. In the lactose challenge, 37.5 g of lactose powder dissolved in 8 oz of whole milk (total lactose content, 50 g) was given. Two baseline breath samples were collected before the challenge, followed by collections every 30 minutes through five hours after ingestion. Volunteers were entered into the study if the concentration of hydrogen in expired air increased 20 ppm or more after the lactose challenge. The screening tests were conducted in the same manner as the tests given on treatment days to allow the subjects to familiarize themselves with the procedures. Volunteers were excluded from the study if the presence of substantial disease was indicated or if they had a history of gastrointestinal disorders other than lactose intolerance.

Subjects were confined in the University of Utah Drug Research Center from the evening before treatment through the completion of breath sampling and questionnaires given five hours after treatment. A standardized meal was served between 1830 and 2030 on the night before, after which the subjects fasted (except for free access to water) until midnight. The subjects then fasted completely, except for the milk challenge, throughout each study period. At 0700 on the two treatment days, the subjects were given three chewable lactase tablets (Dairy-Ease, 3300 FCC units of lactase per tablet, Sterling Health, U.S.A., New York, NY, lot 89031), or three identical-appearing and identical-tasting chewable placebo tablets (lot 89052) in a randomized, double-blind, crossover manner. At the same time, the subjects consumed 8 oz of the milk–lactose powder preparation. The milk was obtained from a single lot. There was a washout period of at least one week (including the study periods) between lactose challenges.

The subjects were monitored for breath hydrogen concentrations, plasma glucose concentrations, symptoms of lactose maldigestion, and adverse reactions during their confinement in the center. Breath hydrogen concentrations were measured within 30 minutes before the lactose challenge (two baseline samples) and every 30 minutes after the challenge through five hours. Plasma samples for glucose concentration determinations were collected before the challenge and 0.25, 0.5, 1, 1.5, 2, and 3 hours afterward. Five hours after consuming the tablets, each patient completed a questionnaire to document subjective impressions about the tablets. Questionnaires were also used to document symptoms of lactose intolerance, including abdominal cramping, bloating, belching, flatulence, audible bowel sounds, vomiting, and loose stools or diarrhea. The symptom questionnaires were completed every eight hours after the lactose challenge until 96 hours had elapsed (including time after discharge from the center). All the tests administered during screening of subjects, except the clinical laboratory tests and physical examination, were replicated during each study period. The physical examination and clinical laboratory tests were repeated at the end of the second study period.

The breath tests were performed with a Quintron model 12 analyzer (Quintron Instrument Company, Milwaukee, WI). Before use, the instrument was calibrated in accordance with instructions supplied by the manufacturer. A standardized gas with a hydrogen concentration of 104 ppm (Quingas standard, Quintron) was used to calibrate the instrument. Standard curves and quality control samples were prepared by diluting the standardized gas. The method was found to be linear, sensitive, accurate, and reproducible within and between daily applications. Standard samples ($n = 5$) showed a linearity of measurements of 0.9999, with coefficients of variation from 0% to 1.3%. A gas-sample storage bag was used for daily preparation and storage of the standards and quality control samples. The 104-ppm standard was transferred to a bag and then diluted with room air to achieve hydrogen concentrations of 79, 52, 30, 15, and 5 ppm.

Standard noncompartmental methods were used for the pharmacokinetic analysis of expired hydrogen and blood glucose concentrations.[7] The observed maximum concentration and the time to the maximum were used in evaluating breath hydrogen and blood glucose. Area-under-the-curve (AUC) calculations were conducted by trapezoidal approximation.[7]

Breath hydrogen concentrations were transformed on the basis of the average baseline value for each patient. Before the statistical analyses, all concentrations less than 5 ppm were set equal to 0 because they were below the limit of the analytical standard curves. The average baseline value was then computed and subtracted from all postchallenge data for each patient. In some cases, hydrogen concentration decreased after a challenge, especially at 0.5 hour after the lactose challenge. The resulting negative values were set equal to 0. (It was subsequently determined that the results were not significantly affected by this minor adjustment.) The maximum increase in hydrogen concentration, time to maximum increase, and hydrogen AUC were compared. The results of the questionnaires, breath tests, and plasma glucose tests were subjected to nonparametric paired statistical analyses with the Wilcoxon signed-ranks test performed by using a standard statistical package for the IBM computer (PC ANOVA and PC Statistician, Human Systems Dynamics, Northridge, CA). The a priori level of significance was set at <0.05.

Results

Twenty-four subjects (15 men and 9 women) with a history of lactose intolerance completed the study. One subject discontinued participation after the first study period for personal reasons. The mean ± S.D. age, weight, and height of the subjects was 30 ± 9 years, 59 ± 21 kg, and 170 ± 7 cm.

Mean breath hydrogen concentrations increased approximately 100 ppm over baseline after the placebo plus lactose challenge (Figure 1). There was no significant difference in the mean ± S.D. maximum breath hydrogen concentration between the lactose challenge during screening and the lactose plus placebo challenge (144 ± 68 versus 139 ± 67 ppm, respectively). Maximum mean breath hydrogen concentrations were significantly lower (by about 60 ppm) after the lactose plus lactase challenge than after the lactose plus placebo challenge (Figure 1). Maximum hydrogen concentration occurred three to four hours after exposure for both the placebo and lactase treatments (Figure 1 and Table 1).

Of the 24 subjects, 21 had lower hydrogen AUC after receiving lactase than after receiving placebo (Table 1). The maximum measured increase in breath hydrogen was lower in 19 of the 24 subjects after lactase treatment.

The results of the product evaluation questionnaire are summarized in Table 2.

Figure 1. Mean breath hydrogen concentrations after a 50-g lactose challenge in 24 lactose-intolerant subjects who were concurrently treated with lactase tablets (lower curve) or placebo tablets (upper curve). The areas under the curves differ significantly ($p < 0.001$). Error bars represent standard errors.

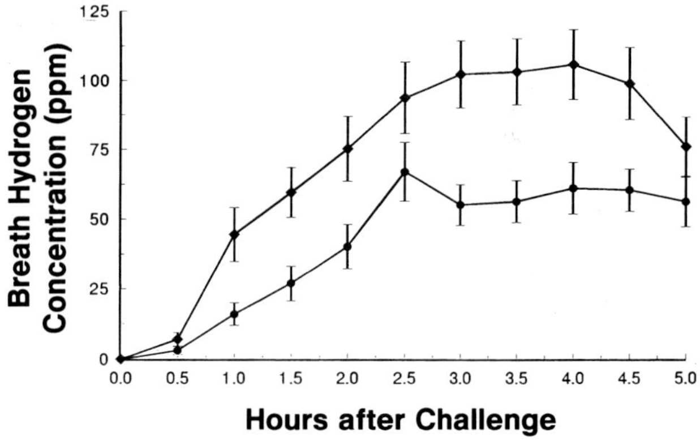

Table 1.
Values for Expired Hydrogen after the Lactose Challenge and Placebo or Lactase Treatment

	Placebo			Lactase		
Patient No.	Maximum Breath Hydrogen Conc. (ppm)	Time to Maximum Conc. (hr)	AUC (ppm · hr)[a]	Maximum Breath Hydrogen Conc. (ppm)	Time to Maximum Conc. (hr)	AUC (ppm · hr)
1	234	5.0	610	105	4.5	210
2	37	3.0	74	48	2.5	90
3	106	3.0	244	137	2.5	321
4	137	4.0	264	157	4.0	208
5	221	3.0	525	154	2.5	426
6	74	3.0	149	2	4.0	2
7	143	4.0	446	44	3.0	108
8	103	1.5	316	56	2.0	97
10	54	4.5	165	0	0.0	0
11	140	4.5	325	107	5.0	275
12	43	2.5	99	50	2.5	106
13	126	3.5	355	118	5.0	316
14	134	4.0	291	103	3.5	232
15	58	4.5	129	28	4.5	53
16	183	3.5	491	124	5.0	267
17	174	2.5	452	93	2.5	197
18	93	4.5	291	112	2.5	227
19	240	3.0	655	168	2.5	438
20	174	2.5	424	114	5.0	296
21	93	1.5	212	43	4.0	136
22	88	5.0	103	14	5.0	4
23	212	4.0	739	147	2.5	335
24	193	4.0	662	132	5.0	414
25	275	4.5	704	74	3.0	209
Mean ± S.D.	139 ± 67	3.5 ± 1.0	363 ± 206	89 ± 51[b]	3.4 ± 1.3	207 ± 133[b]

[a]AUC = area under the hydrogen concentration–time curve.
[b]Significantly different from corresponding value for placebo treatment ($p < 0.001$, Wilcoxon signed-ranks test).

In most subjects (17 subjects after receiving placebo and 19 subjects after receiving lactase), symptoms of lactose intolerance resolved within 24 hours. During the first eight-hour period of symptom evaluation, severity ratings were significantly lower for abdominal cramping, belching, flatulence, and loose stools or diarrhea after the lactase treatment than after the placebo treatment (Table 3). The significant difference in ratings for abdominal cramping and flatulence continued during the second eight-hour period (Table 3). Ratings for bloating differed significantly only during the second eight-hour period, reflecting the relatively delayed presentation of this symptom in persons with lactose intolerance.

After receiving lactase, subjects 1, 7, and 23 had hydrogen AUCs that were more than 300 ppm · hr lower than after they took placebo. These three patients also had much better symptom scores. Symptom ratings on the 5-point scale were ≥2 points less severe for these subjects after lactase than after placebo. Of the three subjects who showed the least change in hydrogen AUC (subjects 2, 3, and 12), two showed little difference in symptoms between treatments. Subject 2, despite showing no difference in hydrogen AUC after the lactase treatment, reported improved symptoms.

There were no significant differences in plasma glucose concentrations between treatments (Table 4). The screening glucose tolerance test showed the expected normal increase in glucose concentration after the 100-g glucose challenge. Glucose concentrations decreased similarly over time after both the lactase and placebo treatments. There was a slight mean increase in plasma glucose 0.5 hour after lactase that was not observed after placebo.

No clinically important findings were observed in the physical examination or laboratory tests that followed the study. Lactose intolerance symptoms of various severities were experienced by all the subjects whether they received placebo or lactase. Other adverse events were minor and included headache (in one patient after placebo and two patients after lactase), lightheadedness (two placebo, one lactase), and muscle stiffness (one placebo).

Table 2.
Results of the Questionnaire in Which Subjects Evaluated the Lactase-Containing and Placebo Tablets

Question and Possible Responses	No. Subjects Making Indicated Response: Placebo Treatment	Lactase Treatment	p^a
Did you like the product?			
Definitely	1	5	0.033
Possibly	7	10	
Somewhat	5	3	
Not at all	11	6	
Would you use the product again?			
Yes	2	10	0.016
Maybe	11	8	
No	11	6	
How did the product taste?			
Excellent	0	0	0.059
Good	7	13	
Satisfactory	13	8	
Terrible	4	3	
Select the phrase that most accurately describes whether you would buy the product:			
Definitely would	1	3	0.016
Probably would	5	8	
Might or might not	6	7	
Probably would not	3	2	
Definitely would not	9	4	

[a]Placebo treatment versus lactase treatment (Wilcoxon signed-ranks test).

Discussion

The results show an efficacy of orally administered lactase similar or superior to that reported previously.[8-10] Although there have been minor differences in the results of lactase studies, there is a relationship between the lactose challenge dose and the dose of lactase required for fewer symptoms and a lower concentration of hydrogen in expired breath. Breath hydrogen concentrations observed after the placebo treatment in this study were approximately 60 ppm higher than those described by DiPalma and Collins[8] after challenge with a solution containing 50 g of lactose and some 80 ppm higher than Moskovitz et al.[9] reported after a 17-g milk challenge. Both groups of researchers found a significantly lower concentration of breath hydrogen after a 500-mg (3300-FCC unit) dose of lactase but no significant reduction after a 250-mg (1650-FCC unit) dose. Onwulata et al.[10] gave 10 lactose-intolerant persons 18 g of whole milk followed by 756 FCC units of lactase and reported a mean decrease in expired hydrogen concentration of only 4 ppm. However, symptom scores for flatulence and diarrhea were reduced. These studies show that lower doses of lactase are less effective in reducing breath hydrogen.

In this study, higher concentrations of breath hydrogen appeared to be associated with a greater severity of intolerance symptoms, especially in patients with high levels of breath hydrogen after the placebo treatment. A liberal approach to adjusting the lactase dose to accommodate the anticipated lactose exposure in foods might enhance effectiveness. The use of lactase doses higher than the 9900 FCC units studied here is not likely to present a risk to lactose-intolerant individuals because lactase is virtually nontoxic; the enzyme is digested in the gut like any protein found in food.

The subjects in this study were presented with a substantial lactose challenge. The 37.5 g of lactose powder was administered in 8 oz of milk, providing the equivalent of a quart of milk in terms of total lactose burden (50 g). Also, no meal was administered before the lactose was given, permitting rapid transit of the lactose from the stomach. This minimized the time available for binding of enzyme and substrate in

Table 3.
Symptom Ratings after the Lactose Challenge and Placebo or Lactase Treatment

	No. Subjects Selecting Indicated Rating[a]												
	Placebo Treatment						Lactase Treatment						
Symptom	0	1	2	3	4	5	0	1	2	3	4	5	p^b
0–8 Hours after Challenge													
Abdominal cramping	9	2	3	3	3	4	15	3	2	1	2	1	0.011
Bloating	11	1	2	5	3	2	13	3	4	2	1	1	0.088
Belching	15	2	5	0	2	0	18	4	1	1	0	0	0.199
Flatulence, gas	1	1	3	10	5	4	4	6	5	6	3	0	0.020
Audible bowel sounds	12	1	2	6	3	0	17	3	1	2	1	0	0.003
Vomiting	23	0	0	0	1	0	24	0	0	0	0	0	0.057
Loose stools or diarrhea	9	2	1	4	7	1	17	2	1	2	2	0	0.012
8–16 Hours after Challenge													
Abdominal cramping	14	3	3	2	1	1	22	1	0	0	1	0	0.028
Bloating	15	1	3	5	0	0	19	3	1	0	1	0	0.039
Belching	19	1	1	2	0	1	22	1	1	0	0	0	0.199
Flatulence, gas	4	5	8	5	2	0	14	7	2	1	0	0	0.002
Audible bowel sounds	15	3	4	1	1	0	20	1	2	1	0	0	0.288
Vomiting	23	1	0	0	0	0	24	0	0	0	0	0	0.319
Loose stools or diarrhea	23	1	0	0	0	0	20	1	0	1	2	0	0.102

[a]On a scale of 0 to 5, where 0 = symptom absent and 5 = symptom severe.
[b]Placebo treatment versus lactase treatment (Wilcoxon signed-ranks test).

Table 4.
Plasma Glucose Values after the Screening Glucose Tolerance Test and after the Lactose Challenge and Lactase or Placebo Treatment

	Mean ± S.D.		
Variable	Glucose Tolerance Test[a]	Lactase Treatment	Placebo Treatment
Plasma glucose concentration (mg/dL)			
0 hr	87.5 ± 9.3	87.2 ± 4.8	87.5 ± 4.8
0.25 hr	111.5 ± 29.6	90.2 ± 7.4	90.5 ± 10.5
0.5 hr	121.8 ± 25.2	94.7 ± 14.5	88.5 ± 11.8
1.0 hr	101.1 ± 38.2	82.0 ± 20.7	81.8 ± 13.2
1.5 hr	82.0 ± 23.9	80.1 ± 12.2	82.4 ± 13.5
2.0 hr	81.8 ± 15.4	79.9 ± 10.4	80.9 ± 11.3
3.0 hr	71.1 ± 17.1	80.8 ± 6.3	82.1 ± 6.8
Maximum plasma glucose concentration (mg/dL)	. . .	99.0 ± 11.2	96.5 ± 11.7
Time to maximum (hr)	. . .	0.6 ± 0.6	0.5 ± 0.5
AUC (mg · hr/dL)[b]	. . .	239.5 ± 27.3	239.6 ± 23.8

[a]Glucose 100 g was administered.
[b]AUC = area under the glucose concentration–time curve.

the stomach and may have limited the breakdown of lactose. The ingestion of a smaller amount of lactose, such as that contained in a glass of milk, a serving of cheese or pizza, or a scoop of ice cream, would probably be associated with a lower incidence and lower severity of symptoms than observed here. Three of the lactase tablets (total dose, 9900 FCC units) would be expected to nearly or totally ablate symptoms in persons with a stomach full of solid food. The ingestion of lactose with a meal has been shown to produce fewer symptoms than lactose ingestion during fasting.[11] Increased gastric emptying time after a meal would allow increased mixing time, greater breakdown of lactose, and delayed, reduced delivery of undigested lactase to the intestine.

The reduced mixing time in the stomach of fasting subjects may also partially explain why plasma glucose concentrations did not increase significantly after lactase treatment. Enzymatic cleavage of lactose into glucose and galactose may have occurred slowly because lactose and lactase were diluted by rapid movement along the gastrointestinal tract. A stomach containing food would be expected to mix enzyme and substrate for prolonged periods. More complete breakdown of lactose would probably lead to higher plasma glucose concentrations than in fasting persons.

A lactose load of 50 g would deliver the equivalent of 26.3 g of glucose, assuming 100% breakdown of the lactose. If increases in plasma glucose after lactose ingestion are proportional to increases seen with the glucose tolerance test, which involves a 100-g glucose challenge, the expected increases in plasma glucose concentration and AUC would be minimal—approximately 12 mg/dL and 6.2 mg · hr/dL. Although monitoring of plasma glucose concentrations is readily available as a test for lactose digestion and absorption, the small increases seen even after as much as 50 g of lactose is consumed make this measure unreliable.[12]

Breath hydrogen analysis is an accepted objective method for identifying lactase deficiency.[5,13] Arola et al.,[12] in comparing various methods for studying lactose intolerance, noted that breath testing for hydrogen may result in some false-negative results when compared with data based on intestinal sampling. Since all the subjects in the present study were entered on the basis of a positive breath test result, the observation of Arola et al. has no bearing on the validity of these findings. Arola et al. also reported a false-positive rate of approximately 3%. False positives could account for the few subjects in the present study who did not respond to lactase. The most common cause of false-positive results is bacterial overgrowth in the small bowel.[12]

The potential for Type I error was increased because the questionnaire data underwent multiple statistical comparisons. A total of 21 tests were performed on the symptom data. With the level of significance set at <0.05., there is, by definition, a 5% probability of Type I error. For 21 tests, it is probable that the results of 5% of the tests (1 of 20) would be erroneously found to be significantly different. However, from a clinical perspective, if there were a significant reduction in a single symptom score without resolution of related components of the symptom complex, this would be viewed as therapeutic failure overall. Significantly lower severity scores after lactase than after placebo were reported for four of the seven symptoms during the first eight-hour period; it is unlikely that this was a statistical artifact. In addition, undue restriction of Type I error leads to increased Type II error. Both lactose challenges were designed to elicit symptoms, increasing the likelihood of Type II error. For these reasons, a correction for multiple testing (i.e., a reduction in the a priori level of significance), was not performed.

Conclusion

Single doses of a chewable lactase tablet reduced the concentration of expired hydrogen and symptoms of lactose intolerance after a lactose challenge.

References

1. Goldberg DM. The enzymology of intestinal disease. *Clin Biochem*. 1987; 20:63-72.
2. Scrimshaw NS, Murray EB. The acceptability of milk and milk products in populations with a high prevalence of lactose intolerance. *Am J Clin Nutr*. 1988; 48 (Suppl 4):1079-159.
3. Hammond JB, Littman A. Disaccharide malabsorption. In: Berk JE, ed. Bochus' gastroenterology. Vol. 3. 4th ed. Philadelphia: Saunders; 1985:1703-17.
4. Grey GM. Milk intolerance due to lactase deficiency. Washington, DC: Clearinghouse Fact Sheet, National Digestive Diseases Education and Information Clearinghouse. Washington, DC: U.S. Department of Health and Human Services; 1985.
5. Solomons NW. Evaluation of carbohydrate absorption: the hydrogen breath test in clinical practice. *Clin Nutr*. 1984; 3:71-8.
6. Olson RE. Efficacy of exogenous lactase for lactose intolerance. *Nutr Rev*. 1988; 46:150-1.
7. Gibaldi M, Perrier D, eds. Pharmacokinetics. 2nd ed. New York: Dekker; 1982.
8. DiPalma JA, Collins MS. Enzyme replacement for lactose malabsorption using a beta-D-galactosidase. *J Clin Gastroenterol*. 1989; 11:290-3.
9. Moskovitz M, Curtis C, Galaver J. Does oral enzyme replacement therapy reverse intestinal lactose malabsorption? *Am J Gastroenterol*. 1987; 82:632-5.
10. Onwulata CI, Rao DR, Vankineni P. Relative efficiency of yogurt, sweet acidophilus milk, hydrolyzed-lactose milk, and a commercial lactase tablet in alleviating lactose maldigestion. *Am J Clin Nutr*. 1989; 49:1233-7.
11. Martini MC, Savaiano DA. Reduced intolerance symptoms from lactose consumed during a meal. *Am J Clin Nutr*. 1988; 47:57-60.
12. Arola H, Koivula T, Jodely H et al. Comparison of indirect diagnostic methods for hypolactasia. *Scand J Gastroenterol*. 1988; 23:351-7.
13. Sategna-Giudetti C, Cruto E, Capobianco P. Breath hydrogen excretion after lactase and whole milk ingestion. *J Clin Gastroenterol*. 1989; 11:287-9.

Bioequivalence of verapamil hydrochloride extended-release pellet-filled capsules when opened and sprinkled on food and when swallowed intact

GARY D. KOZLOSKI, JOSEPH M. DE VITO, JERRY B. JOHNSON, GREGORY B. HOLMES, MARGARET A. ADAMS, AND THOMAS L. HUNT

Abstract: A study was performed to determine whether verapamil hydrochloride administered in extended-release pellet-filled capsules is bioequivalent to the same formulation administered by sprinkling the contents of the capsules onto food.

Thirty-two healthy subjects participated in the randomized, two-way crossover study. In treatment A, the subjects swallowed the contents of a verapamil hydrochloride extended-release pellet-filled capsule, 240 mg, that had been sprinkled on applesauce. In treatment B, the subjects swallowed the same type of capsule intact. Blood samples were drawn at baseline, every hour for 10 hours, and at 12, 15, 24, 30, 36, and 48 hours after each dose administration. The plasma was analyzed for verapamil and norverapamil by high-performance liquid chromatography. The following calculations were performed: AUC_{0-48}, $AUC_{0-\infty}$, C_{max}, t_{max}, and k. Results for the two treatments were compared by analysis of variance.

There were no significant differences between the AUC_{0-48}, $AUC_{0-\infty}$, C_{max}, t_{max}, and k for the two methods of dose administration. For verapamil the differences for all variables were less than 5%, and for norverapamil the differences were less than 4% for all variables except t_{max} (9.5%). The 90% confidence intervals were within acceptable limits for all variables except the norverapamil t_{max} comparison.

Sprinkling the contents of extended-release pellet-filled capsules onto food provides verapamil hydrochloride that is bioequivalent to that obtained from the intact capsules.

Index terms: Calcium antagonists; Capsules; Drug administration; Drug interactions; Equivalency; Food; Pharmacokinetics; Sustained-action medications; Toxicity; Verapamil hydrochloride
Clin Pharm. 1992; 11:539-42

Crushing or chewing extended-release oral dosage forms is not recommended; physical disruption can alter their release properties, resulting in an increased amount of drug available for immediate absorption. This may lead to an increase in adverse effects[1-3] and decreased duration of therapeutic effect. Beaded or pelletized extended-release capsule formulations are an alternative for patients who have difficulty swallowing, because the contents of some capsules can be sprinkled onto a soft food and swallowed without crushing or chewing.[4,5]

Verapamil is a calcium-channel blocker often prescribed for the treatment of essential hypertension. Verapamil hydrochloride is available as a multiparticulate extended-release pellet-filled capsule that incorporates the rate-controlling membrane technology of the Spheroidal Oral Drug Absorption System.[6] Although it has been shown that food has a minimal effect on the rate and extent of absorption of verapamil from this formulation,[7] there are no data that establish its bioequivalence when opened and sprinkled onto food and when swallowed intact. To gather these data, we performed a randomized, single-dose, two-way crossover study.

Methods

Subjects. Thirty-two healthy male volunteers, 18 to 37 years of age, participated in this study. The subjects were selected on the basis of acceptable medical histories, including no alcohol or drug abuse. Their good health was confirmed by a physical examination that included an electrocardiogram, hematology (hemoglobin, hematocrit, red blood cell count, and white blood cell count with differential), urinalysis, and blood chemistries (serum glucose, blood urea nitrogen, serum creatinine, alkaline phosphatase, aspartate aminotransferase, bilirubin, calcium, and phosphorus). The subjects were not allowed to take any prescription or nonprescription medications for 14 days before or during the study period. Alcohol was prohibited from 24 hours before the start of the study until the time the last blood sample was collected. The study protocol was reviewed and approved by an in-

GARY D. KOZLOSKI, PHARM.D., is Manager, Scientific Services, JOSEPH M. DE VITO, PHARM.D., is Associate Director, Pharmacology and Scientific Services, and JERRY B. JOHNSON, PHARM.D., is Director, Scientific and Medical Services, Lederle Laboratories, Pearl River, NY. GREGORY B. HOLMES, PHARM.D., is Associate Director, MARGARET A. ADAMS, PHARM.D., is Director, and THOMAS L. HUNT, M.D., PH.D., is Associate Medical Director, Pharmaco Dynamics Research, Austin, TX.

Address reprint requests to Dr. Kozloski at Scientific and Medical Services, Lederle Laboratories, 401 Middletown Road, Pearl River, NY 10965.

Verelan is manufactured for Lederle Laboratories Division, American Cyanamid Company, Pearl River, NY, by Elan Pharmaceutical Research Corp., Gainesville, GA.

Presented in part at the 26th ASHP Midyear Clinical Meeting, New Orleans, LA, December 9, 1991.

stitutional review board, and all subjects gave written informed consent.

Study Design. This was a randomized, two-way crossover study with a seven-day washout period between the two treatments. In treatment A, each subject swallowed, without chewing, the contents of a verapamil hydrochloride extended-release pellet-filled capsule, 240 mg, that had been opened and sprinkled onto a level tablespoon of applesauce. In treatment B, each subject swallowed an intact verapamil hydrochloride extended-release pellet-filled capsule, 240 mg, immediately after swallowing a tablespoon of applesauce. In both treatments, all doses (Verelan 240 mg, control no. 239-325, Elan Pharmaceutical Research Corp., Gainesville, GA) were administered with 150 mL of water. All subjects fasted for a minimum of 10 hours before and four hours after dose administration. Water was allowed as desired after the four-hour postdose blood sample was taken. Standardized meals were served to all subjects 4, 10, and 14 hours after dose administration. Sitting blood pressures and heart rates were measured at 2, 5, 8, and 24 hours and electrocardiograms were obtained at 8 and 24 hours after dose administration.

Blood samples (10 mL) were drawn by venipuncture at baseline, every hour for 10 hours, and at 12, 15, 24, 30, 36, and 48 hours after dose administration. The plasma was immediately separated by centrifugation and stored at −20 °C until it was analyzed for verapamil and norverapamil concentrations by high-performance liquid chromatography (HPLC).

HPLC Analysis. The concentrations of verapamil and norverapamil were measured by HPLC in which modifications of the methods reported by Todd et al.[8] and Harapat and Kates[9,10] were used. In the method used here, verapamil, norverapamil, and an internal standard (propranolol) were extracted from alkaline plasma into ethyl ether, then back-extracted into dilute acid. One hundred microliters of the dilute-acid aqueous phase was chromatographed on Supelco C_8 (5 μm, 4.6 mm × 25 cm) and Supelguard C_8 columns (Supelco, Bellefonte, PA). The mobile phase was a 45:55 mixture of acetonitrile and 0.01 M sodium acetate, pH 2.0, and the flow rate was 2.0 mL/min. Verapamil, norverapamil, and propranolol were detected by fluorescence (203 nm excitation wavelength, 320 nm emission cut-off filter). The chromatograms were integrated by using the Nelson model 2600 chromatography software (PE Nelson, Norwalk, CT). The minimum quantifiable level was 5.0 ng/mL for both verapamil and norverapamil. This concentration produced a peak height response with a signal-to-noise ratio of approximately 10:1 for both analyses. The assay was calibrated between 5 ng/mL and 500 ng/mL for both verapamil and norverapamil, and the correlation coefficients were 0.9979 and 0.9991, respectively. A linear weighted (1/peak height ratio) least-squares regression analysis was used to quantitate unknown samples.

Interday and intraday precision and accuracy for verapamil and norverapamil were determined by analyzing 50 samples each of the low, medium, and high controls over the course of the analytical work. For verapamil, the coefficients of variation for the precision of the 10-, 50-, and 250-ng/mL controls were 12.7%, 9.84%, and 11.8%, respectively, and the percentages of difference from the theoretical values for each control were 5.30%, 1.20%, and 0.983%, respectively. For norverapamil, the coefficients of variation for the precision of the 10-, 50-, and 250-ng/mL controls were 6.15%, 4.44%, and 5.31%, respectively, and the percent differences from the theoretical values for each control were 4.56%, 0.0314%, and 0.739%, respectively.

Pharmacokinetic and Statistical Analyses. The area under the plasma concentration–time curve from 0 to 48 hours (AUC_{0-48}) was calculated by using the linear trapezoidal method. The area under the plasma concentration–time curve from time zero to infinity ($AUC_{0-\infty}$) was calculated by dividing each individual last detectable plasma concentration by the corresponding elimination rate constant and adding the result to the respective AUC_{0-48} value. Peak plasma concentration (C_{max}), time to maximum plasma concentration (t_{max}), and elimination rate constant (k), were calculated by using Lotus 1-2-3 (version 2.2, Lotus Development Corp., Cambridge, MA). The mean pharmacokinetic values for the two methods of administration were compared for significant differences attributable to dosing days, sequence, subjects within sequence, and formulation by analysis of variance (ANOVA) using the general linear model procedure of SAS (version 5.18, SAS Institute, Inc., Cary, NC). Differences were considered significant at $p < 0.05$. The power to detect a 20% difference from the reference mean and the shortest 90% confidence intervals using the two one-sided t test method were calculated for each variable.

Results

The calculated pharmacokinetic values and a summary of statistical analyses for verapamil and norverapamil for both methods of dose administration are given in Tables 1 and 2, respectively. The mean plasma concentration–time curves for verapamil and norverapamil are shown in Figures 1 and 2, respectively.

There were no significant differences between the two methods of dose administration for the calculated pharmacokinetic values for verapamil and norverapamil. For verapamil, the differences between AUC_{0-48}, $AUC_{0-\infty}$, C_{max}, t_{max}, and k for the two methods of dose administration were less than 5%. For norverapamil, the differences between the two methods of dose administration were less than 4% for AUC_{0-48}, $AUC_{0-\infty}$, C_{max}, and k; for t_{max} the difference was 9.5%.

All 90% confidence intervals for the calculated variables were within acceptable limits (80% to 120%) except for the norverapamil t_{max} comparison (97% to 121%). There were no serious adverse effects, nor were there reports of substantial electrocardiogram abnormalities or changes in blood pressure during either treatment.

Table 1.
Pharmacokinetic Values for Verapamil

Pharmacokinetic Variable	Treatment A (Sprinkled Capsules)[a]	Treatment B (Intact Capsules)[a]	Ratio (A/B) (%)	Power	90% Confidence Interval
C_{max} (ng/mL)	76.21 ± 34.91	80.21 ± 39.21	95.0	80.8	83–107
t_{max} (hr)	8.47 ± 2.03	8.31 ± 1.89	101.9	93.2	92–111
AUC_{0-48} (ng · hr/mL)	1104.66 ± 643.06	1096.62 ± 652.14	100.7	99.2	93–108
$AUC_{0-\infty}$ (ng · hr/mL)	1227.45 ± 651.32	1197.94 ± 678.53	102.5	99.6	94–108
k (hr^{-1})	0.0915 ± 0.0287	0.0914 ± 0.0297	100.1	99.4	93–107

[a]Values are expressed as arithmetic mean ± S.D. Pharmacokinetic values for treatments A and B were not significantly different.

Table 2.
Pharmacokinetic Values for Norverapamil

Pharmacokinetic Variable	Treatment A (Sprinkled Capsules)[a]	Treatment B (Intact Capsules)[a]	Ratio (A/B) (%)	Power	90% Confidence Interval
C_{max} (ng/mL)	78.08 ± 21.92	78.46 ± 22.47	99.5	99.6	93–106
t_{max} (hr)	11.19 ± 3.06	10.22 ± 2.87	109.5	78.1	97–121
AUC_{0-48} (ng · hr/mL)	1729.59 ± 579.21	1698.44 ± 546.42	101.8	99.9	97–107
$AUC_{0-\infty}$ (ng · hr/mL)	1876.16 ± 642.76	1857.75 ± 608.02	101.0	99.9	96–106
k (hr^{-1})	0.0707 ± 0.0147	0.0686 ± 0.0150	103.1	99.9	98–108

[a]Values are expressed as arithmetic mean ± S.D. Pharmacokinetic values for treatments A and B were not significantly different.

Figure 1. Mean plasma verapamil concentrations in 32 subjects given 240-mg doses of verapamil hydrochloride extended-release pellet-filled capsules as the pellets sprinkled on applesauce and as the intact capsule.

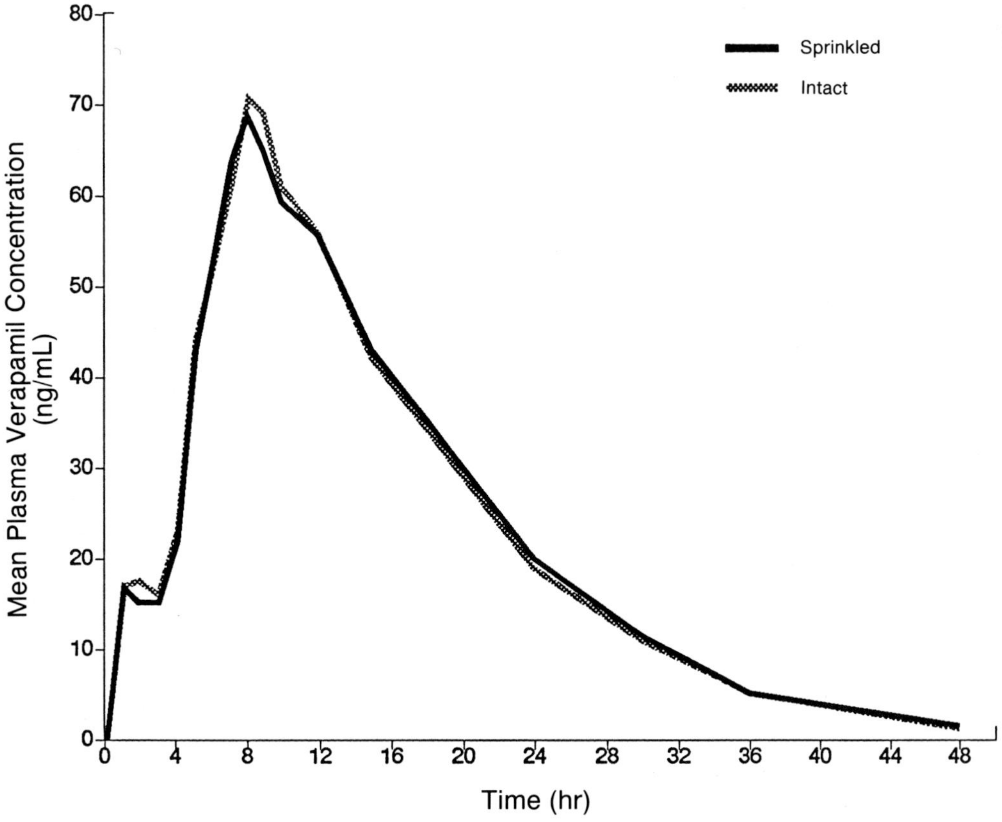

Figure 2. Mean plasma norverapamil concentrations in 32 subjects given 240-mg doses of verapamil hydrochloride extended-release pellet-filled capsules as the pellets sprinkled on applesauce and as the intact capsule.

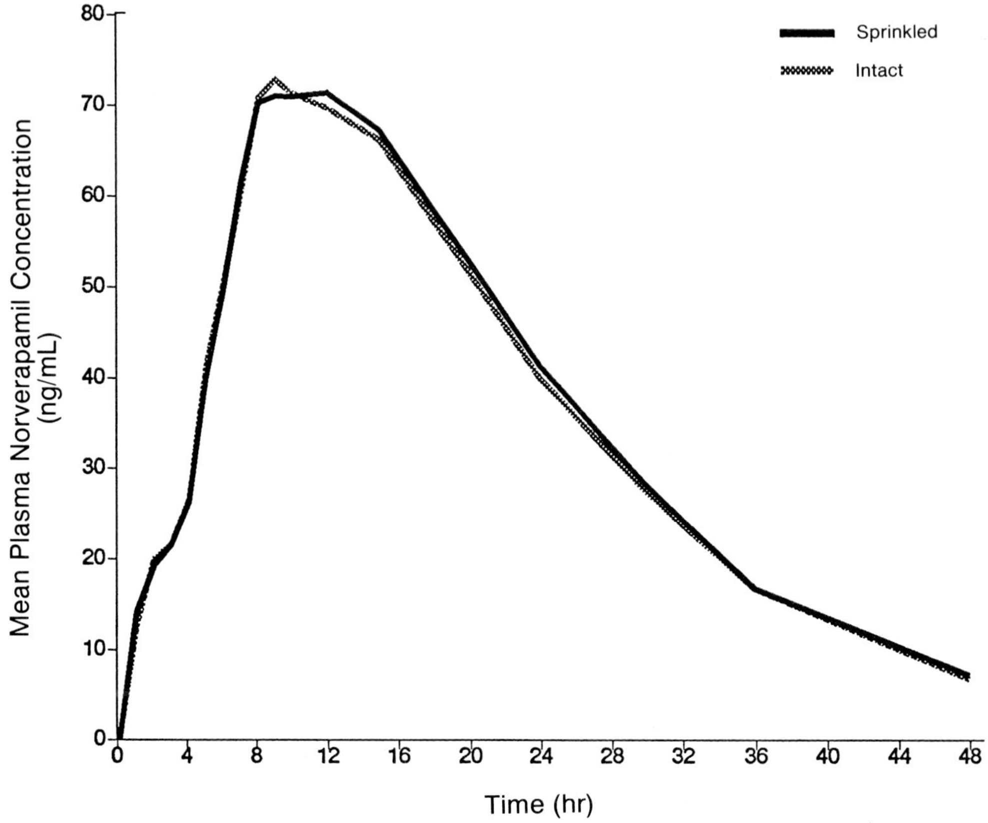

Discussion

Patients who have difficulty swallowing extended-release dosage forms are often switched to immediate-release formulations. For example, commercially available liquid preparations can be prescribed[1] or immediate-release tablets can be crushed or capsules opened and the contents administered with a small amount of liquid or food. However, the higher rate of compliance and increased therapeutic effect that are potential benefits of extended-release formulations may not be obtained with immediate-release preparations.

Pelletized extended-release capsule formulations can be administered on a small amount of food while maintaining the extended-release characteristics of the intact capsule. For verapamil hydrochloride extended-release pellet-filled capsules, we have shown that the pharmacokinetic variables that establish bioequivalence for verapamil hydrochloride and norverapamil are nearly identical when the capsule is swallowed intact and when its contents are sprinkled on applesauce and swallowed without chewing.

Conclusion

Swallowing the contents of extended-release pellet-filled capsules that have been sprinkled onto food provides verapamil hydrochloride that is bioequivalent to that obtained by swallowing the intact capsules.

References

1. Mitchell JF, Pawlicki KS. Oral dosage forms that should not be crushed: 1990 revision. *Hosp Pharm*. 1990; 25:329-35.
2. Shor JB. Crushing medications. *Contemp Longterm Care*. 1986; 9:99.
3. Guttenberg SA. Chemical injury of the oral mucosa from verapamil. *N Engl J Med*. 1990; 323:615.
4. Carrigan PJ, Brinker DR, Cavanaugh JH et al. Absorption characteristics of a new valproate formulation: divalproex sodium-coated particles in capsules (Depakote Sprinkle). *J Clin Pharmacol*. 1990; 30:743-7.
5. Naspitz CK, Sole D. Theophylline serum levels in children with bronchial asthma after administration of slow release theophylline as open or closed capsules. *Respiration*. 1989; 55:210-3.
6. Panoz DE, Geoghegan EJ. U.S. patent 4,863,742. 1989; Sep 5.
7. Devane JG, Kelley JG. Effect of food on the bioavailability of a multiparticulate sustained-release verapamil formulation. *Adv Ther*. 1991; 8:48-53.
8. Todd GD, Bourne DWA, McAllister RG. Measurement of verapamil concentrations in plasma by gas chromatography (GC) and high pressure liquid chromatography. *Ther Drug Monit*. 1980; 2:411-6.
9. Harapat SR, Kates RE. Rapid high pressure liquid chromatographic analysis of verapamil in blood and plasma. *J Chromatogr*. 1979; 170:385-90.
10. Harapat SR, Kates RE. High performance liquid chromatographic analysis of verapamil. II. Simultaneous quantitation of verapamil and its active metabolite, norverapamil. *J Chromatogr*. 1980; 181:484-9.

Complications of home parenteral nutrition

ERIC T. HERFINDAL, LINDA R. BERNSTEIN, ALVIN F. WONG, VALERIE W. HOGUE, AND JEANNE A. DARBINIAN

Abstract: The complications associated with home parenteral nutrition (HPN) and their relationship to length of therapy were studied.

The medical records of 56 patients treated with HPN (age range, 6 months to 82 years) were retrospectively reviewed to study complications associated with HPN.

Of the 56 study patients, 30 (53.6%) had complications related to HPN, 18 (32.1%) had complications not related to HPN, and 8 (14.3%) had no complications. Of the 365 total complications noted, 125 (34.2%) were related to HPN. The mean ± S.D. interval between initiation of HPN and occurrence of a complication was 1.25 ± 1.73 years (mean ± S.D.). Patients were more likely to have fluid or electrolyte complications or glucose intolerance in the first year of therapy and catheter-related complications later in the course of treatment. The first episode of septicemia occurred 2.1 ± 1.8 years (mean ± S.D.) after the initiation of HPN. The risk of developing catheter-related septicemia was higher for patients on long-term HPN therapy and for young patients.

Patients receiving HPN should be carefully monitored for complications such as fluid and electrolyte abnormalities and glucose intolerance, which commonly occur early in the course of therapy; later complications of HPN include catheter-related infection, thrombosis, and breakage or dislodgement.

Index terms: Age; Dosage schedules; Health care; Nutrition; Toxicity
Clin Pharm. 1992; 11:543-8

Home parenteral nutrition (HPN) is a well-established therapy for the nutritional management of patients with severe inflammatory bowel disease,[1] short-bowel syndrome,[2] malabsorption disorders, and immunodeficiency diseases.[3] Oncology patients who need nutritional rehabilitation after chemotherapy, radiotherapy, or surgery are also likely candidates for HPN.[4] These patients typically require many weeks to months of parenteral nutritional support before they can resume normal enteral feeding, whereas some patients with short-bowel syndrome or severe radiation enteritis may require a lifetime of parenteral nutrition.

Before the introduction of HPN, patients often remained hospitalized for prolonged periods to receive parenteral nutrition. The majority of these patients are now managed at home. Home care significantly reduces total medical cost and frees hospital beds in a tertiary-care facility for patients with more acute conditions.[5] In addition, HPN programs have permitted some patients with conditions previously regarded as totally disabling to return to work and lead fully productive lives.[6] It is estimated that more than 4000 patients are receiving partial or complete HPN in the United States.[7] Although there are many advantages of HPN for the patient and the health-care system, there can be many complications leading to serious morbidity and mortality.[8,9]

Numerous studies have characterized the morbidity and mortality associated with HPN.[8-14] Potential complications of therapy can be categorized as mechanical problems related to catheter insertion and maintenance, infection, and metabolic disorders. Existing studies, however, do not document the temporal relationship of these adverse effects to the course of HPN therapy.

The objectives of this study were to delineate the morbidity associated with HPN therapy and to explore whether a relationship exists between HPN-related complications and the length of time on HPN therapy.

Methods

A retrospective review was conducted of the medical records of all patients at University of California San Francisco Medical Center in whom HPN was initiated between 1980 and 1987. A complication was defined as an incident requiring a formalized patient–practitioner encounter, including any clinic visits, hospitalizations, emergency room visits, or home visits. During the study, complications were identified from patients' medical records and reviewed by staff mem-

ERIC T. HERFINDAL, PHARM.D., M.P.H., is Chairman and Professor, School of Pharmacy, Division of Clinical Pharmacy, and Director, Department of Pharmaceutical Services, University of California, San Francisco. LINDA R. BERNSTEIN, PHARM.D., is Associate Clinical Professor, School of Pharmacy, Division of Clinical Pharmacy, and Senior Pharmacist, Department of Pharmaceutical Services, University of California, San Francisco. ALVIN F. WONG, PHARM.D., is Associate Clinical Professor, School of Pharmacy, Division of Clinical Pharmacy, and Pharmacist Specialist, Department of Pharmaceutical Services, University of California, San Francisco. VALERIE W. HOGUE, PHARM.D., is Assistant Professor, Department of Pharmacy Practice, College of Pharmacy and Pharmacal Sciences, Howard University, and Ambulatory Care Clinical Pharmacist, Veterans Affairs Medical Center, Washington, DC; at the time of this study, she was a pharmacy resident at the School of Pharmacy, University of California, San Francisco. JEANNE A. DARBINIAN, M.S., is Clinical Nutritionist, Department of Nutrition and Dietetics, University of California, San Francisco.

Address reprint requests to Dr. Herfindal at the School of Pharmacy, Division of Clinical Pharmacy, Room C-152, University of California, San Francisco, CA 94143-0622.

Funded by the ASHP Research and Education Foundation.

bers of the home nutritional support service. All complications were classified as either related or not related to HPN according to criteria based on the clinical experience of the nutritional support team and accepted medical literature.[7,15] Complications were defined as follows:

1. To be evaluated for fluid, electrolyte, and glucose abnormalities, patient records had to contain the following information: (1) documented evidence of stability on the HPN regimen and normal results for all baseline fluid, electrolyte, and glucose laboratory tests (Table 1) at least two days before discharge from the hospital; (2) daily measurements of weight, fluid intake and output, temperature, and urine glucose concentration recorded by the patient (appendix) throughout the evaluation period; and (3) laboratory determinations monitored at least once monthly (appendix). Fluid, electrolyte, and glucose disturbances were defined as HPN-related when the following corresponding criteria were met: (1) diagnosis of fluid overload or dehydration, supported by clinical and laboratory evidence, that required a change in the HPN solution; (2) diagnosis of electrolyte abnormalities, supported by clinical and laboratory evidence, that required a change in electrolyte solution composition; or (3) diagnosis of hyperglycemia or hypoglycemia, supported by clinical and laboratory evidence, that required a change in HPN dextrose formulation. Patients with known fluid instability, sepsis, or acute changes in their primary disease state that affected their fluid, electrolyte, or glucose requirements were not considered to have HPN-related abnormalities.
2. Baseline liver function tests (LFTs) performed before the start of HPN included aspartate aminotransferase (AST), alanine aminotransferase (ALT), albumin, total protein, total bilirubin, alkaline phosphatase, blood urea nitrogen, clotting times, complete blood count, and platelet count (see Table 1 for normal values). An HPN-related liver abnormality was defined as follows: (1) an abnormal value greater than twice the upper limit of the standard reference value for AST, ALT, alkaline phosphatase, or total bilirubin occurring two or more times on consecutive laboratory determinations; and (2) histologic changes, such as fat infiltration or cholestatic changes, observed on liver biopsy. If LFT abnormalities developed during HPN, specific causes such as sepsis, infectious hepatitis, or an adverse drug reaction were considered and the abnormality was not considered to be HPN-related if the cause of the liver dysfunction was unclear. Patients with preexisting liver disease were not considered to have HPN-related abnormalities.
3. An infectious episode was defined as catheter-related when it met one of the following criteria: (1) microbiologically documented bacterial or fungal abscess or cellulitis localized at the catheter exit site, in the subcutaneous tunnel, or at the entrance of the catheter into the blood vessel; (2) septicemia in which bacterial or fungal microorganisms were isolated only in blood cultures drawn from the catheter and not from simultaneously drawn peripheral vein cultures; (3) septicemia in which identical microorganisms were isolated from blood cultures and from swabs taken from the catheter tip or insertion site; or (4) the existence of a temporal relationship between the use of the catheter, the onset of fever and chills, and the isolation of a microorganism from blood cultures taken during the episode, suggesting catheter release of microorganisms into the bloodstream after manipulation of the catheter. A catheter-related infectious episode was excluded when another definite site of infection was identified or when an infectious episode of unknown source occurred and it was not possible to identify the catheter as the source of the infection.
4. Bacterial overgrowth was defined as a breath hydrogen value (normal, 20 ppm) twice baseline, accompanied by increased malabsorption or diarrhea not attributable to other bowel diseases, that decreased in response to oral antibiotic therapy.[16]
5. HPN-related metabolic bone disease was defined when all of the following criteria were met: (1) complaint of pain in a periarticular bone; (2) abnormal results on histomorphometric analysis of bone biopsy, bone density, and radiographic examination; (3) normal or slightly elevated serum concentrations of calcium, phosphorus, and 25-hydroxycholecalciferol with normal results of parathyroid hormone tests; and (4) the presence of hypercalciuria.
6. Catheter thrombosis was defined by radiographic evidence of thrombus formation at the outlet of the catheter and documentation in the chart of treatment and resolution of the thrombus with fibrinolytic therapy, catheter removal, or both.
7. Catheter dislodgement was defined by radiographic analysis demonstrating catheter malposition compared with baseline radiographic reports of proper catheter placement.
8. Catheter rupture after the start of HPN was defined by chart notation and documentation of repair or removal of the catheter.

Table 1.
Normal Laboratory Values

Hemoglobin	10.5–16.0 g/dL
Hematocrit	35–50%
White blood cells	4.5–10.0 $\times$ 10^3 cells/μL
Platelets	140–450 $\times$ 10^3/μL
Prothrombin time	10.5–12.1 sec
Activated partial thromboplastin time	23–38 sec
Sodium	135–145 meq/L
Potassium	3.5–5.0 meq/L
Chloride	96–106 meq/L
Carbon dioxide	24–32 meq/L
Calcium	8.5–10.5 mg/dL
Phosphorus	3.3–5.0 mg/dL
Magnesium	1.6–2.7 mg/dL
Glucose	60–120 mg/dL
Blood urea nitrogen	10–24 mg/dL
Creatinine	0.4–1.0 mg/dL
Albumin	3.4–4.7 g/dL
Protein	5.6–8.5 g/dL
Alanine aminotransferase	7–39 U/L
Aspartate aminotransferase	7–39 U/L
Alkaline phosphatase	41–133 U/L
Bilirubin, total	0.1–1.2 mg/dL

Standard procedures for HPN therapy are briefly reviewed in the appendix.

The date of the HPN-related complication was recorded and the number of days on therapy was calculated. In analyzing the temporal relationship of the complications, we dealt only with the first occurrence of a complication. This was done because the event of a complication may itself alter the likelihood of any subsequent occurrence of that complication. Several other variables were also recorded, including diagnosis, age, sex, ethnicity, and length of hospitalization.

The primary objective was to determine if there was a relationship between length of therapy and complications. The Kaplan-Meier product limit estimate was used for "survival" curves describing the probability of being complication-free as a function of months after the initiation of HPN services.[17] We did not consider covariates and how they might affect the occurrence of complications. As previously stated, our analysis was based on data from the time of initiation of HPN until the first occurrence of a particular complication for each individual. We chose to interpret catheter sepsis data according to duration of catheter use and calculated the incidence of infections per days of catheter use. This is the most appropriate measure of infection rates associated with long-term use of catheters and we were able to compare our data with values reported in the literature.[8-10,12-14] A Mann-Whitney U test was used to analyze differences between patients with or without sepsis. The a priori level of significance was set at 0.05.

Results

Of the 62 patients in whom HPN was started between 1980 and 1987 at our institution, 56 were included in the final study. Six patients were excluded from the study because of loss to follow-up or missing medical records. Patients were followed during their entire course of HPN or until 1989.

HPN was used for an average duration of 1.02 years (range, 7.3 days to 4.33 years). The indications for HPN were cancer (16 patients), bowel obstruction (13), short-bowel syndrome (12), malnutrition (10), chronic malabsorption (9), immunodeficiency (9), gastrointestinal pseudo-obstruction (6), fistula (6), radiation enteritis (5), inflammatory bowel disease (3), and other (6). Some patients had more than one indication for HPN.

The median age at the initiation of therapy was 27.9 years (range, 6 months to 82 years). The distribution of patients by ethnic group was as follows: white, 73.2%; black, 14.3%; Asian, 3.6%; Hispanic, 3.6%; and unknown, 5.4%.

Of the 56 study patients, 30 (53.6%) had complications related to HPN, 18 (32.1%) had complications not related to HPN, and 8 (14.3%) had no recorded complications. Of the 365 total complications noted, 125 (34.2%) were related to HPN. The mean (± S.D.) interval between initiation of HPN and occurrence of a complication was 1.25 ± 1.73 years. Patients having complications related to HPN did not significantly differ from patients having complications not related to HPN with respect to ethnicity, sex, age, or medical reason for beginning HPN. The average length of stay for the 61 HPN-related hospitalizations was 13.3 ± 13.7 days (mean ± S.D.).

Table 2.
Complications Associated with Home Parenteral Nutrition

Complication	No. (%)
Fluid or electrolyte disturbance	35 (28.0)
Liver abnormalities	24 (19.2)
Infection	
Catheter exit site	18 (14.4)
Systemic	8 (6.4)
Thrombosis	13 (10.4)
Bacterial overgrowth	7 (5.6)
Catheter rupture	7 (5.6)
Catheter dislodgement	4 (3.2)
Osteoporosis	3 (2.4)
Other	6 (12.8)

Fluid or electrolyte disturbances and hyperglycemia were the most frequent complications associated with HPN in our study group, accounting for 28% of all complications (Table 2). The graph in Figure 1 plots the probability of being complication-free as a function of the number of months on HPN. We were specifically interested in knowing, for any given number of months on HPN, what would be the probability of avoiding a particular complication. For example, at the end of the first year, the probability of not having a catheter infection was 0.6; the probability of being free of a fluid or electrolyte disturbance or hyperglycemia was only 0.45. In contrast, the probability of avoiding catheter breakage or dislodgement and thrombosis was 0.85 by the end of the first year.

Seventy catheters were used in the 56 patients and there were 26 catheter-related infections (local infections and septicemia) for a cumulative total of 20,805 catheter-days. However, only eight patients had catheter-related septicemia for an incidence of 0.038/100 catheter-days. The other 18 patients had local infections for an incidence of 0.086/100 catheter-days. *Staphylococcus epidermidis*, the most common organism cultured, was isolated in three patients. *Staphylococcus aureus* and *Candida* species were cultured from two patients. Other organisms found included *Escherichia coli*, *Torulopsis glabrata*, and *Streptococcus faecalis*.

The first episode of septicemia occurred at 2.1 ± 1.8 years (mean ± S.D.) (range, 0.21–5.05 years) after initiation of HPN. The mean ± S.D. age at initiation of HPN was 16.1 ± 14.1 years in patients who developed sepsis and 29.9 ± 24.5 years in those who did not ($p < 0.13$). Patients with sepsis were on HPN significantly longer (2.9 years) than patients without sepsis (0.96 years) ($p < 0.03$).

All patients with sepsis were initially treated empirically with broad-spectrum antimicrobials. The antimi-

Figure 1. Probability of being free of HPN-related complications over time (months). Solid line = fluid, electrolyte, or glucose complication, short dash = breakage or dislodgement of catheter, medium dash = catheter infection, long/medium dash = thrombosis.

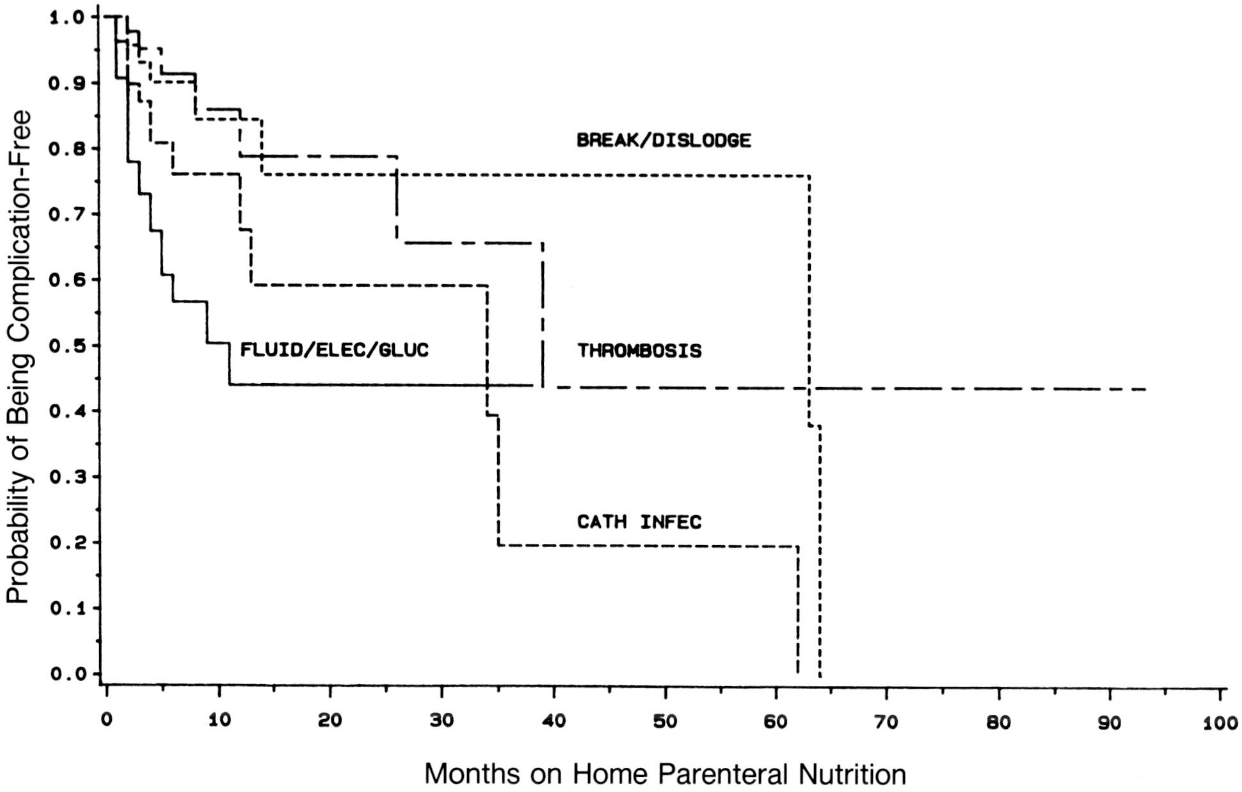

crobial regimen was modified according to blood culture results, and therapy was continued for 7 to 10 days. If the patient did not respond to therapy, the catheter was removed and then replaced 7 to 10 days after the patient became afebrile.

Transient moderate elevations in serum concentrations of alkaline phosphatase, AST, and ALT accounted for 19.2% of all complications and were fully reversed when the parenteral nutrition formulation was manipulated or when HPN therapy was ended. Two patients, who were on HPN for more than two years, had clinical evidence of hepatic steatosis. Three patients had radiographic evidence of osteoporosis, and seven patients were diagnosed as having bacterial overgrowth. These complications were few in number, and temporal probability could not be statistically established.

Discussion

The severe complications associated with HPN therapy can be avoided if clinicians are aware of the importance of monitoring these patients during the complete course of therapy. Our study suggests several interesting trends in the occurrence of HPN-related complications. Earlier in the course of therapy, patients were more likely to have fluid or electrolyte abnormalities or hyperglycemia than the other complications we analyzed. This may be attributed to changes in physical and environmental factors, experienced by the patients at home, that can alter their nutritional requirements.

The risk of catheter-related mechanical failure, infection, and thrombosis increased with the length of time the catheter remained in place. Others have suggested that patients receiving prolonged HPN therapy and possibly younger patients are at greater risk of experiencing a septic complication.[14] Over time, the patients' catheters are subject to an increased number of manipulations, which can increase the chance of contamination or catheter breakage. Very young patients, who are unable to care for themselves, are more susceptible to accidental self-contamination or contamination by the caregiver. The development of catheter thrombus and fibrin sleeve formation has been postulated to be due to (1) the turbulence in the blood flow caused by the catheter and (2) platelet aggregation with subsequent fibrin deposition on the surface of the catheter.[15,18] Catheter thrombosis formed during parenteral nutrition therapy may need to remain in situ for long periods of time before it becomes clinically significant.

Catheter sepsis occurred at a rate of 0.038/100 catheter-days in our study. This finding was favorable compared with the results reported for studies of other HPN populations incorporating pediatric and adult patients (range, 0.15–0.29 per 100 catheter-days) and oncology patients.[14,19-21] The organisms isolated in our patients during episodes of septicemia were consistent with those reported in the literature for these patients.[14,19] This low rate of sepsis is encouraging, and we believe it reflects the concentrated training that the patients receive in aseptic technique and the vested interest and commitment that they have in HPN.

Osteoporosis and bacterial overgrowth occurred in patients who received prolonged HPN therapy (greater than eight months). Aluminum contamination of parenteral nutrient solutions[22,23] and vitamin D deficiency[24,25] are hypothesized as possible etiologies of this problem. Patients receiving long-term HPN typically have little or no oral intake, which may increase the incidence of intestinal bacterial overgrowth. Bacterial overgrowth may lead to further malabsorption, increased risk of bacteremia, and possibly increased incidence of hepatotoxicity.[26] We also found a high incidence of liver function abnormalities, which is in agreement with previous reports.[8,9,27] Two of our patients had severe liver disease and prior liver abnormalities. The mildly affected patients were treated by a decrease in glucose intake for one to three months, which resulted in complete normalization of liver enzyme concentrations.

The primary limitations of the study are the small population size and the use of a single institution as the investigation site. The difficulty of determining whether a complication is HPN-related or simply a manifestation of the patient's disease is an inherent weakness of the study.

Conclusion

HPN effectively provides nutrition to patients who require prolonged parenteral support and causes relatively few severe complications. Complications of HPN can occur throughout the course of therapy; however, fluid or electrolyte abnormalities or glucose intolerance tend to occur in the early months of therapy, whereas catheter infection, thrombosis, and breakage or dislodgement manifest later.

References

1. Ostro MJ, Greenberg, Jeejeeboy KN. Total parenteral nutrition and complete bowel rest in the management of Crohn's disease. *JPEN J Parenter Enteral Nutr*. 1985; 9:280-7.
2. Purdum PP, Kirby DF. Short-bowel syndrome: a review of the role of nutrition support. *JPEN J Parenter Enteral Nutr*. 1991; 15:93-101.
3. Singer P, Rothdopf MM, Kvetan V et al. Risks and benefits of home parenteral nutrition in the acquired immunodeficiency syndrome. *JPEN J Parenter Enteral Nutr*. 1991; 15:75-9.
4. Weiss SM, Worthington PH, Prioleau M et al. Home parenteral nutrition in cancer patients. *Cancer*. 1982; 50:1210-3.
5. Baptista RJ, Blackburn GL, Champagne CD et al. The cost of home parenteral nutrition. *Nutr Clin Pract*. 1987; 2:14-22.
6. Herfindal ET, Bernstein LR, Kudzia K et al. Survey of home nutrition support patients. *JPEN J Parenter Enteral Nutr*. 1989; 13:255-61.
7. Board of Directors, American Society for Parenteral and Enteral Nutrition. Guidelines for use of home total parenteral nutrition. *JPEN J Parenter Enteral Nutr*. 1987; 11:342-4.
8. Steiger E, Srp F. Morbidity and mortality related to home parenteral nutrition in patients with gut failure. *Am J Surg*. 1983; 145:102-5.
9. Stokes MA, Irving MH. Mortality in patients on home parenteral nutrition. *JPEN J Parenter Enteral Nutr*. 1989; 13:172-5.
10. Broviac JW, Scribner BH. Prolonged parenteral nutrition in the home. *Surg Gynecol Obstet*. 1974; 139:24-8.
11. Jeejeebhoy KN, Langer B, Tsallas G et al. Total parenteral nutrition at home in patients surviving four months to five years. *Gastroenterology*. 1976; 71:943-53.
12. Gouttebel MC, Saint-Aubert B, Jonquet O et al. Ambulatory home total parenteral nutrition. *JPEN J Parenter Enteral Nutr*. 1987; 11:475-9.
13. Riella MC, Scribner BH. Five years' experience with a right atrial catheter for prolonged parenteral nutrition at home. *Surg Gynecol Obstet*. 1976; 143:205-8.
14. Decker MD, Edwards KM. Central venous catheter infections. *Pediatr Clin North Am*. 1988; 35:579-612.
15. Costanzo JD, Sastre B, Choux R et al. Mechanism of thrombogenesis during total parenteral nutrition: role of catheter composition. *JPEN J Parenter Enteral Nutr*. 1988; 12:190-4.
16. Ostrander CR, Cohen RS, Hopper AO et al. Breath hydrogen analysis: a review of the methodologies and clinical applications. *J Pediatr Gastroenterol Nutr*. 1983; 2:525-33.
17. Kaplan EL, Meier P. Non-parametric estimation from incomplete observations. *J Am Stat Assoc*. 1958; 53:457-81.
18. Beers TR, Burnes J, Fleming CR. Superior vena caval obstruction in patients with gut failure receiving home parenteral nutrition. *JPEN J Parenter Enteral Nutr*. 1990; 14:474-9.
19. Schroop KP, Ginn-Pease ME, King DR. Catheter-related sepsis: a review of the experience with Broviac and Hickman catheters. *Nutrition*. 1988; 4:195-200.
20. Vargas JH, Ament ME, Berquist WE. Long-term home parenteral nutrition in pediatrics: ten years of experience in 102 patients. *J Pediatr Gastroenterol Nutr*. 1987; 6:24-32.
21. Schmidt-Sommerfeld E, Snyder G et al. Catheter-related complications in 35 children and adolescents with gastrointestinal disease on home parenteral nutrition. *JPEN J Parenter Enteral Nutr*. 1990; 14:148-51.
22. Ott SM, Maloney NA, Klein GL et al. Aluminum is associated with low bone formation in patients on chronic parenteral nutrition. *Ann Intern Med*. 1983; 98:910-4.
23. ASCN/ASPEN Working Group on Standards for Aluminum Content of Parenteral Nutrition Solutions. Parenteral drug products containing aluminum as an ingredient or a contaminant: response to Food and Drug Administration notice of intent and request for information. *JPEN J Parenter Enteral Nutr*. 1991; 15:194-8.
24. Shike M, Harrison JE, Sturtridge WC et al. Metabolic bone disease in patients receiving long-term parenteral nutrition. *Ann Intern Med*. 1980; 92:343-50.
25. Hurley DL, McMahon MM. Long-term parenteral nutrition and metabolic bone disease. *Endocrinol Metab Clin North Am*. 1990; 19:113-31.
26. Fouin-Fortunet H, Le Quernec L, Erlinger S et al. Hepatic alteration during total parenteral nutrition in patient with inflammatory bowel disease: a possible consequence of lithocholate toxicity. *Gastroenterology*. 1982; 82:932-7.
27. Clarke PJ, Ball MJ, Kettlewell MGW. Liver function tests in patients receiving parenteral nutrition. *JPEN J Parenter Enteral Nutr*. 1991; 15:45-59.

Appendix—Standard HPN Procedures

Nutrition: Daily nutrition solutions are mixed under sterile conditions and delivered by our home-care pharmacy. The composition depends on the patient's individual requirements. Caloric requirements are met by the combination of dextrose and lipids. Nitrogen is provided by amino acid solutions (Baxter Healthcare, Deerfield, IL). Electrolytes and trace elements are added to the nutrient solutions based on requirements. Vitamins are added by the patient on a daily basis. Some patients are allowed to eat (except for patients on complete bowel rest or those with high-output fistulas), but daily oral caloric intake is not sufficient to maintain adequate nutrition.

Solution Administration: Nutrient solution is delivered through a subcutaneously tunneled silicone catheter. The flow rate is regulated by an infusion device on an overnight schedule. Some patients infuse their solutions only two to three times a week. Patients are taught to add heparin to the catheter daily using 2 mL of a 100-unit/mL solution of heparin to prevent interluminal thrombosis. A one- to two-week supply of the HPN solutions is delivered and stored under refrigeration (at 4 °C) in the patient's home. The patients are furnished with all the supplies necessary for proper maintenance of the catheter and solutions.

Outpatient Monitoring: Following discharge from the hospital, the patients are seen regularly in our clinic. If patients live outside our area, they are seen by their primary physicians in correspondence with our program. Specialized home therapy nurses from our program also visit the patients in their homes to assess the home environment and to provide advice and encouragement to the patients and their families. The responsibility for the clinical monitoring of the HPN therapy is shared jointly by the patient and the HPN team. The patient monitors and records daily weights, temperature, total fluid intake and output, blood and urine glucose concentrations, and any adverse events. On return visits to the clinic for follow-up (once or twice monthly), the patient is evaluated for progress; for detection of fluid, electrolyte, or nutrient imbalances; for infectious complications; and for metabolic complications. All pertinent laboratory tests are performed, including the following: serum concentrations of electrolytes, glucose, albumin, and creatinine; liver function tests; complete blood count; and prothrombin time. Other laboratory analysis or diagnostic tests are performed when necessary before appropriate changes in the HPN regimen are made. All of the monitoring data are documented in the patient's medical chart and in the patient records kept by the home-therapy pharmacy.

Patient Education: Patients are taught the techniques involved in administration of the nutrient solutions, care of the catheters, aseptic technique, and self-monitoring for progress and adverse effects. During their hospital stay, patients are instructed in HPN therapy by the home nutritional support team. The education process is completed usually within one week. In some cases, care of the patient is undertaken by a family member or a private nurse. All patients give informed consent and demonstrate competence in all HPN techniques before discharge from the hospital. Additionally, the patients must be clinically stable on their parenteral nutrient formulation and medically stable before discharge.

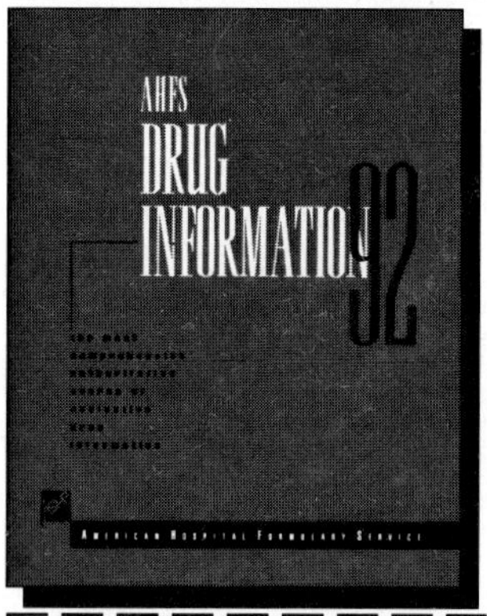

Commentary

New calcium-channel blockers: Improved therapy?

EDMUND V. CAPPARELLI

Clin Pharm. 1992; 11:549-52

In the past few years, several new formulations of calcium-channel-blocking agents have become available for clinical use. Extended-release formulations of nifedipine, diltiazem, and verapamil became available, and new dihydropyridine derivatives—nimodipine, nicardipine, felodipine, and isradipine—were approved by the FDA. Bepridil, a calcium-channel blocker that is chemically unrelated to the other available agents, also recently became available. With the exception of nimodipine, which received approval for a unique indication (subarachnoid hemorrhage), the other drugs are used as antihypertensive and antianginal agents.

The overall use of calcium-channel blockers has also been expanding during this time period. Both the Joint National Committee on Detection, Evaluation, and Treatment of High Blood Pressure[1] and the World Health Organization[2] have recently added calcium-channel blockers to the list of first-line pharmacologic agents for the treatment of hypertension. By increasing the use of calcium-channel blockers and adding these new agents, have we improved therapy by liberating patients from adverse effects, by increasing clinical efficacy, or by enhancing patient compliance?

Adverse Effects

Specific Hazards of Bepridil. Individual classes of calcium-channel blockers tend to possess some group-specific adverse effects. The introduction of a new class of calcium-channel blocker, in bepridil, provides a new group of adverse effects and hemodynamic effects for consideration. Most commonly, bepridil produces some minor adverse effects on the central nervous system (primarily dizziness and tremors) and the gastrointestinal system.

EDMUND V. CAPPARELLI, PHARM.D., is Clinical Pharmacokinetics Specialist, Department of Pharmacy, University of California, San Diego Medical Center, 225 Dickinson Street, Route 8765, San Diego, CA 92103-1990.

Bepridil also possesses class I and III electrophysiologic properties, which has led to evaluation of the drug for the treatment of supraventricular and ventricular arrhythmias.[3-5] To date, the number of patients who have received bepridil for antiarrhythmic therapy is rather limited, and the drug's labeling does not include an indication for this use. Furthermore, recent studies suggest increased mortality with certain antiarrhythmic agents.[6,7] This finding has led to reduced use of antiarrhythmic agents in non-life-threatening arrhythmias. Although these trials studied agents with different electrophysiologic properties than those of bepridil, their results have curtailed enthusiasm for the development of new antiarrhythmic agents.

Because of its class III electrophysiologic properties, bepridil can cause the ventricular tachycardia known as torsade de pointes. This condition occurred in approximately 1% of patients treated with bepridil during United States trials.[8] Characteristics of patients who are at increased risk for torsade de pointes during bepridil therapy include advanced age, hypokalemia, elevated serum bepridil concentrations, and concurrent diuretic therapy.[9] Torsade de pointes may begin up to 10 months after initiation of bepridil therapy, making monitoring for this potentially life-threatening adverse reaction difficult.[9] Agranulocytosis has also been reported in two patients during bepridil therapy. These adverse reactions to bepridil have restricted its labeled indication to use in "patients who have failed to respond optimally to, or are intolerant of, other antianginal medication."[8]

Vasodilatory Effects. The prototypical dihydropyridine, nifedipine, has been associated with frequent vasodilator-mediated adverse effects, including flushing, pedal edema, and headaches. The three new dihydropyridines—nicardipine, felodipine, and isradipine—have also been associated with these adverse effects. Whereas the overall frequency with nicardipine and felodipine appears to be similar to that with nifedipine,[10,11] one double-blind crossover study comparing isradipine with nifedipine demonstrated fewer adverse reactions and increased patient preference for isradipine.[12]

In a comparison between conventional nifedipine and the extended-release nifedipine preparation available in the United States (nifedipine gastrointestinal therapeutic system [GITS]), the extended-release formulation produced fewer adverse reactions.[13] Although large comparative trials with power to detect differences in frequencies of adverse reactions among the new dihydropyridines and nifedipine GITS are lacking, it is doubtful that the frequency of vasodilatory adverse reactions among these agents differs greatly.

Cardiodepression. A major difference among the calcium-channel blocking agents that often influences drug selection is their degree of cardiodepression. Since many patients treated for angina also have left ventricular dysfunction, the ideal calcium-channel blocker would not precipitate heart failure.

Confusing this issue is the widespread perception that nifedipine is not a cardiodepressant. Although reflex sympathetic outflow can lead to increased cardiac output with nifedipine, there is both in vitro and in vivo evidence that nifedipine exerts a direct negative inotropic effect on myocardium.[14,15] Furthermore, in a recent double-blind comparison with isosorbide dinitrate for mild to moderate heart failure, nifedipine resulted in clinical deterioration and more frequent hospitalizations.[16] Therefore, the search for a more vasoselective calcium-channel blocker may be warranted.

In vitro and in vivo studies with nicardipine, felodipine, and isradipine have shown the new dihydropyridines to have less of a direct cardiodepressant effect than nifedipine or the other classes of calcium-channel-blocking agents.[14,17,18] Clinical studies with these new agents in patients with heart failure are scant. However, small studies with both isradipine and felodipine have demonstrated no deterioration in patients with heart failure after one to six months of therapy.[19-21]

These data are encouraging, but there are some indications that precipitation of heart failure with calcium-channel blockers may not entirely relate to their direct cardiodepressant effects. Some studies suggest that clinical deterioration may be related to the tendency of calcium-channel blockers to activate neurohumoral systems (e.g., the sympathetic nervous system and the renin–angiotensin system), which over time leads to increased symptoms of heart failure.[22,23] This may explain the deterioration in clinical status of patients with heart failure who are treated with nicardipine[24] despite indications of little or no in vivo negative inotropic effect with nicardipine.[25] If neurohumoral activation plays a major role in worsening heart failure during calcium-channel blocker therapy, then attempting to develop agents with greater vasoselectivity may not achieve improved tolerance in patients with heart failure.

One small study did suggest that felodipine did not result in neurohumoral activation. However, the high mortality (50%) and higher baseline neurohumoral activation in felodipine-treated patients in this study greatly weaken this claim.[20] In another study, felodipine therapy did increase norepinephrine concentrations in patients with heart failure.[26]

Currently, there is insufficient evidence to support any one of the dihydropyridines over the others on the basis of reduced risk of precipitation or worsening of heart failure, and these agents must be used with caution in patients with left ventricular dysfunction.

Efficacy

Another potential rationale for using one of the newer calcium-channel blockers is increased efficacy. In the treatment of chronic hypertension, new agents and formulations have failed to demonstrate superior efficacy over traditional agents in well-controlled trials. Agents that are approved for the treatment of angina pectoris—nicardipine, nifedipine GITS, and bepridil—have also failed to consistently demonstrate improved efficacy over older agents. In one open-label trial, nifedipine GITS did decrease anginal attack frequency compared with an equal daily dosage of standard-formulation nifedipine.[27] However, this difference was small (less than one attack per week) and may merely reflect differences in patient recording, patient compliance, or bias encountered in an open-label study.

Bepridil's labeling as a second-line antianginal agent implies that it may be effective when other agents have failed. There are few published data to support that inference. Studies comparing the efficacy of bepridil and verapamil demonstrated that bepridil caused minor improvement in exercise duration; however, it did not reduce anginal frequency.[28] Studies comparing bepridil with the β-adrenergic antagonists propranolol and nadolol failed to show any statistically significant differences among drugs in reducing anginal frequency.[29,30]

In the only study that attempted to target patients with refractory angina, bepridil was compared with diltiazem in patients who continued to have frequent angina despite maximum diltiazem hydrochloride dosages (up to 360 mg/day).[31] Despite the fact that subjects had to have an unsatisfactory response to diltiazem, bepridil caused only minor improvement in exercise performance at selected points during therapy and did not reduce the frequency of angina during ambulation. Since the majority of the patients in this study were also taking β-adrenergic antagonists and long-acting nitrates, this trial did demonstrate that bepridil, used in combination with these agents, was relatively well tolerated.

Improved long-term outcomes in coronary-artery disease would be another argument for selecting one of the newer calcium-channel-blocking agents. Many animal studies have shown all classes of calcium-channel blockers to reduce ischemia-induced myocardial damage and to have antiatherogenic properties; however, clinical corroboration of these effects has been sparse.[32,33] Large clinical trials have suggested that morbidity and mortality may be reduced with diltiazem and verapamil in certain post-myocardial-infarction patient populations.[34-37] A trial of nifedipine that used a similar study design failed to show any benefit in post-myocardial-infarction patients.[38] This difference may result from more skillful data manipulation in the verapamil and diltiazem trials. We must await further studies to see if any of the new dihydropyridines can reduce cardiovascular morbidity or mortality in a particular setting.

Patient Compliance

One clear improvement in calcium-channel-blocker therapy that has been established with these new agents and formulations is reduced dosing frequency and improved patient compliance. The standard formulations of verapamil, diltiazem, and nifedipine all require dosage intervals of six to eight hours. Whereas the new dihydropyridines isradipine and nicardipine can be taken two and three times daily, respectively, felodipine can be taken once daily. Nifedipine GITS, which uses an osmotic gradient to "pump" nifedipine out of the tablet at a zero-order rate, can also be taken once daily.[13,39] Extended-release preparations of verapamil and diltiazem have also reduced dosage frequency to once or twice daily. To promote use of these extended-release preparations, manufacturers have priced them competitively and, in some cases, they cost less than their immediate-release counterparts and the newer calcium-channel blockers.

Conclusion

Although we are likely to see more calcium-channel blockers in the near future, all currently available dihydropyridines appear to be effective for their respective cardiovascular indications and to differ primarily in pharmacokinetics. A possible reduction in vasodilatory adverse effects may be seen with the longer-acting dihydropyridines (including nifedipine GITS) because of small peak-to-trough concentration fluctuations. The relative roles of direct cardiodepression and neurohumoral activation in the development of heart failure associated with calcium-channel blockers are unclear. Understanding the contribution of these effects may provide insight into the safe use of calcium-channel blockers in patients with left ventricular dysfunction.

The adverse reactions and electrophysiologic effects of both verapamil and diltiazem differ substantially from those of the dihydropyridines. Therefore, formulary availability of agents from all three classes (dihydropyridines, verapamil-like drugs, diltiazem-like drugs) may be necessary to treat various patients. Bepridil, an agent from a new class of calcium-channel blockers, needs further study to determine if its effectiveness with multiple-drug combinations in the treatment of refractory angina offsets its inherent toxicities.

The development of new calcium-channel blockers has encouraged research into new and expanded roles for calcium-channel blockers in general, yet therapeutic improvements over older agents remain unproven. New insights regarding calcium-channel-blocker therapy, potentially improved patient compliance, and price competition are welcome, but the impetus to replace older calcium-channel blockers with newer ones is not compelling at this time.

References

1. 1988 Joint National Committee. The 1988 report of the Joint National Committee on Detection, Evaluation, and Treatment of High Blood Pressure. *Arch Intern Med.* 1988; 148:1023-38.
2. World Health Organization/International Society of Hypertension Fifth Mild Hypertension Conference. The 1989 guidelines for the management of mild hypertension: memorandum from a WHO/ISH meeting. *J Hypertens.* 1989; 7:689-93.
3. Somberg J, Torres V, Flowers D et al. Prolongation of QT interval and antiarrhythmic action of bepridil. *Am Heart J.* 1985; 109:19-27.
4. Perelman MS, McKenna WJ, Rowland E et al. A comparison of bepridil with amiodarone in the treatment of established atrial fibrillation. *Br Heart J.* 1987; 58:335-44.
5. Roy D, Montigny M, Klein GJ et al. Electrophysiologic effects and long-term efficacy of bepridil for recurrent supraventricular tachycardias. *Am J Cardiol.* 1987; 59:89-92.
6. Coplen SE, Antman EM, Berlin JA et al. Efficacy and safety of quinidine therapy for maintenance of sinus rhythm after cardioversion: a meta-analysis of randomized control trials. *Circulation.* 1990; 82:1106-16.
7. Echt DS, Liebson PR, Mitchell LB et al. Mortality and morbidity in patients receiving encainide, flecainide or placebo: the Cardiac Arrhythmia Suppression Trial. *N Engl J Med.* 1991; 324;781-8.
8. McNeil Consumer Products. Vascor package insert. Fort Washington, PA; 1990 Dec.
9. Manouvrier J, Sagot M, Caron C et al. Nine cases of torsades de pointes with bepridil administration. *Am Heart J.* 1986; 111:1005-7.
10. Maetzel FK, Teufel WE, Griebel A et al. Double-blind, randomized comparative study of the antihypertensive effect of nicardipine slow-release and nifedipine slow-release in hypertensive patients with coronary disease. *Cardiovasc Drugs Ther.* 1991; 5:647-54.
11. Littler WA, Baig MW, Chee D et al. Comparison of felodipine with nifedipine as additions to metoprolol in the treatment of hypertension. *J Cardiovasc Pharmacol.* 1990; 15(Suppl 4):S99. Abstract.
12. Welzel D, Burger KJ. The calcium antagonist isradipine in the therapy of hypertension: a double-blind crossover comparison with nifedipine. *Drugs.* 1990; 40(Suppl 2):60-4.
13. Bittar N. Usefulness of nifedipine for myocardial ischemia and the nifedipine gastrointestinal therapeutic system. *Am J Cardiol.* 1989; 64:F31-4.
14. Schwinger RH, Bohm M, Erdmann E. Negative inotropic activity of the calcium antagonists isradipine, nifedipine, diltiazem and verapamil in diseased human myocardium. *Am J Hypertens.* 1991; 4:S185-7.
15. Packer M, Lee WH, Medina N et al. Comparative negative inotropic effects of nifedipine and diltiazem in patients with severe left ventricular dysfunction. *Circulation.* 1985; 72(Suppl III):III-275. Abstract.
16. Elkayam U, Amin J, Mehra A et al. A prospective, randomized, double-blind, crossover study to compare the efficacy and safety of chronic nifedipine therapy with that of isosorbide dinitrate and their combination in the treatment of chronic congestive heart failure. *Circulation.* 1990; 82:1954-61.
17. Koolen J, Piek J, van Wezel H et al. Relative effects of intracoronary nifedipine and felodipine on myocardial contractility and oxygen consumption. *Circulation.* 1991; 84(Suppl II):II-683. Abstract.
18. Cheng CP, Noda T, Little WC. Comparison of inotropic effect of felodipine, nifedipine, and amlodipine in conscious dogs. *Circulation.* 1991; 84(Suppl II):II-401. Abstract.
19. McGrath BP, Newman R, Older P. Hemodynamic study of short- and long-term isradipine treatment in patients with chronic ischemic congestive heart failure. *Am J Med.* 1989; 86(Suppl 4A):75-80.
20. Kassis E, Amtorp O. Long-term clinical, hemodynamic, angiographic and neurohumoral responses to vasodilation

with felodipine in patients with chronic congestive heart failure. *J Cardiovasc Pharmacol.* 1990; 15:347-52.
21. Tweddel AC, Martin W, McGhie AI et al. Sustained haemodynamic effects of felodipine in patients with chronic cardiac failure. *Br J Clin Pharmacol.* 1988; 25:689-94.
22. Barjon JN, Rouleau JL, Bichet D et al. Chronic renal and neurohumoral effects of the calcium channel blocker nisoldipine in patient with congestive heart failure. *J Am Coll Cardiol.* 1987; 58:122-8.
23. Packer M. Calcium channel blockers in chronic heart failure: the risks of "physiologically rational" therapy. *Circulation.* 1990; 82:2254-7.
24. Gheorghiade M, Hall V, Goldberg AD et al. Long-term clinical and neurohumoral effects of nicardipine in patients with severe heart failure on maintenance therapy with angiotensin converting enzyme inhibitors. *J Am Coll Cardiol.* 1991; 17(Suppl A):A274. Abstract.
25. Rousseau MF, Pouleur H. Calcium antagonism free of negative inotropic effects? A comparison of intracoronary nifedipine and nicardipine. *Circulation.* 1984; 70(Suppl II):A304. Abstract.
26. Kassis E, Amtorp O. Cardiovascular and neurohumoral postural responses and baroreceptor abnormalities during a course of adjunctive vasodilator therapy with felodipine for congestive heart failure. *Circulation.* 1987; 75:1204-13.
27. Vetrovec GW. Once-daily therapy for angina pectoris with nifedipine gastrointestinal therapeutic system. *Am J Med.* 1989; 86(Suppl 1A):28-32.
28. Nielson HR, Krusell LR, Husted SF et al. Bepridil versus verapamil in stable angina pectoris—a controlled clinical trial. *Int J Cardiol.* 1988; 23:357-64.
29. Destors JM, Roissel JP, Philippon AM et al. Controlled clinical trial of bepridil, propranolol and placebo in the treatment of exercise induced angina pectoris. *Fundam Clin Pharmacol.* 1989; 3:597-611.
30. Pflugfelder PW, Human DP, O'Brien PA et al. Comparison of bepridil with nadolol for angina pectoris. *Am J Cardiol.* 1987; 59:1283-8.
31. Singh BN. Comparative efficacy and safety of bepridil and diltiazem in chronic stable angina pectoris refractory to diltiazem: the Bepridil Collaborative Study Group. *Am J Cardiol.* 1991; 68:306-12.
32. Kober G, Schneider W, Kaltenbach M. Can the progression of coronary sclerosis be influenced by calcium antagonists? *J Cardiovasc Pharmacol.* 1989; 13(Suppl 4):S2-6.
33. Fitzpatrick DB, Karmazyn M. Comparative effects of calcium channel blocking agents and varying extracellular calcium concentration on hypoxia/reoxygenation and ischemia/reperfusion-induced cardiac injury. *J Pharmacol Exp Ther.* 1984; 228:761-8.
34. The Multicenter Diltiazem Postinfarction Trial Research Group. The effect of diltiazem on mortality and reinfarction after myocardial infarction. *N Engl J Med.* 1988; 319:385-92.
35. Gibson RS, Boden WE, Theroux P et al. Diltiazem and reinfarction in patients with non-Q-wave myocardial infarction: results of a double-blind randomized multicenter trial. *N Engl J Med.* 1986; 315:423-9.
36. The Danish Study Group on Verapamil in Myocardial Infarction. Effect of verapamil on mortality and major events after acute myocardial infarction (The Danish Verapamil Infarction Trial II–DAVIT II). *Am J Cardiol.* 1990; 66:779-85.
37. The Danish Study Group on Verapamil in Myocardial Infarction. Verapamil in acute myocardial infarction. *Eur Heart J.* 1984; 5:516-28.
38. The Israeli Sprint Study Group. Secondary Prevention Reinfarction Israeli Nifedipine Trial (SPRINT). A randomized interventional trial of nifedipine in patients with acute myocardial infarction. *Eur Heart J.* 1988; 9:354-64.
39. Chung M, Reitberg DP, Gaffney M et al. Clinical pharmacokinetics of nifedipine gastrointestinal therapeutic system: a controlled-release formulation of nifedipine. *Am J Med.* 1987; 83(Suppl 6B):10-4.

DUE Criteria

The DUE Criteria *section of* Clinical Pharmacy *features model drug-use evaluation criteria that may be employed as a component of a comprehensive quality assurance program. The criteria sets are presented in the format used in the ASHP book* Criteria for Drug Use Evaluation. *Some of the criteria sets will have been originally published in that book; others will be presented here for the first time and published in future volumes of the ASHP book. The practitioners who developed a criteria set are acknowledged.*

In selecting drug products for coverage in DUE Criteria, *priority is given to products that have been recently marketed, those that are frequently prescribed, those that have high potential risk associated with their use, and those that are expensive. When feasible, a criteria set will be linked with a* Drug Review *that appears in the same issue.*

These criteria sets are a starting point for the development of DUE Criteria for a specific practice setting. Readers are encouraged to modify the model criteria to fit their own circumstances.

Criteria for use of agents for extrapyramidal adverse effects in adult, adolescent, and child inpatients and outpatients[a]

Element	Standard 100%	Standard 0%	Exception[b] or Critical Preventive/Responsive Measure[c]	Sources of Information
Justification for Use				
1. Treatment of extrapyramidal adverse effects (EPAE) induced by antipsychotic drugs: parkinsonian symptoms, akathisia, or dystonia[1,2] or	X		1A. None	1. History and physical (H&P), intake assessment, progress notes, physician orders
2. Prophylaxis for dystonia in young patient (<45 years old) treated with high-potency antipsychotic agent (with high potential to produce EPAE) or having history of dystonia[2,3]	X		2A. None	2. H&P, intake assessment, progress notes, physician orders
Critical (Process) Indicators				
3. Symptoms of EPAE present and documented in chart, and patient unresponsive to dosage reduction or switch to lower-potency antipsychotic agent[3]	X		3A. Clinical situation prohibits dosage reduction or switch to lower potency antipsychotic agent[3] 3B. Agent for EPAE used prophylactically	3,3A,B. H&P, progress notes, physician orders
4. No history of allergy to prescribed agent for EPAE	X		4A. Alleged drug allergy judged nonallergic in etiology or cannot be corroborated	4,4A. H&P, allergies
5. No history of closed-angle glaucoma or prostatic hypertrophy	X		5A. Amantadine used	5,5A. H&P, progress notes, physician orders

Prepared by Patricia A. Marken, Pharm.D., Assistant Professor of Pharmacy Practice in Psychiatry, Schools of Pharmacy and Medicine, University of Missouri–Kansas City, and Psychopharmacy Specialist, Western Missouri Mental Health Center, Kansas City; and Jeanne R. Ezell, M.S., Director of Pharmacy, Blount Memorial Hospital, Maryville, TN.

Element	Standard 100%	Standard 0%	Exception[b] or Critical Preventive/ Responsive Measure[c]	Sources of Information
6. No history of or current severe ulcerative colitis, obstructive disease of gastrointestinal tract, paralytic ileus, intestinal atony, or cardiospasm[1]	X		6A. Amantadine, β-blocker, or benzodiazepine used	6,6A. H&P, progress notes, physician orders
7. No history of congestive heart failure, sinoatrial node dysfunction, bronchospastic disease, Raynaud's syndrome, or diabetes mellitus[1]	X		7A. Anticholinergic agent, amantadine, or benzodiazepine used	7,7A. H&P, progress notes, physician orders
8. No history of tardive dyskinesia[4]	X		8A. History of tardive dystonia[5] or tardive dyskinesia mixed with EPAE[6] 8B. Beta-blocker or amantadine used	8,8A. H&P, progress notes 8B. H&P, physician orders
9. Diphenhydramine used for patient <3 years old[7]	X		9A. None	9. H&P, progress notes, physician orders
10. Beta-blocker used only for antipsychotic-induced akathisia[2]	X		10A. None	10. Progress notes, physician orders
11. Benzodiazepine used only for antipsychotic-induced akathisia,[8] acute dystonia,[8] tardive dyskinesia,[9] or chronic tardive dystonia[9]	X		11A. None	11. H&P, progress notes, physician orders
12. Risk factors for dystonia documented	X		12A. None	12. H&P, progress notes
13. Serum creatinine concentration measured before amantadine therapy	X		13A. Patient without renal disease who had normal test results within past 6 months	13,13A. H&P, physician orders, laboratory reports
14. Baseline electrocardiogram (ECG) performed	X		14A. Patient on amantadine, anticholinergic agent, or benzodiazepine 14B. Beta-blocker used in patient <40 years of age and without history of cardiac problems 14C. Patient without history of cardiac problems who had normal ECG within past 6 months	14. H&P, physician orders, ECG reports 14A. Physician orders, medication administration record (MAR) 14B. H&P, progress notes, physician orders 14C. H&P, progress notes, ECG reports
15. Appropriate oral dosage (mg/day)[d]: a. Amantadine hydrochloride[1] 100–200 b. Benztropine mesylate[1] 1–8 c. Biperiden hydrochloride[1] 2–6 d. Clonazepam (for akathisia)[10] 1 e. Diphenhydramine hydrochloride[1,3] 75–400 f. Ethopropazine hydrochloride[1,2] 50–600 g. Lorazepam (for akathisia)[8] 1–6 h. Procyclidine hydrochloride[1] 7.5–20 i. Propranolol hydrochloride[8,10] 30–160 j. Trihexyphenidyl hydrochloride[1] 1–15	X		15A. Amantadine hydrochloride up to 400 mg/day in patient not responding to lower dosage[1] 15B. Lower dosage of amantadine hydrochloride in patient with compromised renal function (based on creatinine clearance)[1] 15C. Benztropine mesylate 1–2 mg i.v. or i.m. in patient requiring immediate response[1] 15D. Biperiden lactate 2 mg i.m. or slow i.v. in patient requiring immediate response; dose repeated every 30 minutes if necessary, not to exceed 8 mg/day[1] 15E. Diphenhydramine hydrochloride oral dosage: in child ≤9.1 kg, 6.25–12.5 mg t.i.d. or q.i.d.; in child >9.1 kg, 5 mg/kg/day, not to exceed 300 mg/day[1] 15F. Diphenhydramine hydrochloride 50 mg i.m. or i.v. in adult patient requiring immediate response; total daily dosage not to exceed 400 mg orally, i.m., or i.v. in adult patient[1,2] 15G. Lorazepam 0.025–0.050 mg/kg	15,15A. Physician orders, MAR; progress notes 15B. H&P, laboratory reports, progress notes, physician orders 15C-G. Physician orders, MAR, progress notes

Element	Standard 100%	Standard 0%	Exception[b] or Critical Preventive/ Responsive Measure[c]	Sources of Information
			i.m. in patient with acute dystonia[8]	
16. Antiparkinsonian agent for EPAE used for <3 months[2]	X		16A. Patient reassessed for medication need every 3 months[2]	16,16A. H&P, progress notes
17. Agent for prophylaxis and management of dystonia used for <5 days[2]	X		17A. Recurrence of dystonia	17,17A. H&P, progress notes
18. Agent for EPAE not used with drug having anticholinergic effects	X		18A. Antipsychotics and other agents with anticholinergic adverse effects used if clinically indicated and alternative not available 18B. Benzodiazepine, β-blocker, or amantadine used	18. Physician orders, MAR 18A,B. Physician orders, MAR, progress notes
19. Diphenhydramine not used with monoamine oxidase inhibitor[1]	X		19A. None	19. Physician orders, MAR
Complications				
20. Anticholinergic effects: urinary retention, constipation, blurred vision, dry mouth[1]		X	20A. Identify other drug and nondrug causes 20B. Manage dry mouth with fluids or sugarless candy or gum; manage constipation with diet or bulk-forming laxative[2] 20C. Reduce dosage or discontinue agent for EPAE if possible 20D. If reaction persists, change to agent for EPAE without anticholinergic effects	20. Progress notes, nursing notes 20A,B. Physician orders, MAR, nursing notes, progress notes 20C,D. Physician orders, MAR, progress notes
21. Anticholinergic psychosis, confusion, delirium (caused by anticholinergic agent for EPAE), or psychosis (caused by amantadine)[1]		X	21A. Identify other drug and nondrug causes 21B. Discontinue agent for EPAE; restart at lower dosage if necessary or consider alternative agent 21C. Discontinue all medications with anticholinergic properties 21D. Monitor geriatric patient carefully[2]	21. H&P, progress notes, intake assessment, nursing notes 21A-C. Progress notes, nursing notes, physician orders, MAR 21D. H&P, progress notes, physician orders
22. Gastrointestinal effects: nausea, vomiting[2]		X	22A. Identify other drug and nondrug causes 22B. Administer anticholinergic agent for EPAE with meals[2] 22C. Reduce amantadine dosage[2]	22. Progress notes, nursing notes 22A. Progress notes, physician orders, MAR, nursing notes 22B,C. Physician orders, MAR
23. Cardiovascular effects: tachycardia (caused by anticholinergic agent),[2] postural hypotension (caused by amantadine or β-blocker),[2] heart failure or block (caused by β-blocker), symptomatic bradycardia (caused by β-blocker)[7]		X	23A. Identify other drug and nondrug causes 23B. Reduce dosage or discontinue agent for EPAE if possible 23C. Change to another agent for EPAE 23D. Monitor pulse, blood pressure, and heart rate daily until stable and patient asymptomatic	23. Progress notes, nursing notes, ECG reports, nursing flow sheets 23A. Progress notes, physician orders, MAR, nursing notes 23B,C. Physician orders, MAR, progress notes 23D. Physician orders, MAR, nursing notes, progress notes, nursing flow sheets
24. Livedo reticularis (blue or purple mottling of skin) caused by amantadine		X	24A. Identify other drug and nondrug causes 24B. Discontinue amantadine only if of concern to patient	24. H&P, progress notes 24A,B. Progress notes, physician orders, nursing notes, MAR
Outcome Measures				
25. Treatment: resolution of or decrease in EPAE within 3 months	X		25A. Patient unresponsive to drug therapy; alternative treatment indicated 25B. Patient lost to follow-up 25C. Patient left psychiatric service against medical advice 25D. Patient died (drug-related etiology ruled out)	25. Progress notes, nursing notes 25A. Progress notes, physician orders 25B-D. Progress notes
26. Prophylaxis: no dystonic reaction in young patient on high-potency antipsychotic	X		26A. Patient unresponsive to drug therapy; alternative treatment indicated	26. Progress notes, nursing notes 26A. Progress notes, physician orders

Element	Standard 100%	0%	Exception[b] or Critical Preventive/ Responsive Measure[c]	Sources of Information
agent or with history of dystonias			26B. Patient lost to follow-up 26C. Patient left psychiatric service against medical advice 26D. Patient died (drug-related etiology ruled out)	26B-D. Progress notes

[a] Criteria address justification for use (indications), critical (process) indicators, complications of therapy, and patient outcome. Each criterion consists of an element, a standard, exceptions to the standard, and sources of information. The element is the minimum level of evidence needed to show that patient care was optimal. The standard defines the deviation from an element that is acceptable. If no deviation is acceptable, the standard is 100%. Exceptions are circumstances in which deviation is allowable. Sources of information listed are the most reliable sources. Sources pertaining to an element or exception are identified by the number assigned to the element or exception (e.g., 3,3A).

[b] For justification for use, critical (process) indicators, and outcome measures.

[c] For complications.

[d] Although other benzodiazepines are used for akathisia and tardive dyskinesia (and clonazepam is used for tardive dyskinesia as well as akathisia) and β-blockers other than propranolol are used for EPAE, published information on appropriate dosages is sparse. Higher end of dosage range is avoided or used with caution in elderly patients.

References

1. McEvoy GK, ed. AHFS drug information 90. Bethesda, MD: American Society of Hospital Pharmacists; 1990:581-5, 2146.
2. Perry PJ, Alexander B, Liskow BI. Psychotropic drug handbook, 5th ed. Cincinnati: Harvey Whitney Books; 1988:175-91.
3. Arana GW, Goff DC, Baldessarini RJ. Efficacy of anticholinergic prophylaxis for neuroleptic induced acute dystonia. *Am J Psychiatry*. 1988; 145:993-6.
4. Jeste DV, Lohr JB, Clark K et al. Pharmacological treatments of tardive dyskinesia in the 1980's. *J Clin Psychopharmacol*. 1988; 8: S38-48.
5. Burke RE, Fahn S, Jankovic J et al. Tardive dyskinesia or dystonia: late onset and persistent dystonia caused by antipsychotic drugs. *Neurology*. 1982; 32:1335-46.
6. Friis T, Christensen TR, Gerlach J. Sodium valproate and biperiden in neuroleptic-induced movement disorders. *Biol Psychiatry*. 1983; 18:1085-91.
7. Knoben JE, Anderson PO. Handbook of clinical drug data, 6th ed. Hamilton, IL: Drug Intelligence Publications; 1988:287, 485-6.
8. Ereshefsky L, Richards A. Psychoses. In: Young LY, Koda-Kimble MA, eds. Applied therapeutics: the clinical use of drugs, 4th ed. Vancouver, WA: Applied Therapeutics; 1988:1189-230.
9. Yadalam KG, Korn ML, Simpson GM. Tardive dystonia: four case histories. *J Clin Psychiatry*. 1990; 51:17-20.
10. Bodkin JA. Emerging uses for high-potency benzodiazepines in psychotic disorders. *J Clin Psychiatry*. 1990; 51:41-6.

ASHP journal continuing-education instructions and enrollment form

Instructions

1. The system is flexible. You may select any combination of tests from *AJHP* and *Clinical Pharmacy* to give you the number of credits you need.
2. An answer sheet is published at the end of each installment of the Continuing Education column. This enrollment form is published in the June and December issues of *AJHP* and *CP*.
3. Complete only one enrollment form, but note on the form all the tests you are taking. Staple together all answer sheets for one enrollment.
4. Tests included must have been published within the past 18 months. Once a particular test is included in an enrollment, it may not be included in a subsequent enrollment.
5. The passing score on each test is 70%. Within four weeks of receiving your enrollment, ASHP will mail you a CE certificate or notify you that certain tests were failed. Failed tests may be retaken only one time, without additional cost. There are no refunds for failed tests.
6. ASHP is approved by the American Council on Pharmaceutical Education as a provider of continuing pharmaceutical education (Provider Number 680-204.) Most states that recognize ACPE-approved providers will accept credit earned through journal CE programs; however, since some states have restrictions on the number of credit hours or CE units they will accept toward the total requirement, it is advised that readers check with their respective state board of pharmacy if they are uncertain about the board's regulations.
7. Send your enrollment form, answer sheet(s), and check (made payable to ASHP) to:

ASHP CE
Customer Service Department
American Society of Hospital Pharmacists
4630 Montgomery Avenue
Bethesda, MD 20814

Enrollment Form

Name ______________________________

Address ______________________________

City ______________ State ______________ Zip ________

Fee Schedule

$5/hour

$20 minimum/enrollment

Tests included in this enrollment must have been published within the past 18 months.

Test Number	*Hours of Credit**
________	________
________	________
________	________
________	________
________	________
________	________
________	________
________	________
________	________

Total hours ________

Total fee ($) enclosed ________

(Write additional numbers and hours on a separate sheet and attach it to this form.)

*10 hours = 1.0 C.E.U.

ACPE® *The American Society of Hospital Pharmacists is approved by the American Council on Pharmaceutical Education as a provider of continuing pharmaceutical education*

Current Literature

Drug Reaction Alerts 562

Book Reviews

Combined Modality Cancer Therapy: Radiation and Infusional Chemotherapy 565
Edited by Jacob J. Lokich and John E. Byfield
Reviewed by Richard Slimowitz

Drugs in Gastroenterology 565
Edited by P. C. Braga, M. Guslandi, and A. Tittobello
Reviewed by Curtis E. Haas

Self-study Materials

Concepts in Oncology Therapeutics: A Self-Instructional Course 568
Edited by Rebecca S. Finley
Reviewed by Robert J. Ignoffo

Books Received 570

Starting with this issue of *Clinical Pharmacy*, reviews of self-study materials will appear in a separate section of Current Literature, instead of with reviews of books.

Drug Reaction Alerts

Drug Reaction Alerts focuses primarily on serious, unlabeled reactions to new chemical entities. The citations are compiled monthly from International Pharmaceutical Abstracts, *which covers over 800 pharmacy and health-related journals worldwide. An address for reprints (when available) follows the name of the corresponding author in each citation.*

Pharmacists may use the FDA Adverse Reaction Report form that appears in the January and July issues of Clinical Pharmacy *for submitting reports of adverse drug reactions directly to FDA.*

Aminoglycosides

Jojart G (Korhaz, H-2700 Cegled, Hungary). Sense of smell after **gentamicin** nose-drops. *Lancet*. 1992; 339:313. Case. (patient with *Staphylococcus aureus* strain in nose; applied gentamicin 1.6 mg/mL twice daily to nose for five days; developed burning sensation, nasal congestion, and headache after a few days, then lost sense of smell; withdrawal of gentamicin led to improvement, but sense of smell did not return to normal after six months)

Anorexics

Atanassoff PG, Weiss BM, Schmid ER et al. (Tornic M, Department of Anesthesiology, University Hospital of Zurich, CH-8091 Zurich, Switzerland). Pulmonary hypertension and dexfenfluramine: 1. *Lancet*. 1992; 339:436. Case. (30-year-old woman at 34 weeks' gestation who was obese before conception; received **D-fenfluramine** for six months before conception as adjuvant therapy for obesity and developed pulmonary hypertension; underwent cesarean section and pulmonary hypertension worsened; therapy with alprostadil and diuretic did not lead to improvement; experienced cardiac arrest on day 3, and died on day 4; examination at autopsy revealed hypertrophy on right side of heart and pulmonary arteriopathy)

Roche N, Labrune S, Braun JM et al. (Huchon GJ, Pneumology Service, University de Paris Rene Descartes, Hôpital Ambroise Pare, 92104 Boulogne, France). Pulmonary hypertension and dexfenfluramine: 2. *Lancet*. 1992; 339:436-7. Case. (26-year-old woman; received **D-fenfluramine** 15–30 mg for two months; developed symptoms of pulmonary hypertension after one month; withdrawal of D-fenfluramine led to eventual reversal of symptoms; no rechallenge)

Antineoplastic Agents

Akiyama H, Nakamura N, Nagasaka S et al. (Onozawa Y, Hematology and Endocrinology Division, Tokyo Metropolitan Komagome Hospital, Tokyo 113, Japan). Hypercalcemia due to *all-trans* retinoic acid. *Lancet*. 1992; 339:308-9. Case. (19-

Continued on page 564

Continued from page 562

year-old man with acute promyelocytic leukemia; received **tretinoin** 40 mg/sq m for nine weeks; developed hypercalcemia and decreased serum parathyroid hormone and vitamin D concentrations; withdrawal of tretinoin led to return of serum calcium, parathyroid, and vitamin D concentrations to normal)

Cardiac Drugs

Bero CJ (Department of Pharmacy Service, Milton S. Hershey Medical Center, Penn State University Hospital, 500 University Drive, Hershey, PA 17033). Possible association of pulmonary fibrosis with mexiletine. *DICP Ann Pharmacother.* 1991; 25:1329-31. Case. (75-year-old man; received **mexiletine hydrochloride** 200 mg every eight hours for 13 months; developed symptoms of pulmonary fibrosis after three months; withdrawal of mexiletine did not lead to improvement; patient deteriorated and died from intractable respiratory difficulties 27 days after admission to hospital)

Peterson AM (Department of Pharmacy, Crozer-Chester Medical Center, One Medical Center Boulevard, Upland, PA 19013), Conrad SD, Bell JM. Procainamide-induced pseudo-obstruction in a diabetic patient. *DICP Ann Pharmacother.* 1991; 25:1334-5. Case. (65-year-old man with cardiac arrhythmia and diabetes mellitus; received extended-release **procainamide hydrochloride** 500 mg four times daily for two weeks; developed pseudo-obstruction of bowel; concomitant diltiazem hydrochloride, isosorbide dinitrate, and captopril; conversion of procainamide to i.v. administration did not lead to resolution of symptoms; withdrawal of procainamide led to resolution of symptoms)

Drug Administration Routes

Saltuari L, Marosi MJ, Kofler M et al. (Bauer G, Department of Neurorehabilitation and Department for Seizure Disorders and EEG, University Hospital for Neurology, A-6020 Innsbruck, Austria). Status epilepticus complicating intrathecal **baclofen** overdose. *Lancet.* 1992; 339:373-4. Case. (16-year-old patient with tetraparesis due to brain injury; received baclofen 200–400 μg/day by intrathecal delivery via implanted delivery system; accidentally received baclofen 10 mg by intrathecal delivery when system reservoir was punctured during refill procedure; developed focal motor seizures with left-sided clonic motor activity six hours later; concomitant phenytoin; EEG results were abnormal 2.25 hr later even though seizures were controlled after 1.5 hr; removal of drug reservoir eight hours after accident and drainage of 30 mL of cerebrospinal fluid revealed mean ± S.D. baclofen concentration of 4.27 μg/mL (n = 5); serum samples obtained eight hours after accident contained no trace of baclofen; EEGs resembled preoverdose patterns five days later)

Drug Interactions

Sperber AD, Liel Y. Evidence for interference with the intestinal absorption of **levothyroxine sodium** by **aluminum hydroxide**. *Arch Intern Med.* 1992; 152:183-4. Case. (60-year-old man with hypothyroidism who received maintenance therapy with levothyroxine sodium 0.15 mg/day for five years; received two antacid tablets containing aluminum hydroxide, magnesium hydroxide, and simethicone four times daily for four months as part of clinical trial; serum thyrotropin concentration changed to 36 mU/L and serum thyroxine concentration changed to 103 nM, although no symptoms developed; withdrawal of antacid led to return of serum thyrotropin and thyroxine concentrations to normal two weeks later; positive rechallenge)

Hypotensive Agents

Os I (Department of Nephrology, Ullivol Hospital, Oslo, Norway), Bratland B, Dahlof B et al. Female sex as an important determinant of **lisinopril**-induced cough. *Lancet.* 1992; 339:372. Study. (double-blind, randomized trial; 412 hypertensive patients received lisinopril at a mean dose of 18.8 mg and 416 hypertensive patients received nifedipine at a mean dose of 37.4 mg for 10 weeks after four-week run-in placebo period; more patients randomized to lisinopril than to nifedipine reported cough as adverse effect without specific prompting [8.5% versus 3.1%, p = 0.0009]; nearly three times more women than men spontaneously reported cough as adverse effect of lisinopril [12.6% versus 4.4%, p = 0.0027], but no similar effect from nifedipine [2.8% versus 3.0%]; cough contributed to withdrawal of five women from study; nonsmokers [72%] and smokers [28%] who took lisinopril spontaneously reported similar occurrence of cough [9.5% versus 8.1%])

Tsele E, Chu AC (Unit of Dermatology, Royal Postgraduate Medical School, Hammersmith Hospital, London W12 0NN, England). **Nifedipine** and telangiectasias. *Lancet.* 1992; 339:365-6. Case. (49-year-old man with hypertension; received nifedipine 20 mg/day for eight months; developed telangiectatic rash without infiltration, edema, scaling, or pustules on cheeks and spider nevi on arms; biopsy results of facial tissue showed only elastosis and epidermal atrophy; withdrawal of nifedipine and substitution with atenolol led to slight but definite improvement after two months and disappearance of spider nevi after nine months)

Immunosuppressive Agents

Angelucci E (Division Ematology di Muraglia, e Centro Trapianti Midollo Osseo, Ospedale di Pesaro, 61100 Pesaro, Italy), Mariotti E, Lucarelli G et al. Sudden cardiac tamponade after chemotherapy for marrow transplantation in thalassemia. *Lancet.* 1992; 339:287-9. Study. (cohort; 400 thalassemic patients who received **busulfan** and **cyclophosphamide** as conditioning regimen for bone marrow transplantation; eight patients, aged 4–15 years, developed sudden cardiac tamponade characterized by sudden onset of circulatory shock and cardiac arrest; six of eight patients died, representing 9% of all deaths and 29% of deaths occurring between start of conditioning regimen and 30 days posttransplantation; only effective treatment for sudden cardiac tamponade was fluid removal)

Immunotherapy

Alvarez JS, Sacristan JA, Alsar MJ (Hematology Service, Hospital Marqués de Valdecilla, Santander-Cantabria, Spain). **Interferon alfa-2a**-induced impotence. *DICP Ann Pharmacother.* 1991; 25:1397. Case. (37-year-old man with chronic myelogenous leukemia; received interferon alfa-2a 3 million IU/day by i.m. injection and increased to 9 million IU/day for two months; became impotent; reduction of interferon dosage did not lead to improvement; withdrawal of interferon three months later led to gradual resolution of impotence)

Ben-Chetrit E, Putterman C (Hadassah University Hospital-Ein Kerem, Jerusalem 91120, Israel). Transient neutropenia induced by intravenous **immune globulin**. *N Engl J Med.* 1992; 326:270-1. Case. (36-year-old woman with active systemic lupus erythematosus; received immune globulin 400 mg/kg/day by i.v. infusion for five days for two courses two months apart; developed marked neutropenia after first infusion in each course; concomitant azathioprine and prednisone; neutropenia lasted about five days after each course without substantial changes in hemoglobin concentration or platelet count)

Minerals

Ejima A (Department of Neurology, Institute of Brain Disorders, and Department of Radiology, Tohoku University, School of Medicine, Sendai 980, Japan), Imamura T, Nakamura S et al. **Manganese** intoxication during total parenteral nutrition. *Lancet.* 1992; 339:426. Case. (62-year-old man; received manganese 2.2 mg/day for 23 months as part of essential trace elements in total parenteral nutrient solution; developed parkinsonism with dysarthria, mild rigidity, hypokinesia with masked face, halting gait, and severely impaired postural reflexes; cumulative manganese dose, 1.5 g; whole blood manganese concentration, 3.0–5.6 μg/dL [normal range, 0.4–2.0 μg/dL]; magnetic resonance image scan revealed high signal intensity in basal ganglia and brainstem; withdrawal of trace element supplementation and therapy with biperiden and levodopa led to gradual regression of parkinsonism and blood manganese concentration of 0.5 μg/dL after 15 weeks)

Progestins

Henry K (HIV/AIDS Program, Suite 125, St. Paul–Ramsey Medical Center, 640 Jackson Street, St. Paul, MN 55101), Rathgaber S, Sullivan C et al. Diabetes mellitus induced by **megestrol acetate** in a patient with AIDS and cachexia. *Ann Intern Med.* 1992; 116:53-4. Case. (46-year-old man with AIDS and cachexia; received megestrol acetate for 13 weeks; developed diabetes mellitus; withdrawal of megestrol acetate led to improvement of hyperglycemia; positive rechallenge)

Sympathomimetic Agents

Spitzer WO (McGill University, Purvis Hall, 1020 Pine Avenue West, Montreal, Quebec QC H3A 1A2, Canada). Suissa S, Ernst P et al. Use of **β-agonists** and the risk of death and near death from asthma. *N Engl J Med.* 1992; 326:501-6. Study. (case–control; 129 patients who received asthma medications and who had fatal or near-fatal asthma and 655 matched controls; use of β agonists administered by metered-dose inhaler was associated with increased risk of death from asthma [odds ratio, 2.6 deaths/canister/month]; use of **fenoterol** was associated with odds ratio of 5.4 deaths/canister versus **albuterol** with odds ratio of 2.4 deaths/canister; possible concomitant metaproterenol, terbutaline, theophylline, ipratropium bromide, cromolyn, and beclomethasone)

Book Reviews

Combined Modality Cancer Therapy: Radiation and Infusional Chemotherapy

Edited by Jacob J. Lokich and John E. Byfield.
Published by Precept Press, 160 East Illinois Street, Chicago, IL 60611, 1991. xiv + 250 p. Price $99.

In 1947, Farber successfully used aminopterin to treat five children stricken by acute leukemia; thus began cancer management by antineoplastic drugs. In the past 45 years, approximately 40 new drugs have been used to produce cures for such cancers as testicular cancer, acute myelogenous leukemia, Hodgkin's disease, and Wilms' tumor. Other cancers, in sites such as the breast, prostate, and head and neck, have proved responsive but not curable, and others such as renal and pancreatic cancers have responded poorly.

Although there had been growing interest in the combined use of radiation and antineoplastic drugs, it was not until 1979, when Steel and Peckham proposed guidelines, that experiments were designed. These pioneers proposed four approaches for the use of combined therapy: (1) spatial cooperation, in which radiation treats the primary tumor and antineoplastic drugs treat micrometastases, (2) toxicity independence, in which both treatments can be administered in full doses because the toxicities do not overlap, (3) protection of normal tissues, and (4) enhancement of tumor response.

Radiation is the major modality described in the book, with antineoplastic drugs placed in a secondary role. Although many clinical trials have used these two modalities in combination, major books such as *Cancer: Principles and Practice of Oncology, Third Edition* (edited by DeVita et al.) and *Principles and Practice of Radiation Oncology, Second Edition* (edited by Perez) devote scant attention to this subject; *Combined Modality Cancer Therapy: Radiation and Infusional Chemotherapy* attempts to fill this information void. Lokich, a medical oncologist, has written extensively on the infusion of antineoplastic drugs and has edited two books on the subject. Byfield has contributed more than 40 journal articles on the use of antineoplastic drugs as radiosensitizers. Together these men have edited a modest, readable book for the general audience.

The first chapter, written by Vokes and Weichselbaum, defines the experimental basis for combination therapy; I refer interested readers to the *Journal of Clinical Oncology* (1990; 8:911-34) for an expanded version written by these authors. The second chapter, by Byfield, constitutes the heart of the book; this chapter, a model for clear writing, gives the reader a comprehensive understanding of the use of radiation therapy. The third chapter, by Lokich, entitled "Principles and Practice of Infusional Chemotherapy," is a condensed version of his major work, *Principles and Practice of Infusional Chemotherapy, Second Edition.* Chapters 4–14 describe individual tumors for which trials of combined therapy have been used. Chapter 11 is important because it reviews the treatment of anal cancer and its successful treatment with combined therapies, replacing surgery as the major mode of therapy. The combined therapy approach has resulted in a 75–80% cure rate for this cancer, whereas many of the other tumor treatments have shown only modest responses.

As Lokich acknowledges, radiation and antineoplastic drug infusions are evolving therapies. This book gives the nonradiologist a precise overview of the subject.

Reviewed by Richard Slimowitz, Pharmaceutical Services Division, B-134, University Hospital, University of Medicine & Dentistry of New Jersey, 150 South Orange Avenue, Newark, NJ 07013-2757.

Drugs in Gastroenterology

Edited by P. C. Braga, M. Guslandi, and A. Tittobello.
Published by Raven Press, 1185 Avenue of the Americas, New York, NY 10036, 1991. xi + 533 p. Price $60.

According to its preface, *Drugs in Gastroenterology* is intended to be a single source for profiles on the major gastroenteric drugs. Nearly all the chapters are authored by academic, pharmaceutical industry, or clinical researchers from northern Italy. As a result, many of the drug profiles review drugs not approved for clinical use in the United States; of the 35 chapters that review a specific drug or group of drugs, 16 discuss agents not currently available in this country.

The book is divided into 18 major sections according to pharmacologic activity or clinical application. Five of these sections include a chapter that reviews basic pathophysiology relevant to the drugs profiled in that section. These pathophysiology chapters review diseases related to upper GI motility disorders, gastric acid secretion, gastric mucosal protection, bile secretion, and functional intestinal disorders. Other sections discuss pancreatic enzymes, hormonal agents (e.g., somatostatin), antiflatulants, mesalamine, drugs for treatment of hepatic

Continued on page 568

Current Literature *Continued from page 565*

encephalopathy, antixenobiotics, and the role of enteric microflora and the effects of antimicrobials on these flora.

Each chapter profiles a therapeutic agent and provides its chemical, toxicologic, pharmacologic, pharmacokinetic, clinical, and safety data. Most of these chapters are well referenced, and most of the data are presented in tables; however, some chapters rely on heavily referenced but brief statements. The chapters do not compare drugs in a single pharmacologic class, nor do they compare pharmacologic classes for their use in treating the same disease. For example, five chapters discuss five histamine H_2-receptor antagonists.

A major strength of this book is its compilation of information on many drugs in pharmacologic classes used exclusively to treat gastroenteric diseases. Depending on the reader's interest, another strength of this book could be its collection of chapters that review most of the important gastroenteric drugs available outside the United States.

Weaknesses of the book stem from its organization and the manner in which information is presented. Many chapters lack in-depth or critical evaluation of the clinical literature; this weakness combined with the aforementioned lack of pharmacologic class reviews means there is no discussion of an individual drug's place in therapy relative to similarly effective agents. Many chapters extensively review drug chemistry, toxicology, pharmacology, and pharmacokinetics but provide only brief discussions on clinical use and adverse effects. Thus, usefulness of this book as a clinical handbook is limited.

Drugs in Gastroenterology would not be a valuable reference for most practicing hospital pharmacists in this country. Much of the book addresses agents not approved by the U.S. Food and Drug Administration (FDA), and from a clinical standpoint, the reviews of FDA-approved agents are not uniquely insightful nor extensive in comparison with information available from other primary and secondary literature sources. For pharmacists practicing or conducting research in gastroenterology, this book may provide a valuable review of agents in clinical use in other parts of the world, several of which are under development in the United States.

Reviewed by Curtis E. Haas, Pharm.D., Department of Pharmacy, Rochester General Hospital, 1425 Portland Avenue, Rochester, NY 14621.

Self-study Materials

Concepts in Oncology Therapeutics: A Self-Instructional Course

Edited by Rebecca S. Finley.

Published by the American Society of Hospital Pharmacists, 4630 Montgomery Avenue, Bethesda, MD 20814, 1991. xxiii + 482 p. Price $55, ASHP members; $69, nonmembers.

This softbound book is designed to be a self-study manual for practicing pharmacists and, as the chapter authors suggest, a primer for pharmacy students. The authors of the various chapters are practicing oncology pharmacists, and they have organized this book to provide conceptual and practical information on subjects pertinent to the field of oncology.

The first 4 of 18 chapters lay the groundwork for understanding the basic concepts of cancer. An initial overview of cancer provides a simple but clear discussion of the problem of cancer, its etiology, nomenclature, diagnostic features, and statistics. A good description of tumor-response criteria and the role of various modalities in cancer treatment follows; however, the roles of biologic and hormonal therapies are not included. The essential elements of Phase I–IV clinical trials are discussed. The factors that affect tumor growth are discussed, and the relationship between cytotoxic drug therapy and the cell cycle is clearly explained, including the role of pharmacokinetics, dosage and scheduling, and the circadian rhythm. The issue of dose intensity is not presented, yet this omission does not substantially detract from an otherwise excellent chapter.

The mechanisms of action of cytotoxic agents and most of their important pharmacologic features are discussed after the introductory chapters. Although important drug interactions are presented for most agents, some are not included, such as the pharmacodynamic interaction of fluorouracil and folinic acid. Combination antineoplastic drug therapy and strategies for drug selection are discussed.

Endocrine therapy including regulation of hormone receptors is important in cancers affected by hormonal manipulation. Pharmacologic interventions useful in breast or prostate cancer are presented, including hormonal castration, estrogens, antiestrogens, aminoglutethimide, gonadotropin-releasing hormone, and corticosteroids.

Humoral and cellular immunopathology, recombinant DNA development, and adjuvant systemic therapy are reviewed. The mechanisms of action of the interferons, interleukins, and colony-stimulating factors are briefly described; a more detailed discussion on the clinical role of colony-stimulating factors should have been included. The results of adjuvant systemic therapy in stage 1 breast cancer, early colon cancer, and high-risk osteosarcoma illustrate the usefulness of this therapy in patients with high risk for tumor recurrence.

Methods of drug administration ranging from oral and intravenous to intrathecal, intraperitoneal, and intrapleural are presented, with discussion of potential benefits and hazards of regional administration. This well-done chapter presents enough details for both conceptual understanding and practical usage, such as information on extravasation kits, portable infusion devices, and novel catheters.

Antineoplastic drugs can cause organ system toxicities and nausea and vomiting. Risk factors are delineated for each organ system toxicity, and methods for minimizing adverse effects are outlined in a chapter with good details and practical recommendations. The pathophysiology of emesis and mechanisms for drug-induced emesis are discussed; however, a strategy for the use of combination antiemetic therapy is not presented.

Infection control and pain management are important considerations in the therapy of cancer patients. Predisposing factors for infections, an empiric management strategy for the febrile neutropenic patient, and common infections are presented with good details. The discussion of pain management includes not only the features of traditional analgesics but also adjuvant drugs and alter-

Continued on page 570

Continued from page 569

nate delivery methods. The concepts of pain control in the cancer patient are outlined, along with the comparative pharmacology of commonly used narcotics and non-narcotic analgesics. Nutritive and oncologic emergencies are appropriately presented. Helpful chapters on antineoplastic drug accountability and handling provide information necessary for compliance with guidelines set forth by the Food and Drug Administration and the Occupational Safety and Health Administration; sample forms are presented.

Although *Concepts in Oncology Therapeutics* is not and was not meant to be a comprehensive reference book, it satisfies the established goals. Some chapters provide more detail than others, but overall the content is reasonably balanced. The self-instructional approach provides immediate feedback to the participant. I recommend this book to both instructors and pharmacists who want to develop courses in oncology or update their basic skills in oncology practice.

Reviewed by Robert J. Ignoffo, Pharm. D., FASHP, Division of Clinical Pharmacy, School of Pharmacy, Box 0622, University of California, San Francisco, CA 94143-0622.

Books Received

Books are listed as soon as received; selected books may be reviewed in Book Reviews in subsequent issues.

Basic & Clinical Pharmacology, Fifth Edition, by Bertram G. Katzung. Published by Appleton & Lange, 25 Van Zant Street, East Norwalk, CT 06855, 1992. xiii + 1017 p. Price $34.95.

Endothelin, edited by Gabor M. Rubanyi. Published by Oxford University Press, Inc., 200 Madison Avenue, New York, NY 10016, 1992. xiii + 277 p. Price $70.

Handbook of Basic Pharmacokinetics . . . including Clinical Applications, Fourth Edition, by W. A. Ritschel. Published by Drug Intelligence Publications, Inc., 1241 Broadway, Hamilton, IL 62341, 1992. xxi + 588 p. Price $34.

Handbook of Cancer Chemotherapy, Third Edition, edited by Roland T. Skeel. Published by Little, Brown and Company, 34 Beacon Street, Boston, MA 02108, 1991. xiv + 549 p. Price $29.50.

Urinary Incontinence in Adults. Published by the Agency for Health Care Policy and Research, Public Health Service, U.S. Department of Health and Human Services, 2101 East Jefferson Street, Rockville, MD 20852, 1992. Available at no charge from the Center for Research Dissemination and Liaison, AHCPR Clearinghouse, P.O. Box 8547, Silver Spring, MD 20907. Clinical Practice Guideline (AHCPR #92-0038), xii + 125 p. Quick Reference Guide for Clinicians (AHCPR #92-0041), 27 p. Patient's Guide (AHCPR #92-0040), a 9-page pamphlet.

Advertising Index

American Society of Hospital Pharmacists
AHFS Drug Information 92, 548
Aseptic Preparation of Parenteral Products, 560
ASHP Databases, 569
ASHP Software, 466
Basic Skills in Interpreting Laboratory Data, 479
Clinical Pharmacy, 470
Concepts in Clinical Pharmacokinetics, 558
Concepts in Oncology Therapeutics, 470
Criteria for Drug Use Evaluation, Volumes 1 and 2, 556
Medication Teaching Manual, 463
MedTeach, 528
Amgen Inc.
Epogen, 468-469
Neupogen, 459-462
ASHP Research and Education Foundation
Anticoagulation Clinic Traineeship Program, 563
Institutional, 475
Burroughs Wellcome Company
Exosurf Neonatal, 471-474
Enzon, Inc.
Institutional, 465
Eli Lilly and Company
Hospital Division, 457
International Pharmaceutical Federation (F.I.P.)
Institutional, 464
Roche Laboratories, Division of Hoffmann-La Roche, Inc.
Rocephin, inside back cover, outside back cover
Roerig, A Division of Pfizer Pharmaceuticals
Cefobid, 557-558
Unasyn, 566-568
The Upjohn Company
Zefazone, 480-482
Wyeth-Ayerst Laboratories, Inc.
Ativan Injection, 476-478
Tubex, inside front cover

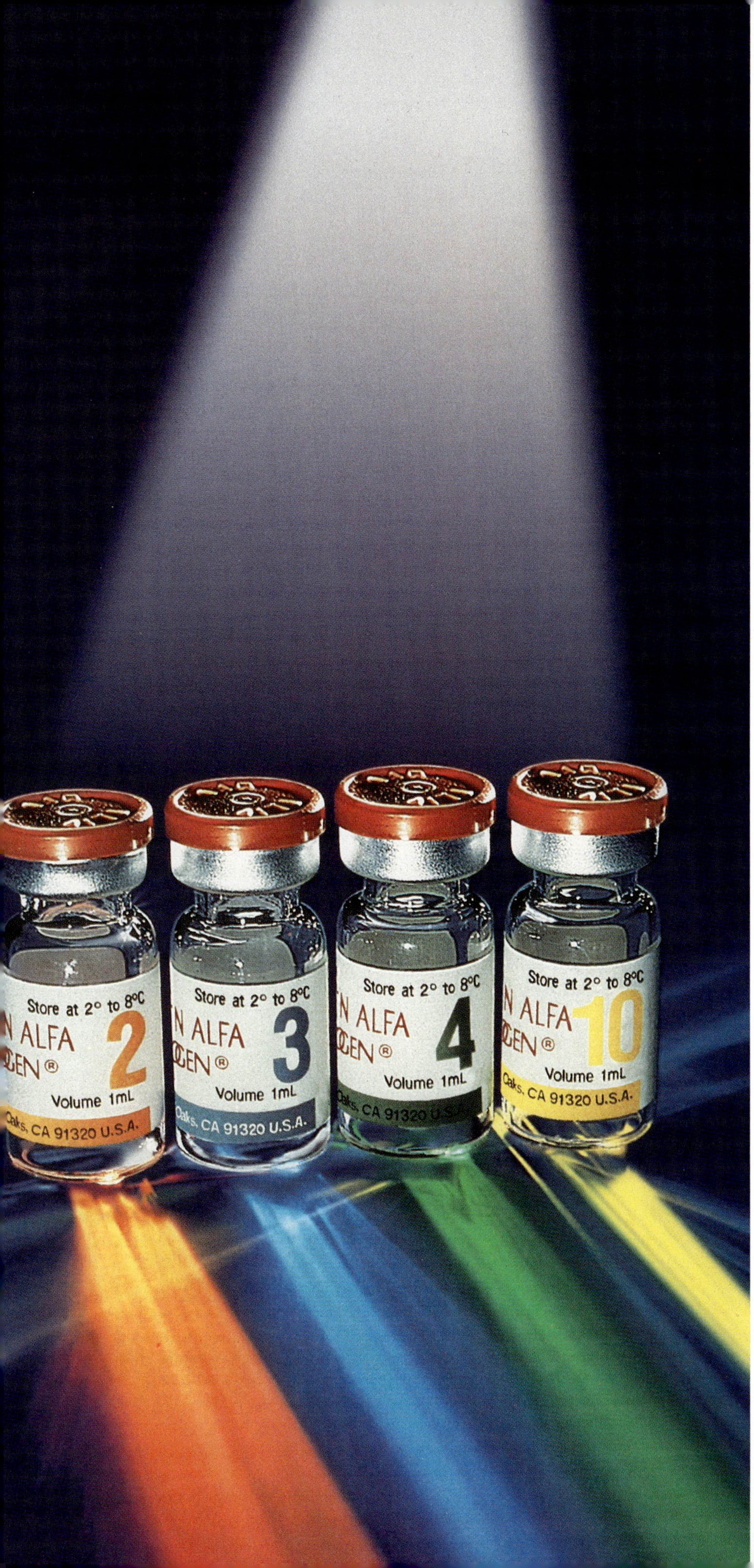
Store at 2° to 8°C
2
Volume 1mL
Caks, CA 91320 U.S.A.
Store at 2° to 8°C
3
Volume 1mL
Oaks, CA 91320 U.S.A.
Store at 2° to 8°C
4
Volume 1mL
Store at 2° to 8°C
10
Volume 1mL
Caks, CA 91320 U.S.A.

News

FDA announces four initiatives for drug approval system 574

Results of ISIS-3 published 576

Pediatrics academy issues new guidelines for acellular pertussis vaccine use 576

News Briefs 576

Upcoming Specialty Meetings 576

FDA announces four initiatives for drug approval system

Four initiatives for streamlining the drug approval process are being implemented by FDA. These changes include the use of outside expert reviewers to reduce the backlog of new drug applications awaiting approval; elimination of duplicate animal testing by the European Community, Japan, and the United States; institution of a parallel-track policy; and a proposed rule that would accelerate the approval of important new drugs through the introduction of such measures as the use of surrogate markers for efficacy.

External Review Program. FDA will begin using experts from outside the government to review certain applications. The program will be implemented in areas where a backlog of applications exists and will include product licensing applications for biologics, new drug applications, and supplements. In general, the products slated for external review will be ones that are not expected to pose problems (e.g., a product that is similar to one already on the market). The contract reviewers will be expected to submit a comprehensive report with a recommendation regarding approval 120 days after receiving the application. FDA will retain oversight and approval authority. The agency will be expected to notify the product sponsor within 180 days of the start of the review as to whether the drug is approvable. The first review by contract experts is expected to begin this summer.

Safety-Test Agreement. By agreement of the European Community, Japan, and the United States, animal safety data obtained in accordance with the requirements of one country can be accepted for review by another. This consensus on the scientific requirements and technical standards for safety testing is expected to reduce both the number of animals used and the time and resources required for completion of safety tests. The draft guidelines will be made public soon.

Parallel Track. The parallel-track policy is intended to increase patient access to treatments for conditions related to human immunodeficiency virus (HIV) infection while the studies required for marketing approval are being performed. The parallel track will be an option for patients with advanced HIV-related diseases who have no satisfactory alternative treatment and cannot participate in the controlled studies. In deciding whether to approve a sponsor's proposal for parallel-track studies, FDA will consider whether the proposal meets predetermined criteria, including criteria establishing that the drug is reasonably safe and has promising effectiveness. According to FDA, the Public Health Service is prepared

Continued on page 576

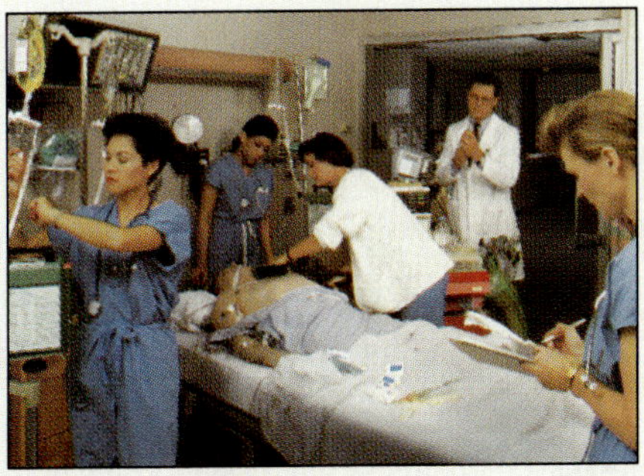

From emergency rooms to patients' rooms—pharmacists are there

Across the nation, pharmacists play a critical role in the day-to-day operation of hospitals. Interacting with physicians and patients when attending rounds is just one part of providing quality health care at the hospital.

From ER to OR to ICU, the experience and knowledge of the pharmacist is needed—and used.

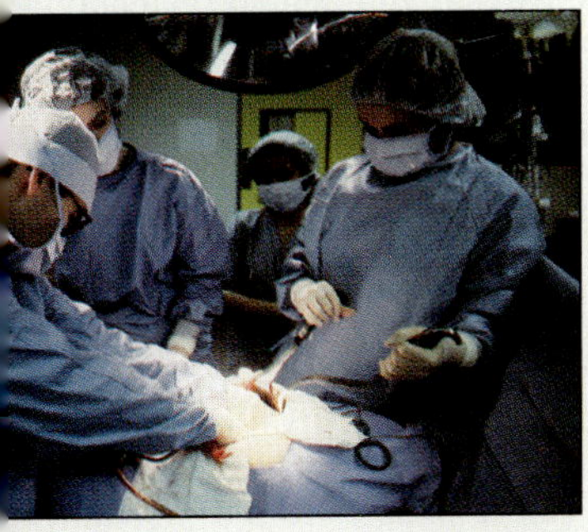

Managing health care costs—pharmacists are there

As a pivotal player in clinical and financial decisions, pharmacists help select the drug therapies used throughout the hospital that not only save lives, but also reduce the cost and length of hospitalizations.

WHEREVER YOU LOOK, YOU'LL FIND A HOSPITAL PHARMACIST

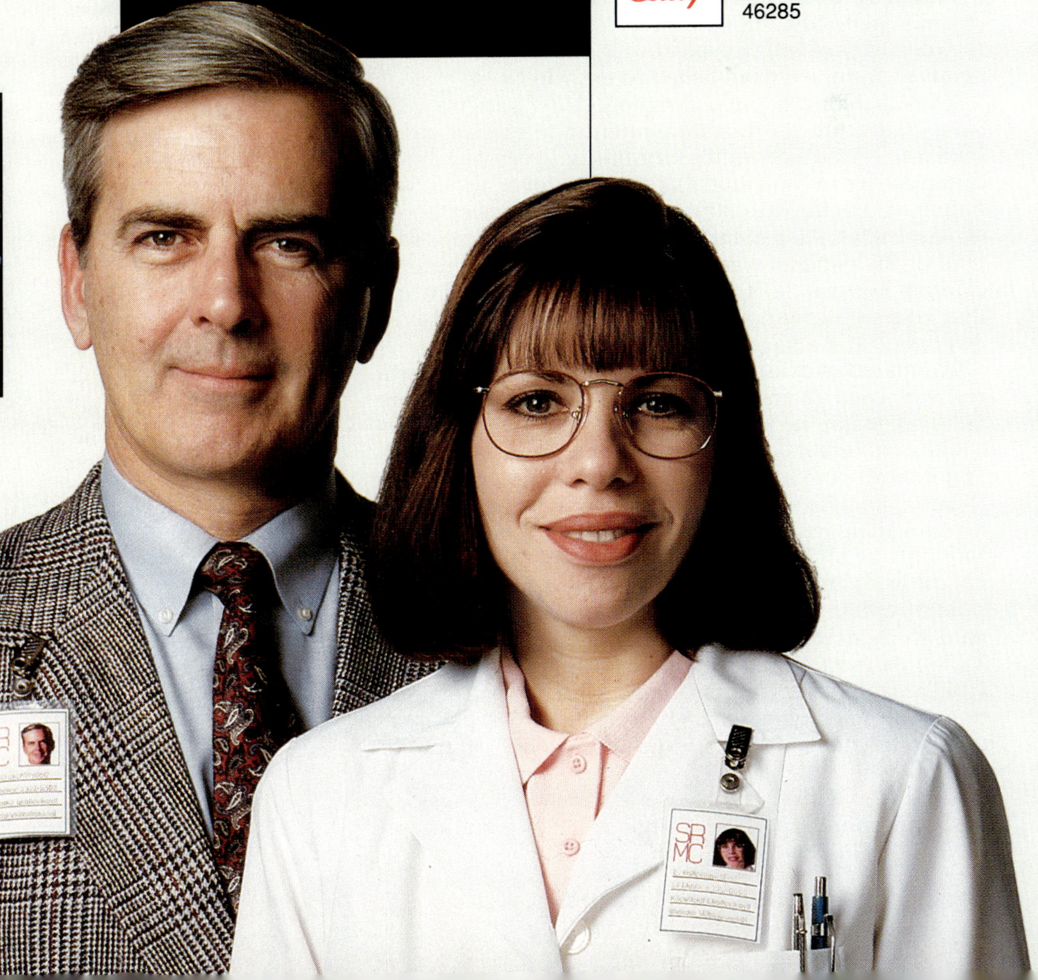

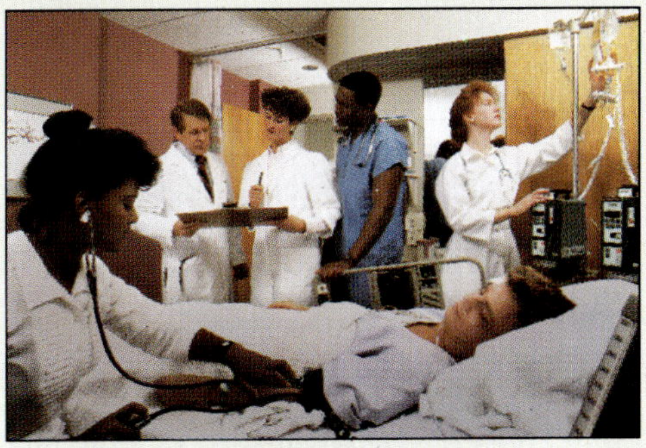

Helping pharmacists nationwide...Lilly is proud to be there

For over 50 years, Lilly has provided innovative products, drug information, and programs to serve hospital pharmacists.

Whether you need specific product information or detailed clinical information, Lilly can help provide answers to your questions.

Working in partnership with hospital pharmacists for over 50 years

Lilly

Eli Lilly and Company
Indianapolis, Indiana
46285

Continued from page 574

to work with groups interested in developing comparable programs for patients with other life-threatening illnesses.

Accelerated Approval. FDA is proposing the use of surrogate endpoints for effectiveness to speed the approval of drugs intended for use by patients with serious or life-threatening illnesses. Under this proposed rule, demonstration of a direct health benefit would not be required for drug approval; an endpoint such as a laboratory measurement or a physical sign that is thought to correspond to a real health benefit would be accepted as an indication of effectiveness. A surrogate marker of disease activity (CD4 cell count) was the primary measure of effectiveness in FDA's decision to approve marketing of didanosine.

Because this rule would result in earlier drug approval, greater emphasis would be placed on postmarketing studies conducted to confirm product efficacy. The procedures would include a streamlined process for drug withdrawal if postmarketing studies failed to confirm drug efficacy or safety problems arose.

The accelerated-approval procedures could also be applied to drugs that are effective for treatment of a serious disease but are highly toxic. In some cases, restricted distribution and imposed clinical tests could be a condition of marketing.

Results of ISIS-3 published

Results of the Third International Study of Infarct Survival (ISIS-3), which compared anistreplase or duteplase, a primarily double-stranded recombinant tissue-type plasminogen activator, with streptokinase and evaluated the concomitant use of aspirin with or without subcutaneous heparin, were published recently in *Lancet*.[1]

Investigators randomly assigned 41,299 patients with suspected acute myocardial infarction to receive streptokinase 1.5 million units infused i.v. over one hour, duteplase 0.6 million units/kg given i.v. over about four hours, or anistreplase 30 units injected i.v. over about three minutes. All patients received aspirin 162 mg/day. Half of the patients were randomly assigned to receive calcium heparin 12,500 units s.c. twice daily (starting four hours after randomization and continuing for seven days or until discharge) in addition to aspirin.

Compared with aspirin alone, the aspirin plus heparin regimen used in the study was associated with more cases of major noncerebral hemorrhage (1.0% versus 0.8%) and cerebral hemorrhage (0.56% versus 0.40%). The overall risk of stroke did not differ significantly. Reinfarction was slightly less common with aspirin plus heparin than with aspirin alone (3.16% versus 3.47%). Mortality at 35 days and at six months of follow-up did not differ significantly for the two treatments.

Anistreplase and streptokinase did not differ with regard to reinfarction (anistreplase, 3.55%; streptokinase, 3.47%) or mortality (anistreplase, 10.5%; streptokinase, 10.6%). Duteplase was associated with fewer reinfarctions than streptokinase (2.93% versus 3.47%), but mortality rates did not differ (duteplase, 10.3%; streptokinase, 10.6%).

Compared with streptokinase, anistreplase was associated with more reports of allergic reactions or noncerebral bleeding (but not of hemorrhage requiring transfusion), and duteplase was associated with fewer allergic reactions and more reports of stroke or noncerebral bleeding (but not of hemorrhage requiring transfusion).

1. Third International Study of Infarct Survival Collaborative Group. ISIS-3: a randomised comparison of streptokinase vs tissue plasminogen activator vs anistreplase and of aspirin plus heparin vs aspirin alone among 41,299 cases of suspected acute myocardial infarction. *Lancet*. 1992; 339:753-70.

Pediatrics academy issues new guidelines for acellular pertussis vaccine use

The American Academy of Pediatrics has recommended that acellular pertussis vaccine be used for the fourth and fifth doses of the pertussis immunization schedule. The series includes doses of pertussis vaccine, given in combination with diphtheria and tetanus toxoids, at the ages of 2, 4, 6, and 15–18 months and 4–6 years. Although either acellular or whole-cell pertussis vaccine would be effective when used for the fourth and fifth doses, the acellular vaccine is associated with a lower incidence of local reactions and other minor adverse effects. The acellular vaccine should not be used for the first three doses, because studies evaluating its safety and immunogenicity when used in this manner have not been completed.

News Briefs

• A clinical practice guideline entitled **"Urinary Incontinence in Adults"** is available from the U.S. Public Health Service Agency for Health Care Policy and Research (AHCPR). A quick reference guide for clinicians and a guide for patients are also available. To order a copy, call the AHCPR Clearinghouse at 800-358-9295 or write to Center for Research Dissemination and Liaison, AHCPR Clearinghouse, P.O. Box 8547, Silver Spring, MD 20907.

• Copies of a report on **orphan drugs in development** can be obtained by writing to Editor, Orphan Drugs in Development, Pharmaceutical Manufacturers Association, 1100 15th Street, N.W., Washington, DC 20005. The report lists the manufacturer, orphan indication(s), and stage of development for 189 drugs. This information is based on PMA-sponsored surveys of government and industry sources.

Upcoming Specialty Meetings

American Association for Cancer Education. Buffalo, NY, October 1–4; contact C. M. Brooks, Ed.D., Box 700, UAB Station, Birmingham, AL 35294; 205-934-3054.

American Academy of Pain Management. Albuquerque, NM, October 8–11; contact AAPM, 3600 Sisk Road, Suite 2D, Modesto, CA 95356; 209-545-0754.

American College of Rheumatology. Atlanta, GA, October 11–15; contact ACR, 60 Executive Park South,

Continued on page 578

News *Continued from page 576*

Suite 150, Atlanta, GA 30329; 404-633-3777.

American Academy of Family Physicians. San Diego, CA, October 15–18; contact AAFP, 8880 Ward Parkway, Kansas City, MO 64114; 816-333-9700.

American Academy of Psychiatry and the Law. Boston, MA, October 15–18; contact AAPL, 819 Park Avenue, Baltimore, MD 21201; 301-539-0379.

Cystic Fibrosis Foundation. Washington, DC, October 15–18; contact C. McPherson, 6931 Arlington Road, Bethesda, MD 20814; 301-951-4422.

Second Congress of the European Association for Palliative Care. Brussels, Belgium, October 19–22; contact C. Deckers, M.D., Radiotherapy Department, Cliniques Universitaires, Saint Luc Avenue Hippocrate 10, 1200 Brussels, Belgium; 32-2-764-4667, (fax) 32-2-764-5322.

American Academy of Child and Adolescent Psychiatry. Washington, DC, October 21–25; contact AACAP, 3615 Wisconsin Avenue, N.W., Washington, DC 20016; 202-966-7300.

Child Neurology Society. New Orleans, LA, October 22–24; contact M. Currey, 475 Cleveland Avenue, Suite 720, St. Paul, MN 55104; 612-641-1584.

American Pain Society. San Diego, CA, October 22–25; contact APS, 5700 Old Orchard Road, First Floor, Skokie, IL 60077; 708-966-5595, (fax) 708-966-9418.

American College of Chest Physicians. Chicago, IL, October 25–29; contact ACCP, 3300 Dundee Road, Northbrook, IL 60062; 708-498-1400.

Letters

Use of surfactant products 583
Elizabeth M. Zola

Value of transdermal fentanyl 584
Dennis W. Joubert
David R. Kohler, Karim A. Calis, and Diane M. Corso

Correction 585

The Letters *column is a forum for rapid exchange of ideas among readers of* Clinical Pharmacy. *Liberal criteria are applied in the review of submissions to encourage contributions to this column.*

The Letters *column includes the following types of contributions: (1) comments, addenda, and minor updates on previously published work, (2) alerts on potential problems related to drug therapy or clinical research, (3) observations or comments on trends in drug therapy or clinical research, and (4) brief expressions of opinion about controversies in drug therapy or clinical research.*

Letters need not be submitted with the journal's manuscript checklist. The following conditions, however, must be adhered to: (1) the body of the letter must be no longer than two typewritten pages, (2) the use of references, tables, and illustrations should be minimized, (3) the authors' names, affiliations, and mailing addresses must be typed at the end of the letter in the format used by Clinical Pharmacy, *and (4) the entire letter (including references, tables, and authors' names) must be typed double-spaced on plain white paper (not letterhead). Following acceptance of a letter, the authors are required to sign an exclusive publication statement and a copyright transferal form.*

Use of surfactant products

Prevost[1] presented a well-researched comparison of surfactant products in the December issue of *Clinical Pharmacy.* I wish to clarify several points about one of the products, beractant intratracheal suspension (Survanta, Ross Laboratories Division of Abbott Laboratories).

One of the major differences between modified natural surfactants, such as Survanta, and totally synthetic products is the protein content. The surfactant-associated proteins are believed to facilitate spreading and adsorption of the phospholipid mixture. Survanta contains the hydrophobic low-molecular-weight surfactant-associated proteins B and C (SP-B and SP-C) but does not contain the hydrophilic high-molecular-weight surfactant-associated protein A (SP-A). Readers may interpret one of Prevost's statements as indicating that SP-A is intentionally removed from Survanta. This is not the case. Rather, because SP-A is water-soluble, it is removed during the manufacturing process, which uses organic-solvent extraction to isolate from minced bovine lung a solution containing phospholipids, neutral lipids, free fatty acids, and hydrophobic protein components.

Less than 5% of the weight (<1.0 mg/mL) of Survanta is accounted for by surfactant-specific proteins. As noted by Prevost, natural human surfactant, in comparison, contains approximately 11% protein. The composition of lung surfactant is relatively constant among mammalian species, with actual surfactant-specific proteins accounting for approximately 2% by weight and contaminating serum proteins accounting for approximately 8% by weight.[2]

Prevost stated that early rescue therapy with Survanta for neonatal respiratory distress syndrome (RDS) is associated with a better outcome than late rescue. Controlled clinical trials of Survanta were not designed to compare the outcomes of early and late rescue and did not specifically demonstrate an association between superior outcome and early surfactant administration.[3,4] Kendig et al.[5] found that very premature infants had a significant survival advantage if they received calf-lung surfactant extract (a modified natural bovine surfactant similar to Survanta) for RDS prophylaxis rather than for rescue therapy.

Finally, Prevost's table indicated that a fractional inspired oxygen concentration (FiO_2) of >0.3 is the criterion for the use of Survanta. The controlled trials of Survanta for rescue therapy required that, for the initial dose to be given, an infant must be diagnosed with RDS severe enough to require mechanical ventilation with an FiO_2 of at least 0.40.[4] Infants could receive up to three additional doses in the first 48 hours after birth, as often as every six hours, if they required mechanical ventilation and an

FiO_2 of at least 0.30.

1. Prevost RR. Comparing surfactant products. *Clin Pharm.* 1991; 10:909,911.
2. Jobe A, Ikegami M. Surfactant for the treatment of respiratory distress syndrome. *Am Rev Respir Dis.* 1987; 136:1256-75.
3. Hoekstra RE, Jackson JC, Myers TF et al. Improved neonatal survival following multiple doses of bovine surfactant in very premature neonates at risk for respiratory distress syndrome. *Pediatrics.* 1991; 88:10-8.
4. Liechty EA, Donovan E, Purohit D et al. Reduction of neonatal mortality after multiple doses of bovine surfactant in low birth weight neonates with respiratory distress syndrome. *Pediatrics.* 1991; 88:19-28.
5. Kendig JW, Notter RH, Cox C et al. A comparison of surfactant as immediate prophylaxis and as rescue therapy in newborns of less than 30 weeks' gestation. *N Engl J Med.* 1991; 324:865-71.

Elizabeth M. Zola, Pharm.D., Clinical Research Manager
Ross Laboratories Division of Abbott Laboratories
625 Cleveland Avenue
Columbus, OH 43215

Value of transdermal fentanyl

In the January issue of *Clinical Pharmacy*, Calis et al.[1] presented an excellent summary of the literature on the transdermal fentanyl delivery system. I disagree, however, with the authors' opinion about the clinical usefulness of this drug product.

The management of pain, especially that associated with terminal cancer, is woefully inadequate in a large percentage of patients. Much of this inadequacy is attributable to unrealistic fears and to ignorance about how to use analgesics properly; the result is that narcotics are prescribed in subtherapeutic dosages.

I believe there are four basic principles of pain management. First, give analgesics aggressively and then decrease the dosage if you have to. Remember that the patient is suffering. Adverse effects are generally manageable and temporary, and addiction is not an issue.

Second, adjust the dosage frequently. Pain changes in intensity, and therapy may have to be altered to control it. Use products that facilitate the adjustment of the analgesic regimen.

Third, therapy doesn't have to be fancy to be effective. Almost any narcotic analgesic, if used properly, will control pain. Stick with a couple of products you like and learn to use them well. As you learn about these products, you will realize that they are quite similar and that you don't need many others.

Fourth, keep costs down. Some of the newer products are very expensive, and your patient already has enough to worry about. Use the more expensive approaches only after others have failed a legitimate trial.

I believe that analgesic therapy is more difficult with transdermal fentanyl than with shorter-acting products. If you use too high a dosage of transdermal fentanyl, the adverse effects persist. Fentanyl is deposited into epidermal storage sites and continues to be absorbed for about 24 hours after the patch is removed. This means that you must be conservative rather than aggressive in using the product. At best, fentanyl patches will provide a basal amount of analgesic that you must supplement with other drugs. I have already seen patients who are treated simultaneously with two or three sizes of the fentanyl patch; these patients are often receiving a short- or long-acting narcotic (sometimes both) as well.

In an experimental setting, many of the deficiencies of transdermal fentanyl can be managed. I fear that, in the true outpatient setting, the disadvantages of the product will not be properly considered and, as a result, the patient will suffer. I recommend that fentanyl patches be prescribed only by physicians who understand the unique pharmacokinetics of the delivery system. Even then, the patches should not be used when other equally effective and less expensive products are available.

1. Calis KA, Kohler DR, Corso DM. Transdermally administered fentanyl for pain management. *Clin Pharm.* 1992; 11:22-36.

Dennis W. Joubert, M.S., Director
Pharmacy Services
Faulkner Hospital
Allandale at Centre Street
Boston, MA 02130

We heartily agree with Mr. Joubert's principles of pain management, but we generally disagree that transdermal fentanyl is difficult to use. We do concur that quick dosage adjustment to the desired level of analgesia is more difficult with transdermal fentanyl than with immediate-release oral formulations or with injectable therapy.

Mr. Joubert describes a scenario in which use of transdermal fentanyl may promulgate a polypharmacy (or, perhaps, polyformulation) approach to pain management. The example of patients who were receiving short- and long-acting narcotics in addition to more than one size of fentanyl patch illustrates an apparent disregard for at least two of Mr. Joubert's tenets of pain management—simplifying the regimen and minimizing costs. Such regimens exemplify an unnecessarily complicated approach to analgesic therapy.

Any drug product has inherent limits to its practical therapeutic application. Mr. Joubert very reasonably advocates mastering the use of a limited number of drug products. To use transdermal fentanyl effectively, one must be aware of the formulation's unique pharmacokinetic characteristics. The delay in achieving steady-state serum concentrations after initial patch application mandates that supplementary analgesics be used during the first 24 hours. In addition, supplementary analgesics may be required during periods of upward dosage adjustment. Conversely, the pharmacodynamic effects of fentanyl diminish very slowly following delivery by any continuous method (e.g., intravenous, subcutaneous, transdermal) and correlate with the attenuated clearance of fentanyl from adipose tissues; thus, downward dosage adjustment is problematical in patients with diminishing analgesic needs.

Patients who frequently and repeatedly require supplemental analgesics for exacerbations of pain are challenging to treat, regardless of whether their basal analgesic staple is an extended-release oral preparation, a continuous infusion, or transdermal fentanyl. The ease with which transdermal fentanyl is employed is directly related to the quality of pain. A fluctuating analgesic requirement is sufficient cause to reconsider using transdermal fentanyl as the sole or primary source of analgesia. Even so, patients with frequent exacerbations of pain may benefit from a delivery system that provides a basal level of analgesia and that precludes the sudden, complete loss of analgesic control that can occur when prompt-release formulations are used. Several investigators have recommended, not condemned, transdermal fentanyl because it provides a basal level of analgesia upon which clinicians can "fine tune" the analgesic regimen with supplemental drugs.

We are not sure how the "true outpatient setting" mentioned by Mr. Joubert differs from any other outpatient oncology clinic. We are accumulating experience using fentanyl patches in the treatment of patients with chronic cancer-related pain. Admittedly, the patients that we consider for treatment with transdermal fentanyl are carefully selected, but our primary criterion is that their analgesic requirements are stable. We agree that an appreciation of the unique pharmacokinetics of the transdermal fentanyl delivery system is a prerequisite for its use but argue that physicians cannot gain clinical experience with the product if it is unavailable or if its use is restricted.

DAVID R. KOHLER, PHARM.D., Oncology Clinical Pharmacy Specialist

KARIM A. CALIS, PHARM.D, Coordinator
Drug Information Service

Department of Pharmacy
Warren G. Magnuson Clinical Center
National Institutes of Health
Building 10, Room 1N-257
Bethesda, MD 20892

DIANE M. CORSO, Immunology Fellow
Department of Pharmacy
Memorial Sloan-Kettering Cancer Center
1275 York Avenue
New York, NY 10021

Correction

Review of 1991 shows 30 new drugs, several important biologics cleared for marketing (March 1992, News). On page 218, the indication for ramipril should have read as follows: angiotensin-converting-enzyme inhibitor for treatment of hypertension.

Oxaprozin: A once-daily nonsteroidal anti-inflammatory drug

LUCINDA G. MILLER

Abstract: The pharmacology, pharmacokinetics, clinical efficacy, adverse effects, and dosage of oxaprozin are reviewed.

Oxaprozin, a nonsteroidal anti-inflammatory drug (NSAID) under consideration for approval by the Food and Drug Administration, is characterized as a propionic acid. By inhibiting cyclo-oxygenase, oxaprozin decreases the formation of prostaglandin (PG) precursors from arachidonic acid, resulting in decreased PG biosynthesis and reduced pain and inflammatory responses. Oxaprozin is well absorbed after oral administration, and peak plasma concentration is reached in three to six hours. Oxaprozin is primarily eliminated by urinary excretion of the unchanged drug. It has a long elimination half-life and persists in synovial fluid.

In clinical studies, oxaprozin was equally or more effective than aspirin and as effective as naproxen in the treatment of rheumatoid arthritis. For treatment of osteoarthritis, oxaprozin was as effective as naproxen and more effective than aspirin or piroxicam. Studies have also shown oxaprozin to be effective therapy for juvenile rheumatoid arthritis and ankylosing spondylitis. Oxaprozin, like other NSAIDs, can cause gastrointestinal adverse effects. Other possible adverse effects include allergic reactions, analgesic nephropathy, hepatotoxicity, and increased bleeding times. For adults, the anticipated daily dosage is 600–1200 mg given as a single dose for rheumatoid arthritis, osteoarthritis, and analgesia. In children, oxaprozin 10–20 mg/kg/day has been used to treat juvenile rheumatoid arthritis.

Oxaprozin is as effective as other NSAIDs and offers once-daily dosing; however, it does not offer any therapeutic advantage over other currently available NSAIDs.

Index terms: Anti-inflammatory agents; Arthritis; Dosage; Dosage schedules; Osteoarthritis; Oxaprozin; Pharmacokinetics; Toxicity
Clin Pharm. 1992; 11:591-603

More than a dozen nonsteroidal anti-inflammatory drugs (NSAIDs) are currently available in the United States.[1] With $1 billion spent annually on 70 million prescriptions for these agents,[2] we will continue to see new NSAIDs enter the market. NSAIDs are involved in a large proportion of the adverse drug reactions reported to the FDA.[a]

This article reviews oxaprozin, the NSAID most recently considered for approval by the FDA.

Oxaprozin was first patented in 1969. It was initially developed by Wyeth Laboratories in the early 1980s, and many of the studies cited in this review were conducted during that time. Wyeth Laboratories chose to devote its attention to other NSAIDs that it was developing at the same time and licensed oxaprozin to G. D. Searle & Company in 1988. G. D. Searle & Company is seeking approval from the FDA, and the company anticipates marketing the drug in 1992. The patent will be extended for five years after FDA approval according to the Drug Price Competition and Patent Term Restoration Act of 1984.

Chemistry

The chemical name for oxaprozin is 4,5-diphenyl-2-oxazolepropranoic acid.[3] As an investigational agent, it was known as WY-21,743. It occurs as a white powder with a molecular weight of 293.[4] Oxaprozin, which has been characterized as a propionic acid, is slightly soluble in alcohol. Other NSAID members of this

LUCINDA G. MILLER, PHARM.D., is Assistant Professor, Department of Family Medicine, Baylor College of Medicine, 5510 Greenbriar Road, Houston, TX 77005.

The assistance of Louis A. Kazal, Jr., M.D., Assistant Professor, Department of Family Medicine, Baylor College of Medicine, in thoughtful review of this paper, and of Connie Finck, in manuscript preparation, is acknowledged.

This is article **680-204-9215** in the **ASHP Continuing Education System**; it qualifies for 1.0 hour of continuing-education credit. See page 641 for learning objectives and test questions.

Figure 1. Chemical structure of oxaprozin.

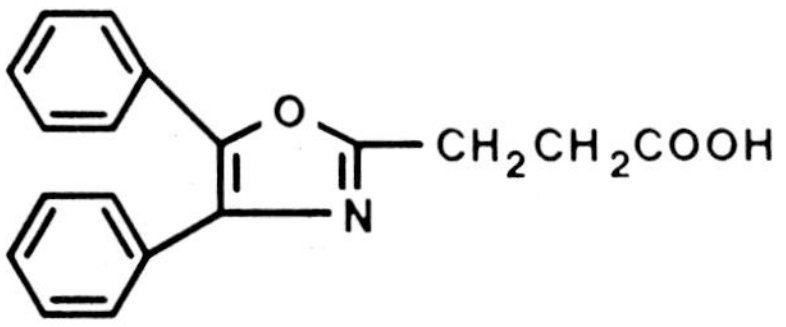

chemical class that are commercially available in the United States include fenoprofen, ibuprofen, and ketoprofen.[1,5] The chemical structure of oxaprozin is shown in Figure 1.

Pharmacology

Inhibition of Prostaglandin Biosynthesis. Oxaprozin possesses anti-inflammatory, antipyretic, and analgesic properties. Similar to other NSAIDs, it inhibits prostaglandin (PG) biosynthesis, thus affecting the intensity of pain and inflammatory responses that are mediated by prostaglandins. Prostaglandins, specifically those in the E and F series, are released during inflammation and appear to sensitize pain receptors to chemical mediators (e.g., bradykinin) and to mechanical stimulation. Thus, inhibition of prostaglandin formation diminishes pain and inflammation; this mechanism explains the analgesic and anti-inflammatory effects of oxaprozin.[6] For a complete review of prostaglandin pharmacology, the reader is referred elsewhere.[7,8]

Oxaprozin and other type I PG inhibitors act by inhibiting cyclo-oxygenase, thereby decreasing the formation of prostaglandin precursors (cyclic endoperoxides) from arachidonic acid (Figure 2).[9] Type II PG inhibitors, including pyrazolones (e.g., phenylbutazone) and oxicams (e.g., piroxicam), inhibit isomerase reductase, thereby reducing the formation of PGE_2 and $PGF_{2\alpha}$, but do not inhibit the formation of cyclic endoperoxides. Because cyclic endoperoxides are uterotoxic substances, type II inhibitors are less effective in the treatment of primary dysmenorrhea.[10] The pharmacology of oxaprozin suggests that this agent would be efficacious in the treatment of primary dysmenorrhea. Oxaprozin does not affect the lipoxygenase pathway,[11] which leads to leukotriene formation.

NSAIDs differ in potency (i.e., the ability to inhibit PG biosynthesis). Because NSAIDs are generally used in equipotent doses, the therapeutic efficacy of these drugs is usually comparable. However, the type and incidence of adverse reactions associated with these agents may differ. For example, indomethacin, one of the most potent NSAIDs, is commonly associated with headaches, hypertension, and renal insufficiency.[1] In contrast, oxaprozin has less effect on renal function and on the central nervous system (CNS).[12] The differences in adverse reactions associated with NSAIDs may reflect their relative potency.

The inhibitory activity of oxaprozin on prostaglandin biosynthesis has been measured by the conversion of arachidonic acid labeled with carbon 14 to ^{14}C-PGE_2 in sheep and mice.[13,14] In sheep, oxaprozin was 40-fold more potent than aspirin and equipotent with naproxen. In mice, oxaprozin was at least 8-fold less potent than most other NSAIDs tested and 12.5-fold more potent than aspirin. Other NSAIDs studied included indomethacin, sulindac, ibuprofen, piroxicam, naproxen, and aspirin. These test results indicate considerable interspecies variation for oxaprozin effects. Postmarketing clinical experience will reveal whether the lesser relative potency of oxaprozin will result in fewer adverse reactions.

Nonprostaglandin Effects. Prostaglandin inhibition does not fully explain NSAID efficacy and adverse effects. Nonprostaglandin effects of NSAIDs have also been investigated. NSAID inhibition of neutrophil activity[14,15] or inhibition of hydrogen peroxide generation by neutrophils has been demonstrated; the latter effect may have implications in free-radical-associated tissue irritation and consequent inflammation.[15,16] NSAIDs may also affect lymphocyte function by unmasking T-cell suppression activity, thereby suppressing production of rheumatoid factor.[17,18]

Some NSAIDs have been shown to protect cartilage by altering connective tissue metabolism.[19] In one study, oxaprozin was shown to inhibit migration of leukocytes into the pleural cavity of rats injected with carrageenan.[20] In a study using mice, oxaprozin inhibited cell-mediated immunity induced by methylated bovine serum albumin.[21]

A marketing strategy being used to show the superior quality of an NSAID over its competitors is the comparison of drug sequestration into synovial fluid. Because NSAIDs are organic acids, they are preferentially sequestered into the synovial tissue of inflamed joints, where they exert a prolonged duration of action.[22] The extent of oxaprozin's sequestration relative to other NSAIDs and whether this difference is clinically significant are unknown.

Pharmacodynamic studies of NSAIDs frequently employ carrageenan-induced rat-paw edema, ultraviolet light-induced inflammation, and adjuvant-induced arthritis. Such data are available for oxaprozin relative to other NSAIDs.[5,20,21] However, data from these studies are not relevant for the use of NSAIDs in rheumatoid arthritis.[23] Gold, an effective therapy for rheumatoid arthritis, has absolutely no effect on these rat models.[23]

Pharmacokinetics

Absorption. Oxaprozin is well absorbed after oral administration, achieving a peak plasma concentration within three to six hours in most patients after a single 1200-mg dose.[24] The mean ± S.D. area under the plasma concentration–time curve (AUC) after a single 600-mg oral dose was 6170 ± 1150 μg · hr/mL, and the mean steady-state plasma concentration after multiple doses (600 mg twice daily) was 200 μg/mL.[25] Plasma

Figure 2. Site of action of oxaprozin in pathway of prostaglandin (PG) biosynthesis. Each set of double hatch marks indicates a site of enzyme inhibition.

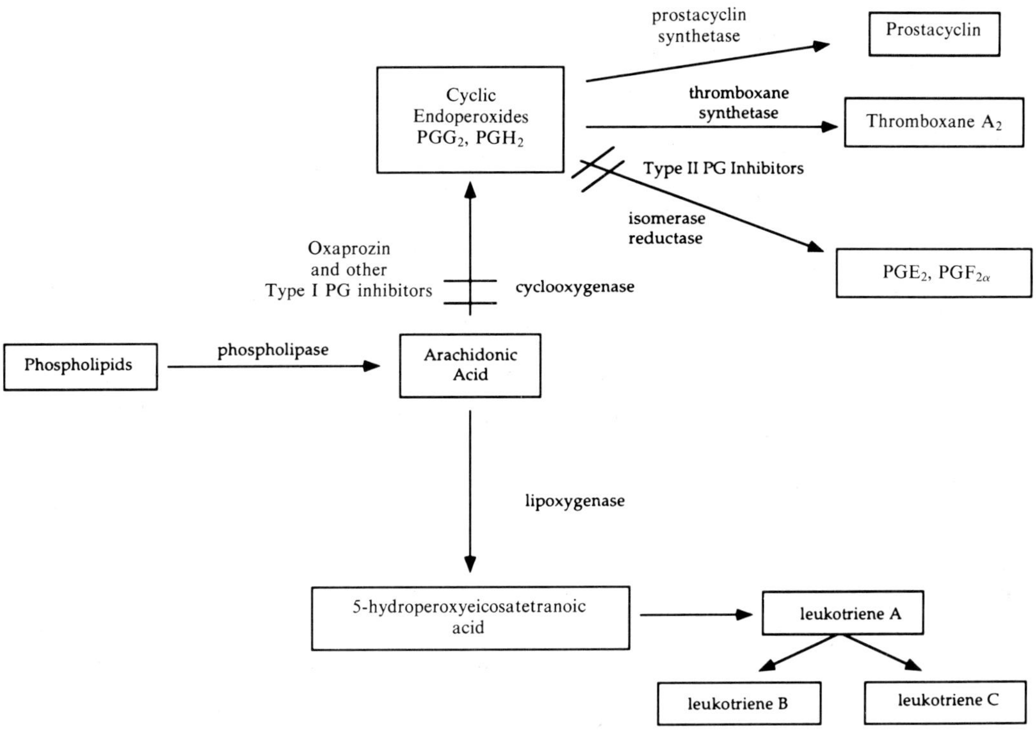

concentrations typically ranged from 50 to 200 μg/mL; however, it is not necessary to monitor plasma drug concentrations during NSAID therapy.

Distribution. Oxaprozin has a small volume of distribution (V): mean, 0.25 L/kg; range, 0.16–0.36 L/kg.[24] This reflects its limited extravascular distribution. The apparent V declines with increasing age, which can be attributed to the decrease in lean body mass relative to total weight in the elderly.[24]

The transsynovial distribution of oxaprozin probably contributes to the efficacy of once-daily dosing. Twelve hours after administration of 1200 mg of oxaprozin, synovial tissue samples yielded 27 μg of oxaprozin per gram of tissue, while corresponding plasma concentrations were considerably lower at 10–17 μg/mL.[26] However, one cannot conclude that, because oxaprozin has limited extravascular distribution, it will be associated with fewer or less severe adverse effects. The tissue concentration of oxaprozin in the gastrointestinal (GI) tract or kidney, for example, is unknown. In fact, one can speculate that the time for which an adverse effect persists may be prolonged because of oxaprozin's long half-life. Clinical observation of many patients is needed to further examine the adverse effect profile of oxaprozin.

Oxaprozin is extensively bound (99.5%) to plasma proteins, primarily albumin.[27] This binding has been described as nonlinear,[27] indicating an increase in the free fraction of drug in plasma (f_u) that is not directly proportional to the increase in the total plasma drug concentration. Within the therapeutic concentration range, however, the binding of oxazoprin remains linear.

Metabolism. The major metabolic pathways for oxaprozin include glucuronidation of the carboxyl group and hydroxylation followed by glucuronidation of the phenyl rings.[25] If oxaprozin glucuronide is excreted in bile, intestinal glucuronidases can reverse the metabolic pathway by deconjugation, which regenerates the parent drug. If the parent drug is then reabsorbed into the enterohepatic circulation, GI toxicity can increase; a similar metabolic pathway has been demonstrated for indomethacin.[28]

Elimination. In rats and dogs, oxaprozin is primarily eliminated by biliary excretion; in humans, it is primarily eliminated by urinary excretion.[28] Biliary excretion of biotransformed drug, however, has resulted in fecal recovery of oxaprozin metabolites more than 48 hours after drug administration.[25] After administration of a single oral dose of oxaprozin 600 mg, greater than 90% is excreted unchanged in the urine.[25]

Oxaprozin follows first-order elimination kinetics with a slow clearance (CL) of 0.08–0.12 L/hr.[25] At steady state, plasma concentrations of oxaprozin are higher than after single-dose administration and are associated with an increase in f_u, which consequently increases the clearance of oxaprozin.[27] In healthy men, oxaprozin CL significantly decreases with age (21–89 years, $r = -0.58$, $p < 0.01$); this correlation is not evident in healthy women[24]

The mean elimination half-life ($t_{1/2}$) of oxaprozin in patients aged 23–89 years was 59 hours (range, 36–92 hours).[24] The $t_{1/2}$ in healthy volunteers appears to be unchanged for doses ranging from 300 to 1200 mg.[29] The long $t_{1/2}$ of oxaprozin has been attributed to extensive protein binding of the drug. Other NSAIDs that are highly protein bound have $t_{1/2}$ values as brief as two hours[1]; therefore, protein binding alone does not explain oxaprozin's prolonged $t_{1/2}$. The low renal clearance of the unchanged drug and the slow rate of metabolism may contribute to its long $t_{1/2}$, which allows once-daily dosing.

Pharmacokinetics in Patients with Renal Disease. Oxaprozin CL, volume of distribution at steady state (V_{ss}), and $t_{1/2}$ for an oral dose did not differ significantly among 15 volunteers who were normal, were renally impaired, or had undergone hemodialysis (five volunteers per group).[30] However, the mean f_u of oxaprozin was 0.08% in the normal group and 0.18% and 0.28% in the renally impaired and hemodialysis groups, respectively. In normal volunteers, intrinsic clearance (CL_{int}) and V were greater than in the other volunteers. The smaller V values in the renally impaired and hemodialysis groups can be attributed to a decrease in oxaprozin tissue binding. In another report,[31] the mean f_u was 0.42%, 0.79%, and 1.03% in normal, renally impaired, and hemodialysis patients, respectively; this finding was also attributed to altered plasma binding in the two latter patient groups.

In 16 patients undergoing hemodialysis who had normal serum albumin concentrations, Audet et al.[32] found a larger CL and V_{ss} for both total and unbound oxaprozin. Consequently, steady-state plasma concentration (C_{ss}) was 40–50% lower in patients on hemodialysis. The $t_{1/2}$ was essentially unchanged with values of 52 hours and 56 hours in normal and dialysis patients, respectively. Because CL_{int} of oxaprozin was not impaired in patients on hemodialysis, the authors concluded that the oxaprozin dose need not be reduced in hemodialysis patients with normal serum albumin concentrations.

Pharmacokinetics in Patients with Liver Disease. Cirrhosis does not appear to affect oxaprozin C and $t_{1/2}$.[33] In one study, a single oral dose of oxaprozin 1200 mg was given to 10 patients with chronic compensated cirrhosis and 10 healthy individuals. The f_u of oxaprozin was significantly greater in the cirrhosis patients (0.084%) than in the healthy individuals (0.065%, $p < 0.01$). The CL of protein-bound oxaprozin was also greater in the cirrhotic patients (0.0026 L/hr/kg) than in the healthy individuals (0.0020 L/hr/kg), but the difference was not statistically significant. C and $t_{1/2}$ did not change. Thus, dosage adjustments for oxaprozin are probably not necessary in patients with hepatic impairment.

Pharmacokinetics in Patients with Congestive Heart Failure. Although protein binding of oxaprozin is altered in patients with congestive heart failure (CHF), no significant change in oxaprozin CL has been observed.[34] In this study, a 1200-mg oral dose of oxaprozin was given to 12 CHF patients aged 26–71 years and 12 healthy individuals. Mean $t_{1/2}$ did not differ significantly in CHF patients (63 hours) compared with healthy individuals (69 hours). However, the apparent V was significantly greater (0.29 versus 0.22 L/kg, $p < 0.05$) and peak C was significantly lower (63 versus 79 µg/mL, $p < 0.01$) in the CHF patients. The f_u of oxaprozin was greater in the CHF patients (0.44% versus 0.25%, $p < 0.01$), resulting in a slightly higher oxaprozin CL in the CHF patients (0.053 versus 0.042 mL/min/kg). The distribution of unbound oxaprozin did not differ significantly between the groups.

Pharmacokinetics and Renal Toxicity. The use of oxaprozin, or any NSAID, in patients with CHF or renal insufficiency is associated with risk of renal toxicity. These patients are dependent on the compensatory local release of prostaglandins to cause vasodilatation of renal vasculature and to maintain renal perfusion. Oxaprozin may diminish or eradicate this compensatory response, resulting in renal toxicity. Avoidance of all NSAIDs in patients with these conditions is advisable.

Clinical Efficacy

Rheumatoid Arthritis. Nine studies to date have established the efficacy of oxaprozin in the treatment of rheumatoid arthritis.[4,35–42] Oxaprozin 1200 mg was found to be of comparable efficacy with a lower incidence of adverse effects than aspirin 3900 mg divided into four equal doses.[4] In studies comparing oxaprozin 1200 mg or 600 mg with aspirin 3900 mg, all drug regimens produced significant improvement from baseline,[35,36] but fewer patients who took oxaprozin withdrew[35] and better results were obtained with the 1200-mg than with the 600-mg dosage,[36] suggesting a dose–response relationship. A similar adverse effect profile was noted for both oxaprozin regimens.[36] A six-month study with 218 patients confirmed the finding of equal efficacy between aspirin and oxaprozin.[37] In a placebo-controlled study of 202 patients, oxaprozin was found superior to aspirin in the treatment of patients who did not respond to aspirin therapy[38]; improvement was noted within one week of oxaprozin administration.

When compared with patients treated with ibuprofen 1200–1800 mg daily, patients treated with daily doses of oxaprozin experienced a significantly shorter duration of morning stiffness ($p < 0.05$).[39] In a study comparing ibuprofen 1200 mg daily (titrated to 1800 mg daily, if necessary) with oxaprozin, oxaprozin was associated with a significant improvement in time to walk 50 feet, duration of morning stiffness, and grip strength for more evaluation periods than ibuprofen.[40] These two studies, however, failed to employ an adequate anti-inflammatory dose of ibuprofen (i.e., 2400 mg daily) to allow a valid comparison.

Oxaprozin 1200 mg and naproxen 500 mg were similarly efficacious in the treatment of 22 rheumatoid arthritis patients who were evaluated for the number of tender joints, number of swollen joints, grip strength, and duration of morning stiffness.[41] A comparison of sulindac 200 mg twice daily with oxaprozin 1200 mg showed that only sulindac significantly improved hand function[42]; neither drug was associated with serious adverse effects.

For rheumatoid arthritis, the efficacy of oxaprozin appears to be similar to that of other NSAIDs that are currently available.

Juvenile Rheumatoid Arthritis. Oxaprozin 10–20 mg/kg/day has been effective in the treatment of juvenile rheumatoid arthritis.[43] In this study, the average patient age was nine years, with a duration of illness at enrollment of three years (range, 1–13 years). Sixty percent of the children demonstrated clinical improvement in disease indices, including number of tender joints, tenderness severity score, number of swollen joints, swelling severity score, duration of morning stiffness, and limited motion assessments. This pediatric oxaprozin dose was found equivalent to an adult dose of 600–1200 mg. Other NSAIDs with labeled indications for juvenile rheumatoid arthritis include naproxen, naproxen sodium, and tolmetin.[44]

Osteoarthritis. The use of oxaprozin in patients with osteoarthritis has been examined in three studies.[45-47] Twenty-four patients with osteoarthritis of the knee or hip were evaluated in a double-blind study comparing oxaprozin 1200 mg daily with naproxen 250 mg three times daily for eight weeks.[45] Once-daily oxaprozin was equivalent to three times daily naproxen as measured by pain intensity, time to walk 15 meters, observer's opinion, and patient's opinion.

When oxaprozin was compared with aspirin in 688 patients for six months, patients with osteoarthritis of the knee or hip responded similarly to both drugs, but patients with cervical spine involvement had significantly greater relief with oxaprozin than with aspirin ($p < 0.05$).[46] In a 90-patient comparison of oxaprozin with piroxicam, a drug with a similar pharmacokinetic profile, physicians ranked symptom improvement as moderate or marked for 53% of patients receiving oxaprozin, compared with 44% of those receiving piroxicam.[47]

Oxaprozin appears to be efficacious in the treatment of osteoarthritis, but more studies are needed.

Postoperative Oral Surgery Pain. When used for postsurgical oral pain, a single dose of oxaprozin 1200 mg has been found to offer more prolonged pain relief than a single dose of aspirin 650 mg or placebo.[48] Patients in both drug-treated groups experienced comparable pain relief during the first four hours. After four hours, oxaprozin provided superior pain relief, reflecting the respective pharmacokinetic profiles of each drug involved.

Two patients receiving oxaprozin and one patient receiving aspirin experienced nausea, vomiting, or both. Whether oxaprozin has a more prolonged effect on bleeding time in these patients remains to be determined.

Ankylosing Spondylitis. Oxaprozin has been evaluated for its efficacy in the treatment of ankylosing spondylitis in two published studies to date.[12,49] In a six-week study of 40 patients, oxaprozin 1200 mg daily and diclofenac sodium 100 mg in divided doses demonstrated comparable efficacy with similar adverse effect profiles[49]; however, oxaprozin offers the convenience of once-daily dosing.

Indomethacin and oxaprozin demonstrated comparable efficacy in 97 patients with ankylosing spondylitis until week 28, when indomethacin was favored. Indomethacin, however, was associated with a greater frequency ($p < 0.05$) of adverse effects (dizziness, vertigo, headache, nausea, and abdominal distress) than oxaprozin.

Hyperuricemia and Acute Gouty Arthritis. Oxaprozin administered as a single 1200-mg dose followed five days later with 300 mg four times daily was compared with a similarly divided regimen of indomethacin 150 mg orally for effect on uric acid concentrations.[50] Indomethacin did not affect either serum or urinary uric acid concentrations, whereas oxaprozin decreased mean ± S.E. serum uric acid concentration from 5.8 ± 0.2 mg/dL to 4.8 ± 0.4 mg/dL ($p < 0.01$) and increased mean ± S.E. 24-hour urinary uric acid concentration from 673 ± 47 mg/24 hr to 825 ± 66 mg/24 hr ($p < 0.01$). Although these differences were statistically significant, clinical significance was minimal because the patients had no symptoms associated with gout. Clinicians treat hyperuricemia only when the patient has symptoms of gout.

Oxaprozin provided relief to 50 patients who presented within 48 hours of the onset of acute gouty arthritis and had hyperuricemia or uric acid crystals in synovial fluid.[51] During the first two days, the patients received oxaprozin 1200 mg in the morning and 600 mg in the evening. The patients then received oxaprozin 1200 mg daily until symptoms were relieved. Eighty-four percent of the patients ($p < 0.001$) reported improvement during the first 24 hours after receiving at least 1800 mg of oxaprozin; five patients discontinued therapy because of an unsatisfactory response.

Until more data are available, it would be prudent to treat hyperuricemia associated with gout by using NSAIDs of known efficacy for this indication, such as indomethacin, naproxen, or phenylbutazone.[44,50]

Tendonitis and Bursitis. Oxaprozin has been found efficacious in a study evaluating its use in the seven-day treatment of 125 patients with acute tendonitis and bursitis.[52] Compared with phenylbutazone 100 mg four times daily, oxaprozin 1200 mg afforded comparable improvement in mean overall pain score, limitation of motion, tenderness on pressure, and pain on motion by the third day of treatment. Thus, oxaprozin represents an alternative NSAID that may be used in the treatment of tendonitis and bursitis.

Behçet's Disease. Oxaprozin was proved efficacious in treating the articular symptoms of Behçet's disease in a small number of patients.[53] Five patients with Behçet's disease were treated with a relatively low dosage of oxaprozin (200 mg twice daily) for 8–12 weeks. Four of the five patients had diminished or resolved articular swelling and pain within two days.

Systemic Lupus Erythematosus and Lupus-like Conditions. Although species-to-species variation limits the generalizability of results from nonhuman trials, oxaprozin 100 mg/kg was found to decrease thymic lymphoid hyperplasia in rats.[54] Similar human studies have not yet been conducted; however, oxaprozin can be expected to have efficacy comparable with that of other NSAIDs in the treatment of systemic lupus erythematosus.

Male Infertility. The use of NSAIDs in the treatment of male infertility has been investigated. PGE_1 and PGE_{12} have an inhibitory effect on spermatogenesis, whereas aspirin and indomethacin, which are cyclooxygenase inhibitors, increase spermatogenesis in mice.[55] Indomethacin has been found to increase follicle-stimulating hormone, luteinizing hormone, sperm count, and sperm motility in a study of 100 oligospermic men (sperm count less than 1–20 million/mL, motility less than 65%, and a minimum of 60% normal sperm cells).[56]

Oxaprozin 600 mg/day has been shown to decrease seminal PG concentrations, but it did not influence sperm motion characteristics and serum hormone concentrations in young healthy men.[57] Ten of the subjects in the study were given indomethacin 25 mg three times daily and experienced similar effects. Given the findings of the aforementioned trial of indomethacin therapy in oligospermic men, one would speculate that the inclusion of healthy volunteers instead of clearly oligospermic men affected the results in the oxaprozin study. Also, if the usual pharmacologic dose of 1200 mg of oxaprozin had been used, the effect on fertility may have been better.

Caution must be used when treating male infertility with indomethacin or oxaprozin. Although Knuth et al.[57] found no negative influence of indomethacin or oxaprozin administered for 14 days on male reproductive function, impotence has been associated with use of extended-release indomethacin. In one case, a 60-year-old man experienced diminished libido and impotence after two to three weeks of treatment with extended-release indomethacin; these effects resolved within one week of drug discontinuation.[58]

Additional data must be collected before NSAIDs such as indomethacin or oxaprozin can be advocated in the treatment of male infertility. Neither drug has FDA-approved labeling for this indication.

Summary. The limited number of studies evaluating oxaprozin indicate that it is equally efficacious as other currently available NSAIDs. Not all of these studies, however, were placebo-controlled, and none of the studies compared oxaprozin with more than one other NSAID. Table 1 provides a summary of the clinical trials of oxaprozin efficacy conducted in humans.

Contraindications

Oxaprozin is contraindicated in any patient with known hypersensitivity to oxaprozin or any other NSAID. There are two types of NSAID allergy. The first type of allergy, which is related to the degree of inhibition of PG synthesis, causes bronchospasm, primarily in patients with asthma.[59] Since all NSAIDs mediate this inhibition of PG synthesis, patients with asthma should avoid all NSAIDs. The second type of allergy, characterized by urticaria, is an allergic response mediated by immunoglobulin E.[60] NSAIDs of a similar structure in the same chemical class should be avoided (e.g., sulindac should be avoided by a patient with a demonstrated allergy to indomethacin). Use of an NSAID of a different class and with a dissimilar structure may be initiated cautiously. When possible, it is preferable to avoid all NSAIDs in these circumstances.

All NSAIDs should be avoided in patients whose liver function test results exceed three times the upper limit of normal.[1] Monitoring for liver function abnormalities in a cost-effective manner remains elusive; liver function test results may increase without accompanying symptoms. Liver function abnormalities may remain unchanged or return to baseline despite continued drug therapy. With these caveats in mind, it is prudent to obtain baseline liver function tests and repeat them every six weeks for the first three months because this is the time when liver toxicity is most likely to manifest.[61] If oxaprozin must be used in patients with hepatic impairment, the dosage need not necessarily be adjusted, but the risk of hepatic injury must be considered.

Adverse Effects

Gastrointestinal Effects. GI effects are perhaps the most troubling adverse effects associated with the use of NSAIDs. Oxaprozin is expected to cause the same but milder GI effects, according to data from company-sponsored studies. Most of the studies have compared oxaprozin with aspirin and have shown that oxaprozin is associated with less GI intolerance; however, this favorable comparison applies to most NSAIDs.[1] Also, most of the oxaprozin data are based on small numbers of patients. Further studies are needed to determine whether oxaprozin has a more favorable profile of GI effects than other NSAIDs.

Fecal blood loss, determined by the use of red blood cells labeled with chromium 51, was evaluated in a four-week study in which 10 patients received oxaprozin 600 mg twice daily, 11 received aspirin 975 mg four times daily, and 8 received placebo for two weeks; all received placebo during the last two weeks.[62] The mean blood loss during week 3 was significantly greater with aspirin (8.8 mL/day) than with oxaprozin (3.3 mL/day) or placebo (1.4 mL/day).

In a crossover gastroscopic study,[63] eight volunteers received 3900 mg of aspirin (975 mg four times daily), 1200 mg of oxaprozin (400 mg three times daily), and placebo (three times daily). Submucosal hemorrhage or mucosal bleeding was observed in seven of eight volunteers taking aspirin and in only two of eight taking oxaprozin ($p = 0.061$).

Table 1.
Summary of Clinical Trials of Oxaprozin Efficacy

Reference	No. Patients	Oxaprozin Dosage (mg/day)	Other NSAID[a] Dosage (mg/day)	Study Design: Placebo-controlled?	Study Design: Duration (wk)	Results
Rheumatoid Arthritis						
4	21	1200	Aspirin 3900	No	12	Equal efficacies
35	212	1200 or 600	Aspirin 3900	No	12	Equal efficacies
36	40	1200 or 600	Aspirin 3900	No	12	Equal efficacies
37	218	1200	Aspirin 3900	No	24	Equal efficacies
38	202	1200	Aspirin 3900	Yes	4	Oxaprozin provided greater patient improvement
39	159	1200	Ibuprofen 1200–1800	Yes	52	Oxaprozin provided greater patient improvement
40	197	1200	Ibuprofen 1200–1800	Yes	52	Oxaprozin provided greater patient improvement
41	22	1200	Naproxen 500	Yes	12	Equal efficacies
42	20	1200	Sulindac 400	No	12	Sulindac provided greater patient improvement
Juvenile Rheumatoid Arthritis						
43	59	10–20 mg/kg/day	. . .	No	12	Efficacious in 60% of patients
Osteoarthritis						
45	24	1200	Naproxen 750	No	8	Equal efficacies
46	688	600 and 1200	Aspirin 2600–3250	No	24	Oxaprozin provided greater patient improvement
47	90	1200	Piroxicam 20	Yes	12	Oxaprozin provided greater patient improvement
Postoperative Oral Surgery Pain						
48	105	1200	Aspirin 650	Yes	8[b]	After 4 hr, oxaprozin provided greater pain relief
Ankylosing Spondylitis						
49	40	1200	Diclofenac sodium 100[c]	No	6	Equal efficacies
12	97	1200–1800	Indomethacin 50–200	No	28	Equal efficacies until week 28, then indomethacin provided greater patient improvement
Hyperuricemia and Acute Gouty Arthritis						
50	12	1200	Indomethacin 150	No	12[d]	Oxaprozin decreased serum uric acid concentration and increased urinary uric acid concentration
51	50	1800 for two days, then 1200	. . .	No	8[d]	Efficacious
Tendonitis and Bursitis						
52	125	1200	Phenylbutazone 400	Yes	7[d]	Equal efficacies
Behçet's Disease						
53	5	400	. . .	No	8–12	Efficacious
Male Infertility						
57	34	600	Indomethacin 75	No	12	Equal efficacies

[a]NSAID = nonsteroidal anti-inflammatory drug.
[b]Hours.
[c]Of diclofenac.
[d]Days.

In a randomized, crossover study of eight healthy male volunteers ingesting 600 mg or 1200 mg of oxaprozin, 50 mg of indomethacin, and 1000 mg of aspirin, oxaprozin was found to have less irritative potency than indomethacin.[64] This finding was based on the model of transmural gastric potential difference, which provides no information on irritation after continuous drug exposure.

In rat studies, oxaprozin caused less GI toxicity and fewer GI lesions than other NSAIDs.[65,66] However, data from animal studies of oxaprozin cannot be generalized to humans.

In an independent analysis of data from several company-sponsored clinical trials (1423 patients), Dahl et al.[67] compared the relative safety of oxaprozin in elderly patients (>60 years) versus nonelderly patients (≤60 years) with rheumatoid arthritis or osteoarthritis. The data, as presented in the published report, suggest that a greater percentage of patients who took oxaprozin had GI intolerance, compared with patients who took ibuprofen or, in some cases, aspirin.

Oxaprozin is expected to have a profile of GI effects similar to that of other NSAIDs, with the following exceptions: (1) enterohepatic recirculation does not occur for oxaprozin, so it may potentially cause less GI upset than indomethacin and (2) the long $t_{1/2}$ of oxaprozin creates the potential for prolonged duration of GI adverse effects that do occur.[68]

Nephrotoxicity. Analgesic nephropathy is a potential complication of therapy with all NSAIDs, including oxaprozin. Renal toxicity caused by NSAID therapy is rare in generally healthy patients.[69] However, patients with CHF, hypertension, atherosclerosis, or diabetes and patients taking diuretics develop a dependence on PG-mediated vasodilation of renal vasculature.[70] Inhibition of PG synthesis caused by NSAID therapy may block this compensatory mechanism, leading to vasoconstriction of the renal vasculature and the development of analgesic nephropathy.

Bonney et al.,[71] evaluated five controlled, double-blind studies of patients with rheumatoid arthritis or osteoarthritis who received oxaprozin, ibuprofen, or aspirin. Of 847 patients who received oxaprozin, 51 (6.0%) developed potentially important increases in blood urea nitrogen (BUN) or serum creatinine concentration; only one patient developed serious elevations in BUN or creatinine concentration. The authors concluded that all three drugs (oxaprozin, ibuprofen, and aspirin) display a high level of renal safety.

In patients receiving oxaprozin or indomethacin, indomethacin but not oxaprozin transiently reduced glomerular filtration rate (GFR) and sodium clearance after multiple doses.[72] After a single dose, however, oxaprozin decreased GFR from 113.7 ± 5.7 mL/min to 98 ± 4.7 mL/min ($p < 0.01$) and decreased sodium clearance from 0.84 ± 0.07 mL/min to 0.61 ± 0.08 mL/min ($p < 0.005$). Both drugs reduced potassium excretion transiently, but only indomethacin caused a sustained change in potassium concentrations; serum potassium concentration rose from 4.32 ± 0.10 meq/L to 4.56 ± 0.11 meq/L ($p < 0.05$) after one week of indomethacin treatment.

Oxaprozin does not affect the kidney as much as indomethacin, a more potent PG synthesis inhibitor. However, oxaprozin should be used with extreme caution or not at all in patients with renal insufficiency.

Hepatotoxicity. Hepatotoxicity caused by therapy with NSAIDs, including oxaprozin, occurs in approximately 5% of patients.[73] Fenamates (e.g., meclofenamate sodium, mefenamic acid) are least often associated with hepatotoxicity, whereas pyrazolones (e.g., phenylbutazone) are most often associated with hepatotoxicity.

The hepatic safety of ibuprofen, aspirin, and oxaprozin in patients with rheumatoid arthritis or osteoarthritis was evaluated[74] in a manner similar to the evaluation of renal safety described previously. Among these three drugs, aspirin accounted for the greatest frequency of drug-related increases in serum aspartate aminotransferase (AST) concentration (5.2%). Of the patients receiving oxaprozin, 3.2% had elevations in serum AST concentrations that were believed to be secondary to drug treatment; none of the 182 patients receiving ibuprofen had elevations in serum AST concentrations related to the drug.

In a review of 1338 patients with rheumatoid disease, Zimmerman[75] found abnormally increased serum AST concentrations in 15.4% of 1135 patients given oxaprozin who had previously normal baseline values. In 1.1% of these patients, the AST values exceeded three times the upper limit of normal; one patient developed anicteric hepatitis.

Oxaprozin is expected to have a hepatotoxicity profile similar to that of other NSAIDs. It is hoped that oxaprozin will not prove as hepatotoxic as phenylbutazone, but initial and periodic monitoring of liver function tests throughout the first three months of therapy is recommended.

Hemostasis. The effect of NSAIDs, including oxaprozin, on bleeding time is of concern for patients suffering trauma or undergoing surgery. Aspirin binds irreversibly to cyclo-oxygenase; thus, new platelet production (requiring 7–12 days) is needed for platelet concentrations of cyclo-oxygenase to return to baseline. Only 20% of normal platelets, however, are required to maintain control of bleeding; therefore, bleeding times generally return to normal within 48 hours of discontinuation of aspirin.[76]

The other NSAIDs reversibly bind to cyclo-oxygenase such that the $t_{1/2}$ of each NSAID determines how long the antiplatelet effects persist. Bleeding times return to baseline less than 24 hours after discontinuation of ibuprofen or indomethacin and two weeks after discontinuation of piroxicam, which has a mean $t_{1/2}$ of 50 hours[77]; however, in a controlled setting with 10 volunteers, piroxicam's effect on platelet aggregation persisted for only two days.[78]

Oxaprozin, which also has a long half-life, may simulate piroxicam's effect on bleeding time. In a study comparing the effect of oxaprozin versus aspirin on hemostasis, both drugs were found to inhibit collagen-induced platelet aggregation to a similar degree.[79] In neither study group, however, was there clinical evidence of bleeding. Although bleeding time was prolonged and a significant decrease in platelet aggregation was noted on day 8 and days 13–16 ($p < 0.003$), the bleeding time remained within normal limits. Caution is advised, however, since oxaprozin does affect bleeding time.

Other Adverse Effects. Other adverse effects that may be associated with the use of oxaprozin include erythematous rash,[79] headache,[4] abdominal distress,[4] tinnitus,[4] hypotension,[38] diarrhea,[44,47] weight loss,[44] vomiting,[44] and dizziness.[52] Phototoxicity manifesting as a vesicular eruption on exposed skin areas also has been described.[45]

Drug Interactions

Anticoagulants. Because oxaprozin is highly protein bound, it may interfere with the protein binding of warfarin and aspirin and potentially cause enhanced anticoagulant effects. A seven-day regimen of oxaprozin 1200 mg daily started in 10 healthy, non-smoking men on the 21st day of warfarin treatment slightly increased mean prothrombin times and serum warfarin concentrations.[80] The authors concluded that, although oxaprozin may cause a modest nonstereoselective inhibition of warfarin metabolites and subsequently increase the prothrombin time slightly in some patients, this effect does not appear to be clinically important, at least for those patients undergoing only two weeks of concomitant therapy.

In contrast, aspirin has been shown to displace oxaprozin from its serum protein binding sites, resulting in increased oxaprozin CL (from 20 mL/min/kg to 26 mL/min/kg, $p < 0.05$) and decreased $t_{1/2}$ (from 45 hours to 40 hours, $p = 0.10$) but no clinical evidence of bleeding.[79] Thus, concomitant therapy with oxaprozin may influence the pharmacokinetic behavior of aspirin or warfarin, but these effects may not be clinically important for hemostasis.

Antihypertensives. Many patients who are being treated with NSAIDs for arthritis may also have hypertension. NSAIDs promote renal retention of sodium, which may attenuate the blood-pressure-lowering effects of many antihypertensive agents.[81] Also, vascular resistance may be increased as a result of reduced PGE_2 excretion associated with NSAID use[70,82]; evaluation of this pharmacodynamic interaction has been hindered by the short duration of the studies. If NSAID therapy is continued for one month, it appears that compensatory mechanisms are activated that attenuate a sustained hypertensive response caused by NSAIDs.[83,84]

Oxaprozin did not affect the antihypertensive effect of metoprolol during a four-week period.[85] The hypertensive patients had been taking metoprolol for an average of four weeks before administration of oxaprozin or placebo. In patients receiving oxaprozin, the systolic blood pressure increased during a 14-day period compared with patients receiving placebo (142.8 mm Hg versus 132.3 mm Hg, $p = 0.004$). However, after four weeks of therapy, the systolic blood pressure was no longer significantly different between the groups. Thus, the effect of oxaprozin on blood pressure appears to be transient, approaching baseline after one month of concomitant therapy with an antihypertensive agent.

Histamine H_2-Receptor Antagonists. Histamine H_2-receptor antagonists can potentially affect the hepatic metabolism of oxaprozin. In a single-dose, four-way crossover study of 12 healthy male volunteers aged 21–46 years (mean, 32 years), oxaprozin oral clearance was significantly lowered by 20% in volunteers receiving concomitant therapy with either cimetidine or ranitidine compared with controls (0.047 mL/min/kg versus 0.059 mL/min/kg).[86] Although this reduction in oxaprozin CL is statistically significant, the changes were small in magnitude and are not expected to be clinically important.

Conjugated Estrogens. Similarly, some studies have investigated whether conjugated estrogens impair the hepatic clearance of oxaprozin. Scavone et al.[87] studied 22 healthy female volunteers aged 21–64 years; 11 had taken conjugated estrogens (at a dosage of at least 0.625 mg/day) for at least three months, and 11 were not taking conjugated estrogens. Both groups received oxaprozin. The mean V, C_{max}, C, and $t_{1/2}$ for the two groups did not differ significantly. The only significant finding was a delay in time to peak serum concentration (t_{max}) in the control group (8.9 hours) compared with the conjugated estrogen group (4.0 hours; $p < 0.05$). The results of this study indicate that oxaprozin CL is not affected by concomitant treatment with conjugated estrogens.

Food. The ingestion of food concomitantly with oxaprozin does not appear to affect the pharmacokinetics of oxaprozin. Chiang et al.[88] studied 12 healthy volunteers who were given a single 1200-mg oral dose of oxaprozin after a standard breakfast. Mean C_{max}, absorption rate constants, and total AUC did not differ significantly for the fasting and postprandial states. Food delayed the onset of absorption from the GI tract (lag time, 24 versus 9 minutes), but it did not affect t_{max}, which was maintained at approximately five hours. These data suggest that oxaprozin can be taken with food (to decrease GI intolerance) without affecting its pharmacokinetic profile.

FDA-Approved Labeling

G. D. Searle & Company is seeking FDA-approved labeling for oxaprozin, under the brand name Daypro, for three indications: rheumatoid arthritis, osteoarthritis, and analgesia. Although preliminary data indicate oxaprozin is effective in the treatment of juvenile rheumatoid arthritis, the manufacturer is currently not seeking approved labeling for this indication. Oxaprozin's pharmacology suggests its efficacy in the treatment of primary dysmenorrhea, but this indication is not being pursued, nor apparently investigated.

Dosage and Administration

The anticipated adult dosage for oxaprozin is 600–1200 mg daily given as a single dose. In children, 10–20 mg/kg/day has been used for juvenile rheumatoid arthritis.[45] In the elderly, every-other-day dosing has been recommended[26]; this regimen offers cost benefits but may prove confusing for elderly patients. If prescribed for patients with renal disease who are experiencing azotemia, the dosage of oxaprozin should begin at 600 mg once daily.[32]

Oxaprozin will be marketed as a 600-mg caplet. Presently, there are no plans to develop a liquid or injectable preparation.[b] Oxaprozin is available in Japan as a nasal spray[89]; there are currently no plans to make this dosage form available in the United States.

Cost

Comparative costs based on the average wholesale price for currently available NSAIDs are provided in

Table 2. As noted in the table, the most expensive NSAID is etodolac (recently marketed in the United States), which is available at a monthly cost of $69.30. Phenylbutazone is the least expensive NSAID at a generic cost of $6.93 per month. These costs reflect a 10-fold range in monthly costs among the NSAIDs themselves and do not include expenditures for attendant costs of therapy, such as costs for misoprostol or sucralfate to treat NSAID-associated GI intolerance. The manufacturer did not provide the anticipated unit cost of oxaprozin and stated that the cost of oxaprozin is similar to that of other NSAIDs.[a]

Instructions to the Patient

The patient should be warned of possible adverse effects associated with oxaprozin, including GI intolerance (nausea, vomiting, and diarrhea), rash, headache, tinnitus, hypotension, and dizziness. Because of reported phototoxicity, sun exposure should be minimized and sunscreens should be employed as needed. The patient should be instructed to consult with a pharmacist or physician before administering oxaprozin with any other drug. If the patient has a history of a hypersensitivity reaction to any NSAID or aspirin, he or she should also avoid oxaprozin. Asthmatics are at greater risk for a hypersensitivity reaction and should be instructed to call their physician at the first sign of allergy.

Comments

The present trend in pharmacologic formulation is to believe that a longer half-life is always preferable because longer dosing intervals improve patient compliance. This concept may be of limited usefulness, however, with NSAIDs. Because of synovial sequestration of NSAIDs and the associated prolonged duration of action, an increase in systemic half-life may not appreciably improve efficacy; however, a longer half-life may contribute disproportionately to the profile of adverse effects. More specifically, the adverse effects experienced may be of longer duration than the adverse effects associated with other NSAIDs that have shorter half-lives. Only clinical experience will prove or disprove this hypothesis.

Oxaprozin appears to be another NSAID comparable in efficacy to currently available NSAIDs. Its long half-life and synovial sequestration support once-daily dosing. Although oxaprozin offers another choice in NSAID therapy, it does not provide any advantage over other currently available NSAIDs.

With the introduction of oxaprozin into the commercial market, pharmacy and therapeutics (P&T) committees may choose to consider, if they have not already, a protocol for unbiased consideration of new NSAIDs for formulary inclusion (Figure 3). In such a protocol, the P&T committee would adopt a policy whereby a new NSAID is not added to the formulary unless (1) it represents a therapeutic advance according to the FDA; (2) it represents an advantageous, unique dosage form (e.g., injectable or liquid preparation); (3) it offers improved compliance (e.g., once-daily or every-other-day dosing); or (4) it represents a substantial cost saving as compared with currently available NSAIDs. Anecdotal experience or manufacturer influence should not be a part of this decision-making process.

Table 2.
Drug Acquisition Costs for 30 Days of NSAID[a] Therapy

Generic Drug	Brand Name Drug	Average Minimum Anti-inflammatory Dosage	Average Wholesale Cost ($)[b] Generic Drug	Brand Name Drug
Phenylbutazone	Butazolidin	100 mg t.i.d.	6.93	48.60
Aspirin		325 mg q.i.d.	7.20	NA
Indomethacin	Indocin	25 mg t.i.d.	9.90	43.20
Ibuprofen	Motrin	400 mg q.i.d.	14.40	21.60
Meclofenamate sodium	Meclomen	100 mg (of meclofenamic acid) b.i.d.	23.40	36.00
Naproxen sodium	Anaprox	275 mg b.i.d.	NA	38.40
Naproxen	Naprosyn	250 mg b.i.d.	NA	38.40
Fenoprofen calcium	Nalfon	300 mg (of fenoprofen) t.i.d.	NA	42.30
Tolmetin sodium	Tolectin	200 mg (of tolmetin) t.i.d.	NA	43.20
Sulindac	Clinoril	150 mg b.i.d.	43.20	51.60
Flurbiprofen	Ansaid	50 mg t.i.d.	NA	48.60
Ketoprofen	Orudis	75 mg b.i.d.	NA	58.20
Piroxicam	Feldene	20 mg daily	NA	58.80
Diclofenac sodium	Voltaren	75 mg b.i.d.	NA	61.50
Oxyphenbutazone	Oxalid	100 mg t.i.d.	62.10	NA
Etodolac	Lodine	100 mg t.i.d.	NA	69.30
Oxaprozin	Daypro	600 or 1200 mg daily	NA	NP[c]

[a]NSAID = Nonsteroidal anti-inflammatory drug.
[b]Based on 1991 *Drug Topics* Redbook Annual Pharmacists' Reference. This is the cost to the pharmacy; prices charged to the patient will vary markedly. NA = drug not available in this form.
[c]NP = Cost not provided by manufacturer, but company spokesperson said that the cost would be similar to that of other NSAIDs (Bruno K, G.D. Searle & Co. Personal communication. 1991 Oct.).

Figure 3. Questions for formulary consideration of new nonsteroidal anti-inflammatory drugs (NSAIDs). At least one question should be answered yes before a new NSAID is added to the institution's formulary.

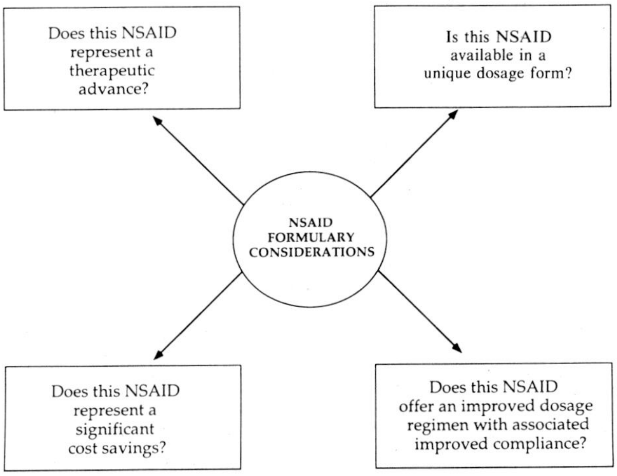

Formulary Considerations

Few data exist that would support adding oxaprozin to an established formulary. Its long half-life would certainly support once-daily dosing, but piroxicam has a similar half-life with a known adverse effect profile and also provides once-daily dosing. The contribution of the long systemic half-life to the adverse effect profile for oxaprozin may not be fully appreciated until it has undergone Phase IV postmarketing surveillance (as was true of zomepirac, suprofen, and benoxaprofen, which have since been removed from the U.S. market). While studies suggest that oxaprozin is equally effective as other NSAIDs (as outlined in Table 1), it does not appear to offer any distinct advantages. Its GI toxicity profile must be evaluated in a larger number of patients and it must be compared with other NSAIDs (as was done by Carson et al.[90]) before it can be determined if oxaprozin causes less GI toxicity than other currently available NSAIDs.

Conclusion

Oxaprozin is a new NSAID with a long half-life averaging 59 hours, which should support once-daily dosing. It will be marketed for the treatment of rheumatoid arthritis and osteoarthritis and for use as an analgesic. Adverse effects include GI irritation, headache, tinnitus, dizziness, phototoxicity, and elevation of liver and renal function indices. Although oxaprozin will represent another alternative within this class, it offers no clear advantage over other currently available NSAIDs.

---

[a]Goetsch R, FDA. Personal communication. 1992 Apr 13.

[b]Bruno K, G. D. Searle & Co. Personal communication. 1991 Oct.

References

1. Miller LG, Prichard JG. Selecting nonsteroidal anti-inflammatory drugs: pharmacologic and clinical considerations. *J Am Board Fam Pract*. 1989; 2:257-71.
2. Baum C, Kennedy DL, Forbes MB. Utilization of nonsteroidal anti-inflammatory drugs. Rockville, MD: Food and Drug Administration, Drug Use Branch, Division of Drug and Biological Product Experience, 1983; publication no. HFN-737.
3. Budarari S, ed. The Merck manual. Rathway, NJ: Merck & Co.; 1989:1095.
4. Reynolds WJ, Shaar SF, Buuk A et al. Oxaprozin: a once daily treatment regimen in rheumatoid arthritis. *J Rheumatol*. 1979; 6:345-50.
5. Rosenthal ME, Begany AJ, Dervinis A et al. Anti-inflammatory properties of 4,5-diphenyloxazole-2-oxazolepropionic acid (oxaprozin). *Agents Actions*. 1974; 4:15-9.
6. Robinson DR. Prostaglandins and the mechanism of action of anti-inflammatory drugs. *Am J Med*. 1983; 10:26-31.
7. Oates JA, FitzGerald GA, Branch RA et al. Clinical implications of prostaglandin and thromboxane A_2 formation (first of two parts). *N Engl J Med*. 1988; 319:689-98.
8. Oates JA, FitzGerald GA, Branch RA et al. Clinical implications of prostaglandin and thromboxane A_2 formation (second of two parts). *N Engl J Med*. 1988; 319:761-7.
9. Moncada S, Flower RJ, Vane JR. Prostaglandins, prostacyclin, thromboxane A_2, and leukotrienes. In: Gilman AG, Goodman LS, Rall TW et al., eds. The pharmacologic basis of therapeutics. New York: Macmillan; 1985:660-73.
10. Dawood MY. Dysmenorrhea. *J Reprod Med*. 1985; 30:154.
11. Lewis AJ. The pharmacologic profile of oxaprozin. *Semin Arthritis Rheum*. 1986; 15(Suppl 2):11-7.
12. Caldwell JR, Altman RD, Burch FX et al. Treatment of ankylosing spondylitis with oxaprozin: a comparison with indomethacin. *Semin Arthritis Rheum*. 1986; 15(Suppl 2):95-100.
13. Flower RJ, Cheung HS, Cushman DW. Quantitative determination of prostaglandins and malondialdehyde formed by the arachidonate oxygenase (prostaglandin synthetase) system of bovine seminal vesicles. *Prostaglandins*. 1973; 4:325-41.
14. Minta JO, Williams MD. Some nonsteroidal anti-inflammatory drugs inhibit the generation of superoxide anions by activated polymorph by blocking ligand-receptor interactions. *J Rheumatol*. 1985; 12:751-7.
15. Abramson S, Korchak HM, Ludewig R et al. Modes of action of aspirin-like drug. *Proc Natl Acad Sci USA*. 1985; 82:7227-31.
16. Kitchen EA, Dawson W, Rainsford KD et al. Inflammation and possible modes of action of anti-inflammatory drugs. In: Rainsford KD, ed. Anti-inflammatory and anti-rheumatic drugs. Vol 1. Inflammation mechanism and action of traditional drugs. Boca Raton, FL: CRC Press; 1985:21-87.
17. Ceuppens JG, Rodriguez MA, Goodwin JS. Nonsteroidal anti-inflammatory agents inhibit the synthesis of IgM rheumatoid factor in vitro. *Lancet*. 1982; 1:528-30.
18. Cush JJ, Lipsky PE, Postelthwaite AE et al. Correlation of serological indicators of inflammation with effectiveness of nonsteroidal anti-inflammatory drug therapy in rheumatoid arthritis. *Arthritis Rheum*. 1990; 33:19-28.
19. Burkhardt D, Ghosh P. Laboratory evaluation of antiarthritic drugs as potential chondroprotective agents. *Semin Arthritis Rheum*. 1987; 17(Suppl 1):3-34.
20. Lewis AJ, Carlson RP, Chang J et al. The pharmacologic profile of oxaprozin, an anti-inflammatory and analgesic agent with low gastrointestinal toxicity. *Curr Ther Res*. 1983; 34:777-94.
21. Lewis J, Parker J, DiLuigi J et al. Immunomodulation of delayed hypersensitivity to methylated bovine serum albumin (MBSA) in mice using subliminal and normal sensitization procedures. *J Immunopharmacol*. 1981-82; 3(3-4):289-307.
22. Cummings NA, Nordby GL. Measurement of synovial fluid pH in normal and arthritic knees. *Arthritis Rheum*. 1966; 9:47-56.
23. Goodwin JS. Mechanism of action of nonsteroidal anti-in-

flammatory drugs. *Am J Med*. 1984; 79(Suppl 1):57-64.
24. Greenblatt DJ, Matlis R, Scavone JM et al. Oxaprozin pharmacokinetics in the elderly. *Br J Clin Pharmacol*. 1985; 19:373-8.
25. Janssen FW, Jusko WJ, Chiang ST et al. Metabolism and kinetics of oxaprozin in normal subjects. *Clin Pharmacol Ther*. 1980; 27:352-62.
26. Kurowski M, Thabe H. The transsynovial distribution of oxaprozin. *Agents Actions*. 1989; 24:458-60.
27. Homon CA, Fluck ER, Janssen FW et al. Protein binding and clearance of oxaprozin, a highly bound anti-inflammatory agent. *Agents Actions*. 1982; 12:211-5.
28. Ruelius HW. Extrapolation from animals to man: predictions, pitfalls, and perspectives. *Xenobiotica*. 1987; 17:255-65.
29. Chiang ST, Lasseter KC, Fluck ER et al. Oxaprozin dose proportionality. *J Clin Pharmacol*. 1984; 24:515-22.
30. Chiang ST, Morrison G, Knowles JA et al. Oxaprozin disposition in renal disease. *Clin Pharmacol Ther*. 1982; 31:509-15.
31. Jusko WJ, Chiang ST. Distribution volume related to body weight and protein binding. *J Pharm Sci*. 1982; 71:649-70.
32. Audet PR, Knowles JA, Troy SM et al. Effect of chronic renal failure on oxaprozin multiple-dose pharmacokinetics. *Clin Pharmacol Ther*. 1988; 44:303-9.
33. Lasseter KC, Chiang ST, Rogers SL et al. Pharmacokinetics of oxaprozin in patients with hepatic impairment. *Clin Res*. 1985; 33:284A.
34. Ochs HR, Greenblatt DJ, Knuchel M. Oxaprozin pharmacokinetics in patients with congestive heart failure. *Arzneim Forsch Drug Res*. 1986; 36:1837-40.
35. Hubsher JA, Ballard IM, Walke BR et al. A multicenter double-blind comparison of oxaprozin and aspirin therapy on rheumatoid arthritis. *J Int Med Res*. 1979; 7:69-76.
36. Jamar R, Dequeker J. Oxaprozin versus aspirin in rheumatoid arthritis. *Curr Med Res Opin*. 1985; 5:433-8.
37. Barber JV, Collins RL, Kitriodou RC et al. The efficacy and safety of single daily doses of oxaprozin in the treatment of rheumatoid arthritis: a comparison with aspirin. *Semin Arthritis Rheum*. 1986; 15(Suppl 2):42-53.
38. Vreede PD, Harper FE, Sheldon WB. Use of oxaprozin in the treatment of aspirin failure in rheumatoid arthritis. *Semin Arthritis Rheum*. 1986; 15(Suppl 2):66-71.
39. Appelrouth DJ, Chodock AL, Miller JL et al. A comparison of single daily doses of oxaprozin with multiple daily doses of ibuprofen for the treatment of rheumatoid arthritis. *Semin Arthritis Rheum*. 1986; 15(Suppl 2):54-8.
40. Poiley JE, Spinkler JS, Clarke JP et al. Nonsteroidal anti-inflammatory drug therapy in rheumatoid arthritis: a comparison of oxaprozin and ibuprofen. *Semin Arthritis Rheum*. 1986; 15(Suppl 2):59-65.
41. Schorn D. A comparison between oxaprozin and naproxen in rheumatoid arthritis. *S Afr Med J*. 1981; 14:768.
42. Zuccallo R, Mackinnon MI, Fraser KM et al. Oxaprozin and sulindac in rheumatoid arthritis: a double-blind comparative trial. *Curr Med Res Opin*. 1983; 38:302-9.
43. Bass JC, Athreya BH, Brewer EJ et al. A once-daily anti-inflammatory drug, oxaprozin, in the treatment of juvenile rheumatoid arthritis. *J Rheumatol*. 1985; 2:384-6.
44. Miller LG, Prichard JG. Current issues in NSAID therapy. *Prim Care*. 1990; 17:589-601.
45. Ginsberg F, Famaey JP. A double-blind, parallel trial of oxaprozin versus naproxen in the treatment of osteoarthritis. *Curr Med Res Opin*. 1984; 10:689-95.
46. Kolodny AL, Klipper AR, Harris BK et al. The efficacy and safety of single daily doses of oxaprozin in the treatment of osteoarthritis: a comparison with aspirin. *Semin Arthritis Rheum*. 1986; 15(Suppl 2):72-9.
47. Powell WR, Miller JL, Sheldon WB. Once-daily oxaprozin and piroxicam compared in osteoarthritis. *Semin Arthritis Rheum*. 1986; 15(Suppl 2):80-5.
48. Winter L, Post A. Double-blind comparison of single oral doses of oxaprozin, aspirin, and placebo for relief of post-operative oral surgery pain. *J Int Med Res*. 1983; 11:308-14.
49. Santa JE, Queiroz MV. Oxaprozin versus diclofenac sodium in the treatment of ankylosing spondylitis. *J Int Med Res*. 1988; 16:150-6.
50. Goldfarb S, Walker BR, Agus ZS. The uricosuric effect of oxaprozin in humans. *J Clin Pharmacol*. 1985; 25:144-8.
51. Mease PJ, Willkens RF. Treatment of acute gout with oxaprozin. *Semin Arthritis Rheum*. 1986; 15(Suppl 2):86-9.
52. Bono RF, Finkel S, Goodman HF et al. Oxaprozin in the treatment of patients with tendonitis and bursitis: comparison with phenylbutazone and placebo. *Semin Arthritis Rheum*. 1986; 15(Suppl 2):90-4.
53. Takeuchi A, Mori M, Hashimoto A et al. Efficacy of oxaprozin in the treatment of articular symptoms of Behçet's disease. *Clin Rheumatol*. 1984; 3:397-9.
54. Carlson RP, Gilman SC, Hodge TG et al. Effects of oral aspirin and oxaprozin in the development of lupus-like disease in MRL/1 mice. *J Immunopharmacol*. 1984; 6:69-78.
55. Abbatiello ER, Kanimsky M, Wersbrath S. The effect of prostaglandins and prostaglandin inhibition on spermatogenesis. *Int J Fertil*. 1975; 20:177-82.
56. Barkay J, Harper-Kerpel S, Ben-Ezra S et al. The prostaglandin inhibitor effect of anti-inflammatory drugs in the therapy of male infertility. *Fertil Steril*. 1984; 42:406-11.
57. Knuth UA, Kuhne J, Crosby J et al. Indomethacin and oxaprozin lower seminal prostaglandin levels but do not influence sperm motion characteristics and serum hormones of young healthy men in a placebo-controlled double-blind trial. *J Androl*. 1989; 10:108-19.
58. Miller LG, Rogers JC, Swee DE. Indomethacin-associated sexual dysfunction. *J Fam Pract*. 1989; 29:210-1.
59. Dahl SC, Katcher BS. Rheumatic diseases. In: Katcher BS, Young LY, Koda-Kimble MA, eds. Applied therapeutics: the clinical use of drugs. Spokane: Applied Therapeutics; 1983:1421-47.
60. Mathison DA, Stevenson DD. Hypersensitivity to nonsteroidal anti-inflammatory drugs: indications and methods for oral challenges. *J Allergy Clin Immunol*. 1979; 64:669-74.
61. Prichard JG, Miller LG. Monitoring of hepatotoxicity secondary to NSAID therapy. *J Am Board Fam Pract*. 1990; 3:142.
62. Lussier LA, Lebel E, Tetreault L. Gastrointestinal blood loss of oxaprozin and aspirin with placebo control. *J Clin Pharmacol*. 1982; 22:173-88.
63. Lanza FL, Hubscher JA, Walker BR. Gastroscopic evaluation of the effect of aspirin and oxaprozin on the gastric mucosa. *J Clin Pharmacol*. 1981; 21:157-61.
64. Lucker PW, Venitz J, Ahrens S et al. Gastric irritation of oxaprozin, a new nonsteroidal anti-inflammatory drug, in comparison to acetylsalicylic acid and indomethacin: a gastric potential difference analysis. *Methods Find Exp Clin Pharmacol*. 1987; 9:469-75.
65. Suwa T, Urano H, Kohno Y et al. Comparative studies on the gastrointestinal lesions caused by several nonsteroidal anti-inflammatory agents in rats. *Agents Actions*. 1987; 21:167-72.
66. Shriver DA, Dove PA, White CB et al. A profile of the gastrointestinal toxicity of aspirin, indomethacin, oxaprozin, phenylbutazone, and fentiazac in arthritic and Lewis normal rats. *Toxicol Appl Pharmacol*. 1977; 42:75-83.
67. Dahl SL, Ward JR. Efficacy and tolerability of oxaprozin in the elderly. *Semin Arthritis Rheum*. 1986; 15(Suppl 2):40-6.
68. Greenblatt DJ, Scavone JM. Pharmacokinetics of oxaprozin and other nonsteroidal anti-inflammatory agents. *Semin Arthritis Rheum*. 1986; 15(Suppl 2):18-26.
69. Sedor JR, Davidson EW, Dunn MJ. Effects of nonsteroidal anti-inflammatory drugs on healthy subjects. *Am J Med*. 1986; 81:58-70.
70. Brown J, Dolery C, Valdez G. Interaction of nonsteroidal anti-inflammatory drugs with antihypertensive and diuretic agents: control of vascular reactivity by endogenous prostanoids. *Am J Med*. 1986; 86(Suppl):43-57.
71. Bonney SL, Northington RS, Hedrich DA et al. Renal safety of two analgesics used over the counter: ibuprofen and aspirin. *Clin Pharmacol Ther*. 1986; 40:373-7.
72. Mitnick DD, Greenberg A, Deoreo PB et al. Effects of two nonsteroidal anti-inflammatory drugs, indomethacin and oxaprozin, on the kidney. *Clin Pharmacol Ther*. 1980; 28:680-9.

73. Lewis JH. Hepatic toxicity of nonsteroidal anti-inflammatory drugs. *Clin Pharm*. 1984; 3:128-38.
74. Freeland GR, Northington RS, Hedrich DA et al. Hepatic safety of two analgesics used over the counter: ibuprofen and aspirin. *Clin Pharmacol Ther*. 1988; 43:473-9.
75. Zimmerman JH. Hepatic effects of oxaprozin. *Semin Arthritis Rheum*. 1986; 15(Suppl 2):35-9.
76. Gardner FH. NSAIDs and bleeding time. *J Am Board Fam Pract*. 1990; 3:71-2.
77. Bowen CA. What are the effects of nonsteroidal anti-inflammatory drugs on platelet function? *US Pharm*. 1987; 12(May):34.
78. Cronberg S, Wallmark E, Soderberg I. Effect on platelet aggregation of oral administration of 10 nonsteroidal analgesics to humans. *Scand J Haematol*. 1984; 33:155-9.
79. Kahn SB, Hubsher JA. Effects of oxaprozin alone or in combination with aspirin on hemostasis and plasma protein binding. *J Clin Pharmacol*. 1983; 23:139-46.
80. Davis LJ, Dayser SR, Hubsher J et al. Effect of oxaprozin on the steady-state anticoagulant activity of warfarin. *Clin Pharm*. 1984; 3:295-7.
81. McGiff JC, Quillery CP. Interaction of nonsteroidal anti-inflammatory drugs and antihypertensives. *JAMA*. 1988; 260:850-1.
82. Wennmulm A, Carlsson I, Edund A et al. Central and peripheral hemodynamic effects of nonsteroidal anti-inflammatory drugs in man. *Arch Toxicol*. 1984; 7(Suppl 1):350-9.
83. Miller LG. Ibuprofen and antihypertensive drugs. *Ann Intern Med*. 1988; 108:485. Letter.
84. Puddey IB, Beilin LJ, Vandongen R et al. Differential effects of sulindac and indomethacin on blood pressure in treated essential hypertensive subjects. *Clin Sci*. 1985; 69:327-36.
85. Halabi A, Linde M, Zeidler H et al. Double-blind study on the interaction of oxaprozin with metoprolol in hypertensives. *Cardiovasc Drugs Ther*. 1989; 3:441-3.
86. Scavone JM, Greenblatt DJ, Matlis R et al. Interaction of oxaprozin with acetaminophen, cimetidine and ranitidine. *Eur J Clin Pharmacol*. 1986; 31:371-4.
87. Scavone JM, Ochs HR, Greenblatt DJ et al. Pharmacokinetics of oxaprozin in females receiving conjugated estrogens. *Eur J Clin Pharmacol*. 1988; 35:105-8.
88. Chiang ST, Knowles JA, Hubsher JA et al. Effects of food on oxaprozin bioavailability. *J Clin Pharmacol*. 1984; 24:381-5.
89. Namiki N, Yokoyama H, Fukuda M et al. Studies on improvement of pharmaceutical preparations prescribed in hospitals. VI. Oxaprozin nasal spray. *Drug Des Deliv*. 1988; 2:311-21.
90. Carson JL, Strom BC, Mose ML et al. The relative gastrointestinal toxicity of the nonsteroidal anti-inflammatory drugs. *Arch Intern Med*. 1987; 147:1054-9.

Ticlopidine: A new platelet aggregation inhibitor

Matthew K. Ito, Alden R. Smith, and Marisa L. Lee

Abstract: The chemistry, pharmacology, pharmacokinetics, clinical efficacy, adverse effects, and dosage of ticlopidine are reviewed.

Ticlopidine appears to inhibit platelet aggregation induced by adenosine diphosphate. Ticlopidine hydrochloride is rapidly absorbed after oral administration, and maximum antiplatelet effects occur one to three hours after the dose. In multicenter, randomized, double-blind trials, ticlopidine was more effective than aspirin or placebo in preventing stroke, myocardial infarction, or death caused by vascular events. Ticlopidine was more effective than aspirin in preventing recurrent transient ischemic attacks after six months of therapy. Ticlopidine has also been used to prevent occlusion and improve patency of aortocoronary bypass grafts, to prevent ischemic ulcers in patients with chronic arterial occlusive disease, and to slow the progression of diabetic microangiopathy. The most serious adverse effect, neutropenia, occurred in about 1% of patients. The most frequently reported adverse effects are diarrhea, nausea, vomiting, and abdominal cramps. Ticlopidine is indicated for reducing the risk of thrombotic stroke in patients who have experienced a minor stroke, transient ischemic attack, or completed thrombotic stroke. The recommended dosage is 500 mg/day in two divided doses taken with food.

Ticlopidine is an alternative agent for the primary and secondary prevention of stroke. Because of the risk of neutropenia and agranulocytosis and the high cost of therapy, ticlopidine should be reserved for patients who are intolerant of or lack benefit from aspirin.

Index terms: Cerebrovascular disorders; Dosage; Mechanism of action; Pharmacokinetics; Platelet aggregation inhibitors; Ticlopidine hydrochloride; Toxicity
Clin Pharm. 1992; 11:603-17

Matthew K. Ito, Pharm.D., is Assistant Professor of Pharmacy Practice and Regional Coordinator, San Diego Program, School of Pharmacy, University of the Pacific, Stockton, CA, and Cardiovascular Pharmacotherapy Specialist, Veterans Affairs Medical Center, San Diego, CA. Alden R. Smith, Pharm.D., is a clinical pharmacist, Rx Relief, Fallbrook, CA; at the time of this report, he was a clinical pharmacy resident, Department of Pharmacy Service, Veterans Affairs Medical Center, San Diego. Marisa L. Lee is a Pharm.D. candidate at the University of Southern California School of Pharmacy, Los Angeles, CA.

Address reprint requests to Dr. Ito at the Cardiovascular Pharmacodynamics Laboratory (119), VA Medical Center, 3350 La Jolla Village Drive, San Diego, CA 92161.

The editorial assistance of Scott T. Johns, Pharm.D., Veterans Affairs Medical Center, San Diego, CA, is acknowledged.

This is article **680-204-9217** in the **ASHP Continuing Education System**; it qualifies for 1.0 hour of continuing-education credit. See page 642 for learning objectives and test questions.

During the past three decades, much attention has been focused on the development of drugs to prevent thromboembolic diseases of the cerebrovascular and cardiovascular systems. Platelets play a major role in the pathogenesis of thromboembolic events. Inhibition of platelet function has provided some protection against thrombogenesis in specific patient subpopulations.[1]

Aspirin administered in dosages ranging from 30 mg to 1.5 g daily has been shown to reduce the number of thromboembolic events occurring in patients who have had minor strokes or transient ischemic attacks.[2-6] Women do not seem to benefit from aspirin to the same extent as men[3,4,7,8]; however, this finding may be a function of the small number of women enrolled in these clinical trials and the evidence that women are less likely than men to experience recurrent strokes.[9] Moreover, aspirin is not beneficial in the treatment of patients with completed stroke.

Aspirin therapy reduces the risk of death or nonfatal myocardial infarction in patients with a history of previous infarction or unstable angina.[10,11] In addition, aspirin 325 mg taken every other day by male physicians reduced the relative risk of fatal and nonfatal myocardial infarctions by almost 50% compared with placebo. However, an increased risk of moderate, severe, or fatal hemorrhagic stroke was observed in physicians receiving aspirin.[12]

Results from clinical trials investigating the efficacy of dipyridamole and sulfinpyrazone in the treatment of cerebrovascular disease and the primary and secondary prevention of myocardial infarction are conflicting at best.[13] Thus, the routine use of these agents is discouraged.

Ticlopidine hydrochloride (Ticlid; Syntex Laboratories, Palo Alto, CA) is a new inhibitor of platelet aggregation. Ticlopidine has a broader mechanism of action than aspirin or dipyridamole. Ticlopidine appears to act by inhibiting platelet aggregation induced by a variety of stimuli, including adenosine diphosphate (ADP). Its effects on stable endoperoxides, thrombin, and platelet-activating factor (PAF) may play a contributory role. Ticlopidine blocks the "primary wave" and "secondary wave" of platelet aggregation, whereas aspirin blocks only the secondary wave.[14] This article reviews the chemistry, pharmacology, pharmacokinetics, adverse effects, and clinical uses of ticlopidine.

Chemistry

Ticlopidine, 5-[(2-chlorophenyl)methyl]-4,5,6,7-tetrahydrothieno-[3,2-*c*]pyridine hydrochloride, is structurally different from aspirin, sulfinpyrazone, and dipyridamole (Figure 1). Ticlopidine was the result of a search for a nonsteroidal nonacidic anti-inflammatory drug. Ticlopidine was shown to have no anti-inflammatory effects, but it possessed platelet antiaggregating properties ex vivo.

Ticlopidine hydrochloride is a white, nonhygroscopic powder with a melting point of 200 °C. Ticlopidine has a pKa of 7.5 at 20 °C and its solubility in water is 61 mg/mL at 23 °C. Ticlopidine is soluble in methanol, ethanol, chloroform, methylene chloride, dimethyl sulfoxide, and polyethylene glycol.[15]

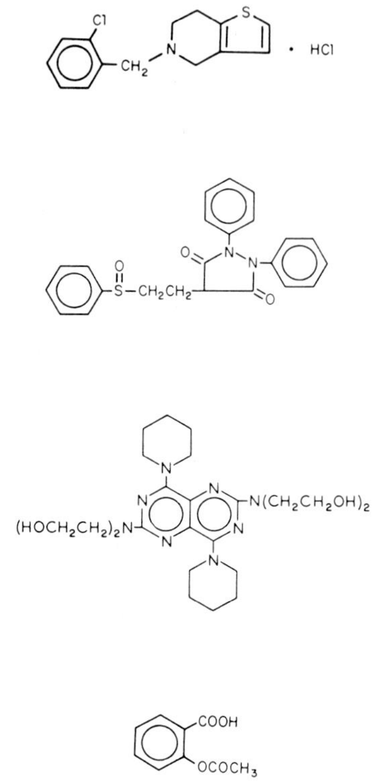

Figure 1. Structures of ticlopidine hydrochloride, sulfinpyrazone, dipyridamole, and aspirin (from top to bottom).

Pharmacology

In areas of rapid blood flow, such as in systemic arteries, thrombus formation is secondary to vascular damage and subsequent interaction of the subendothelium with various blood components, particularly platelets. The biochemical scheme of platelet adhesion and aggregation is illustrated in Figure 2.

Platelets do not adhere to normal endothelium. However, once the endothelium is damaged and subendothelial constituents, such as type I and III collagen, elastin, and von Willebrand factor, are exposed, platelet membranes are altered and platelets attach to the damaged endothelium.

Subsequently, platelets release a growth factor from their alpha-granules that promotes intimal smooth muscle proliferation. During this stage, activated platelet membranes release calcium, causing the platelet to contract and release ADP and serotonin. Additionally, platelet calcium appears to activate platelet phospholipase, leading to the formation of thromboxane A_2. Free circulating ADP contacts the surface of neighboring platelets, leading to an increase in their

Figure 2. Biosynthetic pathways and biochemical events involved in platelet activation. After vascular tissue injury occurs, platelet membranes are activated when they are exposed to subendothelial constituents. Calcium released from these platelets activates phospholipase A_2 and the subsequent formation of prostaglandin I_2 (PGI_2) and thromboxane A_2 (TxA_2) leading to platelet adhesion. Adenosine disphosphate (ADP) released from these activated platelets along with circulating fibrinogen causes other platelets to aggregate. vWF = von Willebrand factor, cAMP = adenosine 3',5'-cyclic phosphate, 5'AMP = 5'-adenosine monophosphate. (Adapted from references 16–20.)

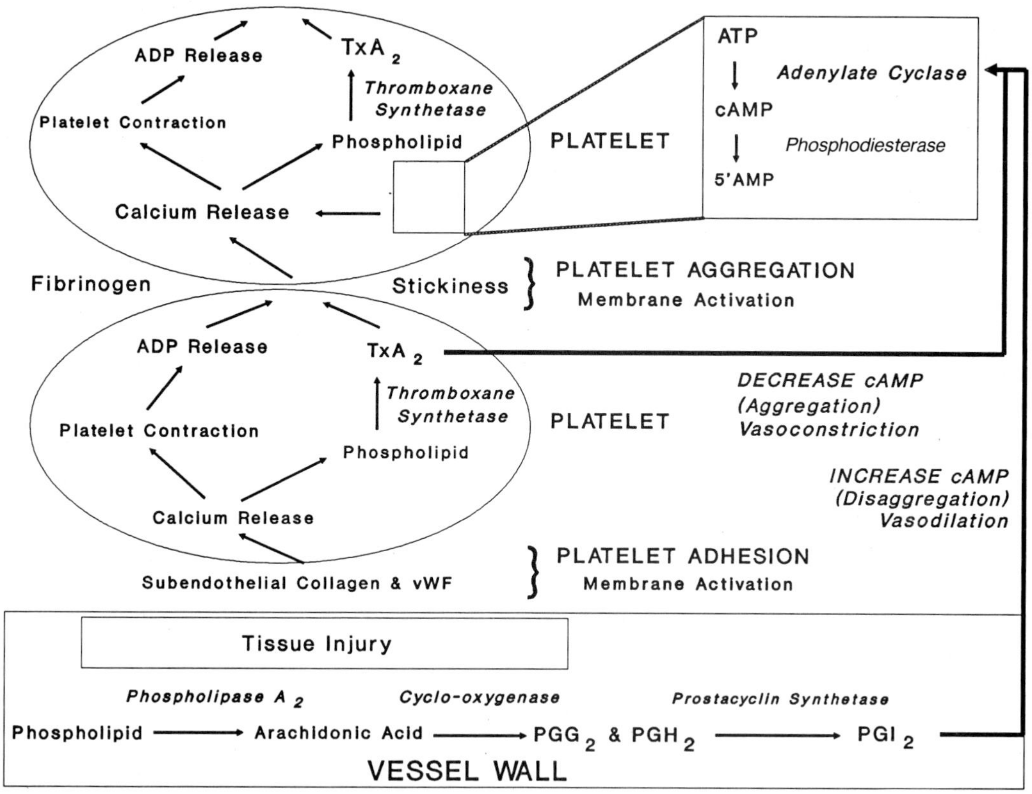

cytoplasmic calcium, ADP, and thromboxane A_2. This results in enhanced platelet "stickiness," which induces platelet aggregation and the formation of a hemostatic plug.[16,17] Epinephrine, serotonin, and vasopressin also promote platelet aggregation.

If blood flow is laminar, ADP and thromboxane A_2 will not accumulate around the adherent platelets; thus, only a thin layer of platelets forms on the endothelium. In contrast, if blood flow is disturbed, platelets can accumulate and aggregate on other adherent platelets. Around the aggregating platelets, the coagulation system is activated, further promoting platelet aggregation through the formation of thrombin. Eventually, the arterial thrombus is stabilized through the formation of fibrin.[16,17,21] Additionally, platelet "stickiness" appears to be dependent on the binding of fibrinogen to platelet membrane receptors. Fibrinogen acts as a bridge connecting neighboring platelets.[16,17]

Concurrently within vessel walls, prostaglandin (PG) I_2 is formed from cyclic endoperoxide. PGI_2 causes platelet disaggregation through the activation of platelet adenylate cyclase. This results in an increase in platelet adenosine 3',5'-cyclic phosphate (cAMP) concentration and a decrease in platelet calcium concentration.

PAF released from platelets, circulating leukocytes, and damaged endothelial cells serves as an additional pathway for platelet activation. PAF has been shown to induce platelet aggregation independent from ADP or thromboxane A_2.[21] The binding of PAF to its receptor appears to unmask cell-surface binding sites for fibrinogen, which promotes platelet aggregation directly.

The exact mechanism by which ticlopidine exerts its inhibitory effects on platelets has yet to be elucidated. Ticlopidine has minimal activity in vitro; however, platelet aggregation is markedly depressed in plasma obtained from primates after oral administration of ticlopidine. Thus, the antiplatelet effects of ticlopidine are likely due to a biotransformation product. Ticlopidine appears to inhibit platelet activity primarily through suppression of ADP-induced platelet aggregation. However, suppression of PAF and thromboxane A_2 and activation of adenylate cyclase may play a contributory role.[22,23]

Effects on Adenosine Diphosphate. Ex vivo and in vivo studies in animals and humans have shown that ticlopidine effectively inhibits the primary and secondary phases of ADP-induced platelet aggregation.[14,23-32] Platelet function in human plasma is disrupted within hours after oral administration of ticlopidine.[25] Maximum inhibition of platelet function appears to occur between five and seven days. Antiplatelet effects persist for up to 96 hours after drug withdrawal and dissipate as new platelets are released into the blood stream.[14,25] Continued disruption of ADP-induced aggregation has also been demonstrated throughout long-term administration (one year) in patients with previous cerebrovascular accidents.[30]

Effects on Binding of Fibrinogen to Platelets. Fibrinogen plays an important role in ADP-induced platelet aggregation. Suspensions of washed human platelets will not aggregate or do so only slightly without the addition of fibrinogen.[18] In ADP-induced aggregation, the interaction of fibrinogen with platelets appears to involve multiple steps in which there is participation of ADP, divalent cations, and fibrinogen.[17] In human platelets treated with ticlopidine, there is a dose-dependent inhibition of fibrinogen binding stimulated by ADP.[33]

In ex vivo platelet binding studies, ticlopidine has been shown to decrease fibrinogen binding of ADP-treated platelets by approximately 68%.[34] This appears to be a result of the direct action of ticlopidine on the platelet receptor for fibrinogen.[34] DiMinno et al.[35] reported that ADP-induced fibrinogen binding ex vivo was inhibited by 90% after seven days of ticlopidine administration. Ticlopidine induced a thrombasthenic state in normal platelets without quantitatively affecting the glycoprotein IIb–IIIa complex (the putative receptor for fibrinogen on the platelet surface).[19,31] In patients with diabetic retinopathy, ticlopidine normalizes the binding of fibrinogen to platelets, presumably by reducing the abnormally high fibrinogen binding.[35]

Effects on cAMP. As depicted in Figure 2, elevations in cAMP result in inhibition of platelet aggregation. Inhibition of adenylate cyclase results in a decrease in cAMP, whereas inhibition of phosphodiesterase enhances platelet disaggregation. Elevated levels of cAMP appear not to be essential for ticlopidine activity. Addition of SQ-22536 (an inhibitor of adenylate cyclase activity) to human platelets did not reverse the inhibition caused by ticlopidine. In contrast, SQ-22536 partially reverses the platelet-inhibiting effects of PGE_1, adenosine, and dipyridamole.[29] However, Ashida and Abiko[28] reported that platelets obtained from ticlopidine-treated rats showed increased basal and PGE_1-stimulated adenylate cyclase activity and prevented reduction in adenylate cyclase activity caused by low concentrations of PGE_2, thus increasing platelet cAMP levels. They also noted that ticlopidine inhibited platelet malondialdehyde formation (a measure of prostaglandin synthesis[36]) induced by thrombin but not by exogenous arachidonic acid.

Effects on Prostaglandins. The effect of ticlopidine on the arachidonic acid cascade is controversial. In vitro, ticlopidine has minimal activity against prostaglandin synthetase (approximately one-sixteenth the potency of aspirin) as measured in human citrated platelet-rich plasma.[24] In washed human platelets pretreated with ticlopidine 50 mmol/L, levels of PGE_2, $PGF_{2\alpha}$, PGD_2, and 6-keto-$PGF_{1\alpha}$ were elevated, while thromboxane B_2 levels were decreased.[37] Other investigators have demonstrated similar findings[38] or no effect on thromboxane B_2 production.[39] However, Bruno et al.[40] reported a dose-dependent inhibition of both thromboxane B_2 production and malondialdehyde formation stimulated by 0.05 U/mL of thrombin in washed platelet-rich plasma.

Effects on Bleeding Time. Like aspirin, ticlopidine increases template bleeding time in humans. Average increases in template bleeding time were 2, 3.5, and 4.7 times baseline in healthy human volunteers treated with 125, 325, and 500 mg per day, respectively. Maximal prolongation of template bleeding time occurred after three to five days of therapy. No hemorrhagic complications were associated with the increased template bleeding times in any of the treatment groups.[41] In patients who received ticlopidine hydrochloride at dosages of 750 mg daily, Duke bleeding times were increased at both 4 and 12 months of therapy.[30] No serious bleeding episodes were observed in these patients.

Effects on Other Blood Components. Ticlopidine is a hydrophobic molecule that binds to the membranes of erythrocytes. In vitro, ticlopidine at concentrations greater than 5×10^{-4} M causes hemolysis of red blood cells and denatures membrane proteins. At pharmacologic concentrations, ticlopidine protects erythrocytes from hemolysis and increases the fluidity of the hydrophobic core of the phospholipid bilayer.[42] In vitro, ticlopidine prevents sickling of erythrocytes by expanding the cell membrane, thus increasing the surface-to-volume ratio. This, in turn, results in partial protection against osmotic lysis. Membrane expansion leads to a secondary dilution of intracellular hemoglobin. It should be noted, however, that the in vitro concentration used in these experiments was 1 mM. Concentrations of only 1 μM are attainable in vivo.

Pharmacokinetics

Absorption. Up to 90% of a single oral dose of ticlopidine hydrochloride is rapidly absorbed.[43] Peak plasma concentrations occur one to three hours after a single oral dose and average 0.3 and 1.9 μg/mL after a single 250-mg and 500-mg dose, respectively. These concentrations increase because of drug accumulation with long-term administration. Individuals receiving 250 mg twice daily for 21 days had a mean peak plasma ticlopidine concentration of 0.9 μg/mL.[44]

Distribution. In healthy volunteers, the distribution half-life of ticlopidine after a single 250-mg or 500-mg dose was 2.0–2.5 hours.[44] Tissue distribution of ticlopidine in humans has not been reported in the literature; however, appreciable concentrations have been detected in kidney, liver, and fat tissue of rats. Greater than 98% of ticlopidine hydrochloride is reversibly bound to serum proteins, primarily albumin.[45]

Metabolism and Elimination. Ticlopidine is active in vitro only at concentrations higher than those achieved with usual dosages. This finding suggests that the activity of ticlopidine is likely due to one or more active metabolites. In animal and human studies using ticlopidine labeled with carbon 14, inhibition of platelet function did not correlate with plasma concentrations of the parent drug after a single dose or at steady state. Ticlopidine is metabolized rapidly and extensively in animals and in humans.[44]

The pattern of metabolism is complicated, but the primary routes of metabolism appear to involve *N*-dealkylation, *N*-oxidation, and oxidation of the thiophene ring. A total of 13 metabolites have been identified, four of which have been identified in humans. Of the 13 metabolites, only the 2-keto derivative of ticlopidine appears to be more active than the parent compound.

The 2-keto metabolite is about eight times more potent than ticlopidine in inhibiting ADP-induced platelet aggregation. The 2-keto metabolite also has a rapid onset of effect in inhibition of ADP-induced platelet aggregation in the rat (10 minutes for the 2-keto derivative, 60 minutes for ticlopidine).[16] So far, the 2-keto metabolite has been isolated only in the bile of ticlopidine-treated rats; further studies are needed to evaluate the importance of the 2-keto derivative in humans.

Less than 1% of ticlopidine is excreted unchanged in the urine.[44,45] The apparent elimination half-life of ticlopidine is 24–36 hours[44,45] after a single oral dose and up to 96 hours after 14 days of repeated dosing.[45]

Pharmacokinetic evaluation of ticlopidine in patients with renal and hepatic dysfunction has not been reported. Because ticlopidine undergoes extensive metabolism,[44] dosage adjustment in patients with renal insufficiency appears not to be necessary. The clearance of ticlopidine decreases with age.[45] The mean area under the serum concentration–time curve calculated during ticlopidine therapy was twofold to threefold greater in elderly volunteers (65–76 years) than in younger volunteers (20–43 years).

Clinical Trials in Humans

Ticlopidine is used to treat a variety of disorders characterized by a dysfunction in platelet adhesion and aggregation. Its role has been evaluated in prevention of ischemic ulcers caused by chronic arterial occlusion; treatment of intermittent claudication, diabetic microangiopathy and nephropathy, or sickle cell disease; maintenance of arteriovenous fistulas in long-term dialysis; improvement of patency after coronary artery bypass grafting; reduction of infarct size after myocardial infarction; and prevention of ischemic events in patients with coronary artery disease. Several large clinical trials have focused attention on the use of ticlopidine in patients with cerebral ischemic disorders caused by thromboembolism.

Cerebrovascular Disease. Ticlopidine has been extensively evaluated in the primary and secondary prevention of stroke and other cerebrovascular events (Table 1).[46-49] The results from multicenter, double-blind trials have shown that ticlopidine is more effective than placebo[49] or aspirin[48] in preventing stroke, myocardial infarction, or death caused by vascular events.

The Canadian–American Ticlopidine Study (CATS) compared ticlopidine with placebo for the rate of stroke, myocardial infarction, or vascular death in patients with a recent thromboembolic stroke (one week to four months before study enrollment).[49] This trial was a multicenter, randomized, double-blind design with treatment follow-up lasting up to three years (mean, 24 months). A total of 1053 patients were enrolled (525 received ticlopidine).

The yearly event rate for stroke, myocardial infarction, or vascular death was 15.3% and 10.8% for the placebo and ticlopidine groups, respectively. This outcome represents a relative risk reduction of 30.2% with ticlopidine ($p = 0.006$). Ticlopidine was beneficial in both men and women; relative risk reduction was

Table 1.
Clinical Trials of Ticlopidine in Cerebrovascular Disease[a]

Reference	No. Patients	Daily Dosage Regimen	Study Design	Duration of Therapy	Outcome
46	165 169	Ticlopidine HCl 200 mg Aspirin 500 mg	R, DB	12 mo	Percentage remaining event-free in first 6 mo: ticlopidine, 80.6%; aspirin, 70.4% (NS) More favorable outcome for ticlopidine; percentages and p values not reported
49	525 528	Ticlopidine HCl 500 mg Placebo	R, DB	3-year follow-up	Risk reduction for stroke, myocardial infarction, or vascular death: 30.2% with ticlopidine ($p = 0.006$)
48	1529 1540	Ticlopidine HCl 500 mg Aspirin 1300 mg	R, DB	2- to 6-yr follow-up	Three-yr event rate for nonfatal stroke and death: ticlopidine, 17%; aspirin, 19%; risk reduction of 12% ($p = 0.048$)
47	66 69	Ticlopidine HCl 300 mg Placebo	R, DB	4 wk	% Patients with good or excellent outcome: ticlopidine, 92%; placebo, 79% ($p < 0.05$)

[a]R = randomized, DB = double-blind, NS = not significant.

28.1% ($p = 0.037$) and 34.2% ($p = 0.045$), respectively. Treatment was discontinued because of adverse reactions in 62 patients receiving ticlopidine, compared with only 15 patients receiving placebo. The most common reasons for discontinuation of ticlopidine were diarrhea and rash. Neutropenia was observed in 11 patients (2.1%) in the ticlopidine group; however, reversal of neutropenia ensued within days after the drug was discontinued.

The Ticlopidine–Aspirin Stroke Study (TASS) involved 56 North American medical centers. This trial was designed to compare the effect of ticlopidine with that of aspirin on the risk of stroke or death.[48] Patients 40 years and older were eligible if, three months before entry into the study, they experienced one or more of the following: transient ischemic attack, amaurosis fugax, reversible ischemic neurologic deficit, or minor stroke. Patients with moderate-to-major stroke or a history of carotid-artery surgery were eligible only if the stroke or surgery occurred more than three months before enrollment in the study and was followed by one of the above events. A total of 3069 patients were enrolled (1529 received ticlopidine), and follow-up lasted for two to six years.

The three-year event rate for nonfatal stroke or death from any cause was 17% for patients receiving ticlopidine and 19% for patients receiving aspirin. This outcome represents a 12% risk reduction associated with the use of ticlopidine ($p = 0.048$). Moreover, the rates for fatal and nonfatal stroke at three years were 10% for patients receiving ticlopidine and 13% for patients receiving aspirin, representing a risk reduction of 21% ($p = 0.024$) with ticlopidine. In concordance with the CATS, a significant risk reduction was observed for both men and women who received ticlopidine.

Diarrhea, rash, urticaria, and neutropenia occurred more frequently in patients receiving ticlopidine ($p < 0.05$); however, gastrointestinal pain, gastritis, gastrointestinal hemorrhage, and peptic ulcers were more prevalent in patients receiving aspirin ($p < 0.05$). The number of patients who prematurely terminated therapy because of an adverse reaction was significantly greater for those receiving ticlopidine (20.9%) than for those receiving aspirin (14.5%). In addition to neutropenia, the only other laboratory abnormality was a statistically significant increase in total serum cholesterol concentration (9%) among patients treated with ticlopidine.

In an earlier trial, Tohgi et al.[46] compared the effect of ticlopidine with that of aspirin on the frequency of transient ischemic attacks in patients with a recent history of transient ischemic attacks. The percentages of patients remaining event-free were similar between the aspirin and ticlopidine groups throughout the first six months of therapy. After six months, the percentage of patients remaining event-free was significantly higher in the ticlopidine group.

Cerebral vasospasm associated with subarachnoid hemorrhage is a cause of increased mortality in patients with cerebral aneurysm. Various chemical mediators have been implicated as the cause of vasospasm, and the mechanisms are thought to be complicated. Ticlopidine has been compared with placebo after surgical repair of ruptured aneurysm.[47] Drug therapy commenced 24 hours after surgery and continued for four weeks.

Results of cerebral angiograms showed that the incidence of severe cerebral vasospasm with neurologic deficit (ticlopidine group, 5%; placebo group, 6%) and mild-to-moderate cerebral vasospasm with neurologic deficit (ticlopidine group, 43%; placebo group, 39%) was similar for both groups. There were three deaths in the ticlopidine group and nine deaths in the placebo group during the three-month evaluation period. The percentage of patients with an "excellent" or "good" outcome was significantly higher in the ticlopidine group (92%) than in the placebo group (79%). In addition, no significant increase in hemorrhagic complications was associated with ticlopidine treatment.

Ischemic Heart Disease. The use of antiplatelet drugs in patients with ischemic heart disease may slow progression of atherogenesis and thrombogenesis.[50,51] Platelets are thought to play an important role in the progression of the pathogenesis and clinical manifestations of coronary artery disease.[20,52] Although the exact mechanism of platelet involvement in the pathogenesis of coronary artery disease is not known, decreased platelet survival, increased adhesiveness of platelets, and hyperaggregability have been observed.[53,54]

Measurement of platelet-specific proteins, such as platelet factor 4 and β-thromboglobulin, provides a method of determining platelet activation in vivo. These proteins have been reported to be elevated in patients with coronary artery disease or those predisposed to its development.[55-57] Ugarte et al.[58] measured plasma concentrations of platelet factor 4 in 12 healthy subjects, 15 patients with angiographically proven coronary artery disease receiving traditional antianginal therapy, and 8 patients with ischemic heart disease treated with both ticlopidine and traditional therapy.

Platelet factor 4 concentrations were significantly lower in the ticlopidine group than in the healthy subjects or the patients receiving only traditional therapy. The authors concluded that the constant platelet activation that occurs in the coronary circulation can be prevented with ticlopidine.

In contrast, a study by Berglund et al.[59] showed that serum concentrations of platelet factor 4, β-thromboglobulin, and fibrinogen in patients with stable angina pectoris were unaffected after eight weeks of treatment with ticlopidine hydrochloride (500 mg daily).

Studies have shown that there is increased platelet reactivity during effort-induced angina in patients with coronary artery disease.[60,61] Reactive platelets release thromboxane A_2, causing coronary artery vasospasm and platelet aggregation.[61,62] In animal studies of artificial coronary artery stenosis, agents that inhibit platelet function have reversed flow reduction caused by platelet aggregates.

Studies assessing the use of ticlopidine in patients with chronic stable angina have failed to show any significant improvement in the objective indices of myocardial ischemia (Table 2).[63,64] These findings agree with earlier studies that demonstrated no improvement in exercise tolerance with use of other platelet inhibitors in patients with chronic stable angina.[66-68]

In contrast, ticlopidine combined with conventional antianginal therapy has been shown to decrease both vascular death and nonfatal myocardial infarction in patients with unstable angina compared with conventional treatment alone.[65] It should be noted that the intent of this trial was not to show that ticlopidine is an alternative to aspirin in reducing vascular death and nonfatal myocardial infarction but rather to evaluate the effects of an antiplatelet agent with a mechanism of action distinctly different from that of aspirin.

Myocardial Infarction. Increased platelet activity and shortened platelet survival have been implicated in the evolution of an acute myocardial infarction.[69,70] The effects of ticlopidine on platelet function, coagulation, fibrinolysis, and infarct size have been evaluated in patients with acute myocardial infarction.[71] Ticlopidine treatment was associated with significantly lower serum concentrations of creatine kinase MB isoenzyme and aspartate aminotransferase, which were used to estimate infarct size. The authors suggest that a smaller infarct size is probable secondary to improved microcirculation in the marginal infarction area. Coagulation and fibrinolysis were unaffected by ticlopidine.

Aortocoronary Saphenous Vein Bypass Grafts. Coronary artery bypass grafting using an autogenous vein is the procedure of choice in patients who require surgery for an obstructed artery. The role of antiplatelet therapy in maintaining graft patency is well recognized. The use of aspirin in combination with dipyridamole has been shown to improve graft pa-

Table 2.
Clinical Trials of Ticlopidine in Ischemic Heart Disease[a]

Reference	No. Patients	Daily Dosage Regimen	Study Design	Duration of Therapy	Outcome
58	12 (Controls)	No therapy	O	48 hr	Serum concentrations of platelet factor 4 decreased in patients receiving ticlopidine ($p < 0.01$)
	15 (CAD)	Traditional therapy (i.e., nitroglycerin)			
	8 (CAD)	Traditional therapy + ticlopidine HCl 500 mg q.d. for 48 hr			
59	21	Ticlopidine HCl 500 mg	R, DB, 2-wk placebo run-in	8 wk	Serum concentrations of platelet factor 4, β-thromboglobulin, and fibrinogen unaffected by ticlopidine
	17	Placebo			
63	30	Ticlopidine HCl 500 mg Placebo	DB, C	4 wk	No significant effect on exercise time, time to ST-segment depression, maximal ST-segment depression, heart rate, or rate–pressure product compared with placebo
64	38	Ticlopidine HCl 500 mg Placebo	R, DB, 2-wk placebo run-in	8 wk	ADP-induced platelet aggregation inhibited by ticlopidine; no difference in exercise tolerance or maximal ST-segment depression compared with placebo
65	314	Ticlopidine HCl 500 mg + conventional antianginal therapy	R, OB	6 mo	Vascular death or nonfatal MI: control, 13.6%; ticlopidine, 7.3%; risk reduction of 46.3% ($p = 0.009$)
	338	Conventional therapy			Fatal and nonfatal MI: control, 10.9%; ticlopidine, 5.1%; risk reduction of 53.2% ($p = 0.006$)

[a]CAD = coronary artery disease, R = randomized, DB = double-blind, C = crossover, OB = observer-blind, MI = myocardial infarction, O = open-label, ADP = adenosine diphosphate.

tency compared with placebo.[72]

The effect of ticlopidine on the patency rates of aortocoronary bypass grafts has been investigated (Table 3).[73-76] Pfluger et al.[75] reported that ticlopidine-treated patients experienced a greater frequency of bleeding without an improvement in graft patency compared with placebo-treated patients. In this study, antiplatelet therapy began three days before surgery and continued for three months after surgery. In contrast, Chevigne et al.[76] and Limet et al.[74] reported increased graft patency rates in ticlopidine-treated patients compared with placebo-treated patients. In both of these trials, treatment was instituted postoperatively and no serious hemorrhagic complications were reported. Rothlin et al.[73] compared ticlopidine with acenocoumarol, an anticoagulant, in the prevention of aortocoronary bypass graft occlusion. The average patency rate per patient was 84% in the group receiving ticlopidine and 82% in the group receiving acenocoumarol.

The results of these studies suggest the following: (1) ticlopidine is as effective as oral anticoagulants for the prevention of aortocoronary bypass graft occlusion, (2) ticlopidine is effective in increasing the patency rate of aortocoronary bypass grafts compared with placebo, and (3) ticlopidine therapy should not be instituted preoperatively because of the increased risk of bleeding complications.

Peripheral Vascular Disease. Peripheral atherosclerotic disease is characterized by intermittent claudication caused by progressive narrowing or vasospasm of a peripheral artery. Platelets release growth factors that stimulate division of vascular smooth muscle cells and enhance the formation of collagen and cholesterol, resulting in the formation of atherosclerotic plaques. Continued platelet adherence to these plaques causes progressive narrowing of the lumen. Moreover, additional narrowing of the vessel lumen can occur as thromboxane A_2 produced in the plaques initiates spasm of the vessel. Serum concentrations of indicators of platelet activation, such as platelet factor 4 and β-thromboglobulin, are elevated in patients with arterial occlusive disorders. Aspirin combined with dipyridamole has been shown to significantly decrease disease progression compared with placebo or aspirin alone.[77]

Ticlopidine has been reported to have beneficial effects on platelet function in patients with arterial oc-

Table 3.
Clinical Trials of Ticlopidine in Aortocoronary Saphenous Vein Bypass Grafts[a]

Reference	No. Patients	Daily Dosage Regimen	Study Design	Duration of Therapy	Outcome
73	78	Ticlopidine HCl 500 mg	R	Started on postoperative day 1 and continued for 3 mo	No significant difference in patency rate: ticlopidine, 84%; acenocoumarol, 82%
	71	Acenocoumarol (adjusted to a prothrombin time of 20–25% of normal)		Started on postoperative day 2 or 3 and continued for 3 mo	
74	87	Ticlopidine HCl 500 mg	R, DB	Started on postoperative day 2 and continued for 3 mo	Graft occlusion rate on day 10: ticlopidine, 7.1%; placebo, 13.4% ($p < 0.05$) Graft occlusion rate on day 180: ticlopidine, 15.0%; placebo, 24.0% ($p < 0.02$)
	86	Placebo		12 mo	Graft occlusion rate on day 360: ticlopidine, 15.9%; placebo, 26.1% ($p < 0.01$)
75	136	Ticlopidine HCl 500 mg	R, DB	Started 3 days before surgery and continued for 3 mo after surgery	Patency rates: ticlopidine, 79%; placebo, 81% Postoperative hemorrhage: ticlopidine, 2364 ± 918 mL; placebo, 1559 ± 218 mL ($p < 0.001$)
	155	Placebo			
76	75	Ticlopidine HCl 500 mg	R, DB	Started on postoperative day 1 and continued for 3 mo	Graft attrition rate excluding discordant biological data: ticlopidine, 7.1%; placebo, 21.8% ($p < 0.02$)
	75	Placebo			

[a]R = randomized, DB = double-blind.

clusive disease of the lower limbs.[78] Several studies have addressed whether ticlopidine favorably affects measures of clinical improvement such as walking distance, Doppler ankle-pressure indices, and epithelial regeneration (Table 4). Two studies[79,80] that assessed the clinical effectiveness of ticlopidine in peripheral atherosclerotic disease failed to demonstrate any clinical benefits. However, other investigators have reported that ticlopidine does provide clinical improvement in patients suffering from peripheral vascular disease.[81-83]

Randi et al.[81] reported that, compared with nicotinate, ticlopidine hydrochloride at higher dosages (750 mg daily), significantly increased walking distance in patients with peripheral atherosclerotic disease. Subsequently, two double-blind placebo-controlled trials using standard dosages of ticlopidine reported significant improvement in walking distance compared with placebo.[82,83]

Additionally, ticlopidine has been reported to improve epithelialization and healing of ischemic leg ulcers in patients with chronic arterial occlusive disease compared with placebo.[84,85]

Most often, intermittent claudification associated

Table 4.
Clinical Trials of Ticlopidine in Peripheral Vascular Disease[a]

Reference	No. Patients	Daily Dosage Regimen	Study Design	Duration of Therapy	Outcome
78	14	Ticlopidine HCl 500 mg Placebo	DB, C	60 days therapy before crossover	ADP-, collagen-, and PAF-induced platelet aggregation inhibited by ticlopidine
79	12	Ticlopidine HCl 500 mg Placebo	SB, C	4 wk of placebo, 4 wk ($n = 6$) or 16 wk ($n = 4$) of ticlopidine, and 4 wk of placebo	No effect on coagulation; ADP-induced platelet aggregation inhibited by ticlopidine; no improvement in walking distance
80	25 26	Ticlopidine HCl 500 mg Placebo	R, DB, 4-wk placebo run-in	1 yr	ADP-, collagen-, and fibrinogen-induced platelet aggregation inhibited by ticlopidine; no change in walking distance, peak and resting calf flow
81	10 10	Ticlopidine HCl 750 mg Nicotinate 900 mg	O	3 mo	Mean ± S.D. percentage increase in walking distance from baseline at 90 days: ticlopidine, 65.2 ± 21.0% ($p = 0.02$); nicotinate, 47.6 ± 26.5% (NS)
82	63 69	Ticlopidine HCl 500 mg Placebo	R, DB	6 mo	Subjective improvement: ticlopidine, 84%; placebo, 44% ($p < 0.001$) Improvement in Doppler studies: ticlopidine, 56%; placebo, 30% ($p < 0.01$)
83	83 86	Ticlopidine HCl 500 mg Placebo	R, DB	6 mo	Improved walking distance: ticlopidine, 56.5%; placebo, 39.7% ($p = 0.02$)
84	93 100	Ticlopidine HCl 500 mg Placebo	R, DB	6 wk	Healing of vascular leg ulcers and subjective improvement significantly greater with ticlopidine
85	14 12	Ticlopidine HCl 1 g for 1 wk followed by 750 mg for 1 wk Placebo	R, DB	2 wk	Improvement in leg ulcers (graded 1–7): ticlopidine, 3.0 ± 2.1; placebo, 5.2 ± 1.9 ($p < 0.05$)
86	338 349	Ticlopidine HCl 500 mg Placebo	R, DB	5 yr	Total mortality: ticlopidine, 18.5%; placebo, 26.1% ($p = 0.015$)

[a]DB = double-blind, C = crossover, SB = single-blind, R = randomized, O = open-label, ADP = adenosine diphosphate, PAF = platelet-activating factor, NS = not significant.

with arteriosclerosis obliterans is a manifestation of a generalized arteriosclerotic process, and mortality usually results from cardiovascular or cerebrovascular pathology. The Swedish Ticlopidine Multicentre Study (STIMS) was a double-blind, placebo-controlled trial designed to determine the effect of ticlopidine on the incidence of myocardial infarction and stroke in 687 patients with intermittent claudication.[86] All patients were monitored and treated for known cardiovascular risk factors, encouraged to abstain from smoking, and asked to not use aspirin-containing products. On-treatment analysis (excludes patients who never received medication or endpoints that occurred more than 15 days after treatment was discontinued) showed that significantly fewer endpoints (i.e., myocardial infarction, stroke, transient ischemic attack) had occurred in the ticlopidine-treated group (47 versus 76, $p = 0.017$). However, intention-to-treat analysis showed that the number of endpoints reached (99 for placebo-treated group versus 89 for ticlopidine-treated group) did not differ significantly between the groups ($p = 0.24$). Similar to the CATS and TASS, diarrhea was the most common adverse effect associated with ticlopidine use; reversible neutropenia was reported in seven patients in this study.[86]

Although results from earlier trials are conflicting, more recent experience suggests that ticlopidine exerts a beneficial effect on ischemic ulcers and pain-free or maximal walking distance and reduces mortality in patients with chronic arterial occlusive disease.

Diabetes Mellitus. Patients with diabetes mellitus suffer from an excess of thromboembolic vascular disorders. The pathogenesis of these thrombotic tendencies involves platelet, coagulative, and fibrinolytic abnormalities. These platelet abnormalities, such as a shortened platelet life span, increased platelet adhesiveness, and an increased sensitivity to platelet aggregants,[87-89] have prompted the investigation of ticlopidine's role in this disease state.

Three studies assessed the effects of ticlopidine and placebo in diabetic patients with regard to blood rheology and platelet function (Table 5).[90-92] Placebo treatment was not associated with any significant change in rheologic or platelet functions; however, treatment with ticlopidine significantly increased the threshold concentration of ADP required for platelet aggregation and significantly lowered the concentration of β-

Table 5.
Clinical Trials of Ticlopidine in Diabetes Mellitus[a]

Reference	No. Patients	Daily Dosage Regimen	Study Design	Duration of Therapy	Outcome
90	21	Ticlopidine HCl 500 mg	PC	12 wk of placebo followed by 12 wk of ticlopidine	Significant decrease in blood viscosity with ticlopidine
91	20	Ticlopidine HCl 400 mg	SB, PC	3 mo of placebo followed by 3 mo of ticlopidine	Significant decrease in blood viscosity, increase in erythrocyte deformability, and decrease in ADP-induced platelet aggregation with ticlopidine; no change in impaired left ventricular function
92	11 11	Ticlopidine HCl 500 mg Placebo	R, DB	6 mo	Significant reduction in platelet aggregation with ticlopidine; no improvement in renal function
93	220 215	Ticlopidine HCl 500 mg Placebo	R, DB	3 yr	In insulin-dependent patients ticlopidine significantly reduced progression of microaneurysms compared with placebo as reflected by the mean ± S.D. microaneurysmal slope: ticlopidine, 0.48 ± 5.79; placebo, 1.44 ± 4.67 ($p = 0.03$) Overall progression of retinopathy less severe in ticlopidine-treated group ($p = 0.04$)

[a]PC = placebo-controlled, SB = single-blind, R = randomized, DB = double-blind, ADP = adenosine diphosphate.

thromboglobulin. Plasma and whole blood viscosity were also significantly lowered. However, these studies failed to demonstrate that short-term (6–12 months) treatment with ticlopidine arrests or alters the progression of diabetic retinopathy,[90] nephropathy,[88,92] neuropathy,[90] or impairment of left ventricular wall motion associated with diabetic cardiomyopathy.[91]

In contrast, the Ticlopidine Microangiopathy of Diabetics (TIMAD) study was designed to determine the effect of long-term treatment with ticlopidine hydrochloride (500 mg daily) on the progression of nonproliferative diabetic retinopathy.[93] Compared with placebo, ticlopidine significantly reduced the yearly progression of microaneurysms in insulin-dependent patients. In patients with non-insulin-dependent diabetes, ticlopidine did not significantly reduce microaneurysm progression. In insulin-dependent patients, the number of patients with new vessel involvement was reduced in the ticlopidine-treated group compared with the placebo-treated group; in non-insulin-dependent patients, no difference was noted between the groups.

The TIMAD study results are consistent with those found in the Dipyridamole–Aspirin Microangiopathy of Diabetics (DAMAD) study[94]; however, results with aspirin and aspirin combined with dipyridamole were favorable in both insulin-dependent and non-insulin-dependent diabetics. In the TIMAD study, new vessel involvement was less common in ticlopidine-treated patients than in placebo-treated patients; however, in the DAMAD study, aspirin (alone or combined with dipyridamole) did not differ from placebo in reducing new vessel involvement.

Other Indications. Ticlopidine has been shown in vitro to have an antisickling effect on red blood cells.[95] Cabannes et al.[96] demonstrated that, among patients with sickle cell disease, those receiving ticlopidine had fewer crises and shorter duration of crises than those receiving placebo. Hematologic examination showed a reduction in serum bilirubin concentration in ticlopidine-treated patients compared with placebo-treated patients. This finding is consistent with ticlopidine's antihemolytic effect. In contrast, Semple et al.[97] were unable to demonstrate an improvement in platelet survival time or a reduction in the number of vaso-occlusive crises in patients with sickle cell disease who were treated with ticlopidine.

The thromboprophylactic effect of ticlopidine was investigated in patients with arteriovenous fistulas for hemodialysis.[98] Of the 36 patients completing this trial, 10 patients, eight of whom received placebo, developed occlusion of their fistula ($p < 0.05$). Other authors have reported a decrease in platelet adhesiveness to dialysis membranes associated with ticlopidine use.[99,100]

The effect of ticlopidine on thromboembolic events in patients with implanted pacemakers programmed in the ventricle-ventricle-inhibit mode has been studied.[101] Significantly fewer thromboembolic events occurred in ticlopidine-treated patients compared with patients who received no treatment. Adverse effects occurred in only 12% of patients treated with ticlopidine; this result is probably due to the lower daily dosage used.

Table 6.
Adverse Effects of Ticlopidine[a]

Adverse Effect	No. (%) Patients CATS	No. (%) Patients TASS
Diarrhea	113 (21.5)	310 (20.4)
Dyspepsia	...	191 (12.6)
Nausea	...	169 (11.1)
Gastrointestinal pain	...	110 (7.2)
Gastritis	...	13 (0.9)
Peptic ulcer	...	12 (0.8)
Bleeding disorders	34 (6.5)	137 (9.0)
Rash	78 (14.9)	180 (11.9)
Urticaria	...	30 (2.0)
Abnormal liver function	23 (4.4)	...
Neutropenia	11 (2.1)	13 (0.9)
Any adverse experience	283 (53.9)	945 (62.3)

[a]Adapted from references 48 and 49. Adverse effects reported in 1228 (60%) of 2046 patients exposed to ticlopidine. CATS = Canadian-American Ticlopidine Study, TASS = Ticlopidine–Aspirin Stroke Study.

Adverse Effects

Adverse effects of ticlopidine are listed in Table 6. In the two largest clinical trials of ticlopidine to date, more than 50% of patients who received the drug experienced an adverse event. The most serious adverse event reported was neutropenia. Neutropenia occurred in approximately 1% of the patients. After the drug was withdrawn, granulocyte counts returned to baseline within three weeks. Ticlopidine-induced agranulocytosis is most likely caused by direct toxicity to marrow cells; however, some believe it is an immunologic reaction.[102]

The adverse effects reported to occur most frequently were those associated with the gastrointestinal tract, including diarrhea, nausea, vomiting, and abdominal cramps. Concomitant administration with food or dosage reduction appears to offer some relief. Other adverse reactions include elevation of liver function test results, skin rashes, and an increase in total serum cholesterol concentration by approximately 9%.

Drug Interactions

Ticlopidine appears to reversibly inhibit the metabolic clearance of theophylline. The pharmacokinetics of theophylline were determined before institution of ticlopidine hydrochloride therapy (250 mg every 12 hours for 10 days), 12 hours after the last dose of ticlopidine on day 10, and one month later. Blood samples were obtained from 10 healthy male volunteers after an overnight fast and administration of 5 mg/kg of theophylline oral solution. Three months later, the same methodology was used to determine theophylline pharmacokinetics in the same subjects after placebo administration. Ticlopidine significantly reduced total body clearance of theophylline compared with baseline; serum theophylline concentrations returned to initial values within 30 days after ticlopidine withdrawal. No change in theophylline clearance was observed during placebo treatment.[103]

An interaction between cyclosporine and ticlopidine in an 18-year-old corticosteroid-dependent boy with nephrotic syndrome has been described.[104] Cyclosporine was administered at a dosage of 5.6 mg/kg/day during periods of relapse, and the resulting mean ± S.D. whole blood cyclosporine concentration was 455 ± 120 ng/mL. Ticlopidine hydrochloride (500 mg daily) was started in a effort to prevent thrombosis. After one month of ticlopidine treatment, the mean cyclosporine concentration fell to 218 ± 83 ng/mL and the boy required an increase in cyclosporine dosage to 7.2 mg/kg/day; however, proteinuria persisted. Ticlopidine was then discontinued and, one week later, his mean cyclosporine concentration increased to 353 ± 103 ng/mL and proteinuria resolved. Six months later, the patient was taking cyclosporine 6.7 mg/kg daily (mean whole blood cyclosporine concentration, 172 ± 33 ng/mL); when he was rechallenged with ticlopidine, his mean whole blood cyclosporine concentration fell to 78 ± 2.7 ng/mL.

Prolongation of bleeding time caused by ticlopidine therapy is reportedly antagonized by both orally and intravenously administered corticosteroids.[105] Ten healthy subjects who received a seven-day course of ticlopidine hydrochloride (250 mg twice daily) as monotherapy were randomly selected to receive concomitant oral prednisone (15 mg twice daily for seven days) or a single 20-mg injection of methylprednisolone given on day 8. All patients ultimately received both corticosteroid treatments separated by a one-week washout period. Both corticosteroid treatments resulted in a significant reduction in bleeding time without affecting ADP-induced platelet aggregation. The proposed mechanism was reduced endothelial prostacyclin secretion resulting from corticosteroid-induced vasoconstriction.

In healthy male subjects, the bioavailability of ticlopidine was assessed when it was administered in the fasting and postprandial states and after antacid administration.[106] After a high-fat breakfast, both the rate and extent of absorption of a single 250-mg dose of ticlopidine hydrochloride were enhanced relative to the fasting state. The relative bioavailability of ticlopidine was increased by 20% after a high-fat meal and decreased by the same amount during antacid treatment.

The effect of ticlopidine combined with aspirin on bleeding time has been assessed.[39,107] Six patients with coronary artery disease were given ticlopidine hydrochloride (250 mg twice daily) for seven days; on the seventh day, they were also given 500 mg of intravenous aspirin.[39] The mean ± S.D. bleeding times at baseline, after seven days of ticlopidine therapy, and after intravenous administration of aspirin were 7.4 ± 0.6, 9.2 ± 0.8, and 15.0 ± 0.7 minutes, respectively. Bleeding times measured during treatment were significantly different ($p < 0.05$) from baseline values. In addition, bleeding time after combined treatment with ticlopidine and aspirin on day 7 was significantly prolonged compared with bleeding time after treatment with ticlopidine alone. No bleeding episodes were reported during the study. Similar effects on bleeding time were demonstrated in patients suffering from transient ischemic attacks.[107] However, hemorrhagic complications were observed in 34.8% of the patients receiving combination therapy compared with 11.8% of patients receiving ticlopidine and 12.5% of patients receiving aspirin.

Dosage and Administration

Ticlopidine hydrochloride is available as a white 250-mg film-coated tablet for oral administration. According to TASS and CATS, the recommended dosage of ticlopidine hydrochloride is 500 mg per day administered in two divided doses, which should be taken with food.[108]

FDA-Approved Labeling

Ticlopidine is indicated for reducing the risk of thrombotic stroke in patients who have experienced a minor stroke, transient ischemic attack, or completed thrombotic stroke. Because of the risk of neutropenia and agranulocytosis, ticlopidine should be reserved for those patients who are intolerant of aspirin.[108]

Contraindications and Use in Pregnancy

Ticlopidine is classified as pregnancy category B according to available animal studies.[15] Studies of rats, mice, and rabbits receiving oral doses of 50, 100, 200, and 400 mg/kg (rats only) have not demonstrated ticlopidine to cause teratogenic effects. At the highest dose in rats, impairment of sternebral calcification and a reduction in fetal growth rate were demonstrated.[15] No controlled studies have been conducted in pregnant women or women who are breast-feeding; therefore, ticlopidine should be used in these patients only if clearly indicated.[108]

Ticlopidine is contraindicated in patients who have experienced an allergic reaction to the drug, individuals with hematologic disorders or a predisposition to serious bleeding problems, and patients with severe hepatic dysfunction.[108]

Instructions for the Patient

Pharmacists should instruct patients to take ticlopidine with food in an effort to reduce gastrointestinal discomfort. Patients should be warned about the risk, although small (about 1.0%), of developing reversible neutropenia. If neutropenia occurs, it usually does so within the first three months of treatment. Patients should be instructed on the importance of keeping their appointments with the physician and any scheduled appointments for blood tests. Patients should be instructed to watch for unusual bruising and prolonged bleeding and to advise other health professionals that they are taking ticlopidine.[108]

Formulary Recommendations

Ticlopidine represents a new class of antiplatelet agents available for clinical use. Clearly, the acquisition cost of ticlopidine will exceed the cost of aspirin, the only other antiplatelet inhibitor proven effective in reducing the risk of threatened stroke and death. The average wholesale price for a bottle of 30 250-mg tablets of ticlopidine hydrochloride is $39.60.[109] In addition, other costs, such as those associated with the monitoring of hematologic and hepatic function, need to be considered.

Ticlopidine appears to be more or at least as effective as aspirin in the primary prevention and the secondary prevention of stroke after a transient ischemic attack or minor stroke. The experience with long-term safety of ticlopidine in the United States is limited. However, clinical trials and animal studies indicate that ticlopidine is relatively nontoxic. Moreover, ticlopidine has been used for many years in other countries. The frequency of agranulocytosis reported to the Ministry of Health and Welfare in Japan was 0.14% (11 of 7933).[110]

The increased cost of therapy with ticlopidine compared with that of aspirin may limit its general use; however, in women, patients who are intolerant to aspirin, and selected individuals in whom aspirin has not offered any benefit, ticlopidine appears to be a reasonable alternative.

The decision to add ticlopidine to the formulary will be institution-specific. We recommend adding ticlopidine to the formulary; however, its use should be restricted to those patients with documented intolerance of or lack of benefit from aspirin.

Conclusion

Ticlopidine, a new platelet aggregation inhibitor, is an alternative agent for the primary and secondary prevention of stroke. Because of the risk of neutropenia and agranulocytosis and the high costs of therapy, ticlopidine should be reserved for patients who are intolerant of or lack benefit from aspirin.

References

1. De Gaetano G, Cerletti C, Dejana E et al. Current issues in thrombosis prevention with antiplatelet drugs. *Drugs*. 1986; 31:517-49.
2. Bousser MG, Eschege E, Haguenau M et al. "AICLA" controlled trial of aspirin and dipyridamole in the secondary prevention of athero-thrombotic cerebral ischemia. *Stroke*. 1983; 14(1):5-14.
3. Canadian Cooperative Study Group. A randomized trial of aspirin and sulfinpyrazone in threatened stroke. *N Engl J Med*. 1978; 299:53-9.
4. Fields WS, Lemak NA, Frankowski RF et al. Controlled trial of aspirin in cerebral ischemia. *Stroke*. 1977; 8:301-16.
5. The Dutch TIA Trial Study Group. A comparison of two doses of aspirin (30 mg vs. 283 mg a day) in patients after a transient ischemic attack or minor stroke. *N Engl J Med*. 1991; 325:1261-6.
6. Antiplatelet Trialists' Collaboration. Secondary prevention of vascular disease by prolonged antiplatelet treatment. *Br Med J*. 1988; 296:320-31.
7. ESPS Group. European stroke prevention study. *Stroke*. 1990; 21:1122-30.
8. UK-TIA Study Group. United Kingdom transient ischemic attack (UK-TIA) aspirin trial: interim report. *Br Med J*. 1988; 296:316-20.
9. Hershey LA. Stroke prevention in women: role of aspirin versus ticlopidine. *Am J Med*. 1991; 91:288-92.
10. Canner PL. Aspirin in coronary heart disease: comparison of six clinical trials. *Isr J Med Sci*. 1983; 19:413-23.
11. Veterans Administration Cooperative Trial: anticoagulation in acute myocardial infarction. *JAMA*. 1973; 225:724-9.
12. The Steering Committee of the Physicians' Health Study Research Group. Preliminary report: findings from the aspirin component of the ongoing Physicians' Health Study. *N Engl J Med*. 1988; 318:262-7.
13. The American-Canadian Cooperative Study Group. Persantine aspirin trial in cerebral ischemia, part II: endpoint results. *Stroke*. 1985; 16:406-15.
14. Thebault J, Blatrix C, Blanchard J et al. Effects of ticlopidine, a new platelet aggregation inhibitor in man. *Clin Pharmacol Ther*. 1975; 18:485-90.
15. Panak E, Maffrand JP, Picard-Fraire C et al. Ticlopidine: a promise for the prevention and treatment of thrombosis and its complications. *Haemostasis*. 1983; 13(Suppl 1):1-54.
16. Packham MA. Platelet function inhibitors. *Thromb Haemost*. 1983; 50:610-9.
17. Fuster V, Chesebro JH. Current concepts of thrombogenesis: role of platelets. *Mayo Clin Proc*. 1981; 56:102-12.
18. Mustard JF, Packham MA, Kinlough-Rathbone RL et al. Fibrinogen and ADP-induced platelet aggregation. *Blood*. 1978; 52:453-66.
19. Nachman RL, Leung LK. Complex formation of platelet membrane glycoproteins IIb and IIa with fibrinogen. *J Clin Invest*. 1982; 69:263-9.
20. Mehta J, Mehta P. Role of blood platelets and prostaglandins in coronary artery disease. *Am J Cardiol*. 1981; 48:366-73.
21. Lecrubier C, Horellou MH, Samama M. Study of platelet aggregation induced by platelet activating factor (PAF) after administration of ticlopidine or aspirin. *Agents Actions*. 1983; 13(1):77-80.
22. Saltiel E, Ward A. Ticlopidine: a review of its pharmacodynamic and pharmacokinetic properties and therapeutic efficacy in platelet-dependent disease states. *Drugs*. 1987; 34:222-62.
23. Hardisty RM, Powling MJ, Nokes TJC. The action of ticlopidine on human platelets. *Thromb Haemost*. 1990; 64:150-5.
24. Bruno J. The mechanisms of action of ticlopidine. *Thromb Res*. 1983; (Suppl IV):59-67.
25. Knudsen JB, Gormsen J. The effect of ticlopidine on platelet function in normal volunteers and in patients with platelet hyperaggregability in vitro. *Thromb Res*. 1979; 16:663-71.
26. Lips JPM, Sixma JJ, Schiphorst ME. The effect of ticlopidine administration to humans on the binding of adenosine diphosphate to blood platelets. *Thromb Res*. 1980; 17:19-27.
27. Tomokawa M, Ashida S, Koji K et al. Anti-thrombotic action of ticlopidine, a new platelet aggregation inhibitor. *Thromb Res*. 1978; 12:1157-64.
28. Ashida S, Abiko Y. Mode of action of ticlopidine in inhibition of platelet aggregation in the rat. *Thromb Haemost*. 1979;

41:436-49.
29. Bruno JJ, Yang D, Taylor LA. Role of platelet c'AMP and prostaglandin synthesis in platelet aggregation inhibition by ticlopidine hydrochloride. *Thromb Haemost*. 1981; 46:66. Abstract.
30. Conard J, Lecrubier C, Scarabin PY et al. Effects of long-term administration of ticlopidine on platelet function and hemostatic variables. *Thromb Res*. 1980; 20:143-8.
31. DiMinno G, Cerbone AM, Mattioli PL et al. Functionally thrombasthenic state in normal platelets following the administration of ticlopidine. *J Clin Invest*. 1985; 75:328-38.
32. David JL, Monfort F, Herion F et al. Compared effects of three dose levels of ticlopidine on platelet function in normal subjects. *Thromb Res*. 1979; 14:35-9.
33. Lee H, Paton RC, Ruan C et al. The in vitro effect of ticlopidine on fibrinogen and factor VII binding to human platelets. *Thromb Haemost*. 1981; 46:590-2.
34. Dunn FW, Soria J, Thomaidis A et al. In vivo effect of ticlopidine on fibrinogen-platelet cofactor activity and binding of fibrinogen to platelets. *Agents Actions*. 1984; 15(Suppl):97-104.
35. DiMinno G, Palladino M, Pannain M et al. Normalization of the abnormally high fibrinogen binding to platelets from retinopathic diabetics. *Thromb Haemost*. 1985; 54:64. Abstract.
36. Smith JB, Ingerman CM, Silver MJ. Malondialdehyde as an indicator of prostaglandin production by human platelets. *J Lab Clin Med*. 1976; 88:167-72.
37. Lagarde M, Ghazi I, Dechavanne M. Effects of ticlopidine on platelet prostaglandin metabolism: possible consequences for prostacyclin production. *Prostaglandins Med*. 1979; 2:433-40.
38. Chap H, Simon MF, Douste-Blazy L. Effect of ticlopidine on arachidonic acid metabolism in platelet phospholipids in vitro. *Biochem Pharmacol*. 1981; 30(12):1463-8.
39. De Caterina R, Sicari R, Bernini W et al. Benefit/risk profile of combined antiplatelet therapy with ticlopidine and aspirin. *Thromb Haemost*. 1991; 65:504-10.
40. Bruno JJ, Chang LF, McSpadden MM et al. The effect of oral ticlopidine on arachidonic acid products in human platelets. *Agents Actions*. 1984; 15(Suppl):76-87.
41. Ellis DJ, Roe RL, Bruno JJ et al. The effects of ticlopidine hydrochloride on bleeding time and platelet function in man. *Thromb Haemost*. 1981; 46:176. Abstract.
42. Daveloose D, Sablayrolles M, Molle D et al. Interaction of ticlopidine with the erythrocyte membrane. *Biochem Pharmacol*. 1982; 31:3949-54.
43. Picard-Fraire C. Pharmacokinetic and metabolic characteristics of ticlopidine in relation to its inhibitory properties on platelet function. *Agents Actions*. 1984; 15(Suppl):68-75.
44. Picard-Fraire C. Ticlopidine hydrochloride: relationship between dose, kinetics, plasma concentration and effect on platelet function. *Thromb Res*. 1983; (Suppl IV):119-28.
45. Teitelbaum P, Gabzuda TG, Koretz SH et al. Pharmacokinetics of ticlopidine hydrochloride in young and old normal adult subjects following single and multiple dosing. *J Pharm Sci*. 1987; 76:599.
46. Tohgi H. The effect of ticlopidine on TIA compared with aspirin: a double blind, twelve-month follow-up study. *Agents Actions*. 1984; 15(Suppl):279-82.
47. Ono H, Mizukami M, Kitamura H et al. Subarachnoid hemorrhage. *Agents Actions*. 1984; 15(Suppl):259-72.
48. Hass WK, Easton JD, Adams HP et al. Ticlopidine Aspirin Stroke Study Group (TASS): a randomized trial comparing ticlopidine hydrochloride with aspirin for the prevention of stroke in high-risk patients. *N Engl J Med*. 1989; 321:501-7.
49. Gent M, Easton JD, Hachinski VC et al. The Canadian-American ticlopidine study (CATS) in thromboembolic stroke. *Lancet*. 1989; 2:1215-20.
50. Lewis HD, Davis JW, Archibald DG et al. Protective effects of aspirin against acute myocardial infarction and death in men with unstable angina. *N Engl J Med*. 1983; 309:396-403.
51. Gitler B, Spielman E. Efficacy of antiplatelet drugs in the maintenance of aortocoronary vein bypass graft patency. *Am Heart J*. 1983; 106:563-70.
52. Moncada S, Vane JR. Arachidonic acid metabolites and the interactions between platelets and blood vessel walls. *N Engl J Med*. 1979; 300:1142-7.
53. Ross R, Glomset JA. The pathogenesis of atherosclerosis. *N Engl J Med*. 1976; 295:420-5.
54. Steele PP, Weily HS, Davies JW et al. Platelet function studies in coronary artery disease. *Circulation*. 1973; 48:1194-200.
55. White CG, Marouf AA. Platelet factor 4 in coronary artery disease. *J Clin Lab Med*. 1981; 97:369-78.
56. Smitherman TC, Milam M, Woo J et al. Elevated beta-thromboglobulin in peripheral venous blood of patients with acute myocardial ischaemia: direct evidence for enhanced platelet reactivity in vivo. *Am J Cardiol*. 1981; 48:395-402.
57. Nichols AB, Owen J, Kaplan KL et al. Fibrinopeptide, platelet factor 4, and beta-thromboglobulin levels in coronary heart disease. *Blood*. 1982; 60:650-4.
58. Ugarte M, Teresa E, Pilar L et al. Intracoronary platelet activation in ischemic heart disease: effects of ticlopidine. *Am Heart J*. 1985; 109:738-43.
59. Berglund U, von Shenck H, Walletin L. Effects of ticlopidine on platelet function in men with stable angina pectoris. *Thromb Haemost*. 1985; 54:808-12.
60. Green LH, Seroppian E, Handin RI. Platelet activation during exercise-induced myocardial ischemia. *N Engl J Med*. 1980; 302:193-7.
61. Kumpuris AG, Luchi RJ, Waddell CC et al. Production of circulating platelet aggregates by exercise in coronary patients. *Circulation*. 1980; 61:62-5.
62. Fox KM, Jonathan A, Selwyn A. Effects of platelet inhibition on myocardial ischaemia. *Lancet*. 1982; 2:727-30.
63. Khurmi NS, Bowles MJ, Raferty EB. Are antiplatelet drugs of value in the management of patients with chronic stable angina? A study with ticlopidine. *Clin Cardiol*. 1986; 9:493-8.
64. Berglund U, Lassvik C, Wallentin L. Effects of the platelet inhibitor ticlopidine on exercise tolerance in stable angina pectoris. *Eur Heart J*. 1987; 8:25-30.
65. Balsano F, Rizzon P, Francsco V et al. Antiplatelet treatment with ticlopidine in unstable angina: controlled multicenter clinical trial. *Circulation*. 1990; 82:17-26.
66. Thaulow E, Dale J, Myrhe E. Effects of a selective thromboxane synthetase inhibitor, dazoxiben, and of acetylsalicylic acid on myocardial ischemia in patients with coronary artery disease. *Am J Cardiol*. 1984; 53:1255-8.
67. Davis JW, Lewis HD, Phillips PE et al. Effect of aspirin on exercise induced angina. *Clin Pharmacol Ther*. 1978; 23:505-10.
68. Frishman WH, Christodoulou J, Weksler B et al. Aspirin therapy in angina pectoris: effects on platelet aggregation, exercise tolerance, and electrocardiographic manifestations of ischaemia. *Am Heart J*. 1976; 92:3-10.
69. Chesebro JH, Fuster V, Byrne J. Improvement of shortened platelet survival half-life from the early to the late phase of myocardial infarction. *Thromb Haemost*. 1981; 46:143. Abstract.
70. Sorkin RP, Tokarsky MJ, Huber-Smith MJ et al. In vivo platelet aggregation and plasma catecholamines in acute myocardial infarction. *Am Heart J*. 1982; 104:1255-61.
71. Knudsen JB, Kjoller E, Skagen K et al. The effect of ticlopidine on platelet functions in acute myocardial infarction. *Thromb Haemost*. 1985; 53:332-6.
72. Chesebro JH, Clements IP, Fuster V et al. A platelet-inhibitor-drug trial in coronary-artery bypass operation: benefit of preoperative dipyridamole and aspirin on early postoperative vein-graft patency. *N Engl J Med*. 1982; 307:73-80.
73. Rothlin ME, Pfluger N, Speiser K et al. Platelet inhibitors versus anticoagulants for prevention of aorto-coronary bypass graft occlusion. *Eur Heart J*. 1985; 6:168-75.
74. Limet R, David JL, Magotteaux P et al. Prevention of aorto-coronary bypass graft occlusion: beneficial effect of ticlopidine on early and late patency rates of venous coro-

nary bypass grafts: a double-blind study. *J Thorac Cardiovasc Surg*. 1987; 94:773-83.
75. Pfluger N, Goebel N, Turina M et al. Influence of the antiaggregant ticlopidine on the patency of aorto-coronary bypass grafts. *Eur Heart J*. 1981; 2:208.
76. Chevigne M, David J-L, Rigo P et al. Effect of ticlopidine on saphenous vein bypass patency rates: a double blind study. *Ann Thorac Surg*. 1984; 37:371-8.
77. Hess H, Ingrisch H, Deichsel G. Drug-induced inhibition of platelet function delays progression of peripheral occlusive arterial disease: a prospective double-blind arteriographically controlled trial. *Lancet*. 1985; 1:415-9.
78. Davi G, Pinto A, Francavilla S et al. Inhibition of platelet function by ticlopidine in atherosclerosis obliterans of the lower limbs. *Thromb Res*. 1985; 40:275-81.
79. Kirstein P, Jogestrand T, Johnsson H et al. Antiaggregatory, physiological and clinical effects of ticlopidine in subjects with peripheral atherosclerosis. *Atherosclerosis*. 1980; 36:471-80.
80. Aukland A, Hurlow RA, George AJ et al. Platelet inhibition with ticlopidine in atherosclerotic intermittent claudication. *J Clin Pathol*. 1982; 35:740-3.
81. Randi ML, Fabris F, Crociani ME et al. Effects of ticlopidine on blood fibrinogen and blood viscosity in peripheral atherosclerotic disease. *Arzneimittelforschung*. 1985; 35:1847-9.
82. Cloarec M, Caillard P, Mouren X. Double-blind clinical trial of ticlopidine versus placebo in peripheral atherosclerotic disease of the legs. *Thromb Res*. 1986; (Suppl VI):160. Abstract.
83. Arcan AJ, Destors JM. Controlled clinical trial of ticlopidine in patients suffering from intermittent claudication. *Thromb Res*. 1986; (Suppl VI):159. Abstract.
84. Katsumura T, Mishima Y, Kamiya K et al. Therapeutic effect of ticlopidine, a new inhibitor of platelet aggregation, on chronic arterial occlusive diseases, a double-blind study versus placebo. *Angiology*. 1982; 33:357-67.
85. Bourde C, Eschwege E, Verry M. Controlled clinical trial of an antiaggregating agent, ticlopidine, in vascular ulcers of the leg. *Thromb Haemost*. 1981; 46:91.
86. Janzon L, Bergqvist D, Boberg J et al. Prevention of myocardial infarction and stroke in patients with intermittent claudication; effects of ticlopidine: results from STIMS, the Swedish Ticlopidine Multicentre Study. *J Intern Med*. 1990; 227:301-8.
87. Tindall H, Paton RC, Zuzel M et al. Platelet life-span in diabetics with and without retinopathy. *Thromb Res*. 1981; 21:641-8.
88. Bern MM. Platelet function in diabetes mellitus. *Diabetes*. 1978; 27:342-50.
89. Fuller JH, Keen H, Jarret RJ et al. Haemostatic variables associated with diabetes and its complications. *Br Med J*. 1979; 2:964-6.
90. Neumann V, Cove DH, Shapiro LM et al. Effect of ticlopidine on platelet function and blood rheology in diabetes mellitus. *Clin Hemorheol*. 1983; 3:13-21.
91. Shapiro LM, Cove DH, Trethowan N et al. Clinical trials of an antiplatelet agent, ticlopidine, in diabetes mellitus. *Curr Med Res Opin*. 1983; 8:518-23.
92. Nyberg G, Larsson O, Westberg NG et al. A platelet aggregation inhibitor—ticlopidine—in diabetic nephropathy: a randomized double blind study. *Clin Nephrol*. 1984; 21:184-7.
93. The TIMAD Study Group. Ticlopidine treatment reduces the progression of nonproliferative diabetic retinopathy. *Arch Ophthalmol*. 1990; 108:1577-83.
94. The DAMAD Study Group. Effects of aspirin alone and aspirin plus dipyridamole in early diabetic retinopathy: a multicenter randomized controlled clinical trial. *Diabetes*. 1989; 38:491-8.
95. Sablayrolles M, Wajcman H, Castaigne JP et al. Membrane expansion as a mechanism explaining the antisickling effect of ticlopidine observed in vitro. *Am J Hematol*. 1985; 18(2):121-30.
96. Cabannes R, Lonsdorfer J, Castaigne JP et al. Clinical and biological double-blind-study of ticlopidine in preventive treatment of sickle cell disease crises. *Agents Actions*. 1984; 15(Suppl):199-212.
97. Semple MJ, Al-Hasani SF, Kioy P et al. A double-blind trial of ticlopidine in sickle cell disease. *Thromb Haemost*. 1984; 51:303-6.
98. Grontoft K, Mulec H, Gutierrez A et al. Thromboprophylactic effect of ticlopidine in arteriovenous fistulas for haemodialysis. *Scand J Urol Nephrol*. 1985; 19:55-7.
99. Kobayashi K, Maeda K, Koshikawa S et al. Antithrombotic therapy with ticlopidine in chronic renal failure patients on maintenance hemodialysis: a multicenter collaborative double blind study. *Thromb Res*. 1980; 20:255-61.
100. Maeda J, Usuda M, Kawaguchi S et al. Effects of ticlopidine in thrombotic obstruction of A-V shunts and on dialysance of artificial kidneys. *Artif Organs*. 1980; 4:30-3.
101. Fazio S, Santomauro M, Cittadini A et al. Efficacy of ticlopidine in the prevention of thromboembolic events in patients with VVI pacemakers. *PACE*. 1991; 14:168-73.
102. Ono K, Kirohara K, Yoshihara M et al. Agranulocytosis caused by ticlopidine and its mechanism. *Am J Hematol*. 1991; 37:239-42.
103. Colli A, Buccino G, Cocciolo M et al. Ticlopidine-theophylline interaction. *Clin Pharmacol Ther*. 1988; 41:358-62.
104. Birmele B, Lebranchu T, Bagros PH et al. Interaction of cyclosporin and ticlopidine. *Nephrol Dial Transplant*. 1991; 6:150-1.
105. Thebault J, Blatrix C, Blanchard J et al. A possible method to control prolongation of bleeding time under antiplatelet therapy with ticlopidine. *Thromb Haemost*. 1982; 48:6-8.
106. Shah J, Fratis A, Ellis D et al. Effects of food and antacid on absorption of orally administered ticlopidine hydrochloride. *J Clin Pharmacol*. 1990; 30:733-6.
107. Uchiyama S, Stone R, Nagayama T et al. Combination therapy with low dose aspirin and ticlopidine in cerebral ischemia. *Stroke*. 1989; 20:1643-7.
108. Syntex Laboratory. Ticlid package insert. Palo Alto, CA; 1991 Nov.
109. Drug Topics redbook annual pharmacists' reference. Sifton DW, ed. Montvale, NJ: Medical Economics; 1992.
110. Japan Pharmaceutical Information Center (JPC). Ticlopidine hydrochloride. In: Drugs in Japan: ethical drugs. Tokyo: Yakugyoujihou; 1989:653.

Therapy Update

Long-term dobutamine therapy for refractory congestive heart failure

KERRY K. PICKWORTH

Abstract: The proposed benefit of long-term dobutamine therapy is explained, relevant clinical trials are described, and recommendations for this treatment are discussed.

Dobutamine increases cardiac contractility and causes vasodilation with little change in heart rate. It is routinely administered for short periods to relieve exacerbations of congestive heart failure (CHF) in hospitalized patients. Sustained effects have been seen with dobutamine infusions, although the known properties of the drug do not explain these effects. Long-term dobutamine therapy can lessen the symptoms of CHF and improve exercise tolerance and cardiac function. Nine published reports showed consistent improvement in 77 patients treated with multiple infusions of dobutamine. At Ohio State University, long-term dobutamine therapy (typically 5.0–7.5 μg/kg/min infused continuously) is used in patients with refractory CHF and those awaiting heart transplantation. Because the therapy does not prolong survival in most patients, specific endpoints of therapy should be determined for each patient. Because it may cause sudden death, patients receiving this therapy must be carefully monitored.

Long-term use of dobutamine infusion lessens the symptoms of CHF but does not prolong survival.

Index terms: Cardiac drugs; Clinical studies; Dobutamine; Dosage; Dosage schedules; Heart failure; Injections
Clin Pharm. 1992; 11:618-24

Congestive heart failure (CHF) develops in approximately 400,000 persons yearly in the United States.[1,2] Drug therapy for CHF primarily involves diuretics, vasodilators, and inotropic agents. The availability of immunosuppressive agents has allowed heart transplantation to become a treatment alternative for a select group of patients.

Oral inotropic agents have not altered the mortality associated with CHF, and patients with the syndrome generally become refractory to treatment with such agents. Repeated hospitalization and the administration of i.v. medications may be necessary to control symptoms.

Dobutamine is given routinely for short periods to relieve exacerbations of CHF in hospitalized patients, but the long-term use of dobutamine is less well accepted. The clinical experience that has accumulated in the past several years allows some conclusions to be made about the latter form of therapy. This review provides an explanation for the proposed benefit of long-term dobutamine therapy, describes the relevant clinical trials, and discusses recommendations for this treatment.

Properties of Dobutamine

Receptor Activity. The dextrorotatory enantiomer of dobutamine is a β_1- and β_2-adrenergic agonist and an α-adrenergic antagonist.[3-5] The levorotatory enantiomer is a potent α-adrenergic agonist. Because dobutamine is available as a racemic mixture, the α-adrenergic properties of the two enantiomers offset each other, and the mixture's net effect is to increase cardiac contractility (through β_1-adrenergic stimulation) and cause vasodilation (through β_2-adrenergic stimulation) with little change in heart rate (HR).

Pharmacokinetics. The pharmacokinetic properties of dobutamine have been well defined through investigations involving patients with CHF.[6,7] Dobutamine has a mean ± S.D. elimination half-life of 2.4 ± 0.7

KERRY K. PICKWORTH, PHARM.D., is Clinical Assistant Professor, Cardiology, College of Pharmacy, The Ohio State University, Columbus.

Address reprint requests to Dr. Pickworth at The Ohio State University Hospital, Room 368 Doan Hall, 410 West Tenth Avenue, Columbus, OH 43210.

minutes in patients with CHF consistent with functional class 4 of the New York Heart Association (NYHA) classification system. (NYHA functional classes range from 1 to 4, with 4 representing severely symptomatic CHF.) In these patients, plasma dobutamine concentration increases linearly with the rate of drug administration; this suggests linear first-order elimination. Dobutamine is rapidly metabolized by catechol-*O*-methyltransferase to 3-*O*-methyldobutamine, which becomes conjugated before being excreted in the urine.[8] Small amounts of dobutamine may be found in the bile as dobutamine glucuronide. Both metabolites are inactive. Thus, the long-lasting effects of dobutamine that are described in this review cannot be explained by prolonged presence of the drug in serum.

Hemodynamic Effects. Dobutamine is effective in alleviating the symptoms of CHF when given in dosages ranging from 2.5 to 15 μg/kg/min.[9-14] (All dosages in this review are expressed in terms of dobutamine; the drug is administered as the hydrochloride salt.) Dobutamine infusion in patients with NYHA class-3 or class-4 CHF has been associated with an increase in myocardial contractility and resultant increases in stroke volume and cardiac output (CO). Dobutamine reduces systemic vascular resistance and pulmonary capillary wedge pressure (PCWP), with resultant reductions in afterload and preload, respectively. HR and blood pressure (BP) are affected minimally.

Dobutamine also improves renal function.[13] This effect is caused by the enhancement of renal perfusion that results from the dobutamine-associated increase in CO.

Tolerance. Dobutamine's receptor-site interactions increase concentrations of adenosine 3',5'-cyclic phosphate (cAMP) through activation of adenylate cyclase. Although cAMP concentrations increase rapidly with initial administration of a β-adrenergic agonist, the concentrations soon return to baseline levels despite continued presence of the drug, and drug tolerance occurs. Some investigators have suggested that the elevated serum norepinephrine concentrations that are typical in patients with CHF cause down-regulation of β-receptors.[15-18]

Dobutamine tolerance was studied in 20 patients with idiopathic congestive cardiomyopathy (NYHA functional class 3 or 4).[19] Dobutamine was infused initially at 2.5 μg/kg/min i.v., and the dosage was increased by 2.5 μg/kg/min every 30 minutes until a dosage of 10 μg/kg/min was attained. The dosage was lowered if the BP or HR exceeded 120% of the baseline value or if premature ventricular contractions occurred more than 12 times per minute. The effect of dobutamine on CO, HR, and pre-ejection period divided by left ventricular ejection time (PEP/LVET) was significantly less after 72 and 96 hours of infusion than it was during the first 2 hours of infusion. Dobutamine's effect on mortality and functional class was not studied.

The Therapy Update *section provides concise analytical reviews of narrowly defined, important topics in pharmacotherapy. Priority is given to articles that focus on new or emerging standards in drug therapy. Articles are not intended to be comprehensive reviews of drugs or of disease states and their treatment.*

Initial Evidence of Sustained Benefit

Long-term use of dobutamine is based on early investigations that suggested prolonged drug effects. Leier et al.[13] gave dobutamine 10–15 μg/kg/min i.v. for 72 hours to 25 patients with severe CHF (NYHA functional class 4). The mean cardiac index (CI) improved from 1.97 to 3.33 L/min/sq m. Ejection fraction (EF) and stroke volume also increased, and PEP/LVET and PCWP decreased; all of these changes were significant. Indicators of left ventricular function remained improved 30 minutes after the infusion was stopped, and 17 patients maintained an improvement of one NYHA functional class for one week.

Unverferth et al.[20] conducted a study that included 38 patients who had nonischemic cardiomyopathy and whose average NYHA functional class was 3.8. The mean ± S.D. baseline EF and CI were 0.25 ± 0.02 and 2.0 ± 0.1 L/min/sq m, respectively. Dobutamine infusion was started at a dosage of 2.5 μg/kg/min i.v. and increased to a dosage that kept the HR and systolic BP under 120% of the baseline value, PCWP under 140% of the baseline value, and frequency of premature ventricular contractions under 12/min (maximum dosage, 15 μg/kg/min). This dosage was maintained for 72 hours. All measures of cardiovascular function improved during the infusion. The mean NYHA functional class was 2.74 and 3.12 two days and four weeks after completion of the infusion, respectively. An improvement in NYHA functional class was maintained by 43% of the patients 10 weeks after the infusion.

In another study, Unverferth et al.[21] gave 23 patients with nonischemic cardiomyopathy a 72-hour dobutamine infusion (mean ± S.D. dosage, 11.1 ± 3.4 μg/kg/min). Eleven patients had an improvement in NYHA functional class two months after the infusion, and three maintained clinical improvement after six months.

In a double-blind study, Liang et al.[22] randomly assigned 15 patients with nonischemic cardiomyopathy (NYHA functional class 3 or 4) to receive either dobutamine (mean dosage, 25.3 μg/kg/min) or 5% dextrose injection for 72 hours. Dobutamine was initiated at 2.5 μg/kg/min and increased at 20-minute intervals until (1) CO increased to twice the baseline value, (2) HR increased by 25 beats per minute, or (3) BP rose to 15 mm Hg over the baseline value. After four weeks, six of the eight patients who received dobutamine remained improved by at least one NYHA functional class. In the control group of seven patients, two improved by one functional class, four remained unchanged, and one experienced clinical deterioration. EF and exercise tolerance improved significantly in the dobutamine group but remained unchanged in the control group.

Conditioning Effect

The sustained benefit in exercise tolerance seen in patients who have received a 72-hour dobutamine infusion suggests a conditioning effect similar to that seen with exercise training.[23] Physical conditioning enables an individual to respond to the same workload with less effort. The cardiovascular system adapts and delivers more oxygen, and peripheral tissues respond by enhancing the capacity of skeletal muscle to extract oxygen. Repetitive sympathetic stimulation of the heart causes a decrease in heart rate and an increase in myocardial contractility.

The conditioning effect was investigated in 24 healthy men who were randomized to receive one of three treatments for 17 days.[24] The first treatment was infusion of 250 mL of 0.9% sodium chloride injection i.v. for two hours daily. The second treatment was dobutamine i.v. for two hours daily. Dobutamine was given at dosages sufficient to increase resting HR by 20% for one hour, by 40% for 45 minutes, and by 60% for 15 minutes; the mean ± S.D. dosages were 17 ± 4, 26 ± 9, and 34 ± 10 μg/kg/min, respectively. The third treatment was exercise on a stationary bicycle for two hours daily to achieve the same HR goals set for the second group. Except for the two hours of exercise, complete bed rest was maintained for all three groups. Oxygen consumption during maximal exercise fell significantly in the group that received 0.9% sodium chloride injection but was unchanged in the dobutamine and exercise groups. The HR increase in response to exercise was unchanged in the exercise group, mildly increased in the dobutamine group, and significantly increased in the group treated with 0.9% sodium chloride injection. The investigators concluded that dobutamine infusion produces an effect that resembles physical conditioning and prevents deconditioning during bed rest.

Investigations Using Endomyocardial Biopsy

The mitochondrial effects of dobutamine were studied in 16 patients with congestive cardiomyopathy.[25] Endomyocardial biopsy specimens were taken before and after three days of bed rest and then 4–18 hours after completion of a three-day dobutamine infusion. The maximum dobutamine dosage was 15 μg/kg/min and was adjusted to keep the HR and BP below 120% of baseline values, PCWP below 140% of the baseline value, and frequency of premature ventricular contractions below 12/min. The study variables were (1) the number of electron-dense particles per 100 mitochondria, (2) the crista:matrix ratio, and (3) the average mitochondrial size. Electron-dense particles result from precipitation or denaturation of protein in mitochondria and are usually more numerous in degenerating myocardial cells. Cristae house the enzymes of oxidative phosphorylation and are the site of adenosine 5'-triphosphate (ATP) generation in the mitochondria; the crista:matrix ratio is relatively low in the failing heart. Swelling of mitochondria in the failing heart accounts for their relatively large average size in diseased myocardium. The three days of bed rest had no effect on the mitochondrial variables, but there was a significant decrease in the number of electron-dense particles and a significant increase in the crista:matrix ratio after dobutamine infusion. The change in mitochondrial size was the most specific indicator of overall clinical improvement, but mean mitochondrial size did not change significantly after dobutamine infusion.

In another study, endomyocardial biopsy was performed to measure tissue adenine nucleotide content in six patients before and after three days of bed rest and after a three-day dobutamine infusion.[21] The dobutamine dosage criteria were identical to those used in the study described above. Coronary blood flow is diminished in congestive cardiomyopathy because of elevated diastolic and systolic coronary filling pressures. Hypoperfusion of the subendocardium leads to increased concentrations of adenosine 5'-diphosphate and adenosine 5'-monophosphate and a decreased concentration of ATP. Over time, the depressed ATP concentration leads to further impairment of diastolic and systolic performance, possible myocardial cell death, and the replacement of cells by subendocardial fibrosis. The ATP:creatine ratio did not change after bed rest but rose significantly after dobutamine infusion. The authors concluded that the increased coronary blood flow and the lowered ventricular and diastolic coronary pressures caused by dobutamine led to improved perfusion of the subendocardium.

Reports of Multiple Dobutamine Infusions

Investigators have studied the use of multiple short-term dobutamine infusions in the treatment of refractory CHF. Early case reports led to several small clinical trials, most of which had no control patients (Table 1).[26-34] Several factors must be considered in evaluating and comparing these reports and in applying their findings to a realistic clinical situation.

Cause and Severity of Disease. The reports differed in the cause of patients' cardiomyopathy. Compared with patients with nonischemic cardiomyopathy, patients with ischemic cardiomyopathy are more likely to develop dobutamine-induced anginal pain and ventricular ectopy; dobutamine dosage must be lowered in the presence of ischemic cardiomyopathy to minimize these complications.[20,21] Patients with ischemic cardiomyopathy were involved in all but one clinical trial in Table 1, and this fact must be considered when comparing the frequency of adverse effects

Table 1.
Reports of Long-term Dobutamine Therapy for Congestive Heart Failure[a]

Reference	No. Patients	Age (yr)	No. in FC 4	Type of Cardiomyopathy	Baseline Cardiac Index (L/min/sq m)	Dobutamine Dosage (μg/kg/min)	Setting	Outcome	Adverse Effects
Clinical Trials									
26	17 M, 9 F	52	3	Nonischemic	2.1	7.4–8.7 for 4 hr/wk for 24 wk	Clinic	Improved ET; improved FC in 12 pts.	Ventricular tachycardia (1 pt.)
27	13 M	62	4	Ischemic in 9 pts.	1.6	7.5 for 48 hr/wk	Clinic	Improved FC in 6 pts.; 10 died	Sudden death (6 pts.)
28, 29	10 M, 11 F	55	16	Ischemic in 10 pts.	1.8	7.1 for 48 hr/wk (11 pts.) or continuously (8 pts.)	Home	Improved FC in all; 20 died	Extravasation (3 pts.); sudden death (3 pts.)
30	9 M, 2 F	54	11	Ischemic in 6 pts.	1.5	5.0 continuously, then decreased to 24 hr/wk (6 pts.); or 5.0 for 2–6 days/wk (5 pts.)	Home	Improved FC in all; 4 died; 7 weaned to oral drugs	...
Case Reports									
31	1 M, 2 F	51	3	Nonischemic	...	1.5–8.0 for 4 days/wk for 3–4 wk, then 48 hr/wk	Home	Increased EF from ≤0.15 to 0.27	Angina, PVCs
32	1 M	19	1	Viral	1.6	6.0 for 48 hr/wk	Hospital	Increased EF from 0.15 to 0.17; improved FC; transplant	...
33	1 M	68	1	Ischemic	2.1	5.0 for 48 hr/wk	Home	Increased BP, EF, FC; pt. died	Extravasation
34	1 M	76	1	Ischemic	...	10.0 for 36 hr/wk	...	Improved FC and ET; pt. died	...

[a] FC = New York Heart Association functional class, M = male, F = female, ET = exercise tolerance, EF = ejection fraction, PVCs = premature ventricular contractions, BP = blood pressure. Mean values are given for reports involving more than one patient.

among trials.

Patients in NYHA functional class 3 tend to have a better prognosis and a better overall response to therapy than patients in functional class 4. Despite aggressive treatment, patients in functional class 4 succumb to their disease sooner than those in functional class 3. Thus, differences in disease severity may have affected outcome among the trials. In addition, patients with a relatively high baseline CI may be healthier and, thus, have a better long-term prognosis than patients with a lower baseline CI.

Concurrent Medications. Concurrent administration of digoxin and furosemide was common in early studies, which were conducted before the beneficial effect of vasodilators was fully appreciated; concurrent treatment with vasodilators was common in the more recent trials. One group of investigators gave dopamine to promote diuresis.[28,29] Antiarrhythmic therapy also varied among studies. In one trial, two of three surviving patients were receiving amiodarone, which may have prevented sudden death.[27] Amiodarone may also be inotropic and may benefit patients with CHF.[35]

Although anticoagulants were mentioned in only two dobutamine trials,[30,32] many patients died of complications associated with embolic phenomena.[27-9,33,34] Many clinicians prescribe anticoagulants in patients with dilated cardiomyopathy because of the high risk of systemic and pulmonary embolism. Thus, the influence of anticoagulation in the dobutamine trials may have been an important factor in the outcome of the studies.

Choice of Therapeutic Endpoints. To date, the only known indicator of prolonged survival in patients with severe CHF is a decrease in mortality rate.[36] In the dobutamine studies, however, NYHA functional class was the most commonly used outcome variable. The assignment of functional class depends on the judgment of individual researchers and reflects patients' symptoms only. Many trials involved the measurement of hemodynamic variables (e.g., CO, PCWP, EF, systemic vascular resistance, systolic time intervals, PEP/LVET) during the initial adjustment of dobutamine dosage, but measurements were generally not repeated after weeks of therapy. Leier et al.[26] repeated echocardiograms, exercise tolerance tests, and functional class determinations every two weeks. They also included a control group, but the study was not blinded. Krell et al.[27] used mortality as an endpoint but did not have a control group.

Dobutamine Administration. Maximum dobutamine dosages in the cited trials were those that produced an increase in CO of at least 25% or those above which no further increase in CO occurred. Dosages were decreased if ventricular ectopy increased or if the HR increased by more than 40% of the baseline value. The duration and frequency of dobutamine administration varied, but the most common regimen was continuous infusion for 48 hours once a week.

Whether patients were hospitalized during infusion also varied among studies. Although outpatient dobutamine administration may contribute to an improvement in quality of life and minimize costs and the number of hospitalizations, dobutamine infusions that are given at home (and are thus not monitored closely) may cause sudden death in patients with CHF.[37] Among the reports cited in this review, dobutamine was given at home in four, at a heart-failure clinic in two, in the hospital in one, and at an undisclosed site in one.

Dobutamine in outpatients was generally given via a portable infusion pump and a venous access catheter. The most common complication related to the pump or catheter was catheter-site infection, which generally required a 10-day course of oral antimicrobial therapy (without hospitalization). Catheter thrombosis occurred in two patients despite anticoagulant therapy.[30] Infusion-pump failure occurred six times in one trial and was thought to have been caused by inadvertent pinching of the outflow tubing when the pump housing was closed.[29] One of two patients in whom dobutamine was given via an implantable infusion device developed necrosis of the tissue surrounding the site of catheter insertion into the external jugular vein; this was attributed to dobutamine infiltration into the subcutaneous tissue.[33] Four other instances of dobutamine-associated local tissue necrosis occurred in two other trials.[29,33]

One obstacle to the use of dobutamine in outpatients is the drug solution's instability when stored for more than 48 hours.[38,39] Patients in the studies relied on a home infusion-care company or a nearby clinic to deliver an adequate supply of fresh drug solution. Dobutamine is stable for at least 24 hours in peritoneal dialysis solution,[40] but there are insufficient data to support the use of intraperitoneal dobutamine administration.

Hemodynamic Complications. Dobutamine-associated hemodynamic complications were generally minimal in the cited trials. Tolerance (i.e., an increase in symptoms of CHF and a reduction in EF) developed in 4 of 21 patients in one study.[29] The four patients had received 96-hour dobutamine infusions. In two of the patients, infusion therapy was withheld for 7–10 days before being resumed at the same dosage for 48 hours at a time. In the other two patients, the infusion duration was simply reduced to 48 hours. Resolution of congestive symptoms occurred in all four patients.

Leier et al.[26] described one patient who developed ventricular tachycardia while receiving dobutamine 10 μg/kg/min; dobutamine was withdrawn, and the patient required cardioversion and hospitalization. In an early case report, the dosage of dobutamine had to be reduced after a patient experienced anginal pain and an increase in frequency of premature ventricular contractions.[31]

Miller et al.[30] assessed arrhythmia by using Holter monitoring before, during, and 24 hours after dobutamine infusion. Antiarrhythmic drug therapy was begun in patients who had a substantial number of ventricular couplets or ventricular tachycardia during baseline assessment or during infusion. No patients underwent electrophysiologic testing, but 5 of 11 were treated with amiodarone. The investigators used an attenuated dosage of dobutamine (5 μg/kg/min) because of the drug's arrhythmogenic potential.

Outcome. There was a consistent improvement in patients' functional class among the reviewed trials. Two groups of investigators found significant increases in exercise tolerance, as measured by treadmill testing.[26,34]

The most surprising data came from two studies in which 10 of 13 and 20 of 21 patients died despite improvement in functional class and relief of symptoms; nine of the deaths were sudden.[27-29] One possible explanation for the deaths is that the patients in these trials were more severely ill than those in other studies. Another possibility is that long-term stimulation (by dobutamine) of a heart that is already exposed to high concentrations of catecholamines is detrimental.[41]

Dies et al.[42] conducted a double-blind randomized study involving 60 patients with refractory CHF (NYHA functional class 3 or 4) to investigate the possible detrimental effects of dobutamine. Patients were given a 48-hour infusion of dobutamine (mean dosage, 8.1 μg/kg/min) or placebo once weekly; the protocol called for 24 weeks of infusion. Patients who failed to respond (seven in the placebo group and one in the dobutamine group) were crossed over to receive the other infusion. Symptoms improved in both groups, but 20 patients died and the trial was stopped prematurely. Of the patients who died, 5 had received placebo alone, 13 had received dobutamine alone, and 2 had been crossed over from the placebo group to receive dobutamine. In patients receiving dobutamine, there was an association between mortality and the presence of four or more episodes of ventricular tachycardia per day.

Clinical Experience with Long-term Dobutamine Therapy

Long-term dobutamine therapy is used at our institution as a palliative measure in patients whose CHF is refractory to maximal therapy with oral medications. We have found that dobutamine therapy attenuates the symptoms of CHF much as i.v. morphine lessens pain in patients with terminal cancer. In patients awaiting heart transplantation, long-term dobutamine infusion is used until a donor heart becomes available. Because dobutamine is arrhythmogenic, infusion therapy is initiated in the hospital. Dobutamine is typically infused continuously (not intermittently) at a dosage of 5.0–7.5 µg/kg/min, and infusion may last as long as eight months. Constant electrocardiographic monitoring is accomplished via telemetry, and serum electrolyte concentrations, urine output, and medications are also monitored carefully. We have found that potassium and magnesium must frequently be given i.v. to supplement routine oral electrolyte administration.

Summary and Recommendations

Clinical trials of long-term dobutamine therapy have not shown this form of treatment to be ideal but have suggested guidelines for its use.

Long-term dobutamine therapy lessens symptoms of CHF and improves functional class, exercise tolerance, and EF. However, because this therapy does not prolong survival in most patients, other specific endpoints of therapy should be determined for each patient.

Patients must be monitored carefully, at least during the initial adjustment of dosage, because dobutamine is arrhythmogenic and can cause sudden death. Outpatient dobutamine administration may contribute to an improvement in quality of life and may be less expensive than hospital treatment, but it is not without risk.

It is possible that dobutamine therapy may prolong survival in some patients (e.g., those with nonischemic cardiomyopathy, those in NYHA functional class 3 [rather than class 4], and those awaiting transplantation). Further studies must be performed to identify these patients.

The maintenance dosage of dobutamine (usually 5.0–7.5 µg/kg/min) should be based on the response to initial dosage adjustment. The optimal dosage regimen is unknown, but the most common has been a 48-hour infusion once a week.

The role of concurrent medications (e.g., amiodarone) in decreasing the adverse effects of dobutamine is not established and should be further investigated.

Conclusion

Long-term use of dobutamine infusion lessens the symptoms of CHF but does not prolong survival.

References

1. Smith WM. Epidemiology of congestive heart failure. *Am J Cardiol.* 1985; 55:3A-8A.
2. Parmley WW. Pathophysiology and current therapy of congestive heart failure. *J Am Coll Cardiol.* 1989; 13:771-85.
3. Ruffolo RR, Yaden EL. Vascular effects of the stereoisomers of dobutamine. *J Pharmacol Exp Ther.* 1983; 224:46-50.
4. Ruffolo RR, Spradin TA, Pollock GD et al. Alpha- and beta-adrenergic effects of the stereoisomers of dobutamine. *J Pharmacol Exp Ther.* 1981; 219:447-52.
5. Tuttle RR, Mills J. Dobutamine: development of a new catecholamine to selectively increase cardiac contractility. *Circ Res.* 1975; 36:185-96.
6. Kates RE, Leier CV. Dobutamine pharmacokinetics in severe heart failure. *Clin Pharmacol Ther.* 1978; 24:537-41.
7. Leier CV, Unverferth DV, Kates RE. The relationship between plasma dobutamine concentrations and cardiovascular responses in cardiac failure. *Am J Med.* 1979; 66:238-42.
8. Murphy PJ, Williams TL, Kau DLK. Disposition of dobutamine in the dog. *J Pharmacol Exp Ther.* 1976; 119:423-31.
9. Jewitt D, Birkhead J, Mitchell A et al. Clinical cardiovascular pharmacology of dobutamine, a selective inotropic catecholamine. *Lancet.* 1974; 2:363-7.
10. Akhtar N, Mikulic E, Cohn JN et al. Hemodynamic effect of dobutamine in patients with severe heart failure. *Am J Cardiol.* 1975; 36:202-5.
11. Andy JJ, Curry CL, Ali N et al. Cardiovascular effects of dobutamine in severe congestive heart failure. *Am Heart J.* 1977; 94:175-82.
12. Loeb HS, Khan M, Klodnycky ML et al. Hemodynamic effects of dobutamine in man. *Circ Shock.* 1975; 2:29-35.
13. Leier CV, Webel J, Bush CA. The cardiovascular effects of the continuous infusion of dobutamine in patients with severe cardiac failure. *Circulation.* 1977; 56:468-72.
14. Bendersky R, Chatterjee K, Parmley WW et al. Dobutamine in chronic ischemic heart failure: alterations in left ventricular function and coronary hemodynamics. *Am J Cardiol.* 1981; 48:554-8.
15. Cohn JN. The sympathetic nervous system in heart failure. *J Cardiovasc Pharmacol.* 1989; 14(Suppl 5):S57-61.
16. Packer M. Is activation of the sympathetic nervous system beneficial or detrimental to the patient with congestive heart failure? Lessons learned from clinical trials with beta adrenergic agonists and antagonists. *J Cardiovasc Pharmacol.* 1989; 14(Suppl 5):S38-43.
17. Bristow MR, Kantrowitz NE, Ginsberg R et al. Beta adrenergic function in heart muscle disease and heart failure. *J Mol Cell Cardiol.* 1985; 17:41-52.
18. Bristow MR, Port JD, Hershberger RE et al. The beta adrenergic receptor-adenylate cyclase complex as a target for therapeutic intervention in heart failure. *Eur Heart J.* 1989; 10:45-54.
19. Unverferth DV, Blanford M, Kates RE et al. Tolerance to dobutamine after a 72 hour continuous infusion. *Am J Med.* 1980; 69:262-6.
20. Unverferth DV, Magorien RD, Lewis RP et al. Long-term benefit of dobutamine in patients with congestive cardiomyopathy. *Am Heart J.* 1980; 100:622-30.
21. Unverferth DV, Magorien RD, Altschuld R et al. The hemodynamic and metabolic advantages gained by a three-day infusion of dobutamine in patients with congestive cardiomyopathy. *Am Heart J.* 1983; 106:29-34.
22. Liang CS, Sherman LG, Doherty JU et al. Sustained improvement of cardiac function in patients with congestive heart failure after short-term infusion of dobutamine. *Circulation.* 1984; 69:113-9.
23. Liang CS, Tuttle RR, Hood WB et al. Conditioning effects of chronic infusions of dobutamine: comparison with exercise training. *J Clin Invest.* 1979; 64:613-9.
24. Sullivan MJ, Binkley PF, Unverferth DV et al. Prevention of bedrest-induced physical deconditioning by daily dobutamine infusions: implications for drug-induced physical conditioning. *J Clin Invest.* 1985; 76:1632-42.
25. Unverferth DV, Leier CV, Magorien RD et al. Improvement of human myocardial mitochondria after dobutamine: a quantitative ultrastructure study. *J Pharmacol Exp Ther.* 1980; 215:527-32.
26. Leier CV, Huss P, Lewis RP et al. Drug-induced conditioning

in congestive heart failure. *Circulation*. 1982; 65:1382-7.
27. Krell MJ, Kline EM, Bates ER et al. Intermittent ambulatory dobutamine infusion in patients with severe congestive heart failure. *Am Heart J*. 1986; 112:787-91.
28. Roffman DS, Applefeld MM, Grove WR et al. Intermittent dobutamine hydrochloride infusion in outpatients with chronic congestive heart failure. *Clin Pharm*. 1985; 4:195-9.
29. Applefeld MM, Newman KA, Sutton FJ et al. Outpatient dobutamine and dopamine infusion in the management of chronic heart failure. Clinical experience in 21 patients. *Am Heart J*. 1987; 114:589-95.
30. Miller LW, Merkle EJ, Herrmann V. Outpatient dobutamine for end-stage congestive heart failure. *Crit Care Med*. 1990; 18:S30-3.
31. Applefeld MM, Newman KA, Grove WR et al. Intermittent, continuous outpatient dobutamine infusion in the management of congestive heart failure. *Am J Cardiol*. 1983; 51:455-8.
32. Hodgson JM, Aja M, Sorkin RP. Intermittent, ambulatory dobutamine infusion for patients awaiting cardiac transplantation. *Am J Cardiol*. 1984; 53:375-6.
33. Berger M, McSherry CK. Outpatient dobutamine using a totally implantable infusion pump for refractory congestive heart failure. *Chest*. 1985; 88:295-6.
34. Van der Brande P, Van Mieghem W, Demedts M. Intermittent dobutamine infusion in severe congestive heart failure in elderly patients. *Gerontology*. 1990; 36:49-54.
35. Hamer AW, Arkles B, Johns J. Beneficial effects of low dose amiodarone in patients with congestive cardiac failure: a placebo-controlled trial. *J Am Coll Cardiol*. 1989; 14:1768-74.
36. Rude RE, Grossman W, Colucci WS et al. Problems in assessment of new pharmacologic agents for the heart failure patient. *Am Heart J*. 1981; 102:584-90.
37. Miller LW. Outpatient dobutamine for refractory congestive heart failure: advantages, techniques, and results. *J Heart Lung Transplant*. 1991; 10:482-7.
38. Kirschenbaum HL, Aronoff W, Perentesis GP et al. Stability of dobutamine hydrochloride in selected large-volume parenterals. *Am J Hosp Pharm*. 1982; 39:1923-5.
39. Eli Lilly and Company. Dobutrex package insert. Indianapolis, IN; 1991 Feb.
40. Gora ML, Visconti JV, Seth S et al. The stability of dobutamine hydrochloride in peritoneal dialysis solutions. *Am J Hosp Pharm*. 1991; 48:1234-7.
41. LeJemtel TH, Sonnenblick EH. Should the failing heart be stimulated? *N Engl J Med*. 1984; 310:1384-5. Editorial.
42. Dies F, Krell MJ, Whitlow P et al. Intermittent dobutamine in ambulatory outpatients with chronic cardiac failure. *Circulation*. 1986; 74(Suppl 2):38. Abstract.

Research

Influence of sucralfate on the detection of occult blood in simulated gastric fluid by two screening tests

JONATHAN S. HOLMAN AND JILL A. SHWED

Abstract: The influence of sucralfate on the detection of occult blood in simulated gastric fluid by two screening tests was investigated.

Two simulated gastric solutions (pH 1.2 and 4.1) containing sucralfate 2.5 or 10 mg/mL were spiked with fresh whole blood (hemoglobin concentration, 15.7 g/dL) to achieve a blood concentration of 1 or 5 μL/mL. Fifty-microliter samples were applied to separate Hemoccult and Gastroccult test slides, which were read by a blinded evaluator at 60, 120, and 180 seconds after the addition of developer. Any trace of blue in the test area was considered a positive result. Sucralfate-free simulated gastric fluid spiked with blood served as a positive control, and fluid with or without sucralfate and containing no blood served as a negative control.

No false-positive or false-negative results were obtained with Gastroccult. Hemoccult yielded false-positive results in 3 of 20 determinations at 60 seconds for solution containing sucralfate 10 mg/mL (pH 1.2) and 13 of 20 determinations at 60 seconds for solution containing sucralfate 2.5 mg/mL (pH 1.2). All the results with Hemoccult were positive when the slides were read at 120 and 180 seconds. Also, all the results for the negative controls were positive at 120 seconds. Hemoccult did not produce any false-negative results.

False-positive results occurred when Hemoccult was used to test simulated gastric fluid that had a low pH (1.2) and contained sucralfate. Gastroccult did not yield false-positive results.

Index terms: Drug interactions; Gastrointestinal drugs; Occult blood; Sucralfate; Tests, laboratory
Clin Pharm. 1992; 11:625-7

The detection of occult blood can be important in the early recognition of gastric trauma or deteriorating gastric conditions.[1] Hemoccult (SmithKline Diagnostics, Inc., San Jose, CA) and Gastroccult (SmithKline Diagnostics) are two guaiac slide tests commonly used to screen for blood in various gastrointestinal fluids and stool. Both tests use filter paper treated with natural guaiac resin and a developing solution of hydrogen peroxide and denatured ethyl alcohol. A positive result is produced when hemoglobin catalyzes the oxidation reaction of α-guaiaconic acid to a blue quinone structure by the peroxide reagent.[2,3] This turns the test paper blue. The result is considered positive regardless of the intensity of the color.

Knowledge of the factors that may alter the sensitivity and specificity of these screening tests allows one to use them more reliably. Various factors, including pH and the presence of drugs (e.g., rifampin, cimetidine, antacids, bismuth salts), metal ions, peroxidase-containing foods, and ascorbic acid, have been associated with erroneous results.[4] Hauser et al.[5] evaluated the effect of cimetidine on the sensitivity of Hemoccult when testing gastric fluid. False-positive results were observed with cimetidine concentrations of ≥15 mg/mL, regardless of the pH of the gastric solution or the form of cimetidine (liquid, tablet, stock solution, or injectable). The authors concluded that the interference was concentration dependent. Conversely, Schentag[6] found a false-positive reaction with Hemoccult when testing dissolved cimetidine tablets but not with cimetidine stock solution or blank

JONATHAN S. HOLMAN, PHARM.D., is Critical Care Pharmacist, St. Vincent's Medical Center, Jacksonville, FL; at the time of this study he was a doctor of pharmacy degree candidate, Medical University of South Carolina (MUSC), Charleston. JILL A. SHWED, PHARM.D., is Assistant Professor, Department of Hospital Pharmacy Practice and Administration, MUSC.

Address reprint requests to Dr. Shwed at the College of Pharmacy, Medical University of South Carolina, 171 Ashley Avenue, Charleston, SC 29425.

Published as an abstract of a paper accepted for the 12th Annual Meeting of the American College of Clinical Pharmacy.

Supported by the Doctor of Pharmacy Candidate Research Fund, Department of Hospital Pharmacy Practice and Administration, College of Pharmacy, Medical University of South Carolina, Charleston.

nasogastric aspirates. He concluded that the interference was due to the presence of FD&C blue lake no. 2. Subsequently, Demise et al.[7] did not detect an interference with Hemoccult or Gastroccult by several drug products that contain blue dyes, including cimetidine. They did caution that a "blue staining" occurred with several products when the tests were evaluated outside the 60-second time limit recommended by the manufacturer.

Antacids have also been found to alter the sensitivity of these tests. Gogel et al.[4] reported that Hemoccult was less sensitive when used to test gastric contents neutralized with an antacid containing both magnesium and aluminum than when used to test gastric contents neutralized with an antacid containing aluminum alone. However, directly conflicting results were obtained by Layne et al.,[8] who observed that Hemoccult was less sensitive when gastric contents were neutralized with an aluminum-containing antacid than with an antacid containing both aluminum and magnesium. The exact mechanism of the interaction with antacids is unknown; however, the manufacturer of Gastroccult and Hemoccult recognizes the possibility for interference and advises users to avoid sampling gastric contents immediately after the administration of antacids or cimetidine.[2,3]

Sucralfate has demonstrated an effectiveness comparable or superior to that of antacids and histamine H_2-receptor antagonists in the prophylaxis of upper gastrointestinal bleeding from stress-related mucosal damage.[9-12] The absence of occult blood was one measure of effectiveness in these evaluations. In the study reported here, we sought to determine if sucralfate, an aluminum-containing compound, interferes with the detection of occult blood in simulated gastric fluid by Gastroccult or Hemoccult.

Methods

Preparation of Solutions. Two batches of simulated gastric fluid were prepared by dissolving 2 g of sodium chloride and 3.2 g of pepsin (Fisher Scientific, Pittsburgh, PA) in distilled water.[13] The pH was adjusted with 1*N* hydrochloric acid to obtain two solutions of pH 1.2 and 4.1. Sufficient distilled water was added to dilute each solution to 1000 mL. Both solutions were then placed in an oven and warmed to 37 °C. Commercially available 1-g sucralfate tablets (Carafate, Marion Merrell Dow, Inc., Kansas City, MO, lot K02983) were weighed, and appropriate portions were added to 50 mL of each solution to achieve final sucralfate concentrations of 2.5 or 10 mg/mL. These concentrations were selected to approximate possible sucralfate concentrations in the gastric contents of fasting individuals treated with this agent. The 50-mL solutions were then spiked with 100 or 500 µL of fresh whole blood (hemoglobin concentration, 15.7 g/dL) to obtain solutions containing 1 µL of blood per milliliter (hemoglobin concentration, 313 µg/mL) or 5 µL/mL (1554 µg/mL). These concentrations of blood were chosen so that comparisons could be made with documented sensitivity data for Hemoccult and Gastroccult.[2,3] The solutions were maintained at 37 °C on a warming plate during the additions of blood and sucralfate and were continuously mixed with a magnetic stirrer until samples were removed and tested by Hemoccult (lot 1009) and Gastroccult (lot 20498). Simulated gastric fluid spiked with blood served as a positive control, and simulated gastric fluid with or without sucralfate served as a negative control. The pH of all solutions was measured with a pH meter (Ionalyzer model 811, Orion Research Inc., Cambridge, MA) before and after the addition of blood or sucralfate or both.

The concentrations of sucralfate and blood in the control and test solutions are summarized in Table 1.

Testing with Hemoccult and Gastroccult. Fifty-microliter samples of the test and control solutions were applied to separate Hemoccult and Gastroccult test slides, which were developed according to the manufacturer's guidelines[2,3] and read by one blinded evaluator. A result was considered positive if there was any trace of blue in the test area and negative if there was no such color change. All slides were evaluated 60 seconds after the addition of developer (in accordance with the manufacturer's guidelines), as well as at 120 and 180 seconds.

Results

No false-positive or false-negative results were obtained with Gastroccult. With Hemoccult, we obtained false-positive results in 3 (15%) of 20 determinations at 60 seconds when the solution contained sucralfate 10 mg/mL and had a pH of 1.2. All 20

Table 1.
Concentrations of Sucralfate and Blood in the Simulated Gastric Fluids Studied

pH	No. Samples Tested	Sucralfate (mg/mL)	Blood (µL/mL)
Positive Controls			
1.2	10	0	1
1.2	10	0	5
4.1	10	0	1
4.1	10	0	5
Negative Controls			
1.2	20	0	0
1.2	20	10	0
1.2	20	2.5	0
4.1	20	0	0
4.1	20	10	0
4.1	20	2.5	0
Test Solutions			
1.2	20	10	1
1.2	20	2.5	1
1.2	20	10	5
1.2	20	2.5	5
4.1	20	10	1
4.1	20	2.5	1
4.1	20	10	5
4.1	20	2.5	5

outcomes were positive when the slides were read at 120 and 180 seconds. We obtained false-positive results in 13 (65%) of 20 determinations at 60 seconds when the solution contained sucralfate 2.5 mg/mL (pH 1.2); all results were positive when the slides were read after the 60-second time point. In addition, the results for all the negative controls (sucralfate, no blood) were positive at 120 seconds. No false-negative results were obtained with Hemoccult. The mean change in pH for all solutions was ≤0.7 after the addition of blood, sucralfate, or both.

Discussion

The findings of this study suggest that Gastroccult is more reliable than Hemoccult for detecting occult blood in gastric aspirate. Gastroccult is formulated with buffers for greater sensitivity at low pH and with binders for increased selectivity for hemoglobin in samples containing high drug and metal ion concentrations and foods containing peroxidases. In practice, however, Hemoccult is also used for this purpose.

The reliability of Hemoccult used on specimens with a low pH has previously been questioned. Layne et al.[8] observed poor sensitivity of Hemoccult to blood in acidic gastric fluid. Negative results were obtained even when the blood concentration was as high as 40 µL per milliliter of unbuffered gastric fluid. An evaluation of 381 samples of gastric aspirate with various degrees of acidity was conducted by SmithKline Diagnostics.[2] For samples with a pH of <2, Hemoccult and Gastroccult accurately detected blood at a concentration of 1–2 µL/mL in 15% and 70% of the samples, respectively. The Gastroccult product information claims that the test is capable of reliably detecting hemoglobin at concentrations of 0.3–0.5 µg/mL at pH 1–9.[2] Rosenthal et al.[14] were able to detect blood at a 2-µL/mL concentration in gastric fluid at pH 3 when using Gastroccult; however, they obtained negative results for blood concentrations of <1 µL/mL. In our investigation, interference with the sensitivity of Hemoccult and Gastroccult was not seen at whole blood concentrations of 1 and 5 µL/mL.

Neither concentration of sucralfate (2.5 or 10 mg/mL) limited the detection of blood in simulated gastric fluid (i.e., there were no false-negative results). This observation is noteworthy in light of the widespread use of occult blood testing as an endpoint of prophylactic therapy in patients at risk for stress-related mucosal damage. In clinical trials, occult blood is rarely used as the sole indicator of efficacy; however, in practice it may very well be. Our results indicate that if occult blood is present at a detectable level, sucralfate will not hinder its detection.

The false-positive results obtained with Hemoccult for solutions with a pH of 1.2 are difficult to explain. False-positive reactions are thought to be due to oxidation of guaiaconic acid or interference by dyes. Sucralfate itself or the presence of FD&C red dye no. 30 or FD&C blue lake dye no. 1 in the tablet formulation may potentiate the color change at low pH. The reaction does not appear to be concentration dependent; false-positive results were observed at both concentrations. When false-positive results were obtained, the initially faint blue increased in intensity 60–120 seconds after the addition of the developer. Thus the results were dependent on when the slides were read. The results for all negative controls became positive within 120 seconds. Had we not adhered to the manufacturer's guidelines, the false-positive rate for Hemoccult would have been 100%.

On the basis of these results, we recommend using Gastroccult to test for occult blood in gastric aspirates when patients are receiving sucralfate. Clinicians should be aware of the potential for false-positive results when using Hemoccult under these circumstances. The manufacturer's guidelines should always be adhered to in the use and interpretation of these tests.

Conclusion

False-positive results occurred when Hemoccult was used to test simulated gastric fluid that had a low pH (1.2) and contained sucralfate. Gastroccult did not yield false-positive results.

References

1. Priebe HJ, Skillman JJ, Bushnell LS et al. Antacid versus cimetidine in preventing acute gastrointestinal bleeding. *N Engl J Med*. 1980; 302:425-30.
2. SmithKline Diagnostics, Inc. Gastroccult package insert. San Jose, CA; 1989 Jan.
3. SmithKline Diagnostics, Inc. Hemoccult package insert. San Jose, CA; 1990 Apr.
4. Gogel HK, Tandberg D, Strickland RG. Substances that interfere with guaiac tests: implications for gastric aspirate testing. *Am J Emerg Med*. 1989; 7:474-80.
5. Hauser AR, Quigley ML, Driever CW et al. More on false positive "Hemoccult" reaction with cimetidine. *N Engl J Med*. 1981; 304:847-8.
6. Schentag JJ. False-positive "Hemoccult" reaction with cimetidine. *N Engl J Med*. 1980; 303:108.
7. Demise JJ, Nelson LA, Lawson LA et al. Effect of drug products containing blue dye on Hemoccult and Gastroccult tests. *Am J Hosp Pharm*. 1987; 44:356-7.
8. Layne EA, Mellow MH, Lipman TO. Insensitivity of guaiac slide tests for detection of blood in gastric juice. *Ann Intern Med*. 1981; 94:774-6.
9. Borrero E, Bank S, Margolis I et al. Comparison of antacid and sucralfate in the prevention of gastrointestinal bleeding in patients who are critically ill. *Am J Med*. 1985; 79(Suppl 2C):55-61.
10. Tryba M. Prophylaxis of stress ulcer bleeding: a meta analysis. *J Clin Gastroenterol*. 1991; 13(Suppl 2):s44-s55.
11. Cannon LA, Heiselman D, Gardner W et al. Prophylaxis of upper gastrointestinal tract bleeding in mechanically ventilated patients. *Arch Intern Med*. 1987; 147:2101-6.
12. Tryba M. Sucralfate versus antacids or H2 antagonists for stress ulcer prophylaxis: a meta-analysis on efficacy and pneumonia rate. *Crit Care Med*. 1991; 19:942-9.
13. The United States pharmacopeia, 22nd rev., and The National Formulary, 17th ed. Rockville, MD: The United States Pharmacopeial Convention; 1990:1788.
14. Rosenthal P, Thompson J, Singh M. Detection of occult blood in gastric juice. *J Clin Gastroenterol*. 1984; 6:119-21.

Research Note

Safety and tolerability of an intravenous immune globulin at various concentrations in 5% dextrose injection or sterile water for injection

KENNETH B. MILLER, DAVID P. SCHENKEIN, AND RICHARD L. WASSERMAN

Clin Pharm. 1992; 11:628-31

The introduction of i.v. immune globulin (IGIV) in the United States in 1981 heralded dramatic progress in the management of immunodeficiency and immunoregulatory disorders.[1] IGIV is widely used today to treat primary immunodeficiencies (e.g., X-linked hypogammaglobulinemia, severe combined immunodeficiency, common variable immunodeficiency) and idiopathic thrombocytopenic purpura.[2-5] IGIV is finding application in secondary immunodeficiency states, such as chronic lymphocytic leukemia, bone marrow transplantation, autoimmune diseases, Kawasaki disease, neonatal sepsis, burn injury, and human immunodeficiency virus infection in pediatric patients.[2-7]

Lyophilized forms of IGIV may offer more flexibility in preparation and administration than do forms that require no reconstitution. The specific needs of patients may make it desirable to individualize the choice of the diluent used to reconstitute lyophilized IGIV. For example, a clinician might want to avoid using 0.9% sodium chloride injection as an IGIV diluent when treating a sodium-restricted patient. In addition, giving large volumes of fluid with IGIV may not be advisable for all patients. Thus, administering IGIV at relatively high concentrations may be preferred for patients sensitive to fluid overload.

Until recently, the package labeling for Sandoglobulin (Sandoz) IGIV indicated that 3% and 6% solutions should be prepared with 0.9% sodium chloride injection.[8] Current labeling indicates that an IGIV solution with a concentration of up to 12% can be prepared with 0.9% sodium chloride injection, 5% dextrose injection (D5W), or sterile water for injection (SWFI).[9] Use of the 12% concentration is recommended only after patients have tolerated lower concentrations.[9]

We conducted a study to determine the safety and tolerability of Sandoglobulin at various concentrations in either D5W or SWFI.

Methods. The study was an open-label assessment of Sandoglobulin reconstituted with SWFI or D5W and given in IGIV concentrations ranging from 6% to 12%. It was conducted in the outpatient units of New England Medical Center and Baylor University Medical Center.

Patients with primary or secondary immunodeficiency disease or an immunodeficiency secondary to a therapeutic intervention were eligible. Patients had to have been stabilized for at least one month on a standard IGIV regimen given at a dosage sufficient to maintain a trough serum immunoglobulin G concentration of >300 mg/dL when IGIV was given every two weeks. Patients with a history of adverse reactions to an IGIV preparation were excluded.

The protocol was approved by the institutional review board at each study center, and written informed consent was obtained from all patients. Before entry, all patients received a physical examination and had their immunodeficiency disorders documented.

Sandoglobulin (lots 7.371.246, 6.370.240, 8.371.131, and 8.370.114 at New England Medical Center and lots

KENNETH B. MILLER, M.D., is Associate Professor of Medicine, Tufts University School of Medicine, Boston, MA, and Director of the Bone Marrow Transplant Service, New England Medical Center Hospital, Boston. DAVID P. SCHENKEIN, M.D., is Assistant Professor of Medicine, Tufts University School of Medicine. RICHARD L. WASSERMAN, M.D., is Assistant Chief, Department of Pediatrics, Baylor University Medical Center, Dallas, TX, and Clinical Assistant Professor, Department of Pediatrics, University of Texas Southwestern Medical Center at Dallas.

Address reprint requests to Dr. Miller at the Division of Hematology–Oncology, New England Medical Center, 15 Kneeland Street, Box 168, Boston, MA 02111.

The assistance of Tammy Fisher, R.N., and Heide Temples, R.N., is acknowledged.

Supported by a research grant from Sandoz Pharmaceuticals Corporation.

Dr. Wasserman is a paid consultant to Sandoz Pharmaceuticals Corporation.

After acceptance of this paper, the editors and authors learned that the 13 patients from New England Medical Center are described in another paper (Miller KB, Schenkein DP, Fogaren T. An assessment of the safety and tolerability of immune globulin intravenous [human] Sandoglobulin prepared in sterile water or 5% dextrose at various concentrations. *Semin Hematol.* 1992; 29 [Suppl 2]:in press).

0.371.159, 8.371.131, and 8.370.114 at Baylor University Medical Center) was reconstituted with either SWFI or D5W by pharmacists (at New England Medical Center) or nurses (at Baylor University Medical Center). The IGIV dose was individualized for patients with common variable immunodeficiency and was 500 mg/kg for patients who had undergone bone marrow transplantation. On day 1, patients received 6% IGIV reconstituted with SWFI or D5W. The diluent was selected at random. An infusion rate of 2.0 mg/kg/min was used throughout the study unless poor drug tolerability dictated a rate reduction. On day 15, patients who had tolerated 6% IGIV were given 9% IGIV (at Baylor University Medical Center) or 8% or 9% IGIV (at New England Medical Center, depending on the pharmacist's technique) prepared with the diluent that was used for the first infusion. If the 8% or 9% solution was tolerated, a 12% solution, prepared in the same diluent, was given on day 29. Patients at New England Medical Center who tolerated the 12% solution could, at the discretion of the investigator, be crossed over to receive IGIV in the alternate diluent (starting at an IGIV concentration of 6%).

Supine systolic blood pressure (SBP), supine diastolic blood pressure (DBP), oral temperature, radial pulse, and respiratory rate were measured before, halfway through, and every 15 minutes (up to one hour) after each infusion. If a serious adverse reaction occurred, the infusion was stopped and the patient was removed from the study.

For each IGIV concentration and diluent, the paired Student's *t* test was used to compare differences between (1) baseline and midinfusion and (2) baseline and one-hour-postinfusion vital signs. The a priori level of significance was <0.05.

Results. Eight female and 15 male patients (aged 2–57 years) were enrolled (Table 1); 10 had been stabilized with a regimen of Sandoglobulin in 0.9% sodium chloride injection, and 13 had been stabilized with a regimen of Gamimune N (Miles–Cutter) in D5W. Of the 13 patients at New England Medical Center, four did not cross over to receive the alternate diluent either because continued IGIV therapy was not indicated or because adverse effects necessitated withdrawal from the study. Sandoglobulin doses for the patients with common variable immunodeficiency ranged from 101 to 508 mg/kg (mean, 259 mg/kg). The mean infusion time for all patients was approximately three hours (Table 2).

Ninety-four IGIV infusions were initiated; two were stopped because of adverse reactions (Table 3). A 26-year-old patient who had undergone bone marrow transplantation experienced no adverse effects when IGIV (in SWFI) was given in lower concentrations but developed severe rigors, moderate chills, clammy feelings, and sweats (with no temperature elevation) 15 minutes after infusion of 12% IGIV in SWFI was begun. The infusion was discontinued, and symptoms were treated with meperidine hydrochloride 50 mg i.v. The symptoms abated, and the patient was withdrawn from the study. In addition, a 49-year-old man with common variable immunodeficiency had difficulty breathing and developed sweats during his initial study infusion, with 6% IGIV in SWFI. Decreasing the infusion rate did not alleviate the symptoms. With continued infusion, the patient developed itching, hives, nausea, and vomiting. The infusion was halted, and the patient was treated with oral diphenhydramine and hydrocortisone and removed from the study.

Symptomatic adverse reactions occurred during

Table 1.
Patient Characteristics and Sandoglobulin Diluent[a]

Age (yr)	Sex	Diagnosis	Sandoglobulin Diluent
New England Medical Center			
57	M	BMT	SWFI, then D5W
53	M	BMT	SWFI, then D5W
49	M	CVID	SWFI only
40	F	BMT	D5W, then SWFI
37	M	BMT	SWFI, then D5W
36	M	BMT	SWFI, then D5W
35	M	BMT	D5W only
25	M	BMT	SWFI only
25	F	BMT	D5W only
21	F	BMT	SWFI, then D5W
20	F	BMT	SWFI, then D5W
20	M	CVID	SWFI, then D5W
18	F	BMT	SWFI, then D5W
Baylor University Medical Center			
47	F	CVID	D5W only
43	F	CVID	D5W only
39	M	CVID	D5W only
13	M	CVID	D5W only
8	M	CVID	SWFI only
6	M	CVID	SWFI only
6	M	CVID	SWFI only
4	F	CVID	D5W only
3	M	CVID	SWFI only
2	M	CVID	SWFI only

[a] BMT = immunodeficiency after bone marrow transplantation, SWFI = sterile water for injection, D5W = 5% dextrose injection, CVID = common variable immunodeficiency.

Table 2.
Sandoglobulin Infusion Times

Sandoglobulin Concentration[a]	*n*	Infusion Time (min) Mean	Range
New England Medical Center			
6% in SWFI	11	197	20–480
8% or 9% in SWFI	10	202	45–510
12% in SWFI	10	185	15–465
6% in D5W	11	167	6–360
8% or 9% in D5W	11	155	60–330
12% in D5W	11	119	60–240
Baylor University Medical Center			
6% in SWFI	5	215	165–240
9% in SWFI	5	210	120–240
12% in SWFI	5	209	120–235
6% in D5W	5	187	165–270
9% in D5W	5	158	120–195
12% in D5W	5	189	124–265

[a] SWFI = sterile water for injection, D5W = 5% dextrose injection.

Table 3.
Dosages of and Adverse Reactions to Sandoglobulin[a]

Sandoglobulin Concentration and Diluent	*n*	Mean Dose (mg/kg)	No. Patients with Adverse Reactions: Anaphylactoid	Rate-Related	DBP Decrease >15 mm Hg	Oral Temperature Increase >0.7 °C
6% in SWFI	16	387	1[b]	0	0	1
8% or 9% in SWFI	15	470	0	0	0	2
12% in SWFI	15	394	0	1[c]	2	1
6% in D5W	16	421	0	0	2	1
8% or 9% in D5W	16	408	0	1[d]	1	1
12% in D5W	16	399	0	1[e]	0	4

[a] DBP = diastolic blood pressure, SWFI = sterile water for injection, D5W = 5% dextrose injection.
[b] Sweating, difficulty breathing, hives, itching, nausea, and vomiting. The infusion was stopped, and the patient received no further doses in either diluent.
[c] Rigors, chills, clammy feeling, sweats. The infusion was stopped, and the patient did not cross over to receive Sandoglobulin in D5W.
[d] Headache and abdominal pain, which disappeared with continued infusion.
[e] Chills and fever, which decreased when flow rate was reduced.

two other infusions. A four-year-old girl with common variable immunodeficiency developed a mild headache and abdominal pain during infusion of 9% IGIV in D5W; these symptoms disappeared as the infusion continued. A 13-year-old boy with common variable immunodeficiency complained of moderate chills and a mild fever when he received 12% IGIV in D5W; these symptoms resolved after the infusion rate was slowed.

The data for the 8% and 9% infusions did not differ significantly and were combined for further analysis. There were no significant changes in SBP, pulse, respiratory rate, or oral temperature associated with the administration of IGIV in any concentration or diluent. The change in DBP between baseline and one-hour-postinfusion readings was not significant when data from both study centers were combined. However, at Baylor University Medical Center, the mean ± S.D. DBP dropped by 9.2 ± 3.1 mm Hg in patients receiving 6% IGIV in D5W ($p = 0.04$) and by 15.2 ± 5.0 mm Hg in patients receiving 12% IGIV in SWFI ($p = 0.0008$). DBP fell by >15 mm Hg in five instances. DBP in one patient receiving IGIV in D5W dropped by 20 mm Hg during the final phase of infusion when the rate was increased from 90 to 125 mg/min. No infusions were stopped because of hypotension, and DBP returned to normal in 30 minutes in all cases.

In only one instance did the oral temperature exceed 38.0 °C after an infusion. This occurred in a patient who had received 12% IGIV in D5W, and the temperature returned to normal in 30 minutes. Another patient's temperature exceeded 37.8 °C before each infusion, but it fell slightly after IGIV infusion.

Discussion. This study demonstrates that Sandoglobulin diluted in D5W or SWFI and in concentrations of up to 12% can be given safely to patients with primary and secondary immunodeficiencies.

The few adverse reactions that we observed were similar to those previously associated with administration of commercially available IGIV preparations. Such reactions are generally mild and nonanaphylactic.[1,2-5] They occur in <10% of patients, usually appear during or within an hour after the infusion, and may include back or abdominal pain, nausea and vomiting, chills, fever, headache, myalgia, and fatigue. Other reactions are anaphylactoid and are characterized by flushing, dizziness, hypotension, chest tightness, and dyspnea. The anaphylactoid reactions may be caused by an interaction between the infused antibodies and free antigens in the patient.[3,10] Adverse reactions can be minimized or prevented by slowing the initial infusion rate; premedicating with aspirin, diphenhydramine, or acetaminophen; or temporarily interrupting the infusion. True anaphylactic reactions to IGIV therapy are rare.[3,4] Some patients can tolerate one IGIV product but not another.[11]

Administration of 3% or 6% IGIV in 0.9% sodium chloride injection has been associated with minimal toxicity. Adverse reactions to Sandoglobulin occur in <1% of patients who are not immunodeficient.[11] If the initial infusion rate exceeds the manufacturer's recommendation, adverse reactions occur in approximately 10% of agammaglobulinemic or hypogammaglobulinemic patients who have not been treated previously with IGIV or whose last treatment was more than eight weeks before.[12]

Our findings suggest that patients who tolerate lower concentrations of IGIV will usually tolerate Sandoglobulin in concentrations up to 12% (in either D5W or SWFI). Our study confirms and extends the results of a recent report that Sandoglobulin, in concentrations of up to 12%, can be given safely to patients with primary disorders of humoral immunity.[12] That study showed that patients could tolerate Sandoglobulin infusion rates that were 2 to 10 times more rapid than standard recommended rates.

Flexibility in allowable concentrations and infusion rates can reduce the time required to deliver large IGIV doses. It takes four to eight hours to deliver currently recommended doses if 3% or 6% solutions are given at recommended rates. In our study, the average infusion took three hours. A reduction in infusion time could mean less time lost from school or employment by the patient and less time spent by health-care professionals monitoring infusions. The ability to individualize the diluent could give the practitioner more freedom in timing doses of IGIV and could affect the clinical status of the patient.

Our results do not necessarily apply to other IGIV preparations. Sandoglobulin is supplied as a lyophilized protein powder; if sodium chloride is to be included in the solution, it must be contained in the diluent. Other products incorporate sodium chloride in the lyophylate and, therefore, cannot be prepared as a high-protein, low-osmolarity solution. Other differences among products are the size of the donor pool, the mode of fractionation, pH, specific antibody titers, and immunoglobulin subclass distribution.[2,4,5] Thus, IGIV products should be prepared and used in accordance with the manufacturers' instructions.

Conclusion. When reconstituted with D5W or SWFI, Sandoglobulin can be given safely in concentrations up to 12% to immunocompromised patients who have previously tolerated lower concentrations.

References

1. Ammann AJ, Ashman RF, Buckley RH et al. Use of intravenous γ-globulin in antibody immunodeficiency: results of a multicenter controlled trial. *Clin Immunol Immunopathol.* 1982; 22:60-7.
2. Knapp MJ, Colburn PA. Clinical uses of intravenous immune globulin. *Clin Pharm.* 1990; 9:509-29.
3. Buckley RH, Schiff RI. The use of intravenous immune globulin in immunodeficiency diseases. *N Engl J Med.* 1991; 325:110-7.
4. ASHP Commission on Therapeutics. ASHP therapeutic guidelines for intravenous immune globulin. *Clin Pharm.* 1992; 11:117-36.
5. Berkman SA, Lee ML, Gale RP. Clinical uses of intravenous immunoglobulins. *Semin Hematol.* 1988; 2:140-58.
6. Stiehm ER. New uses for intravenous immune globulin. *N Engl J Med.* 1991; 325:123-5. Editorial.
7. National Institute of Child Health and Human Development Intravenous Immunoglobulin Study Group. Intravenous immune globulin for the prevention of bacterial infections in children with symptomatic human immunodeficiency virus infection. *N Engl J Med.* 1991; 325:73-80.
8. Sandoz Pharmaceuticals. Sandoglobulin package insert. East Hanover, NJ; 1989 Mar.
9. Sandoz Pharmaceuticals. Sandoglobulin package insert. East Hanover, NJ; 1991 Aug.
10. Cunningham-Rundles C, Day NR, Wahn V et al. Reactions to intravenous gammaglobulin infusions and immune complex formation. In: Nydegger UE, ed. Immunohemotherapy: a guide to immunoglobulin prophylaxis and therapy. London: Academic Press; 1981:447-9.
11. Peerless AG, Stiehm ER. Intravenous gammaglobulin for reaction to intramuscular preparation. *Lancet.* 1983; 2:461. Letter.
12. Schiff RI, Sedlak D, Buckley RH. Rapid infusion of Sandoglobulin in patients with primary humoral immunodeficiency. *J Allergy Clin Immunol.* 1991; 88:61-7.

Grand Rounds

Warfarin-induced intramural hematoma of the small intestine

MINYON L. AVENT, BRUCE R. CANADAY, AND WILLIAM T. SAWYER

Abstract: A case of warfarin-induced intramural hematoma and hemorrhagic infarction of the small intestine is described, and the literature on this adverse effect is reviewed.

A 32-year-old white woman who had been receiving warfarin and carbamazepine came to a clinic complaining of lower back and stomach pain. She had a history of iliofemoral deep venous thromboses and seizures. A pelvic sonogram showed a large quantity of fluid present. Her prothrombin time (PT) was 29.2 sec. Her hemoglobin concentration and hematocrit were within the normal ranges. The patient was admitted to the hospital when her back pain increased and she vomited. The warfarin was discontinued. On day 5 the patient was still having abdominal pain and nausea. Her hemoglobin concentration and hematocrit had fallen to 6.6 g/dL and 20%, although her PT had decreased to 12.5 sec. On the same day, the patient underwent an exploratory laparotomy, and an indurated and ischemic area of jejunum was found and resected. The pathology report indicated the presence of hemorrhage and infarction consistent with an anticoagulant-related disorder.

About 100 cases of intramural hematoma of the small intestine induced by anticoagulant therapy have been reported. Most patients are white males about 60 years of age. The sites most frequently involved are the duodenum and proximal jejunum. Symptoms include constipation, nausea, vomiting, and abdominal pain. Laboratory test and radiological findings are fairly nonspecific, but when found together in a patient receiving an anticoagulant, the diagnosis can be made with some confidence. Management may be complicated by the bleeding disorder, the intestinal obstruction if present, and the original indication for warfarin therapy.

A patient who has abdominal pain and a prolonged PT while receiving an anticoagulant may have intramural hematoma of the small intestine. Surgery should be contemplated only if the patient's status does not improve when the drug is withdrawn.

Index terms: Anticoagulants; Carbamazepine; Hematoma; Toxicity; Warfarin sodium
Clin Pharm. 1992; 11:632-5

Hemorrhagic complications associated with oral anticoagulant therapy have been well documented. Hematuria, cutaneous ecchymosis, epistaxis, and gingival bleeding are common but usually are of limited severity.[1,2] More serious bleeding events, involving the intestinal tract, adrenal glands, brain and epidural space, and pericardium occur much less frequently.[1,2]

Oral anticoagulant-induced intramural hematoma of the small intestine is relatively uncommon but may be associated with serious complications, such as obstruction of the small bowel,[3-6] intestinal infarction and necrosis,[7-10] and, rarely, death.[3,6] The syndrome includes hemorrhage into the bowel wall, the peritoneal cavity, or the retroperitoneal space.[6]

We describe a case of warfarin-induced intramural hematoma and hemorrhagic infarction of the small intestine and review the literature on this adverse effect.

MINYON L. AVENT, PHARM.D., is Pharmacy Resident, Department of Pharmacy, Moses H. Cone Memorial Hospital, Greensboro, NC; when this article was written she was a Pharm.D. degree student, School of Pharmacy, University of North Carolina (UNC), Chapel Hill, NC. BRUCE R. CANADAY, PHARM.D., is Clinical Professor, School of Pharmacy, UNC, and Director of Pharmacy Programs, Wilmington Area Health Education Center, Wilmington, NC. WILLIAM T. SAWYER, M.S., FASHP, is Associate Professor, School of Pharmacy, UNC.

Address reprint requests to Dr. Canaday at the Wilmington Area Health Education Center, 2131 South 17th Street, Wilmington, NC 28402.

The assistance of Peter Ungaro, M.D., is acknowledged.

This is **article 680-204-9214** in the **ASHP Continuing Education System**; it qualifies for 1.0 hour of continuing-education credit. See page 640 for learning objectives and test questions.

Case Report

A 32-year-old white woman came to the outpatient clinic of a regional medical center complaining of left lower back pain and stomach pain of three days' duration. The pain was not exacerbated by food and was relieved by acetaminophen. The patient had experienced no nausea or vomiting until the day she came to the clinic. She had had watery stools, which were exacerbated by food, for many months.

The patient had experienced two previous episodes of left iliofemoral deep venous thrombosis and had a history of seizures. Three months before appearing in the clinic she had been hospitalized for right flank pain and right lower quadrant pain, which also began three days before the admission. On that earlier admission the patient had reported taking warfarin sodium 20 mg/day and carbamazepine 200 mg p.o. b.i.d. The prothrombin time (PT) was 34.2 seconds (control time, 12.1 sec; International Sensitivity Index [ISI], 2.83; and International Normalized Ratio [INR], 18.4). During the five months before that admission, her anticonvulsant therapy had been changed on three separate occasions and it had been noted that the patient altered her anticonvulsant medication and missed several clinic appointments. Also, adequate anticoagulation was difficult to achieve. Her PTs varied from 20.5 sec (control, 12.0 sec; ISI, 2.83; INR, 4.55) to 34.2 sec (control, 12.1 sec; ISI, 2.83; INR, 18.4) when she was taking warfarin sodium 20 mg/day and from 14.7 sec (control, 11.2 sec; ISI, 2.83; INR, 2.16) to 29.2 sec (control, 12.0 sec; ISI, 2.83; INR, 12.39) when she was taking warfarin sodium 17.5 mg/day. Diagnostic studies, including abdominal ultrasound, intravenous pyelography, and abdominal computed tomography (CT), produced negative results. Her symptoms improved greatly despite continued warfarin therapy, and the patient was discharged with a diagnosis of mesenteric adenitis. At discharge she was receiving warfarin sodium 17.5 mg/day and carbamazepine 200 mg b.i.d. and had a PT of 19.1 sec (control, 12.0 sec).

On coming to the clinic during the latest episode, the patient reported taking warfarin sodium 17.5 mg/day and carbamazepine 300 mg p.o. b.i.d. Her PT was 29.2 sec (control, 12.0 sec; ISI, 2.83; INR, 12.39). No pertinent family or social historical data were elicited. Physical examination revealed an elevated pulse (108 beats/min) and diffuse abdominal pain without guarding, which caused the patient to lie in the fetal position.

The results of blood tests were within normal limits, including a hemoglobin concentration of 14.1 g/dL (normal, 12–16 g/dL) and a hematocrit of 41.9% (37–47%). Serum chemistry values were within normal limits, except for a cholesterol concentration of 243 mg/dL (normal, 120–200 mg/dL), an alkaline phosphatase concentration of 153 U/L (44–135 U/L), a lactate dehydrogenase concentration of 656 U/L (301–580 U/L), a γ-glutamyltransferase concentration of 146 U/L (8–69 U/L), and an albumin concentration of 2.9 g/dL (3.5–4.8 g/dL). Urinalysis showed the presence of 20–25 red blood cells per high-power field.

The outcome of intravenous pyelography was negative. CT of the abdomen was negative for a retroperitoneal hematoma but did reveal a small left ovarian cyst. A sonogram of the pelvis showed the presence of a large quantity of fluid.

While she was undergoing her initial evaluation at the clinic, the patient's back pain increased, and she complained of nausea and vomited once. The vomitus was without blood or "coffee ground" material. She was then admitted to the medical center for observation and further evaluation. Her warfarin therapy was discontinued and she was hydrated with intravenous fluids. Vitamin K was not administered. Her hemoglobin concentration and hematocrit declined after admission to 12.6 g/dL and 37.5%, respectively, on day 2; 9.5 g/dL and 28.4% on day 3; and 8.0 g/dL and 23.9% on day 4. On day 5 the patient was still experiencing abdominal pain, epigastric discomfort, and occasional nausea. Her hemoglobin concentration and hematocrit had fallen to 6.6 g/dL and 20%, although her PT had decreased to 12.5 sec (control, 12.0 sec). On that day the patient underwent an exploratory laparotomy for possible resection of a ruptured ovarian cyst. The laparotomy revealed a normal right ovary with a few follicular cysts, and a 1.5–2-cm corpus luteum was noted on the left ovary, but there was no active bleeding. Further exploration revealed an indurated and ischemic area of small bowel. A 35-cm segment of hemorrhagic and vasculitic bowel and associated mesentery was resected from the mid-jejunum. The pathology report indicated the presence of "hemorrhage and infarction consistent with an anticoagulant-related disorder." The postoperative course was uneventful, and the patient was discharged on day 12 with orders to take carbamazepine 300 mg b.i.d.

Papers in the Grand Rounds *section are patient case reports and literature review combined in a way that gives them high educational value. The papers lead off with a well-documented case report of an unusual drug experience (e.g., adverse drug reaction or other unexpected drug response, experimental use of a drug). The case generally deals with a difficult therapeutic problem or dilemma that is commonly encountered but may be overlooked or misunderstood. (Esoteric or rare occurrences of minor importance do not make good* Grand Rounds *material.) A literature review puts the case in perspective with previously reported similar cases and alternative treatments. The review is integrated with related discussion of the case being reported.*

CP *readers are encouraged to use* Grand Rounds *for educational group discussions. For this purpose, discussion questions are printed at the end of* Grand Rounds *papers.*

Occurrence of Anticoagulant-Induced Intramural Hematoma

Approximately 100 cases of intramural hematoma of the small intestine associated with anticoagulant therapy have been reported in the Western literature.[5,6] Stanton et al.[6] reviewed 65 of these cases, of which 30 were managed with surgical resection. Pathological evidence of necrosis was found in only one of these 30 cases. Bowel necrosis due to intestinal hematoma is quite unusual.[7-10] The average age of anticoagulant-treated patients developing intramural hematoma is 60 years, 70% of the patients are male, and 90% are Caucasian.[6] Generally the patients are receiving anticoagulants because of previous myocardial infarction or cerebrovascular disease.[6]

The most common sites for intramural hematoma of the small intestine are the duodenum and proximal jejunum.[4,5,11] A sudden increase in intra-abdominal pressure causes stretching and retraction of the bowel wall capable of producing tears in the submucosal blood vessels.[11] However, the exact pathogenesis of intramural hematoma associated with anticoagulant therapy is not known, and there is no evidence that trauma is a factor.

Signs, Symptoms, and Diagnosis

The symptoms of anticoagulant-induced intramural hematoma of the small bowel are usually gradual in onset, increasing in severity over several days, and include constipation, nausea, vomiting, abdominal pain, and other features of partial or complete intestinal obstruction.[4,6,12-14] As many as half the patients may initially be asymptomatic, since the symptoms depend on the rapidity of the onset of bleeding and its amount.[4]

Laboratory test findings are also nonspecific. They can include anemia,[5,11,12,15] elevated serum bilirubin[15] and amylase[5,15] concentrations, and leukocytosis.[5,11] The PT is usually markedly elevated.[3,5,12,14,16] Although excessive anticoagulant therapy most commonly contributes to intramural hematoma, this complication may also appear in patients whose therapy is well controlled.[1,14,17]

The results of radiological tests are also somewhat nonspecific. Roentgenographic signs that have been observed include (1) gastric dilatation; (2) a distended proximal bowel with or without air–fluid levels in the proximal duodenum and little or no air in the distal bowel, consistent with paralytic ileus or obstruction; (3) displacement of the greater curvature of the stomach or adjacent bowel, if the hematoma is large enough; and (4) gas trapped in the involved bowel, which may show luminal narrowing, "scalloping," and thumb-printing.[18] Although roentgenographic and ultrasound studies have resulted in the detection of intramural hematoma, the most definitive diagnostic procedure is a barium study of the upper GI tract.[4,5,19] The findings depend on the extent of hemorrhage, presence of intestinal secretions, and presence of mucosal edema.[20] Colonoscopy may also be useful if the results of the barium study are indeterminate or if there is recurrent bleeding.[21]

Because of their nonspecific nature, neither the clinical nor the laboratory and radiological features are in themselves diagnostic of intramural hematoma, but when these features are found together in a patient receiving anticoagulant therapy, the diagnosis can usually be made with confidence.[12] However, differential diagnoses should include gastrointestinal hemorrhage, intestinal obstruction, paralytic ileus, an inflammatory lesion, a palpable mass, and peritonitis.[2]

A barium study of the upper GI tract was not performed in this patient because there were signs and symptoms of intestinal obstruction. There were also reservations about performing an endoscopic procedure on a patient with an unknown site of bleeding and excessively prolonged PTs.

The radiological workup of the patient included abdominal ultrasound and a CT scan. With both, knowledge of the time between the onset of bleeding and the procedure is critical to interpretation.[22] Initially, the hematoma appears hyperdense compared with the surrounding tissue. As the clot ages, it becomes isodense and then hypodense, mimicking a cystic lesion.[22] The uncertainty of the time of onset of bleeding in this patient may well explain the lack of definitive findings.

An attempt was made to rule out the most likely abdominal complications of oral anticoagulation therapy (i.e., gastrointestinal hemorrhage and bowel obstruction due to hemorrhage),[2] but there were features of the case that should also have suggested intramural hematoma. The patient was receiving warfarin, had abdominal pain, and had laboratory test findings suggestive of a bleeding episode. Although her hemoglobin concentration and hematocrit were within the normal ranges on admission, they declined markedly during the hospital stay. The PT ratios measured on both hospital admissions (2.8 and 2.4) were also markedly elevated, and the corresponding INR values (18.4 and 12.39, with an ISI of 2.83) were substantially above the INR range of 2.0–3.0 recommended for the management of deep venous thrombosis.[23]

The patient's anticoagulant therapy had been difficult to manage. Carbamazepine may have enhanced her warfarin metabolism and accounted for the relatively high warfarin requirements,[24] but noncompliance may also have contributed to the variability in PTs.

Management

The management of patients with proved or suspected warfarin-induced intramural hematoma of the small intestine presents challenges. Three aspects of management merit particular attention: (1) the bleeding disorder, (2) the intestinal obstruction when present, and (3) the original indication for warfarin therapy.[12] When the diagnosis of intramural hematoma is not in doubt, these patients are best treated conservatively, as they are usually poor surgical candidates by virtue of their underlying disease and their vulnerability to serious postoperative complications.[3,5,6,12] In addition, provided that the tendency to bleed is controlled, the clinical condition often resolves rapidly within a few days,[6,12,19] and the radiological features resolve completely in three weeks.[12] Treatment, therefore, consists of discontinuing the anticoagulant therapy, administering intravenous fluids, and providing nasogastric drainage.[5,12,19]

If the patient does not improve with conservative therapy within 72 hours,[12] or symptoms worsen (e.g., pain increases), surgery should be considered, principally to rule out other disease.[5,12,16] The patient reported here showed no improvement by the fifth hospital day, despite the discontinuation of warfarin therapy and conservative management. In addition, the hematocrit and the hemoglobin level continued to decline. Therefore, surgical exploration was considered necessary.

The continuation of anticoagulant therapy after successful treatment of an intramural hematoma is controversial. The decision to resume treatment with the anticoagulant should be based on the nature of the underlying disease, whether the event is thought to be idiosyncratic or dose related, and, if it is a dose-related problem, on the ability of the patient to follow a proper treatment regimen.[25] Warfarin therapy was discontinued in the patient because the risk of a further hemorrhagic episode associated with warfarin was considered to be greater than the potential benefit of treating the underlying vascular disease. After two previous episodes with similar clinical signs and symptoms, and in view of the prolonged PT measured during anticoagulant therapy, this risk was deemed unacceptable. Also, the patient had received five months of warfarin treatment since her last episode of deep venous thrombosis. Other treatment options, such as the administration of subcutaneous heparin, were considered, but since the treatment of venous thrombosis lasts six weeks to six months,[23] it was believed that the patient had probably received adequate anticoagulant therapy.

Conclusion

Intramural hematoma of the small intestine should be considered in the differential diagnosis of a patient who has abdominal pain and a prolonged PT while receiving anticoagulant therapy. The condition is best managed conservatively, but surgery should be contemplated if the patient's status does not improve when the anticoagulant is withdrawn.

Discussion Questions

1. Describe the signs and symptoms associated with intramural hematoma of the small intestine.
2. Describe the typical laboratory and radiological findings associated with warfarin-induced intramural hematoma.
3. Recommend appropriate treatment for a patient with warfarin-induced intramural hematoma.
4. Identify the benefits and risks of resuming anticoagulation therapy after the resolution of warfarin-induced intramural hematoma.

References

1. Pastor BH, Resnick ME, Rodman T. Serious hemorrhagic complications of anticoagulant therapy. *JAMA*. 1962; 180:747-51.
2. Gilbert AE, Jorgenson NC. Small bowel obstruction due to hemorrhage secondary to anticoagulant therapy. *Am J Surg*. 1960; 99:945-8.
3. Askey JM. Small bowel obstruction due to intramural hematoma during anticoagulant therapy. *Calif Med*. 1966; 104:449-53.
4. Birns MT, Katon RM, Keller M. Intramural hematoma of the small intestine presenting with major upper gastrointestinal hemorrhage. Case report and review of the literature. *Gastroenterology*. 1979; 77:1094-100.
5. Hughes CE, Conn J, Sherman JO. Intramural hematoma of the gastrointestinal tract. *Am J Surg*. 1977; 133:276-9.
6. Stanton PE, Wilson JP, Lamis PA et al. Acute abdominal conditions induced by anticoagulant therapy. *Am Surg*. 1974; 40:1-14.
7. Zer M, Chaimoff CH, Dintsman M. Anticoagulant ileus with intestinal necrosis. *Isr J Med Sci*. 1972; 8(Feb):154-7.
8. Morley AP. Obstruction of terminal small bowel and anticoagulant therapy. *South Med J*. 1970; 63:342-4.
9. Segaul AI, Mills M, Wertheimer HM. Intramural hematoma of the small intestine as a complication of anticoagulant therapy. *Am J Surg*. 1964; 107:891-4.
10. Levine S, Whelan TJ. Small bowel infarction due to intramural hematoma during anticoagulant therapy. *Arch Surg*. 1967; 95:245-8.
11. Devroede GJ, Tirol FT, LoRusso VA et al. Intramural hematoma of the duodenum and jejunum. *Am J Surg*. 1966; 112:947-54.
12. Lloyd DA, Immelman EJ, Wright MGE. Anticoagulant induced intramural haematoma of the bowel. *S Afr Med J*. 1973; 47:734-8.
13. Goldfarb WB. Coumarin-induced obstruction. *Ann Surg*. 1965; 161:27-34.
14. Beamish RE, McReath ND. Intestinal obstruction complicating anticoagulant therapy. *Lancet*. 1961; 2:390-2.
15. Jones WR, Hardin WJ, Davis JT et al. Intramural hematoma of the duodenum: a review of the literature and case report. *Ann Surg*. 1971; 173:534-44.
16. Daniel TM, Jones RH, Dryer TM et al. Small bowel intramural hematoma secondary to Coumadin anticoagulation. *N C Med J*. 1975; 36(May):289-91.
17. Meyer CH, Otteni F, Hollender LF. Intestinal occlusion due to an intramural haematoma of the small intestine. A rare complication of anti-coagulant treatment. *Chir Gastroenterol*. 1972; 6:64-72.
18. Sears AD, Hawkins J, Kilgore BB et al. Plain roentgenographic findings in drug-induced intramural hematoma of the small bowel. *Am J Roentgenol*. 1964; 91:808-13.
19. Azizkhan R, Piepgrass W, Wilhelm MC. Anticoagulant-induced hematomas of the small intestine. *South Med J*. 1982; 75:242-4.
20. Eiland M, Han SY, Hicks GM. Intramural hemorrhage of the small intestine. *JAMA*. 1978; 239:139-42.
21. Wilcox CM, Truss CD. Gastrointestinal bleeding in patients receiving long-term anticoagulant therapy. *Am J Med*. 1988; 84:683-90.
22. Raghavendra BN, Grieco AJ, Balthazar EJ et al. Diagnostic utility of sonography and computed tomography in spontaneous mesenteric hematoma. *Am J Gastroenterol*. 1982; 77:570-3.
23. Hirsh J, Levine MN. The optimal intensity of oral anticoagulant therapy. *JAMA*. 1987; 258:2723-6.
24. Baciewicz AM. Carbamazepine drug interactions. *Ther Drug Monit*. 1986; 8:305-17.
25. Crisler C, Stafford ES, Zuidema GD. Intestinal obstruction in patients receiving anticoagulants. *Surg Clin North Am*. 1970; 50:1009-13.

Drug Experience

Straightforward reports of unusual drug experiences are included in this section. These may be confirmations of previously reported drug experiences or brief apparent first reports. While selected references may be cited, the purpose of a Drug Experience *report is not to present an extensive review of the literature.*

A related section, Grand Rounds, *includes papers that are well-documented patient case reports with a thorough review of the important literature to help put the case in perspective.*

Sucralfate-associated aluminum toxicity in a patient with renal failure: Treatment with deferoxamine

David I. Min and John A. D'Elia

Clin Pharm. 1992; 11:636-9

Aluminum intoxication can be a serious problem in patients with end-stage renal failure who are receiving long-term dialysis.[1] Aluminum accumulates in a variety of tissues, including the brain and bone,[2,3] and aluminum excess has been associated with encephalopathy, osteomalacia, and microcytic anemia.[4] The early symptoms of encephalopathy consist of a mixed dysarthria and apraxia and may afflict dialysis patients who receive excessive aluminum.[5] With time and increasing aluminum loads, neurological symptoms grow to include asterixis, myoclonus, dementia, focal seizures, and a characteristically abnormal electroencephalogram (EEG).[4] The aluminum-related bone diseases most commonly involve skeletal bone pain, muscle weakness, and fractures.[3]

Sucralfate is a basic aluminum salt of sucrose sulfate, which is widely used to treat peptic ulcer disease and gastritis. Like aluminum hydroxide gel, it also can be used as a phosphate binder in the gastrointestinal tract.[6] Serum aluminum concentration appears not to differ between patients with normal renal function who are taking sucralfate and those who are not.[7]

We describe a patient who was receiving continuous ambulatory peritoneal dialysis (CAPD), experienced worsening symptoms of aluminum toxicity with a substantially elevated serum aluminum concentration after taking sucralfate, and was treated with deferoxamine mesylate.

Case Report. A 43-year-old, 51-kg white woman with a 23-year history of insulin-dependent diabetes mellitus was brought to the emergency room with intense pain due to an apparent shoulder fracture after falling. On admission to the hospital she experienced some shortness of breath, occasional palpitations, mild nausea, vomiting, and mental confusion. She had no fever and denied having any chest pain, abdominal pain, or dyspnea. Her medical history included multiple diabetic complications, in particular end-stage renal failure, retinopathy, and neuropathy. She had been receiving CAPD for more than three years.

Since beginning CAPD, she had been taking two 500-mg aluminum hydroxide capsules three times a day with each meal to control her serum phosphate level and occasionally aluminum hydroxide gel for gastritis symptoms. Four months before this admission she experienced an episode of acute mental status changes and was hospitalized. Her serum aluminum concentration at that time was 6.7 μmol/L (180 μg/L) (normal, <0.37 μmol/L [10 μg/L], measured by flameless atomic absorption spectrometry). Since then, all treatment with aluminum hydroxide products had been discontinued, and calcium carbonate two tablets (500 mg per tablet) with each meal was started for the control of serum phosphate. At the same time, sucralfate 1 g four times daily p.o. was started to treat her continuous gastritis symptoms.

On the day of the current admission, her laboratory values were within normal limits except for the following: blood urea nitrogen concentration, 61 mg/dL (normal, 5–24 mg/dL); serum creatinine concentration, 12.6 mg/dL (0.5–1.3 mg/dL); serum alkaline phosphatase concentration, 164 U/L (16–106 U/L); hemoglobin concentration, 9.9 g/dL (12–15 g/dL); hematocrit, 30.7% (36–44%); mean corpuscular vol-

David I. Min, Pharm.D., M.S., is Assistant Professor, Department of Pharmacy Practice, College of Pharmacy and Allied Health Professions, Northeastern University, Boston, MA. John A. D'Elia, M.D., is Assistant Professor, Department of Medicine, Harvard Medical School, Boston; Nephrologist, Division of Nephrology, New England Deaconess Hospital, Boston; and Senior Physician, John Cook Renal Unit, Joslin Diabetic Center, Boston.

Address reprint requests to Dr. Min at the Department of Pharmacy Practice, College of Pharmacy and Allied Health Professions, Northeastern University, 114 Mugar Hall, 360 Huntington Avenue, Boston, MA 02115.

Presented in part at the 26th Annual ASHP Midyear Clinical Meeting, New Orleans, LA, December 12, 1991.

ume, 77.7 cu µm (82–98 cu µm); and serum aluminum concentration, 12.3 µmol/L, or 331 µg/L. Chest x-ray films were clear, but a roentgenogram of the right upper extremity showed a fracture of the humeral head. The patient's medications on admission included captopril 12.5 mg p.o. three times daily, sucralfate 1 g p.o. four times daily, subcutaneous insulin, an oral multivitamin, and oral aspirin as needed for pain. A lumbar puncture was performed because of her fluctuating mental status. It revealed a white blood cell count of 1/cu mm (normal, 0–8/cu mm), a total protein concentration of 78 mg/dL (15–45 mg/dL), and a glucose concentration of 226 mg/dL (40–80 mg/dL). The concurrent blood glucose concentration was 559 mg/dL (60–110 mg/dL). Computed tomography of her head revealed an old lacunar infarct and a new left internal capsular infarct with no evidence of intracranial hemorrhage. A neurological examination revealed no focal deficits, and an EEG was consistent with diffuse metabolic encephalopathy. Her mental status fluctuated widely, and she had episodes of severe confusion, dysarthria, and mild asterixis.

A 2-g i.v. infusion of deferoxamine mesylate was initiated, but the patient's systolic blood pressure dropped from 100 mm Hg to 80 mm Hg, and the infusion had to be stopped. On the next day, 18 hours after the infusion, her aluminum concentration had increased to 21.7 µmol/L (585 µg/L). Her sucralfate was replaced by ranitidine 150 mg (as the hydrochloride salt) p.o. two times daily for treatment of her gastritis symptoms, and calcium carbonate was continued to control serum phosphate levels.

The route of deferoxamine administration was changed from i.v. to intraperitoneal. Deferoxamine mesylate 1 g was placed in the portion of peritoneal dialysis solution to be used for the overnight dwell. After 27 nightly doses of intraperitoneal deferoxamine, the patient developed peritonitis with *Klebsiella oxytoca*; CAPD was discontinued and hemodialysis with an aluminum-free dialysis solution was begun. Deferoxamine mesylate 500 mg i.v. was given during the last hour of the first (four-hour) hemodialysis period. Since she tolerated this well, the dose of deferoxamine mesylate was increased to 750 mg i.v. three times a week during hemodialysis. On day 3 of this series of i.v. deferoxamine doses, the patient's regimen was supplemented with epoetin alfa 2000 units i.v. three times a week and ferrous sulfate 325 mg p.o. three times a day to treat the anemia and the possible deferoxamine-induced iron loss. During the three-month hospitalization, the serum aluminum concentration gradually decreased to 4.5 µmol/L (122 µg/L) (Table 1), and mental status improved slowly and stabilized. The patient was then transferred to a local rehabilitation hospital and received deferoxamine for four more months in the dialysis clinic.

Discussion. Most cases of aluminum toxicity in dialysis patients are associated with aluminum from medical sources, including aluminum-contaminated dialysis solutions and aluminum-containing antacids given to control serum phosphate levels.[8] Currently in most dialysis units in the United States, aluminum-free dialysis solution is used and aluminum levels in the solution are monitored. This virtually eliminates the risk of aluminum toxicity from an aluminum-contaminated dialysis solution.[9]

Table 1.
Association of Serum Aluminum Concentration with Sucralfate and Deferoxamine Therapy in the Patient

No. Days after Sucralfate Therapy Begun[a]	Cumulative Dose of Deferoxamine Mesylate (g)[b]	Serum Aluminum Concentrations[c]	
		µmol/L	µg/L
3	0	6.7	180
60	0	13.7	370
118	1.00	12.3	331
119	2.00	21.7	585
151	28.25	10.2	275
170	31.25	6.9	187
181	34.25	6.0	161
193	38.00	5.3	144
216	44.75	4.5	122

[a]Sucralfate therapy was discontinued on day 119.
[b]Deferoxamine was given i.v. on day 118, intraperitoneally (in peritoneal dialysis solution) on days 119–145, and i.v. (during hemodialysis) after day 145.
[c]Normal concentration, <0.37 µmol/L (<10 µg/L).

Of the various aluminum-salt antacids available, aluminum hydroxide is the most commonly used for symptomatic relief of peptic ulcer disease. Because of the ability of aluminum hydroxide to bind dietary phosphorus and decrease its absorption in the gastrointestinal tract, it is common practice to use products containing this salt to control serum phosphate concentrations in patients with chronic renal failure.

Despite the long-held notion that aluminum salts are unabsorbable, a number of studies have demonstrated that a substantial amount of aluminum can be absorbed after oral intake of aluminum-containing products. Kaehny et al.[10] measured plasma aluminum concentrations in 13 healthy subjects by using flameless atomic absorption spectrometry. Antacids containing four different salts—aluminum hydroxide, aluminum carbonate, dihydroxyaluminum aminoacetate, and aluminum phosphate (2.2 g of elemental aluminum for three days for each salt)—were used in this study. All salts except aluminum phosphate were associated with significant increases in plasma aluminum concentrations and urinary aluminum excretion. Brahm[11] found that among uremic patients not undergoing dialysis, those who had taken aluminum hydroxide had significantly higher serum aluminum levels than those who had not used the aluminum products.

Our patient had typical symptoms of aluminum-induced encephalopathy (severe mental confusion, dysarthria, and asterixis) and bone disease (severe pain and a humeral fracture), as well as microcytic anemia. The possible sources of the aluminum load in this patient were (1) peritoneal dialysis solutions, (2) previous aluminum hydroxide therapy, and (3) sucralfate therapy.

Current peritoneal dialysis solutions are an unlikely source of aluminum because of the aluminum-free purified water being used. Our patient had received aluminum hydroxide gel for more than three years and subsequently had an elevated serum aluminum concentration (180 μg/L) and mild toxicity. However, in most cases serum aluminum levels and symptoms of toxicity improve after treatment with these products is discontinued.[6,12] Despite the withdrawal of all aluminum hydroxide products, this patient's encephalopathy worsened and her serum aluminum levels doubled, indicating substantial aluminum intake from another source.

Aluminum accounts for 20.69% of the molecular weight of sucralfate, which is typically given at a dosage of 1 g four times a day for four to eight weeks in the treatment of duodenal ulcer.[8,13] This corresponds to a potential intake of 827.6 mg of aluminum per day. Sucralfate dissociates into aluminum and sucrose sulfate at the low pH of the stomach, and the dissociated aluminum can serve as a source of bioavailable aluminum.[14] In patients with chronic renal failure, gastrointestinal absorption of aluminum appears to increase because of an abnormal intestinal wall and increased circulating parathyroid hormones.[15]

There are conflicting reports regarding the absorption of aluminum after oral intake of sucralfate. When sucralfate was administered to humans[7] or rats[16] with normal renal function, no significant increase in plasma aluminum was detected. However, analysis of the animal tissue did reveal increased aluminum concentrations from sucralfate.[16] While serum aluminum seems unlikely to reflect the total body burden of aluminum because aluminum is strongly tissue bound, it appears to be a good indicator of the risk of clinical aluminum toxicity.[17,18] McCarthy et al.[17] suggested that serum aluminum concentrations above 3.7 μmol/L (100 μg/L) indicate aluminum toxicity because a majority of dialysis patients with serum aluminum concentrations above that value develop microcytic anemia and osteomalacia. Winney et al.[18] reported that a plasma aluminum concentration above 7 μmol/L was associated with a high risk of clinical aluminum toxicity.

Because plasma aluminum concentrations are a relatively poor indicator of total body aluminum, a deferoxamine infusion test is used to determine the aluminum burden and to diagnose aluminum-related bone disease. Our patient's first dose of deferoxamine was such a test. The infusion test can be carried out by administering deferoxamine mesylate 2 g or 40 mg/kg i.v. over two hours; plasma aluminum levels are measured before and 36–48 hours after the infusion.[19] If the plasma aluminum concentration increases more than 14.8 μmol/L, the patient is likely to have aluminum-related bone disease. When the increment is less than 7.4 μmol/L, it is unlikely that aluminum-related bone disease is present. When the increment in plasma aluminum is between 7.4 and 14.8 μmol/L, patients generally have substantially elevated bone aluminum; however, they may or may not have histological features of aluminum-related bone disease.

Several cases of possible sucralfate-induced aluminum toxicity in patients receiving extended dialysis have been reported.[20,21] Robertson et al.[20] observed a relapse in bone pain and seizures in a 13-year-old dialysis patient with a previous history of biopsy-proved osteomalacia attributed to aluminum carbonate gel therapy despite deferoxamine therapy. Before her relapse, the patient had received sucralfate 1 g three times daily for six months for the treatment of gastritis. After the discontinuation of sucralfate therapy and continuation of chelation therapy with deferoxamine, plasma aluminum concentrations fell from 30 μmol/L to 1.1 μmol/L, and the symptoms resolved.

Removal of aluminum is difficult because of its large volume of distribution and high degree of protein binding.[22] Aluminum is 95% bound in plasma, possibly to transferrin.[2] The chelating agent deferoxamine, which carries FDA-approved labeling for the treatment of iron intoxication, has been successfully used to treat aluminum overload in dialysis patients. Deferoxamine has a high affinity for iron and aluminum. Intravenous doses of deferoxamine 2–10 g produce a rapid increase in serum aluminum because of the mobilization of aluminum from tissues to plasma, which facilitates the removal of aluminum by dialysis.[19,23] Molitoris et al.[23] found that deferoxamine administered by intramuscular and intraperitoneal routes had clinical effects like those of intravenous deferoxamine but fewer adverse effects. This chelator facilitates the excretion of aluminum from bone, as well as other tissues.[24]

The long-term administration of deferoxamine to uremic patients with dialysis-associated encephalopathy led to improvements in dysarthria, apraxia, overall intellectual function, and EEG abnormalities, as seen in our patient.[25] Because deferoxamine can remove iron from the body, patients need iron supplementation and close monitoring of iron stores during deferoxamine therapy. Our patient received iron supplementation and epoetin therapy and maintained normal iron stores. The ideal dosage of deferoxamine for the treatment of aluminum toxicity has not been established, although 1–2 g three times a week has been the dosage most reported in the literature.[19,23-25] Deferoxamine therapy may have to be continued for several months before serum aluminum levels fall and symptoms improve.

Conclusion. Sucralfate induced or worsened aluminum toxicity in a patient with renal failure. The patient improved after being treated with deferoxamine.

References

1. Alfrey AC, LeGendre GR, Kaehny WD. The dialysis encephalopathy syndrome: possible aluminum intoxication. *N Engl J Med*. 1976; 294:184-8.

2. Alfrey AC. Aluminum metabolism. *Kidney Int*. 1986; 29(Suppl 18):8-11.
3. Cournot-Witmer G, Plachot JJ, Bourdeau A et al. Effect of aluminum on bone and cell localization. *Kidney Int*. 1986; 29(Suppl 18):37-40.
4. Alfrey AC. Dialysis encephalopathy. *Kidney Int*. 1986; 29(Suppl 18):53-7.
5. Rosenbeck JC, McNeil MR, Lemme ML. Speech and language findings in a chronic hemodialysis patient: a case report. *J Speech Hear Disord*. 1975; 40:245-52.
6. Leung ACT, Henderson IS, Halls DJ et al. Aluminium hydroxide versus sucralfate as a phosphate binder in uraemia. *Br Med J*. 1983; 286:1379-81.
7. Kinoshita H, Kumaki K, Nakano K et al. Plasma aluminum levels of patients on long term sucralfate therapy. *Res Commun Chem Pathol Pharmacol*. 1980; 35:515-8.
8. Lione A. Aluminum toxicology and the aluminum-containing medications. *Pharmacol Ther*. 1985; 29:255-85.
9. Sideman S, Manor D. The dialysis dementia syndrome and aluminum intoxication. *Nephron*. 1982; 31:1-10.
10. Kaehny WD, Hegg AP, Alfrey AC. Gastrointestinal absorption of aluminum from aluminum-containing antacids. *N Engl J Med*. 1977; 296:1389-90.
11. Brahm M. Serum-aluminum in nondialyzed chronic uremic patients before and during treatment with aluminum-containing phosphate-binding gels. *Clin Nephrol*. 1986; 25:231-5.
12. Masselot JP, Adhemar JP, Jaudon MC et al. Reversible dialysis encephalopathy: role for aluminium-containing gels. *Lancet*. 1978; 2:1386-7.
13. Martin F, Farley A, Gagnon M et al. Comparison of the healing capacities of sucralfate and cimetidine in the short-term treatment of duodenal ulcer: a double blind randomized trial. *Gastroenterology*. 1982; 82:401-5.
14. Nakazawa S, Nagashima R, Samloff IM. Selective binding of sucralfate to gastric ulcer in man. *Dig Dis Sci*. 1981; 26:297-300.
15. Ihle BU, Becker GJ. Gastrointestinal absorption of aluminum. *Am J Kidney Dis*. 1985; 6:302-5.
16. Burnatowska-Hledin MA, Mayor GH. The effects of sucralfate ingestion on serum and specific tissue aluminum concentration in normal rats. *Clin Toxicol*. 1984; 22:87-93.
17. McCarthy JT, Milliner DS, Kurtz SB et al. Interpretation of serum aluminum values in dialysis patients. *Am J Clin Pathol*. 1986; 86:629-36.
18. Winney RJ, Cowie JF, Robson JS. What is the value of plasma/serum aluminum in patients with chronic renal failure? *Clin Nephrol*. 1985; 24(Suppl 1):S2-S8.
19. Coburn JW, Norris KC. Diagnosis of aluminum-related bone disease and treatment of aluminum toxicity with deferoxamine. *Semin Nephrol*. 1986; 6(Suppl 1):12-21.
20. Robertson JA, Salusky IB, Goodman WG et al. Sucralfate, intestinal aluminum absorption, and aluminum toxicity in a patient on dialysis. *Ann Intern Med*. 1989; 111:179-81.
21. Campistol JM, Cases A, Botey A et al. Acute aluminum encephalopathy in an uremic patient. *Nephron*. 1989; 51:103-6.
22. Kaehny WD, Alfrey AC, Holman RE et al. Aluminum transfer during hemodialysis. *Kidney Int*. 1977; 12:361-5.
23. Molitoris BA, Alfrey PS, Miller NL et al. Efficacy of intramuscular and intraperitoneal deferoxamine for aluminum chelation. *Kidney Int*. 1987; 31:986-91.
24. Malluche HH, Smith AJ, Abrfo K et al. The use of deferoxamine in the management of aluminum accumulation in bone of patients with renal failure. *N Engl J Med*. 1984; 311:140-1.
25. Arze RS, Parkinson IS, Cartlidge NEF et al. Reversal of aluminium dialysis encephalopathy after desferrioxamine treatment. *Lancet*. 1981; 2:1116. Letter.

CP Continuing Education

The ASHP Continuing-Education System gives readers a self-assessment mechanism for selected articles in Clinical Pharmacy *and* AJHP. *It allows readers to obtain continuing-education credit for these articles.*

For the purpose of CE-credit enrollment, a blank answer sheet is published at the end of each installment of the column for the CE articles in that issue. An enrollee accumulates these answer sheets until the enrollment is submitted, using the form that is published in the June and December issues of Clinical Pharmacy *and in the June and December issues of* AJHP. *Any combination of tests within an 18-month period, from both* Clinical Pharmacy *and* AJHP, *may be included in an enrollment. More complete details about enrollment in the system appear in the semiannual enrollment form.*

Article 680-204-9214 (see page 632)
Qualifies for 1.0 hour of CE credit

Warfarin-induced intramural hematoma of the small intestine

Learning Objectives

After studying this article, the reader should be able to

1. Describe the demographic and anatomical setting in which warfarin-induced intramural hematoma of the small intestine is most likely to occur.
2. Describe the signs and symptoms of intramural hematoma.
3. Describe the laboratory and radiological findings associated with warfarin-induced intramural hematoma.
4. Recommend a treatment regimen for a patient with warfarin-induced intramural hematoma.
5. Identify the benefits and risks of resuming warfarin therapy after warfarin-induced intramural hematoma has resolved.

Self-assessment Questions

For each question there is only one best answer.

1. The typical patient described in the medical literature as suffering warfarin-induced intramural hematoma of the small intestine is a
   a. 40-year-old white man.
   b. 60-year-old white man.
   c. 40-year-old black woman.
   d. 60-year-old black man.
2. Intramural hematoma typically occurs in the
   a. Duodenum.
   b. Proximal jejunum.
   c. Ileum.
   d. Alternatives a and b only are correct.
3. Symptoms that commonly accompany warfarin-induced intramural hematoma include
   a. Dizziness, headache, and nausea.
   b. Nausea, vomiting, and abdominal pain.
   c. Shortness of breath, fever, and vomiting.
   d. Calf tenderness, nausea, and vomiting.
4. Laboratory findings commonly associated with warfarin-induced intramural hematoma include
   a. A high hemoglobin concentration and hematocrit and a prolonged prothrombin time.
   b. A low hemoglobin concentration and hematocrit and a normal prothrombin time.
   c. A low hemoglobin concentration and hematocrit and a prolonged prothrombin time.
   d. A high hemoglobin concentration and hematocrit and a normal prothrombin time.
5. A roentgenographic sign associated with intramural hematoma is
   a. Flattening of the diaphragm.
   b. Free air in the peritoneum.
   c. Gas trapped in the involved section of bowel.
   d. None of the above alternatives is correct.
6. One technique that may be useful in the diagnosis of intramural hematoma is
   a. Diagnostic ultrasound.
   b. Computed tomography.
   c. Barium study of the upper GI tract.
   d. All of the above alternatives are correct.
7. Clinical resolution of warfarin-induced intramural hematoma
   a. Often occurs within a few days after withdrawal

Current Literature

Drug Reaction Alerts 652

Book Review

The Biochemical Basis of Neuropharmacology, Sixth Edition 655
Jack R. Cooper, Floyd E. Bloom, and Robert H. Roth
Reviewed by Martha P. Fankhauser

Books Received 655

Drug Reaction Alerts

Drug Reaction Alerts focuses primarily on serious, unlabeled reactions to new chemical entities. The citations are compiled monthly from International Pharmaceutical Abstracts, *which covers over 800 pharmacy and health-related journals worldwide. An address for reprints (when available) follows the name of the corresponding author in each citation.*

Pharmacists may use the FDA Adverse Reaction Report form that appears in the January and July issues of Clinical Pharmacy *for submitting reports of adverse drug reactions directly to FDA.*

Androgens

Rosner F, Khan MT. Renal cell carcinoma following prolonged **testosterone** therapy. *Arch Intern Med.* 1992; 152:426, 429. Case. (22-year-old man with ambiguous genitalia that were surgically corrected in infancy; received oral and injectable testosterone therapies for at least two years after surgeries; developed renal cell carcinoma that had widely metastasized by time of diagnosis; died within a few weeks of diagnosis)

Antineoplastic Agents

Bentley CR, Davies G, Aclimandos WA (Ophthalmology Department, King's College Hospital, London SE5 9RS, England). **Tamoxifen** retinopathy: rare but serious complication. *Br Med J.* 1992; 304:495-6. Case. (72-year-old woman with breast cancer and diabetes mellitus; received tamoxifen 40 mg daily for five years after radiotherapy; complained of blurred vision after one year, which worsened during subsequent four years; misdiagnosed with diabetic retinopathy; further examination of visual problem revealed similarity to previously reported cases of tamoxifen-induced retinal toxicity; withdrawal of tamoxifen did not change visual acuity after six months)

O'Brien ME, Tonge K, Blake P et al. (Wiltshaw E, Department of Medicine, Royal Marsden Hospital, London SW3 6JJ, England). Blindness associated with high-dose **carboplatin**. *Lancet.* 1992; 339:558. Cases. (two women, aged 60 and 61 years, with advanced epithelial ovarian cancer and impaired renal function; received high-dose carboplatin for total doses of 720 and 900 mg; developed sudden-onset cortical blindness; improved gradually during week after onset of blindness; 61-year-old woman continued carboplatin therapy without further episodes of blindness)

Weiss KS (Kaiser Permanente Medical Center, Cleveland, OH 44130). Nephrotic range of proteinuria and interferon therapy. *Ann Intern Med.* 1992; 116:347. Case. (64-year-old man with malignant melanoma; received **interferon gamma** 0.01 mg/sq m three times weekly by i.v. injection for four weeks; developed proteinuria with urine protein concentration in range usually associated with nephrotic syndrome; withdrawal of interferon gamma led to resolution of proteinuria after one week)

Continued on page 654

Continued from page 652

Antivirals

Herskowitz A (The Johns Hopkins School of Hygiene, Department of Immunology and Infectious Diseases, 615 N. Wolfe Street, Room 5017D, Baltimore, MD 21205), Willoughby SB, Baughman KL et al. Cardiomyopathy associated with antiretroviral therapy in patients with HIV infection: a report of six cases. *Ann Intern Med.* 1992; 116:311-3. Cases. (five men and one woman, aged 25–50 years, with human immunodeficiency virus and helper T-cell count <100/sq mm; received **zidovudine** for 7–23 months; three patients who also had AIDS developed cardiac dysfunction, which improved after withdrawal of zidovudine; four of six patients developed new or further depression of cardiac function after replacement of zidovudine with **didanosine** or with didanosine plus **zalcitabine** [ddC]; withdrawal of zidovudine led to rapid improvement in cardiac function in four patients; two patients developed skeletal myositis along with myocarditis during zidovudine therapy; positive rechallenge in two patients)

Contamination

Ayliffe W (Manchester Royal Eye Hospital, Manchester M13 9PH, England), Haeney M, Roberts SC et al. Uveitis after antineutrophil cytoplasmic antibody contamination of immunoglobulin replacement therapy. *Lancet.* 1992; 339:558-9. Case. (nine-year-old boy with X-linked agammaglobulinemia; received **immune globulin** 0.2 g/kg every two weeks by i.v. injection and increased to 0.4 g/kg every two weeks; developed decreased vision with granulomatous uveitis in left eye within three months of dose increase; replacement of immune globulin formulation with one not contaminated with antineutrophil cytoplasmic antibodies and therapy with systemic prednisolone led to improvement in visual acuity and resolution of cellular infiltrate; therapy with topical prednisolone led to control of persistent mild anterior uveitis)

Drug Abuse

Screaton GR (Department of Medicine, University College Hospital, London WC1E 6AU, England), Singer M, Cairns HS et al. Hyperpyrexia and rhabdomyolysis after MDMA (ecstasy) abuse. *Lancet.* 1992; 339:677-8. Cases. (three 19-year-old men; abused **methylenedioxymethamphetamine**; developed hyperpyrexia with subsequent rhabdomyolysis and disseminated intravascular coagulation; therapy with rapid cooling and forced diuresis led to full neurological recovery in two men; further neurological deterioration in third man led to death; one man who recovered developed a severely impaired gait because of muscle loss)

Fetal Death

Dearlove JC, Betteridge TJ, Henry JA (Guy's Hospital, London SE1 9RT, England). Stillbirth due to intravenous **amphetamine**. *Br Med J.* 1992; 304:548. Case. (34-week-old female fetus of 29-year-old pregnant mother with history of amphetamine abuse; mother intravenously injected amphetamine 500 mg; two hours after injection, fetal heart rate was 90–100 beats/min and subsequently decreased further; approximately 24 hours after injection, 3-kg fetus born stillborn; umbilical cord blood and infant plasma amphetamine concentrations were 0.11 and 0.09 mg/L, respectively; mother developed acute tubular necrosis but recovered without hemodialysis and refused postpartum follow-up)

Immunotherapy

Chazerain P, Meyer O, Kahn MF (Xavier Bichet Medical School, 75018 Paris, France). Rheumatoid arthritis-like disease after alpha-interferon therapy. *Ann Intern Med.* 1992; 116:427. Cases. (three patients, aged 42–64 years, with chronic myeloproliferative disorder or chronic active autoimmune hepatitis; received **interferon alfa-2a** or **interferon alfa-2b**; developed polyarthritis; withdrawal of interferon alfa and therapy with corticosteroids led to improvement of symptoms in two patients; therapy with prednisone and azathioprine did not lead to resolution of symptoms in third patient)

Penicillins

Fairley CK (Department of Sociology and Preventive Medicine, Monash University, Alfred Hospital, Prahran, Victoria 3181, Australia), Boyd I, Purcell P et al. Flucloxacillin jaundice. *Lancet.* 1992; 339:679. Study. (case series; 17 men and 34 women in whom **floxacillin** was sole drug suspected of causing cholestatic jaundice; mean age, 58 years; mean duration of floxacillin therapy, 14.9 days; mean onset latency for development of cholestasis, 22.6 days after start of floxacillin therapy; mean daily floxacillin dose, 2.2 g; total of 131 cases of cholestasis reported to adverse-drug-reaction registry, but not all could be determined to be caused by floxacillin)

Platelet Aggregation Inhibitors

Baker PN, Williamson JG (Rosie Maternity Hospital, Cambridge CB2 2NQ, England), Louden KA. Possible low-dose-**aspirin**-induced gastropathy. *Lancet.* 1992; 339:550. Cases. (two women, aged 28 and 30 years; received aspirin 60 or 75 mg/day; one woman, with no history of peptic ulceration, received aspirin for 10 days as part of study of cyclo-oxygenase-dependent platelet reactivity; developed melena two weeks after repeat of 10-day course 12 months later; healing duodenal ulcer noted at gastroscopy and treated with cimetidine; other woman, at 10 weeks' gestation, received aspirin for pregnancy-induced hypertension; developed epigastric pain and melena 19 weeks later; therapy with blood transfusions and i.v. ranitidine did not allow continuation of pregnancy; decelerations in fetal heart rate led to cesarean section and delivery of live 680-g baby girl; small superficial gastric ulcer and mild gastritis seen at gastroscopy of mother; therapy with cimetidine and alginic acid led to uneventful recovery)

Prolactin Inhibitors

Merola B, Sarnacchiaro F, Colao A et al. (Lombardi G, Department of Endocrinology and Institute of Pharmacology, II School of Medicine, University of Naples, 80131 Naples, Italy). Allergy to ergot-derived dopamine agonists. *Lancet.* 1992; 339:620. Case. (26-year-old man with hyperprolactinemia; received single dose of **bromocriptine** 2.5 mg; immediately developed allergic manifestations with headache and vomiting; replacement of bromocriptine with **lisuride**, another ergot-derived dopamine agonist, led to allergic reaction; replacement with **quinagolide** 0.075 mg, a non-ergot-derived dopamine agonist, led to no adverse effects or allergic reactions and serum prolactin concentration decreased from 163 to 12 ng/mL; continued therapy with quinagolide led to serum prolactin concentrations in normal range with restoration of gonadal function)

Skin and Mucous Membrane Preparations

McIvor A (Wellesley Hospital, Toronto, Ontario M5R 1A8, Canada). Fatal toxic epidermal necrolysis associated with **etretinate**. *Br Med J.* 1992; 304:548. Case. (65-year-old man with psoriatic arthropathy and non-insulin-dependent diabetes; received etretinate 25 mg twice daily for 16 days; developed ulcers on mucous membranes and erythematous blisters on skin; skin tissue biopsy confirmed fatal toxic epidermal necrolysis; concomitant ultraviolet-B light therapy, coal tar preparations, indomethacin, and chlorpropamide; therapy with broad-spectrum antimicrobials and transfer to intensive-care unit did not lead to improvement; developed pseudomonal septicemia with pancytopenia and died)

Sympatholytic Agents

Varkey S (Rotherham District General Hospital, Rotherham S60 2UD, England). Overdose of **yohimbine**. *Br Med J.* 1992; 304:548. Case. (38-year-old man with impotence and insulin-dependent diabetes; self-poisoned with yohimbine 350 mg;

developed atrial fibrillation with ventricular response of 150 beats/min, retrograde amnesia that would last four days, and rectal temperature of 35.5 °C 25 hours after ingestion of yohimbine; recovered without specific therapy)

Teratogenicity

Camera G (Center for Human Genetics, Galliera Hospital, 16128 Genoa, Italy), Pregliasco P. Ear malformation in baby born to mother using **tretinoin** cream. *Lancet*. 1992; 339:687. Case. (2.62-kg baby girl born after 41 weeks' gestation; mother applied 0.05% tretinoin cream during month before her last menstruation and during first 11 weeks of pregnancy; baby born with crumpled hypoplastic ear and atresia of external auditory meatus on right side)

Tranquilizers

Cates M, Lusk K, Wells BG et al. (West M, Memphis Mental Health Institute, Memphis, TN 38105). Nonleukopenic neutropenia in a patient treated with **clozapine**. *N Engl J Med*. 1992; 326:840-1. Case. (29-year-old woman with chronic disorganized schizophrenia; received clozapine 25–112.5 mg/day for 15 days; developed nonleukopenic neutropenia; neutrophil count decreased by more than 50% from day 7 to day 14, while white blood cell count remained stable and within normal limits; clozapine withdrawn)

Book Review

The Biochemical Basis of Neuropharmacology, Sixth Edition

By Jack R. Cooper, Floyd E. Bloom, and Robert H. Roth. Published by Oxford University Press, Inc., 200 Madison Avenue, New York, NY 10016, 1991. xi + 454 p. Price $45 (hardback), $24.95 (softbound).

First published in 1970, this book is one of the most popular basic reviews of neuropharmacology for students, clinicians, and scientists. It can usually be found in the private libraries of specialists in neuropharmacology, psychiatry, or neurology, because it reviews the basics of neurotransmitters and drug actions in the central nervous system (CNS).

In the sixth edition, several chapters have been updated and reorganized, and new information about peptides and receptor subtypes has been added; the only new chapter is a reinstated one on neuropharmacology and cellular mechanisms of learning and memory. The first six chapters include a general introduction and cover the basics of neuropharmacology. The well-written overview of biochemistry provides a complete description of the nerve cell and the steps for synaptic transmission. The chapter on molecular neuropharmacology discusses biological engineering and molecular-cloning methods. The review of CNS metabolism presents the interrelationships of neurochemicals and neurotransmitters and describes biochemical pathways and hereditary diseases with defects in amino acid, lipid, or carbohydrate metabolism. The excellent chapter on neuronal receptors gives new information about receptor subtypes for such receptors as adrenergic, dopaminergic, serotonergic, and cholinergic. The overview of synaptic transmission discusses changes in presynaptic and postsynaptic modulation and explains current knowledge of secondary messenger systems.

The next six chapters provide excellent reviews of neurotransmitter systems (amino acids, acetylcholine, norepinephrine and epinephrine, dopamine, serotonin and histamine, and neuroactive peptides). Each chapter includes schematics of neuronal pathways, information about neurotransmitter synthesis and metabolism, and illustrations of neurons and receptors. The models of neurons are helpful for understanding the possible sites of drug action. For each type of neuron, medications are listed that may affect neurotransmitter biosynthesis, storage, release, presynaptic or postsynaptic receptor interaction, reuptake, and metabolism. Each chapter includes recently published references and recommends review articles about the neurotransmitter system.

The book reflects the authors' enormous efforts to review the basics of neuropharmacology at a level that is understandable and applicable to clinical practitioners. It provides a complete and current update of neurotransmitters, nerve cell transmission, CNS disease states, and medications with CNS activity. Considering its reasonable price, *The Biochemical Basis of Neuropharmacology* is one of the best resources available to pharmacists who want a concise review that updates their knowledge of neuropharmacology.

Reviewed by Martha P. Fankhauser, M.S., Department of Pharmacy Practice, College of Pharmacy, The University of Arizona Health Sciences Center, Tucson, AZ 85721.

Books Received

Books are listed as soon as received; selected books may be reviewed in Book Reviews in subsequent issues.

Clinical Primer of Psychopharmacology: A Practical Guide, Second Edition, by Donald M. Pirodsky and Jerry S. Cohn. Published by McGraw-Hill, Inc., 1221 Avenue of the Americas, New York, NY 10020, 1992. xiii + 129 p. Price $19.95.

Clinical Pharmacology: Basic Principles in Therapeutics, Third Edition, edited by Kenneth L. Melmon, Howard F. Morrelli, Brian B. Hoffman et al. Published by McGraw-Hill, Inc., 1221 Avenue of the Americas, New York, NY 10020, 1992. xv + 1141 p. Price $49.95.

Compendium of Pharmaceuticals and Specialties, Twenty-seventh Edition, Carmen M. E. Krogh, editor-in-chief. Published by the Canadian Pharmaceutical Association, 1785 Alta Vista Drive, Ottawa, Ontario K1G 3Y6, Canada, 1992. xv + 1546 p. Price $100 + $10 shipping and handling per copy.

Pharmaceutical Biotechnology: A Programmed Text, edited by S. William Zito. Published by Technomic Publishing Company, Inc., 851 New Holland Avenue, Box 3535, Lancaster, PA 17604, 1992. x + 177 p. Price $45.

Advertising Index

American Lung Association
Institutional, 578
American Society of Hospital Pharmacists
AHFS Drug Information 92, 656
ASHP Membership, 647-648
ASHP Software, 653
Basic Skills in Interpreting Laboratory Data, 585
Clinical Pharmacy, 586
Criteria for Drug Use Evaluation, Volumes 1, 2, and 3, 656
Drug Information on CD, 578
Medication Errors: A Closer Look, 617
Medication Teaching Manual, 643
Publications Services Catalogue, 579
Rx Triage, 631
Safe Handling of Cytotoxic and Hazardous Drugs, 624
Amgen Inc.
Epogen, 573
ASHP Research and Education Foundation
Anticoagulation Clinic Traineeship Program, 651
Burroughs Wellcome Company
Exosurf Neonatal, 587-590
Enzon, Inc.
Institutional, 577
Eli Lilly and Company
Hospital Division, 575
SmithKline Beecham
Timentin, inside back cover, outside back cover
UMI Article Clearinghouse
Microform Reproductions, 585
The Upjohn Company
Zefazone, 580-582
Wyeth-Ayerst Laboratories, Inc.
Ativan Injection, 644-646
Tubex, inside front cover

News

FDA approves release of recombinant interleukin-2 product 669

Federal task force revises recommendations for PCP prophylaxis 670

News Briefs 670

Upcoming Specialty Meetings 670

FDA approves release of recombinant interleukin-2 product

Aldesleukin (Proleukin, Cetus Oncology Corporation), a human recombinant interleukin-2 product, has been approved by FDA for the treatment of adults with metastatic renal cell carcinoma.

Immunologic effects of aldesleukin include activation of cellular immunity with lymphocytosis, eosinophilia, and thrombocytopenia and production of cytokines, including tumor necrosis factor, interleukin-1, and gamma interferon. The mechanism of antitumor activity is unknown.

An objective response was seen in 37 (15%) of the 255 patients with metastatic renal cell carcinoma who were treated through clinical trials; there were 9 complete responses and 28 partial responses. The median duration of response was 23.2 months (range, 1–50 months). Both the response to treatment and the frequency of adverse reactions were related to performance status. Candidates for therapy should have normal cardiac, pulmonary, hepatic, and central nervous system function.

Serious adverse reactions are common. Drug-related deaths occurred in 11 (4%) of the 255 patients treated through clinical trials. The most frequently reported serious reactions are hypotension (85%), renal dysfunction with oliguria or anuria (76%), dyspnea (54%) or pulmonary congestion (52%), and mental status changes (73%). Capillary leak syndrome can occur.

Aldesleukin is contraindicated in patients with abnormal results on thallium stress tests or pulmonary function tests. Patients who experience certain serious adverse reactions should not be retreated with aldesleukin; these include sustained ventricular tachycardia; cardiac rhythm disturbances not controlled or unresponsive to management; recurrent chest pain with electrocardiographic changes, documented angina, or myocardial infarction; pericardial tamponade; intubation for more than 72 hours; renal dysfunction requiring dialysis for more than 72 hours; coma or toxic psychosis lasting for more than 48 hours; repetitive or difficult-to-control seizures; bowel ischemia or perforation; or gastrointestinal bleeding that requires surgery.

Dosage recommendations for aldesleukin in the treatment of metastatic renal cell carcinoma call for a 28-dose course of therapy. Aldesleukin 600,000 IU/kg (0.037 mg/kg) is infused intravenously over 15 minutes every eight hours for a total of 14 doses. Nine days later, this schedule is repeated. Response should be evaluated about four weeks after the 28-dose treatment course is completed. If the tumor is smaller and retreatment is not contraindicated, additional courses may be given. At least seven weeks should elapse between hospital discharge and retreatment. In clinical trials, this dosage schedule was modified frequently because of toxicity; patients received a median of 20 of 28 scheduled doses.

Proleukin is supplied in packs of 10 single-use vials containing 22×10^6 IU of lyophilized aldesleukin.

Federal task force revises recommendations for PCP prophylaxis

A task force of the U.S. Public Health Service has updated its recommendations for prophylaxis against *Pneumocystis carinii* pneumonia (PCP) in adults and adolescents infected with human immunodeficiency virus (HIV). The recommendations now name trimethoprim/sulfamethoxazole (TMP/SMX) as the preferred agent for primary and secondary prophylaxis. Recommendations issued by the task force in 1989 did not identify either pentamidine or TMP/SMX as preferred therapy. Coadministration of leucovorin with TMP/SMX is no longer recommended.

Primary prophylaxis is recommended for patients with a CD4+ T-lymphocyte count of <200 cells/μL and for patients with constitutional symptoms such as thrush or an unexplained fever of >100 °F (37.8 °C) for at least two weeks, regardless of CD4+ T-lymphocyte count. Primary prophylaxis should be lifelong. Secondary prophylaxis is indicated in any patient who has recovered from an episode of PCP. Before any prophylactic regimen is started, active pulmonary diseases that require treatment (e.g., tuberculosis, PCP, or histoplasmosis) should be excluded.

Recommended regimens for prophylaxis are (1) TMP/SMX 160 mg/800 mg given once daily seven days each week, (2) pentamidine 300 mg given once each month via a Respirgard II nebulizer (Marquest, Englewood, CO), or (3) pentamidine 60 mg given every two weeks via a Fisoneb nebulizer (Fisons, Rochester, NY) (after a loading regimen of five 60-mg doses given over two weeks).

TMP/SMX is the preferred treatment for patients who have had no serious reactions to trimethoprim or sulfa drugs. Data regarding other drugs were insufficient for the task force to recommend their use, but other drugs may be considered if neither of the recommended drugs can be given. The task force members disagreed on whether patients who have experienced non-life-threatening reactions to TMP/SMX can be safely rechallenged with TMP/SMX. Aerosolized pentamidine is contraindicated in patients who have developed hypoglycemia, pancreatitis, arrhythmia, or severe hypotension after treatment with any form of pentamidine.

Despite compliance with the prescribed prophylactic regimen, breakthrough episodes can occur. Although data are lacking, some task force members choose to treat these episodes with a different agent (i.e., intravenous pentamidine for patients receiving TMP/SMX prophylaxis and TMP/SMX for patients receiving aerosol pentamidine prophylaxis). The choice of prophylactic regimen after a breakthrough episode should be based on the same considerations that guided the original decision.

1. Centers for Disease Control. Recommendations for prophylaxis against *Pneumocystis carinii* pneumonia for adults and adolescents infected with HIV. *MMWR*. 1992; 41(RR-4):1–12.

News Briefs

- **Chlorodeoxyadenosine** is being made available under a treatment IND protocol for use by patients with hairy cell leukemia who cannot participate in ongoing clinical trials. The drug is administered as a continuous seven-day intravenous infusion; one course of therapy is given. For more information, call the National Cancer Institute at 301-496-5725.

- Novo Nordisk Pharmaceuticals Inc. has notified pharmacists of the potential for problems with the **NovolinPen Dial-A-Dose insulin delivery device** when patients rely on an audible "click" to set the insulin dose; after wear on the device, the sound may disappear. The company warns that visually impaired patients should not rely on the sound and should not use the device without assistance. To exchange their devices for the newest model, current users of the NovolinPen may contact Novo Nordisk, 800-727-6500.

- An **intravenous formulation of ofloxacin** (Floxin I.V., McNeil Pharmaceutical) has been introduced; it is supplied in 50-mL flexible containers (200 mg of ofloxacin in solution) and in 10- and 20-mL vials, 100-mL bottles, and 100-mL flexible containers (each containing 400 mg of ofloxacin in solution). Dosage recommendations for the oral and intravenous formulations are identical.

- An article published in the April 23, 1992, issue of *The New England Journal of Medicine* (1992; 326:1153-7) provides additional analysis of the preclinical and clinical studies of **HA-1A** (Centoxin, Centocor); the report includes new information presented at an FDA advisory committee meeting in September 1991. The authors summarize alternative analyses presented at that meeting by FDA analysts and critically review the available data. They conclude that HA-1A should remain experimental until a second randomized, placebo-controlled trial confirms the drug's efficacy in patients with presumed gram-negative bacteremia who are in septic shock.

- A subcommittee of the American Heart Association has issued a statement that provides strategies for **promoting cardiovascular health for all children** as a part of routine pediatric care; the report was published in the April 1992 issue of *Circulation*.

- A viscous solution of **diazepam for rectal administration** (Diastat, Upsher-Smith) has been granted orphan drug status for treatment of uncontrolled, severe epilepsy.

Upcoming Specialty Meetings

Association of Clinical Scientists. Santa Barbara, CA, November 11–15; contact F. W. Sunderman, Jr., M.D., Department of Laboratory Medicine, University of Connecticut School of Medicine, Farmington, CT 06030; 203-679-2328.

American College of Allergy and Immunology. Chicago, IL, November 14–18; contact ACAI, 800 East Northwest Highway, Suite 1080, Palatine, IL 60067; 708-359-2800.

American Geriatrics Society. Washington, DC, November 15–18; contact AGS, 700 Lexington Avenue, Suite 300, New York, NY 10021; 212-308-1414.

American Heart Association. New Orleans, LA, November 16–19; contact AHA, 7320 Greenville Avenue, Dallas, TX 75231; 214-706-1335.

Assistant Professor/Lecturer
The Wellesley Hospital/Faculty of Pharmacy
Doctor of Pharmacy Program
University of Toronto

Applications are invited for two assistant professor/lecturer positions associated with the Doctor of Pharmacy program at the University of Toronto. The positions are offered jointly by the Department of Pharmaceutical Services at The Wellesley Hospital and the Faculty of Pharmacy at the University of Toronto. The primary site of employment will be The Wellesley Hospital, with one position involved in family practice and the other involved with general internal medicine.

- **Family Practice Position**: Working in the family practice clinics, the candidate would develop and maintain a strong clinical pharmacy practice, providing pharmaceutical care in a multidisciplinary setting to a diverse patient population.
- **General Internal Medicine Position**: This position would involve provision of pharmaceutical care to one inpatient medical care unit. Follow-up of patients in an ambulatory-care clinic environment would also be expected. Expertise in infectious disease would be an asset or an expectation for development.

Each candidate would be responsible to serve as preceptor to up to eight Doctor of Pharmacy students per year for one-month rotations in their practice setting and to provide up to two months of instruction in the Advanced Therapeutics Course of the program. Approximately 80% of each individual's time would relate to teaching and clinical service while the balance of time would relate to the hospital's specific needs, which may include research, and/or provision of continuing education to hospital staff. Qualified applicants should possess a Doctor of Pharmacy degree plus a minimum of one year of experience in a relevant specialty area, or another degree with sufficient experience to provide comparable expertise. These positions will interest self-motivated pharmacists capable of problem-based teaching and working collaboratively with the health-care team. Applications will be considered by the Faculty and The Wellesley Hospital beginning August 1, 1992. For further information, contact Nancy Winslade or Andrea Cameron, Director of Pharmaceutical Services, The Wellesley Hospital, 416-926-4840.

Applicants should submit a current curriculum vitae and arrange to have three letters of reference sent to Dr. Nancy Winslade, Director of the Pharm.D. Program, Faculty of Pharmacy, University of Toronto, 19 Russell Street, Toronto, Ontario M5S 2S2, Canada; 416-978-4241. EOE.

CLINICAL PHARMACY SERVICES COORDINATOR

VHA of Southern New England, a regional alliance of hospitals in Connecticut, is seeking applicants for the position of Clinical Pharmacy Services Coordinator.

This unique position offers growth opportunities for an innovative pharmacist to work with 13 hospitals in a regional system to 1) coordinate marketing strategies and programs to reduce drug costs, 2) develop and maintain selected comparative statistics and DUE reports, and 3) develop and maintain clinical modules for the advancement of pharmacy practice at the staff level.

Candidates must have a Pharm.D. or M.S. degree, with a residency or fellowship preferred, and at least five years of clinical pharmacy experience. Excellent communication and management skills are required. Salary commensurate with experience. Equal Opportunity Employer.

Please send résumé to
Linda Poniatoski
VHA of Southern New England, Inc.
74 Scott Swamp Road
Farmington, CT 06032

Therapy Consultation

The Therapy Consultation *section provides brief advice, in question-and-answer format, on how to handle specific drug-therapy problems. Readers are invited to submit questions, which will be referred to a consultant for an answer. The problems should not be highly specialized or unusual, nor should they be mundane. Questions are answered briefly, based largely on the judgment and personal experience of the consultant, although selected references may be cited to substantiate the consultant's advice.*

Assistance in identifying Therapy Consultation *topics is provided by the drug information centers at Medical College of Virginia Hospitals, Richmond; University of California Medical Center, San Diego; and University of Michigan Medical Center, Ann Arbor.*

Use of ursodiol in a patient with biliary cirrhosis

Question: A patient with biliary cirrhosis is experiencing severe pruritus. Use of ursodiol to relieve pruritus has been suggested. What is the rationale for this suggestion? Should the drug be given? If so, what dosage should be used?

Answer: *Function of Ursodiol.* Severe pruritus frequently occurs in patients with primary or secondary biliary cirrhosis. This pruritus is thought to result from elevated serum levels of bile acids that accumulate secondary to hepatobiliary obstruction (cholestasis).

The hallmark of primary biliary cirrhosis (PBC) is progressive destruction of the small and intermediate intrahepatic ducts. This destruction is thought to be secondary to immunologic attack, although the exact etiology is yet unproven. Secondary biliary cirrhosis results from prolonged biliary obstruction caused by strictures, carcinoma, gallstones, or biliary atresia.

The cholestasis that ensues is thought to contribute to the resultant biochemical, histologic, and physiologic derangements observed. The hydrophobic bile acids, deoxycholic, chenodeoxycholic, and cholic acids, are found in relatively larger quantities in the bile acid pool than is ursodeoxycholic acid (ursodiol), the most hydrophilic bile acid. This is key, because the hydrophobicity of those accumulated bile acids appears to correlate with their ability to solubilize membrane lipids and cause cytotoxic hepatic damage. The bile acid pool, composed mainly of potentially hepatotoxic bile acids, is elevated 20–40 fold in biliary cirrhosis.

The rationale for the use of ursodiol is to increase the hydrophilicity of the bile acid pool, thereby decreasing the cytotoxic potential. The effect of ursodiol on the total bile acid pool is variable; however, it has been clearly demonstrated that with repeated administration ursodiol becomes the major bile acid in the plasma, with concurrent reductions in the more toxic chenodeoxycholic and cholic acids. Ursodiol may also have a favorable impact on reducing immunologic responses that may be the etiology of certain diseases. Because of these potential benefits, ursodiol has also been studied for other liver diseases such as chronic hepatitis[1,2] and chronic graft versus host disease.[3]

Effects on Pruritus. Eight studies of PBC specifically evaluated pruritus as an outcome measure; ursodiol was associated with a beneficial effect in all of these studies, but the degree of benefit varied. Matsuzaki et al.,[4] in an open trial of ursodiol at a dosage of 1800 mg/day, reported abolishment of pruritus after only one month of therapy in six of seven patients who had reported that symptom before starting therapy. In another open trial, Osuga et al.[1] used a much smaller dosage of ursodiol, 600 mg/day; one month into treatment, these investigators also demonstrated diminished pruritus in all five patients who had reported it before therapy began. Combined results from two other open trials and one placebo-controlled, crossover study, involving a total of 18 patients complaining of pruritus, demonstrated that ursodiol therapy with dosages ranging from 750 mg/day to 15 mg/kg/day resulted in the absence of pruritus in 12 patients and a reduction of pruritus in 4 of the remaining 6 patients.[5-7]

In two double-blind, placebo-controlled trials using ursodiol for PBC, a trend toward decreased pruritus, but no significant reduction, was demonstrated.[8,9] In both trials, the lack of statistical significance was mainly due to a large placebo effect. In a study by Poupon et al.,[8] more than 130 persons with PBC were randomized to receive either 13–15 mg/kg/day of ursodiol or placebo; a 22% decrease in the incidence of pruritus was seen in the ursodiol group, but a similar 13% decrease was seen in the placebo group. A smaller study by Oka et al.[9] showed similar results; four of nine patients receiving ursodiol 600 mg/day reported decreased or resolved pruritus, but so did two of seven members of the placebo group.

Although statistical significance of ursodiol's benefit for pruritus may be obscured by the large placebo effect, the clinical significance of benefit is evident when all eight studies are examined. In addition to its potential benefits for pruritus, ursodiol administration for PBC also appears to confer significant benefits in terms of both biochemical (aspartate aminotransferase, alanine aminotransferase, alkaline phosphatase, γ-glutamyl transferase, and total bilirubin) and histologic outcomes.[1,4-12]

Conclusion. In this patient with severe pruritus due to biliary cirrhosis, a trial of ursodiol seems warranted. Its potential benefit and virtual lack of adverse effects (infrequent diarrhea or transient exacerbation of pruritus) compare favorably with other agents with very narrow therapeutic indices that have been evaluated for treatment of PBC (corticosteroids, azathioprine, penicillamine, and cyclosporine).

Dosages of ursodiol in studies for PBC have usually ranged from 600 to 1800 mg/day; the most frequently used dosage is 13 to 15 mg/kg/day. However, in one study that did not examine pruritus, significant improvement in biochemical indices was found when ursodiol 250 mg/day was used for two months. Despite ursodiol's lack of adverse effects, it seems prudent to begin treatment with a dosage of 600 to 900 mg/day, since this therapy is not guided by conclusive comparative clinical trials. If required, the dosage may be increased to near 1800 mg/day.

1. Osuga T, Tanaka N, Matsuzaki Y et al. Effect of ursodeoxycholic acid in chronic hepatitis and primary biliary cirrhosis. *Dig Dis Sci*. 1989; 34(12, Suppl):49S-51S.
2. Podda M, Ghezzi C, Battezzati PM et al. Ursodeoxycholic acid for chronic liver diseases. *J Clin Gastroenterol*. 1988; 10(Suppl 2):S25-S31.
3. Fried RH, Murakami CS, Fisher LD et al. Ursodeoxycholic acid treatment of refractory chronic graft-versus-host disease of the liver. *Ann Intern Med*. 1992; 116:624-9.
4. Matsuzaki Y, Tanaka N, Osuga T et al. Improvement of biliary enzyme levels and itching as a result of long-term administration of ursodeoxycholic acid in primary biliary cirrhosis. *Am J Gastroenterol*. 1990; 85:15-23.
5. Bateson MC, Ross PE, Diffey BL. Ursodeoxycholic acid in primary biliary cirrhosis. *Lancet*. 1989; 1:898-9. Letter.
6. Poupon R, Poupon RE, Calmus Y et al. Is ursodeoxycholic acid an effective treatment for primary biliary cirrhosis? *Lancet*. 1987; 1:834-6.
7. Batta AK, Salen G, Arora R et al. Effect of ursodeoxycholic acid on bile acid metabolism in primary biliary cirrhosis. *Hepatology*. 1989; 10:414-9.
8. Poupon RE, Eschwege E, Poupon R et al. Ursodeoxycholic acid for the treatment of primary biliary cirrhosis. Interim analysis of a double-blind multicentre randomized trial. *J Hepatology*. 1990; 11:16-21.
9. Oka H, Toda G, Ikeda Y et al. A multi-center double-blind controlled trial of ursodeoxycholic acid for primary biliary cirrhosis. *Gastroenterol Jpn*. 1990; 25:774-80.
10. Kao JH, Lai MY, Lin JT et al. Therapeutic effect of ursodeoxycholic acid on early-stage primary biliary cirrhosis. *J Formosan Med Assoc*. 1991; 90:970-4.
11. Poupon RE, Balkau B, Eschwege E et al (UDCA-PBC Study Group). A multicenter, controlled trial of ursodiol for the treatment of primary biliary cirrhosis. *N Engl J Med*. 1991; 324:1548-54.
12. Podda M, Ghezzi C, Battezzati PM et al. Ursodeoxycholic acid for chronic liver diseases. *J Clin Gastroenterol*. 1988; 10(Suppl 2):S25-S31.

THOMAS G. VONDRACEK, PHARM.D.
Pharmacotherapy Specialty Resident in Adult Medicine

CHARLES F. SEIFERT, PHARM.D., BCPS
Associate Professor of Adult Medicine

College of Pharmacy
University of Oklahoma Health Sciences Center
Oklahoma City, OK 73190

Letters

Use of cytomegalovirus immune globulin 674
David R. Snydman

Potential interaction between terfenadine and macrolide antibiotics 675
Linda M. Cortese, Darrel C. Bjornson

The Letters *column is a forum for rapid exchange of ideas among readers of* Clinical Pharmacy. *Liberal criteria are applied in the review of submissions to encourage contributions to this column.*

The Letters *column includes the following types of contributions: (1) comments, addenda, and minor updates on previously published work, (2) alerts on potential problems related to drug therapy or clinical research, (3) observations or comments on trends in drug therapy or clinical research, and (4) brief expressions of opinion about controversies in drug therapy or clinical research.*

Letters need not be submitted with the journal's manuscript checklist. The following conditions, however, must be adhered to: (1) the body of the letter must be no longer than two typewritten pages, (2) the use of references, tables, and illustrations should be minimized, (3) the authors' names, affiliations, and mailing addresses must be typed at the end of the letter in the format used by Clinical Pharmacy, *and (4) the entire letter (including references, tables, and authors' names) must be typed double-spaced on plain white paper (not letterhead). Following acceptance of a letter, the authors are required to sign an exclusive publication statement and a copyright transferal form.*

Use of cytomegalovirus immune globulin

I found ASHP's guidelines for the use of i.v. immune globlin (IGIV),[1] which appeared in the February issue of *Clinical Pharmacy*, to be quite comprehensive, detailed, and well done. However, they only briefly mentioned the use of cytomegalovirus (CMV) immune globulin (human) to reduce the risk of CMV disease in CMV-seronegative recipients of kidneys from seropositive donors. Studies have provided sufficient data to support FDA's licensing of CMV immune globulin for the prevention of primary CMV disease in renal transplant recipients.[2]

There are relatively few data to support the use of unselective IGIV in patients with renal transplants. The ASHP guidelines cited studies by Steinmuller et al.[3,4]; however, one of those studies was actually uncontrolled and used historical data to establish the frequency of febrile CMV-related illness.

Although I recognize that the ASHP guidelines were developed to address the use of unselective IGIV, they should have mentioned that CMV immune globulin is available, is cost-effective when used for the prevention of primary CMV disease in recipients of kidney transplants,[5] and has this indication in its approved product labeling.

Some manufacturers of unselective IGIV have been touting the "CMV titer" of their product. The ASHP guidelines correctly pointed out that, without standardized techniques, direct comparison of products based on antibody titers is invalid. Brands and lots of IGIV vary in their CMV antibody titer. This is not the case for CMV immune globulin, which consistently has five to eight times as much CMV antibody titer as unselective IGIV. Thus, CMV immune globulin is the "gold standard" when the CMV antibody titer is considered and when the issue is clinical usefulness for CMV prophylaxis.

Recommendations for the use of any biologic product should be based on the results of prospective, randomized, controlled trials in which the endpoints and study hypotheses are predefined. The studies of unselective IGIV in solid-organ transplantation have consistently failed to meet these criteria.

1. ASHP Commission on Therapeutics. ASHP therapeutic guidelines for intravenous immune globulin. *Clin Pharm.* 1992; 11:117-36.
2. Nightingale SL. CMV-IGIV approved. *JAMA.* 1990; 264:168.
3. Steinmuller DR, Graneto D, Swift C et al. Use of intravenous immunoglobulin prophylaxis for primary cytomegalovirus infection post living-related-donor renal transplantation. *Transplant Proc.* 1989: 21:2069-71.
4. Steinmuller DR, Novick AC, Streem SB et al. Intravenous immunoglobulin infusions for the prophylaxis of secondary cytomegalovirus infection. *Transplantation.* 1990; 49:68-70.
5. Tsevat J, Snydman DR, Pauker SG et al. Which renal transplant

patients should receive cytomegalovirus immunoglobulin? A cost-effectiveness analysis. *Transplantation.* 1991;52:259-65.

DAVID R. SNYDMAN, M.D., Director
Clinical Microbiology
New England Medical Center Hospitals
750 Washington Street
Boston, MA 02111

Potential interaction between terfenadine and macrolide antibiotics

The review of clarithromycin and azithromycin by Piscitelli et al.[1] in the the February issue of *Clinical Pharmacy* did not mention what may be an important potential drug interaction. This interaction involves terfenadine and the macrolide antibiotics.

Terfenadine undergoes extensive hepatic metabolism, probably by the cytochrome P-450 oxidative pathway; thus, its metabolism may be reduced by drugs, such as some macrolide antibiotics, that inhibit the P-450 system. The current product labeling for terfenadine recommends against the concurrent use of terfenadine and troleandomycin and states that the concurrent use of terfenadine and other macrolide antibiotics should be approached with caution.[2]

Inhibition of the P-450 system during terfenadine therapy may have serious clinical consequences. Monahan et al.[3] reported the occurrence of torsade de pointes in a patient who was taking terfenadine and ketoconazole. The authors suggested that ketoconazole, which inhibits the P-450 pathway, decreased the metabolism of terfenadine and that an elevated serum terfenadine concentration caused the arrhythmia. They added that other drugs that inhibit the P-450 pathway, such as cimetidine and erythromycin, might have similar effects on terfenadine concentrations. Eller and Okerholm[4] subsequently confirmed that ketoconazole inhibits the metabolism of terfenadine. Honig et al.[5] showed that erythromycin alters terfenadine metabolism and that the resultant accumulation of terfenadine is associated, in certain individuals, with altered cardiac repolarization.

Terfenadine may not interact with all macrolide antibiotics. Nevertheless, a potential interaction between terfenadine and the macrolides clarithromycin and azithromycin should be kept in mind until studies prove that such interactions do not occur.

1. Piscitelli SC, Danziger LH, Rodvold KA. Clarithromycin and azithromycin: new macrolide antibiotics. *Clin Pharm.* 1992; 11:137-52.
2. Marion Merrell Dow, Inc. Seldane package insert. Kansas City, MO; 1990 Jul.
3. Monahan BP, Ferguson CL, Killeavy ES et al. Torsades de pointes occurring in association with terfenadine use. *JAMA.* 1990; 264:2788-90.
4. Eller MG, Okerholm RA. Pharmacokinetic interaction between terfenadine and ketoconazole. *Clin Pharmacol Ther.* 1991; 49:130. Abstract.
5. Honig PK, Zamani K, Woosley RL et al. Erythromycin changes terfenadine pharmacokinetics & electrocardiographic pharmacodynamics. *Clin Pharmacol Ther.* 1992; 51:156. Abstract.

LINDA M. CORTESE, M.S., Clinical Research Pharmacist
LTC DARREL C. BJORNSON, PH.D., Clinical Research Pharmacist

Henry M. Jackson Foundation
Walter Reed Army Medical Center
Building #1, Ward 11
Washington,DC 20307-5001

Drug Review

Pravastatin: A new drug for the treatment of hypercholesterolemia

PAUL W. JUNGNICKEL, KIMBERLY A. CANTRAL, AND PIERRE A. MALOLEY

Abstract: The chemistry, pharmacology, pharmacokinetics, clinical trials, adverse effects, role in lipid-lowering therapy, and dosage and administration of pravastatin are reviewed.

Pravastatin sodium is a new 3-hydroxy-3-methylglutaryl-coenzyme A (HMG-CoA) reductase inhibitor for the treatment of hypercholesterolemia. Its structural formula is similar to those of lovastatin and simvastatin, but it is active in the parent form. It competitively inhibits HMG-CoA reductase, reduces hepatic cellular cholesterol synthesis, increases the expression of hepatic low-density lipoprotein (LDL) receptors, and reduces hepatic very low-density lipoprotein (VLDL) synthesis.

Pravastatin has been demonstrated to reduce cholesterol in patients with familial and nonfamilial polygenic hypercholesterolemia and patients with diabetes mellitus. In doses of 10–40 mg/day, pravastatin has been shown to reduce total cholesterol by 15–30% and LDL cholesterol by 15–40%. It also increases high-density lipoprotein cholesterol by 2–20% and reduces triglycerides. It is generally well tolerated, with few adverse effects reported in clinical trials.

Pravastatin reduces LDL cholesterol and increases HDL cholesterol comparably to lovastatin but possibly with fewer adverse effects. Further studies and clinical use will be needed to confirm potential differences in adverse effect profiles between the two drugs.

Index terms: Antilipemic agents; Clinical studies; Dosage; Hypercholesterolemia; Pharmacokinetics; Pravastatin sodium; Toxicity
Clin Pharm. 1992; 11: 677-89

Hypercholesterolemia is a recognized independent risk factor for coronary heart disease (CHD). The recently published report from the National Cholesterol Education Program Expert Panel on Detection, Evaluation, and Treatment of High Blood Cholesterol in Adults[1] advocates intensified efforts to identify and treat patients with elevated low-density lipoprotein (LDL) cholesterol concentrations. Drug therapy is recommended for patients whose LDL cholesterol concentrations are not adequately lowered by dietary modifications.

Pharmacologic lowering of LDL cholesterol concentration has been shown in several primary[2,3] and secondary[4-7] intervention trials to decrease the occurrence of CHD and to prevent or delay CHD progression; regression of atherosclerotic lesions has been demonstrated in some patients.[4] However, the lipid-lowering drugs most commonly used in these trials, nicotinic acid (niacin) and bile acid-binding resins, produce adverse effects that may limit the degree of cholesterol lowering that can be achieved in many patients.[2-8]

The 3-hydroxy-3-methylglutaryl-coenzyme A (HMG-CoA) reductase inhibitors represent a new class of drugs that have potent LDL cholesterol-lowering effects and are well tolerated.[9] Mevastatin, a fungal metabolite produced by *Penicillium citrinum*, was discovered in 1976.[10] Lovastatin (Mevacor, Merck Sharp & Dohme), marketed in September 1987, was the first HMG-CoA reductase inhibitor introduced in the United States. Pravastatin (Pravachol, Bristol-Myers Squibb; CS-514; SQ-31,000; eptastatin) and simvastatin (Zocor, Merck Sharp & Dohme) are new additions to this class. Pravastatin is the subject of this review.

Chemistry

Pravastatin is formed by microbial transformation by the microorganism *Nocardia autotrophica*. Its struc-

PAUL W. JUNGNICKEL, M.S., KIMBERLY A. CANTRAL, PHARM.D., and PIERRE A. MALOLEY, PHARM.D., are Assistant Professors, Pharmacy Practice, University of Nebraska Medical Center, Omaha.
Address reprint requests to Mr. Jungnickel at the College of Pharmacy, University of Nebraska Medical Center, 600 South 42nd Street, Omaha, Nebraska 68198-6045.
The secretarial assistance of Sharon M. Dunbar, the clerical assistance of Karla Kube, and the graphics assistance of Marvin C. Pankaskie, Ph.D., and Scott A. Swigart, Pharm.D., are acknowledged.
Supported by a grant from Bristol-Myers Squibb Company.

tural formula is shown in Figure 1 along with those of lovastatin and simvastatin. The dihydroxyheptanoic acid moiety is the substrate analogue that interacts with the active site of HMG-CoA reductase. The decalin ring interacts with the binding site. Pravastatin sodium is chemically designated as [1*S*-[1α(β*S**,δ*S**),2α, 6α,8β(*R**),8α]]-1,2,6,7,8,8a-hexahydro-β,δ,6-trihydroxy-2-methyl-8-(2-methyl-1-oxobutoxy)-1-naphthaleneheptanoic acid, monosodium salt. Its empirical formula is $C_{23}H_{35}NaO_7$ and its molecular weight is 446.52.[11]

Pravastatin is a hygroscopic, crystalline powder that is freely soluble in water (>300 mg/mL) and methanol, slightly soluble in isopropanol, and practically insoluble in acetone, acetonitrile, chloroform, and ether.[11]

Pravastatin is active in the parent form, whereas lovastatin exists as an inactive lactone prodrug that must be converted in vivo to the active hydroxyacid form.[12] Pravastatin is relatively hydrophilic because of the hydroxyl group at the 6 position of the decalin ring and the open acid form of the substrate analogue (Figure 1). In contrast, lovastatin and simvastatin are lipophilic because of the presence of a methyl group at this position; simvastatin contains an additional methyl group on the isobutyl side chain.[13]

Figure 1. Structural formulas of pravastatin, lovastatin, and simvastatin. Boxes indicate notable differences among the drugs.

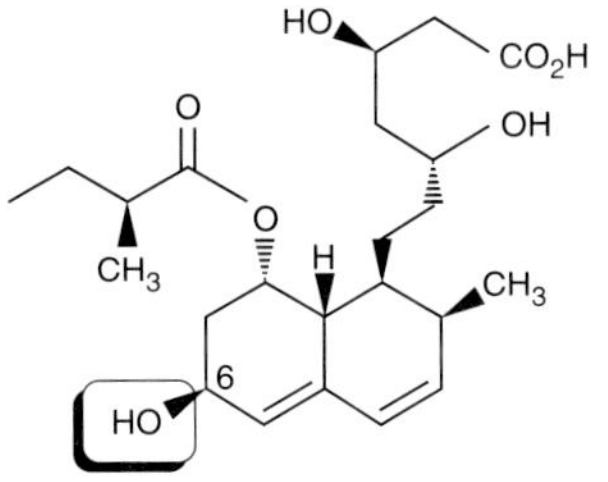

Pravastatin

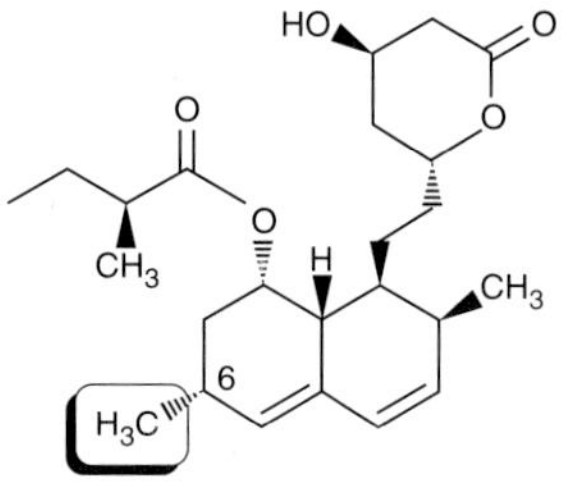

Lovastatin

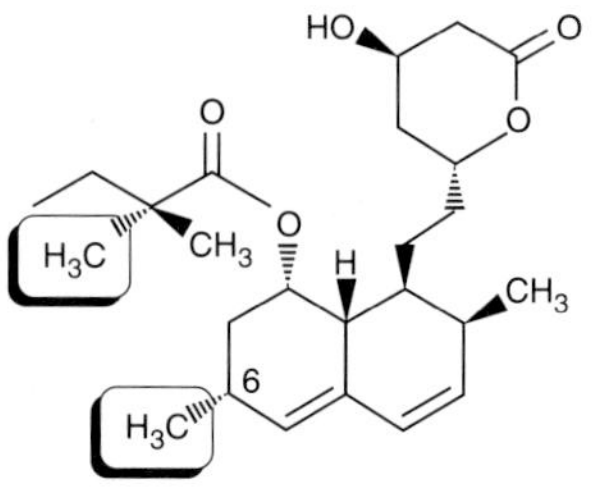

Simvastatin

Pharmacology

Knowledge of basic lipoprotein metabolism and CHD pathogenesis is necessary to understand the clinical pharmacology of the HMG-CoA reductase inhibitors. Such topics are beyond the scope of this article, however, and readers are referred to several reviews for this information.[14-18] Like the other agents in this class, pravastatin reversibly and competitively inhibits HMG-CoA reductase, the rate-limiting enzyme responsible for the conversion of HMG-CoA to mevalonate, the precursor of cholesterol and other sterols (Figure 2).[12,19] The resultant partial depletion of cellular cholesterol leads to increased production (up-regulation) of LDL receptors. Thus, the primary effect of pravastatin is to increase the clearance of LDL, very-low-density lipoprotein (VLDL), and VLDL remnants.[20,21] A secondary effect, related to the inhibition of cholesterol synthesis, is interference with hepatic VLDL synthesis, resulting in an indirect reduction of LDL concentration.[21,22]

The precise contribution of each of the above mechanisms to the pharmacologic action of the HMG-CoA reductase inhibitors is still being elucidated. Bilheimer et al.[23] demonstrated increased receptor-mediated LDL catabolism in patients with heterozygous familial hypercholesterolemia (FH) who were treated with lovastatin. In these patients, lovastatin had little effect in reducing the rate of LDL production. However, in pa-

Figure 2. The cholesterol biosynthesis pathway. Pravastatin inhibits HMG-CoA reductase, decreasing cholesterol biosynthesis. Acetyl-CoA = acetyl-coenzyme A; HMG-CoA = 3-hydroxy-3-methylglutaryl-coenzyme A.

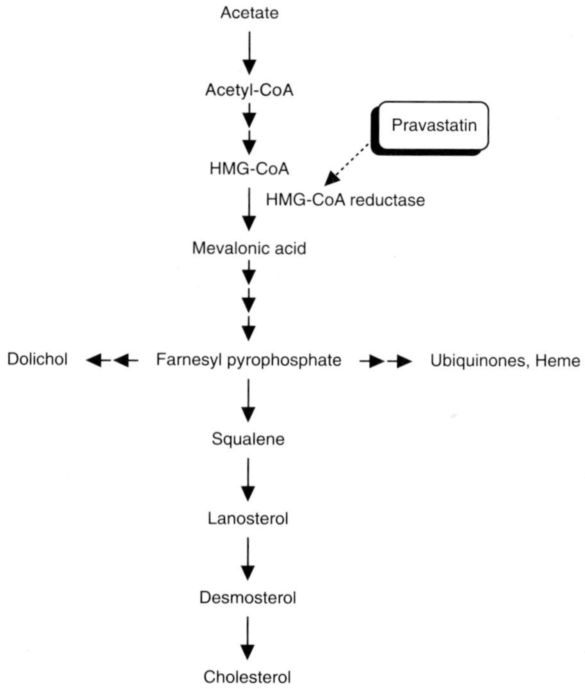

tients with adequate numbers of LDL receptors (i.e., patients who do not have FH), inhibition of lipoprotein formation seemed to play a more important role. Two recent studies with pravastatin in patients with moderate nonfamilial hypercholesterolemia (non-FH) support up-regulation of LDL receptors as the predominant mechanism of action.[21,24] Increased high-density lipoprotein (HDL) cholesterol concentrations have also been observed as a result of treatment with HMG-CoA reductase inhibitors,[20] although the precise mechanism is unknown.

Human cholesterol balance studies have shown incomplete blockade of total body cholesterol synthesis following administration of an HMG-CoA reductase inhibitor.[20] Thus, cholesterol synthesis remains sufficient to meet basal requirements for steroidogenesis and cell-membrane formation.

Pravastatin was found to reduce biliary cholesterol concentrations in six patients with heterozygous FH.[25] After receiving pravastatin sodium 40 mg/day for eight weeks, patients exhibited a 23% decrease in cholesterol saturation index of fasting gallbladder bile and a 24% reduction of biliary cholesterol. Biliary bile acid composition was unchanged. These results suggest that pravastatin therapy does not promote gallstone formation and may actually facilitate gallstone dissolution.

Animal and in vitro studies have shown that pravastatin acts selectively by inhibiting cholesterol synthesis in the liver and ileum, the major sites of de novo cholesterol synthesis, while sparing cholesterol synthesis at peripheral tissue sites.[26-28] In vitro studies have shown that hepatocytes have a specific transport mechanism for uptake of HMG-CoA reductase inhibitors but that pravastatin does not readily pass through the lipophilic membranes of nonhepatic cells.[29] In several animal studies, lovastatin and pravastatin inhibited cholesterol synthesis to a similar extent in the liver while extrahepatic tissues were much more resistant to cholesterol-synthesis inhibition by pravastatin than by lovastatin.[13,30] In addition, the pravastatin concentration needed to inhibit cholesterol synthesis by 50% (IC_{50}) in cultured human fibroblasts was 90–180 times higher than in primary hepatocytes. This contrasts with lovastatin and simvastatin, which have similar IC_{50} concentrations in fibroblasts and hepatocytes.[30] Differential transport mechanisms appear to account for this, with lipophilic lovastatin and simvastatin apparently entering extrahepatic cells by passive diffusion.[28] In addition, other animal studies have demonstrated that concentrations of pravastatin needed to inhibit cholesterol synthesis in the intact ocular lens are 100 times greater than for lovastatin or simvastatin.[31]

A study was conducted in 12 healthy male subjects who received single oral doses of pravastatin sodium (40 mg) or lovastatin (40 mg) for five consecutive days to compare penetration of the two drugs into the central nervous system.[32] In this study, pravastatin was not detected in the cerebrospinal fluid; lovastatin was detected at low concentrations that have been associated with HMG-CoA reductase inhibition.

While the tissue selectivity and cellular specificity of pravastatin have been clearly demonstrated in laboratory studies, the implications in terms of possible clinical benefits in humans are not known.

Pharmacokinetics

Most of the available data on pravastatin pharmacokinetics are derived from single- and multiple-dose studies conducted in healthy volunteers[22,33-35] after administration of radiolabeled ^{14}C-pravastatin. Oral absorption averages 34%, and bioavailability of the parent drug is approximately 18%.[35] The hepatic extraction ratio is approximately 0.66.[36] Thus, the low bioavailability of orally administered pravastatin can be attributed to extensive first-pass hepatic extraction. Consequently, most of an oral dose is delivered directly to the primary site of pharmacologic activity (i.e., the liver).

Food appears to decrease the bioavailability of pravastatin by approximately one third.[34] This may be due to degradation of pravastatin to inactive metabolites in the acidic environment of the stomach. Despite the decrease in systemic bioavailability, administration of pravastatin with food does not compromise its lipid-lowering effects. No differences in efficacy were seen between pravastatin sodium 20 mg twice daily administered with meals (LDL cholesterol decreased by 36.3%) and the same dosage administered one hour before meals (LDL cholesterol decreased by 36.4%).[34]

Steady-state pharmacokinetic parameters for oral pravastatin are summarized in Table 1.[22] Peak serum concentrations of pravastatin are dose dependent and are reached at approximately one hour; the volume of distribution at steady state is approximately 0.5 L/kg. Plasma protein binding is 55–60%.

The major active metabolite of pravastatin is SQ-31,906 (3-α-hydroxy isomeric metabolite). Its HMG-CoA reductase inhibitory activity is 1/10 to 1/40 that

Table 1.
Mean Steady-State Pharmacokinetic Variables in Healthy Volunteers following Twice-Daily Doses of Pravastatin Sodium for 12 Days[a]

	Dose		
Variable[b]	10 mg ($n = 8$)	20 mg ($n = 8$)	40 mg ($n = 8$)
$AUC_{0\text{-}24}$ (ng · hr/mL)	22.0	43.7	92.6
C_{max} (ng/mL)	9.2	19.0	43.0
t_{max} (hr)	1.3	1.1	1.3
$t_{½}$ (hr)	2.0	1.6	1.7
Protein binding (%)	57.3	55.0	57.8
CUE (% of dose)	6.8	5.5	6.4

[a]Adapted from reference 22, with permission.
[b]$AUC_{0\text{-}24}$ = area under the plasma concentration–time curve from 0 to 24 hours; C_{max} = maximum plasma concentration; t_{max} = time to reach C_{max}; $t_{½}$ = elimination half-life from plasma; protein binding = binding to plasma proteins at 1.5 hours; CUE = cumulative urinary excretion over 24 hours.

of pravastatin.[37] A second metabolite, SQ-31,945 (3-α,5-β,6-β-trihydroxy isomeric metabolite), has 1/3000 the activity of the parent drug. Pravastatin differs from lovastatin in that the parent drug is responsible for most of the HMG-CoA reductase activity in plasma.[37] With lovastatin, approximately 75% of the activity is due to active metabolites.[37]

Pravastatin and its metabolites are excreted in the urine and feces; unchanged pravastatin and SQ-31,906 are the predominant components.[22,35] Renal clearance of pravastatin is estimated at 47% of total clearance; nonrenal clearance is 53%.[35] After an oral radiolabeled dose, 71% is excreted in the feces and 20% in the urine. Negligible amounts of pravastatin and its major metabolite are excreted in the breast milk of lactating women.[35] Because of the potential for serious adverse reactions in infants, pravastatin, like other HMG-CoA reductase inhibitors, is contraindicated in nursing mothers.[38]

Age does not appear to significantly affect the pharmacokinetics of pravastatin. Similar parameters were found when pravastatin pharmacokinetics were studied in 15 elderly (ages 65–75 years) and 10 young (ages 19–31 years) healthy male subjects.[33,39] The elimination half-life was 2.0 hours in the elderly subjects, compared with 1.6 hours in the younger group. A slight increase in the area under the concentration–time curve (AUC) and a decrease in urinary excretion were noted in the elderly group. The short half-life in the elderly subjects suggests little potential for pravastatin accumulation, and pravastatin is recommended for dosing once daily.

Types of Hypercholesterolemia

Familial Hypercholesterolemia. FH can be classified as either heterozygous or homozygous.[40] Heterozygous FH is estimated to affect one in 500 people in the general population, while the homozygous form occurs in approximately one in 1,000,000. Individuals with heterozygous FH typically have very high LDL cholesterol levels (greater than 200 mg/dL), tendon xanthomas (particularly over the Achilles tendon), and evidence of CHD, often appearing early in adulthood. The basis of their disease is the presence of only half the normal number of functional LDL receptors. Therefore, dietary management alone usually is not sufficient to control cholesterol levels, and combination drug therapy is frequently needed. Homozygous FH occurs in patients who lack both genes for LDL receptors and are therefore unable to clear cholesterol from their plasma via LDL receptor-mediated mechanisms. HMG-CoA reductase inhibitors would not be expected to be as effective in homozygous FH patients because they lack the ability to synthesize functional LDL receptors.

Nonfamilial Hypercholesterolemia. Most hypercholesterolemic patients do not have FH; instead, the elevation in their cholesterol is due to dietary indiscretion, heritable disorders of lipid metabolism other than FH, or both of these factors. Approximately one third of patients with non-FH do not respond adequately to dietary therapy and require drug therapy of varying intensities.

Preclinical Evaluation

Before efficacy studies were undertaken in humans, pravastatin was evaluated in a variety of animal species, including Watanabe heritable hyperlipidemic (WHHL) rabbits, an animal model for FH.[13,41] In WHHL rabbits, pravastatin sodium 50 mg/kg/day reduced serum cholesterol (28%; $p < 0.001$ versus control) and triglycerides (16%; $p < 0.05$ versus control) and substantially prevented coronary atherosclerosis and peripheral deposition of cholesterol.[42] The frequency of coronary atherosclerosis was 42% in placebo-treated animals, compared with 19% in animals treated with pravastatin ($p < 0.01$). The frequency of xanthomas in digital joints was 90% with placebo and 58% with pravastatin ($p < 0.005$).

Clinical Trials

A variety of clinical trials have been conducted in healthy volunteers and in hypercholesterolemic patients to assess the efficacy of pravastatin.[21,22,24,39,43-71] These trials have shown pravastatin to have potent effects in reducing total and LDL cholesterol concentrations. Effects on HDL cholesterol and triglycerides have been favorable but more variable.

Studies in Healthy Volunteers. A double-blind, placebo-controlled dose-response study was performed in 36 healthy (normocholesterolemic) volunteers.[22] Subjects received pravastatin or placebo for 10 consecutive days. Pravastatin sodium dosages of 10, 20, and 40 mg twice daily reduced total cholesterol by 18.2%, 23.3%, and 29.6%, respectively, and decreased LDL cholesterol by 13.0%, 28.1%, and 40.0%, respectively. HDL cholesterol did not change significantly.

Another study compared the effects of pravastatin sodium 20 mg twice daily or placebo for seven days in 10 healthy volunteers.[43] Total cholesterol decreased by 18.6% and LDL cholesterol decreased by 22.7%. The triglyceride concentration decreased, but the change was not significant. HDL cholesterol decreased slightly in both groups, possibly because the subjects were inactive during the testing period.

Studies Involving Non-FH. Saito et al.[44] gave placebo or pravastatin sodium (10 or 20 mg/day for eight weeks) to 108 patients with non-FH. No significant changes in any lipid variable were found in 23 placebo-treated patients. In the 41 patients receiving pravastatin sodium 10 mg/day, the drug reduced total cholesterol by 17.1% (286 ± 6 [mean ± S.E. pretreatment] to 237 ± 5 mg/dL [mean ± S.E. posttreatment]) and LDL cholesterol by 26.2% (202 ± 8 to 149 ± 6 mg/dL). In 44 patients treated with pravastatin sodium 20 mg/day, total cholesterol was reduced by 21.7% (276 ± 5 to 216 ± 4 mg/dL) and LDL cholesterol was reduced by 32.3% (189 ± 6 to 128 ± 4 mg/dL). The nonsignificant changes caused by pravastatin in triglycerides (1–3%) did not appear to be dose dependent. Increases in HDL cholesterol concentrations varied and also were not dose dependent. Similar lipoprotein alterations were observed in two smaller studies.[21,24]

Yoshino et al.[64] studied 36 patients with either type IIA hyperlipidemia (increased LDL cholesterol) or type IIB hyperlipidemia (increased LDL and VLDL cholesterol and VLDL triglycerides). No significant change in serum triglycerides occurred in patients with type IIA hyperlipidemia after 10–30 mg/day of pravastatin sodium. However, triglyceride concentrations significantly decreased (by approximately 20%) in patients with type IIB hyperlipidemia who received similar doses. Thus, patients with higher baseline triglyceride concentrations appear to demonstrate a greater response to pravastatin.

In two other studies, pravastatin decreased total and LDL cholesterol and apolipoprotein B in all evaluable patients but increased HDL cholesterol and decreased triglycerides only in patients with type IIB hypercholesterolemia.[65,66] Yoshino et al.[66] suggested that pravastatin enhances the removal of LDL precursors via LDL receptors, which would compensate for the overproduction of VLDL that exists in patients with type IIB hyperlipidemia. Alternatively, pravastatin may simply decrease the production of VLDL by the liver.[24] Since patients with type IIA hyperlipidemia do not have elevated VLDL levels, VLDL may be produced and removed at a basal rate. Thus, in these patients pravastatin or any HMG-CoA reductase inhibitor would not be expected to lower triglyceride levels.

In general, hypercholesterolemic patients are asked to follow a low-fat diet (e.g., American Heart Association [AHA] Step I diet) before lipid-lowering medication is initiated, and to maintain this diet during drug therapy. The effects of an AHA Step I diet in addition to treatment with pravastatin have been studied. After 16 weeks of therapy, a significantly greater increase in serum HDL cholesterol (mean, 8 mg/dL; $p < 0.05$) was observed when an AHA Step I diet was used in conjunction with pravastatin therapy as compared with the increase (mean, 4 mg/dL; not significant) when pravastatin was administered to patients on a control diet.[67] However, LDL cholesterol reductions were essentially the same in both groups: 31% in the dietary control group and 27% in the group receiving the AHA diet. Although the additional lipid-modifying effects of dietary restrictions were not pronounced in the study, a low-fat, low-cholesterol diet is a prudent approach and is recommended by the National Cholesterol Education Program.[1]

Studies Involving FH. Pravastatin was studied in 13 patients with heterozygous FH who were first treated with a cholesterol-reducing diet for four weeks, followed by the addition of pravastatin sodium 5 mg twice daily for six weeks and then 10 mg twice daily for an additional six weeks.[46] After the dietary phase, initial mean ± S.E. total and LDL cholesterol concentrations were 360 ± 20 and 278 ± 21 mg/dL, respectively. Significant decreases in total cholesterol (18%; $p < 0.001$) and LDL cholesterol (26%; $p < 0.001$) were observed with pravastatin sodium 5 mg twice daily; after the dosage increase, the total reductions in total and LDL cholesterol were 26% and 33%, respectively. HDL cholesterol increased significantly (16%) with pravastatin sodium 5 mg twice daily but did not increase further with the higher dosage.

LDL apheresis also can be used to normalize cholesterol concentrations in patients with FH who do not respond to drug therapy. Even if this procedure is repeated frequently (every two weeks), the reduction in total and LDL cholesterol may not be adequate to prevent the long-term consequences of hypercholesterolemia. Mabuchi et al.[47] reported additional decreases in total cholesterol concentrations of 14.5% when pravastatin sodium 10 mg twice daily was administered to patients with FH who were receiving LDL apheresis. This decrease is much smaller than that normally observed in patients with FH who are not undergoing LDL apheresis (25%). A possible explanation for this phenomenon is that apheresis may stimulate endogenous cholesterol synthesis, and higher doses of pravastatin may be needed to overcome this increased production. Pravastatin had no effect on HDL cholesterol or triglycerides in this study.

When the combination of LDL apheresis and pravastatin was compared with combinations of LDL-apheresis and cholestyramine or probucol, all three combinations prolonged the interval between LDL-apheresis treatments (the time required for total cholesterol to return to 250 mg/dL).[68] Pravastatin prolonged the interval for the longest period (39 days), followed by cholestyramine (27 days), and probucol (15 days).

Studies in Mixed Hypercholesterolemic Populations. A number of studies have established the efficacy of pravastatin in combined groups of patients with FH and non-FH. Nakaya et al.[49] evaluated pravastatin in 37 hypercholesterolemic patients. After a four-week placebo phase (in which patients followed their usual diet), patients received pravastatin sodium doses of 2.5, 10, or 20 mg twice daily; reductions in total cholesterol of 11.1%, 18.8%, and 25.3%, respectively, were observed after four weeks of pravastatin (all $p < 0.01$ versus baseline). LDL cholesterol was reduced by 16.7% (mean ± S.E., 203 ± 21 to 169 ± 17 mg/dL) with 2.5 mg twice daily, by 28.8% (191 ± 15 to 136 ± 13 mg/dL) with 10 mg twice daily, and by 37.3% (177 ± 15 to 111 ± 12 mg/dL) with 20 mg twice-daily (all $p < 0.01$ versus baseline). HDL cholesterol concentrations increased with all three regimens, but a significant increase (11.8%) was noted only with the 20 mg twice daily regimen ($p < 0.05$). Lipid alterations were maximal after three to four weeks of treatment and returned to baseline within two weeks of discontinuing pravastatin.

Similar therapeutic effects were found in a multicenter double-blind dose-response study involving 268 patients.[50] Pravastatin sodium doses of 5, 10, or 20 mg twice daily were administered to patients already receiving a low-fat, low-cholesterol diet. Lipid-modifying effects were maximal at four weeks and were sustained throughout the 12-week study. Respective reductions in total cholesterol were 12.9%, 17.4%, and 23.3% (all $p < 0.001$ versus baseline and placebo). Mean LDL cholesterol was reduced by 16.7% (228 to 190 mg/dL) with 5 mg twice daily, by 22.4% (246 to 191 mg/dL) with 10 mg twice daily, and by 30.3% (228 to 159 mg/dL) with 20 mg twice daily (all $p < 0.001$). Reductions in triglycerides (11.0–15.4%) and increases in HDL cholesterol (5.6–6.7%) occurred with all pravastatin regimens (all $p < 0.05$) and did not appear to be dose dependent.

The comparative effectiveness of once- versus twice-daily pravastatin was demonstrated in an eight-week, double-blind, placebo-controlled trial in 188 patients.[51] Patients were randomized to receive placebo or pravastatin sodium in doses of 40 mg every morning, 40 mg every night, or 20 mg twice daily, all in conjunction with a cholesterol-lowering diet. Similar reductions in total cholesterol (all $p < 0.001$ versus baseline and placebo) were achieved with the three regimens: 22.9% with 40 mg every morning, 25.6% with 40 mg every night, and 27.0% with 20 mg twice daily. LDL cholesterol was reduced by 29.7% (mean ± S.E., 246 ± 10 to 173 ± 8 mg/dL), 32.2% (245 ± 11 to 166 ± 9 mg/dL), and 33.6% (247 ± 10 to 164 ± 8 mg/dL), respectively, with the three regimens (all $p < 0.001$). Each regimen produced significant elevations in HDL cholesterol (4.1–8.2%) and reductions in triglycerides (10.6–24.5%) (all $p < 0.05$ versus baseline).

Jones et al.[52] found similar efficacy for once-daily pravastatin in a dose-ranging study involving 107 patients. After a six-week dietary stabilization period and a four-week placebo lead-in period, patients received an eight-week course of placebo or pravastatin sodium in doses of 5, 10, 20, or 40 mg at bedtime. Dose-dependent reductions of total cholesterol (14.3%, 16.2%, 23.9%, and 25.1%) and LDL cholesterol (19.2%, 22.4%, 32.4%, and 34.1%) were seen with the four pravastatin regimens (all $p < 0.05$ versus baseline and placebo). Increases in HDL cholesterol (2.4–11.7%) and reductions in triglycerides (11.4–23.9%) were not dose dependent and not all were statistically significant. Similar lipid-lowering effects have been shown in several smaller studies.[53,69,70] In one study, beneficial lipoprotein alterations were maintained over a two-year period in 10 patients.[53]

Comparative Trials. Pravastatin has been compared with simvastatin in an open-label trial.[54] After a four-week stabilization period on a lipid-lowering diet, patients received either pravastatin sodium 5 mg twice daily or simvastatin 2.5 mg daily for three months. Baseline lipid levels for the two treatment groups were matched before treatment; the study included 13 patients with type IIA and 12 patients with type IIB hyperlipidemia in each group. Pravastatin reduced total and LDL cholesterol by 17% (mean ± S.D., 279 ± 36 to 232 ± 30 mg/dL) and 28% (189 ± 42 to 137 ± 30 mg/dL), respectively. The reductions were similar for simvastatin: 20% (280 ± 46 to 225 ± 38 mg/dL) and 26% (184 ± 55 to 137 ± 38 mg/dL). Reductions for both drugs were statistically significant (all $p < 0.001$ versus baseline). Both drugs produced significant elevations in HDL cholesterol (12% with pravastatin, 6% with simvastatin, $p < 0.05$). Triglycerides were not significantly altered in either group.

Pravastatin also has been compared with simvastatin and lovastatin in a six-week, parallel, open-label continuation of short-term controlled studies in patients with primary hypercholesterolemia.[62] After a six-week stabilization (dietary lead-in) phase, patients received one of the three HMG-CoA reductase inhibitors in a dose of 20 mg twice daily for six months. Pravastatin reduced total cholesterol and triglycerides by 28.2% and 6.0%, respectively; lovastatin by 25.5% and 17.4%, respectively; simvastatin by 30.2% and 19.6%, respectively. Reductions in total cholesterol for all three drugs were significant when compared with baseline values. Pravastatin, lovastatin, and simvastatin increased HDL cholesterol concentrations by 8.0%, 9.7%, and 2.3%, respectively; these changes were not significant.

Pravastatin has also been compared with probucol.[56] After three months of therapy with probucol 250 mg two or three times daily, only five of nine patients experienced a decrease (mean, 10.2%) in total cholesterol (mean ± S.E., 325 ± 17 to 292 ± 17 mg/dL), while all nine patients receiving pravastatin 10 or 20 mg/day experienced a significant decrease in this lipid fraction (mean, 16.0%; 331 ± 29 to 278 ± 20; $p < 0.05$).

Probucol has previously been shown to decrease HDL cholesterol; this was demonstrated in eight of nine patients in this study.[56] However, for the group, the difference was not significant. Pravastatin increased HDL cholesterol in eight of nine patients treated, and produced a significant increase for the group as compared with baseline (15.9%; $p < 0.05$).

The Italian Multicenter Pravastatin Study I evaluated pravastatin sodium 40 mg daily at bedtime and gemfibrozil 600 mg twice daily in primary hypercholesterolemia (both non-FH and FH).[55] After eight weeks of dietary stabilization, patients were randomized to receive one of the two regimens in a double-blind, placebo-controlled manner; 360 patients completed the full 24 weeks of drug treatment. Pravastatin produced significantly greater reductions in total and LDL cholesterol than gemfibrozil (both $p < 0.001$). The respective reductions in total and LDL cholesterol with pravastatin were 23.3% (mean ± S.D., 354 ± 54 to 275 ± 54 mg/dL) and 29.6% (280 ± 56 to 197 ± 55 mg/dL). With gemfibrozil, the reductions were 14% (350 ± 54 to 301 ± 63 mg/dL) and 16% (272 ± 56 to 229 ± 54 mg/dL). Both regimens reduced total and LDL cholesterol concentrations more in the patients with non-FH than in the patients with FH (both $p < 0.05$). Elevations of HDL cholesterol concentrations with gemfibrozil (13%) were significantly greater than with pravastatin (5%) ($p < 0.05$). Reductions of triglyceride concentrations with gemfibrozil (37%) were significantly greater than with pravastatin (5%) ($p < 0.01$). Baseline mean triglyceride levels were 132 mg/dL and 140 mg/dL for pravastatin and gemfibrozil, respectively.

A smaller double-blind parallel trial has also compared pravastatin sodium 20 mg b.i.d. with gemfibrozil 600 mg b.i.d. in patients with FH.[48] Pravastatin reduced total (23.6% versus 18.1%) and LDL (28.2% versus 21.4%) cholesterol concentrations more than gemfibrozil (all $p < 0.001$ versus baseline). Both drugs increased HDL cholesterol, but the change was only significant for gemfibrozil.

Pravastatin was compared with the bile acid-binding resin cholestyramine in a 12-week, double-blind, placebo-controlled trial in 120 patients with FH.[45] After an 8- to 10-week period during which patients received a low-fat, low-cholesterol diet, patients were treated with pravastatin plus placebo resin, cholestyramine plus placebo pravastatin, or double placebo. Pravastatin sodium was dosed at 10 mg twice daily for six weeks, followed by 20 mg twice daily for six more weeks. Cholestyramine was dosed at the highest tolerable dose up to 24 g/day. After 12 weeks, pravastatin reduced total cholesterol by 23% (mean ± S.D., 383 ± 74 to 296 ± 59 mg/dL) and LDL cholesterol by 28% (316 ± 74 to 228 ± 59 mg/dL) ($p < 0.001$ versus placebo). Cholestyramine reduced total cholesterol by 24% (373 ± 74 to 284 ± 67 mg/dL) and LDL cholesterol by 30% (307 ± 68 to 216 ± 68 mg/dL). HDL concentrations were increased more by pravastatin (9%) than by cholestyramine (3%) ($p < 0.05$). Triglyceride concentrations were not changed with either regimen.

Another study compared pravastatin sodium 40 mg every night and cholestyramine 8 g twice daily in a mixed hypercholesterolemic population (FH and non-FH) with type IIA hypercholesterolemia.[57] After 12 weeks, respective total and LDL cholesterol concentrations were reduced by 24.3% and 30.7% with pravastatin versus 21.1% and 25.1% with cholestyramine ($p < 0.05$ versus baseline for all reductions). HDL cholesterol concentrations increased by 22.2% with pravastatin ($p < 0.001$), while the 10.9% increase with cholestyramine was not significant. Pravastatin significantly reduced triglyceride concentrations (11.8%, $p < 0.01$), while the 7.7% increase in triglyceride concentration with cholestyramine was not significant.

Studies Involving Combination Therapy. Because of their complementary mechanisms of action, a bile acid-binding resin combined with pravastatin would seem advantageous. Several studies have evaluated this combination, with LDL cholesterol generally reduced by 45–55%. Pravastatin also blunts the tendency for resins to increase triglycerides.[45,58]

Hoogerbrugge et al.[63] administered pravastatin sodium 40 mg daily to 40 patients with heterozygous FH. After eight weeks, total and LDL cholesterol concentrations were reduced by 28% and 33% (both $p < 0.01$). Colestipol hydrochloride (up to 30 g/day) or cholestyramine (up to 24 g/day) was then added for patients whose LDL cholesterol remained above 195 mg/dL. This resulted in additional total and LDL cholesterol reductions of 8% and 12%, respectively (both $p < 0.01$, combination versus pravastatin monotherapy). In 22 control patients receiving a resin plus placebo, total cholesterol was reduced by 17% and LDL cholesterol by 22%.

Similar results have been found in other studies. Pan et al.[39] used combination therapy of cholestyramine 24 g/day with pravastatin sodium 5 mg, 10 mg, or 20 mg, given two times a day, in 33 hypercholesterolemic white males. LDL cholesterol was reduced by 47–56%. In another study, pravastatin sodium 40 mg/day combined with cholestyramine 24 g/day reduced LDL cholesterol by 51% (mean, 237 to 117 mg/dL).[71]

In a two-year, double-blind crossover study in 14 patients with primary hypercholesterolemia, the addition of colestipol hydrochloride 30 g/day to pravastatin sodium 40 mg/day produced significantly reduced total and LDL cholesterol compared with baseline (41.8% and 50.8%, both $p < 0.003$).[58] In contrast, the addition of probucol 1 g/day produced detrimental lipoprotein alterations compared with pravastatin monotherapy. The addition of probucol did not enhance the LDL cholesterol reduction seen with pravastatin alone (32.7% with combination therapy versus 38.0% with pravastatin alone), but did reduce HDL cholesterol significantly (19.1% with combination therapy versus 2.1% with pravastatin alone).

Clinical trials to evaluate the efficacy of pravastatin in combination with nicotinic acid and a fibric-acid derivative are now in various stages of completion.[72]

Studies in Diabetic Patients. Pravastatin has been evaluated in two studies involving patients with hypercholesterolemia secondary to noninsulin-dependent diabetes mellitus (NIDDM). Yoshino et al.[59] treated nine patients with pravastatin 5 mg twice daily and one patient with 10 mg twice daily. Mean reductions in total and LDL cholesterol of 15.4% (mean ± S.E., 262.4 ± 9.3 to 221.9 ± 9.7 mg/dL) and 15.7% (157.7 ± 14.3 to 132.9 ± 8.9 mg/dL), respectively, were seen after 12 months of treatment. The reductions in LDL cholesterol were not significant until six months. LDL cholesterol concentrations were further decreased after 12 months of pravastatin therapy.

Patients with NIDDM usually have an increase in LDL cholesterol production as well as an increase in LDL cholesterol catabolism. Because pravastatin stimulates the catabolism of LDL cholesterol, it may not be as effective in lowering the LDL cholesterol in these patients, who already have an increased turnover, but this requires specific evaluation. Alternatively, the investigators hypothesized that the glycosylation of LDL cholesterol may have interfered with the ability of pravastatin to decrease LDL cholesterol concentrations. HDL cholesterol significantly increased (9.1%) after one month but returned to baseline with continued therapy.

A previously published study by the same group demonstrated a significant decrease in LDL cholesterol concentrations when pravastatin sodium 5 mg twice daily was administered to eight patients with NIDDM.[60] Total cholesterol concentrations decreased by 18.6% (mean, 291 to 237 mg/dL), while LDL cholesterol concentrations decreased by 16.9% (183 to 152 mg/dL). A significant increase in HDL cholesterol (8.5%) was also found. Triglyceride concentrations were significantly decreased in both studies (24.2–26.9%). No effect on fasting blood glucose or hemoglobin A_{1c} was found.

Pravastatin has also been compared with probucol in treating hypercholesterolemic patients with diabetes.[61] Four men and three women received probucol 250 mg twice daily for three months, followed by a four-week washout period, then pravastatin sodium 10 mg/day for three months. The two drugs did not differ significantly in their ability to lower total cholesterol; mean reductions were 18.4% (mean ± S.E., 331 ± 11 to 270 ± 12 mg/dL) with probucol and 17.2% (320 ± 35 to 265 ± 23 mg/dL) with pravastatin. However, pravastatin significantly increased the HDL cholesterol concentration (19.0%), while no significant change was noted with probucol therapy.

Adverse Effects

Although only recently introduced to the marketplace, the HMG-CoA reductase inhibitors have been generally well tolerated. Nevertheless, there is concern over potential toxicities that may occur with more widespread and long-term use of these agents. This concern stems in part from experience with triparanol (MER-29), which was withdrawn in 1962. Toxic adverse effects, including cataracts and ichthyosis, occurred because triparanol blocked the late stages of cholesterol synthesis, resulting in accumulation of lipid-soluble precursors such as desmosterol.[73-76] In contrast, HMG-CoA reductase inhibitors block cholesterol synthesis at a much earlier stage, in which the precursors are water soluble and readily eliminated via alternate metabolic pathways.[74] Thus, such adverse effects are unlikely with this class of drugs.

The toxicities of pravastatin and lovastatin appear to be qualitatively similar, although initial data suggest that pravastatin may produce some adverse effects less frequently.

Frequency of Adverse Reactions. Pravastatin has been evaluated in more than 14,000 hypercholesterolemic patients worldwide (McGovern M, Bristol-Myers Squibb Company. Personal communication, 1992 June 16).[77] Safety data were recently reported for 1142 patients who received pravastatin in six long-term multicenter clinical trials in the United States.[77] Clinical data to date show pravastatin to be well tolerated by most patients. The results of other smaller clinical trials have demonstrated adverse-effect profiles similar to those found in the U.S. multicenter trials.[21,24,43,49,53-57,59-61,66,68-70]

In short-term placebo-controlled trials (average duration of four months), 19.6% of the patients receiving pravastatin reported adverse reactions, compared with 20.9% of those receiving placebo.[77,78] Table 2 lists the frequency of adverse events that occurred at rates of 2% or greater with pravastatin treatment during these trials. Rash was the only adverse effect that occurred significantly more frequently ($p < 0.05$) in patients treated with pravastatin than in patients treated with placebo. During the long-term extensions of these studies, the frequency of adverse effects did not increase. Of the 1100 patients treated with pravastatin monotherapy for a mean duration of 15 months, 3.2% discontinued treatment because of adverse drug experiences (average rate of 0.2% per month).[77] In contrast, the discontinuation rate was 4.5% (0.5% per month) for 243 patients who were treated with bile acid-binding resins for a mean duration of 10 months. During the placebo-controlled portions of these studies (mean duration of four months), discontinuation rates were not significantly different (1.6% with pravastatin and 1.2% with placebo).

When all 1142 patients are considered (mean duration of 18 months pravastatin treatment), including patients who concomitantly received other lipid-lowering agents (mostly bile acid-binding resins), the rate of discontinuation was 4.3% (0.2% per month).[77] The most common reasons for discontinuation of pravastatin were nonspecific gastrointestinal complaints (1.4%) and asymptomatic hepatic aminotransferase elevations (1.0%).

Skeletal Muscle. The development of muscle toxicity has been a concern with HMG-CoA reductase inhib-

Table 2.
Adverse Reactions to Pravastatin or Placebo Reported with Frequencies of 2% or More during Short-Term Placebo-Controlled Clinical Trials[a]

Reaction	Frequency (%) Pravastatin ($n = 900$)	Placebo ($n = 411$)
Gastrointestinal		
Nausea or vomiting	6.2	5.8
Diarrhea	5.2	4.9
Constipation	3.9	6.8
Abdominal pain	3.2	5.1
Flatulence	2.9	3.6
Musculoskeletal		
Muscular or skeletal pain	6.9	8.0
Central Nervous System		
Headache	4.6	3.9
Dizziness	2.6	2.7
Respiratory		
Upper respiratory infection	4.7	5.8
Rhinitis	3.3	3.9
Cardiovascular		
Cardiac chest pain	2.8	2.9
Dermatologic		
Rash	3.3[b]	1.2
General		
Fatigue	3.1	2.9
Noncardiac chest pain	2.6	1.9

[a]Adapted from reference 78, with permission.
[b]Significantly different from corresponding frequency for placebo ($p < 0.05$).

itor therapy, although the mechanism by which these drugs induce myopathy is not known.[79] Myopathy, defined as muscle pain or weakness combined with a creatine kinase (CK) elevation of 10 times the upper limit of normal or greater, occurred in 17 of approximately 4000 patients in lovastatin clinical trials through March 1988 (0.4%).[9] The occurrence of myopathy was markedly increased by concomitant therapy with cyclosporine (28%), gemfibrozil (5%), or niacin (2%). Erythromycin also reportedly induced myopathy when it was initiated in patients receiving lovastatin therapy.[80,81] Pierce et al.[79] reported 12 cases of myopathy, some of which progressed to rhabdomyolysis, in patients receiving the combination of gemfibrozil and lovastatin. CK increased to concentrations ranging from 1,000–148,000 IU/L (mean 30,886 IU/L, median 15,250 IU/L). One patient died from cardiogenic shock that occurred one month after recovery from the initial episode. Rhabdomyolysis severe enough to produce renal failure has also been reported in two patients who had undergone cardiac transplantation, both receiving lovastatin and concomitant cyclosporine and one also receiving niacin.[82,83]

Data from the large postmarketing Expanded Clinical Evaluation of Lovastatin (EXCEL) study suggest that with lovastatin monotherapy, musculoskeletal toxicity is less frequent, milder, and possibly dose related.[84] Five cases of reversible myopathy were reported (0.1%), with four of the cases occurring in patients receiving 40 mg two times daily (0.2% for this dose). No patients developed renal failure.

Data from clinical trials suggest that muscle toxicity occurs less frequently with pravastatin than with lovastatin. Among 1142 pravastatin-treated patients, only one case of possible drug-induced myopathy was found.[77] However, before treatment, this 50-year-old woman had a CK of 373 IU/L (normal, 21–169 IU/L) and arthritis. The patient did not experience rhabdomyolysis or renal failure. In an additional 3500 patients treated worldwide with pravastatin in clinical trials, there have been no definitive cases of pravastatin-caused myopathy.[77] One patient developed myopathy when clofibrate was added to well-tolerated pravastatin therapy.[38] The myopathy resolved when clofibrate was discontinued and pravastatin was continued.

In the placebo-controlled trials, there were no significant differences in the frequency of CK elevations to values greater than four times the upper limit of normal between pravastatin-treated (4.3%) and placebo-treated (2.5%) patients.[77] The frequency of CK elevations was also similar in patients receiving pravastatin or resin monotherapy.

Pravastatin has been used clinically with cyclosporine in 25 patients with no observation of myopathy.[85] Myopathy was also not seen in studies of pravastatin in combination with gemfibrozil and in combination with niacin.[77,86]

Liver. Thirteen (1.1%) of 1142 pravastatin-treated patients experienced asymptomatic aminotransferase elevations to greater than three times the upper limit of normal on more than one occasion.[77] About half had confounding factors for the increases or experienced resolution of the enzyme abnormalities while continuing pravastatin. Patient populations tended to have small, dose-dependent mean elevations in aminotransferases that plateaued at eight weeks. These same elevations occurred in patients treated with bile acid-binding resins.[77,78]

Similar frequencies of persistent aminotransferase elevations have been found in lovastatin clinical trials[87] (1.9%) and the EXCEL study (0.7%).[84] In the EXCEL study, a significant dose-related trend for persistently elevated aminotransferases was found. The rates were 0.1% with 20 mg every night, 0.9% with either 40 mg every night or 20 mg twice daily, and 1.5% with 40 mg twice daily. Evaluation of a similar phenomenon with pravastatin would require further study.

Eye. Concern regarding possible cataractogenic effects associated with HMG-CoA reductase inhibitors developed after lens opacities were reported in an early lovastatin clinical trial.[88] However, no patient in that trial developed a change in visual acuity, and subsequent large-scale controlled trials have shown no such change. In the 8245-patient EXCEL study, no cataractogenic effect of lovastatin was observed in patients receiving 20–80 mg/day for 48 weeks.[80,89]

Pravastatin has not been associated with the development of cataracts in clinical studies to date.[77] This has been shown using slit-lamp examination and the Lens Opacity Classification System of Chylack et al.[90]

Insomnia. Schaefer[91] has reported insomnia in 9 of 51 patients taking lovastatin and none of 33 patients taking pravastatin. Newman et al.[77] reported low rates of sleep disturbances with both pravastatin and placebo. A sophisticated sleep-laboratory study has shown that lovastatin was associated with significant increases in wake time after onset of sleep and a significant increase in stage 1 sleep, whereas pravastatin was not.[92] Further study will be needed to evaluate the clinical relevance of this finding.

Drug Interactions

No clinically significant drug interactions have been reported in patients receiving pravastatin therapy. Cholestyramine has been shown to alter pravastatin systemic bioavailability.[39] When cholestyramine was administered one hour after pravastatin, steady-state AUC decreased by 18–49%, but the efficacy of pravastatin was not reduced. Decreases in LDL cholesterol of 47–56% were similar to those commonly achieved with combined administration of bile acid-binding resins and HMG-CoA reductase inhibitors, and much greater than that achieved with resins administered as monotherapy. Any potential for a drug interaction should be minimized by administering these drugs as recommended (i.e., the bile acid-binding resin before meals and pravastatin as a once-daily bedtime dose).

The bioavailability of pravastatin was not altered when it was coadministered with probucol, gemfibrozil, aspirin, nicotinic acid, or a combination of aspirin and nicotinic acid in healthy subjects.[36]

Coadministration of pravastatin and warfarin for six days in healthy volunteers resulted in no alteration in the bioavailability of pravastatin, the plasma protein binding of warfarin, or the prothrombin time.[36]

Pravastatin has been shown not to increase the prothrombin time in patients receiving warfarin in a controlled clinical trial.[72] In contrast, lovastatin has been associated with elevated prothrombin times, bleeding, or both, in at least 10 patients receiving concomitant warfarin.[93] Lovastatin and its principal active metabolite are highly protein bound (both more than 95%).[63] The lower degree of protein binding with pravastatin should minimize the risk of highly protein-bound drugs, such as warfarin, being displaced from plasma protein-binding sites, thus minimizing the potential for interactions.[72]

Administration of pravastatin sodium for four weeks in doses of 5–20 mg twice daily has been shown to not alter antipyrine elimination half-life or clearance, suggesting that pravastatin should not affect the metabolism of other drugs metabolized by the cytochrome P-450 system.[94] Coadministration of propranolol hydrochloride (40 mg twice daily) with pravastatin sodium or lovastatin (single 20-mg doses) in healthy volunteers reduced the mean serum AUC of the HMG-CoA reductase inhibitors, but these changes were not thought to be clinically significant.[95] Further clinical experience will be useful in fully assessing the drug interaction profile of pravastatin.

Role of Pravastatin in Lipid-Lowering Therapy

Guidelines for the treatment of hypercholesterolemia have been established by the National Cholesterol Education Program Adult Treatment Panel.[1] Drug therapy is recommended for patients who have an LDL cholesterol of 190 mg/dL or greater despite an adequate trial of dietary management or for high-risk patients (those with definite CHD or at least two other CHD risk factors) who have an LDL cholesterol greater than 160 mg/dL after a period of dietary restriction. The guidelines currently recognize bile acid-binding resins (cholestyramine and colestipol) and nicotinic acid as first-line agents because of their established relative safety with long-term use and demonstrated effectiveness in reducing CHD risk. Reductions in LDL cholesterol of up to 30% are achievable using monotherapy with resins or nicotinic acid. Limitations of these drugs include adverse effects that often result in poor patient compliance with the dosages that are required for optimal LDL cholesterol lowering.[8]

HMG-CoA reductase inhibitors are more potent and better tolerated than either bile acid-binding resins or nicotinic acid. Mean LDL cholesterol reductions of up to 45% are achievable with usual doses. Recently, the Familial Atherosclerosis Treatment Study (FATS) demonstrated the combination of lovastatin and colestipol to be effective in inhibiting progression and inducing regression of coronary lesions.[96] The results of the EXCEL study[80,84] provide additional information to help resolve safety concerns about this class of drugs.

The guidelines of the National Cholesterol Education Program have focused primarily on lowering LDL cholesterol, although an addendum[97] and the recently published Helsinki Heart Study[98] have emphasized the importance of raising HDL cholesterol in patients with high LDL cholesterol and low HDL cholesterol. In patients receiving gemfibrozil, multivariate analysis demonstrated an independent association between increases in HDL cholesterol and reduction in CHD risk.[99] A similar benefit associated with increasing HDL cholesterol was identified in the Lipid Research Clinics Coronary Primary Prevention Trial[100] and the National Heart, Lung, and Blood Institute Type II Coronary Intervention Study.[5,7] However, these studies employed cholestyramine, a drug that produces much smaller increases in HDL cholesterol. In the FATS trial, increases in HDL cholesterol were found to be independently correlated with angiographically demonstrated regression of coronary lesions.[96] Although a similar HDL effect was not seen in the University of California, San Francisco, Arteriosclerosis Specialized Center of Research Intervention Trial, a positive effect of lipid-lowering treatment on lesion regression was observed in both women and men.[101]

For patients with elevated LDL cholesterol and low HDL cholesterol (less than 35 mg/dL), consideration should be given to directing drug therapy at both lipoprotein fractions, although decreasing LDL cholesterol should remain the priority.[97] Nicotinic acid is capable of increasing HDL cholesterol 10–20% or more and, for patients able to tolerate its potential adverse effects, it can be an inexpensive and useful drug.[8] The HDL cholesterol-elevating capacity of gemfibrozil is approximately 10–15%. Although it is better tolerated than nicotinic acid, gemfibrozil's modest LDL cholesterol-lowering effect makes it useful primarily to those patients who do not require large reductions in LDL cholesterol. HMG-CoA reductase inhibitors produce smaller and more variable increases in HDL cholesterol when compared with nicotinic acid and gemfibrozil. However, for patients who require large reductions in LDL cholesterol, the HMG-CoA reductase inhibitors will generally produce an apparently beneficial increase in HDL cholesterol. If even greater decreases in LDL cholesterol are required, HMG-CoA reductase inhibitors can be effectively combined with bile acid-binding resins.

The relative advantages of pravastatin over lovastatin cannot be accurately assessed at this time. Clinical studies have demonstrated the two drugs to be comparable in cholesterol-lowering ability. Initial studies suggest that pravastatin may have a lower frequency of some adverse effects, but more clinical experience is needed to substantiate this possibility. Protein-binding considerations may be important in patients receiving multiple drug therapies. The average wholesale price of pravastatin is lower than that of lovastatin, which may translate into a savings for the patient.[102]

Dosage and Administration

The recommended starting dosage of pravastatin sodium is 10 or 20 mg once daily at bedtime.[38] The dosage range is 10 to 40 mg per day. An initial dosage of 20 mg administered at bedtime is usual. Individualization will be required, depending on the amount of cholesterol lowering required and the response to therapy. Similar reductions in LDL cholesterol occur whether pravastatin is administered with food or in the fasting state; thus, pravastatin may be administered without regard to meals. Once-daily administration in the evening appears to be marginally more effective than once-daily administration in the morning, perhaps because hepatic cholesterol is synthesized mainly at night.

Pravastatin seems to have little hepatotoxic potential but, until more long-term data are available, periodic monitoring of aminotransferases is recommended. It is important to consider that small increases in hepatic enzymes occurring within the first six months of cholesterol-lowering therapy may be due to alterations in hepatic metabolism rather than specific hepatotoxic drug effects.[9]

Instructions for the Patient

Patients receiving pravastatin should be advised that control of elevated cholesterol and other CHD risk factors is a long-term process. Pravastatin is not a substitute for adherence to a cholesterol-lowering diet. Both diet and drug therapy are important parts of a cholesterol control program. The importance of keeping follow-up appointments with their physicians should be stressed to patients.

Patients receiving concomitant bile acid-binding resins should be instructed on scheduling of doses to prevent reduced absorption of pravastatin. However, if pravastatin is administered at bedtime, possible interactions may be avoided. As with any drug, patients taking pravastatin should be instructed to report any unusual symptoms.

Conclusion

Pravastatin is a new HMG-CoA reductase inhibitor for the treatment of primary hypercholesterolemia. Reductions in LDL cholesterol and increases in HDL cholesterol are similar to those produced by lovastatin. Although both agents are well tolerated, data from clinical trials suggest that pravastatin may have a better adverse-effect profile than lovastatin. Further long-term clinical trials and use are needed to substantiate this possibility.

References

1. Expert Panel. Report of the National Cholesterol Education Program Expert Panel on Detection, Evaluation, and Treatment of High Blood Cholesterol in Adults. *Arch Intern Med.* 1988; 148:36-69.
2. Lipid Research Clinics Program. The Lipid Research Clinics Coronary Primary Prevention Trial results. I. Reduction in incidence of coronary heart disease. *JAMA.* 1984; 251:351-64.
3. Lipid Research Clinics Program. The Lipid Research Clinics Coronary Primary Prevention Trial results. II. The relationship of reduction in incidence of coronary heart disease to cholesterol lowering. *JAMA.* 1984; 251:365-74.
4. Blankenhorn DH, Nessim SA, Johnson RL et al. Beneficial effects of combined colestipol–niacin therapy on coronary atherosclerosis and coronary venous bypass grafts. *JAMA.* 1987; 257:3233-40.
5. Brensike JF, Levy RI, Kelsey SF et al. Effects of therapy with cholestyramine on progression of coronary arteriosclerosis: results of the NHLBI Type II Coronary Intervention Study. *Circulation.* 1984; 69:313-24.
6. Canner PL, Berge KG, Wenger NK et al. Fifteen-year mortality in Coronary Drug Project patients: long-term benefit with niacin. *J Am Coll Cardiol.* 1986; 8:1245-55.
7. Levy RI, Brensike JF, Epstein SE et al. The influence of changes in lipid values induced by cholestyramine and diet on progression of coronary artery disease: results of the NHLBI Type II Coronary Intervention Study. *Circulation.* 1984; 69:325-37.
8. Illingworth DR. Lipid-lowering drugs: an overview of indications and optimum therapeutic use. Drugs. 1987; 33:259-79.
9. Tobert JA. Efficacy and long-term adverse effect pattern of lovastatin. *Am J Cardiol.* 1988; 62:28J-34J.
10. Endo A, Kuroda M, Tanzawa K. Competitive inhibition of 3-hydroxy-3-methylglutaryl coenzyme A reductase by ML-236A and ML-236B, fungal metabolites having hypocholesterolemic activity. *FEBS Lett.* 1976; 72:323-6.
11. Arai M, Serizawa N, Terahara A et al. Pravastatin sodium (CS-514), a novel cholesterol-lowering agent which inhibits HMG-CoA reductase. *Annu Rep Sankyo Res Lab.* 1988; 40:1-38.
12. Hoeg JM, Brewer HB Jr. 3-Hydroxy-3-methylglutaryl-coenzyme A reductase inhibitors in the treatment of hypercholesterolemia. *JAMA.* 1987; 258:3532-6.
13. Tsujita Y, Kuroda M, Shimada Y et al. CS-514, a competitive inhibitor of 3-hydroxy-3-methylglutaryl coenzyme A reductase: tissue-selective inhibition of sterol synthesis and hypolipidemic effect on various species. *Biochem Biophys Acta.* 1986; 877:50-60.
14. Brown MS, Goldstein JL. A receptor-mediated pathway for cholesterol homeostasis. *Science.* 1986; 232:34-7.
15. Goldstein JL, Kita T, Brown MS. Defective lipoprotein receptors and atherosclerosis. Lessons from an animal counterpart of familial hypercholesterolemia. *N Engl J Med.* 1983; 309:288-96.
16. Grundy SM. Cholesterol and coronary heart disease. A new era. *JAMA.* 1986; 256:2849-58.
17. Ross R. The pathogenesis of atherosclerosis—an update. *N Engl J Med.* 1986; 314:488-500.
18. Schaefer EJ, Levy RI. Pathogenesis and management of lipoprotein disorders. *N Engl J Med.* 1985; 312:1300-10.
19. Tobert JA. New developments in lipid-lowering therapy: the role of inhibitors of hydroxymethylglutaryl-coenzyme A reductase. *Circulation.* 1987; 76:534-8.
20. Grundy SM. HMG-CoA reductase inhibitors for treatment of hypercholesterolemia. *N Engl J Med.* 1988; 319:24-33.
21. Reihner E, Rudling M, Stahlberg D. Influence of pravastatin, a specific inhibitor of HMG-CoA reductase on hepatic metabolism of cholesterol. *N Engl J Med.* 1990; 323:224-8.
22. Pan HY, Funke PT, Willard DA et al. Pharmacokinetics, pharmacodynamics, and safety of pravastatin sodium, a

potent inhibitor of HMG-CoA reductase, in healthy volunteers. In: LaRosa JC, ed. New advances in the control of lipid metabolism: focus on pravastatin. New York, NY: Royal Society of Medicine Services Ltd.; 1989:9-21.
23. Bilheimer DW, Grundy SM, Brown MS et al. Mevinolin stimulates receptor-mediated clearance of low density lipoprotein from plasma in familial hypercholesterolemia heterozygotes. *Trans Am Assoc Physicians*. 1983; 96:1-9.
24. Vega GT, Krauss RM, Grundy SM. Pravastatin therapy in primary moderate hypercholesterolemia: changes in metabolism of apolipoprotein B-containing lipoproteins. *J Intern Med*. 1990; 227:81-94.
25. Hoogerbrugge-vd Linden N, de Rooy FWM, Jansen H et al. Effect of pravastatin on biliary lipid composition and bile acid synthesis in familial hypercholesterolemia. *Gut*. 1990; 31:348-50.
26. Scott WA, Mahoney EM, Moseley ST. Mechanism of action and differential pharmacology of pravastatin, a hydrophilic and selective HMG-CoA reductase inhibitor. In: LaRosa JC, ed. New advances in the control of lipid metabolism: focus on pravastatin. New York, NY: Royal Society of Medicine Services Ltd.; 1989:1-8.
27. Maher VMG, Thompson GR. HMG-CoA reductase inhibitors as lipid-lowering agents: five years experience with lovastatin and an appraisal of simvastatin and pravastatin. *Q J Med*. 1990; NS74:165-75.
28. Mahoney EM, Child MJ, Smith-Monroy EM. Differential transport of pravastatin and lovastatin by hepatocytes and fibroblasts. *Circulation*. 1990; 82:III-6. Abstract.
29. Roth BD, Bocan TMA, Blankley CJ et al. Relationship between tissue selectivity and lipophilicity for inhibitors of HMG-CoA reductase. *J Med Chem*. 1991; 34:463-6.
30. Koga T, Shimada Y, Kuroda M et al. Tissue-selective inhibition of cholesterol synthesis in vivo by pravastatin sodium, a 3-hydroxy-3-methylglutaryl coenzyme A reductase inhibitor. *Biochem Biophys Acta*. 1990; 1045:115-20.
31. Mosley ST, Kalinowski SS, Schafer BL et al. Tissue-selective acute effects of inhibitors of 3-hydroxy-3-methylglutaryl coenzyme A reductase on cholesterol biosynthesis in lens. *J Lipid Res*. 1989; 30:1411-20.
32. Botti RE, Triscari J, Pan HY et al. Concentrations of pravastatin and lovastatin in cerebrospinal fluid in healthy subjects. *Clin Neuropharmacol*. 1991; 14:256-61.
33. Pan H, Funke P, Waclawski A et al. Comparative pharmacokinetics of pravastatin, an HMG CoA reductase inhibitor, in healthy elderly and young subjects. *J Clin Pharmacol*. 1989; 29:848. Abstract.
34. Pan H, DeVault A, Glaess S et al. Effects of food on the pharmacokinetics of pravastatin, an HMG-CoA reductase inhibitor. *Arteriosclerosis*. 1988; 8:588a. Abstract.
35. Singhvi SM, Pan HY, Morrison RA et al. Disposition of pravastatin sodium, a tissue-selective HMG-CoA reductase inhibitor, in healthy subjects. *Br J Clin Pharmacol*. 1990; 29:239-43.
36. Pan HY. HMG-CoA reductase inhibitors: clinical pharmacology. In: Gotto AM Jr, Mancini M, Richter WO, eds. Treatment of severe hypercholesterolemia in prevention of coronary heart disease—2. Proceedings 2nd international symposium, Munich 1989. Basel: Karger; 1990:66-70.
37. Pan HY, DeVault AR, Wang-Iverson D et al. Comparative pharmacokinetics and pharmacodynamics of pravastatin and lovastatin. *J Clin Pharmacol*. 1990; 30:1128-35.
38. Bristol-Myers Squibb. Pravachol prescribing information. Princeton, NJ: 1992.
39. Pan HY, DeVault AR, Swites BJ et al. Pharmacokinetics and pharmacodynamics of pravastatin alone and with cholestyramine in hypercholesterolemia. *Clin Pharmacol Ther*. 1990; 48:201-7.
40. McKenney JM. Lovastatin: a new cholesterol-lowering agent. *Clin Pharm*. 1988; 7:21-36.
41. Yoshino G, Kazumi T, Kasama T et al. Effect of CS-514 (pravastatin) on VLDL-triglyceride kinetics in rats. *Atherosclerosis*. 1988; 73:191-5.
42. Watanabe Y, Ito T, Shiomi M. Preventive effect of pravastatin sodium, a potent inhibitor of 3-hydroxy-3-methylglutaryl coenzyme A reductase, on coronary atherosclerosis and xanthoma in WHHL rabbits. *Biochem Biophys Acta*. 1988; 960:294-302.
43. Nakaya N, Homma Y, Tamachi H et al. The effect of CS-514, an inhibitor of HMG-CoA reductase, on serum lipids in healthy volunteers. *Atherosclerosis*. 1986; 61:125-8.
44. Saito Y, Goto Y, Nakaya N et al. Dose-dependent hypolipidemic effect of an inhibitor of HMG-CoA reductase, pravastatin (CS-514), in hypercholesterolemic subjects: a double blind test. *Atherosclerosis*. 1988; 72:205-11.
45. Wiklund O, Angelin B, Fager G et al. Treatment of familial hypercholesterolemia: a controlled trial of the effects of pravastatin or cholestyramine therapy on lipoprotein and apolipoprotein levels. *J Intern Med*. 1990; 228:241-7.
46. Mabuchi H, Kamon N, Fujita H et al. Effects of CS-514 on serum lipoprotein lipid and apolipoprotein levels in patients with familial hypercholesterolemia. *Metabolism*. 1987; 36:475-9.
47. Mabuchi H, Fujita H, Michishita I et al. Effects of CS-514 (eptastatin), an inhibitor of 3-hydroxy-3-methylglutaryl coenzyme A (HMG-CoA) reductase, on serum lipid an dapolipoprotein levels in heterozygous familial hypercholesterolemic patients treated by low density lipoprotein (LDL)-apheresis. *Atherosclerosis*. 1988; 72:183-8.
48. Franceschini G, Sirtori M, Vaccarino V et al. Plasma lipoprotein changes after treatment with pravastatin and gemfibrozil in patients with familial hypercholesterolemia. *J Lab Clin Med*. 1989; 114:250-9.
49. Nakaya N, Homma Y, Tamachi H et al. The effect of CS-514 on serum lipids and apolipoproteins in hypercholesterolemic subjects. *JAMA*. 1987; 257:3088-93.
50. Hunninghake DB, Knopp RH, Schonfeld G et al. Efficacy and safety of pravastatin in patients with primary hypercholesterolemia: I. a dose-response study. *Atherosclerosis*. 1990; 85:81-9.
51. Hunninghake DB, Mellies MJ, Goldberg AC et al. Efficacy and safety of pravastatin in patients with primary hypercholesterolemia: II. once-daily versus twice-daily dosing. *Atherosclerosis*. 1990; 85:219-27.
52. Jones PH, Farmer JA, Cressman MD et al. Once-daily pravastatin in patients with primary hypercholesterolemia: a dose-response study. *Clin Cardiol*. 1991; 14:146-51.
53. Yoshino G, Matsushita M, Iwai M et al. Two-year study on the effect of pravastatin (CS-514) on plasma lipoprotein and apolipoprotein concentrations in hypercholesterolemic patients. *Curr Ther Res*. 1989; 46:144-52.
54. Yoshino G, Kazumi T, Matsushita M et al. Comparison of the effects of pravastatin and simvastatin in hypercholesterolemic subjects. *Curr Ther Res*. 1990; 48:259-67.
55. Crepaldi G, Baggio G, Area M et al. Pravastatin vs gemfibrozil in the treatment of primary hypercholesterolemia: The Italian Multicenter Pravastatin Study I. *Arch Intern Med*. 1991; 151:146-52.
56. Yoshino G, Kazumi T, Uenoyama R et al. Effect of eptastatin (CS-514) on hypercholesterolemic patients: comparison with probucol. *Curr Ther Res*. 1986; 40:1017-21.
57. Bard JM, Parra HJ, Douste-Blazy P et al. Effect of pravastatin, an HMG CoA reductase inhibitor, and cholestyramine, a bile acid sequestrant, on lipoprotein particles defined by their apolipoprotein composition. *Metabolism*. 1990; 39:269-73.
58. Kostis JB, Wilson AC, Tannenbaum AK et al. Long-term combination therapy of primary hypercholesterolemia with pravastatin. *Circulation*. 1989; 80:II-128. Abstract.
59. Yoshino G, Kazumi T, Iwai M et al. Long-term treatment of hypercholesterolemic non-insulin dependent diabetics (NIDDM) with pravastatin (CS-514). *Atherosclerosis*. 1989; 75:67-72.
60. Yoshino G, Kazumi T, Kasama T et al. Effect of CS-514, an inhibitor of 3-hydroxy-3-methylglutaryl coenzyme A reductase, on lipoprotein and apolipoprotein in plasma of

hypercholesterolemic diabetics. *Diabetes Res Clin Pract.* 1986; 2:179-81.
61. Yoshino G, Kazumi T, Uenoyama R et al. Probucol versus eptastatin in hypercholesterolemic diabetics. *Lancet.* 1986; 2:740-1. Letter.
62. Ditschuneit HH, Kuhn K, Ditschuneit H. Comparison of different HMG-CoA reductase inhibitors. *Eur J Clin Pharmacol.* 1991; 40(suppl l):S27-32.
63. Hoogerbrugge N, Mol MJTM, Van Dormaal JJ et al. The efficacy and safety of pravastatin, compared to and in combination with bile acid resins, in familial hypercholesterolemia. *J Intern Med.* 1990; 228:261-6.
64. Yoshino G, Kazumi T, Iwai M et al. CS-514 suppresses plasma triglyceride in hypertriglyceridemic subjects without modifying a lipoprotein structural model. *Horm Metab Res.* 1987; 19:513-4.
65. Kazumi T, Yoshino G, Kasama T. Effects of CS-514, a new inhibitor of HMG-CoA reductase, on plasma lipids, lipoproteins and apoproteins in patients with primary hypercholesterolemia. *Horm Metab Res.* 1986; 18:654-5.
66. Yoshino G, Kazumi T, Iwai M et al. Effects of CS-514 on plasma lipids and lipoprotein composition in hypercholesterolemic subjects. *Atherosclerosis.* 1988; 71:95-101.
67. Rubenfire M, Blevins RD, Orringer C et al. The effect of dietary intervention on response to pravastatin in hypercholesterolemic patients. *J Am Coll Cardiol.* 1988; 11:41A. Abstract.
68. Homma Y, Tamachi H, Nakaya N. Normalization of plasma lipoprotein levels in heterozygous familial hypercholesterolemia by combined treatment with plasmapheresis and medication. *Arteriosclerosis.* 1987; 7:514A. Abstract.
69. Saku K, Sasaki J, Arakawa K. Long-term effect of CS-514 (HMG-CoA reductase inhibitor) on serum lipids, lipoproteins, and apoproteins in patients with hypercholesterolemia. *Curr Ther Res.* 1987; 42:491-500.
70. Saxenhofer H, Weidmann P, Riesen WF et al. Therapeutic efficacy of the HMG-CoA reductase inhibitor pravastatin in hyperlipidemia type II. *Eur J Clin Pharmacol.* 1990; 39:101-5.
71. Betteridge DJ. Clinical efficacy of pravastatin. In: LaRosa JC, ed. New advances in the control of lipid metabolism: focus on pravastatin. New York, NY: Royal Society of Medicine Services Ltd.; 1989:23-8.
72. Catalano P. Pravastatin safety: an overview. In: Wood C, ed. Lipid management: pravastatin and the differential pharmacology of HMG-CoA reductase inhibitors. Royal Society of Medicine Round Table Series No. 16. Oxford: Alden Press; 1990:26-31.
73. Achor RWP, Winklemann RK, Perry HO. Cutaneous side effects from the use of triparanol (MER-29): preliminary data on ichthyosis and loss of hair. *Mayo Clin Proc.* 1961; 36:217-28.
74. Illingworth DR, Bacon S. Treatment of heterozygous familial hypercholesterolemia with lipid-lowering drugs. *Arteriosclerosis.* 1989; 9(Suppl l):I121-34.
75. Kirby TJ. Cataracts produced by triparanol (MER/29). *Trans Am Ophthalmol Soc.* 1967; 65:493-543.
76. Laughlin RC, Carey TF. Cataracts in patients treated with triparanol. *JAMA.* 1962; 181:339-40.
77. Newman TJ, Kassler-Taub KB, Gelarden RT et al. Safety of pravastatin in long-term clinical trials in the United States. *J Drug Dev.* 1990; 3(Suppl 2):275-81.
78. Catalano PM, Masonson HN, Newman TJ et al. Clinical safety of pravastatin. In: LaRosa JC, ed. New advances in the control of lipid metabolism: focus on pravastatin. New York, NY: Royal Society of Medicine Services Ltd.; 1989:35-8.
79. Pierce LR, Wysowski DK, Gross TP. Myopathy and rhabdomyolysis associated with lovastatin—gemfibrozil combination therapy. *JAMA.* 1990; 264:71-5.
80. Mantell G, Burke T, Staggers J. Extended clinical safety profile of lovastatin. *Am J Cardiol.* 1990; 66:11B-15B.
81. Ayanian JZ, Fuchs CS, Stone RM. Lovastatin and rhabdomyolysis. *Ann Intern Med.* 1988; 109:682-3. Letter.
82. East C, Alivizatos PA, Grundy SM et al. Rhabdomyolysis in patients receiving lovastatin after cardiac transplantation. *N Engl J Med.* 1988; 318:47-8. Letter.
83. Norman DJ, Illingworth DR, Munson J et al. Myolysis and acute renal failure in a heart-transplant recipient receiving lovastatin. *N Engl J Med.* 1988; 318:46-7. Letter.
84. Bradford RH, Shear CL, Chremos AN et al. Expanded clinical evaluation of lovastatin (EXCEL) study results. I. Efficacy in modifying plasma lipoproteins and adverse event profile in 8245 patients with moderate hypercholesterolemia. *Arch Intern Med.* 1991; 151:43-9.
85. Yoshimura N, Oka T, Yasumura T et al. Efficacy and safety of a hydrophilic HMG-CoA reductase inhibitor, pravastatin, in the management of hypercholesterolemia of renal transplant recipients treated with CoA, Az and steroid (abstract 122). 9th International Symposium on Atherosclerosis, October 6–11, 1991; Rosemont, IL. Abstract.
86. Wiklund O, Angelin B, Bergman M et al. Comparison of pravastatin and gemfibrozil and the combination for the treatment of hypercholesterolemia. *Arteriosclerosis and Thrombosis.* 1991; 11:1459a-1460a. Abstract.
87. Merck Sharp & Dohme. Mevacor prescribing information. West Point, NJ: 1991.
88. Lovastatin Study Group II. Therapeutic response to lovastatin (mevinolin) in nonfamilial hypercholesterolemia. A multicenter study. *JAMA.* 1986; 256:2829-34.
89. Laties AM, Keates EU, Taylor HR et al. The human lens after 48 weeks of treatment with lovastatin. *N Engl J Med.* 1990; 323:683-4. Letter.
90. Chylack LT Jr, Leske MC, Sperduto R et al. Lens opacity classification system. *Arch Ophthalmol.* 1988; 106:330-4.
91. Schaefer EJ. HMG-CoA reductase inhibitors for hypercholesterolemia. *N Engl J Med.* 1988; 319:1222. Letter.
92. Vgontzas AN, Kales A, Bixler EO et al. Effects of lovastatin and pravastatin on sleep efficiency and sleep stages. *Clin Pharmacol Ther.* 1991; 50:730-7.
93. Tobert JA, Shear CL, Chremos AN et al. Clinical experience with lovastatin. *Am J Cardiol.* 1990; 65:23F-6F.
94. Pan HY, Swanson BN, DeVault AR et al. Antipyrine elimination is not affected by chronic administration of pravastatin (SQ 31,000), a tissue-selective HMG-CoA reductase inhibitor. *Clin Res.* 1988; 36:368A. Abstract.
95. Pan HY, Triscari J, DeVault AR et al. Pharmacokinetic interaction between propranolol and the HMG-CoA reductase inhibitors pravastatin and lovastatin. *Br J Clin Pharmacol.* 1991; 31:665-70.
96. Brown G, Albers JJ, Fisher LD et al. Regression of coronary artery disease as a result of intensive lipid-lowering therapy in men with high levels of apolipoprotein B. *N Engl J Med.* 1990; 323:1289-98.
97. Grundy SM, Goodman DS, Rifkind BM et al. The place of HDL in cholesterol management: a perspective from the National Cholesterol Education Program. *Arch Intern Med.* 1989; 149:505-10.
98. Frick MH, Elo O, Haapa K et al. Helsinki Heart Study: primary-prevention trial with gemfibrozil in middle-aged men with dyslipidemia. Safety of treatment, changes in risk factors and incidence of coronary heart disease. *N Engl J Med.* 1987; 317:1237-45.
99. Manninen V, Elo MO, Frick MH et al. Lipid alterations and decline in the incidence of coronary heart disease in the Helsinki Heart Study. *JAMA.* 1988; 260:641-51.
100. Gordon DJ, Knoke J, Probstfield JL et al. High-density lipoprotein cholesterol and coronary heart disease in hypercholesterolemic men: the Lipid Research Clinics Coronary Primary Prevention Trial. *Circulation.* 1986; 74:1217-25.
101. Kane JP, Malloy MJ, Ports TA et al. Regression of coronary atherosclerosis during treatment of familial hypercholesterolemia with combined drug regimens. *JAMA.* 1990; 264:3007-12.
102. Sifton DW, ed. Drug topics red book 1992. Montvale, NJ: Medical Economics Data; 1992:384,470.

Therapy Review

Treatment of nonsteroidal anti-inflammatory drug-induced gastropathy

DONALD R. MILLER

Abstract: The etiology, natural history, epidemiology, prevention, and treatment of nonsteroidal anti-inflammatory drug (NSAID)-induced gastrointestinal (GI) effects are reviewed.

Current evidence suggests that NSAIDs cause acute cellular damage by a topical effect that is exacerbated by impaired healing. Although acute gastric injury from NSAIDs is rapid and almost uniform from patient to patient, not all patients develop serious chronic injury. Some adaptation to the effects of NSAIDs does occur.

Endoscopic studies have found that 14–31% of long-term NSAID users have gastric or duodenal ulcers. Data on individual drugs are inconsistent, but they suggest that enteric-coated aspirin, salsalate, and ibuprofen cause the lowest incidence of GI hemorrhage. Preventive measures tested to date include reduction in gastric acid production (histamine H_2-receptor antagonists) and attempts to increase mucosal defenses (sucralfate or misoprostol). Misoprostol is the only drug with FDA-approved labeling for prevention of NSAID-induced gastropathy. NSAID-related ulcers heal in most patients within two to three months when they are treated with H_2-receptor antagonists with or without antacid, omeprazole, or misoprostol.

In patients with multiple risk factors, prophylaxis with misoprostol would be appropriate unless the clinician is concerned solely about reactivation of a duodenal ulcer, in which case an H_2-receptor antagonist would also be appropriate. Full-dose treatment with H_2-receptor antagonists, omeprazole, or misoprostol will heal NSAID-induced ulcers, even when NSAID therapy is continued.

Index terms: Anti-inflammatory agents; Gastrointestinal drugs; Misoprostol; Omeprazole; Toxicity; Ulcers

Clin Pharm. 1992; 11:690-704

Nonsteroidal anti-inflammatory drugs (NSAIDs) have been in use for nearly a century—ever since aspirin was introduced in 1899.[1] However, during the past two decades there has been a huge increase in the sale of NSAIDs.[2] This increase is related to both an aging population more likely to have an indication for NSAIDs and aggressive marketing of newer NSAIDs for indications ranging from simple pain relief to dysmenorrhea to rheumatoid arthritis. In 1985, NSAIDs were used to treat 3 million Americans daily, at a yearly cost of more than $1 billion.[2]

Gastrointestinal (GI) adverse effects from NSAIDs have long been recognized. In fact, aspirin (acetylsalicylic acid) was synthesized to reduce the GI irritation caused by salicylic acid.[1] Although aspirin appeared to be an improvement, cases of GI hemorrhage due to aspirin were described after World War I,[3] and aspirin's ability to cause gastric bleeding was documented in 1938 by gastroscopic observations in 16 patients.[4] Despite this information, as late as 1980 some authors expressed doubt that aspirin could cause clinically important GI hemorrhage.[1] During the 1980s both retrospective and prospective studies confirmed an association between NSAID use and GI bleeding. Interest in the subject reached a new high in 1987, when the FDA required a class warning on NSAID labeling that states there is a 2–4% annual incidence of serious GI reactions due to NSAIDs.[5] One report estimated that NSAID-related gastropathy accounts for 2,600 deaths and 20,000 hospitalizations per year in patients with rheumatoid arthritis.[6]

These data might suggest that the use of NSAIDs be re-evaluated in light of the dangers described. Is it time to panic? In this review, I evaluate and put in

DONALD R. MILLER, PHARM.D., is Associate Professor of Pharmacy, North Dakota State University, and Clinical Pharmacist, Veterans Affairs Medical Center, Fargo, ND.

Addrss reprint requests to Dr. Miller at the College of Pharmacy, North Dakota State University, Fargo, ND 58105-5055.

This is **article 680-204-9221** in the **ASHP Continuing Education System**; it qualifies for 1.0 hour of continuing-education credit. See page 731 for learning objectives and test questions.

perspective the problem of NSAID-induced GI damage and provide recommendations for minimization of the risk.

Etiology of NSAID-Induced Gastropathy

Terms such as "gastropathy" or even NSAID-related gastric "injury" are vague and do not adequately reflect the complex variety of effects that NSAIDs may have. Lesions associated with NSAIDs, in order of increasing severity, include mucosal erythema and edema, local hemorrhages (variously classified as friability, petechiae, or ecchymoses), erosions, and ulcers.[7] Only ulcers, which by definition have depth, are likely to erode into a blood vessel or perforate. NSAIDs do not produce inflammatory changes in the mucosa but rather cause focal lesions in the midst of otherwise normal mucosa.[7] Although early damage most frequently occurs in the stomach, petechiae, erosions, and ulcers also can be found in the duodenum.[8] In fact, NSAIDs can cause lesions anywhere in the GI tract, from esophagus to colon.[9,10] The etiology is a combination of both local and systemic effects. The severity of damage depends on subject-to-subject variability and factors such as gastric pH, drug dose, and duration of exposure. In this review, I will discuss the effects of NSAIDs on only the stomach and duodenum.

When aspirin is ingested in a single oral dose, extensive disruption of superficial mucosal cells of the gastric fundus and antrum is seen within 10 minutes, in both animals and humans.[3,11] Subepithelial erosions and hemorrhage are evident in healthy volunteers within 15–30 minutes.[3,11,12] Complete recovery in surface cells occurs within six hours,[11] whereas gross recovery takes five to seven days.[12]

Davenport[13,14] theorized that GI injury begins with penetration of drug into the mucosa, which causes dysfunction of the mucosal barrier and permits back diffusion of hydrogen ions. The hydrogen ions then cause additional injury, inflammation, and bleeding. His theory is supported by the fact that all marketed NSAIDs are lipophilic, which allows them to readily penetrate the mucosa, and are weak acids, which allows them to accumulate in gastric epithelial cells by an "ion-trapping" mechanism.[15] Thus, NSAIDs may not cause bleeding by themselves, but rather they may simply break the mucosal barrier, allowing acid to diffuse into mucosal cells and destroy capillaries and venules.[13,14] The drugs also must penetrate the mucosa first; they do not cause damage from outside the cell. Exactly how NSAID accumulation damages mucosal cells is unclear, but the net consequence is an increase in membrane permeability.[15]

Direct Topical Effects. There is much evidence that NSAID-related damage is partly due to direct superficial effects. Uncoated aspirin tablets cause more extensive acute damage than suspensions or solutions, and damage occurs wherever the aspirin contacts gastric mucosa.[3,16] Drugs administered in nonacidic prodrug form, such as sulindac, cause less acute damage than most NSAIDs.[15,17] Enteric coatings also protect the stomach from the topical effects of NSAIDs. These coatings have been shown to substantially reduce gastric mucosal bleeding due to aspirin, even though gastric mucosal prostaglandin E_2 synthesis is inhibited similarly by coated and uncoated tablets.[18] Enteric coating also reduces the prevalence of chronic gastric damage due to aspirin.[19] NSAIDs can induce lesions in the buccal mucosa[15] or esophagus[20] by direct contact. Aspirin and indomethacin also have been documented to increase basal and maximally stimulated gastric acid secretion.[15]

Role of Prostaglandin Inhibition. Prostaglandins are synthesized by the GI mucosa and affect blood flow and secretion of mucus and bicarbonate ions. They also decrease gastric acid secretion.[20] Prostaglandins dramatically protect the gastric mucosa from acute ethanol-induced injury by mechanisms independent of the inhibition of acid secretion. This effect has been called "cytoprotection," although "mucosal protection" has been suggested as a more appropriate term because surface epithelial cells are still damaged despite protection of deeper layers.[21]

All NSAIDs inhibit the activity of cyclo-oxygenase, the enzyme that catalyzes formation of prostaglandins from arachidonic acid. They do not block the response to exogenous prostaglandins.[22] Inhibition of prostaglandin production does not cause mucosal injury by itself, but it does reduce tolerance to new insults. For example, in rats, injected aspirin (despite 95% inhibition of mucosal prostaglandin production) causes no damage unless bile salts are present simultaneously.[23] Thus, prostaglandin inhibition is a secondary, but additive, mechanism of NSAID-induced GI damage. If inhibition of prostaglandin synthesis were not present, mucosal cells would probably recover from the topical insult more easily.[15] Prostaglandin analogues, such as misoprostol, are effective in reducing the frequency of acute gastric injury as well as the long-term rate of gastric ulcer development due to NSAIDs.[24] In addition to protecting the gastric mucosa from injury, prostaglandins help to heal existing ulcers by increasing proliferation of epithelial cells at the edge of the ulcer. Thus, NSAIDs also reduce the healing ability of the mucosa.[25]

The systemic effects of NSAIDs are illustrated by the ability of indomethacin suppositories to cause as much gastric damage as capsules and the ability of aspirin or ketorolac tromethamine to cause bleeding when given intravenously.[21,26,27]

Role of Modifying Factors. Acid plays an important role in permitting development of NSAID-induced gastric damage. Lower stomach pH allows more NSAID to be in an unionized, lipophilic form, permitting greater penetration into mucosal cells. In dogs, bleeding from aspirin is related to the concentration of acid in the stomach,[14] and in dogs and humans, gastric injury is minimal when the gastric pH is greater than 5.[14,15,28] Histamine H_2-receptor antagonists do not reliably prevent development of NSAID-related gastric ulcers,[7] and continued use of NSAIDs impairs healing of gastric ulcers by ranitidine hydrochloride, but not by omeprazole.[29] These data imply that substantial acid inhibition is required to heal or protect NSAID-damaged mucosa.

Traditionally, patients have been advised to take NSAIDs with food, but there are no data to prove this advice is sound. In fact, limited data suggest that gastric erosions due to aspirin are not reduced by a concurrent meal and that food may actually be counterproductive by inducing acid secretion.[30]

Helicobacter pylori colonization of gastric epithelium has been reported to be a risk factor for spontaneous development of peptic ulcer disease. However, only about half of NSAID-induced ulcers are associated with *H. pylori* compared with almost all non-NSAID-induced ulcers.[21] This suggests that NSAIDs damage the GI independently of *H. pylori*. NSAID-induced damage does not result in increased susceptibility to *H. pylori* infection,[31,32] and mucosal damage from NSAIDs is no greater in *H. pylori*-colonized patients than in noncolonized patients.[33] Colonization may even somewhat protect the mucosa from NSAIDs by increasing polymorphonuclear cells in the mucosa.[31] However, one study found that *H. pylori*-colonized patients were more likely to have dyspeptic symptoms due to NSAIDs.[34] The frequency of *H. pylori* infection in patients with arthritis is similar to that in age-matched persons without arthritis.[31,34]

The indication for which NSAIDs are used appears to have a possible role in determining susceptibility to ulcers. Some authors found the incidence to be no different in patients with rheumatoid arthritis than in patients with osteoarthritis.[31,35] However, other researchers found less duodenal damage in patients with rheumatoid arthritis than in patients with osteoarthritis,[36] whereas some epidemiologic data indicate a greater risk of GI bleeding in patients with rheumatoid arthritis than in patients with osteoarthritis.[6] Mucosal damage is increased with higher doses of most NSAIDs,[13] and use of multiple NSAIDs is more damaging than use of a single drug.[35,37] In summary, current evidence suggests that NSAIDs cause acute cellular damage by a topical effect that is exacerbated by impaired healing. The degree of damage also depends on gastric acidity.

Clinical Features

Compared with spontaneous peptic ulcers, NSAID-induced ulcers are more likely to be in the stomach, may be less acid dependent, and are more often asymptomatic.[19,38-40] Histologically, spontaneous gastric ulcers are surrounded by a wide field of nonerosive gastritis, whereas NSAID-related ulcers are likely to be found in the midst of normal mucosa.[7,21] Patients taking NSAIDs frequently complain of nausea or abdominal discomfort. However, the presence of subjective dyspepsia with NSAID therapy does not predict blood loss[16] or the severity of gastric damage observed objectively through an endoscope.[8,19,31,35,38] The exact etiology of NSAID-associated dyspepsia is unknown. It cannot be explained by the presence of *H. pylori* gastritis,[31] although dyspepsia may be somewhat more common in patients who are serologically positive for *H. pylori*.[31,34]

The prevalence of dyspepsia also varies widely from study to study (7–60%), probably depending on the methods used to assess it and the type of population being studied.[39] Conversely, many patients with gastric ulcers who take NSAIDs are completely asymptomatic.[19,40] The elderly may be even more likely to have silent ulcers.[21,41] Graham et al.[31] found that the positive predictive value of NSAID-related dyspepsia for the presence of an ulcer was only 26%, whereas the negative predictive value was 93%. One study suggests that 58% of the complications from NSAID-induced ulcers are silent, versus 25% of the complications from spontaneous ulcers.[42] Therefore, even large NSAID-induced ulcers often may go undetected because patients do not complain of classic ulcer symptoms.

Natural History

Although acute gastric injury from NSAIDs is rapid and almost uniform from patient to patient, not all patients develop serious chronic injury. To determine how aspirin-related injury develops over time, Graham et al.[12] gave aspirin 2.6 g/day to 12 healthy volunteers for one or seven days. Gastroscopy was performed after days 1, 2, 4, and 8 and every other day thereafter until damage resolved. Submucosal hemorrhage or focal erosions, or both, developed in all subjects after one day. With continuous aspirin administration, injury reached its maximum within three days and then lessened, so that the damage at day 8 was less than the damage after day 1. It also took longer for damage to resolve after one day of aspirin use than after seven days of aspirin use. Thus, it appeared that gastric adaptation to the effects of aspirin developed.[12]

The ultimate damage to the gastric mucosa is probably a dynamic process balancing the intrinsic toxicity of NSAIDs against the adaptive, protective mechanisms of the mucosa.[16] Similar signs of gastric adaptation have been noted for aspirin and ibuprofen by Lanza.[8] Adaptation may result from prostaglandin-mediated mechanisms, but other processes may also be involved.[15] The process of adaptation, or stimulation of healing factors, probably begins rapidly, as illustrated by the fast resolution of acute, superficial damage caused by NSAIDs. A process called restitution allows migration of existing gastric epithelial cells along the basement membrane to fill in defects left by sloughing of other cells.[15,21] Gastric erosions can wax and wane spontaneously, even during continuous NSAID use.[38] The development of an ulcer may reflect a failure of adaptation or local susceptibility to damage, or both. The presence of microbleeding or small mucosal hemorrhages and erosions has no proven value for predicting the development of chronic ulcers.[16,21]

Adaptation is also illustrated by the ability of ulcers to heal despite continued NSAID therapy. Duodenal and gastric ulcers have been shown to heal well when ranitidine hydrochloride, omeprazole, or sucralfate is administered, even when NSAID therapy is continued, although healing is somewhat slower than it is when NSAID therapy is stopped.[29,43,44]

Just how quickly NSAIDs can cause serious ulcer complications is unknown, but complications have been reported within days of starting therapy.[44] Some gastroscopic studies[24,36] but not all[35] have found that development of new ulcers is more common during the first month of observation than during the second or third month. This finding may be consistent with an adaptation effect. A meta-analysis of studies of NSAID-induced ulcer epidemiology also found that serious complications are most common during the first month of use, and the incidence declines thereafter.[45]

Thus, erosions and mucosal hemorrhages occur at the onset of NSAID therapy and either heal rapidly if the drug is discontinued or gradually diminish over time as mucosal adaptation develops. These lesions are diffuse, occurring anywhere in the stomach. Chronic ulcers emerge within the first three months after therapy is begun, occur mostly in the antrum, and occur despite mucosal adaptation.[7] Complications associated with NSAIDs may arise from duodenal ulcers as often as from gastric ulcers.[21]

Assessment of GI Toxicity

Techniques for Assessing GI Toxicity. The true measure of drug safety is its record in everyday use. Three methods are commonly used to evaluate and compare the GI adverse effects of NSAIDs, each of which has weaknesses.

Microbleeding studies measure the number of red blood cells labeled with radioactive chromium that appear in the stool before and after drug exposure. This technique requires meticulous methods to obtain accurate results. For example, chromium is excreted into bile, and salicylate stimulates that secretion; fecal blood loss can also come from the lower GI tract. Therefore, increased appearance of chromium in the stool after administration of aspirin may not indicate bleeding from the GI mucosa. One could also question the relevance of short-term chromium-labeling studies to long-term NSAID toxicity.[16]

The gold standard for detecting and evaluating GI lesions is viewing them through an endoscope. Endoscopy can be done before and after drug administration, or a healthy group not exposed to NSAIDs can be used for comparison. Despite the apparent objectivity of this method, some difficult distinctions must be made among degrees of damage. Lesions associated with NSAIDs may be described as erythema, edema, mucosal hemorrhage, erosions, or ulcers. In an effort to include all lesions, many investigators give numerical values to each type of lesion and total them up to get a score for each patient. However, these scoring systems are subjective and subject to error.[7] Ulcers are typically defined as three-dimensional, circumscribed mucosal defects, often covered with an exudate, of at least a certain size. Lesions not meeting these criteria are called erosions. Depth of a lesion is particularly hard to evaluate visually, especially if the lesion is filled with exudate. The chance that a given lesion is an ulcer (i.e., has depth) increases with its size. However, the specific cutoff for using size as a criterion is arbitrary and not consistent among studies.[7,21] These decisions become critical in determining the prevalence of NSAID-related ulcers by endoscopy. The distinction between ulcers and other types of lesions is important because only ulcers are likely to cause clinically important hemorrhage.[21] Another issue is the duration of endoscopic studies. Acute gastritis associated with single doses of NSAIDs may not indicate chronic toxicity of the drugs, especially in view of the gastric adaptation that develops with continued administration of NSAIDs.[16,46]

The third technique for assessing toxicity is epidemiology, or observation of large populations. Case reports are the simplest observational technique; however, they suffer from the lack of a control group, making causal inferences difficult. Case series are too small to arrive at reliable conclusions. Case–control studies and cohort studies can provide useful information, owing to the large numbers of patients typically studied; however, they are prone to biasing factors and cannot establish causality.

Thus, all three techniques have drawbacks, but together they can provide an excellent framework for assessing the GI toxicity of NSAIDs.

Microbleeding Studies. Hundreds of microbleeding studies have been performed to assess the GI toxicity of NSAIDs.[16] Typically, a new NSAID is compared with plain aspirin tablets. No studies have evaluated more than a few NSAIDs at the same time, so assessing the relative toxicity among NSAIDs is virtually impossible based on this literature. Compared with aspirin, newer NSAIDs generally cause less bleeding.[16] However, these studies may be biased by the previously discussed effect of salicylate on biliary excretion of chromium, by the short duration of the studies and the small samples typically used, and by the choice of plain aspirin instead of enteric-coated or rapidly soluble forms.[16]

Another approach to assessing microbleeding is to do gastric washings and quantitate the amount of blood recovered. Using this technique, Prichard et al.[47] showed that bleeding from aspirin was dose related. As little as 75 mg/day of aspirin increases mucosal bleeding, but the increase is not as great as that seen with 300 mg or 2400 mg/day of aspirin.

It is worth noting that despite the microbleeding

induced by NSAIDs, the blood loss is typically not enough to cause a positive stool guaiac test result for occult blood. Clinicians should not assume that a positive guaiac test result can be explained by NSAID use; rather, they should look for the existence of underlying GI pathology.[48]

Endoscopic Studies. Endoscopic studies have many of the same limitations as microbleeding studies, namely, small samples and the inability to simultaneously compare more than a few NSAIDS. Many studies have quantified the prevalence of GI lesions after long-term NSAID therapy. For example, Larkai et al.[49] examined 65 patients taking one of eight NSAIDs continuously for at least six weeks. Using strict, conservative definitions of gastroduodenal lesions, they found normal mucosa in only one third of the patients; 45% had hemorrhages, 54% had erosions, and 15% had ulcers (abnormal mucosa could have more than one lesion).

Caruso and Bianchi Porro[35] performed a study of 164 patients with rheumatoid arthritis and 85 patients with osteoarthritis. Baseline endoscopy showed no active lesions in any patient, and each patient was treated with one or more NSAIDs, in accordance with clinical practice. Therapy with corticosteroids was also allowed. Endoscopy was repeated after 3 to 6 months of treatment for all patients and also at 12 months when possible or if a patient complained of new GI complications. Gastric lesions (defined as erosions or ulcers) occurred in 23% of the patients taking a single drug (including corticosteroids) and in 51% receiving multiple-drug treatment. Prevalence did not vary with the duration of treatment or with the disease being treated. Among patients taking a single drug, lesions developed most frequently with aspirin (presumably plain) at a rate of 50% (13 of 26 patients). Incidences of lesions with other NSAIDs were indomethacin, 30% (6 of 20 patients); ketoprofen, 27% (3 of 11 patients); naproxen, 27% (3 of 11 patients); diclofenac sodium, 20% (2 of 10 patients); ibuprofen, 18% (3 of 17 patients); sulindac, 11% (2 of 19 patients); and diflunisal, 10% (2 of 20 patients).

In general, the prevalence of lesions was dose related but poorly correlated with subjective GI complaints. Peptic ulcer recurred in 11 of 24 (46%) patients who had evidence of a healed ulcer at baseline. Although this is the largest comparative endoscopic study published to date, it still suffers from small numbers of patients per drug and the fact that the assignment of NSAID was not randomized.[35] In a study of the ability of ranitidine hydrochloride to prevent NSAID-related ulcers, Ehsanullah et al.[36] found a higher incidence of ulcers with piroxicam (12 of 75 patients; 16%) than with naproxen (14 of 161 patients; 9%) or diclofenac sodium (1 of 17 patients; 6%).

Lanza et al.[37] compared the effects of ibuprofen, indomethacin, naproxen, aspirin, and placebo on the gastric mucosa of 40 healthy volunteers randomly assigned to receive one drug for seven days. More severe injury was seen with aspirin 3.9 g/day, indomethacin 100 or 150 mg/day, and naproxen 750 mg/day than with ibuprofen 1600 or 2400 mg/day or naproxen 500 mg/day. Lanza's group has done many other studies with similar study designs.[8] In summary, these studies have shown that all NSAIDs can cause chronic GI damage. There tended to be less damage with sulindac, a prodrug, and with enteric-coated aspirin. Ibuprofen generally was associated with mild injury, whereas plain aspirin caused the most damage. In general, the severity of mucosal damage is dose related.[8]

Several endoscopic studies have shown that enteric-coated aspirin causes less damage than plain or buffered tablets. Silvoso et al.[19] performed endoscopy on 82 patients with rheumatic disease who had been receiving aspirin therapy for at least three months. The prevalence of ulcers in these patients was 23% with regular aspirin, 31% with buffered tablets, 6% with enteric-coated aspirin, and 0% in healthy controls. Serum salicylate concentrations were similar in all aspirin users. Lanza's group[50] found that enteric-coated aspirin granules provided similar gastric protection in a short-term study.

In various studies, the prevalence at any given time of ulcers in long-term NSAID users varied from 14% to 31% (mean, 25%).[7,21] Gastric ulcers have been found in 8% to 18% (mean, 13%) of patients and duodenal ulcers in 0% to 19% (mean, 11%) of patients.[7] If duodenal ulcer and gastric ulcer have a prevalence in the general population of about 1.4% and 0.28%, respectively, then the relative risk of duodenal ulcer in NSAID users is eight times the risk of duodenal ulcer in the general population and the relative risk of gastric ulcer is 46 times that in the general population.[7] It is impossible to know from these studies how many ulcers were present before therapy and were simply activated by NSAIDs, compared with the number of ulcers caused solely by drug therapy. The most common site of gastric ulcers is the antrum, although they also can occur in the gastric body and fundus.[21] Prevalence in these studies is highly dependent on the diagnostic criteria used for ulcer.[7,21]

Endoscopic studies cannot determine the relative risk of complicated ulcers with much certainty, because many ulcers are clinically silent and serious bleeding complications are much more rare than ulcers are.

Epidemiologic Studies. *Case–Control Studies.* Only population-based (epidemiologic) studies can follow large enough numbers of patients to obtain a reasonable estimate of the true risk of complications from NSAIDs. Endpoints that can be followed easily, without invasive studies, are the rates of upper GI bleeding and of fatalities due to GI hemorrhage.

In case–control studies, investigators with access to appropriate data assemble all the persons with the endpoint of interest (cases). Another group of persons is then assembled; they are as similar as possible to the cases except they do not have the endpoint of interest (control group). The two groups are then contrasted with respect to their prior use of NSAIDs or other potential risk factors for the endpoint. Because case–control studies are retrospective, they may suffer from incomplete or inaccurate data on risk factor exposures, or they may be biased by confounding variables associated with the risk factors. For example, if patients believe that NSAIDs can cause ulcers, then they will be more likely to recall NSAID use and their physicians may be more likely to pursue a history of NSAID use than would be the case with control patients. Case–control studies may also suffer from diagnostic bias in their assumption that all possible cases have been found and that all control subjects are truly free of the endpoint. An apparent causal relationship between NSAIDs and ulcers can be falsely inferred if patients use NSAIDs to treat symptoms of pain associated with ulcers.[51] The bias in case–control studies tends to overestimate relative risk.[24,52] Despite their disadvantages, case–control studies can assemble very large numbers of cases, particularly in automated databases, and therefore have excellent power to detect associations between risk factors and endpoints.

At least 18 case–control studies[42,53-69] of NSAIDs and upper GI bleeding have been reported in the past decade (Table 1). Estimates of risk ratio have varied widely because of differences in study population, outcome measures, time frame of drug use, ascertainment of NSAID exposure, and other factors. The risk ratios for aspirin have ranged from 1.0 (indicating no risk) to 29.5, and the risk ratios for nonaspirin NSAIDs have ranged from 1.1 to 13.6. On the whole, however, a consistent association between NSAID use and development of GI complications has been found.

Cohort Studies. A cohort study identifies a group of similar persons without disease (for example, people enrolled in a state Medicaid program) who vary in exposure to a risk factor and follows them prospectively over time. The disease rates in the exposed and nonexposed groups are then compared to calculate a risk ratio. These studies frequently use data routinely collected in large databases, such as insurance programs, and are less prone to bias or error in data collection. However, these studies can still suffer from diagnostic bias—physicians may look more carefully for ulcers if they know the patient has taken NSAIDs. Computerized case selection of GI events can be subject to misclassification. Information on duration of NSAID exposure in these studies is hard to verify, and infrequent use of NSAIDs in the population reduces a study's power to detect an association between drug use and disease. Because exposure to NSAIDs is not randomly allocated, NSAID users may be sicker or more prone to ulcer development than nonusers. Risk ratios from cohort studies[6,70-76] have been consistently lower than those from case–control studies (Table 1).

Experimental Studies. Experimental studies are able to infer causality and obtain more accurate estimates of risk than obtained from case–control and cohort studies, because subjects are randomly assigned to groups and are blinded as to treatment. Two experimental studies[77,78] of aspirin for prevention of myocardial infarction provided enough data to estimate the risk of GI bleeding in patients taking aspirin compared with patients taking placebo.

Analysis of Epidemiologic Data. Meta-analyses (systematic, quantitative strategies for reviewing and summarizing literature) of all available data have been reported, and individual studies have been compared and critiqued with respect to quality.[45,52] These summaries have allowed a good estimate of the overall relative risks. Specific results varied because each meta-analysis pooled different studies. The analyses conclude that NSAID users in general are at approximately three times greater relative risk than nonusers for developing serious GI events. When analysis is restricted to cohort studies, the relative risk may be closer to two[52]; however, biases in cohort studies may tend to underestimate the true risk by overestimating the duration of NSAID exposure.[21,45]

A distinction between relative risk and absolute risk should be made. For example, if the actual event rate of GI hemorrhage among non-NSAID users is 1 event per 100,000 persons and it is 3 per 100,000 among NSAID users, then the *relative* risk is 3.0 and the *absolute* risk is 2 excess events per 100,000 users. Clearly, this magnitude of absolute risk would not justify widespread concern. Alternatively, if the actual event rate in nonusers is 1 per 100, the same relative risk of 3.0 would increase the event rate in users to 3 per 100 or a 2% increase in absolute risk. Case–control studies cannot determine absolute risk, information that is critical to analysis of this problem; however, cohort studies can.

One of the cohort studies performed is by the ARAMIS (American Rheumatism Association Medical Information System) investigators.[6,76] This is a long-term cohort study in which 17 centers from North America contribute long-term follow-up data on enrolled patients. A specific database in this system is the ARAMIS Post-Marketing Surveillance Program, which analyzes drug adverse effects among these patients. Analysis of this database containing information on about 2000 patients with rheumatoid arthritis calculated a relative risk of 5.2 for GI hospitalization among patients who used NSAIDs compared with nonusers. Furthermore, the prospective nature of the study allowed calculation of an annual 1.5% absolute risk of a GI hospitalization among patients with rheumatoid arthritis who use NSAIDs versus an annual 0.32% absolute risk for patients with rheumatoid arthritis who do not use NSAIDs. The authors extrapolated this calculation to estimate that if there are 2 million patients with rheumatoid arthritis in the United States, then there would be 20,000 excess hospitalizations per year.[6]

Unfortunately, these extrapolations are probably overestimates, because patients with rheumatoid arthritis who see tertiary-care rheumatologists (the group that comprises much of the database) are likely to be sicker than most patients with rheumatoid arthritis. The investigators' own data confirm that severe rheumatoid arthritis in itself is a risk factor for NSAID-induced GI bleeding.[6,76]

From available cohort studies, Gabriel et al.,[45] estimated the prevalence of serious GI events at only 1 per 1000 patient-years in NSAID users. Prospectively obtained data from the Aspirin Myocardial Infarction Study found an incidence of 5 hospitalizations per 1000 patient-years with 1 g of aspirin daily.[78] However, in a study of elderly Tennessee Medicaid enrollees, the rate of hospitalization for ulcer disease was 23 per 1000 patient-years in NSAID users compared with 5.6 per 1000 patients-years in nonusers.[69] The discrepancies in estimates of absolute risk probably reflect the different populations studied. The lowest absolute risks were derived from younger, healthier health-maintenance-organization populations, whereas the higher estimates were derived from older, sicker populations.

Several studies provide data on exposure to individual NSAIDs. According to Gabriel et al.,[45] the summary odds ratios for individual drugs are piroxicam, 11.12 (95% confidence interval [CI], 6.19–20.23); indomethacin, 4.69 (95% CI, 2.97–7.41); aspirin, 3.38 (95% CI, 2.26–5.01); naproxen, 2.84 (95% CI, 1.68–4.82); and ibuprofen, 2.27 (95% CI, 1.85–2.80). According to Hawkey's meta-analysis,[52] the pooled relative risk in

Table 1.
Nonsteroidal Anti-inflammatory Drugs (NSAIDs) and Relative Risk of Gastropathy[a]

Reference, Year	Study Design and Comments	Relative Risk
Case–Control Studies		
42, 1987	NSAID use in 235 patients with perforated PU versus 1246 unmatched hospital controls	13.7[b]
53, 1981	Analgesic (aspirin plus acetaminophen) use in 127 outpatients diagnosed with GU or DU matched with community controls	29.5[b] for GU after heavy analgesic use
54, 1982	Heavy analgesic use in 99 patients with GU compared with 180 community controls	23.4[b] for women with GU
55, 1982	Aspirin use before admission in 346 matched pairs of hematemesis or melena cases and controls	9.3[b] for DU; 3.3 for GU
56, 1974	Heavy, regular aspirin use in 220 inpatients with upper GI bleeding or new onset of PU compared with 14,813 controls	3.4[b] for GU
57, 1985	Analgesic use in 104 patients with chronic GU compared with 208 community controls	7.4–13.6[b] for GU after NSAID (not aspirin) use 6.8–11.3[b] after aspirin use
58, 1988	NSAID use in 225 outpatients with new onset of GU compared with 411 age- and sex-matched community controls	2.3–5.4[b] after NSAID (not aspirin) use 2.6–5.0[b] after aspirin use
59, 1986	Analgesic use in 180 patients with endoscopically verified DU or GU matched with clinic controls	1.1 for DU and 5.0[b] for GU after NSAID (not aspirin) use 1.0 for DU and 3.0 for GU after aspirin use
60, 1986	NSAID (not aspirin) use at admission in 230 inpatients >60 years of age with bleeding DU or GU compared with two control groups	2.7[b] for DU; 2.8–3.7[b] for GU
61, 1985	NSAID use in 269 patients with perforated PU compared with 269 age- and sex-matched hospital controls	11.5[b] in patients >65 years of age; 2.3 in patients <65 years of age
62, 1986	NSAID use in 57 patients hospitalized with upper GI bleeding compared with 123 age- and sex-matched controls	3.1[b]
63, 1987	NSAID use in 80 patient deaths related to PU compared with 160 matched hospital controls	1.2 after aspirin use 1.1 after NSAID (not aspirin) use
64, 1988	Aspirin use in 230 inpatients ≥60 years of age with bleeding DU or GU compared with two age- and sex-matched control groups	3.0–3.4[b] for DU; 2.0–3.3[b] for GU
65, 1988	NSAID use (outpatient prescriptions) in 122 Medicaid recipients ≥60 years of age with fatal ulcer or with hospitalization for upper GI bleeding compared with 3897 matched controls	7.9[b] for DU; 4.2[b] for GU
66, 1988	NSAID use in 57 patients hospitalized for hematemesis or melena compared with 2417 controls	9.1[b] after NSAID (not aspirin) use 5.6–15.0[b] after aspirin use
67, 1991	NSAID use in 161 patients with upper GI bleeding versus hospitalized age- and sex-matched controls	7.4[b] after NSAID (not aspirin) use 2.2[b] after aspirin use
68, 1991	NSAID use in 875 cases of upper GI bleeding matched with 2682 hospital controls	7.2[b] after aspirin use 4.9–19.1[b] after NSAID (not aspirin) use
69, 1991	NSAID use in 1415 Medicaid recipients >65 years of age hospitalized for PU compared with 7063 matched controls	4.1[b] after NSAID (not aspirin) use

Continued on next page

Table 1 (continued)

Reference, Year	Study Design and Comments	Relative Risk
Cohort Studies		
70, 1987	Computerized hospital admission and outpatient pharmacy charge records; upper GI bleeding (excluding DU bleeding) and 90-day exposure to NSAIDs (excluding aspirin) for patients ≥65 years of age; 300,000-member HMO	1.4
71, 1987	Computerized Medicaid hospitalization and outpatient pharmacy charge records; upper GI bleeding and 30-day exposure to NSAIDs (excluding aspirin); 91,770 study patients	10.5[b]
72, 1987	Computerized hospital admission and outpatient pharmacy charge records; perforated PU and 90-day exposure to NSAIDs (excluding aspirin); 300,000-member HMO	1.6
73, 1988	Computerized hospital admission and prescription records; fatal upper GI bleeding, perforations, and 30-day NSAID exposure; 1,000,000-member Canadian province plan	5.3[b] for women ≥75 years of age
74, 1989	Computerized Medicaid hospitalization and outpatient pharmacy charge records; GI adverse effects (including ulcer) and 90-day exposure to NSAIDs; 73,355 study patients	1.9[b] for DU; 2.8[b] for GU
75, 1989	Computerized registry of patients in Tayside region of Scotland; hospitalization after GI-related events before and after NSAID exposure; 25,959 patients and 25,959 controls	1.59[b] after NSAID use
6, 1989 and 76, 1991	Cohort of 2747 rheumatoid arthritis patients followed prospectively for an average of 4 years at 5 centers; GI hospitalizations and deaths and 6-month exposure to NSAIDs	5.2[b]
Experimental Studies		
77, 1989	Randomized, double-blind, placebo-controlled trial of 22,071 male physicians receiving aspirin 325 mg every other day or placebo for 5 years	1.2 for PU
78, 1990	Randomized, double-blind, placebo-controlled study of 4524 subjects receiving aspirin 1 g/day or placebo for 3 years	10.7[b] for men with DU; 9.1[b] for men with GU

[a]GU = gastric ulcer, DU = duodenal ulcer, PU = peptic ulcer. NSAID may include aspirin unless otherwise stated. Modified with permission from reference 21.

[b]The lower limit of the 95% confidence interval is greater than 1.0, or $p < 0.05$ for statistical test.

case–control studies for aspirin is 4.67 compared with 4.03 for nonaspirin NSAIDs, but the overall risk for nonaspirin NSAIDs is 1.5 in cohort studies.

An individual cohort study providing extensive analysis of GI risks for individual drugs was done by Carson et al.[79] They found sulindac and tolmetin sodium (not analyzed by Gabriel et al.[45]) to have the highest risk among seven nonaspirin NSAIDs. Limited data on piroxicam did not show an abnormally high risk. The ARAMIS database recently reported a toxicity index for NSAIDs that included GI ulcers.[80] Enteric-coated aspirin, salsalate, and meclofenamic acid were the safest drugs for the GI tract. Sulindac also caused a low incidence of ulcers. Piroxicam and ibuprofen had intermediate GI toxicity, whereas fenoprofen calcium, ketoprofen, and tolmetin sodium had high GI toxicity.[80] In a Tennessee Medicaid population, ibuprofen was the safest NSAID and meclofenamate sodium and tolmetin sodium had a high incidence of problems.[69] Postmarketing data reported to the FDA showed higher rates of GI toxicity for piroxicam and tolmetin sodium and lower rates for ibuprofen and meclofenamic acid.[38]

To date, the epidemiologic data on individual drugs are not consistent enough to establish that any one drug is safer or more dangerous for the GI tract than any other drug. However, trends suggest that tolmetin sodium is one of the more dangerous drugs, whereas enteric-coated aspirin, salsalate, and ibuprofen are good choices for safety.

Many of the studies provide fairly consistent data on risk factors for GI events. Although the causal relationship of individual factors has not been established by a prospective, controlled trial, the consistency observed argues for a real relationship.

Risk appears to decrease with duration of use.[45,69,71] The summary odds ratios for less than one month of exposure is 8.0 (95% CI, 6.37–10.06); for one to three months, 3.31 (95% CI, 2.27–4.82); and for longer than three months, 1.92 (95% CI, 1.19–3.13).[45] These changes could be consistent with a mucosal adaptation effect.[52] However, Kurata and Abbey[78] found no evidence of a decrease in risk over a three-year period with low-dose aspirin.

Age is an important risk factor.[6,41,42,61,71,72,76,81] The relative risk of a GI event for elderly patients (defined as more than 60 or 65 years of age, depending on the study) is 5.52 compared with 1.65 for nonelderly patients.[45] Furthermore, the risk of GI surgery for elderly individuals is at least 10 times that for nonelderly individuals.[45] Sex is not a significant influence on GI risk.[45,76,78] However, concomitant corticosteroid use[6,35,45,76,82] and history of prior GI events[35,36,45,49,71,76] each roughly double the risk. Additional risk factors for GI complications appear to be smoking,[6,60] use of multiple NSAIDs,[35,36] and higher NSAID doses.[8,35,37,47,56,69,71,76] A review of risk factors has been done by Agrawal.[83]

Additional data on risk factors come from the ARAMIS database, in which a multivariate risk factor model was used.[76] The factor most predictive of risk in the model was an age of more than 47 years. Additional risk was present at an age of more than 63 years and an age of more than 75 years. Other risk factors were duration of rheumatoid arthritis, concurrent prednisone use, high disability index, NSAID dose, and previous GI adverse effects of NSAIDs. Rheumatoid arthritis itself also appeared to be a risk factor compared with osteoarthritis.[76,81] Risk factors are not necessarily additive or synergistic, but seem to follow a complex model.[76] The most important risk factors appear to be increased age, prior upper GI problems, and increased disability.[76]

We can conclude from observational studies that there is a true risk of serious GI events associated with NSAIDs. The overall relative risk is somewhere between 1.5 and 5.0, but specific subgroups are at higher risk. The absolute risk of a serious GI diagnosis among NSAID users probably varies from about 1 event per 1000 person-years in fairly young, occasional users to about 15 events per 1000 person-years in patients who have several risk factors. Although these events are fairly uncommon from an epidemiologic point of view, they account for a large percentage of all GI bleeds seen by gastroenterologists.[38,69]

Prophylaxis of Gastropathy

Because NSAIDs are definitely linked to development of serious GI side effects, and patients at higher risk can be identified, it seems logical to prevent damage before it occurs. Preventive measures tested to date include reduction in gastric acid production (H_2-receptor antagonists) and attempts to increase mucosal defenses (sucralfate or misoprostol). These measures have been evaluated both in short-term (one week or less) and long-term (four weeks or more) studies.

Short-term Studies. McCarthy[7] reviewed the efficacy of drug therapy at preventing acute gastroduodenal damage from NSAIDs (that is, damage observed hours to seven days after drug administration). Among the H_2-receptor antagonists, cimetidine was studied most often. Conventional doses of cimetidine (300 or 400 mg) taken concurrently with aspirin ingestion markedly reduce the development of lesions. The benefit of cimetidine when given with indomethacin in one study[84] was less than the benefit generally seen when cimetidine is given with aspirin.[74] When given with tolmetin sodium, cimetidine protected 63% of the subjects, but misoprostol 200 µg four times daily protected 93% of healthy volunteers.[85]

The protective effect of sucralfate in short-term studies has not been impressive. Sucralfate tended to protect the duodenum better than the stomach.[7,86] Sucralfate was inferior to both cimetidine and misoprostol when their protective effects were directly compared.[7,86]

Misoprostol has been markedly effective in protecting against gastric damage in short-term studies of healthy volunteers.[7,86] In a direct comparison, misoprostol was superior to cimetidine against tolmetin-induced gastric damage over a six-day period; however, the drugs were equally effective at protecting the duodenum.[85] Similarly, misoprostol was superior to sucralfate against aspirin-induced damage in the stomach but not in the duodenum.[87]

Thus, sucralfate has the weakest short-term protective efficacy of the drugs studied. H_2-receptor antagonists are fairly effective, at least against aspirin-induced damage. Unfortunately, the ability of these drugs to protect against acute damage does not seem to correlate with the ability to protect against chronic ulcers. Based on assessment of gastric damage, misoprostol appears to be the most effective agent; however, it is no better than cimetidine or sucralfate at protecting the duodenum.

Long-term Studies. In view of the relationship between gastric acid production and development of spontaneous or NSAID-induced peptic ulcers, one would expect antisecretory drugs to be highly efficacious in preventing chronic ulcers.

Three groups of researchers[36,88,89] each evaluated oral ranitidine 150 mg (as the hydrochloride salt) twice daily in patients who received NSAID therapy and had no lesions in the stomach or duodenum at baseline. Endoscopy was repeated at four-week intervals (Table 2). The studies were consistent in finding no advantage of ranitidine hydrochloride over placebo in preventing gastric ulcers but finding a significant reduction in the incidence of duodenal ulcers. Ranitidine hydrochloride had little effect on the overall number of endoscopically important lesions, and it did not reduce dyspepsia. In a meta-analysis of the three studies mentioned above plus an unpublished multicenter European study, the pooled data indicated a 6% risk of duodenal ulcers after four weeks of taking placebo versus a 1% risk after four weeks of taking ranitidine hydrochloride.[93]

Roth et al.[90] studied the effect of oral cimetidine 400 mg at bedtime compared with placebo in 36 patients who had gastric lesions due to NSAIDs that earlier improved with full-dose (300 mg four times daily) cimetidine. NSAID therapy continued during the

Table 2.
Studies of Interventions to Prevent Ulcers Related to NSAID Use[a]

Ref.	Study Sample	Duration	Intervention	Ulcer Prevalence at End of Study (%)
36	263 RA or OA patients	8 wk	Ranitidine 150 mg[b] b.i.d.	7.5 PU, 6 GU, 1.5 DU
			Placebo	14 PU, 6 GU, 8DU
88	43 healthy men	4 wk	Ranitidine 150 mg[b] b.i.d.	0 GU, 0 DU
			Placebo	0 GU, 5 DU
89	144 patients	8 wk	Ranitidine 150 mg[b] b.i.d.	10 GU, 0 DU
			Placebo	12 GU, 8 DU
90	26 patients with healed GU	10 mo	Cimetidine 400 mg at bedtime	8 GU
			Placebo	7 GU
24	293 OA patients	3 mo	Misoprostol 100 μg q.i.d.	5.6 GU
			Misoprostol 200 μg q.i.d.	1.4 GU
			Placebo	21.7 GU
91	253 OA patients	3 mo	Misoprostol 200 μg q.i.d.	1.6 GU
			Sucralfate 1 g q.i.d.	16 GU
92	374 RA or OA patients	12 wk	Misoprostol 200 μg q.i.d.	1.1 DU
			Placebo	6.5 DU

[a]NSAID = nonsteroidal anti-inflammatory drug, RA = rheumatoid arthritis, OA = osteoarthritis, PU = peptic ulcer, GU = gastric ulcer, DU = duodenal ulcer.
[b]As the hydrochloride salt.

study. Maintenance therapy with cimetidine was no better than placebo in preventing the worsening of lesions in 26 patients who finished 12 months of maintenance treatment; however, the status of 10 dropouts was not reported.[91]

Some open-label studies of ulcer healing with H_2-receptor antagonist therapy suggest that continued prophylactic therapy after healing is associated with a low recurrence rate (6–16% per year) despite continued NSAID use.[94-97]

The only drug with FDA-approved labeling for prevention of NSAID-induced gastropathy is misoprostol. A key study in the approval of this drug was done by Graham et al.[24] A total of 420 patients with osteoarthritis and abdominal pain due to ibuprofen, piroxicam, or naproxen were randomized to receive placebo, misoprostol 100 μg four times daily, or misoprostol 200 μg four times daily. Concurrent treatment could include up to four antacid tablets daily during the first week. By the end of three months, 21.7% of the patients receiving placebo had developed a new gastric ulcer (defined as a lesion of ≥3 mm in diameter), compared with 5.6% of the patients receiving low-dose misoprostol and 1.4% of the patients receiving high-dose misoprostol. Misoprostol was no more effective than placebo at decreasing the frequency of abdominal pain, but a majority of patients in all groups were pain free after three months. The incidence of duodenal ulcers was very low (2.8%), with no differences among groups; however, duodenal ulcers were not specifically evaluated. Misoprostol did not reduce the efficacy of NSAID treatment, but it did frequently cause diarrhea.

A subsequent study using nearly identical entry criteria and study design compared the prophylactic efficacy of misoprostol 200 μg four times daily with that of sucralfate 1 g four times daily.[91] Two hundred fifty-three patients completed the study protocol; 1.6% of the patients randomized to receive misoprostol developed a gastric ulcer (≥3 mm in diameter) compared with 16% of the patients receiving sucralfate. A similar advantage for misoprostol over sucralfate was seen when ulcers of ≥5 mm in diameter were used as the endpoint (0.8% incidence with misoprostol versus 9.2% incidence with sucralfate). Duodenal ulcers were too rare ($n = 3$) to make a conclusion about the relative efficacy of the drugs. No conclusion could be reached about duodenal ulcers in the foregoing studies; however, a recently published abstract has reported that misoprostol can also prevent NSAID-induced duodenal ulcers.[92]

It appears that sucralfate may be ineffective, because its gastroprotective effect is partly prostaglandin mediated and pretreatment with an NSAID abolishes the gastric mucosal prostaglandin synthesis induced by sucralfate.[91,98] H_2-receptor antagonists reduce development of duodenal ulcers but not gastric ulcers. Only misoprostol appears to prevent both.

Unfortunately, we do not know what effect misoprostol has on preventing peptic ulcers after the first three months. We also do not know whether misoprostol will prevent ulcer complications such as gastric hemorrhage. The misoprostol studies excluded patients with a history of gastric ulcer or its complications; thus, the benefit of misoprostol in this very high risk group could be greater or less than that suggested by available data. Development and prevention of gastric ulcers may be more related to mucosal defense mechanisms, which are highly influenced by prostaglandins, whereas duodenal ulcers are more acid dependent.

Cost-effectiveness Considerations for Prophylaxis. Providing a medication such as misoprostol to all patients receiving NSAIDs exposes them to considerable cost (about \$60–\$80/month) and potential adverse effects, particularly diarrhea, to prevent an NSAID-induced adverse reaction that may never happen. A formal cost-effectiveness analysis has shown that misoprostol therapy can reduce costs, if the drug is priced reasonably (<\$1.74/day) and it successfully prevents typical complications of gastric ulcers.[99] However, these conclusions are based on misoprostol's ability to prevent endoscopic lesions of uncertain importance. This ability does not ensure similar reductions in serious GI bleeding. Another study[100] calculated that it would be necessary to spend $667,400 for misoprostol to prevent the loss of one year of life due to a fatal GI event among all NSAID users; misoprostol was cost-effective only for persons with a history of GI bleeding. The latter study has been criticized for ignoring reductions in morbidity and changes in quality of life.[101]

Even if misoprostol is cost-effective during the first three months of NSAID use, there are no data on its long-term effectiveness, and the complication rate due to NSAIDs may decrease with long-term use.[45,69,99] All cost-effectiveness estimates are hampered by lack of data on the true long-term reduction in GI events provided by misoprostol. Another drawback of these estimates is the assumption that misoprostol is completely safe. Apart from the inconvenience of diarrhea, if misoprostol causes a serious problem (such as spontaneous abortion) even occasionally, its degree of cost-effectiveness is greatly altered.[102]

In conclusion, the wisdom of using misoprostol routinely to reduce NSAID-associated complications is still unclear, but most authorities would strongly advocate selective use.[102,103] For the time being, prophylaxis with misoprostol is justifiable for patients at high risk of GI complications, particularly those with a history of GI hemorrhage or those who could not tolerate GI hemorrhage without a substantial risk of mortality. The optimal duration of the prophylaxis is unknown, but it would be required for at least the first three months of NSAID use.[24,91,92] No other drug can be recommended at this time. H_2-receptor antagonists can prevent duodenal ulcers but not gastric ulcers.

Treatment of Established Disease

Dyspepsia. Caldwell[104] performed an open-label study of sucralfate's ability to relieve abdominal discomfort in 22 patients who were taking a variety of NSAIDs. Sucralfate appeared to be effective at reducing the frequency of heartburn and epigastric pain, burning, and "distress." Consequently, he and others organized a multicenter, double-blind, randomized trial of sucralfate 1 g four times daily compared with placebo in 143 symptomatic NSAID users.[105] A two-week placebo run-in phase was done to eliminate placebo responders. Although sucralfate-treated patients did experience significant decreases in symptom frequency and intensity, placebo-treated patients also improved. The data on symptoms favored sucralfate over placebo, but the difference between treatments was of questionable clinical relevance. Endoscopic grades improved over a six-week period in patients receiving sucralfate, but the mean scores at the end of six weeks were identical in the sucralfate- and placebo-treated groups.

Bijlsma[106] studied cimetidine 400 mg at bedtime compared with placebo in 127 patients with NSAID-related dyspepsia but no endoscopic evidence of GI damage. Over a four-week period both cimetidine-treated and placebo-treated groups experienced a substantial decline in symptoms despite continued NSAID treatment; however, cimetidine was statistically superior to placebo. Cimetidine was particularly helpful in relieving heartburn and upper abdominal pain. Patients in whom endoscopy showed lesions also had symptomatic relief when they took cimetidine at bedtime, but relief took longer to achieve than it did in lesion-free patients.

Misoprostol, in contrast, does not decrease abdominal symptoms associated with NSAIDs, possibly because it can induce new symptoms on its own.[44,91] The value of antacids alone in treating dyspepsia has not been well studied.[7]

In all studies, dyspepsia caused by NSAIDs declines over time in placebo-treated groups. This decline may be due to a pure placebo effect, or it may suggest that tolerance or adaptation to dyspepsia develops over time. Although some authors have recommended prophylactic therapy for patients who experience abdominal pain while receiving NSAID therapy,[6,24] abdominal pain does not predict a clinically important lesion in the GI tract. Dyspepsia should not be the sole reason to begin prophylactic treatment.[49,86]

Chronic Ulcers. A number of studies have investigated the ability of drugs to heal NSAID-induced ulcers (Table 3). NSAID therapy was frequently continued during the study. Fairly good rates of ulcer healing were achieved with H_2-receptor antagonists despite continued NSAID use. Erosions were more likely to heal than ulcers,[94] and ulcers of <5 mm in diameter were more likely to heal within two months than larger ulcers.[107] Two studies evaluated the importance of discontinuing NSAID therapy during treatment.

Lancaster-Smith et al.[44] treated a group of 190 patients who had NSAID-related peptic ulcers with oral ranitidine 150 mg (as the hydrochloride salt) twice daily. Patients were randomly assigned to continue therapy with an NSAID or to stop it. Patients were endoscopically monitored at 4, 8, and 12 weeks. At all time periods, higher ulcer-healing rates were observed in the patients who stopped NSAID therapy, and duodenal ulcers healed faster than gastric ulcers. However, at 12 weeks 79% of the gastric ulcers and 92% of the duodenal ulcers had healed in patients who received ranitidine hydrochloride while continuing to receive an NSAID.

In a more complex study design, Manniche et al.[43] did a randomized, single-blind study in 67 patients who had ulcers of >3 mm in diameter (51 patients with duodenal ulcers, 14 with gastric ulcers, and 2 with both). Patients were treated for nine weeks with either oral ranitidine 150 mg (as the hydrochloride salt) twice daily or sucralfate 1 g four times daily. NSAID therapy was discontinued in half of the patients and maintained in half. At nine weeks 25 of 30 (83%) ulcers had healed in patients receiving sucralfate versus 27 of 32 (84%) in patients receiving ranitidine. When NSAID therapy was stopped, 91% of all ulcers healed versus 77% when NSAID therapy was continued. For

Table 3.
Studies on Healing of Ulcers Related to NSAID Use[a]

Ref.	No. Patients	Duration	Continuation of NSAID Therapy	Intervention	Healing Efficacy (%)
107	18	2 mo	Yes	Antacids plus cimetidine 300 mg q.i.d.	55 GU
				Antacids alone	45 GU
95	70	6 wk	No	Antacids plus cimetidine 300 mg q.i.d.	66 GU
				Antacids alone	25 GU
108	27	6 wk	Yes	Antacids plus cimetidine 300 mg q.i.d.	65 PU
				Antacids alone	50 PU
94	79	8 wk	Yes	Cimetidine 800 mg at bedtime	74 GU, 85 DU
109	56	12 wk	Yes	Ranitidine 150 mg[b] b.i.d.	90 GU, 85 DU
44	190	12 wk	Yes	Ranitidine 150 mg[b] b.i.d.	79 GU, 92 DU
			No	Ranitidine 150 mg[b] b.i.d.	100 GU, 100 DU
43	62	9 wk	Variable	Ranitidine 150 mg[b] b.i.d.	84 PU
				Sucralfate 1 g q.i.d.	83 PU
29	68	8 wk	Yes	Omeprazole 20 mg daily	82 GU
				Omeprazole 40 mg daily	95 GU
				Ranitidine 150 mg[b] b.i.d.	53 GU
110	239	8 wk	Yes	Misoprostol 200 μg q.i.d.	67 PU
				Placebo	26 PU
111	30	4 wk	Yes	Omeprazole 20 mg daily	100 PU
				Sucralfate 1 g q.i.d.	64 PU

[a]NSAID = Nonsteroidal anti-inflammatory drug, GU = gastric ulcer, PU = peptic ulcer, DU = duodenal ulcer.
[b]As the hydrochloride salt.

gastric ulcers alone, 6 of 7 (86%) healed when NSAID therapy was stopped, and 3 of 6 (50%) healed when NSAID therapy was continued.

In contrast to the last study, Caldwell et al.[105] showed minimal healing of mucosal lesions (the actual number of ulcers could not be discerned) in sucralfate-treated patients compared with placebo-treated patients. Sucralfate also has been found inferior to omeprazole with respect to ulcer-healing ability.[111]

Walan et al.[29] performed a controlled study of omeprazole, either 20 mg or 40 mg daily, versus oral ranitidine 150 mg (as the hydrochloride salt) twice daily for treatment of gastric ulcer. The study included a subgroup of 68 patients who continued using NSAIDs. At eight weeks the healing rates were 95% in patients receiving 40 mg of omeprazole, 82% in patients receiving 20 mg of omeprazole, and 53% in patients receiving ranitidine hydrochloride. The patients who received omeprazole while continuing to use NSAIDs had healing rates almost as good as those of patients who did not continue to use NSAIDs, but healing rates were significantly impaired in patients who received ranitidine hydrochloride while continuing to use NSAIDs. Bianchi Porro et al.[111] found a 100% healing rate in patients who were treated with 20 mg of omeprazole daily for four weeks, even when NSAID therapy was continued.

The efficacy of misoprostol in healing gastroduodenal lesions was tested by Roth et al.[110] Patients with rheumatoid arthritis continued to receive therapy with uncoated aspirin while randomized to receive misoprostol 200 μg four times daily (123 patients) or placebo (116 patients). After eight weeks, misoprostol was statistically superior to placebo at healing all levels of mucosal injury; the ulcer healing rate was 67% in misoprostol-treated patients and 26% in placebo-treated patients.

These data suggest that NSAID-related ulcers heal in most patients within two to three months when they are treated with H_2-receptor antagonists with or without antacids, omeprazole, or misoprostol. The efficacy of sucralfate is less clear. Omeprazole seems to be the drug of choice when NSAID therapy needs to be continued.[29,111] Ulcers heal despite continued NSAID therapy but heal faster when NSAID therapy is stopped. Larger ulcers are more resistant to healing than small ones. Healing of NSAID-induced ulcers is impaired by gastric acid, and a high degree of acid suppression (e.g., with omeprazole 40 mg/day) may be the most effective method of treating such ulcers. A reasonable approach to NSAID-induced ulcers would be to discontinue NSAID therapy at least temporarily, if possible, and treat the patient with one of the previously discussed drugs for eight weeks; endoscopy should be repeated at that time for gastric ulcers.[103]

For maintenance therapy of healed ulcers, some of the aforementioned studies found a low recurrence rate when patients were maintained on NSAIDs plus H_2-receptor antagonists. However, no study has prospectively done endoscopic surveillance of all patients regardless of symptoms. The best advice for now may be to continue treatment doses of H_2-receptor antagonists for as long as NSAIDs are needed.[7,103] Additional trials are needed to determine misoprostol's ability to heal and maintain remission of NSAID-induced ulcers; however, its adverse-effect profile makes it less attractive than other alternatives.[103]

Discussion

Despite the enormous literature on NSAID-related gastropathy, there are still important gaps in our knowledge. First, it is unclear just how or how often acute, superficial GI lesions caused by NSAIDs progress to chronic ulcers. Second, although there is little doubt that NSAIDs may cause serious GI bleeding, more precise knowledge of the relative and absolute risks is needed so that we can make more rational cost–benefit decisions on how to prevent major GI bleeds. It is reassuring to note that even among patients with rheumatoid arthritis, who often use NSAIDs, deaths from GI disease account for only 4% of all mortality.[112] Third, it is unknown whether prophylaxis with misoprostol will reduce the incidence of GI hemorrhage, not just the formation of ulcers. If misoprostol does prevent hemorrhage, the question of length of therapy needs to be answered.

To answer the question posed at the beginning of this review, I do not believe it is time to panic. However, one should recognize that the use of NSAIDs, like the use of all drugs, carries a risk of morbidity. Based on available information, certain conclusions and recommendations can be made to minimize morbidity. NSAIDs should not be used unless there is a clear-cut need for them. Acetaminophen can be used to treat most patients with osteoarthritis, which is the most common indication for long-term NSAID therapy.[113] Alternatively, the lowest possible NSAID dose should be used, and the patient should be asked to change modifiable risk factors, such as smoking or alcohol use. Only one drug should be used at a time.

Conclusion

In patients who take NSAIDs and are at low risk for development of an ulcer, no additional specific prophylactic measures seem justified. In patients with multiple risk factors, prophylaxis with misoprostol would be appropriate unless the clinician is concerned solely about reactivation of a duodenal ulcer, in which case an H_2-receptor antagonist would also be appropriate. To date, it is impossible to conclude that any one NSAID is definitely safer or more dangerous than any other NSAID; however, ibuprofen, salsalate, and enteric-coated aspirin all seem to be reasonably safe choices.

If an ulcer is discovered during NSAID treatment, NSAID therapy need not be discontinued if it is therapeutically appropriate. Full-dose treatment with an H_2-receptor antagonist, omeprazole, or misoprostol will heal such ulcers; continued full-dose therapy may decrease the risk of recurrence. Antiulcer treatment for dyspepsia alone is not justified; however, persistent dyspepsia may require a medical workup for gastrointestinal pathology.

References

1. Krantz JC, White JM. Aspirin: four score and more. *South Med J*. 1980; 73:1630-4.
2. Baum C, Kennedy DL, Forbes MB. Utilization of nonsteroidal antiinflammatory drugs. *Arthritis Rheum*. 1985; 28:686-92.
3. Rainsford KD. Aspirin and the salicylates. London: Butterworth; 1984: 148-271.
4. Douthwaite AH, Lintott GAM. Gastroscopic observation of the effects of aspirin and certain other substances on the stomach. *Lancet*. 1938; 2:1222-5.
5. Anon. *FDC Reports*. 1987; 49(Nov 29):8-9.
6. Fries JF, Miller SR, Spitz PW et al. Toward an epidemiology of gastropathy associated with nonsteroidal antiinflammatory drug use. *Gastroenterology*. 1989; 96(Suppl):647-55.
7. McCarthy DM. Nonsteroidal antiinflammatory drug-induced ulcers: management by traditional therapies. *Gastroenterology*. 1989; 96(Suppl):662-74.
8. Lanza FL. Endoscopic studies of gastric and duodenal injury after the use of ibuprofen, aspirin, and other nonsteroidal anti-inflammatory agents. *Am J Med*. 1984; 77(Suppl 1):19-24.
9. Lanas A, Hirschowitz BI. Significant role of aspirin use in patients with esophagitis. *J Clin Gastroenterol*. 1991; 13:622-7.
10. Gibson GR, Whitacre EB, Ricotti CA. Colitis induced by nonsteroidal anti-inflammatory drugs: report of four cases and review of the literature. *Arch Intern Med*. 1992; 152:625-32.
11. Baskin WN, Ivey KJ, Krause WJ et al. Aspirin-induced ultrastructural changes in human gastric mucosa: correlation with potential difference. *Ann Intern Med*. 1976; 85:299-303.
12. Graham DY, Smith JL, Dobbs SM. Gastric adaptation occurs with aspirin administration in man. *Dig Dis Sci*. 1983; 28:1-6.
13. Davenport HW. Gastric mucosal injury by fatty acid and acetylsalicylic acids. *Gastroenterology*. 1964; 46:245-53.
14. Davenport HW. Salicylate damage to the gastric mucosal barrier. *N Engl J Med*. 1967; 276:1307-12.
15. Schoen RT, Vender RJ. Mechanisms of nonsteroidal anti-inflammatory drug-induced gastric damage. *Am J Med*. 1989; 86:449-58.
16. Graham DY, Smith JL. Aspirin and the stomach. *Ann Intern Med*. 1986; 104:390-8.
17. Graham DY, Smith JL, Holmes GI et al. Nonsteroidal anti-inflammatory effect of sulindac sulfoxide and sulfide on gastric mucosa. *Clin Pharmacol Ther*. 1985; 38:65-70.
18. Hawthorne AB, Mahida YR, Cole AT et al. Aspirin-induced gastric mucosal damage: prevention by enteric-coating and relation to prostaglandin synthesis. *Br J Clin Pharmacol*. 1991; 32:77-83.
19. Silvoso GR, Ivey KJ, Butt JH et al. Incidence of gastric lesions in patients with rheumatic disease on chronic aspirin therapy. *Ann Intern Med*. 1979; 91:517-20.
20. Heller SR, Fellows IW, Ogilvie AL et al. Nonsteroidal antiinflammatory drugs and benign esophageal stricture. *Br Med J*. 1982; 285:167-78.
21. Soll AH, Weinstein WM, Kurata J et al. Nonsteroidal anti-inflammatory drugs and peptic ulcer disease. *Ann Intern Med*. 1991; 114:307-19.
22. Isenberg JI, Smedfors B, Johansson C. Effect of graded doses of intraluminal H^+, prostaglandin E_2, and inhibition of endogenous prostaglandin synthesis on proximal duodenal bicarbonate secretion in unanesthetized rats. *Gastroenterology*. 1985; 88:303-7.
23. Ligumsky M, Golanska EM, Hansen DG et al. Aspirin can inhibit gastric mucosal cyclo-oxygenase without causing lesions in rat. *Gastroenterology*. 1983; 84:756-61.
24. Graham DY, Agrawal NM, Roth SH. Prevention of NSAID-induced gastric ulcer with misoprostol: multicentre, double-blind, placebo-controlled trial. *Lancet*. 1988; 2:1277-80.
25. Levi S, Goodlad RA, Lee CY et al. Inhibitory effect of non-steroidal anti-inflammatory drugs on mucosal cell proliferation associated with gastric ulcer healing. *Lancet*. 1990; 336:840-3.
26. Hansen TM, Matzen P, Madsen P. Endoscopic evaluation of the effect of indomethacin capsules and suppositories on the gastric mucosa in rheumatic patients. *J Rheumatol*. 1984; 11:484-7.
27. Mielants H, Veys EM, Varbruggen G et al. Salicylate-induced gastrointestinal bleeding: comparison between soluble buffered, enteric-coated, and intravenous administration. *J Rheumatol*. 1979; 6:210-8.

28. Bowen BK, Krause WJ, Ivey KJ. Effect of sodium bicarbonate on aspirin-induced damage and potential difference changes in human gastric mucosa. *Br Med J.* 1977; 2:1052-5.
29. Walan A, Bader JP, Classen M et al. Effect of omeprazole and ranitidine on ulcer healing and relapse rates in patients with benign gastric ulcers. *N Engl J Med.* 1989; 320:69-75.
30. Cole AT, Brundell S, Hudson N et al. Ranitidine, aspirin, food, and the stomach. *Br Med J.* 1992; 304:544-5.
31. Graham DY, Lidsky MD, Cox AM et al. Long-term nonsteroidal antiinflammatory drug use and *Helicobacter pylori* infection. *Gastroenterology.* 1991; 100:1653-7.
32. Maxton DG, Srivastava ED, Whorwell PJ et al. Do nonsteroidal antiinflammatory drugs or smoking predispose to *Helicobacter pylori* infection? *Postgrad Med J.* 1990; 66:717-9.
33. Lanza FL, Evans DG, Graham DY. Effect of *Helicobacter pylori* infection on the severity of gastroduodenal mucosal injury after the acute administration of naproxen or aspirin to normal volunteers. *Am J Gastroenterol.* 1991; 86:735-7.
34. Jones ST, Clague RB, Eldridge J et al. Serologic evidence of infection with *Helicobacter pylori* may predict gastrointestinal intolerance to nonsteroidal anti-inflammatory drug treatment in rheumatoid arthritis. *Br J Rheumatol.* 1991; 30:16-20.
35. Caruso I, Bianchi Porro G. Gastroscopic evaluation of anti-inflammatory agents. *Br Med J.* 1980; 280:75-8.
36. Ehsanullah RSB, Page MC, Tildesley G et al. Prevention of gastroduodenal damage induced by nonsteroidal anti-inflammatory drugs: controlled trial of ranitidine. *Br Med J.* 1988; 297:1017-21.
37. Lanza FL, Royer GL, Nelson RS et al. The effects of ibuprofen, indomethacin, aspirin, naproxen and placebo on the gastric mucosa of normal volunteers. *Dig Dis Sci.* 1979; 24: 923-8.
38. Butt JH, Barthel JS, Moore RA. Clinical spectrum of the upper gastrointestinal effects of nonsteroidal anti-inflammatory drugs. *Am J Med.* 1988; 84(Suppl 2A):5-14.
39. Gabriel SE, Bombardier C. NSAID induced ulcers: an emerging epidemic? *J Rheumatol.* 1990; 17:1-3.
40. Shallcross TM, Heatley RV. Effect of nonsteroidal anti-inflammatory drugs on dyspeptic symptoms. *Br Med J.* 1990; 300:368-9.
41. Clinch D, Banerjee AK, Ostick G. Absence of abdominal pain in elderly patients with peptic ulcer. *Age Ageing.* 1984; 13:120-3.
42. Armstrong CP, Blower AL. Nonsteroidal anti-inflammatory drugs and life-threatening complications of peptic ulceration. *Gut.* 1987; 28:527-32.
43. Manniche C, Malchow-Moller A, Andersen JR et al. Randomized study of the influence of nonsteroidal anti-inflammatory drugs on the treatment of peptic ulcer in patients with rheumatic disease. *Gut.* 1987; 28:226-9.
44. Lancaster-Smith MJ, Jaderberg ME, Jackson DA. Ranitidine in the treatment of nonsteroidal anti-inflammatory drug associated gastric and duodenal ulcers. *Gut.* 1991; 32:252-5.
45. Gabriel SE, Jaakkimainen L, Bombardier C. Risk for serious gastrointestinal complications related to use of nonsteroidal anti-inflammatory drugs: a meta-analysis. *Ann Intern Med.* 1991; 115:787-96.
46. Carson JL, Strom BL. The gastrointestinal side effects of the nonsteroidal anti-inflammatory drugs. *J Clin Pharmacol.* 1988; 28:554-9.
47. Prichard PJ, Kitchingman GK, Walt RP et al. Human gastric mucosal bleeding induced by low dose aspirin, but not warfarin. *Br Med J.* 1989; 298:493-6.
48. Bahrt KM, Korman LY, Nashel DJ. Significance of a positive test for occult blood in stools of patients taking anti-inflammatory drugs. *Arch Intern Med.* 1984; 144:2165-6.
49. Larkai EN, Smith JL, Lidsky MD et al. Gastroduodenal mucosa and dyspeptic symptoms in arthritic patients during chronic nonsteroidal anti-inflammatory drug use. *Am J Gastroenterol.* 1987; 82:1153-8.
50. Lanza FL, Rack MF, Wagner GS et al. Reduction in gastric mucosal hemorrhage and ulceration with chronic high-level dosing of enteric-coated aspirin granules two and four times a day. *Dig Dis Sci.* 1985; 30:509-12.
51. Avila MH, Walker AM, Romieu I et al. Choice of nonsteroidal anti-inflammatory drug in persons treated for dyspepsia. *Lancet.* 1988; 2:556-9.
52. Hawkey CJ. Non-steroidal anti-inflammatory drugs and peptic ulcers: facts and figures multiply, but do they add up? *Br Med J.* 1990; 300:278-84.
53. Piper DW, McIntosh JH, Ariotti DE et al. Analgesic ingestion and chronic peptic ulcer. *Gastroenterology.* 1981; 80:427-32.
54. Piper DW, McIntosh JH, Greig M et al. Environmental factors and chronic gastric ulcer. A case control study of the association of smoking, alcohol and heavy analgesic ingestion with the exacerbation of chronic gastric ulcer. *Scand J Gastroenterol.* 1982; 17:721-9.
55. Coggon D, Langman MJ, Spiegelhalter D. Aspirin, paracetamol, and haematemesis and melaena. *Gut.* 1982; 23:340-4.
56. Levy M. Aspirin use in patients with major upper gastrointestinal bleeding and peptic-ulcer disease: a report from the Boston Collaborative Drug Surveillance Program, Boston University Medical Center. *N Engl J Med.* 1974; 290:1158-62.
57. McIntosh JH, Byth K, Piper DW. Environmental factors in aetiology of chronic gastric ulcer: a case control study of exposure variables before the first symptoms. *Gut.* 1985; 26:789-98.
58. McIntosh JH, Fung CS, Berry G et al. Smoking, nonsteroidal anti-inflammatory drugs, and acetaminophen in gastric ulcer: a study of associations and of the effects of previous diagnosis on exposure patterns. *Am J Epidemiol.* 1988; 128:761-70.
59. Duggan JM, Dobson AJ, Johnson H et al. Peptic ulcer and non-steroidal anti-inflammatory agents. *Gut.* 1986; 27:929-33.
60. Somerville K, Faulkner G, Langman M. Non-steroidal anti-inflammatory drugs and bleeding peptic ulcer. *Lancet.* 1986; 1:462-4.
61. Collier DSJ, Pain JA. Non-steroidal anti-inflammatory drugs and peptic ulcer perforation. *Gut.* 1985; 26:359-63.
62. Bartle WR, Gupta AK, Lazor J. Nonsteroidal anti-inflammatory drugs and bleeding peptic ulcer. A case-control study. *Arch Intern Med.* 1986; 146:2365-7.
63. Henry DA, Johnston A, Dobson AJ et al. Fatal peptic ulcer complications and the use of nonsteroidal anti-inflammatory drugs, aspirin and corticosteroids. *Br Med J.* 1987; 295:1227-9.
64. Faulkner G, Prichard P, Somerville K et al. Aspirin and bleeding peptic ulcers in the elderly. *Br Med J.* 1988; 297:1311-3.
65. Griffin MR, Ray WA, Schaffner W. Nonsteroidal anti-inflammatory drug use and death from peptic ulcer in elderly persons. *Ann Intern Med.* 1988; 109:359-63.
66. Levy M, Miller DR, Kaufman DW et al. Major upper gastrointestinal tract bleeding: relation to the use of aspirin and other nonnarcotic analgesics. *Arch Intern Med.* 1988; 148:281-5.
67. Holvoet J, Terriere L, Van Hee W et al. Relation of upper gastrointestinal bleeding to nonsteroidal anti-inflammatory drugs and aspirin: a case-control study. *Gut.* 1991; 32:730-4.
68. Laporte JR, Carné X, Vidal X et al. Upper gastrointestinal bleeding in relation to previous use of analgesics and nonsteroidal anti-inflammatory drugs. *Lancet.* 1991; 337:85-9.
69. Griffin MR, Piper JM, Daugherty JR et al. Nonsteroidal anti-inflammatory drug use and increased risk for peptic ulcer disease in elderly persons. *Ann Intern Med.* 1991; 114:257-63.
70. Beard K, Walker AM, Perera DR et al. Nonsteroidal anti-inflammatory drugs and hospitalization for gastroesophageal bleeding in the elderly. *Arch Intern Med.* 1987; 147:1621-3.
71. Carson JL, Strom BL, Soper KA et al. The association of nonsteroidal anti-inflammatory drugs with upper gastrointestinal tract bleeding. *Arch Intern Med.* 1987; 147:85-8.
72. Jick SS, Perera DR, Walker AM et al. Non-steroidal anti-inflammatory drugs and hospital admission for perforated

peptic ulcer. *Lancet*. 1987; 2:380-2.

73. Guess HA, West R, Strand LM et al. Fatal upper gastrointestinal hemorrhage or perforation among users and nonusers of nonsteroidal anti-inflammatory drugs in Saskatchewan, Canada, 1983. *J Clin Epidemiol*. 1988; 41:35-45.
74. Bloom BS. Risk and cost of gastrointestinal side effects associated with nonsteroidal anti-inflammatory drugs. *Arch Intern Med*. 1989; 149:1019-22.
75. Beardon PH, Brown SV, McDevitt DG. Gastrointestinal events in patients prescribed nonsteroidal anti-inflammatory drugs: a controlled study using record linkage in Tayside. *Q J Med*. 1989; 71:497-505.
76. Fries JF, Williams CA, Bloch DA et al. Nonsteroidal anti-inflammatory drug-associated gastropathy: incidence and risk factor models. *Am J Med*. 1991; 91:213-22.
77. Steering Committee of the Physicians' Health Study Research Group. Final report on the aspirin component of the ongoing Physicians' Health Study. *N Engl J Med*. 1989; 321:129-35.
78. Kurata JH, Abbey DE. The effect of chronic aspirin use on duodenal and gastric ulcer hospitalizations. *J Clin Gastroenterol*. 1990; 12:260-6.
79. Carson JL, Strom BL, Morse ML et al. The relative gastrointestinal toxicity of the nonsteroidal anti-inflammatory drugs. *Arch Intern Med*. 1987; 147:1054-9.
80. Fries JF, Williams CA, Bloch DA. The relative toxicity of nonsteroidal anti-inflammatory drugs. *Arthritis Rheum*. 1991; 34:1353-60.
81. Llewellyn JG, Prichard MH. Influence of age and disease state in nonsteroidal anti-inflammatory drug associated gastric bleeding. *J Rheumatol*. 1988; 15:891-4.
82. Piper JM, Ray WA, Daugherty JR et al. Corticosteroid use and peptic ulcer disease: role of nonsteroidal anti-inflammatory drugs. *Ann Intern Med*. 1991; 114:737-40.
83. Agrawal N. Risk factors for gastrointestinal ulcers caused by nonsteroidal anti-inflammatory drugs. *J Fam Pract*. 1991; 32:619-24.
84. Rachmilewitz D, Polak D, Eliakim R et al. Cimetidine significantly decreased indomethacin-induced gastroduodenal mucosal damage. *Gastroenterology*. 1986; 90:1596. Abstract.
85. Lanza FL, Aspinall RL, Swabb EA et al. Double-blind placebo-controlled endoscopic comparison of the mucosal protective effects of misoprostol versus cimetidine on tolmetin-induced mucosal injury to the stomach and duodenum. *Gastroenterology*. 1988; 95:289-94.
86. Elliot DP. Preventing upper gastrointestinal bleeding in patients receiving nonsteroidal anti-inflammatory drugs. *DICP Ann Pharmacother*. 1990; 24:954-8.
87. Lanza F, Peace K, Gustitus L et al. A blinded endoscopic comparative study of misoprostol versus sucralfate and placebo in the prevention of aspirin-induced gastric and duodenal ulceration. *Am J Gastroenterol*. 1988; 83:143-6.
88. Berkowitz JM, Rogenes PR, Sharp JT et al. Ranitidine protects against gastroduodenal mucosal damage associated with chronic aspirin therapy. *Arch Intern Med*. 1987; 147:2137-9.
89. Robinson MG, Griffen JW, Bowers J et al. Effect of ranitidine on gastroduodenal mucosal damage induced by nonsteroidal anti-inflammatory drugs. *Dig Dis Sci*. 1989; 34:424-8.
90. Roth SH, Bennett RE, Mitchell CS et al. Cimetidine therapy in nonsteroidal anti-inflammatory drug gastropathy: double-blind long-term evaluation. *Arch Intern Med*. 1987; 147:1798-801.
91. Agrawal NM, Roth S, Graham DY et al. Misoprostol compared with sucralfate in the prevention of nonsteroidal anti-inflammatory drug-induced gastric ulcer: a randomized, controlled trial. *Ann Intern Med*. 1991; 115:195-200.
92. Graham DY, Stromatt SC, Jaszewski R et al. Prevention of duodenal ulcer in arthritics who are chronic NSAID users: a multicenter trial of the role of misoprostol. *Gastroenterology*. 1991; 100:A75. Abstract.
93. Robinson M, Mills RJ, Euler AR. Ranitidine prevents duodenal ulcers associated with nonsteroidal anti-inflammatory drug therapy. *Aliment Pharmacol Ther*. 1991; 5:143-5.
94. Bijlsma JW. Treatment of NSAID-induced gastrointestinal lesions with cimetidine: an international multicentre collaborative study. *Aliment Pharmacol Ther*. 1988; 2(Suppl):85-96.
95. Loludice TA, Saleem T, Lang JA. Cimetidine in the treatment of gastric ulcer induced by steroidal and nonsteroidal anti-inflammatory agents. *Am J Gastroenterol*. 1981; 75:104-10.
96. Croker JR, Cotton PB, Boyle AC et al. Cimetidine for peptic ulcer in patients with arthritis. *Ann Rheum Dis*. 1980; 39:275-8.
97. O'Laughlin JC, Silvoso GR, Ivey KJ. Healing of aspirin-associated peptic ulcer disease despite continued salicylate ingestion. *Arch Intern Med*. 1981; 141:781-3.
98. Stern AI, Ward F, Hartley G. Protective effect of sucralfate against aspirin-induced damage to the human gastric mucosa. *Am J Med*. 1987; 83(Suppl 3B):83-5.
99. Hillman AL, Bloom BS. Economic effects of prophylactic use of misoprostol to prevent gastric ulcer in patients taking nonsteroidal anti-inflammatory drugs. *Arch Intern Med*. 1989; 149:2061-5.
100. Edelson JT, Tosteson ANA, Sax P. Cost-effectiveness of misoprostol for prophylaxis against nonsteroidal anti-inflammatory drug-induced gastrointestinal tract bleeding. *JAMA*. 1990; 264:41-7.
101. Gabriel SE. Is misoprostol prophylaxis indicated for NSAID induced adverse gastrointestinal events? An epidemiologic opinion. *J Rheumatol*. 1991; 18:958-61.
102. Jones MP, Schubert ML, Smith JL. What do you recommend for prophylaxis in an elderly woman with arthritis requiring NSAIDs for control? *Am J Gastroenterol*. 1991; 86:264-8.
103. Loeb DS, Ahlquist DA, Talley NJ. Management of gastroduodenopathy associated with the use of nonsteroidal anti-inflammatory drugs. *Mayo Clin Proc*. 1992; 67:354-64.
104. Caldwell JR. Sucralfate in the relief of gastrointestinal symptoms associated with nonsteroidal anti-inflammatory drugs. *South Med J*. 1985; 78:938-40.
105. Caldwell JR, Roth SH, Wu WC et al. Sucralfate treatment of nonsteroidal anti-inflammatory drug-induced gastrointestinal symptoms and mucosal damage. *Am J Med*. 1987; 83(Suppl 3B):74-82.
106. Bijlsma JWJ. Treatment of endoscopy-negative NSAID-induced upper gastrointestinal symptoms with cimetidine: an international multicentre collaborative study. *Aliment Pharmacol Ther*. 1988; 2(Suppl):75-83.
107. O'Laughlin JC, Silvoso GK, Ivey KJ. Resistance to medical therapy of gastric ulcers in rheumatic disease patients taking aspirin. A double-blind study with cimetidine and follow-up. *Dig Dis Sci*. 1982; 27:976-80.
108. Davies J, Collins AJ, Dixon AS. The influence of cimetidine on peptic ulcer patients with arthritis taking anti-inflammatory drugs. *Br J Rheumatol*. 1986; 25:54-8.
109. Farah D, Sturrock RD, Russell RI. Peptic ulcer in rheumatoid arthritis. *Ann Rheum Dis*. 1988; 47:478-80.
110. Roth S, Agrawal N, Mahowald M et al. Misoprostol heals gastroduodenal injury in patients with rheumatoid arthritis receiving aspirin. *Arch Intern Med*. 1989; 149:775-9.
111. Bianchi Porro G, Santalucia F, Petrillo M. Omeprazole vs sucralfate in the treatment of NSAID-induced gastric and duodenal ulcer. *Gut*. 1990; 31:A1175. Abstract.
112. Pincus T, Griffin M. Gastrointestinal disease associated with nonsteroidal anti-inflammatory drugs: new insights from observational studies and functional status questionnaires. *Am J Med*. 1991; 91:209-12.
113. Bradley JD, Brandt KD, Katz BP et al. Comparison of an anti-inflammatory dose of ibuprofen, an analgesic dose of ibuprofen, and acetaminophen in the treatment of patients with osteoarthritis of the knee. *N Engl J Med*. 1991; 325:87-91.

Endocrine complications associated with human immunodeficiency virus infection

JOSEPH V. ETZEL, JOSEPH M. BROCAVICH, AND MICHAEL TORRE

Abstract: The causes and management of endocrine disorders associated with human immunodeficiency virus (HIV) infection are reviewed.

Endocrine disorders observed in HIV-positive patients include adrenal abnormalities, hyporeninemic hypoaldosteronism, pituitary insufficiency, pancreatic abnormalities, thyroid and parathyroid disorders, and testicular abnormalities. Opportunistic pathogens implicated in these disorders include cytomegalovirus, *Cryptococcus*, *Toxoplasma*, mycobacteria, *Candida*, and *Aspergillus*. Neoplasms such as Kaposi's sarcoma and lymphoma can also cause endocrine abnormalities. Several drugs used in patients with the acquired immunodeficiency syndrome (AIDS) are associated with the development of endocrine disorders. These drugs include ketoconazole, itraconazole, rifampin, vidarabine, pentamidine, trimethoprim–sulfamethoxazole, didanosine, and ganciclovir. Severe patient debilitation can contribute to the development of endocrine abnormalities.

Monitoring of adrenal gland function may be prudent in HIV-infected patients who have nonspecific symptoms of adrenal insufficiency. If adrenal insufficiency is diagnosed, replacement therapy with oral hydrocortisone is required. Administration of fludrocortisone can rapidly alleviate the signs and symptoms of hyporeninemic hypoaldosteronism. Fluid restriction is the first step in managing the pituitary abnormality known as the syndrome of inappropriate secretion of antidiuretic hormone. Drug-induced endocrine abnormalities often resolve after withdrawal of the offending agent.

Endocrine complications in HIV-infected patients may be caused by infection, malignancy, or drugs. Adjusting or instituting drug therapy may be necessary to control symptomatic endocrine abnormalities.

Index terms: Anti-infective agents; Antibiotics; Antifungals; Antivirals; Endocrine diseases; HIV infections; Toxicity
Clin Pharm. 1992; 11:705-13

Most treatment modalities used in the management of patients afflicted with the acquired immunodeficiency syndrome (AIDS) have been focused on its primary manifestations. Researchers have tried to prevent further spread of the human immunodeficiency virus (HIV) by developing effective antiviral agents and identifying new therapies with improved activity against the common secondary opportunistic infections and malignancies.[1] In the past, endocrine abnormalities have not been considered common manifestations of this disease process. Recently, however, alterations in endocrine function are being reported with increasing frequency in patients with AIDS.[2,3]

The most common pathologic and potentially clinically important endocrine disorder observed in patients with AIDS involves adrenocortical abnormalities.[2-8] In addition, hyporeninemic hypoaldosteronism, pituitary insufficiency, pancreatic abnormalities, thyroid gland dysfunction, and testicular abnormalities have been reported secondary to organ invasion by infectious organisms, adverse effects of drug therapy, and severe patient debilitation. Although these endocrine disorders have not been widely observed in most HIV-infected patients, they may become a clinically important problem and may require treatment.

In this review we describe the causes and management of endocrine disorders associated with HIV-infection.

JOSEPH V. ETZEL, PHARM.D., is Assistant Clinical Professor of Pharmacy, St. John's University, Jamaica, NY, and Clinical Coordinator of Adult Internal Medicine, Nassau County Medical Center (NCMC), East Meadow, NY. JOSEPH M. BROCAVICH, PHARM.D., is Associate Clinical Professor of Pharmacy, St. John's University, and Clinical Coordinator of Infectious Diseases, NCMC. MICHAEL TORRE, M.S., is Clinical Professor of Pharmacy, St. John's University, and Clinical Coordinator of Endocrinology, NCMC.

Address reprint requests to Dr. Etzel at the College of Pharmacy and Allied Health Professions, St. John's University, Grand Central and Utopia Parkways, Jamaica, NY 11439.

The Therapy Update *section provides concise analytical reviews of narrowly defined, important topics in pharmacotherapy. Priority is given to articles that focus on new or emerging standards in drug therapy. Articles are not intended to be comprehensive reviews of drugs or of disease states and their treatment.*

Adrenal Abnormalities

Structural abnormalities associated with the adrenal glands have frequently been noted at autopsy of patients with AIDS.[9-12] These pathologic changes primarily result from opportunistic infections,[9-12] malignancies,[9,10] or chronic illness.[10,12]

Infection-Associated Abnormalities. The most common pathogen isolated in these patients has been cytomegalovirus.[9-12] This organism has been associated with adrenal changes of varying degree in more than 50% of the patients studied postmortem.[9-12] Other common organisms include *Cryptococcus neoformans*,[10-12] *Mycobacterium avium–intracellulare*,[10,12] *Mycobacterium tuberculosis*,[11] and *Toxoplasma*.[11] The primary malignancy involving this gland is Kaposi's sarcoma.[9,10] Although a substantial number of patients in these postmortem series had pathologic involvement of the adrenal gland, most did not have the clinical manifestations commonly associated with adrenal insufficiency.[9-12]

The extent to which clinical adrenal insufficiency occurs in HIV-infected patients is unclear. Many patients with AIDS develop nonspecific symptoms such as weight loss, fever, diarrhea, anorexia, fatigue, nausea, vomiting, hypotension, and orthostasis. These symptoms may be consistent with adrenal suppression; however, in many cases, this potential diagnosis may not be investigated.[7,8,10,11]

Evaluation of adrenal function has shown that most HIV-infected patients have normal to somewhat elevated basal cortisol levels, although depressed levels have also been noted. [2-5,7,13-15] Increased production of cortisol may be due to the stress of HIV infection or the associated complications of this disease.[3,7]

Merenich et al.[2] compared the adrenal function of 40 asymptomatic HIV-infected patients and 27 HIV-negative controls. These investigators found that although the infected individuals had basal and corticotropin-stimulated cortisol levels and basal aldosterone levels that were in the normal range, these levels were significantly lower than those in the HIV-negative controls. Similarly, Mulhall et al.[15] compared adrenal function in 40 homosexual men, 20 who were HIV positive and 20 who were seronegative. Although both groups had normal mean baseline cortisol concentrations (417 nmol/L in the seronegative group versus 423 nmol/L in the seropositive group) and normal mean cosyntropin-stimulated cortisol concentrations (933 nmol/L in the seronegative group versus 796 nmol/L in the seropositive group), there was a significant reduction in the maximum cortisol level ($p = 0.019$) and cortisol rise ($p = 0.004$) in the patients who were HIV positive.[15]

These data suggest that although no patient in either of these studies had symptoms of adrenal insufficiency, subtle changes may exist in adrenal gland function even in asymptomatic HIV-infected patients.[2,15]

Blunted or low-normal responses to the intravenous administration of cosyntropin 0.25 mg have been reported occasionally in both HIV-positive and AIDS patients.[3,4,7] Dobs et al.[3] studied 39 males with AIDS who had normal mean basal cortisol levels; 36 (92%) responded appropriately to corticotropin stimulation. However, a "blunted response" to corticotropin was noted in the remaining three patients.

Likewise, Membrano et al.[4] evaluated the response to cosyntropin of 74 patients with AIDS and 19 male patients with AIDS-related complex (ARC). These investigators also enrolled 25 healthy volunteers to serve as a control group. The patients with AIDS had significantly higher mean ± S.D. basal cortisol levels than the patients with ARC and the healthy controls (433 ± 28 mmol/L versus 295 ± 25 and 298 ± 22 mmol/L; $p < 0.001$). In spite of the elevated basal cortisol level noted in the AIDS patients, their mean ± S.D. 60-minute cortisol level in response to cosyntropin was significantly lower than that of the controls (726 ± 30 versus 855 ± 33 nmol/L; $p < 0.05$). The mean stimulated cortisol level for patients with ARC was also suppressed (618 ± 28 nmol/L). The authors reported that 54% of the AIDS patients had a low-normal response to cosyntropin and, as such, possessed marginal adrenal function. Additionally, four patients with AIDS (5%) had chemically confirmed adrenal insufficiency. The authors presumed that the adrenal abnormalities occurred secondary to HIV or other opportunistic infections.

Greene et al.[7] prospectively evaluated 20 patients with AIDS who had symptoms consistent with adrenal insufficiency. Of these, four had chemical evidence of adrenal suppression manifested by lower-than-expected basal cortisol levels and a lack of response to cosyntropin stimulation. Two patients also had elevated corticotropin levels, and one had a below-normal basal aldosterone level. When treated with corticosteroids, all patients showed marked clinical improvement. The exact cause of the adrenal suppression could not be elucidated, but it probably resulted from an opportunistic infection of the adrenal gland or was secondary to medications the patients had received that have been shown to cause adrenal failure (rifampin in three patients and ketoconazole in two patients).[7] Compared with other studies cited, this study substantially differs in the frequency (20%) of documented adrenal insufficiency, but it must be reiterated that all patients involved in this study were suspected initially of having abnormal adrenal function.

Drug-Induced Abnormalities. Drug therapy also may cause adrenal insufficiency in the AIDS population. Ketoconazole, an antifungal agent commonly prescribed for the treatment of oral or esophageal candidiasis in patients with AIDS, can cause a reversible decrease in the synthesis of cortisol and aldosterone in the adrenal gland by a dose-related interference with the cytochrome P-450 enzyme system.[16-22]

When administered to patients with normal adrenal function, single doses of 400–600 mg of ketoconazole have been shown to transiently decrease adrenal secretion of cortisol for 8 to 16 hours after corticotropin stimulation.[16-19] However, chemically confirmed adrenal insufficiency and frank adrenal crisis also have been rarely associated with ketoconazole therapy in patients without AIDS, even at dosages as low as 400 mg daily.[21,22] The acute hypoadrenalism noted in these patients is usually manifested within the first week of ketoconazole therapy.[21,22] In addition, the adrenal insufficiency may be persistent, requiring cortisol replacement for several years after the discontinuation of ketoconazole therapy.[22] Despite these findings, clinically evident adrenal insufficiency is not manifested in most patients unless other ailments are present that may interfere with the compensatory physiological responses responsible for maintaining adequate plasma cortisol concentrations.[22]

Some clinicians suggest that multiple daily doses of ketoconazole may be more likely to result in adrenal insufficiency than once-daily dosage regimens; the former regimen may result in the continuous blockade of steroidogenesis without allowing adrenal recovery during any part of the day.[22]

Itraconazole, an investigational antifungal agent structurally related to ketoconazole, was originally thought to lack the adrenal-suppressive effects associated with ketoconazole.[23] However, one case of adrenal suppression in a patient with AIDS was noted during high-dose (600 mg/day) itraconazole therapy for the treatment of a systemic mycosis.[24] The patient had a reduced response to corticotropin stimulation after two weeks of itraconazole therapy. The response was further reduced after six weeks of therapy, when the patient began to exhibit symptoms consistent with adrenal insufficiency (i.e., weakness, fatigue, and orthostasis). A dosage reduction to 400 mg daily resulted in resolution of the patient's clinical symptoms as well as improvement in his corticotropin-stimulated cortisol level.[24]

A third antimicrobial agent, rifampin, also has been implicated in precipitating adrenal insufficiency.[25-29] It has been documented that this agent possesses important enzyme-inducing properties that affect the hepatic microsomal (cytochrome P-450) drug-metabolizing system.[30] Rifampin's enzyme induction can lead to increased metabolism of other drugs and endogenous substances (e.g., cortisol) that are affected by the cytochrome P-450 system.[25]

A number of cases of adrenal crisis secondary to rifampin administration have been reported, primarily in patients without AIDS. These patients were either receiving exogenous corticosteroid therapy[25,26] or had presumptive marginal adrenal function secondary to *Mycobacterium tuberculosis* infection.[27,28] All patients received oral rifampin 600 mg daily.[25-28] Symptoms of adrenal crisis developed most frequently within one to two weeks of initiation of therapy.[25,27,28] In one patient the onset of symptoms occurred at seven weeks, but symptoms reappeared within two weeks after discontinuation of therapy and subsequent rechallenge with the drug.[27] All patients responded well to supraphysiological doses of corticosteroids and mineralocorticoid therapy. The dosage of these agents was then tapered over time to an appropriate maintenance regimen.[25-28]

Ediger and Isley[29] reported a case of rifampin-induced adrenal insufficiency in a patient with AIDS. This patient initially had been screened and found to have normal adrenal function but developed clinical evidence of adrenal failure while receiving rifampin therapy.[29] Further studies of the effect of rifampin on adrenal function in patients with AIDS are warranted.

Monitoring and Management. Although it has been suggested that all HIV-infected patients undergo periodic tests to determine basal cortisol levels and responsiveness to cosyntropin stimulation,[12] the current data seem to suggest that this routine screening is unnecessary.[7,15] However, monitoring of adrenal function may be prudent in HIV-infected patients who have nonspecific symptoms of adrenal insufficiency.[7] This monitoring may be especially useful in patients with documented cytomegalovirus or mycobacterial infections, those with Kaposi's sarcoma, and those receiving adrenosuppressive agents such as ketoconazole or rifampin. Once a diagnosis of adrenal insufficiency is made, therapy with oral hydrocortisone, approximately 20 mg in the morning and 10 mg in the evening, is required. Fludrocortisone acetate 0.1 mg p.o. per day is frequently added to provide adequate mineralocorticoid activity.[31] Other corticosteroids may occasionally be substituted at equipotent doses. After initiation, therapy should be individualized based on patient response.[31] Because critically ill patients often require higher cortisol levels, supraphysiological doses of corticosteroids, equivalent to 150 to 200 mg of cortisol daily, should be administered in times of stress or severe infection.[4]

Hyporeninemic Hypoaldosteronism

Hyporeninemic hypoaldosteronism has been observed in patients with AIDS and should be suspected as a possible cause of persistent hyperkalemia in HIV-positive patients.[32] This disorder is characterized by hyperkalemia, hyponatremia, orthostatic hypotension, and mild metabolic acidosis in patients with normal serum levels of basal cortisol, corticotropin-stimulated cortisol, and aldosterone.[32]

Patients with hyporeninemic hypoaldosteronism have low baseline renin and aldosterone levels that fail to increase substantially after stimulation with furosemide. Although the exact cause of this disorder is unclear, management of symptomatic hyperkalemia involves treatment with an agent possessing mineralocorticoid activity. Kalin et al.[32] demonstrated that the administration of fludrocortisone acetate 0.1–0.2 mg p.o. daily can rapidly alleviate the signs and symptoms of hyporeninemic hypoaldosteronism. These authors stressed the need to differentiate hyporeninemic hypoaldosteronism from adrenal insufficiency because therapeutic management of the disorders differs substantially, and inappropriate drug therapy may worsen the patient's prognosis.

Pituitary Abnormalities

Destruction of pituitary tissue has rarely been described in association with AIDS. Cytomegalovirus has been implicated as a cause in at least one patient.[33] Milligan et al.[34] reported a second case in a patient with central nervous system toxoplasmosis who had anterior panhypopituitarism. This patient had deficiencies of corticotropin, growth hormone, prolactin, thyrotropin, luteinizing hormone, and follicle-stimulating hormone. Multiple hormone replacement would be required in such a patient.[34]

Hyponatremia has been common in hospitalized patients with AIDS. The exact cause of this reduction in serum sodium is unclear.[35] In an attempt to assess potential causes, Agarwal et al.[36] evaluated 103 consecutive patients with AIDS who were admitted to the hospital with opportunistic infections. Thirty-six patients had a serum sodium concentration less than 130 meq/L. Volume depletion was noted in 12 of the 36 patients, with complete resolution of symptoms occurring after appropriate rehydration. Additionally, one patient was found to have adrenal insufficiency.

The remaining 23 hyponatremic patients had findings that were consistent with the syndrome of inappropriate secretion of antidiuretic hormone (SIADH), defined as the presence of (1) low plasma osmolality in the setting of adequate hydration and (2) concentrated urine with a high sodium concentration without any associated disease process or diuretic therapy.[36] Plasma concentrations of arginine vasopressin (AVP) also were determined for 11 of these patients. In all 11 patients the AVP plasma concentrations were found to be inappropriately elevated. This AVP abnormality was not found in a control group of 50 patients without AIDS who had opportunistic infections.[36] The authors concluded that, in the patients with SIADH, the disorder was secondary to the opportunistic infections, which primarily affected the lungs and central nervous system. SIADH persisted in two patients after completion of treatment for their acute illness.

In another study evaluating hyponatremia in patients with AIDS, Vitting et al.[37] demonstrated that more than 50% of assessed patients had a serum sodium concentration of 133 meq/L or less. Sixteen patients were evaluated prospectively, and five had a low serum osmolality and a high urine osmolality. Plasma AVP concentrations determined in 14 of 15 patients were substantially elevated in the presence of low serum osmolality. Four patients in this study met the criteria for SIADH. The cause of SIADH in these patients may have been active pulmonary disease, central nervous system infections, or opiate administration.[37] The twelve remaining patients had other nonpituitary causes to explain their hyponatremia.

SIADH occurs in other immunocompromised populations as a result of various infections[38,39] or associated drug therapy.[40-42] One agent associated with SIADH that has a limited role in managing AIDS is vidarabine, an alternative antiviral agent used in treating disseminated herpes zoster. Semel and McNerney[40] reported three cases of SIADH in patients with disseminated herpes zoster. Vidarabine therapy was initiated in two patients who had normal serum sodium concentrations. A low serum sodium concentration, a low plasma osmolality, and increased urine osmolality were noted after 2 days of vidarabine treatment in one patient and after 13 days in the other. Both patients also developed lethargy. Vidarabine therapy was discontinued, and acyclovir therapy and fluid restriction were instituted. Signs and symptoms of SIADH improved dramatically over several days after discontinuation of vidarabine therapy.[40] A similar case implicating this agent was reported by Ramos et al.[41] Although the temporal sequence described by these authors supported vidarabine's role in the development of SIADH, the effect of disseminated herpes zoster or other disease processes cannot be ruled out. The third patient described by Semel and McNerney[40] did not receive vidarabine and still developed SIADH. Ingraham et al.[39] also reported a case of SIADH that developed without vidarabine therapy. Close monitoring of appropriate signs and symptoms of SIADH may be prudent with vidarabine therapy.

Pentamidine, an antiprotozoal agent used to treat *Pneumocystis carinii* pneumonia, has been implicated to cause SIADH in one patient.[42] The same report described a second patient who developed profound hyponatremia during pentamidine therapy. The temporal sequences of these reactions were not evaluable, but the authors reported that this adverse effect resolved over eight days in one patient and that the other patient was discharged; there was no comment as to outcome.

The exact association between pentamidine and SIADH is unclear. Cases of SIADH associated with pneumonias and central nervous system infections have been reported.[38] Additionally, Agarwal et al.[36] noted that SIADH developed in five patients who received pentamidine therapy, yet these authors did not consider whether a temporal sequence existed between therapy with this agent and development of SIADH. This effect of pentamidine on the development of SIADH needs to be evaluated further.

In patients who do develop SIADH, careful assessment of the cause is paramount. Fluid restriction is the first step in managing the syndrome.[43] In determining whether to discontinue therapy with an offending agent, the clinician should weigh the risks and benefits and consider the availability of alternative therapy. Patients who are unresponsive to fluid restriction may benefit from treatment with demeclocycline hydrochloride at doses of 600–1200 mg p.o. daily in four divided doses.[43]

Pancreatic Abnormalities

Alterations of pancreatic function in patients with AIDS are not well documented. Opportunistic infections, malignancies, and drug therapy all have been shown to adversely affect the pancreas.

Pancreatic abnormalities have been noted in approximately 50% of patients with AIDS examined at autopsy.[44-46] The primary etiologies associated with pancreatic lesions are (1) opportunistic infections with cytomegalovirus,[44-46] *Cryptococcus*,[45,46] *Toxoplasma gondii*,[44,45] mycobacteria,[46-48] *Candida*,[45] and *Aspergillus*[49] and (2) neoplasms, namely, Kaposi's sarcoma and lymphoma.[44,46] Like symptoms of adrenal insufficiency in patients with AIDS, clinical symptoms of pancreatitis or altered glucose control were not noted in most patients who had postmortem pathologic abnormalities.[44,45] However, reports implicating HIV as a direct cause of insulin-dependent diabetes mellitus in two patients[50] and as the suspected cause of diabetes in a child with chronic pancreatitis[51] should be noted. Additionally, asymptomatic hyperamylasemia and hyperlipasemia are being seen more frequently in patients with AIDS who are evaluated for pancreatic function.[44,45,52]

Drug-associated effects on the pancreas have been found to be more clinically important than infection-associated effects. Agents used in HIV-infected patients that have been implicated include pentamidine, trimethoprim–sulfamethoxazole, and didanosine.[52-68]

Pentamidine has been associated with several episodes of acute pancreatitis characterized by abdominal pain or elevations in serum amylase and lipase concentrations, or both. The mean ± S.D. onset of symptoms in these patients was 10.5 ± 3.7 days (range, 6–21 days) from initiation of pentamidine therapy.[52-56] Additionally, elevations in serum creatinine concentration were frequently associated with the development of pancreatitis; however, changes in glucose control were reported in only two patients, both of whom died.[53,54] Evaluation of pancreas autopsy specimens in four patients showed extensive pentamidine-induced necrosis. Other causes of necrosis, such as infections and malignancy, were not identified.[44,53,54,56]

No data currently exist to support the theory that pentamidine-associated acute pancreatitis is dose related. If patients receiving this agent develop clinical findings consistent with inflammation of the pancreas, the drug should be discontinued and alternative therapy should be initiated. Adjunctive therapy is usually not necessary because symptoms usually resolve after withdrawal of pentamidine.[52,55,56] However, pentamidine has been implicated as the cause of death in two cases of fatal acute pancreatitis.[53,54]

Didanosine, an antiretroviral agent, has been frequently associated with the development of acute pancreatitis.[57] Yarchoan et al.[58] reported the development of acute pancreatitis in 5 (9%) of 58 patients (three severe cases and two mild cases). These authors postulated that this effect may be dose related and that it occurs primarily when doses exceed 9.6 mg/kg/day.

Lambert et al.[59] reported the development of pancreatitis in 5 (14%) of 37 patients treated with didanosine. Signs and symptoms consisted of abdominal pain, nausea and vomiting, and substantial elevations in serum amylase and lipase levels. Three patients required hospitalization. The mean ± S.D. duration of didanosine therapy before the development of symptoms in these patients was 105 ± 23.2 days. Symptoms resolved over one to three weeks. Pancreatitis redeveloped on rechallenge with the same dosage of didanosine in one patient. Three other patients who were rechallenged at the same or lower dosages remained asymptomatic. Three of the five patients who developed pancreatitis were also receiving aerosolized pentamidine. Other clinical trials have demonstrated similar frequencies and outcomes of pancreatitis associated with didanosine.[60-63] Although all patients described in these trials recovered from this adverse effect, fatal cases of acute pancreatitis secondary to didanosine have been reported.[50,64]

Recommendations to minimize the risk of pancreatitis during didanosine therapy include counseling the patient about the avoidance of alcohol, withholding didanosine in patients with a history of pancreatitis, and withholding the drug when a patient is receiving systemic pentamidine or sulfonamide-containing agents for the treatment of *Pneumocystis carinii* pneumonia.[63] It is further recommended that didanosine be withheld for an additional week after the completion of anti-*Pneumocystis* therapy. Periodic monitoring of serum amylase and triglyceride levels is also recommended, and didanosine therapy should be discontinued when these values increase substantially above baseline. Last, all patients need to be counseled about the potential signs and symptoms of pancreatitis; they should be instructed to discontinue therapy immediately and seek medical assistance if pancreatitis is suspected.

One case of symptomatic pancreatitis associated with trimethoprim–sulfamethoxazole has been reported in the literature.[67] Symptoms and laboratory findings consistent with pancreatitis began one week after therapy with the drug product was begun and continued until the therapy was stopped after 60 days. Within hours after withdrawal of the drug, abdominal complaints abated, and serum amylase levels decreased over the next two weeks. Therapy with the drug product was suspended for a month and then restarted. Within 72 hours, the patient had symptoms and laboratory values consistent with acute pancreatitis. Brivet et al.[44] described postmortem findings of an edematous pancreas in a patient who had received trimethoprim–sulfamethoxazole. Premortem clinical findings of pancreatitis for this patient were not reported. Although only two cases of pancreatitis associated with trimethoprim–sulfamethoxazole have been reported, the diagnosis should be considered in patients who develop abdominal symptoms during therapy.

Abnormalities in glucose regulation in patients with AIDS have occurred most commonly as the result of pentamidine administration.[42,65,68] Hypoglycemia, which results from the destruction of pancreatic beta cells and the subsequent release of insulin, occurs in up to 33% of patients receiving the drug.[42] Hypoglycemia may be mild or life threatening (blood glucose of <25 mg/dL) and has been reported to occur from one day to several weeks after the initiation of pentamidine therapy.[42,65,66] The management of hypoglycemia is determined by the severity and duration of the reaction. Severe reactions unresponsive to traditional therapy may be treated with intravenous glucose[65] or with diazoxide 100 mg p.o. every six hours for three days.[68] In many instances, the destruction of the beta cells by pentamidine is extensive, and permanent diabetes mellitus develops. If this occurs, lifelong insulin therapy is required for glucose control[42,66]; oral sulfonylureas have no role in this setting.

Abnormalities in glucose regulation in HIV-infected patients who are receiving pentamidine may be associated with the development of pentamidine-associated nephrotoxicity.[65] Stahl-Bayliss et al.[65] revealed that the prevalence of nephrotoxicity was greater in patients who developed hypoglycemia than in those who did not (100% compared with 38%; $p < 0.01$). These investigators suggested that pentamidine may accumulate in patients with kidney dysfunction, resulting in a dose-dependent effect on the pancreas. However, further investigation of this hypothesis is required before such a causal relationship can be definitely established.

Megestrol acetate therapy has been associated with the development of frank diabetes mellitus in one patient with AIDS.[69] The patient, who had been receiving the drug for approximately eight weeks for its appetite-stimulating effects, had no other identifiable cause for the signs and symptoms of diabetes. Glucose control became normal after withdrawal of the drug and worsened after rechallenge.

Thyroid and Parathyroid Disorders

Patients with HIV infection may have altered thyroid function secondary to invasion of the gland by opportunistic infections or neoplasms. Organisms that have most commonly been implicated to affect the thyroid include cytomegalovirus[9,33] and *Pneumocystis carinii*.[70-72] Kaposi's sarcoma has also been noted in autopsy specimens.[33]

Pneumocystis carinii caused thyroid dysfunction in two patients receiving aerosolized pentamidine as prophylaxis against *Pneumocystis carinii* pneumonia.[70,71] Such dissemination of the organism outside of the lungs is an important risk associated with the use of aerosolized pentamidine. Two weeks of systemic anti-*Pneumocystis* therapy led to a reduction in thyroid size in one case.[70] Although opportunistic infections may affect the thyroid gland, clinical manifestations of abnormal thyroid function are probably uncommon.[2,3]

The "euthyroid sick syndrome," characterized by alterations in thyroid hormone concentrations in the absence of thyroid gland dysfunction, is frequently encountered in patients with chronic debilitating nonthyroidal conditions, including AIDS.[73,74] This syndrome is generally characterized by decreased triiodothyronine (T_3) serum concentrations secondary to diminished peripheral conversion of thyroxine (T_4) to T_3. However, depending on the severity of the patient's overall clinical condition, this syndrome may also be manifested by a low free T_3 index and a low serum T_4 concentration in the absence of hypothyroidism.[73,74] When the euthyroid sick syndrome is suspected, thyroid hormone replacement is not indicated. Hormone therapy is not beneficial in this situation and may, in fact, be detrimental.[75]

Merenich et al.[2] evaluated thyroid function in 40 asymptomatic HIV-infected male subjects and 27 seronegative controls. No acute thyroid illnesses attributed to HIV infection were noted during this study. No differences in thyroid-function-test results were observed between the two groups with the exception of lower mean basal T_3 levels in the seropositive patients compared with the controls, a finding consistent with the euthyroid sick syndrome.

Dobs and associates[3] evaluated thyroid function in 70 ambulatory HIV-positive men classified as being asymptomatic or as having ARC or AIDS. No significant differences in mean thyroid hormone concentrations were observed among the three groups or in comparison with laboratory control subjects. However, two patients with AIDS (4.5%) and two patients with ARC (33%) had low serum T_4 concentrations. The authors suggested that the failure to show findings consistent with the euthyroid sick syndrome in this population was secondary to these individuals being ambulatory. Debilitated, hospitalized patients are the ones who usually develop this syndrome.

In a prospective evaluation of 66 patients with AIDS and 14 patients with ARC, Tang and Kaptein.[76] determined that these individuals often had altered thyroid hormone serum concentrations as the result of nonthyroidal illnesses. All 80 patients had clinical euthyroidism; however, one patient with AIDS and *Pneumocystis carinii* pneumonia was found to have subclinical hypothyroidism secondary to thyroid dysfunction. A majority of the patients had laboratory values consistent with the euthyroid sick syndrome: 60% had low T_3 levels, and an additional 4% had low serum free T_4 concentrations with no symptoms and with normal thyroid function, as determined by normal thyrotropin levels and normal responses to stimulation with thyrotropin-releasing hormone. In general, it was found that patients with AIDS did not differ substantially from those with ARC with regard to serum thyroid function. The investigators concluded that abnormal thyroid hormone levels are commonly encountered in patients with AIDS and ARC and are primarily the result of nonthyroidal illness.

LoPresti and associates[77] evaluated serum thyroid hormone concentrations in 56 HIV-infected patients; 26 were hospitalized with AIDS and *Pneumocystis carinii* pneumonia, 10 were asymptomatic outpatients, 10 were outpatients with ARC, and 10 were outpatients with AIDS. The investigators discovered that abnormalities in thyroid hormone concentrations are fairly common in HIV-infected patients. It was found that elevated concentrations of thyroxine-binding globulin and a progressive decline in reverse T_3 concentration were associated with advancing HIV disease. In addition, low serum T_3 concentrations were associated with a poor outcome in patients suffering from *Pneumocystis carinii* pneumonia.

Alterations in serum calcium concentrations may be observed in HIV-infected patients. Zaloga et al.[78] reported two cases of hypercalcemia and low parathyroid hormone levels associated with disseminated cytomegalovirus infection. Hypercalcemia in this instance was corrected after the administration of calcitonin.

Alterations in serum calcium concentrations also may be noted in patients receiving medications for the treatment of opportunistic infections associated with HIV.[79-81] In rare instances pentamidine caused hypocalcemia when used in the treatment of *Pneumocystis carinii* pneumonia.[79,80] In addition, foscarnet, an antiviral agent used in the treatment of cytomegalovirus retinitis, caused alterations in serum phosphorus and calcium concentrations secondary to the drug's deposition into bone tissue.[80,81]

Testicular Abnormalities

Evaluations of the testes of HIV-infected men have demonstrated infiltration by a number of infectious pathogens including cytomegalovirus, *Mycobacterium avium–intracellulare*, and *Toxoplasma*.[82,83]

Testicular abnormalities have been observed in patients who have AIDS with or without opportunistic infections and malignancies.[3,5,82,83] Central hypogonadism is common in men with HIV infection, and it may be the first apparent endocrine abnormality noted in these patients.[3] In a study of 70 asymptomatic HIV-infected men, gonadal dysfunction was observed in 50% of those with AIDS and 44% of those with ARC. In addition, 67% and 33% of patients with AIDS had decreased libido and impotence, respectively.[3] The same authors noted decreased testosterone levels in 24 (38%) of 63 individuals known to be HIV seropositive. Luteinizing hormone levels were also low in 18 of these 24 hypogonadal patients.

Abnormal testosterone levels were observed in a study by Villette and coworkers[5] involving seven asymptomatic HIV-infected patients and six patients with AIDS. Although mean testosterone levels were similar for the asymptomatic HIV-infected patients and the healthy control subjects, a significant decrease was found in the mean testosterone levels in AIDS patients compared with controls.[5]

The cause of these testicular abnormalities in HIV-infected men is unclear. They may be the result of HIV infection of the testes or of alterations in the function of the hypothalamic–pituitary–testicular axis that occur in patients suffering from malnutrition or other critical illnesses.[5] When these alterations occur, a factor other than corticotropin stimulates an increase in corticosteroid synthesis, causing a "metabolic shift" that results in decreased production of androgen.[5]

Prolonged treatment with medications such as ganciclovir, which is used for cytomegalovirus retinitis, may be associated with suppression of testosterone synthesis.[84] In animal models, ganciclovir has been shown to inhibit spermatogenesis. Although 10 patients who received a short course (14 days) of this agent had decreased mean serum testosterone concentrations at the completion of therapy compared with the concentrations at baseline (12.3 nmol/L versus 18.2 nmol/L, respectively), the difference was not significant.[84] However, failure to demonstrate statistical significance in such a situation may be because of the small sample size of the study or the relatively short duration of the ganciclovir therapy. Longer courses of therapy with ganciclovir may predispose HIV-infected patients to abnormalities in serum testosterone concentrations.

Other medications commonly used to treat patients with AIDS have been associated with testicular and androgenic abnormalities. Ketoconazole has caused a significant decrease in the secretion of testosterone, resulting in decreased serum concentrations of both free and bound hormone.[85,86] In patients receiving high-dose ketoconazole (800–1200 mg/day) for more than four months, testosterone production may be below normal for the entire day and can result in decreased libido, impotence, oligospermia, and gynecomastia.[17] The hypogonadism caused by ketoconazole is reversible when drug therapy is discontinued.[17] Although acyclovir, an antiviral agent used in the treatment of herpes simplex, has been shown to decrease spermatogenesis in animals, this effect has not been observed when the drug is used clinically in humans.[87]

Eventually, supplementation with androgens may prove to be effective in improving the sexual function of some HIV-infected patients.

Conclusion

Endocrine complications in patients infected with HIV may be caused by infection, malignancy, or drugs. Adjusting or instituting drug therapy may be necessary to control symptomatic endocrine abnormalities.

References

1. Groopman JE. Current advances in the diagnosis and treatment of AIDS: an introduction. *Rev Infect Dis*. 1990; 12:908-11.
2. Merenich JA, McDermott MT, Asp AA et al. Evidence of endocrine involvement early in the course of human immunodeficiency virus infection. *J Clin Endocrinol Metab*. 1990; 70:566-71.
3. Dobs AS, Dempsey NA, Ladenson PW et al. Endocrine disorders in men infected with HIV. *Am J Med*. 1988; 84:611-6.
4. Membrano L, Irony I, Dere W et al. Adrenal cortical dysfunction in acquired immunodeficiency syndrome. *J Clin Endocrinol Metab*. 1987; 65:482-7.
5. Villette JM, Courin P, Doinel C et al. Circadian variations in plasma levels of hypophyseal, adrenocortical and testicular hormones in men infected with human immunodeficiency virus. *J Clin Endocrinol Metab*. 1990; 70:572-7.
6. Falkenbach A, Schmidt K, Helm EB et al. Adrenal insufficiency in AIDS. *South Med J*. 1989; 82:1195. Letter.
7. Greene LW, Cole W, Greene JB et al. Adrenal insufficiency as a complication of the acquired immunodeficiency syndrome. *Ann Intern Med*. 1984; 101:497-9.
8. Klein RS, Mann DN, Friedland GH et al. Adrenocortical function in the acquired immunodeficiency syndrome. *Ann Intern Med*. 1983; 99:566. Letter.
9. Welch K, Finkbeiner W, Alpers CE et al. Autopsy findings in the acquired immune deficiency syndrome. *JAMA*. 1984; 252:1152-9.
10. Glasgow BJ, Steinsapir KD, Anders BSK et al. Adrenal pathology in the acquired immune deficiency syndrome. *Am J Clin Pathol*. 1985; 84:594-7.
11. Bricaire F, Marche C, Zoubi D et al. Adrenocortical lesions and AIDS. *Lancet*. 1988; 1:881. Letter.
12. Tapper ML, Rotterdam HZ, Lerner CW et al. Adrenal necrosis in the acquired immunodeficiency syndrome. *Ann Intern Med*. 1984; 100:239-41.
13. Hilton CW, Harrington PT, Prasad C et al. Adrenal insufficiency in the acquired immunodeficiency syndrome. *S Med J*. 1988; 81:1493-5.
14. Verges B, Chavanet P, Kisterman JP et al. Adrenocortical lesions and HIV infection. *Lancet*. 1988; 1:1345. Letter.
15. Mulhall BP, Fieldhouse S, Deam D. Adrenocortical lesions and HIV infection. *Lancet*. 1988; 1:1345. Letter.
16. Pont A, Williams PL, Loose DS et al. Ketoconazole blocks adrenal steroid synthesis. *Arch Intern Med*. 1982; 97:370-2.
17. Pont A, Grayhill R, Craven PC et al. High dose ketoconazole therapy and adrenal and testicular function in humans. *Arch Intern Med*. 1984; 144:2150-3.
18. White MC, Kendall-Taylor P. Adrenal hypofunction in patients taking ketoconazole. *Lancet*. 1985; 1:44-5.
19. Bradbrook ID, Gillies HC, Morrison PJ et al. Effects of single and multiple doses of ketoconazole on adrenal function in normal subjects. *Br J Clin Pharmacol*. 1988; 20:163-5.
20. McCance DR, Ritchie CM, Sheridan B et al. Acute hypoadrenalism and hepatotoxicity after treatment with ketoconazole. *Lancet*. 1987; 1:573. Letter.
21. Khosla S, Wolfson JS, Demerjian Z et al. Adrenal crisis in the setting of high-dose ketoconazole therapy. *Arch Intern Med*. 1989; 149:802-4.
22. Best TR, Jenkins JK, Murphy FY et al. Persistent adrenal insufficiency secondary to low-dose ketoconazole therapy. *Am J Med*. 1987; 82:676-80.
23. Phillips P, Braybill JR, Fetchick R et al. Adrenal responses to corticotropin during therapy with itraconazole. *Antimicrob Agents Chemother*. 1987; 31:647-9.
24. Sharkey PK, Rinaldi MG, Dunn JF et al. High-dose itraconazole in the treatment of severe mycoses. *Antimicrob Agents Chemother*. 1991; 35:707-13.
25. Kyriazopoulou V, Parparousi O, Vagenakis AG. Rifampicin-induced adrenal crisis in Addisonian patients receiving corticosteroid replacement therapy. *J Clin Endocrinol Metab*. 1984; 59:1204-6.
26. Edwards OM, Courtenay-Evans RJ, Galley JM et al. Changes in cortisol metabolism following rifampicin therapy. *Lancet*. 1974; 2:549-50.
27. Elansary EH, Earis JE. Rifampicin and adrenal crisis. *Br Med J*. 1983; 286:1861-2.
28. Wilkins EGL, Hnizdo E, Cope A. Addisonian crisis induced by treatment with rifampicin. *Tubercle*. 1989; 70:69-73.
29. Ediger SK, Isley WL. Rifampicin-induced adrenal insufficiency in the acquired immunodeficiency syndrome: difficulties in diagnosis and treatment. *Postgrad Med J*. 1988; 64:405-6.
30. Miguet JP, Mavier P, Soussy CJ et al. Induction of hepatic microsomal enzymes after brief administration of rifampicin in man. *Gastroenterology*. 1977; 72:924-6.
31. Fitzgerald PA, Copeland PM. Adrenal disorders. In: Fitzgerald PA, ed. Handbook of clinical endocrinology. 2nd ed. Norwalk, CT: Appleton and Lange; 1992:227-89.
32. Kalin MF, Poretsky L, Seres DS et al. Hyporeninemic-hypoaldosteronism associated with acquired immune deficiency syndrome. *Am J Med*. 1987; 82:1035-8.
33. Frank TS, LiVolsi VA, Connor AM. Cytomegalovirus infection of the thyroid in immunocompromised adults. *Yale J Biol Med*. 1987; 60:1-8.
34. Milligan SA, Katz MS, Craven PC et al. Toxoplasmosis presenting as panhypopituitarism in a patient with the acquired immune deficiency syndrome. *Am J Med*. 1984; 77:760-4.
35. Humphreys MH, Schoenfeld PY. Renal complications in patients with the acquired immune deficiency syndrome (AIDS). *Am J Nephrol*. 1987; 7:1-7.
36. Agarwal A, Soni A, Ciechanowsky M et al. Hyponatremia in patients with the acquired immunodeficiency syndrome. *Nephron*. 1989; 53:317-21.
37. Vitting KE, Gardenswartz MH, Zabetakis PM et al. Frequency of hyponatremia and nonosmolar vasopressin release in the acquired immunodeficiency syndrome. *JAMA*. 1990; 263:973-8.
38. Robertson GL, Aycinena P, Zerbe RL. Neurogenic disorders of osmoregulation. *Am J Med*. 1982; 72:339-53.
39. Ingraham IE, Estes NAM, Bern MM et al. Disseminated varicella-zoster virus infection with the syndrome of inappropriate antidiuretic hormone. *Arch Intern Med*. 1983; 143:1270-1.
40. Semel JD, McNerney JJ Jr. SIADH during disseminated herpes varicella-zoster infections: relationship to vidarabine therapy. *Am J Med Sci*. 1986; 291:115-18.
41. Ramos E, Timmons RF, Schimpff SC. Inappropriate antidiuretic hormone following adenine arabinoside administration. *Antimicrob Agents Chemother*. 1979; 15:142-4.
42. Andersen R, Boedicker M, Ma M et al. Adverse reactions associated with pentamidine isoethionate is AIDS patients: recommendations for monitoring therapy. *Drug Intell Clin Pharm*. 1986; 20:862-8.
43. Culpepper RM, Hebert SC, Andreoli TE. The posterior pituitary and water metabolism. In: Wilson JD, Foster DW, eds. Williams' textbook of endocrinology. 7th ed. Philadelphia: Saunders; 1985:614-52.
44. Brivet R, Coffin B, Bedossa P et al. Pancreatic lesions in AIDS. *Lancet*. 1987; 2:570-1. Letter.
45. Zazzo JR, Pichon F, Regnter B. HIV and the pancreas. *Lancet*. 1987; 2:1212-3. Letter.
46. Bricaire F, Marche C, Zoubi D et al. HIV and the pancreas. *Lancet*. 1988; 1:65-6. Letter.
47. Berson BD, Mendelson DS, Janus CL. Tuberculosis abscess of the pancreas in AIDS: CT findings. *Mount Sinai J Med*. 1989; 56:297-9.
48. Cappell MS, Javeed M. Pancreatic abscess due to mycobacteria associated with the acquired immunodeficiency syndrome. *J Clin Gastroenterol*. 1990; 12:423-9.
49. Bhatt B, Cappell MS. A peripancreatic abscess containing *Aspergillus* in a patient with the acquired immunodeficiency

syndrome. *Am J Gastroenterol*. 1990; 85:1200. Letter.
50. Vendrell J, Nubiola A, Goday A et al. HIV and the pancreas. *Lancet*. 1987; 2:1212. Letter.
51. Torre D, Montanari M, Paolo G et al. HIV and the pancreas. *Lancet*. 1987; 2:1212. Letter.
52. Slavin MB, Brocavich JM, Torre MS et al. Prospective evaluation of pentamidine-associated pancreatitis. Paper presented at 25th Annual ASHP Midyear Clinical Meeting. Las Vegas, NV: 1990 Dec 5.
53. Salmeron S, Petitpretz P, Katlama C et al. Pentamidine and pancreatitis. *Ann Intern Med*. 1986; 105:140-1. Letter.
54. Zuger A, Wolf BZ, El-Sadr W et al. Pentamidine-associated fatal acute pancreatitis. *JAMA*. 1986; 256:2383-5.
55. Murphey SA, Josephs AS. Acute pancreatitis associated with pentamidine therapy. *Arch Intern Med*. 1981; 141:56-8.
56. O'Neil MG, Selub SE, Hak LJ. Pancreatitis during pentamidine therapy in patients with AIDS. *Clin Pharm*. 1991; 10:56-9.
57. Bristol-Myers Squibb. Videx package insert. Princeton, NJ; 1991 Oct.
58. Yarchoan R, Pluda JM, Thomas RV et al. Long-term toxicity/activity of 2',3'-dideoxyinosine in AIDS or AIDS-related complex. *Lancet*. 1990; 336:526-9.
59. Lambert JS, Seidlin M, Reichman RC et al. 2',3'-Dideoxyinosine (DDI) in patients with the acquired immunodeficiency syndrome or AIDS-related complex. *N Engl J Med*. 1990; 322:1333-40.
60. Valentine FT, Seidlin M, Hochster H et al. Phase I study of 2',3'-dideoxyinosine: experience with 19 patients at New York University Medical Center. *Rev Infect Dis*. 1990; 12:S534-S539.
61. Dolin R, Lambert JS, Morse GD et al. 2',3'-Dideoxyinosine in patients with AIDS or AIDS-related complex. *Rev Infect Dis*. 1990; 12:S540-S551.
62. Cooley TP, Kunches LM, Saunders CA et al. Treatment of AIDS and AIDS-related complex with 2',3'-dideoxyinosine given once daily. *Rev Infect Dis*. 1990; 12:S552-S560.
63. Yarchoan R, Mitsuya H, Pluda JM et al. The National Cancer Institute phase I study of 2',3'-dideoxyinosine administration in adults with AIDS or AIDS-related complex: analysis of activity and toxicity profiles. *Rev Infect Dis*. 1990; 12:S522-S533.
64. Bouvet E, Casalino E, Prevost MH et al. Fatal case of 2',3'-dideoxyinosine-associated pancreatitis. *Lancet*. 1990; 336:1515. Letter.
65. Stahl-Bayliss CM, Kalman CM, Laskin OL. Pentamidine-induced hypoglycemia in patients with the acquired immune deficiency syndrome. *Clin Pharmacol Ther*. 1986; 39:271-5.
66. Bouchard PH, Sal P, Reach G et al. Diabetes mellitus following pentamidine-induced hypoglycemia in humans. *Diabetes*. 1982; 31:40-5.
67. Antonow DR. Acute pancreatitis associated with trimethoprim–sulfamethoxazole. *Ann Intern Med*. 1986; 104:363-5.
68. Henry K, Rathgaber S, McCabe K. Diabetes mellitus induced by megestrol acetate in a patient with AIDS and cachexia. *Ann Intern Med*. 1992; 116:53-4.
69. Fitzgerald DS, Young IS. Reversal of pentamidine-induced hypoglycaemia with oral diazoxide. *J Trop Med Hyg*. 1984; 87:15-9.
70. Drucker DJ, Bailey D, Rotstein L. Thyroiditis as the presenting manifestation of disseminated extrapulmonary *Pneumocystis carinii* infection. *J Clin Endocrinol Metab*. 1990; 71:1663-5.
71. Ragni MV, Dekker A, DeRubertis FR et al. *Pneumocystis carinii* infection presenting as necrotizing thyroiditis and hypothyroidism. *Am J Clin Pathol*. 1991; 95:489-93.
72. Gallant JE, Enriquez RE, Cohen KL et al. *Pneumocystis carinii* thyroiditis. *Am J Med*. 1988; 84:303-6.
73. Chopra IJ, Hershman JM, Pardridge WM et al. Thyroid function in nonthyroidal illnesses. *Ann Intern Med*. 1983; 98:946-57.
74. Slag MF, Morley JE, Elson MK et al. Hypothyroxinemia in critically ill patients as a predictor of increased mortality. *JAMA*. 1981; 245:43-5.
75. Brent GA, Hershman JM. Thyroxine therapy in patients with severe nonthyroidal illnesses and low serum thyroxine concentrations. *J Clin Endocrinol Metab*. 1986; 63:1-8.
76. Tang WW, Kaptein EM. Thyroid hormone levels in the acquired immunodeficiency syndrome (AIDS) or AIDS-related complex. *West J Med*. 1989; 151:627-31.
77. LoPresti JS, Fried JC, Spencer CA et al. Unique alterations of thyroid hormone indices in the acquired immunodeficiency syndrome (AIDS). *Ann Intern Med*. 1989; 110:970-5.
78. Zaloga GP, Chernow B, Eil C et al. Hypercalcemia and disseminated cytomegalovirus infection in the acquired immunodeficiency syndrome. *Ann Intern Med*. 1985; 102:331-3.
79. Wharton JM, Coleman DL, Wofsy CB et al. Trimethoprim–sulfamethoxazole or pentamidine for *Pneumocystis carinii* pneumonia in the acquired immunodeficiency syndrome. *Ann Intern Med*. 1986; 105:37-44.
80. Youle MS, Clarbour J, Gazzard B et al. Severe hypocalcemia in AIDS patients treated with foscarnet and pentamidine. *Lancet*. 1988; 1:1455-6. Letter.
81. Jacobson MA, O'Donnell JJ, Mills J. Foscarnet treatment of cytomegalovirus retinitis in patients with the acquired immunodeficiency syndrome. *Antimicrob Agents Chemother*. 1989; 33:736-41.
82. Chabon AB, Stenger RJ, Grabstald H. Histopathology of testis in acquired immune deficiency syndrome. *Urology*. 1987; 29:683-5.
83. DePaepe ME, Guerrieri C, Waxman M. Opportunistic infections of the testis in the acquired immunodeficiency syndrome. *Mount Sinai J Med*. 1990; 57:25-9.
84. Chachoua A, Dieterich D, Krasinski K et al. 9-(1,3-Dihydroxy-2-propoxymethyl) guanine (ganciclovir) in the treatment of *Cytomegalovirus* gastrointestinal disease with the acquired immunodeficiency syndrome. *Ann Intern Med*. 1987; 107:133-7.
85. Pont A, Williams PL, Azhar S et al. Ketoconazole blocks testosterone synthesis. *Arch Intern Med*. 1982; 142:2137-40.
86. Santen RJ, Van den Bossche H, Symoens J et al. Sites of action of low dose ketoconazole on androgen biosynthesis in men. *J Clin Endocrinol Metab*. 1983; 57:732-6.
87. Douglas JM, Davis LG, Remington ML et al. A double-blind controlled trial of chronically administered oral acyclovir on sperm production in men with frequently recurrent genital herpes. *J Infect Dis*. 1988; 157:588-93.

Commentary

Are antiarrhythmic drugs obsolete?

JAMES E. TISDALE AND CHARLES R. WEBB

Clin Pharm. 1992; 49:714-26

Since publication of the results of the Cardiac Arrhythmia Suppression Trial (CAST),[1] clinical use of available antiarrhythmic drugs[2,3] and preclinical development of new antiarrhythmic agents have undergone intense re-evaluation. Several studies have shown that treatment with certain antiarrhythmic drugs has no significant effect on mortality in specific patient populations,[4-8] while CAST[1] and various meta-analyses[9-13] have shown that treatment of some patients with certain antiarrhythmic drugs may actually increase mortality. These data, coupled with the potentially life-threatening proarrhythmic effects of antiarrhythmic agents,[14] the relatively high frequency of other adverse effects associated with antiarrhythmic drugs,[15] and the availability of effective nonpharmacologic treatments for preventing arrhythmia-induced sudden cardiac death[16] and curing selected supraventricular arrhythmias,[17-19] have prompted some authors to suggest that nonpharmacologic options may be the therapies of choice in some patients with arrhythmias.[20-23]

Does this mean that antiarrhythmic drugs are obsolete? The purpose of this commentary is to review the problems associated with antiarrhythmic drug therapy, advantages and disadvantages of nonpharmacologic alternatives to drugs for the treatment of cardiac arrhythmias, and current indications for pharmacologic treatment of arrhythmias.

Problems Associated with Antiarrhythmic Drugs

Adverse Effects. The overall frequency of adverse effects associated with antiarrhythmic drug therapy is substantial; intolerance often results in discontinuation of therapy (Table 1).[24-61] Adverse effects caused by antiarrhythmic agents may be noncardiac or cardiac.

Noncardiac adverse effects include gastrointestinal-tract disturbances such as nausea, vomiting, and diarrhea and are most commonly associated with quinidine, mexiletine, and bretylium but may also occur as a result of therapy with procainamide and amiodarone.[24-35,43,50,51] Central nervous system adverse effects such as blurred vision, tremors, dizziness, and confusion are commonly caused by class IB antiarrhythmic agents like lidocaine, mexiletine, and tocainide and occasionally by class IC agents like flecainide.[40-45] Quinidine is associated with cinchonism (tinnitus, blurred vision, lightheadedness, tremor, flushing), rash, and drug fever.[24] Disopyramide commonly causes anticholinergic adverse effects such as blurred vision, dry mouth, constipation, and urinary retention.[37-39] Amiodarone is associated with pneumonitis and pulmonary fibrosis, thyroid dysfunction (hyperthyroidism or hypothyroidism), tremor, peripheral neuropathy, corneal microdeposits, skin discoloration, and photosensitivity.[51] Quinidine and amiodarone have been reported to cause hepatotoxicity.[24,51] A syndrome resembling systemic lupus erythematosus has been reported in association with procainamide,[62] and several antiarrhythmic drugs have been reported to cause serious adverse hematologic effects such as neutropenia or agranulocytosis (procainamide, tocainide), thrombocytopenia (quinidine), and aplastic or hemolytic anemia (tocainide, quinidine).[24,43,63]

Cardiac adverse effects associated with antiarrhythmic agents include worsening of existing arrhythmias and the initiation of new arrhythmias.[14] In particular, quinidine, procainamide, disopyramide, and amiodarone may precipitate torsade de pointes, a polymorphic ventricular tachycardia preceded by a prolonged QT interval and a long–short initiating sequence of R-R intervals on the surface electrocardiogram (ECG) and characterized by a QRS axis that appears to twist around the isoelectric baseline.[14,64] Intravenous administration of quinidine, procainamide, and bretylium may result in hypotension.[50,65,66] In addition, disopyramide, flecainide, β-adrenergic blocking agents, and verapamil have negative inotropic activity and may precipitate or exacerbate symptoms in patients with a history of congestive

JAMES E. TISDALE, PHARM.D., is Assistant Professor, College of Pharmacy and Allied Health Professions, Wayne State University, Detroit, MI, and Coordinator, Education and Training, Department of Pharmacy Services, Henry Ford Hospital (HFH), Detroit. CHARLES R. WEBB, M.D., is Director, Cardiac Electrophysiology, HFH, and Assistant Clinical Professor of Medicine, School of Medicine, University of Michigan, Ann Arbor.

Address reprint requests to Dr. Tisdale at the College of Pharmacy and Allied Health Professions, Wayne State University, 328 Shapero Hall, Detroit, MI 48202.

Table 1.
Frequency of Adverse Effects Associated with Antiarrhythmic Drugs Available in the United States

Drug[a]	Overall Frequency (%)	% Patients Requiring Discontinuation of Therapy
Class IA		
Quinidine[24-32]	14–92	5–36
Procainamide[33-35]	52–61	41–61
Disopyramide[25,36-39]	16–70	10–25
Class IB		
Lidocaine[40-42]	6–35	2–15
Mexiletine[43]	47–65	30
Tocainide[43]	40	10–20
Class IC		
Flecainide[43-45]	7–30	11–13
Propafenone[46]	21–32	3–7
Moricizine[47]	20–25	9
Class II		
β-adrenergic receptor blockers[48,49]	9–17	2–7
Class III		
Bretylium[50]	50	10
Amiodarone[51]	25–93	1–26
Verapamil[52]	7–40	1–8
Diltiazem[53-56]	2–10	1–7
Unclassified Agents		
Digoxin[57-60]	8–23	8–23
Adenosine[61]	15–100	. . .

[a]Drug classification based on references 2 and 3.

heart failure.[36,48,67]

Interactions of Antiarrhythmic Agents with Drugs and Devices. Antiarrhythmic agents are associated with pharmacokinetic interactions with other drugs (Table 2)[43,46,61,65,68-80] that may result either in elevated plasma concentrations of the affected agent and subsequent toxicity or in reduced plasma concentrations of the affected agent and apparent loss of efficacy. Pharmacodynamic drug interactions may also occur. For example, amiodarone administered with a class IA drug, with bepridil, or with certain antidepressant or antipsychotic agents may excessively prolong the QT interval and increase the risk of torsade de pointes.[64,81,82] Combination therapy with β blockers and digoxin or calcium-channel blockers may result in additive suppressive effects on the sinoatrial and atrioventricular (AV) nodes, resulting in bradycardia or AV-nodal block or both.[78] Furthermore, methylxanthine compounds such as theophylline and caffeine inhibit the pharmacologic activity of adenosine by competitively binding to purine receptors.[61]

In addition to interacting with drugs, antiarrhythmic agents can affect the performance of devices such as external defibrillators, automatic implantable cardioverter–defibrillators (ICDs), and pacemakers. The administration of encainide, flecainide, quinidine, lidocaine, or amiodarone increases the defibrillation threshold in animals.[83] Case reports and studies in humans have associated mexiletine, amiodarone, and moricizine with elevated defibrillation thresholds in patients with ICDs.[83,84] Quinidine, procainamide, flecainide, β blockers, and verapamil have also been reported to increase the threshold for impulse capture or to impair impulse-sensing ability in patients with pacemakers.[84,85] A recent report suggested that class IC antiarrhythmic agents may increase the amount of energy required for successful electrical cardioversion of atrial fibrillation.[86] Therefore, some antiarrhythmic drugs may have detrimental effects on the ability of devices to adequately sense the rhythm of the heart, pace the heart, or convert atrial or ventricular fibrillation to sinus rhythm.

Limited Benefit in Specific Patient Populations. Antiarrhythmic drug therapy has been found to be of limited benefit in studies of specific patient populations with certain cardiac arrhythmias.

Despite long-term benefits in some patients, class I antiarrhythmic drugs and amiodarone are successful at rendering inducible ventricular tachycardia noninducible in only 25–40% of patients undergoing serial electrophysiologic drug testing.[87,88] In addition, patients with a left ventricular ejection fraction of ≤30% are less likely to respond to antiarrhythmic drug therapy during serial electrophysiologic testing than patients without severe left ventricular dysfunction.[89] In other words, efficacy is less likely for those at higher risk.

Aronow et al.[4] prospectively studied the influence of therapy with quinidine or procainamide on mortality in elderly patients (mean age, 82 years) with coronary artery disease and complex ventricular arrhythmias as detected by Holter monitoring. The majority of the patients were initially treated with quinidine; several patients (3.2%) with a history of intolerance to quinidine were given procainamide. Of 406 patients who were initially treated with either drug, 186 had to discontinue treatment because of adverse effects; this group was used as the control group. There were no differences between groups in the occurrence of sudden cardiac death, all cardiac deaths, or deaths due to all causes.

It is well established that frequent or complex ventricular ectopy in patients who have survived acute myocardial infarction (MI) is associated with increased mortality.[90,91] However, studies of the long-term administration of tocainide and mexiletine for suppressing ventricular ectopy in patients after acute MI have shown no significant effect of such treatment on mortality.[5-8] In a meta-analysis, Teo et al.[10] evaluated 53 randomized, controlled trials of class I and III antiarrhythmic drugs used after MI and reviewed several overviews of the effects of class II and IV antiarrhythmic agents for prevention of mortality after acute MI. The analysis included data collected from over 90,000 patients. Prophylactic antiarrhythmic drug therapy with class IA, IB, III, and IV antiarrhythmic agents had no effect on mortality after acute MI.[10] Other reviews of data from clinical trials of prophylactic antiarrhythmic drug therapy after the hospital phase of acute MI also failed to show any significant survival benefit.[92-95]

Table 2.
Pharmacokinetic Drug Interactions Associated with Antiarrhythmic Agents[43,46,61,65,68-80]

Antiarrhythmic Drug	Interacting Drug	Interaction[a]
Quinidine	Digoxin	Increased serum digoxin conc.
	Procainamide	Increased serum procainamide conc.
	Warfarin	Prolonged prothrombin time
	Phenytoin, rifampin	Decreased serum quinidine conc.
Procainamide	Cimetidine, ranitidine, trimethoprim	Increased serum procainamide conc.
Disopyramide	Phenytoin	Decreased serum disopyramide conc.
Lidocaine	Cimetidine, β blockers	Increased serum lidocaine conc.
Mexiletine	Cimetidine	Increased serum mexiletine conc.
	Phenytoin	Decreased serum mexiletine conc.
	Theophylline	Increased serum theophylline conc.
Flecainide	Digoxin	Increased serum digoxin conc.
	Cimetidine	Increased serum flecainide conc.
	Propranolol	Increased serum flecainide and propranolol conc.
Propafenone	Digoxin	Increased serum digoxin conc.
	Warfarin	Prolonged prothrombin time
	Metoprolol	Increased serum metoprolol conc.
Moricizine	Cimetidine	Increased serum moricizine conc.
	Theophylline	Decreased serum theophylline conc.
β blockers	Verapamil	Increased serum conc. of metoprolol, propranolol, atenolol
Amiodarone	Digoxin	Increased serum digoxin conc.
	Quinidine	Increased serum quinidine conc.
	Procainamide	Increased serum procainamide conc.
	Warfarin	Prolonged prothrombin time
	Flecainide	Increased serum flecainide conc.
Verapamil	Digoxin	Increased serum digoxin conc.
	Quinidine	Increased serum quinidine conc.
	Theophylline	Increased serum theophylline conc.
	Carbamazepine	Increased serum carbamazepine conc.
	Cyclosporine	Increased blood cyclosporine conc.
	Rifampin	Decreased serum verapamil conc.
Diltiazem	Carbamazepine	Increased serum carbamazepine conc.
	Cyclosporine	Increased blood cyclosporin conc.
Digoxin	Antacids, kaolin–pectin, cholestyramine, colestipol, sulfasalazine, neomycin	Decreased serum digoxin conc.
	Erythromycin, tetracycline, spironolactone, indomethacin, ibuprofen, diclofenac	Increased serum digoxin conc.
Adenosine	Dipyridamole	Increased blood adenosine conc.

[a]Interactions have not been duplicated (i.e., an interaction is listed for flecainide–digoxin but not for digoxin–flecainide).

In summary, antiarrhythmic agents are ineffective in a substantial proportion of patients with ventricular tachyarrhythmias that are inducible during baseline electrophysiologic testing and may be less effective in patients with left ventricular dysfunction. Quinidine does not influence the incidence of mortality in elderly patients with coronary artery disease and complex ventricular ectopy, and most antiarrhythmic agents do not decrease mortality in patients with ventricular ectopy after acute MI.

Adverse Effect on Mortality in Specific Patient Populations. A meta-analysis of 10 randomized, controlled trials of empirical antiarrhythmic drug therapy after acute MI showed significantly higher mortality in patients who received antiarrhythmic drugs than in control groups.[11] In addition, an analysis of studies that included 6177 survivors of MI randomized to receive class IB antiarrhythmic agents and 6076 patients receiving placebo revealed increased mortality in the treatment group.[12]

Morganroth and Goin[13] published a meta-analysis of four parallel trials in which the efficacy and safety of quinidine (n = 502 patients) for the treatment of benign and potentially life-threatening ventricular arrhythmias were compared with the efficacy and safety of flecainide (n = 141), mexiletine (n = 246), tocainide (n = 67), and propafenone (n = 53). Mortality was significantly higher in the patients who received quinidine.

The CAST data[1] provide the most convincing evidence that prophylactic use of certain antiarrhythmic agents may be dangerous in specific patient populations. CAST was a randomized, double-blind, multicenter study designed to determine if the suppression of ventricular premature depolarizations (VPDs) with antiarrhythmic drugs would decrease mortality after acute MI. Individuals with sustained or symptomatic ventricular arrhythmias were excluded. Initially, two oral dosages of up to three drugs—encainide, flecainide, and moricizine—were evaluated by Holter monitoring for their efficacy at suppressing VPDs. Patients in whom VPDs were successfully suppressed by one of these agents were randomly assigned to receive either the efficacious drug or placebo. Statistical analysis was performed on the basis of the intention-to-treat principle. The primary endpoint evaluated was death from arrhythmia.

In April 1989 the CAST safety and monitoring board recommended that the encainide and flecainide arms of the study be stopped because mortality in patients receiving either of these drugs was significantly higher than in patients receiving placebo (Figure 1).[96] Although the moricizine arm of the study was allowed to continue (as CAST-II), this trial was also prematurely terminated because (1) patients treated with moricizine had a higher rate of cardiac-related mortality during the first two weeks of drug administration than those who received placebo and (2) prolongation of the study was unlikely to result in a demonstrable long-term survival benefit.[97] Teo and colleagues[10] also found that prophylactic treatment of post-MI patients with class IC antiarrhythmic drugs is associated with significantly higher mortality compared with control groups. While these results should not be extrapolated to antiarrhythmic drugs of other classes nor to other patient populations, it is clear that therapy with encainide, flecainide, or moricizine is contraindicated in patients with a history of MI and that routine VPD suppression with antiarrhythmic drugs in asymptomatic patients after MI is unfounded and may be harmful.

Coplen et al.[9] reviewed six randomized, controlled trials, which included a total of 808 patients, to evaluate the efficacy and safety of quinidine for long-term maintenance of sinus rhythm after cardioversion of atrial fibrillation. Although quinidine therapy was significantly more effective than no treatment for the maintenance of sinus rhythm, mortality in patients receiving quinidine (2.9%) was more than three times higher than in the control group (0.8%) ($p < 0.05$). These data should be interpreted with caution, however, as the total number of deaths in each group was small, the cause of death was not identified in several patients, and at least one death (a suicide) in the treatment group was probably unrelated to the quinidine therapy.

In yet another clinical population, a meta-analysis of 14 randomized, controlled studies showed that routine prophylactic administration of lidocaine to patients with acute MI resulted in higher mortality than in the control group.[98]

In summary, there is no evidence that empirical prophylaxis with antiarrhythmic drugs after acute MI in asymptomatic patients has a positive influence on survival, and evidence from CAST and several meta-analyses indicates that such treatment may be harmful. In addition, quinidine therapy in patients with benign or potentially life-threatening ventricular arrhythmias or atrial fibrillation and routine prophylactic administration of lidocaine in patients with acute MI may affect mortality adversely.

Efficacy and Safety of Nonpharmacologic Treatment Modalities

ICDs. The automatic implantable cardioverter–defibrillator is a device that monitors the heart continuously, identifies tachyarrhythmias, and delivers an electrical countershock to restore normal rhythm.[99] The ICD, which was approved for clinical use in 1985, is composed of a lead system and a pulse generator (Figure 2). The lead system is implanted surgically via a midline sternotomy or left thoracotomy, and the leads are tunneled through the diaphragm to the pulse generator, which is implanted in a pocket under abdominal subcutaneous fat.[100] The ICD is programmed to deliver a countershock in response to a predetermined ventricular rate. This device appears to be substantially more effective at preventing sudden cardiac death in susceptible patients than antiarrhythmic drug therapy; one-year survival rates in patients with ICDs range from 88% to 95%.[101] However, the efficacy of ICD therapy for the prevention of sudden cardiac

Figure 1. Survival among 1455 patients randomly assigned to receive encainide or flecainide or matching placebo in the Cardiac Arrhythmia Suppression Trial. The cause of death was cardiac arrhythmia or cardiac arrest. Reprinted from reference 1, with permission.

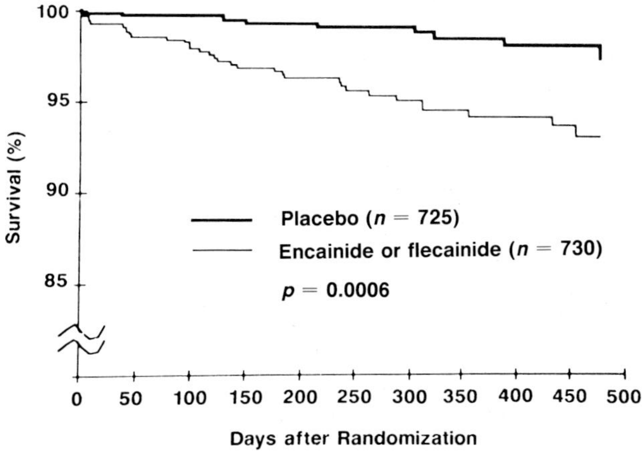

Figure 2. Components of an automatic implantable cardioverter–defibrillator: pulse generator, lead system, and ventricular patches. Reprinted with permission of Cardiac Pacemakers, Inc., St. Paul, MN.

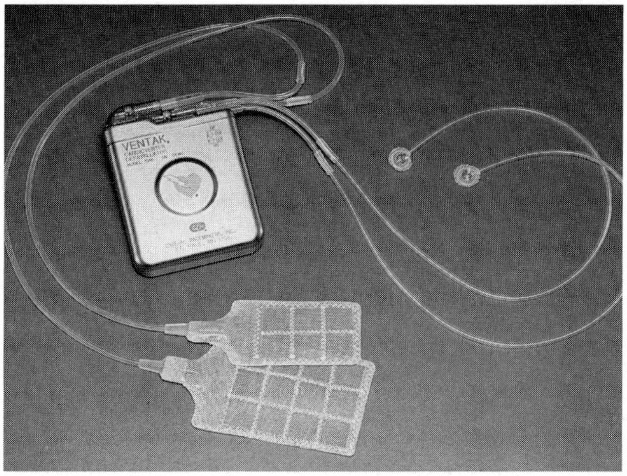

death has not yet been compared with that of antiarrhythmic drug therapy guided by electrophysiologic testing in a randomized trial.

Disadvantages of ICD therapy include the fact that implantation requires major surgery, during which mortality is approximately 1%.[100] In addition, while these devices respond to arrhythmias, they do not prevent them from occurring. For this reason, ICD implantation does not necessarily obviate the need for antiarrhythmic drug therapy; 49–69% of patients with these devices also receive antiarrhythmic agents in an attempt to reduce the frequency of discharges and to prevent hemodynamic collapse before therapeutic discharge of the device.[102,103] Other disadvantages include patient discomfort during cardioversion episodes and the need for patients to make bimonthly follow-up visits for the purpose of monitoring the shock frequency, testing battery function, and rejuvenating the capacitor plates. The most serious long-term complication of ICD therapy is infection, which is reported in 2–3% of patients.[100] Also, some patients may receive inappropriate shocks for non-life-threatening supraventricular tachyarrhythmias and nonsustained ventricular tachycardia, which is another reason for concomitant administration of antiarrhythmic drugs in some patients.[102,103]

More sophisticated ICDs are under development and investigation. These newer devices are expected to minimize the problem of inappropriate discharges through the use of programmed arrhythmia-detection algorithms, which are intended to prevent defibrillation as a response to non-life-threatening arrhythmias and by terminating some arrhythmias through such techniques as overdrive pacing.[104]

ICD therapy is expensive; hospital inpatient charges for ICD implantation average $50,000.[100]

Antitachycardia Pacemakers. Overdrive atrial or ventricular pacing has been attempted for the suppression of some ventricular tachyarrhythmias and is considered a mainstay of therapy for torsade de pointes.[64] Overdrive atrial pacing is also effective for the termination of supraventricular arrhythmias. Antitachycardia pacemakers are effective at terminating supraventricular tachycardia in 93% of patients at one year and in 78% of patients at five years after implantation.[104] Efficacy rates in patients with ventricular tachycardia are reported to be 78% at one year and 55% at five years.[104]

Limitations of these devices include the induction of atrial fibrillation or flutter in up to 30% of patients in whom pacing is used to terminate supraventricular tachycardias.[104] In addition, these devices may promote the degeneration of ventricular tachycardia into ventricular fibrillation; such degeneration has been reported in more than one third of patients in whom pacing has been used to terminate ventricular tachycardia in the electrophysiology laboratory.[105] For this reason, the use of these devices has been limited in patients with ventricular tachyarrhythmias. However, concurrent implantation of antitachycardia pacemakers and internal defibrillators is occasionally performed, and devices that incorporate both into one unit are under investigation. Therefore, the role of antitachycardia devices is likely to expand, although not to the exclusion of pharmacologic therapy.[104]

Catheter Ablation. Catheter ablation is a procedure in which electrode catheters are inserted into the heart transvenously and electrical energy is delivered to interrupt or permanently modify impulse conduction in a localized area from which an arrhythmia originates or that is determined to be an essential part of a reentrant circuit as identified by electrophysiologic mapping.[17,106] The original technique used was high-voltage direct current (DC) catheter ablation, during which currents and voltages often exceeding 50 A and 3000 V, respectively, are delivered to destroy a critical portion of a reentrant arrhythmia circuit.[106] Disadvantages of this technique include complications such as electromechanical dissociation, AV-nodal block, bradycardia, and ventricular perforation. Recently, radiofrequency catheter ablation, which involves the use of alternating current in frequencies from 30 kHz to 300 MHz, was introduced.[106] Potential advantages of radiofrequency ablation include the fact that, unlike DC catheter ablation, the procedure requires no general anesthesia. In addition, the frequency of complications, such as acute proarrhythmia, hemodynamic compromise, and cardiac perforation, appears to be lower than for DC ablation.[106]

Catheter ablation of the AV node with DC or radiofrequency techniques or with ethanol infusion (currently an investigational treatment) is performed for the management of supraventricular tachycardias that are refractory to drug therapy and unresponsive to antitachycardia pacing or surgery.[106] The disadvantage of this approach for the management of atrial fibrillation is that patients usually require the concomitant implantation of a permanent pacemaker. However, with the availability of newer rate-responsive pacemakers, symptomatic improvement may be achieved. Occasionally the AV node is modified rather than ablated, allowing an acceptable rate of conduction in the absence of an artificial pacemaker. However, with current techniques, the results of such a procedure are unpredictable. Conversely, in patients with AV-nodal reentrant tachycardia, the slow pathway in the AV node may be selectively ablated, and pacemakers may be required in only a small percentage of patients.

The most promising application of radiofrequency catheter ablation may be in the management of arrhythmias associated with accessory AV conduction pathways (e.g., Wolff–Parkinson–White syndrome). Accessory conduction pathways have been selectively destroyed in 93–99% of patients, with a complication rate of approximately 2% and no mortality.[17,18] Complications of this procedure in these patients include transient or permanent AV-nodal blockade, pericarditis, cardiac tamponade, and acute MI.[17,18] In view of these recent data, radiofrequency catheter ablation is a reasonable choice as first-line therapy in patients with arrhythmias associated with accessory conduction pathways.[107]

Catheter ablation has also been used to cure refractory ventricular tachyarrhythmias; success rates range from 30% to 90%.[106] However, the complication rate for this procedure in patients with ventricular arrhythmias is 10–15%, and the mortality rate is as high as 7%.[106]

Surgery. Surgical resolution of arrhythmias may be considered for patients with recurrent tachycardias refractory to antiarrhythmic drugs and other nonpharmacologic forms of therapy. Surgery can be considered if the myocardial tissue responsible for generating or propagating the arrhythmia can be identified by electrophysiologic mapping and if the area can be surgically ablated without compromising ventricular function.[19] Before the recent publication of data describing the high success rate and low complication rate of radiofrequency catheter ablation, surgery was the nonpharmacologic treatment of choice in patients with Wolff–Parkinson–White syndrome. Surgical ablation in these patients has been associated with success rates of >90% and a mortality rate of approximately 1%.[19] Surgery is not widely used for the management of patients with supraventricular tachycardias that are not associated with accessory conduction pathways.

Surgery has been used to treat patients with ventricular tachyarrhythmias.[108] However, the mortality rate during surgery for ventricular tachycardia ranges from 5% to 17%, depending on the location and extent of the myocardium responsible for the tachycardia, the involvement of papillary muscle, the skill of the surgeon, the available operative instrumentation, and the accuracy of electrophysiologic mapping.[109-113] Surgical resection is less desirable in patients with several ventricular arrhythmogenic foci, as each one requires individual mapping and resection. The ventriculotomy itself may heal as an arrhythmogenic scar. Use of this technique is limited to those ventricular arrhythmias that are hemodynamically stable and can be mapped before and during surgery. The short-term success of this technique is somewhat limited; 13–33% of patients continue to have inducible ventricular tachycardia after surgery.[109-113] Therefore, arrhythmia surgery in such patients is associated with substantial risk, high cost, and limited short-term success. Surgery is recommended only for patients with life-threatening ventricular tachyarrhythmias who do not have New York Heart Association functional class III or IV heart failure and in whom antiarrhythmic drugs have been unsuccessful.[108]

Current Indications for Antiarrhythmic Drug Therapy

Despite problems associated with antiarrhythmic drugs and the availability of nonpharmacologic forms of arrhythmia therapy, antiarrhythmic agents are effective for the treatment of a variety of cardiac arrhythmias, may have advantages over nonpharmacologic options, and in some cases are the only available treatment modality. Therefore, antiarrhythmic drugs remain the therapy of choice for a number of arrhythmias (Table 3).

Atrial Fibrillation. Drug therapy is the treatment of choice for the control of ventricular rate in patients with paroxysmal or chronic atrial fibrillation and has been associated with improvements in symptoms and the sense of well-being.[114] Relative blockade of impulse conduction through the AV node may be achieved with digoxin, calcium-channel blockers (verapamil or diltiazem), β blockers, or combinations of these agents.[114] Drug therapy with class IA agents is effective for the conversion of atrial fibrillation to sinus rhythm in hemodynamically stable patients with recent-onset or paroxysmal atrial fibrillation, and therapy with class IA or IC antiarrhythmic drugs is

Table 3.
Therapeutic Options for Selected Cardiac Arrhythmias[a]

Arrhythmia	First-Line Therapy	Alternative Therapy
APDs	AA drugs	None
Atrial fibrillation or flutter		
Termination	AA drugs, CV, or ODP[b]	None
Rate control (short-term)	AA drugs	None
Prevention or rate control (long term)	AA drugs	RF AVN ablation and PM[c]
AVNRT	AA drugs or slow AVN CP ablation	RF AVN ablation and PM
AVRT	AA drugs or AP ablation	Surgery
VPDs	AA drugs	None
NSVT	AA drugs	None
VT		
Termination	AA drugs, OPD, or CV	None
Prevention	AA drugs, ICD, or both	ATPM,[d] surgery[e]
VF		
Termination	ED	AA drugs with ED
Prevention, inducible VT	AA drugs, ICD, or both	None
Prevention, no inducible VT	ICD	None
SCD, no inducible arrhythmias	ICD	None

[a]APDs = atrial premature depolarizations, AA = antiarrhythmic, CV = electrical cardioversion, ODP = overdrive pacing, RF = radiofrequency, AVN = atrioventricular (AV) node, PM = permanent pacemaker, AVNRT = AV-nodal reentrant tachycardia, CP = conduction pathway, AVRT = atrioventricular reentrant tachycardia involving an accessory conduction pathway, AP = accessory pathway outside AV node, VPDs = symptomatic ventricular premature depolarizations, NSVT = nonsustained ventricular tachycardia, VT = sustained ventricular tachycardia, ICD = implantable cardioverter–defibrillator, ATPM = anti-tachycardia pacemaker, VF = ventricular fibrillation, ED = electrical defibrillation, SCD = sudden cardiac death.

[b]ODP for termination of atrial flutter only.

[c]Surgery is investigational treatment.

[d]In conjunction with ICD therapy.

[e]Surgery is an option in patients with coronary artery disease or left ventricular dysfunction but is contraindicated in New York Heart Association functional class III or IV heart failure.

effective for the maintenance of sinus rhythm after cardioversion.[115,116]

Despite meta-analytic evidence that quinidine therapy is associated with increased mortality in patients with atrial fibrillation,[9] it is premature to conclude that quinidine should no longer be used to maintain sinus rhythm in such patients, since quinidine has been shown to be effective for this purpose[9] and since the effect of other antiarrhythmic agents on mortality in this population is unknown. Amiodarone is also effective for the maintenance of sinus rhythm in patients with atrial fibrillation, but the frequency of adverse effects associated with this agent, the good long-term prognosis of patients with this arrhythmia, and the need for extended therapy dictate that amiodarone therapy be reserved for patients with atrial fibrillation that is refractory to conventional drug therapy.[117] However, preliminary evidence suggests that amiodarone hydrochloride in relatively low doses (200 mg/day) may be effective for the suppression of atrial fibrillation, thereby reducing the potential for toxicity.[118] Further investigation into the efficacy of low-dose amiodarone in atrial fibrillation is needed.

Atrial Flutter. Like atrial fibrillation, atrial flutter may be paroxysmal or chronic, and the primary goals of therapy are control of ventricular rate and conversion to and maintenance of sinus rhythm. Since drug therapy is often unsuccessful for the conversion of atrial flutter to sinus rhythm, DC cardioversion and rapid atrial pacing are considered alternatives for achieving this therapeutic goal.[119] However, drugs such as β blockers, calcium-channel blockers, and digoxin are useful for controlling the ventricular response.[119] In addition, antiarrhythmic drug therapy is the treatment of choice for the long-term maintenance of sinus rhythm. Class IA agents are considered the first line of therapy, and class IC drugs may be effective as well.[45,119-121] Rarely, however, class IC agents have been reported to cause atrial flutter in patients being treated for atrial fibrillation or other arrhythmias.[122] Amiodarone has been shown to be effective for maintenance of sinus rhythm but is reserved for patients with atrial flutter that is refractory to other antiarrhythmic agents.[119]

Reentrant Paroxysmal Supraventricular Tachycardia (PSVT). PSVT may be due to reentry within the AV node or mediated by an accessory pathway between the atrium and ventricle that is outside the AV node (as in Wolff–Parkinson–White syndrome). The major therapeutic goals are the termination of symptomatic episodes and the prevention of recurrent episodes. Antiarrhythmic drugs are considered the treatment of choice for the termination of episodes of AV-nodal reentrant tachycardia in hemodynamically stable patients who do not respond to vagal maneuvers such as carotid massage.[123] The intravenous administration of verapamil has been reported to terminate 80–85% of such episodes within five minutes.[124,125] The efficacy of adenosine for the termination of PSVT is similar to that of verapamil, but adenosine has the advantages of a shorter duration of action and a lower frequency of hypotension.[126] Recurrent episodes may be prevented by catheter ablation of the slow AV-nodal conduction pathway. However, antiarrhythmic agents are also effective for the prevention of recurrent PSVT and are preferred by some patients. Drug therapy to prevent recurrent episodes of PSVT is directed at interrupting slow antegrade AV-nodal impulse conduction (with such drugs as digoxin, β blockers, and calcium-channel blockers) or at interrupting rapid retrograde AV-nodal conduction (with class IA antiarrhythmic drugs).[123] Class IC agents impair conduction through both limbs of the reentrant circuit and are also effective. Combinations of agents directed at inhibiting conduction over both AV-nodal pathways are often used. Finally, amiodarone therapy may be effective, but it is reserved for patients who do not respond to drugs with a lower potential for toxicity.[123]

In patients with PSVT due to reentry mediated by an extranodal accessory pathway, radiofrequency and DC catheter ablation are reasonable first-line therapies.[107] However, the long-term success and safety of these approaches are uncertain, and drug therapy may be preferred by some patients. Class IA agents, which impair impulse conduction over the accessory pathway, and class IC agents, which inhibit conduction through the AV node and the accessory pathway, are effective.[127] Drugs that inhibit AV-nodal conduction may be effective, but in patients who have short refractory periods in the accessory pathway and a propensity for atrial fibrillation, these agents may facilitate conduction over the accessory pathway and cause ventricular fibrillation.[127] This risk may be assessed during electrophysiologic study. Once again, amiodarone may be effective but is reserved for patients who do not respond adequately to agents with a lower potential for toxicity.[128]

VPDs. Few data exist to support the treatment of asymptomatic VPDs, and CAST showed that suppression of asymptomatic VPDs after MI with encainide or flecainide increases mortality.[1] However, symptomatic VPDs may require treatment with antiarrhythmic drugs. Agents in classes I, II, and III are effective for the suppression of VPDs; the selection of an agent is usually based on the adverse-effect profiles of available agents and is guided by Holter monitoring. Because of their efficacy and comparatively low frequency of adverse effects, β blockers are often used as first-line agents.[129] Encainide and flecainide are contraindicated in patients with ischemic heart disease or a history of MI.[1] Since β blockers reduce mortality after acute MI, drugs in this class should be considered the agents of choice for the suppression of symptomatic VPDs in this patient population.[49,130] It is not known if the beneficial effect of β blockers on mortality after acute MI is related to their antiarrhythmic effects.[131]

Although there are no data indicating that suppression of VPDs favorably influences mortality following acute MI, preliminary data suggest that amiodarone therapy may reduce the incidence of sudden death in these patients. Burkart et al.[132] randomized 312 patients with complex VPDs after acute MI to receive individualized antiarrhythmic drug therapy guided by ambulatory ECG monitoring, amiodarone hydrochloride 1000 mg/day for five days followed by 200 mg/day, or no antiarrhythmic therapy. Primary endpoints of this study were total mortality and arrhythmic events, which were defined as sudden cardiac death, sustained ventricular tachycardia, and ventricular fibrillation. Patients were monitored for one year. Mortality and arrhythmic events were significantly less frequent in the amiodarone-treated group than in the control group. Individualized antiarrhythmic therapy did not significantly influence mortality or arrhythmia-associated events.

In a pilot study to determine the feasibility of a larger multicenter trial, Cairns and colleagues[133] evaluated the efficacy of amiodarone for the reduction of VPDs and mortality in 77 patients experiencing complex VPDs after acute MI. In this double-blind study, patients were randomized in a 2:1 ratio to receive amiodarone hydrochloride 10 mg/kg/day for three weeks followed by 300–400 mg/day, or placebo. The patients were observed for an average of 20 months. The overall rate of mortality in patients treated with amiodarone was 10.4%, which was substantially lower than the 20.7% rate in the placebo group (risk reduction, 50%). Although the sample size was too small for a significant difference in mortality to be identified, a strong trend was demonstrated. It is premature to advocate amiodarone therapy in patients with VPDs after acute MI, but the preliminary data are promising, and a multicenter trial is under way to prospectively evaluate the influence of amiodarone on mortality in patients with complex ventricular ectopy following acute MI.[133]

Nonsustained Ventricular Tachycardia (NSVT). NSVT is a series of at least three consecutive VPDs lasting less than 30 seconds and ending spontaneously.[134] NSVT may cause palpitations or near-syncope. Survivors of acute MI have been shown to be at higher risk of sudden death if NSVT is documented by 24-hour Holter monitoring.[90] The relative risk in other patient populations is not known.

Symptomatic NSVT requires antiarrhythmic drug therapy guided by Holter monitoring or electrophysiologic testing, depending primarily on the presence and severity of underlying structural heart disease.[135] Treatment of asymptomatic NSVT remains controversial. It has been suggested that patients with NSVT who have a left ventricular ejection fraction of <40% and late electrical potentials detected during signal-averaged ECG should undergo electrophysiologic testing; the results would guide the decision to initiate antiarrhythmic drug therapy.[135]

Sustained Ventricular Tachycardia. Sustained ventricular tachycardia lasts 30 seconds or longer and requires intentional termination because of hemodynamic instability.[136] The treatment of choice for hemodynamically unstable ventricular tachycardia is synchronized electrical cardioversion.[137] However, intravenous administration of antiarrhythmic drugs remains the treatment of choice for the management of acute hemodynamically stable sustained or symptomatic ventricular arrhythmias.[137] Lidocaine is considered the best drug for terminating ventricular tachycardia and for prevention in patients experiencing recurrent episodes in the hospital.[137,138] Intravenous procainamide is recommended when acute ventricular tachycardia is refractory to lidocaine therapy.[137,139] These agents have similar efficacies, but procainamide is considered a second-line drug because of its propensity to cause hypotension when administered intravenously.[139]

Patients with sustained ventricular tachycardia for which no underlying cause can be found and corrected may require prolonged antiarrhythmic drug therapy guided by electrophysiologic testing.[135] Antiarrhythmic drugs favorably influence the prognosis in patients in whom a drug has been shown to suppress inducible ventricular tachycardia during electrophysiologic testing. Swerdlow et al.[140] reported that patients with sustained ventricular tachycardia or ventricular fibrillation who received long-term treatment with an antiarrhythmic drug that rendered previously inducible ventricular tachycardia noninducible had a significantly higher rate of survival than patients for whom an effective drug could not be identified. Other investigators have also found that the long-term administration of a drug that suppresses inducible ventricular tachycardia during electrophysiologic testing reduces arrhythmia recurrence and mortality.[89,141-144] Waller et al.[144] observed significantly lower mortality in patients with sustained ventricular tachycardia or ventricular fibrillation who received long-term therapy with an antiarrhythmic drug that suppressed inducible ventricular tachycardia compared with patients for whom an effective drug could not be identified. In addition, these investigators determined that long-term therapy with a drug that reduced the rate or eliminated the symptoms of a still-inducible ventricular tachycardia also significantly reduced mortality.[144] In summary, antiarrhythmic drug therapy is the treatment of choice in patients with recurrent sustained ventricular tachycardia for whom an effective drug can be identified by electrophysiologic testing.

Ventricular Fibrillation. Asynchronous electrical defibrillation is the treatment of choice for the termination of ventricular fibrillation.[137] However, intravenous antiarrhythmic drugs are indicated for facilitating termination of resistant ventricular fibrillation. Lidocaine is considered the best drug for this indication.[137] Bretylium is also efficacious, and it has been shown to be effective in patients in whom lidocaine therapy is unsuccessful.[145]

Patients who have been resuscitated from an out-of-hospital cardiac arrest in the absence of acute MI, exacerbation of congestive heart failure, electrolyte imbalance, or some other reversible cause require therapy to prevent subsequent episodes. Sudden cardiac death is usually due to ventricular fibrillation.[146] ICD therapy is the treatment of choice in patients in whom arrhythmias are not inducible during electrophysiologic testing. However, in patients in whom arrhythmias are inducible and who do not wish to undergo major surgery, antiarrhythmic drug therapy is a reasonable alternative. Although recent data are contradictory,[22,147] several studies have shown that long-term administration of effective antiarrhythmic therapy guided by electrophysiologic studies favorably influences the frequency of recurrent cardiac arrest and the mortality rate in survivors of an out-of-hospital cardiac arrest.[89,148,149]

Diagnosis of Wide-QRS-Complex Tachyarrhythmias. Wide-QRS-complex tachycardias are often misdiagnosed on the basis of interpretation of the surface ECG alone. If a patient with PSVT is misdiagnosed as having ventricular tachycardia, lidocaine may be mistakenly administered, and appropriate treatment may be delayed. On the other hand, if a patient with ventricular tachycardia is misdiagnosed as having PSVT, verapamil may be mistakenly administered, which may result in hypotension or cardiac arrest.[150]

Adenosine has been used successfully to differentiate ventricular tachycardia from PSVT when the diagnosis could not be made with confidence based on the surface ECG. The predictive accuracy of adenosine for this indication has been reported to be 92%.[151] Therefore, adenosine may be extremely useful for diagnosing wide-QRS-complex tachycardias, facilitating rapid and effective treatment, and avoiding potentially dangerous interventions. Alternatively, intravenous procainamide is often recommended for managing wide-QRS tachycardias, as it may be effective for the termination of ventricular tachycardia or PSVT and does not result in hemodynamic deterioration in patients with Wolff–Parkinson–White syndrome.[152,153]

Discussion

Antiarrhythmic drug therapy is associated with a number of clinical problems. The frequency of adverse effects may be high, pharmacokinetic and pharmacodynamic interactions may occur, and these agents may impair the efficacy of electrical antiarrhythmic devices. Antiarrhythmic agents have been shown to be of limited efficacy in certain patient populations, and some agents have proved dangerous in specific clinical situations and should be avoided. In particular, antiarrhythmic agents should not be administered empirically for the treatment of asymptomatic VPDs in patients after acute MI.

Nonpharmacologic forms of antiarrhythmic therapy are available, and some of these, such as catheter ablation and ICDs, have become the treatments of choice for some cardiac arrhythmias. However, despite the availability of effective forms of nonpharmacologic therapy and the problems associated with antiarrhythmic drug therapy, antiarrhythmic drugs are not obsolete. Some nonpharmacologic therapies, such as ICDs, are expensive. Other nonpharmacologic options, such as surgery for ventricular tachycardia, are not only expensive but are associated with high rates of mortality. The long-term efficacy and safety of catheter ablation remain uncertain. Antiarrhythmic agents are currently the safest and most effective treatment for some cardiac arrhythmias and are preferred over invasive procedures by many patients.

Although nonpharmacologic treatments for cardiac arrhythmias will no doubt continue to be developed and will become more sophisticated, antiarrhythmic drugs are unlikely to become obsolete in the foreseeable future. However, the endpoints of drug efficacy may change. For example, many patients with ICDs receive long-term therapy with antiarrhythmic drugs to reduce the frequency of shocks. New endpoints for antiarrhythmic drug efficacy may therefore include reducing the frequency of discharges in patients with ICDs and thereby prolonging ICD battery life.

Future trends may also include the development of antiarrhythmic drugs that are more effective and less toxic and that do not influence defibrillation or pacing thresholds. New methods of delivering antiarrhythmic drugs are under study, including the retrograde infusion of agents directly into the coronary sinus of the heart[154] and the implantation of pumps in the heart to automatically infuse antiarrhythmic drugs during detected arrhythmias.[155]

Conclusion

Despite the availability of effective nonpharmacologic forms of antiarrhythmic therapy, drugs are likely to remain important for the treatment of cardiac arrhythmias. The challenge for clinicians is to select those drugs and dosages that maximize benefit and minimize toxicity for individual patients. The challenge for investigators is to develop antiarrhythmic agents that are more effective and induce fewer adverse effects than currently available drugs.

References

1. Cardiac Arrhythmia Suppression Trial (CAST) Investigators. Preliminary report: effect of encainide and flecainide on mortality in a randomized trial of arrhythmia suppression after myocardial infarction. *N Engl J Med.* 1989; 321:406-12.
2. Vaughan Williams EM. A classification of antiarrhythmic actions reassessed after a decade of new drugs. *J Clin Pharmacol.* 1984; 24:129-47.
3. Vaughan Williams EM. Classification of the antiarrhythmic action of moricizine. *J Clin Pharmacol.* 1991; 31:216-21.
4. Aronow WS, Mercando AD, Epstein S et al. Effect of quinidine or procainamide versus no antiarrhythmic drug on sudden cardiac death, total cardiac death, and total death in elderly patients with heart disease and complex ventricular arrhythmias. *Am J Cardiol.* 1990; 66:423-8.
5. Rydén L, Arnman K, Conradson T-B et al. Prophylaxis of ventricular tachyarrhythmias with intravenous and oral tocainide in patients with and recovering from acute myocardial infarction. *Am Heart J.* 1980; 100:1006-12.

6. Bastian BC, Macfarlane PW, McLauchlan JH et al. A prospective randomized trial of tocainide in patients following myocardial infarction. *Am Heart J*. 1980; 100:1017-22.
7. Chamberlain DA, Julian DG, Boyle DM et al. Oral mexiletine in high-risk patients after myocardial infarction. *Lancet*. 1980; 2:1324-7.
8. Impact Research Group. International mexiletine and placebo antiarrhythmic coronary trial: I. Report on arrhythmia and other findings. *J Am Coll Cardiol*. 1984; 4:1148-63.
9. Coplen SE, Antman EM, Berlin JA et al. Efficacy and safety of quinidine therapy for maintenance of sinus rhythm after cardioversion. A meta-analysis of randomized control trials. *Circulation*. 1990; 82:1106-16.
10. Teo K, Yusuf S, Furberg C. Effect of antiarrhythmic drug therapy on mortality following myocardial infarction. *Circulation*. 1990; 82:III-197. Abstract.
11. Hine LK, Laird NM, Hewitt P et al. Meta-analysis of empirical long-term antiarrhythmic therapy after myocardial infarction. *JAMA*. 1989; 262:3037-40.
12. Anderson JL. Reassessment of benefit–risk ratio treatment algorithms for antiarrhythmic drug therapy after the Cardiac Arrhythmia Suppression Trial. *J Clin Pharmacol*. 1990; 30:981-9.
13. Morganroth J, Goin JE. Quinidine-related mortality in the short-to-medium-term treatment of ventricular arrhythmias. A meta-analysis. *Circulation*. 1991; 84:1977-83.
14. McCollam PL, Parker RB, Beckman KJ et al. Proarrhythmia: a paradoxic response to antiarrhythmic agents. *Pharmacotherapy*. 1989; 9:144-53.
15. Mehta D, Saxena A. Safety of use of antiarrhythmic drugs. *Indian Heart J*. 1990; 42:445-50.
16. Kay GN, Plumb VJ, Dailey SM et al. Current role of the automatic implantable cardioverter–defibrillator in the treatment of life-threatening ventricular arrhythmias. *Am J Med*. 1990; 88:25N-34N.
17. Jackman WM, Wang X, Friday KJ et al. Catheter ablation of accessory atrioventricular pathways (Wolff-Parkinson-White syndrome) by radiofrequency current. *N Engl J Med*. 1991; 324:1605-11.
18. Calkins H, Sousa J, El-Atassi R et al. Diagnosis and cure of the Wolff-Parkinson-White syndrome or paroxysmal supraventricular tachycardias during a single electrophysiologic test. *N Engl J Med*. 1991; 324:1612-8.
19. Klein GJ, Guiraudon GM, Sharma AJ et al. Surgery for tachycardia: indications and electrophysiologic assessment. *Circulation*. 1987; 75(Suppl 3):186-9.
20. Lehmann MH, Steinman RT, Schuger CD et al. The automatic implantable cardioverter defibrillator as antiarrhythmic treatment modality of choice for survivors of cardiac arrest unrelated to acute myocardial infarction. *Am J Cardiol*. 1988; 62:803-5.
21. Prystowsky EN, Katz A, Knilans TK. Ventricular arrhythmias: risk stratification and approach to therapy after the Cardiac Arrhythmia Suppression Trial (CAST). *PACE*. 1990; 13:1480-7.
22. Sousa J, Rosenheck S, Calkins H et al. Results of electrophysiologic testing and long-term prognosis in patients with coronary artery disease and aborted sudden death. *Am Heart J*. 1991; 122:1001-6.
23. Salperno DM. Quinidine. Worse than adverse? *Circulation*. 1991; 84:2196-8.
24. Cohen IS, Jick H, Cohen S. Adverse reactions to quinidine in hospitalized patients: findings based on data from the Boston Collaborative Drug Surveillance Program. *Prog Cardiovasc Dis*. 1977; 20:151-63.
25. Arif M, Laidlaw JC, Oshrain C et al. A randomized, double-blind parallel group comparison of disopyramide phosphate and quinidine in patients with cardiac arrhythmias. *Angiology*. 1983; 34:393-400.
26. Fenster PE, Hanson CD. Mexiletine and quinidine in ventricular ectopy. *Clin Pharmacol Ther*. 1983; 34:136-42.
27. Flecainide–Quinidine Research Group. Flecainide versus quinidine for treatment of chronic ventricular arrhythmias. A multicenter clinical trial. *Circulation*. 1983; 67:1117-23.
28. Singh JB, Rasul AM, Shah A et al. Efficacy of mexiletine in chronic ventricular arrhythmias compared with quinidine: a single-blind, randomized trial. *Am J Cardiol*. 1984; 53:84-7.
29. Morganroth J, Oshrain C, Steele PP. Comparative efficacy and safety of oral tocainide and quinidine for benign and potentially lethal ventricular arrhythmias. *Am J Cardiol*. 1985; 56:581-5.
30. Wasty N, Saksena S, Barr MJ. Comparative efficacy and safety of oral cibenzoline and quinidine in ventricular arrhythmias: a randomized cross-over study. *Am Heart J*. 1985; 110:1181-8.
31. Chandraratna PAN. Comparison of acebutolol with propranolol, quinidine, and placebo: results of three multicenter arrhythmia trials. *Am Heart J*. 1985; 109:1198-204.
32. Morganroth J, Somberg JC, Pool PE et al. Comparative study of encainide and quinidine in the treatment of ventricular arrhythmias. *J Am Coll Cardiol*. 1986; 7:9-16.
33. Kosowsky BD, Taylor J, Lown B et al. Long-term use of procaine amide following acute myocardial infarction. *Circulation*. 1973; 47:1204-10.
34. Winkle RA, Gradman AH, Fitzgerald JW et al. Antiarrhythmic drug effect assessed from ventricular arrhythmia reduction in the ambulatory electrocardiogram and treadmill test: comparison of propranolol, procainamide and quinidine. *Am J Cardiol*. 1978; 42:473-80.
35. Giardina E-GV, Fenster PE, Bigger JT et al. Efficacy, plasma concentrations and adverse effects of a new sustained release procainamide preparation. *Am J Cardiol*. 1980; 46:855-62.
36. Podrid PJ, Schoeneberger A, Lown B. Congestive heart failure caused by oral disopyramide. *N Engl J Med*. 1980; 302:614-7.
37. Lerman BB, Waxman HL, Buxton AE et al. Disopyramide: evaluation of electrophysiologic effects and clinical efficacy in patients with sustained ventricular tachycardia or ventricular fibrillation. *Am J Cardiol*. 1983; 51:759-64.
38. Zema MJ. Serum drug concentrations and adverse effects in cardiac patients after administration of a new controlled-release disopyramide preparation. *Ther Drug Monit*. 1984; 6:192-8.
39. Bauman JL, Gallastegui J, Strasberg B et al. Long-term therapy with disopyramide phosphate: side effects and effectiveness. *Am Heart J*. 1986; 111:654-60.
40. Lie KI, Wellens HJ, van Capelle FJ et al. Lidocaine in the prevention of primary ventricular fibrillation. A double-blind, randomized study of 212 consecutive patients. *N Engl J Med*. 1974; 291:1324-6.
41. Rademaker AW, Kellen J, Tam YK et al. Character of adverse effects of prophylactic lidocaine in the coronary care unit. *Clin Pharmacol Ther*. 1986; 40:71-80.
42. Wyse DG, Kellen J, Rademaker AW. Prophylactic versus selective lidocaine for early ventricular arrhythmias of myocardial infarction. *J Am Coll Cardiol*. 1988; 12:507-13.
43. Kreeger RW, Hammill SC. New antiarrhythmic drugs: tocainide, mexiletine, flecainide, encainide, and amiodarone. *Mayo Clin Proc*. 1987; 62:1033-50.
44. Nappi JM, Anderson JL. Flecainide: a new prototype antiarrhythmic agent. *Pharmacotherapy*. 1985; 5:209-21.
45. Anderson JL, Jolivette DM, Fredell PA. Summary of efficacy and safety of flecainide for supraventricular arrhythmias. *Am J Cardiol*. 1988; 62:62D-66D.
46. Chow MSS, Lebsack C, Hilleman D. Propafenone: a new antiarrhythmic agent. *Clin Pharm*. 1988; 7:869-77.
47. Kennedy HL. Noncardiac adverse effects and organ toxicity of moricizine during short- and long-term studies. *Am J Cardiol*. 1990; 65:47D-50D.
48. Greenblatt DJ, Koch-Weser J. Adverse reactions to β-adrenergic receptor blocking drugs: a report from the Boston Collaborative Drug Surveillance Program. *Drugs*. 1974; 7:118-29.
49. Beta-blocker Heart Attack Trial Research Group. A randomized trial of propranolol in patients with acute myocardial

infarction. I. Mortality results. *JAMA*. 1982; 247:1707-14.
50. Anderson JL. Bretylium tosylate: profile of the only available class III antiarrhythmic agent. *Clin Ther*. 1985; 7:205-24.
51. Wilson JS, Podrid PJ. Side effects from amiodarone. *Am Heart J*. 1991; 121:158-71.
52. Lewis JG. Adverse reactions to calcium antagonists. *Drugs*. 1983; 25:196-222.
53. McGraw BF, Walker SD, Hemberger JA et al. Clinical experience with diltiazem in Japan. *Pharmacotherapy*. 1982; 2:156-61.
54. Gibson RS, Boden WE, Theroux P et al. Diltiazem and reinfarction in patients with non-Q-wave myocardial infarction. Results of a double-blind, randomized, multicenter trial. *N Engl J Med*. 1986; 315:423-9.
55. Frishman WH, Zawada ET, Smith LK et al. Comparison of hydrochlorothiazide and sustained-release diltiazem for mild-to-moderate systemic hypertension. *Am J Cardiol*. 1987; 59:615- 23.
56. Opie LH. Clinical use of calcium channel antagonist drugs. Boston: Kluwer Academic; 1989.
57. Gotsman MS, Schrire V. Toxicity—a frequent complication of digitalis therapy. *S Afr Med J*. 1966; 40:590-3.
58. Shapiro S, Slone D, Lewis GP et al. The epidemiology of digoxin. A study in three Boston hospitals. *J Chronic Dis*. 1969; 22:361-71.
59. Beller GA, Smith TW, Abelmann WH et al. Digitalis intoxication: a prospective clinical study with serum level correlations. *N Engl J Med*. 1971; 284:989-97.
60. Mahdyoon H, Battilana G, Rosman H et al. The evolving pattern of digoxin intoxication: observations at a large urban hospital from 1980 to 1988. *Am Heart J*. 1990; 120:1189-94.
61. Parker RB, McCollam PL. Adenosine in the episodic treatment of paroxysmal supraventricular tachycardia. *Clin Pharm*. 1990; 9:261-74.
62. Blomgren SE, Condemi JJ, Vaughan JH. Procainamide-induced lupus erythematosus. Clinical and laboratory observations. *Am J Med*. 1972; 52:338-48.
63. Ellrodt AG, Murata GH, Riedinger MS et al. Severe neutropenia associated with sustained-release procainamide. *Ann Intern Med*. 1984; 100:197-201.
64. Raehl CL, Patel AK, LeRoy M. Drug-induced torsade de pointes. *Clin Pharm*. 1985; 4:675-90.
65. Cosín-Aguilar J, Hernandiz-Martinez A. The clinical usefulness of the antiarrhythmic drug quinidine. *Eur Heart J*. 1987; 8(Suppl A):1-9.
66. Lima JJ, Goldfarb AL, Conti DR et al. Safety and efficacy of procainamide infusions. *Am J Cardiol*. 1979; 43:98-105.
67. Chew CYC, Hecht HS, Colett JT et al. Influence of severity of ventricular dysfunction on hemodynamic responses to intravenously administered verapamil in ischemic heart disease. *Am J Cardiol*. 1981; 47:917-22.
68. Hughes B, Dyer JE, Schwartz AB. Increased procainamide plasma concentrations caused by quinidine: a new drug interaction. *Am Heart J*. 1987; 114:908-9.
69. Twum-Barima Y, Carruthers SG. Quinidine–rifampin interaction. *N Engl J Med*. 1981; 304:1466-9.
70. Kosoglou T, Vlasses PH. Drug interactions involving renal transport mechanisms: an overview. *DICP Ann Pharmacother*. 1989; 23:116-22.
71. Willis PW. The clinical scope of disopyramide seven years after introduction—an overview. *Angiology*. 1987; 38:165-73.
72. Pieper JA, Rodman JH. Lidocaine. In: Evans WE, Schentag JJ, Jusko WJ, eds. Applied pharmacokinetics. Principles of therapeutic drug monitoring. 2nd ed. Spokane, WA: Applied Therapeutics; 1986:639-81.
73. Ueno K, Miyai K, Kato M et al. Mechanism of interaction between theophylline and mexiletine. *DICP Ann Pharmacother*. 1991; 25:727-9.
74. Lewis GP, Holtzman JL. Interaction of flecainide with digoxin and propranolol. *Am J Cardiol*. 1984; 53:52B-7B.
75. Mann HJ. Moricizine: a new class I antiarrhythmic. *Clin Pharm*. 1990; 9:842-52.
76. Lesko LJ. Pharmacokinetic drug interactions with amiodarone. *Clin Pharmacokinet*. 1989; 17:130-40.
77. Schlanz KD, Myre SA, Bottorff MB. Pharmacokinetic interactions with calcium channel antagonists (part I). *Clin Pharmacokinet*. 1991; 21:344-56.
78. Schlanz KD, Myre SA, Bottorff MB. Pharmacokinetic interactions with calcium channel antagonists (part II). *Clin Pharmacokinet*. 1991; 21:448-60.
79. Barbarash RA, Bauman JL, Fischer JH et al. Near-total reduction in verapamil bioavailability by rifampin: electrocardiographic correlates. *Chest*. 1988; 94:955-9.
80. Rodin SM, Johnson BF. Pharmacokinetic interactions with digoxin. *Clin Pharmacokinet*. 1988; 15:227-44.
81. Tisdale JE. Combination antiarrhythmic therapy. *Conn Med*. 1989; 53:101-5.
82. Prystowsky EN. Effects of bepridil on cardiac electrophysiologic properties. *Am J Cardiol*. 1992; 69:63D-7D.
83. Gottlieb CD, Horowitz LN. Potential interactions between antiarrhythmic medication and the automatic implantable cardioverter defibrillator. *PACE*. 1991; 14(part 2):898-904.
84. Tworek DA, Nazari J, Ezri M et al. Interference by antiarrhythmic agents with function of electrical cardiac devices. *Clin Pharm*. 1992; 11:48-56.
85. Reiffel JA, Coromilas J, Zimmerman JM et al. Drug–device interactions: clinical considerations. *PACE*. 1985; 8(part 1):369- 73.
86. Guarnieri T, Tomaselli G, Griffith LSC et al. The interaction of antiarrhythmic drugs and the energy for cardioversion of chronic atrial fibrillation. *PACE*. 1991; 14:1007-12.
87. Rae AP, Greenspan AM, Spielman SR et al. Antiarrhythmic drug efficacy for ventricular tachyarrhythmias associated with coronary artery disease as assessed by electrophysiologic studies. *Am J Cardiol*. 1985; 55:1494-9.
88. Wellens HJJ, Brugada P, Stevenson WG. Programmed electrical stimulation: its role in the management of ventricular arrhythmias in coronary heart disease. *Prog Cardiovasc Dis*. 1986; 29:165-80.
89. Wilber DJ, Garan H, Finkelstein D et al. Out-of-hospital cardiac arrest. Use of electrophysiologic testing in the prediction of long-term outcome. *N Engl J Med*. 1988; 318:19-24.
90. Bigger JT, Fleiss JL, Kleiger R et al. The relationship among ventricular arrhythmias, left ventricular dysfunction and mortality in the 2 years after myocardial infarction. *Circulation*. 1984; 69:250-8.
91. Mukharji J, Rude RE, Poole KE et al. Risk factors for sudden death after acute myocardial infarction: two-year follow-up. *Am J Cardiol*. 1984; 54:31-6.
92. May GS, Eberlein KA, Furberg CD et al. Secondary prevention after myocardial infarction: a review of long-term trials. *Prog Cardiovasc Dis*. 1982; 24:331-52.
93. Furberg CD. Effect of antiarrhythmic drugs on mortality after myocardial infarction. *Am J Cardiol*. 1983; 52:32C-6C.
94. Gottlieb SH, Achuff SC, Mellits ED et al. Prophylactic antiarrhythmic therapy of high-risk survivors of myocardial infarction: lower mortality at 1 month but not at 1 year. *Circulation*. 1987; 75:792-9.
95. Gheorghiade M, Goldstein S. Arrhythmia suppression in postmyocardial infarction patients with special notation to Cardiac Arrhythmia Suppression Trial. *Prog Cardiovasc Dis*. 1991; 33:213-8.
96. Bigger JT. The events surrounding the removal of encainide and flecainide from the Cardiac Arrhythmia Suppression Trial (CAST) and why CAST is continuing with moricizine. *J Am Coll Cardiol*. 1990; 15:243-5.
97. Greene HL, Roden DM, Katz RJ et al. The Cardiac Arrhythmia Suppression Trial: first CAST . . . then CAST-II. *J Am Coll Cardiol*. 1992; 19:894-8.
98. Hine LK, Laird NM, Hewitt P et al. Meta-analytic evidence against prophylactic use of lidocaine in acute myocardial infarction. *Arch Intern Med*. 1989; 149:2694-8.
99. Mirowski M. The automatic implantable cardioverter–defibrillator; an overview. *J Am Coll Cardiol*. 1985; 6:461-6.
100. Cannom DS. Automatic implantable cardioverter defib-

rillator. In: Horowitz LN, ed. Current management of arrhythmias. Philadelphia: Decker; 1991:417-23.
101. Winkle RA. State-of-the-art of the AICD. *PACE*. 1991; 14(part 2):961-6.
102. Kelly PA, Cannom DS, Garan H et al. The automatic implantable cardioverter–defibrillator: efficacy, complications and survival in patients with malignant ventricular arrhythmias. *J Am Coll Cardiol*. 1988; 11:1278-86.
103. Winkle RA, Mead RH, Ruder MA et al. Long-term outcome with the automatic implantable cardioverter–defibrillator. *J Am Coll Cardiol*. 1989; 13:1353-61.
104. Klein LS, Miles WM, Zipes DP. Antitachycardia devices: realities and promises. *J Am Coll Cardiol*. 1991; 18:1349-62.
105. Roy D, Waxman HL, Buxton AE et al. Termination of ventricular tachycardia: role of ventricular tachycardia cycle length. *Am J Cardiol*. 1982; 50:1346-50.
106. Hindricks G, Borggrefe M, Haverkamp W et al. Catheter ablation. In: Horowitz LN, ed. Current management of arrhythmias. Philadelphia: Decker; 1991:373-8.
107. Leather RA, Leitch JW, Klein GJ et al. Radiofrequency catheter ablation of accessory pathways: a learning experience. *Am J Cardiol*. 1991; 68:1651-5.
108. Ferguson TB, Cox JL. Antiarrhythmic surgery: ventricular arrhythmias. In: Horowitz LN, ed. Current management of arrhythmias. Philadelphia: Decker; 1991:382-91.
109. Ostermeyer J, Borggrefe M, Breithardt G et al. Direct operations for the management of life-threatening ischemic ventricular tachycardia. *J Thorac Cardiovasc Surg*. 1987; 94:848- 61.
110. Kron IL, Lerman BB, Nolan SP et al. Sequential endocardial resection for the surgical treatment of refractory ventricular tachycardia. *J Thorac Cardiovasc Surg*. 1987; 94:843-7.
111. Kehoe R, Zheutlin T, Finkelmeier B et al. Visually directed endocardial resection for ventricular arrhythmia: long term outcome and functional status. *J Am Coll Cardiol*. 1985; 5:497. Abstract.
112. Miller JM, Gottlieb CD, Hargrove WC et al. Factors influencing operative mortality in surgery for ventricular tachycardia. *Circulation*. 1988; 78:II-44. Abstract.
113. Swerdlow CD, Mason JW, Stinson EB et al. Results of operations for ventricular tachycardia in 105 patients. *J Thorac Cardiovasc Surg*. 1986; 92:105-13.
114. Lewis RV. Atrial fibrillation. The therapeutic options. *Drugs*. 1990; 40:841-53.
115. Bauernfeind RA, Welch WJ. New hope in atrial fibrillation. *J Am Coll Cardiol*. 1990; 15:708-9.
116. Anderson JL, Gilbert EM, Alpert BL et al. Prevention of symptomatic recurrences of paroxysmal atrial fibrillation in patients initially tolerating antiarrhythmic therapy. A multicenter, double-blind, crossover study of flecainide and placebo with transtelephonic monitoring. *Circulation*. 1989; 80:1557-70.
117. Gold RL, Haffajee CI, Charos G et al. Amiodarone for refractory atrial fibrillation. *Am J Cardiol*. 1986; 57:124-7.
118. Ward DE, Camm AJ, Spurell RAJ. Clinical antiarrhythmic effects of amiodarone in patients with resistant paroxysmal tachycardias. *Br Heart J*. 1980; 44:91-5.
119. Waldo AL. Atrial flutter. In: Horowitz LN, ed. Current management of arrhythmias. Philadelphia: Decker; 1991:58-64.
120. Van Gelder IC, Crijns HJGM, Van Gilst WH et al. Efficacy and safety of flecainide acetate in the maintenance of sinus rhythm after electrical cardioversion of chronic atrial fibrillation or atrial flutter. *Am J Cardiol*. 1989; 64:1317-21.
121. Crijns HJ, Van Gelder IC, Van Gilst WH et al. Serial antiarrhythmic drug treatment to maintain sinus rhythm after electrical cardioversion for chronic atrial fibrillation or atrial flutter. *Am J Cardiol*. 1991; 68:335-41.
122. Feld GK, Chen P-S, Nicod P et al. Possible atrial proarrhythmic effects of class IC antiarrhythmic drugs. *Am J Cardiol*. 1990; 66:378-83.
123. Huycke EC, Sung RJ. Paroxysmal reentrant supraventricular tachycardia without preexcitation: pharmacologic therapy. In: Horowitz LN, ed. Current management of arrhythmias. Philadelphia: Decker; 1991:74-80.
124. Rinkenberger RL, Prystowsky EN, Heger JJ et al. Effects of intravenous and chronic oral verapamil administration in patients with supraventricular tachyarrhythmias. *Circulation*. 1980; 62:996-1010.
125. Sung RJ, Elser B, McAllister RG. Intravenous verapamil for termination of re-entrant supraventricular tachycardias. *Ann Intern Med*. 1980; 93:682-9.
126. DiMarco JP, Miles W, Ahktar M et al. Adenosine for paroxysmal supraventricular tachycardia: dose ranging and comparison with verapamil. *Ann Intern Med*. 1990; 113:104-10.
127. Cain ME, Lindsay BD. Preexcitation syndromes: diagnostic and management strategies. In: Horowitz LN, ed. Current management of arrhythmias. Philadelphia: Decker; 1991: 91-103.
128. Feld GK, Nademanee K, Weiss J et al. Electrophysiologic basis for the suppression by amiodarone of orthodromic supraventricular tachycardias complicating pre-excitation syndromes. *J Am Coll Cardiol*. 1984; 3:1298-307.
129. Morganroth J. Ventricular premature complexes and unsustained ventricular tachycardia: noninvasive approach. In: Horowitz LN, ed. Current management of arrhythmias. Philadelphia: Decker; 1991:138-41.
130. Norwegian Multicenter Study Group. Timolol-induced reduction in mortality and reinfarction in patients surviving acute myocardial infarction. *N Engl J Med*. 1981; 304:801-7.
131. Frishman WH, Lazar EJ. Reduction of mortality, sudden death and non-fatal reinfarction with beta-adrenergic blockers in survivors of acute myocardial infarction: a new hypothesis regarding the cardioprotective action of beta-adrenergic blockade. *Am J Cardiol*. 1990; 66:66G-70G.
132. Burkart F, Pfisterer M, Kiowski W et al. Effect of antiarrhythmic therapy on mortality in survivors of myocardial infarction with asymptomatic complex ventricular arrhythmias: Basel antiarrhythmic study of infarct survival (BASIS). *J Am Coll Cardiol*. 1990; 16:1711-8.
133. Cairns JA, Connolly SJ, Gent M et al. Post-myocardial infarction mortality in patients with ventricular premature depolarizations. Canadian amiodarone myocardial infarction arrhythmia trial pilot study. *Circulation*. 1991; 84:550-7.
134. Buxton AE, Marchlinski FE, Flores BT et al. Nonsustained ventricular tachycardia in patients with coronary artery disease: role of electrophysiology study. *Circulation*. 1987; 75:1178-85.
135. McCollam PL, Parker RB. Evaluation and treatment of ventricular arrhythmias: an update. *Clin Pharm*. 1991; 10:195-205.
136. Kastor JA. Ventricular tachycardia. *Clin Cardiol*. 1989; 12:586-99.
137. American Heart Association. Textbook of advanced cardiac life support. 2nd ed. Dallas: American Heart Association; 1987.
138. Griffith MJ, Linker NJ, Garratt CJ et al. Relative efficacy and safety of intravenous drugs for termination of sustained ventricular tachycardia. *Lancet*. 1990; 336:670-3.
139. Harrison DC, Sprouse JH, Morrow AG. The antiarrhythmic properties of lidocaine and procaine amide. Clinical and physiologic studies of their cardiovascular effects in man. *Circulation*. 1963; 28:486-91.
140. Swerdlow CD, Winkle RA, Mason JW. Determinants of survival in patients with ventricular tachyarrhythmias. *N Engl J Med*. 1983; 308:1436-42.
141. Horowitz LN, Josephson ME, Farshidi A et al. Recurrent sustained ventricular tachycardia. 3. Role of the electrophysiology study in selection of antiarrhythmic regimens. *Circulation*. 1978; 58:986-97.
142. Mason JW, Winkle RA. Accuracy of the ventricular tachycardia-induction study for predicting long-term efficacy and inefficacy of antiarrhythmic drugs. *N Engl J Med*. 1980; 303:1073-7.
143. Horowitz LN, Spielman SR, Greenspan AM et al. Ventricular arrhythmias: use of electrophysiologic studies. *Am Heart J*. 1983; 106:881-6.
144. Waller TJ, Kay HR, Spielman SR et al. Reduction in sudden

death and total mortality by antiarrhythmic therapy evaluated by electrophysiologic drug testing: criteria of efficacy in patients with sustained ventricular tachyarrhythmia. *J Am Coll Cardiol.* 1987; 10:83-9.

145. Holder DA, Sniderman AD, Fraser G et al. Experience with bretylium tosylate by a hospital cardiac arrest team. *Circulation.* 1977; 55:541-4.
146. Greene LH. Sudden arrhythmic cardiac death—mechanisms, resuscitation and classification: the Seattle perspective. *Am J Cardiol.* 1990; 65:4B-12B.
147. Poole JE, Mathisen TL, Kudenchuk PJ et al. Long-term outcome in patients who survive out of hospital ventricular fibrillation and undergo electrophysiologic studies: evaluation by electrophysiologic subgroups. *J Am Coll Cardiol.* 1990; 16:657-65.
148. Ruskin JN, DiMarco JP, Garan H. Out-of-hospital cardiac arrest. Electrophysiologic observations and selection of long-term antiarrhythmic therapy. *N Engl J Med.* 1980; 303:607-13.
149. Benditt DG, Benson DW, Klein GJ et al. Prevention of recurrent cardiac arrest: role of provocative electropharmacologic testing. *J Am Coll Cardiol.* 1983; 2:418-25.
150. Buxton AE, Marchlinski FE, Doherty JU et al. Hazards of intravenous verapamil for sustained ventricular tachycardia. *Am J Cardiol.* 1987; 59:1107-10.
151. Faulds D, Chrisp P, Buckley MM-T. Adenosine. An evaluation of its use in cardiac diagnostic procedures, and in the treatment of paroxysmal supraventricular tachycardia. *Drugs.* 1991; 41:596-624.
152. Wellens HJJ. The wide QRS tachycardia. *Ann Intern Med.* 1986; 104:879. Editorial.
153. Levitt MA. Supraventricular tachycardia with aberrant conduction versus ventricular tachycardia: differentiation and diagnosis. *Am J Emerg Med.* 1988; 6:273-7.
154. Karagueuzian HS, Ohta M, Drury JK et al. Coronary venous retroinfusion of procainamide: a new approach for the management of spontaneous and inducible sustained ventricular tachycardia during myocardial infarction. *J Am Coll Cardiol.* 1986; 7:551-63.
155. Cammilli L, Mugelli A, Grassi G et al. Implantable pharmacological defibrillator (AIPhD): preliminary investigations in animals. *PACE.* 1991; 14(part 2):381-6.

DUE Criteria

The DUE Criteria *section of* Clinical Pharmacy *features model drug-use evaluation criteria that may be employed as a component of a comprehensive quaity assurance program. The criteria sets are presented in the format used in the ASHP book* Criteria for Drug Use Evaluation. *Some of the criteria sets will have been originally published in that book; others will be presented here for the first time and published in future volumes of the ASHP book. The practitioners who developed a criteria set are acknowledged.*

In selecting drug products for coverage in DUE Criteria, *priority is given to products that have been recently marketed, those that are frequently prescribed, those that have high potential risk associated with their use, and those that are expensive. When feasible, a criteria set will be linked with a Drug Review that appears in the same issue.*

These criteria sets are a starting point for the development of DUE criteria for a specific practice setting. Readers are encouraged to modify the model criteria to fit their own circumstances.

Criteria for use of adenosine in adults with paroxysmal supraventricular tachycardia[a]

Element	Standard 100%	Standard 0%	Exception[b] or Critical Preventive/ Responsive Measure[c]	Sources of Information
Justification for Use 1. Conversion of paroxysmal supraventricular tachycardia (PSVT) to sinus rhythm when at least one of the following conditions is met[1-7]: a. PSVT does not respond to a cumulative verapamil hydrochloride dose of 10 mg or to a cumulative dose of <10 mg if hypotension (systolic blood pressure <90 mm Hg or diastolic blood pressure <70 mm Hg) develops b. Use of verapamil is contraindicated because of at least one of the following conditions: (1) Hypotension (systolic blood pressure <90 mm Hg or diastolic blood pressure <70 mm Hg) (2) Signs or symptoms of congestive heart failure (e.g., jugular venous distention, third heart sound, pulmonary congestion, edema) (3) Left ventricular ejection fraction <0.40 (4) Pretreatment with i.v. β-adrenergic blocker c. Possibility that PSVT is associated with accessory bypass tracts is	X		1A. None	1. Electrocardiogram (ECG), history and physical (H&P), physician orders, progress notes, medication administration record (MAR)

Prepared by Enid Morales, Pharm.D., Assistant Professor, Department of Pharmacy Practice, College of Pharmacy, Rutgers University, Piscataway, NJ, and Patrick L. McCollam, Pharm.D., Assistant Professor, Department of Clinical Pharmacy, College of Pharmacy, Medical University of South Carolina, Charleston.

Presented in part at the 26th Annual ASHP Midyear Clinical Meeting, New Orleans, LA, December 9, 1991.

Element	Standard 100%	Standard 0%	Exception[b] or Critical Preventive/ Responsive Measure[c]	Sources of Information
supported by at least one of the following[3,5-7]: (1) History of preexcitation syndrome (2) Presence of accessory pathway diagnosed by electrophysiologic study or previous adenosine challenge (3) Evidence of preexcitation on ECG or				
2. Production of atrioventricular (AV) block to aid in diagnosis of latent preexcitation syndrome in patient with both of the following[3,7,8]: a. ECG showing sinus rhythm without evidence of preexcitation b. Documented episodes of tachyarrhythmias or	X		2A. None	2. ECG, H&P, physician orders, progress notes
3. Production of AV block to aid in the identification of supraventricular tachyarrhythmias in patients with both of the following[7,9,10]: a. ECG suggestive of (but not diagnostic for) PSVT, atrial fibrillation, or atrial flutter b. Contraindications to verapamil (see element 1b) or	X		3A. Presence of an accessory pathway (see element 1c)[4,11]	3. ECG, H&P, physician orders, progress notes 3A. ECG, H&P, progress notes
4. Production of AV block to aid in determining origin of regular wide-complex tachycardia (QRS duration >0.12 sec)[10,11]	X		4A. None	4. ECG, H&P, physician orders, progress notes
Critical (Process) Indicators				
5. No evidence of second- or third-degree AV block or sick sinus syndrome[5]	X		5A. Presence of functional atrial pacemaker[5]	5. ECG, H&P, progress notes 5A. ECG, H&P, progress notes
6. No history of hypersensitivity to adenosine[5]	X		6A. None	6. H&P, progress notes, nursing notes
7. No current evidence of atrial fibrillation or atrial flutter[5]	X		7A. Patient treated for justification 3 or 4	7. ECG, H&P, physician orders, progress notes 7A. ECG, H&P, physician orders, progress notes
8. ECG monitored continuously during adenosine administration[5]	X		8A. None	8. ECG, physician orders, progress notes, nursing notes
9. Initial adenosine dose: 6 mg i.v. given over 1–2 sec[1,5]	X		9A. Patients receiving dipyridamole should receive 1/4 of the dose (1.5 mg)[9,12,13]; patients who have undergone cardiac transplantation should receive 1/5 to 1/3 of the dose (1–2 mg)[9,14]; lower doses are advised for patients receiving carbamazepine and asthmatic patients,[5,9] and for central administration, but no specific recommendations are available in the literature	9. Physician orders, progress notes, nursing notes, MAR 9A. H&P, progress notes, nursing notes, MAR
10. Second and third doses of 12 mg i.v. (each) given 1–2 min after previous dose if needed[1,5]	X		10A. Patients receiving dipyridamole should receive 1/4 of the dose (3 mg)[9,12,13]; patients who	10. Physician orders, progress notes, nursing notes, MAR 10A. H&P, progress notes, nursing notes, MAR

Element	Standard 100%	Standard 0%	Exception[b] or Critical Preventive/ Responsive Measure[c]	Sources of Information
			have undergone cardiac transplantation should receive 1/5 to 1/3 of the dose (2.5–4 mg)[9,14]; lower doses are advised for patients receiving carbamazepine and asthmatic patients,[5,9] and for central administration, but no specific recommendations are available in the literature	
11. Each dose followed by rapid flush of 0.9% sodium chloride injection (10 mL)[1,5]	X		11A. None	11. Physician orders, progress notes, nursing notes, MAR
Complications				
12. Cardiovascular: sinus arrest, atrial fibrillation (in patient without atrial fibrillation), symptomatic AV block, chest pain, facial flushing, headache, sweating, hypotension[1,5,7,10]		X	12A. No corrective measures necessary because complications are rapidly self-limiting[1-5]; treatment of prolonged cardiovascular complications should be individualized (cardioversion, digoxin, β-adrenergic blockers, fluids)	12. ECG, progress notes, nursing notes 12A. ECG, physician orders, progress notes, nursing notes, MAR
13. Noncardiac: dyspnea, hyperventilation, chest pressure, head pressure, lightheadedness, dizziness, blurred vision, heaviness in arms, nausea[1,5,7,10]		X	13A. No corrective measures necessary because complications are rapidly self-limiting	13. ECG, progress notes, nursing notes 13A. Physician orders, progress notes, nursing notes, MAR
Outcome Measures				
14. Restoration of sinus rhythm	X		14A. Patient treated for justifications 2–4	14. ECG, progress notes, nursing notes 14A. ECG, H&P, physician orders, progress notes
15. Positive identification of arrhythmia or of preexcitation	X		15A. Patient treated for justification 1	15. ECG, progress notes, nursing notes 15A. ECG, H&P, physician orders,

[a]Criteria address justification for use (indications), critical (process) indicators, complications of therapy, and patient outcome. Each criterion consists of an element, a standard, exceptions to the standard, and sources of information. The element is the minimum level of evidence needed to show that patient care was optimal. The standard defines the deviation from an element that is acceptable. If no deviation is acceptable, the standard is 100%. Exceptions are circumstances in which deviation is allowable. Sources of information listed are the most reliable sources. Sources pertaining to an element or exception are identified by the number assigned to the element or exception (e.g., 5, 5A).

[b]For justification for use, critical (process) indicators, and outcome measures.

[c]For complications.

References

1. DiMarco JP, Miles W, Akhtar M et al. Adenosine for paroxysmal supraventricular tachycardia: dose ranging and comparison with verapamil. *Ann Intern Med.* 1990; 113:104-10.
2. Rankin AC, Rae AP, Oldroyd KG et al. Verapamil or adenosine for the immediate treatment of supraventricular tachycardia. *Q J Med.* 1990; 274:203-8.
3. Garratt C, Linker N, Griffith M et al. Comparison of adenosine and verapamil for termination of paroxysmal supraventricular tachycardia. *Am J Cardiol.* 1989; 64:1310-6.
4. Rankin AC, McGovern BA. Adenosine or verapamil for the acute treatment of supraventricular tachycardia? *Ann Intern Med.* 1991; 114:513-5.
5. Fujisawa Pharmaceutical Company. Adenocard package insert. Deerfield, IL; 1990 Nov.
6. DiMarco JP, Sellers TD, Berne RM et al. Adenosine: electrophysiologic effects and therapeutic use for terminating paroxysmal supraventricular tachycardia. *Circulation.* 1983; 68:1254-63.
7. DiMarco JP, Sellers TD, Lerman BB et al. Diagnostic and therapeutic use of adenosine in patients with supraventricular tachyarrhythmias. *J Am Coll Cardiol.* 1985; 6:417-25.
8. Garrat CJ, Antoniou A, Griffith MJ et al. Use of intravenous adenosine in sinus rhythm as a diagnostic test for latent preexcitation. *Am J Cardiol.* 1990; 65:868-73.
9. Lerman BB, Belardinelli L. Cardiac electrophysiology of adenosine. *Circulation.* 1991; 83:1499-509.
10. Rankin AC, Oldroyd KG, Chong E et al. Value and limitations

of adenosine in the diagnosis and treatment of narrow and broad complex tachycardias. *Br Heart J*. 1989; 62:195-203.

11. Griffith MJ, Linker NJ, Ward DE et al. Adenosine in the diagnosis of broad complex tachycardia. *Lancet*. 1988; 1:672-5.
12. Lerman BB, Wesley RC, Belardinelli L. Electrophysiologic effects of dipyridamole on atrioventricular nodal conduction and supraventricular tachycardia: role of endogenous adenosine. *Circulation*. 1989; 80:1536-43.
13. Watt AH, Webster BJ, Passani SL et al. Intravenous adenosine in the treatment of supraventricular tachycardia: a dose-ranging study and interaction with dipyridamole. *Br J Clin Pharmacol*. 1986; 21:227-30.
14. Ellenbogen KA, Thames MD, DiMarco JP et al. Electrophysiologic effects of adenosine in the transplanted human heart: evidence of supersensitivity. *Circulation*. 1990; 81:821-8.

Current Literature

Drug Reaction Alerts 735

Book Review

Manual of Antibiotics and Infectious Diseases, Seventh Edition 742
By John E. Conte, Jr., and Steven L. Barriere
Reviewed by Kyle Vance-Bryan

Books Received 742

Drug Reaction Alerts

Drug Reaction Alerts focuses primarily on serious, unlabeled reactions to new chemical entities. The citations are compiled monthly from International Pharmaceutical Abstracts, *which covers over 800 pharmacy and health-related journals worldwide. An address for reprints (when available) follows the name of the corresponding author in each citation.*

Pharmacists may use the FDA Adverse Reaction Report form that appears in the January and July issues of Clinical Pharmacy *for submitting reports of adverse drug reactions directly to FDA.*

Antibiotics

McDonald BJ (Bone Marrow Transplant Unit [119], Veterans Affairs Medical Center, 1660 S. Columbian Way, Seattle, WA 98108), Singer JW, Blanco JA. Toxic epidermal necrolysis possibly linked to **aztreonam** in bone marrow transplant patients. *Ann Pharmacother.* 1992; 26:34-5. Cases. (two men, aged 23 and 32 years, who underwent bone marrow transplantation; 23-year-old man with acute lymphocytic leukemia received aztreonam 2 g every eight hours by i.v. injection for 19 days, starting two days before transplantation; 32-year-old man with diffuse non-Hodgkin's lymphoma received aztreonam 2 g every eight hours by i.v. injection for 11 days, starting three days after transplantation; developed symptoms of toxic epidermal necrolysis; concomitant vancomycin; skin tissue biopsies consistent with toxic epidermal necrolysis or graft-versus-host disease in 23-year-old man and consistent with toxic epidermal necrolysis in 32-year-old man; withdrawal of aztreonam and therapy with pigskin graft to 23-year-old man and silver sulfadiazine cream to 32-year-old man led to stabilization of symptoms but death from infectious complications; examination at autopsy of 32-year-old man showed no evidence of graft-versus-host disease)

Wagner BK, Heaton AH (Pharmacy Services, United Hospital, 333 N. Smith Avenue, St. Paul, MN 55102), Flink JR. **Cefotetan disodium**-induced hemolytic anemia. *Ann Pharmacother.* 1992; 26:199-200. Case. (46-year-old woman; received cefotetan disodium 2 g every 12 hours for two doses as chemoprophylaxis for postoperative infection; developed fulminant hemolytic anemia with respiratory failure and acute renal failure; received initial exposure to cefotetan disodium seven months before; concomitant metronidazole, fluoxetine, lorazepam, meperidine, oxazepam, and ranitidine; withdrawal of cefotetan disodium and therapy with plasmapheresis led to successful treatment of hemolysis, but patient also required intubation and hemodialysis; patient died 25 days later)

Antidepressants

Hemlock C (Department of Psychiatry, Beth Israel Medical Center, Fierman Hall, 9th Floor, 317 E. 17th Street, New York, NY 10003), Rosenthal JS, Winston A. **Fluoxetine**-induced psoriasis. *Ann Pharmacother.* 1992; 26:211-2. Cases. (two women, aged 42 and 61 years, with depression; received fluoxetine hydrochloride 20–40 mg/day for 6 or 12 months; developed raised, reddish, scabbing lesions on wrists, elbows, or shins that were unresponsive to topical hydrocortisone and that appeared to decrease in size when exposed to sunlight; 42-year-old woman concomitantly received imipramine and alprazolam; 61-year-old woman concomitantly received lovastatin, triamterene plus hydrochlorothiazide, levothyroxine sodium, and enalapril maleate; tapering of fluoxetine dosage to 20 mg every third day in 61-year-old woman led to resolution of lesions; continuation of fluoxetine 40 mg/day in 42-year-old woman led to occasional intermittent development of psoriatic lesions)

Antidotes

Bonfiglio MF (Department of Pharmacy Services, Akron City Hospital, 525 E. Market Street, Akron, OH 44309), Traeger SM, Hulisz DT et al. Anaphylactoid reaction to intravenous **acetylcysteine** associated with electrocardiographic abnormalities. *Ann Pharmacother.* 1992; 26:22-5. Case. (20-year-old woman who ingested 20 tablets containing propoxyphene 65 mg plus acetaminophen 650 mg; received acetylcysteine 150 mg/kg by i.v. infusion followed by 150 mg/kg by continuous i.v. infusion over next 20 hours; developed severe anaphylactoid reaction with abnormal ECG findings and chest pain; concomitant ingestion of 10–15 tablets of methocarbamol 500 mg; serum acetaminophen concentration at least 16 hours postingestion was 38.2 μg/mL; discontinuation of acetylcysteine and therapy with diphenhydramine led to relief of symptoms)

Antilipemic Agents

Wallace CS, Mueller BA (Purdue University Pharmacy Program Office, OPW 224, Wishard Memorial Hospital, 1001 W. 10th Street, Indianapolis, IN 46202). **Lovastatin**-induced rhabdomyolysis in the absence of concomitant drugs. *Ann Pharmacother.* 1992; 26:190-2. Case. (60-year-old man with hypercholesterolemia; received lovastatin 40 mg/day for 14 months; complained of weakness, malaise, myalgia, and two-week loss of appetite; concomitant aspirin, enalapril maleate, prazosin hydrochloride, furosemide, colchicine, allopurinol, and isophane insulin; withdrawal of lovastatin and colchicine and therapy with hemodialysis led to resolution of complaints; no rechallenge)

Antineoplastic Agents

Miller LJ (Division of Pharmacy, University of Texas M. D. Anderson Cancer Center, 1515 Holcombe Boulevard, Box 90, Houston, TX 77030), Eaton VE. **Ifosfamide**-induced neurotoxicity: case report and review of the literature. *Ann Pharmacother.* 1992; 26:183-7. Case. (56-year-old man with follicular, mixed-cell non-Hodgkin's lymphoma; received ifosfamide 1.33 g/sq m/day by continuous i.v. infusion for three days; exhibited somnolence, confusion, disorientation, hand and leg tremors, and blank stares; concomitant mesna, etoposide, and fluconazole and single dose of mitoxantrone on day 1 of ifosfamide therapy; discontinuation of combined infusion of ifosfamide and mesna and therapy with amphotericin B for suspected fungal pneumonia did not lead to improvement of symptoms; progressed from unresponsive mental state to one of agitation and nonstop nonsensical verbalization; therapy with haloperidol led to resolution of symptoms)

Murphy CP (Department of Pharmacy, Humana Hospital, University of Louisville, 530 S. Jackson Street, Louisville, KY 40202), Harden EA, Thompson JM. Generalized seizures secondary to high-dose **busulfan** therapy. *Ann Pharmacother.* 1992; 26:30-1. Cases. (two patients, 17-year-old man with chronic myelogenous leukemia in chronic phase and 28-year-old woman with acute promyelocytic leukemia in first complete remission, in preparative regimen for allogeneic bone marrow transplantation; received oral busulfan 1 mg/kg four times daily for 5 doses [man] or 15 doses [woman]; experienced generalized tonic–clonic seizure that resolved spontaneously; concomitant trimethoprim plus sulfamethoxazole, allopurinol, immune globulin, norethindrone acetate, and acyclovir sodium; unenhanced computed tomographic scan of brain normal)

Antivirals

Chen JL (Pharmacy Department, Montefiore Medical Center, 111 E. 210 Street, Bronx, NY 10467), Brocavich JM, Lin AY. Psychiatric disturbances associated with **ganciclovir** therapy. *Ann Pharmacother.* 1992; 26:193-5. Case. (45-year-old woman with AIDS, cytomegalovirus retinitis, and mild renal dysfunction; received ganciclovir 5 mg/kg every 12 hours by i.v. injection for 15 days; complained of nightmares and developed visual hallucinations and severe agitation; concomitant ketoconazole, folic acid, docusate sodium, clotrimazole, and multivitamin product; withdrawal of ganciclovir and therapy with haloperidol led to resolution of problems; positive rechallenge; concomitant therapy with haloperidol led to continued ganciclovir therapy without further episodes of visual hallucinations)

Benzodiazepine Antagonists

Seebach J, Jost R (Department of Internal Medicine, University Hospital, 8091 Zurich, Switzerland). **Flumazenil**-induced psychotic disorder in hepatic encephalopathy. *Lancet.* 1992; 339:488-9. Case. (38-year-old woman with hepatic encephalopathy; received oral flumazenil 25 mg twice daily for 48 hours; developed progressive anxiety, restlessness, insomnia, and crying fits accompanied by verbal attacks, aggressiveness, panic, disorientation, and hallucinations; withdrawal of flumazenil led to resolution of psychotic state within 12 hours)

Drug Interactions

Dillard ML, Fink RM (Johnson City Medical Center Hospital, 400 State of Franklin Road, Johnson City, TN 37604), Parkerson R. **Ciprofloxacin–phenytoin** interaction. *Ann Pharmacother.* 1992; 26:263. Case. (78-year-old man who received maintenance therapy with phenytoin 300 mg/day for control of seizures; received ciprofloxacin 400 mg every 12 hours by i.v. injection for two weeks for treatment of left pulmonary lobe abscess secondary to aspiration pneumonia; experienced breakthrough seizures; serum phenytoin concentrations decreased from 14.7 mg/L to 6.3 mg/L after one day of ciprofloxacin therapy and to 4.8 mg/L after two days; therapy with increased phenytoin dosage of 500 mg/day led to control of seizures; serum phenytoin concentration was 13.7 mg/L one day after completion of ciprofloxacin therapy; continued phenytoin therapy at 500 mg/day)

Frenia ML, Long KS (Department of Pharmacy Practice and Administration, College of Pharmacy, Busch Campus, Rutgers, The State University of New Jersey, P.O. Box 789, Piscataway, NJ 08855). **Methotrexate** and nonsteroidal antiinflammatory drug interactions. *Ann Pharmacother.* 1992; 26:234-7. Case. (74-year-old woman with rheumatoid arthritis controlled by methotrexate 7.5 mg/wk; received **flurbiprofen** 100 mg/day for one to two weeks for additional control of rheumatoid arthritis; developed acute GI bleeding; concomitant folic acid, digoxin, gemfibrozil, dipyridamole, and iron supplement; blood test results revealed anemia, neutropenia, and thrombocytopenia; therapy with packed red-blood-cell and platelet transfusions, folic acid, vitamin K, sucralfate, and ranitidine led to positive response)

Grasela TH (Center for Pharmacoepidemiology Research, State University of New York at Buffalo, School of Pharmacy, 319 Cooke Hall, Buffalo, NY 14260), Dreis MW. An evaluation of the **quinolone–theophylline** interaction using the Food and Drug Administration spontaneous reporting system. *Arch Intern Med.* 1992; 152:617-21. Study. (case series; 48 reports of adverse reactions attributed to simultaneous administration of theophylline and ciprofloxacin [39] or norfloxacin [9] obtained from FDA's Spontaneous Reporting System; 25 women and 23 men; mean ± S.D. age, 68.4 ± 18.5 years; mean percent-

Continued on page 741

Continued from page 736

age change in blood theophylline concentration after addition of quinolone, 114% [range, 32–308%]; 14 [36%] patients who received ciprofloxacin and 3 [33%] patients who received norfloxacin experienced a seizure)

Serpa MD, Cossolias J, McGreevy MJ (Grossmont Hospital, 5555 Grossmont Center Drive, La Mesa, CA 91942). **Moricizine–warfarin:** a possible drug interation. *Ann Pharmacother.* 1992; 26:127. Case. (69-year-old woman who received maintenance therapy with warfarin 7.5 mg/day after mitral valve replacement; received moricizine 300 mg three times daily for four days; developed right-upper-quadrant abdominal pain, hematuria, and blood emesis; concomitant digoxin, captopril, and prednisone; prothrombin times increased from 15–20 sec to 41 sec after start of moricizine therapy; withdrawal of warfarin and moricizine and therapy with oral phytonadione led to prothrombin time of 14 sec; restarted on warfarin 2.5 mg/day)

Gastrointestinal Drugs

Humphries JE (Department of Pathology, University of Virginia Health Science Center, Box 214, Charlottesville, VA 22908). Thrombocytopenia associated with **famotidine** in a hemophiliac. *Ann Pharmacother.* 1992; 26:262. Case. (23-year-old man with hemophilia and dyspepsia; received famotidine 40 mg/day for 11 days; developed shoulder pain after minor fall and received anti-inhibitor coagulant complex, meperidine, and promethazine; blood test results revealed thrombocytopenia; no evidence of bleeding; concomitant intermittent acetaminophen plus oxycodone hydrochloride and aluminum hydroxide; withdrawal of famotidine led to reversal of thrombocytopenia within one day)

Hypotensive Agents

Jonville AP (Clinical Pharmacology Service, Hôpital Bretonneau, 37044 Tours, France), Echenberger J, Dutertre JP et al. **Urapidil** and enuresis. *Lancet.* 1992; 339:688. Cases. (two women, aged 76 and 80 years, with refractory hypertension; received urapidil 30 or 60 mg/day; 76-year-old woman developed enuresis at rest and worsened stress incontinence; 80-year-old woman developed persistent enuresis at rest and upon stress; withdrawal of urapidil led to disappearance of symptoms after 48 hours; positive rechallenge with another brand of urapidil in 80-year-old woman)

McCloskey LW, Psaty BM, Koepsell TD et al. Level of blood pressure and risk of myocardial infarction among treated hypertensive patients. *Arch Intern Med.* 1992; 152:513-20. Study. (case–control; 912 hypertensive patients, aged 30–79 years, receiving **antihypertensive drugs** through an HMO, 175 of whom experienced myocardial infarction [MI] during study; J-shaped relationship between most recently measured diastolic blood pressure and risk of MI; lowest risk of MI [1.0] occurred at diastolic blood pressure of 84 mm Hg; 2.07 [95% confidence interval, 0.86–5.01] relative risk of MI at 60 mm H; 1.45 [95% confidence interval, 1.02–2.06] relative risk of MI at 100 mm Hg; linear relationship between treated systolic blood pressure and risk of MI; optimum target range for diastolic blood pressure in treated patients was 84–90 mm Hg)

Roentgenographic Agents

Tardy B, Guy C, Barral G et al. (Bertrand JC, Department of Emergency Medicine, Toxicology, and Radiology, Hôpital Bellevue, Saint-Etienne 42023, France). Anaphylactic shock induced by intravenous **gadopentetate dimeglumine**. *Lancet.* 1992; 339:494. Case. (40-year-old man; received gadopentetate dimeglumine 0.1 mM/kg by i.v. injection as contrast agent for magnetic resonance imaging scan; developed anaphylactic shock; therapy with methylprednisolone and oxygen did not lead to improvement; therapy with i.v. gelatin fluid and methylprednisolone led to clinical improvement)

Topical Preparations

Evans RJ (Royal Infirmary of Edinburgh, Edinburgh EH3 9YW, Scotland). Acute anaphylaxis due to topical **chlorhexidine acetate**. *Br Med J.* 1992; 304:686. Case. (19-year-old man with burn; applied topical preparation containing 0.5% chlorhexidine acetate; developed acute anaphylaxis; removal of chlorhexidine acetate preparation and therapy with oxygen, i.v. colloids, antihistamines, nebulized β agonists, and corticosteroids led to complete recovery)

Trattner A (Kedumim, D.N. Shomron, 44856 Israel), Ingber A. Topical treatment with **minoxidil** 2% and smoking intolerance. *Ann Pharmacother.* 1992; 26:198-9. Cases. (two men, aged 21 and 42 years, who smoked 20 and 40 cigarettes/day, respectively; applied topical 2% minoxidil twice daily for two to three weeks as therapy for alopecia; experienced unpleasant taste sensation when smoking without other alterations in taste or changes in appetite; withdrawal of minoxidil led to disappearance of smoking intolerance within two to three days; positive rechallenge; both men chose to continue long-term therapy with topical minoxidil and discontinue smoking)

Toxicity

Bowlby HA, Elanjian SI (Indiana University Hospital, Indianapolis, IN 46202). Necrosis caused by extravasation of **arginine hydrochloride**. *Ann Pharmacother.* 1992; 26:263-4. Case. (eight-year-old boy; received 74 mL of 120-mL dose of 10% arginine hydrochloride 500 mg/kg as diagnostic agent to stimulate production and release of growth hormone; developed puffiness at injection site on right foot and discomfort; concomitant divalproex sodium and levothyroxine sodium; immediate dis-

Continued on page 742

Continued from page 741

continuation of arginine hydrochloride did not halt rapid development of blisters and full-thickness necrosis that required debridement and subsequent skin grafting)

Book Review

Manual of Antibiotics and Infectious Diseases, Seventh Edition

By John E. Conte, Jr., and Steven L. Barriere.

Published by Lea & Febiger, 200 Chester Field Parkway, Malvern, PA 19355-9725, 1992. xvi + 419 p. Price $29.95.

Few disciplines in medical practice change as rapidly as the area of infectious diseases. The emergence of relatively new problems such as AIDS and Lyme disease, the re-emergence of old diseases such as tuberculosis, and the availability of an ever-increasing number of pharmacotherapeutic agents for prevention as well as treatment of infectious processes have contributed to rapid change in this field.

Health-care practitioners involved in day-to-day patient-care decisions related to infectious diseases will welcome the arrival of this book. The content, format, and style make the book potentially valuable to house staff, specialists, and various health-science students including interns.

Compared with other available books on antimicrobials and infectious diseases, this book is unique; it can serve as a single source for useful information that normally can be found only by perusing several reference books. Included are antimicrobial monographs that explain clinical use, dosage, adverse reactions, and important drug interactions; empirical and established infection treatment recommendations; guidelines for the use of prophylactic antimicrobials; and availability and clinical use of immunobiologic agents.

This seventh edition has been enhanced considerably over the sixth edition. Obsolete drugs have been deleted, and information on several new agents has been added. The tabulated data on microbiological susceptibility have been expanded, and footnotes provide helpful clinical comments. Sections on chemoprophylaxis, tuberculosis screening and treatment, prevention of *Haemophilus influenzae* type B infection, and availability and use of immunobiologics have been lengthened. Where relevant, advisory committee recommendations for prophylaxis and use of immunobiologics have been included; for example, the recommendation of the Immunization Practices Advisory Committee on measles prevention. The increased number of tables and the enhanced formats of many tables enable the rapid retrieval of practical information, which can be extremely important to the clinician at the patient's bedside. Updated bibliographies for each section reflect new information; throughout the text, references have been added that are valuable to the occasional reader who needs more background information.

As a specialist in critical care and infectious diseases, I found the sixth edition of this book to be a valuable and much used component of my reference library. The monographs, the recommendations for empirical treatment, and the section on immunobiologics were very useful; my criticisms included inadequate bibliographies and insufficient use of tables. I consider the seventh edition to be a considerable improvement.

I highly recommend this new edition as a valuable, affordable, and timely resource for clinically relevant infectious disease information. Few currently available books provide such breadth of practical knowledge under a single cover. Clinical practitioners at any level of training or experience who make decisions related to infectious diseases will find this book very useful.

Reviewed by Kyle Vance-Bryan, Pharm.D., Section of Clinical Pharmacy, St. Paul–Ramsey Medical Center, 640 Jackson Street, St. Paul, MN 55101-2595.

Books Received

Books are listed as soon as received; selected books may be reviewed in Book Reviews in subsequent issues.

Handbook of Psychotropic Drugs. Published by Springhouse Corporation, 1111 Bethlehem Pike, Springhouse, PA 19477, 1992. ix + 308 p. Price $24.95.

Pharmacology, edited by Theoharis C. Theoharides. Published by Little, Brown and Company, 34 Beacon Street, Boston, MA 02108, 1992. x + 651 p. Price $26.

Polymers in Medicine: Biomedical and Pharmaceutical Applications, edited by Raphael M. Ottenbrite and Emo Chiellini. Published by Technomic Publishing Company, Inc., 851 New Holland Avenue, Box 3535, Lancaster, PA 17604, 1992. vii + 258 p. Price $68.

Advertising Index

American Society of Hospital Pharmacists
ASHP Membership, 733-734
Clinical Pharmacy, 671
Concepts in Immunology and Immunotherapeutics, 664
Concepts in Oncology Therapeutics, 675
Criteria for Drug Use Evaluation, Volumes 1, 2, and 3, 730
The Elements of Quality in Pharmaceutical Care, 732
Handbook on Injectable Drugs, 7th Edition, 676
QARx 3.0, 726
Resource Book on Progressive Pharmaceutical Services, 2nd Edition, 741
Amgen Inc.
Epogen, 659
Neupogen, 737-740
Burroughs Wellcome Company
Exosurf Neonatal, 665-668
Elsevier Science Publishers
Pharmacotherapy: A Pathophysiologic Approach, Second Edition, 673
Roche Laboratories, Division of Hoffmann-La Roche, Inc.
Rocephin, inside back cover, outside back cover
Roerig, A Division of Pfizer Pharmaceuticals
Cefobid, 663-664
University of Toronto
Position Available, 671
VHA of Southern New England
Position Available, 671
Wyeth-Ayerst Laboratories, Inc.
Ativan Injection, 660-662
Tubex, inside front cover

News

Zalcitabine approved under accelerated drug review policy 747

Adverse effects prompt withdrawal of temafloxacin 747

Talley to succeed Zellmer as editor of *AJHP* and *Clinical Pharmacy* 750

News Briefs 750

Upcoming Specialty Meetings 750

Correction 750

Zalcitabine approved under accelerated drug review policy

Zalcitabine (dideoxycytidine [ddC]; Hivid, Roche Laboratories) has been approved for marketing under FDA's proposed accelerated drug review policy. The drug is indicated for use in combination with zidovudine in adults with advanced human immunodeficiency virus (HIV) infection (CD4 cell count of ≤300/cu mm) who have significant clinical or immunologic deterioration.

The labeled indication is based on two small studies in which patients who had not previously received zidovudine therapy were treated with zidovudine alone (not at the currently recommended dosage) or in combination with zalcitabine. Increases in CD4 cell counts were larger and more sustained with the combination regimen. Data on clinical endpoints (e.g., survival, frequency of opportunistic infections, or progression of HIV infection) are not available. The zalcitabine product labeling states that zidovudine monotherapy should still be considered as initial treatment for HIV-infected adults who show evidence of impaired immunity. According to Roche, six clinical studies of the combination regimen are ongoing.

Data on the adverse effect profile of zalcitabine are based mainly on use as monotherapy. The most common adverse reaction is peripheral neuropathy, which has occurred in 17% to 31% of clinical trial participants who received the drug. Other commonly reported adverse effects are nausea, oral ulcers, headache, and fatigue. Fatal cases of pancreatitis have been reported with zalcitabine alone or in combination with zidovudine.

The recommended dosage of zalcitabine is 0.75 mg every eight hours given in combination with zidovudine 200 mg every eight hours. Hivid is available as 0.375- and 0.75-mg tablets in bottles of 100. Roche has estimated the average monthly cost (to the wholesaler) of Hivid therapy at $152.

Adverse effects prompt withdrawal of temafloxacin

In early June, Abbott Laboratories halted distribution of temafloxacin (Omniflox) and recalled all drug supplies from U.S. and foreign markets because of serious adverse reactions. Since mid-February, when the drug was introduced in the United States, FDA had received approximately 50 reports of serious reactions, including three deaths. Reports included hemolytic anemia and other blood cell abnormalities; renal dysfunction, with dialysis required in about one half of cases; hepatic dysfunction; and several cases of severe hypoglycemia, especially in elderly persons with decreased renal function.

Continued on page 750

AMGEN®

There's More To EPOGEN® (Epoetin alfa) Than Epoetin Alfa.

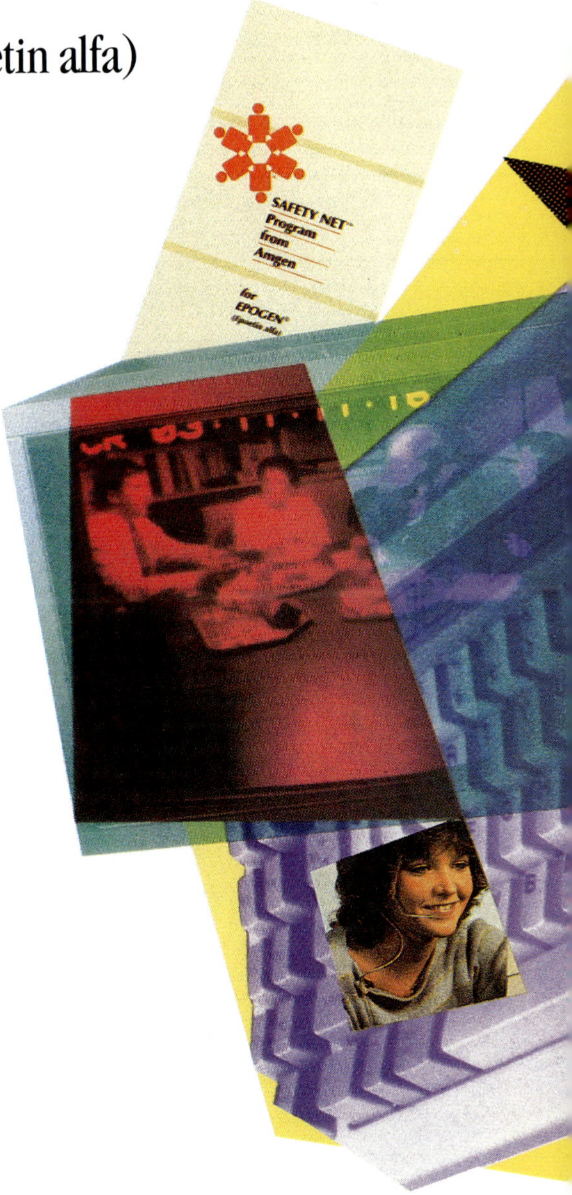

When you specify EPOGEN® (Epoetin alfa), you also get a comprehensive support system. That's important, because the depth and quality of professional support is a significant element in long-term clinical success.

Here's just a glimpse of how much more there is behind EPOGEN® technology:

- **Professional Services**
  A multidisciplinary team of experts to answer your clinical and product-related questions and to help you ensure proper usage of EPOGEN®.
- **Clinical Support Services**
  On-site consultation, inservice training and speaker programs.
- **Professional Education Programs**
  A wide variety of educational programs for the pharmacist, physician, staff and the patient. This includes continuing-education accredited programs.
- **SAFETY NET™ Program**
  Free replacement EPOGEN® for underinsured patients with a financial need.
- **Amgen Reimbursement Hotline**
  Immediate access to reimbursement experts with the most up-to-date information about the evolving reimbursement guidelines.

There simply is no comparable source of professional support. That's not surprising because EPOGEN® is a lot more than just a drug. It's a way of life.

For more information about EPOGEN® support services, call 1-800-77-AMGEN.

EPOGEN®
(EPOETIN ALFA)
RECOMBINANT

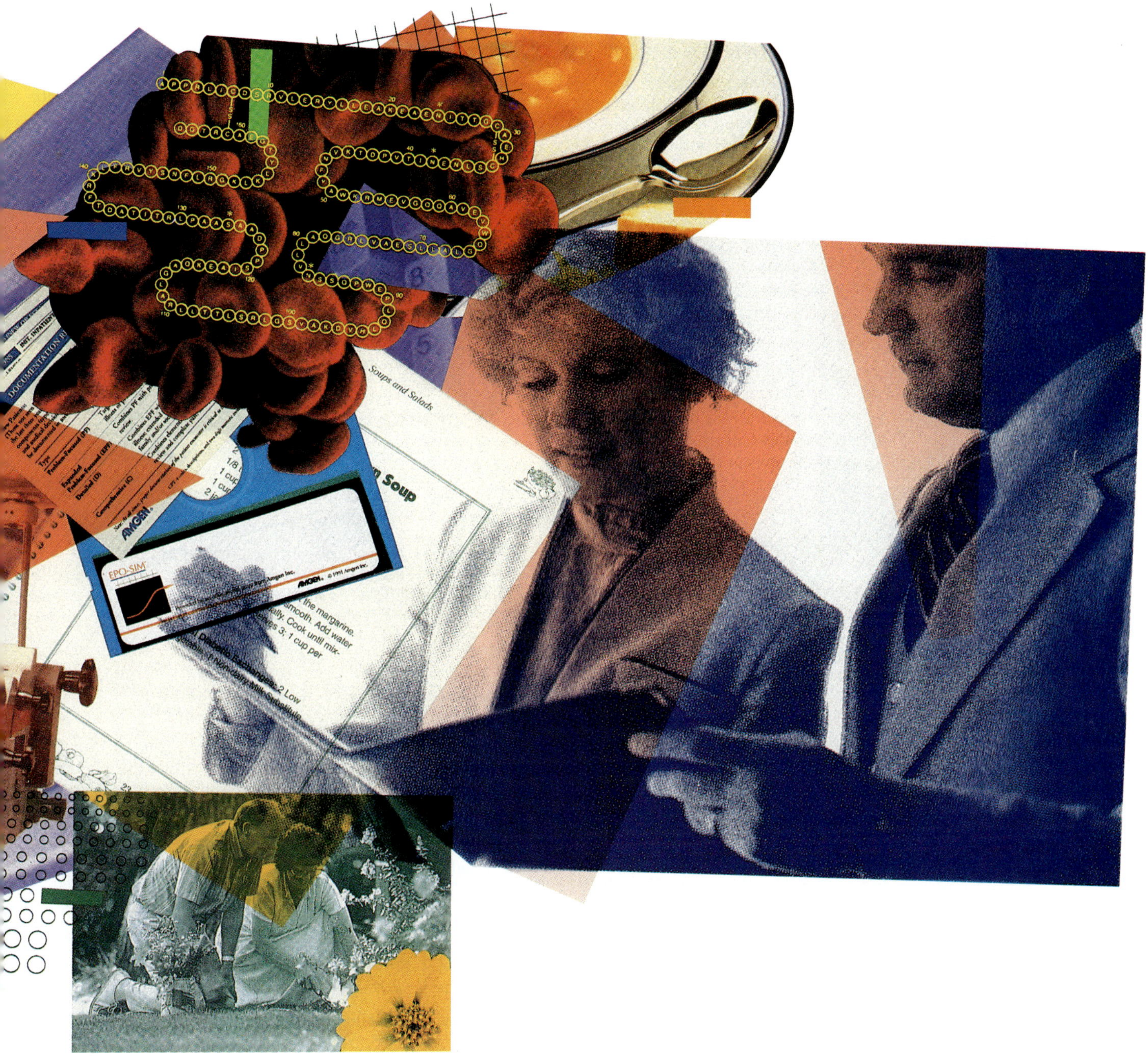
Soups and Salads
Soup
AMGEN
EPO-SIM

Continued from page 747

Allergic reactions causing life-threatening respiratory distress were also reported.

Talley to succeed Zellmer as editor of *AJHP* and *Clinical Pharmacy*

C. Richard Talley has been promoted from Managing Editor to Editor, *American Journal of Hospital Pharmacy* and *Clinical Pharmacy*, effective with the October 1992 issues.

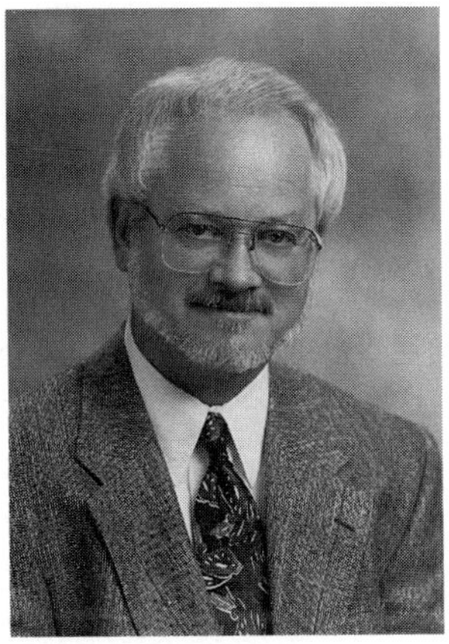

C. Richard Talley

Before joining the editorial staff of *AJHP* in 1978, Talley was Assistant Director of Pharmacy at Harris Hospital in Fort Worth, Texas. He became Managing Editor of *AJHP* in 1981 and of *Clinical Pharmacy* in 1982. In his new post, he will continue as director of the 15-member Communication Services Division, a position he has held since July 1985.

Current editor William A. Zellmer will continue on the ASHP staff in his position as Vice President, Professional and Government Affairs. Editor of *AJHP* since 1974, Zellmer will now become Editor at Large, writing a new column to be called "At Large." He has been editor of *Clinical Pharmacy* since it was founded in 1982.

News Briefs

- **Ketorolac tromethamine** (Toradol, Syntex) is now available as an oral 10-mg tablet for limited-duration, as-needed use for pain management; the recommended dosage is 10 mg every four to six hours as needed.

- An investigational live, attenuated **varicella vaccine** is available at no charge to children with acute lymphocytic leukemia who meet specified criteria for use, including no clinical history of varicella and continuous remission for at least 12 months; for more information, contact Dr. Jo White at Merck Research Laboratories, 215-834-2554.

- Limited supplies of **streptomycin and aminosalicylic acid** are available from the Centers for Disease Control (CDC) for use by (1) patients with active tuberculosis that is resistant to isoniazid and rifampin and (2) patients with active tuberculosis in areas where resistant strains are predominant and whose susceptibility results are not yet known. The drugs can be obtained from the Clinical Research Branch, Division of Tuberculosis Elimination, National Center for Prevention Services, CDC, 404-639-2530. Clinicians should be prepared to provide a brief medical history and a recent serum creatinine concentration result (to obtain streptomycin). Both drugs are expected to be available from U.S. companies later this year.

- Centocor has begun a new randomized, double-blind, placebo-controlled trial of **HA-1A** in patients with septic shock and presumed gram-negative bacteremia; the endpoint of the trial will be mortality after 14 days. Since June 30, Centocor's compassionate-use program for HA-1A has been limited to children.

- A clinical practice guideline entitled **"Pressure Ulcers in Adults: Prediction and Prevention"** is available from the U.S. Public Health Service Agency for Health Care Policy and Research (AHCPR). A quick reference guide for clinicians and a guide for patients are also available. To order a copy, call the AHCPR Publications Clearinghouse at 800-358-9295 or write to Guidelines, P.O. Box 8547, Silver Spring, MD 20907.

- **"Hypertension and the Brain,"** an article from the National High Blood Pressure Education Program of the National Heart, Lung, and Blood Institute, was published in the May 1992 issue of *Archives of Internal Medicine*; the review describes the harmful effects of high blood pressure on the brain and cerebral circulation and summarizes the benefits of antihypertensive therapy.

Upcoming Specialty Meetings

Gene Therapy. Washington, DC, September 10–11. Contact International Business Communications USA Conferences Inc., 8 Pleasant Street, Building D, South Natick, MA 01760, 508-650-4700, (fax) 508-653-1627.

Cancer Pain Management 1992: Challenges and Strategies. Oakbrook, IL, September 12. Contact Educational Affairs, Loyola University, 2160 South First Street, Maywood, IL 60153; 708-216-3236.

10th Annual Psychopharmacology Update. Boston, MA, October 9–10. Contact Office of Continuing Education, Tufts University School of Medicine, 136 Harrison Avenue, Boston, MA 02111; 617-956-6579.

The Diabetic Eye. Sacramento, CA, October 10. Contact Office of Continuing Medical Education, UC Davis Medical Center, 2701 Stockton Boulevard, Sacramento, CA 95817; 916-734-5390, (fax) 916-736-0188.

Anesthesiology Update. Monterey, CA, November 6–8. Contact Office of Continuing Medical Education, UC Davis Medical Center, 2701 Stockton Boulevard, Sacramento, CA 95817; 916-734-5390, (fax) 916-736-0188.

National Kidney Foundation Annual Meeting. Baltimore, MD, November 11–15. Contact NKF, Inc., 30 East 33rd Street, New York, NY 10016; 212-889-2210.

American Society of Hematology. Anaheim, CA, December 4–8. Contact D. I. Feinstein, M.D., Healthcare Consultation Center, School of Medicine, University of Southern California, Suite 601, 1510 San Pablo Street, Los Angeles, CA 90033; 202-857-1118.

Correction

Parenteral nutrition in pediatric patients (May 1988, Therapy Review). On page 354 in Table 2, the daily requirements of elemental magnesium for neonates and for infants and children should be 0.5 meq/kg and 0.2–0.4 meq/kg, respectively.

Therapy Consultation

The Therapy Consultation *section provides brief advice, in question-and-answer format, on how to handle specific drug-therapy problems. Readers are invited to submit questions, which will be referred to a consultant for an answer. The problems should not be highly specialized or unusual, nor should they be mundane. Questions are answered briefly, based largely on the judgment and personal experience of the consultant, although selected references may be cited to substantiate the consultant's advice.*

Assistance in identifying Therapy Consultation *topics is provided by the drug information centers at Medical College of Virginia Hospitals, Richmond; University of California Medical Center, San Diego; and University of Michigan Medical Center, Ann Arbor.*

Diabetes control during bowel cleansing with PEG–electrolyte solution

Question: A patient with diabetes mellitus must undergo bowel cleansing with polyethylene glycol (PEG)–electrolyte lavage solution before a gastrointestinal examination. Management of the patient's blood glucose is difficult because he must fast, perhaps for 11 hours or longer, before the procedure. Management is further complicated because the manufacturer of the lavage solution warns against concomitant administration of sugar-containing products with the lavage solution because of the potential for explosive gas formation. Can you suggest any guidelines for caring for this patient?

Answer: Product information for PEG-electrolyte solution warns against the administration of any sugar-containing products with the lavage.[1] This warning is based on a fatal case of colonic explosion that occurred during polypectomy.[2] In that case, large quantities of mannitol were used as the lavage solution. It was suspected that hydrogen and methane, produced by fermentation of this nonabsorbable carbohydrate by colonic bacteria, were ignited by the electrocautery.

This warning appears to complicate the management of patients with diabetes mellitus, because hypoglycemia must be prevented during the long periods of fasting required. However, when the patient is prepared in the usual manner—with a residue-free diet, overnight fast, cathartics, and enemas—hydrogen and methane concentrations are far below explosive levels.[3] The carbohydrates used to correct hypoglycemia would be rapidly absorbed and leave little residue in the bowel for fermentation. Thus, the risk of severe hypoglycemia if carbohydrates are not administered outweighs the risk of explosion from the ingestion of carbohydrate before the procedure. If electrocautery is not used, there is absolutely no risk of explosion.

Preparation of the patient for the examination depends on three factors: (1) Does the patient have insulin-dependent or insulin-requiring diabetes, or is the patient being treated with oral sulfonylureas? (2) What insulin regimen is the patient using? and (3) What is the patient's degree of glycemic control.

Day before Procedure. On the day before the procedure, patients receiving oral hypoglycemic agents require no change in their current regimen.

Patients who require insulin therapy should omit any evening dose of short-acting insulin on the day before the procedure but administer the usual dose of intermediate-acting insulin. Patients who receive multiple insulin injections and have a fasting blood glucose concentration of less then 140 mg/dL may need to reduce the evening dose of intermediate-acting insulin. Blood glucose concentration should be monitored every three to four hours. Supplemental doses of rapid-acting insulin should be administered as indicated by blood glucose monitoring. Non-residue liquids should be used to supplement calories and treat hypoglycemia. The patient can supplement calories with appropriate amounts of clear juice every hour. Alternatively, the evening calories can be replaced with a supplement such as Ensure[4] (two 240-mL cans = approximately 500 kcal), with the patient ingesting one-half can approximately every three hours after lavage is complete.

Day of Examination. On the day of the examination, the patient receiving an oral hypoglycemic agent should omit the morning dose and take the dose after the procedure when fasting is no longer required. The fluid ad-

Continued on page 752

Therapy Consultation *Continued from page 751*

ministered to maintain intravenous access should be dextrose free. Blood glucose concentration should be monitored before and after the procedure. Dextrose should be administered intravenously as needed. Supplemental rapid-acting insulin should be administered as indicated by blood glucose concentration.[5] Give 4 units of human regular insulin s.c. if the blood glucose concentration is 250–300 mg/dL, 6 units if the concentration is 300–400 mg/dL, and 8 units if the concentration is >400 mg/dL.

For the patient requiring insulin therapy, give one half of the usual morning dose of intermediate-acting insulin on the day of the examination. A patient whose blood glucose concentration is >200 mg/dL may be able to tolerate the full dose of intermediate-acting insulin. The fluid administered to maintain intravenous access should be 5% dextrose and 0.45% sodium chloride injection. Blood glucose concentration should be monitored before, during, and after the procedure until the patient is no longer fasting. Glucose should be administered orally or dextrose administered intravenously as indicated. If the blood glucose concentration before the procedure is <90 mg/dL, give 10–15 g of liquid glucose source orally. Recheck the blood glucose concentration in 10 minutes and administer another dose of oral glucose source if needed. During the procedure, change the infusion rate or solution composition as required based on glucose concentration and pre-existing cardiovascular or renal disease. Administer s.c. doses of rapid-acting insulin as required. Suggested supplemental doses of rapid-acting insulin[5] are as follows: no insulin if blood glucose concentration is <200 mg/dL, 4 to 6 units of human regular insulin if the concentration is 200–299 mg/dL, 6 to 8 units if the concentration is 300–399 mg/dL, and 8 to 10 units if the concentration is ≥400 mg/dL.

If the examination is to be performed in the afternoon, it may be possible to administer the lavage on the morning of the examination, shortening the fasting period and minimizing the need to adjust insulin doses.

Conclusion. There are many approaches to the regulation of blood glucose; however, all require attention to the patient's status.

1. Reed & Carnick. Manufacturer's prescribing information for Colyte. Jersey City, NJ; 1991 Nov.
2. Bigard MA, Gaucher P, Lassalle C. Fatal colonic explosion during colonoscopic polypectomy. *Gastroenterology.* 1979; 77:1307-10.
3. Bond JH, Levitt MD. Colonic gas explosion—is a fire extinguisher necessary? *Gastroenterology.* 1979; 77:1349-50.
4. Ross Laboratories. Manufacturer's product information for Ensure. Columbus, OH; 1991 Jul.
5. Shuman CR. Controlling diabetes during surgery. *Diabetes Spectrum.* 1989; 2:263-9.

TERESA MCMAHON, PHARM.D., CDE
Diabetes Specialist
Department of Pharmacy and I.V. Therapy and Benaroya Diabetes Center
Virginia Mason Medical Center
Seattle, WA 98101

Drug Review

Lomefloxacin and temafloxacin: Two new fluoroquinolone antimicrobials

WILLIAM T. SYMONDS AND DAVID E. NIX

Abstract: The chemistry, mechanism of action, antimicrobial spectrum, pharmacokinetics, clinical efficacy, safety, drug interactions, and dosage and administration of lomefloxacin and temafloxacin, two new antimicrobials, are presented.

Lomefloxacin and temafloxacin exhibit activity comparable to that of ciprofloxacin against the Enterobacteriaceae. Lomefloxacin has only modest activity against common gram-positive organisms. Temafloxacin exhibits increased activity against the streptococci and moderate activity against many anaerobes, as compared with ciprofloxacin. Lomefloxacin and temafloxacin have only moderate antipseudomonal activity. Their elimination half-lives are 6–10 hours and they have good oral absorption, excellent penetration into many tissues and fluids, and a better drug-interaction profile than other similar agents.

Lomefloxacin has demonstrated comparable efficacy to other therapies in the treatment of lower respiratory-tract infections and urinary-tract infections (UTIs) and for prophylaxis before surgical procedures in the urinary tract. Temafloxacin has been shown to be effective in the treatment of lower respiratory-tract infections, infections of the skin and associated structures, uncomplicated and complicated UTIs, bacterial prostatitis, and gonococcal and nongonococcal urethritis and cervicitis. The most frequent adverse effects with lomefloxacin are gastrointestinal upset and headache; with temafloxacin, gastrointestinal complaints. Lomefloxacin's dosage is 400 mg p.o. daily for 10 days for treatment of acute bacterial exacerbations in chronic bronchitis or simple cystitis and for 14 days for treatment of complicated UTIs.

Lomefloxacin is a new oral fluoroquinolone that is indicated for the treatment of various bacterial infections. Temafloxacin, another new fluoroquinolone, appeared to have some favorable characteristics but was withdrawn from the market.

Index terms: Dosage; Drug interactions; Lomefloxacin hydrochloride; Mechanism of action; Pharmacokinetics; Quinolones; Temafloxacin hydrochloride; Toxicity

Clin Pharm. 1992; 11: 753-66

Lomefloxacin (Maxaquin, Searle) and temafloxacin (Omniflox, Abbott) are fluoroquinolone antimicrobials developed through structural modifications to the basic quinolone nucleus. Because of these modifications, these agents have several potential advantages over other fluoroquinolones, including improved pharmacokinetic profiles, enhanced antimicrobial activity, and the absence of any significant drug interaction with theophylline or caffeine. Clinical trials of both agents have focused on various infections, such as those involving the lower respiratory tract and the urinary tract; these studies have highlighted the drugs' efficacy in comparison with current therapies. This review provides an overview of these two agents in comparison with other members of the fluoroquinolone class and discusses the clinical use of these agents.

FDA approval for marketing occurred in January 1992 for temafloxacin and in February 1992 for lomefloxacin. In June 1992 temafloxacin was recalled by its manufacturer because of severe adverse effects that were reported in the first three months of marketing.

Chemistry

Newer fluoroquinolones were developed with the goals of attaining high oral bioavailability, enhancing their activity against gram-positive organisms and anaerobes, reducing hepatic metabolism, prolonging the terminal elimination half-life to allow once-daily administration, and minimizing drug interactions.

WILLIAM T. SYMONDS, PHARM.D., is Research Fellow, The Clinical Pharmacokinetics Laboratory, Millard Fillmore Hospital, State University of New York at Buffalo. DAVID E. NIX, PHARM.D., is Assistant Director, The Clinical Pharmacokinetics Laboratory, Millard Fillmore Hospital, and Clinical Assistant Professor of Pharmacy, State University of New York at Buffalo.

Address reprint requests to Dr. Nix at The Clinical Pharmacokinetics Laboratory, Millard Fillmore Hospital, 3 Gates Circle, Buffalo, NY 14209.

This is article **680-204-9225** in the **ASHP Continuing Education System**; it qualifies for 1.0 hour of continuing-education credit. See page 814 for learning objectives and test questions.

There are few locations on the quinolone nucleus that can be modified to achieve these goals. However, in lomefloxacin and temafloxacin, key structural modifications to the quinolone nucleus provide advantages over other quinolones (Figure 1). These two agents differ structurally from one another by substitutions at positions 1 and 8 on the quinolone nucleus.[1] Lomefloxacin has a fluorine atom at position 8, which enhances metabolic stability and reduces metabolic drug interactions[2]; temafloxacin has a hydrogen atom at this position. Position 1 on lomefloxacin is occupied by an ethyl group; temafloxacin has a difluorinated phenyl group at this position, which enhances its activity against gram-positive organisms and increases its aqueous solubility. This substituent also appears to limit metabolic drug interactions with temafloxacin. In contrast, ciprofloxacin contains a cyclopropyl group at position 1, which increases its antibacterial potency against *Pseudomonas aeruginosa* and some Enterobacteriaceae. The α-methyl group on temafloxacin's piperazine substituent provides increased lipid solubility.

Lomefloxacin hydrochloride has a molecular weight of 387.81 and is only slightly soluble in water. Temafloxacin hydrochloride has a molecular weight of 453.85 and is soluble in water at concentrations of up to 5.6 mg/mL.[3] Dosages of lomefloxacin and temafloxacin are expressed in terms of the base, although both drugs are administered as the hydrochloride salt.

Mechanism of Action

The exact mechanism by which quinolones kill bacteria has not been completely characterized. The mechanism is thought to involve binding of the drug to DNA gyrase (also known as topoisomerase IIA) and subsequent inhibition of the enzyme's activity.[4] This enzyme causes the relaxation or introduction of negative supercoils in bacterial DNA. Other investigators have determined that quinolones bind directly to bacterial DNA and rapidly form a DNA gyrase–quinolone–DNA complex.[5] This complex formation leads to an immediate decrease in DNA synthesis and activation of the bacterial DNA repair mechanism.[4] The bacterium ceases division, and numerous proteins associated with cell repair accumulate inside the cell. However, the exact event causing cell death remains to be elucidated.

Figure 1. Chemical structures of lomefloxacin, temafloxacin, and ciprofloxacin.

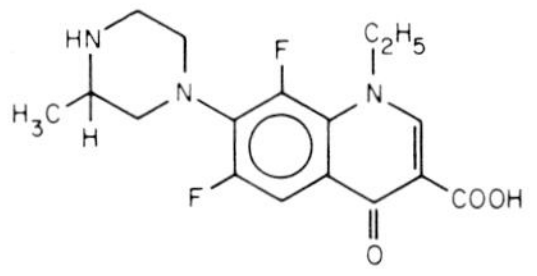

Lomefloxacin

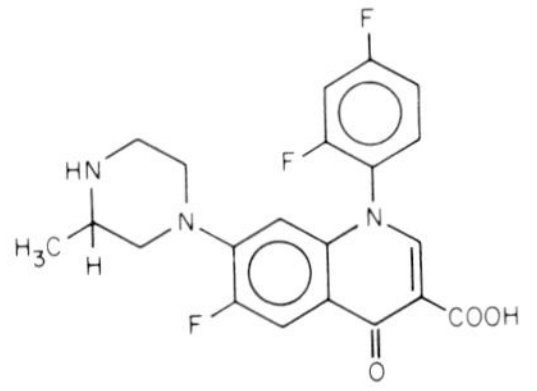

Temafloxacin

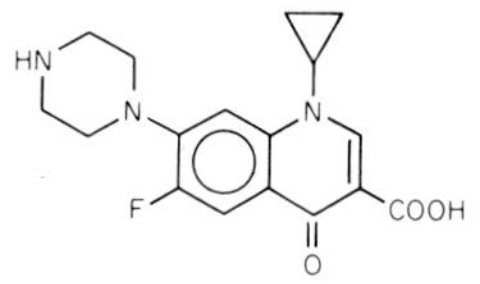

Ciprofloxacin

Antimicrobial Activity

As with other quinolones, the bactericidal activities of lomefloxacin and temafloxacin are unaffected by the bacterial growth phase (logarithmic or stationary); this property is in contrast to the β-lactams. The minimum inhibitory concentration (MIC) is generally similar to the bactericidal concentrations for lomefloxacin and temafloxacin.[3,6] Like other fluoroquinolones, the antimicrobial activity of lomefloxacin and temafloxacin is decreased in an acidic medium and in the presence of divalent cations, such as magnesium. Thus, the activity of both agents is decreased in normal urine. MICs of lomefloxacin for certain Enterobacteriaceae and *Ps. aeruginosa* are slightly increased in the presence of a high bacterial inoculum (10^7 colony-forming units [CFU]/mL).[7]

Both agents exhibit a substantial postantibiotic effect, the clinical significance of which is unknown.[7-10] Susceptibility testing by standard dilution techniques with both lomefloxacin and temafloxacin should be interpreted as follows: MIC of ≤2 μg/mL = susceptible, MIC of 4 μg/mL = intermediate, and MIC of ≥8 μg/mL = resistant.[11] Disks used in disk-susceptibility testing contain lomefloxacin 10 μg or temafloxacin 5 μg. Results for lomefloxacin should be interpreted based on the inhibition-zone diameter: ≥22 mm = susceptible, 19–21 mm = intermediate, and ≤18 mm = resistant. When temafloxacin is tested by this method, ≥16 mm = susceptible, 13–15 mm = intermediate, and ≤12 mm = resistant.[12] MICs for lomefloxacin, temafloxacin, and ciprofloxacin against selected organisms are presented in Table 1.

Gram-Positive Aerobic Organisms. Lomefloxacin has marginal activity against *Staphylococcus aureus*, including methicillin-resistant strains, but slightly better activity against *Staphylococcus epidermidis*.[13] Temafloxacin seems to be one to two times more active against staphylococcal strains than lomefloxacin. Temafloxacin exhibits significantly better activity against streptococcal species than lomefloxacin. Temafloxacin has comparable activity to ciprofloxacin against enterococcus. Temafloxacin appears to be more active against pneumococcal strains, including those with decreased

Table 1.
Median MIC_{50} and MIC_{90} for Lomefloxacin, Temafloxacin, and Ciprofloxacin against Selected Organisms[a]

Organism	Drug[b]	MIC_{50} (μg/mL)	MIC_{90} (μg/mL)
Escherichia coli	L	0.06	0.25
	T	0.06	0.12
	C	0.015	0.06
Klebsiella pneumoniae	L	0.25	0.5
	T	0.5	1.0
	C	0.03	0.25
Enterobacter cloacae	L	0.5	0.5
	T	0.25	0.25
	C	0.015	0.03
Proteus mirabilis	L	0.25	0.5
	T	0.25	0.5
	C	0.03	0.06
Serratia marcescens	L	0.5	2.0
	T	2.0	4.0
	C	0.12	0.5
Citrobacter diversus	L	0.12	0.12
	T	0.25	0.5
	C	≤0.008	≤0.008
Pseudomonas aeruginosa	L	2.0	4.0
	T	1.0	4.0
	C	0.12	0.5
Xanthomonas maltophilia	L	8.0	8.0
	T	1.0	8.0
	C	4.0	8.0
Aeromonas hydrophilia	L	0.06	0.12
	T	0.12	0.5
	C	<0.008	0.06
Providencia stuartii	L	1.0	2.0
	T	0.25	0.5
	C	0.12	0.25
Acinetobacter calcoaceticus	L	0.78	6.25
	T	0.12	0.25
	C	0.25	1.0
Haemophilus influenzae	L	0.06	0.12
	T	0.015	0.03
	C	<0.008	0.015
Chlamydia trachomatis	L	2.0	4.0
	T	0.125	0.25
	C	0.5	1.0
Staphylococcus aureus (methicillin-susceptible)	L	1.0	1.0
	T	0.25	0.25
	C	0.5	1.0
Staphylococcus aureus (methicillin-resistant)	L	1.0	2.0
	T	0.25	0.5
	C	0.5	1.0
Staphylococcus epidermidis (methicillin-susceptible)	L	0.5	1.0
	T	0.25	0.5
	C	0.125	0.25
Staphylococcus epidermidis (methicillin-resistant)	L	0.5	1.0
	T	0.25	0.5
	C	0.25	0.5
Staphylococcus saprophyticus	L	2.0	4.0
	T	0.5	0.5
	C	0.5	0.5
Streptococcus pneumoniae (penicillin-susceptible)	L	4.0	8.0
	T	0.5	1.0
	C	0.5	2.0
Streptococcus pneumoniae (penicillin-resistant)	L	8.0	NA[c]
	T	0.06	0.12
	C	0.5	2.0
Streptococcus pyogenes	L	4.0	8.0
	T	0.5	1.0
	C	0.5	1.0
Enterococcus faecalis	L	4.0	8.0
	T	1.0	2.0
	C	1.0	2.0

[a]Adapted from references 7–10, 13, 14. MIC_{50} = minimum inhibitory concentration for 50% of isolates; MIC_{90} = minimum inhibitory concentration for 90% of isolates.
[b]L = lomefloxacin, T = temafloxacin, C = ciprofloxacin.
[c]NA = not available.

susceptibility to penicillins.[14]

Gram-Negative Aerobic Organisms. Lomefloxacin and temafloxacin exhibit marked activity against the Enterobacteriaceae, with few exceptions. These agents' MICs against the Enterobacteriaceae are two to four times higher than ciprofloxacin's, with temafloxacin one to two times more active than lomefloxacin. However, both agents should be more than adequate in the treatment of infections caused by most Enterobacteriaceae, because achievable serum and tissue concentrations greatly exceed their MICs.[7,8,10] Against *Ps. aeruginosa* strains, both agents exhibit only marginal activity, with the MIC for 90% of isolates (MIC_{90}) equal to 4.0 µg/mL, whereas ciprofloxacin maintains an MIC_{90} of 0.5 µg/mL. *Xanthomonas maltophilia* was found to be resistant to both agents, with an MIC_{90} of 8.0 µg/mL.[7,8] Disk-susceptibility tests should not be used to determine susceptibility of *X. maltophilia*, because false positives are common.

Respiratory Pathogens. Lomefloxacin and temafloxacin both have excellent activity against most respiratory pathogens, including *Haemophilus influenzae*, *Moraxella catarrhalis*, *Legionella pneumophilia*, and *Klebsiella pneumoniae*.[13] However, many agents that inhibit *Legionella* spp. in vitro are not effective in vivo. Clinical studies will be required to support this use. Lomefloxacin is approximately three times less active against *Streptococcus pneumoniae* than temafloxacin and ciprofloxacin.[10]

Both agents display excellent activity against *Bordetella pertussis* and *Bordetella parapertussis*, while maintaining only marginal activity against *Mycoplasma pneumoniae* and *Mycobacterium tuberculosis* isolates.[15-18]

Genital and Intestinal Pathogens. The fluoroquinolones have been viewed as a therapeutic alternative in the treatment of sexually transmitted bacterial diseases. While lomefloxacin provides excellent activity against *Neisseria gonorrhoeae*, it maintains only marginal activity against other clinically important genital pathogens.[19,20] Temafloxacin provides excellent coverage against *N. gonorrhoeae* and is also very active against *Chlamydia trachomatis* and *Mycoplasma hominis*. Both lomefloxacin and temafloxacin have only marginal activity when tested against clinical isolates of *Ureaplasma urealyticum*.[18,21,22]

Lomefloxacin and temafloxacin have excellent activity against most of the common intestinal pathogens, including *Shigella* spp., *Salmonella* spp., *Yersinia enterocolitica*, *Campylobacter* spp., *Aeromonas hydrophilia*, and *Vibrio* spp.[23] There is evidence that temafloxacin may have marginal activity against *Helicobacter pylori*.[24] However, regardless of the in vitro susceptibility results, the use of quinolones in the treatment of *Helocobacter pylori*-associated gastritis is questionable because of limited clinical success.[25]

Anaerobic Pathogens. As seen with most other quinolone antimicrobials, lomefloxacin has no appreciable activity against anaerobic pathogens.[8] In contrast, temafloxacin inhibits the growth of many anaerobes at clinically achievable concentrations. Although few in vitro studies have been performed, temafloxacin appears to inhibit most strains tested at or near 4.0 µg/mL.[26,27] However, temafloxacin's role in the treatment of anaerobic or mixed aerobic–anaerobic infections must be scrutinized in animal studies and controlled clinical studies.

Resistance. The new fluoroquinolones do not have the same problems with bacterial resistance as early quinolones, such as nalidixic acid, to which resistance developed frequently during therapy. The in vitro development of mutants resistant to newer fluoroquinolones is extremely low at 4–8 times the MIC, concentrations which are normally encountered in clinical practice.[3,8,28] The mechanisms by which bacteria become resistant to these agents involve spontaneous mutations of subunit A of bacterial DNA gyrase, changes in the outer membrane proteins that affect the drug's ability to permeate the cell membrane,[29] or an energy-dependent drug-efflux mechanism.[30] Fortunately, the fluoroquinolones are not affected by bacterial enzymes such as β-lactamases. Resistance is chromosomally mediated and is generally not transferable between bacteria via plasmids. However, cross-resistance among the quinolones does occur and rarely may extend to other drug classes, depending on the bacterium involved.[29]

Resistance during therapy with ciprofloxacin has been observed most frequently when *Ps. aeruginosa* or *Staph. aureus* have been involved. These organisms typically have initial MICs ranging from 0.5 to 2.0 µg/mL (which are near the limit of susceptibility) at the onset of therapy, thereby becoming resistant after only one or two stepwise mutations. In addition, infections involving methicillin-resistant *Staph. aureus* display an even higher emergence of resistance during therapy both for localized infections and for the eradication of the methicillin-resistant *Staph. aureus* carrier state.[31]

Pharmacokinetics

Clinical studies examining the pharmacokinetic properties of lomefloxacin and temafloxacin have involved both high-performance liquid chromatography (HPLC) and microbiological analytical methods. However, there are few published assay procedures (bioassay or HPLC) for lomefloxacin[32-35] and temafloxacin.[36-38] Lomefloxacin serum concentrations determined by bioassay and HPLC have been similar.[35] Although definitive data concerning the correlation between microbiologic analytical methods and HPLC for temafloxacin have not been published, the two methods would probably yield similar results, as no active metabolites have been discovered for temafloxacin. Comparative pharmacokinetic values for ciprofloxacin, lomefloxacin, and temafloxacin are presented in Table 2.

Bioavailability. Lomefloxacin seems to be absorbed rapidly following oral administration to healthy volunteers, with an absolute bioavailability of >95%.[11] Mean ± S.D. peak serum concentrations were 1.88 ±

Table 2.
Comparative Pharmacokinetic Variables[a] Following Multiple Oral Dosing of Ciprofloxacin, Lomefloxacin, and Temafloxacin[39-43]

Variable	Ciprofloxacin 500 mg Twice Daily	Lomefloxacin 400 mg Once Daily	Temafloxacin 400 mg Twice Daily
C_{SSmax} (μg/mL)	3.5 ± 0.3	2.8 ± 0.4	5.3 ± 1.2
t_{max} (hr)	1.0 ± 0.4	1.5 ± 1.5	2.7 ± 1.9
CL (mL/min)	483.4 ± 207.8	258.6 ± 15.2	169 ± 58
CL_R (mL/min)	358.4 ± 135.8	166.5 ± 19.1	99 ± 33
$t_{1/2}$ (hr)	4.7 ± 1.2	7.8 ± 1.4	9.0 ± 1.9
V_β (L/kg)	2.0 ± 0.0	1.7 ± 0.5	2.5 ± 1.0

[a]Mean ± S.D.
[b]C_{SSmax} = maximum serum concentration at steady state, t_{max} = time to peak concentration, CL = total drug clearance, CL_R = renal drug clearance, $t_{1/2}$ = elimination half-life, V_β = terminal-phase volume of distribution.

0.29 μg/mL after a lomefloxacin dose of 200 mg, 3.43 ± 0.62 μg/mL after a 400-mg dose, 5.02 ± 1.11 μg/mL after a 600-mg dose, and 5.42 ± 0.68 μg/mL after an 800-mg dose.[40] The mean ± S.D. steady-state maximum concentration achieved after multiple oral dosing of lomefloxacin 400 mg once daily for seven days was 2.8 ± 0.43 μg/mL. Although the peak serum concentrations were not proportional to the dose administered—the lower dosages exhibited the highest normalized serum concentrations—the area under the concentration–time curve (AUC) was proportional to the dose administered. Thus, the bioavailability was consistent for each of the different dosages.[44] The absorption of lomefloxacin is not markedly affected by food intake; only the time to peak concentration was altered (delayed by one hour) after standard and high-fat meals, and the extent of absorption was similar with or without food.[45]

Temafloxacin also appears to be well absorbed after oral administration, with an absolute bioavailability of approximately 93%.[46] After administration of single oral doses of temafloxacin to healthy adult volunteers, mean ± S.D. peak serum concentrations were 0.98 ± 0.3 μg/mL after a 100-mg dose, 1.61 ± 0.6 μg/mL after a 200-mg dose, 2.43 ± 0.6 μg/mL after a 400-mg dose, 3.87 ± 0.7 μg/mL after a 600-mg dose, 4.54 ± 1.0 μg/mL after an 800-mg dose, and 6.67 ± 0.7 μg/mL after a 1000-mg dose. After multiple doses of 600 mg twice daily, temafloxacin reached a steady-state serum concentration of 6.2 ± 1.8 μg/mL, approximately 1 μg/mL for every 100 mg administered.[40] As with lomefloxacin, the peak serum concentrations did not increase proportionally with increased doses, and the time to peak concentration doubled from 1.25 hours after the 100-mg dose to 2.5 hours after the 1000-mg dose. In contrast, the AUC was proportional to the dose, suggesting that the extent of the absorption is independent of the dose administered.[47]

In Phase I studies examining the bioavailability of orally administered temafloxacin (200 mg, 400 mg, and 600 mg) with and without food, the AUC was slightly higher in nonfasting subjects than in fasting subjects. Because of enhanced dissolution, the hydrochloride-salt form may be more completely absorbed when food delays gastric emptying.[48]

Distribution. In general, quinolone antimicrobials, including lomefloxacin and temafloxacin, are distributed throughout the body into most tissues and fluids.[49] After a single 400-mg oral dose of lomefloxacin, the mean ± S.D. apparent volume of distribution was 2.5 ± 0.7 L/kg in healthy volunteers.[50] Because lomefloxacin has been targeted for treatment of acute bacterial exacerbations of chronic bronchitis, its penetration into lung tissues has been extensively studied. After the administration of 400 mg of lomefloxacin daily for four days, mean ± S.D. drug concentrations in the epithelial lining fluid (ELF) reached 8.8 ± 1.0 μg/mL (with a mean ± S.D. ELF:serum ratio of 2.8 ± 0.4), which is slightly higher than the bronchial-tissue concentration of 5.6 ± 0.6 μg/g. Lomefloxacin concentrations within the alveolar macrophages (AM) reached 54.6 ± 8.1 μg/g with an AM:ELF ratio of 6.6 ± 0.9.[51] In 20 patients undergoing prostatic resection, the median lomefloxacin concentration in the central zone of the prostate gland was 5.4 μg/g, in comparison with median serum levels of 2.4 μg/mL and a resultant mean ± S.D. tissue:serum concentration ratio of 2.2 ± 0.6.[33]

Concentrations attained in interstitial fluid have also been determined after mechanical induction of suction blisters.[36] After a single 400-mg oral dose of lomefloxacin, the mean ± S.D. peak blister-fluid concentration was 3.5 ± 0.7 μg/mL at 2.7 ± 0.8 hours, and the peak serum concentration was 4.7 ± 1.2 μg/mL at 1.0 ± 0.5 hours. After attainment of peak concentrations, the serum and blister-fluid concentrations remained remarkably similar. The mean percentage of penetration into the blister fluid was 100%.

Since lomefloxacin is primarily eliminated by renal excretion, urinary drug concentrations are quite high. Urine obtained over 24–48 hours after a single 400-mg dose of lomefloxacin exhibited a mean concentration of 31.0 μg/mL. Although bacterial susceptibility is lower in urine than in broth media, urinary drug concentrations are sufficient to inhibit most urinary pathogens for at least 24 hours.[36]

After oral administration of temafloxacin, the mean ± S.D. apparent volume of distribution was 149 ± 20 L, which greatly exceeds the volume of body water.[47]

After a dosage of 600 mg of temafloxacin twice daily for three days, mean ± S.D. concentrations in bronchial tissue were 14.9 ± 1.8 μg/g with a tissue:serum ratio of 1.6 ± 0.1, while temafloxacin concentrations in the ELF reached 26.3 ± 3.6 μg/mL with an ELF:serum ratio of 3.1 ± 0.3. Drug concentrations within the AM reached 79.2 ± 11.0 μg/g with an AM:ELF ratio of 5.7 ± 2.2.[51]

Temafloxacin also reaches moderately high concentrations in the prostate gland. After multiple oral 400-mg doses of temafloxacin administered every 12 hours, mean ± S.D. prostate tissue concentrations reached a maximum of 3.9 ± 2.8 μg/g 12 hours after the final dose, with a prostate tissue:serum ratio of 1.5 ± 0.8.[52] Temafloxacin penetrates well into bone tissue, with a peak concentration approximately equal to the peak serum concentration[53]; into tonsils, with a tonsillar tissue:serum ratio of 2.8 ± 0.9 at four hours[54]; and into suction-blister fluid, with a blister fluid:serum AUC ratio of 1.05.[55]

As expected, temafloxacin also reaches high concentrations in the urine. Shortly after a single 600-mg oral dose of temafloxacin, the maximum urinary drug concentration ranged from 168 to 672 μg/mL and remained between 1 and 5 μg/mL after 96 hours.[56] Temafloxacin concentrations found in the bile were 5 to 10 times higher than the corresponding serum concentrations;[38] however, biliary excretion is not a major elimination route.

Elimination. Most of an oral dose of either lomefloxacin or temafloxacin administered to healthy volunteers is excreted renally, with nonrenal mechanisms accounting for only a small fraction of total body clearance. After a single 400-mg oral dose of lomefloxacin or temafloxacin, the apparent total clearance and the renal clearance of both agents were highly correlated with creatinine clearance. The mean ± S.D. renal clearance of lomefloxacin was reported to be 199.5 ± 54.9 mL/min,[50] which exceeds the glomerular filtration rate and suggests active tubular secretion. Temafloxacin had a mean renal clearance of 125 mL/min, which more closely approximates the glomerular filtration rate.[44]

The nonrenal clearance of lomefloxacin and temafloxacin is mediated by both hepatic and (to a greater extent) extrahepatic mechanisms. Because metabolism of these agents accounts for a negligible fraction of nonrenal clearance, it appears that transintestinal elimination accounts for most of the nonrenal clearance, as is the case with other quinolones.[57,58] Both lomefloxacin and temafloxacin have a glucuronide conjugate as their major metabolite.[41,59] Temafloxacin also undergoes oxidative metabolism of its piperazinyl moiety to form both ethylenediamine- and methylethylenediamine-substituted metabolites.[41]

Effects of Renal Disease. Based on the percentage of drug eliminated unchanged in urine, the pharmacokinetics of both lomefloxacin and temafloxacin would be expected to be greatly influenced by decreases in renal function.

The pharmacokinetics of lomefloxacin have been studied in both healthy subjects and patients with varying degrees of renal impairment. Upon administration of a single 400-mg oral dose of lomefloxacin to healthy volunteers and renally compromised patients, significant differences were noted in the elimination-rate constant, terminal elimination half-life, $AUC_{0-\infty}$, apparent total body clearance, renal clearance, and apparent nonrenal clearance.[59] The mean ± S.D. half-life was 8.1 ± 2.2 hours in healthy subjects and 44.3 ± 14.0 hours in anuric patients. A direct relationship existed between creatinine clearance, renal clearance, and apparent total body clearance. Less than 3% of the administered dose was recovered in the dialysate after four hours of hemodialysis.

The pharmacokinetics of temafloxacin have been characterized in both healthy subjects and patients with impaired renal function. After a single 400-mg oral dose of temafloxacin, the mean ± S.D. terminal elimination half-life was 10.6 ± 2.4 hours in healthy subjects and 24.6 ± 7.3 hours in anuric patients.[41] Renal clearance and apparent total body clearance were significantly correlated with creatinine clearance, but nonrenal clearance did not vary with renal function. Less than 10% of the dose administered was recovered in the dialysate after four hours of hemodialysis.

On the basis of these studies, investigators have suggested dosage reductions in patients whose creatinine clearances are below 40 mL/min/1.73 sq m for lomefloxacin[59] and below 40 mL/min for temafloxacin.[41] Manufacturers' dosing recommendations for lomefloxacin will be discussed in a later section. No supplemental doses are necessary for either agent in patients undergoing hemodialysis.

Use in the Elderly. The pharmacokinetics of both lomefloxacin and temafloxacin have been analyzed in elderly patients.[60,61] While the two agents exhibit pharmacokinetic differences between young and elderly patients, they are not large enough to warrant dosage adjustment on the basis of increasing age alone. However, dosage adjustment is needed in patients with renal dysfunction beyond the normal age-related decline.

Clinical Experience

Numerous clinical investigations in the United States and abroad have examined the efficacy of lomefloxacin in the treatment of acute bacterial exacerbations in chronic bronchitis and urinary-tract infections (complicated and uncomplicated) and as prophylaxis before transurethral surgery. Temafloxacin has been evaluated in lower respiratory-tract infections (in acute exacerbations of chronic bronchitis and in pneumonia), genitourinary-tract infections (bacterial prostatitis, urinary-tract infections, and sexually transmitted bacterial diseases), and infections involving the skin and skin structures.

Acute Bacterial Exacerbations in Chronic Bronchitis. The treatment of acute bacterial exacerbations of chronic bronchitis ideally requires antimicrobial agents that are effective against *H. influenzae, M. catarrhalis*, and *Strep. pneumoniae*. Once-daily dosing of lomefloxacin (400 mg) has proved effective in patients with gram-negative infections but has limited activity against *Strep. pneumoniae*.[62] Temafloxacin has been used in higher doses (600 mg twice daily) and has exhibited greater activity against *Strep. pneumoniae* than most other fluoroquinolone antimicrobials.[13,51]

Lomefloxacin and amoxicillin have been evaluated in a worldwide, multicenter comparative study of the treatment of acute bacterial exacerbations in patients with chronic bronchitis.[63-66] The study included 525 patients, who received either 400 mg of lomefloxacin p.o. once daily or 500 mg of amoxicillin (as the trihydrate) p.o. every eight hours. The clinical response rates (cure plus improvement) for lomefloxacin was 93.6% and for amoxicillin was 82.8%. Bacterial eradication was achieved in 84.8% of the lomefloxacin treatment group and 78.5% of the amoxicillin group. Most clinical isolates were gram-negative, with only the United Kingdom center reporting a substantial percentage of *Strep. pneumoniae* (16.7%). Lomefloxacin 400 mg p.o. once daily has also been compared with cefaclor 250 mg p.o. given every eight hours for 7–10 days.[67] In this investigation, the three most prevalent pathogens were gram-negative, while *Strep. pneumoniae* accounted for approximately 10% of infections in each group. Lomefloxacin produced bacterial eradication (81.8%) and clinical success (80.0%) significantly more often than cefaclor did (62.7% and 64.7%, respectively, $p < 0.05$), based on intent-to-treat analysis. Although both agents achieved equivalent clinical success rates against the subgroup of pathogens susceptible to both agents, lomefloxacin eradicated a higher percentage of all pathogens than cefaclor did ($p = 0.002$). Lomefloxacin was as effective as amoxicillin and cefaclor in these trials, but more cases involving *Strep. pneumoniae* are needed to fully assess lomefloxacin's potential in this population. Cefaclor treatment was associated with bacterial persistence in 9 of 35 isolates of *H. influenzae* and 1 of 4 isolates of *Ps. aeruginosa*.

The results of six clinical trials of temafloxacin versus ciprofloxacin in patients with acute bacterial exacerbations of chronic bronchitis have been summarized.[68] In this analysis, evaluable patients had pathogens susceptible to both agents, and temafloxacin and ciprofloxacin had similar overall clinical response rates (93% versus 92%). Temafloxacin was superior in relation to overall bacterial eradication, with 98% eradication versus 92% with ciprofloxacin ($p < 0.01$). Upon further analysis by individual pathogen, *Strep. pneumoniae* was 100% eradicated in the temafloxacin group versus 78% in the ciprofloxacin group ($p < 0.001$).

Community-Acquired Pneumonia. The antimicrobial of choice for the empirical therapy of community-acquired pneumonia has traditionally been a penicillin derivative, such as amoxicillin, because of that group's activity against *Strep. pneumoniae* and *H. influenzae*. Although penicillin resistance among *Strep. pneumoniae* isolates in the United States is not a major problem, resistant strains are being isolated with increasing frequency in other parts of the world. Isolates of *H. influenzae* that produce β-lactamase are also appearing more frequently. Thus, alternative antimicrobial agents are needed in patients who cannot tolerate penicillins or when resistant organisms are suspected.

Temafloxacin has been compared with amoxicillin in the treatment of community-acquired pneumonia.[69] No significant differences were observed between the two treatment groups; the overall response rate was 88.5% in the temafloxacin group versus 86.2% in the amoxicillin group. Subgroup analysis by pathogen showed no differences between the pneumococcal group and the nonpneumococcal group for either agent. Thus, temafloxacin is as effective as amoxicillin, and it may be a good alternative in countries where penicillin resistance is a concern.

Temafloxacin has also been compared with cefotaxime, an injectable third-generation cephalosporin.[70] In this trial, clinical cure rates were 89% for temafloxacin and 92% for cefotaxime, with more than 90% of the patients in both treatment groups achieving bacteriological cure.

Controversy surrounds the use of any fluoroquinolone in documented or suspected pneumococcal pneumonia, as the number of patients studied with proven serious infections (bacteremia) is small. Although temafloxacin has greater activity than other agents, further experience with bacteremic cases is needed.

Skin and Skin-Structure Infections. To effectively treat infections of the skin, an antimicrobial agent must be active against gram-positive organisms, such as *Staph. aureus* and *Streptococcus* spp. When treating more complicated skin infections, activity against gram-negative organisms and anaerobes is also necessary. Temafloxacin is active against most of the common organisms involved. To date, lomefloxacin has not been evaluated in the treatment of these infections in the United States.

When temafloxacin was compared with cefadroxil in mild to moderately severe skin infections, both agents elicited similar clinical response rates (>96%).[71] However, the two agents differed significantly in eradicating the *Staph. epidermidis* subgroup, with temafloxacin eradicating 100% and cefadroxil eradicating 80.6%. Thus, temafloxacin appears to be at least as efficacious as cefadroxil in the treatment of skin infections. In patients likely to be infected with anaerobic pathogens, the addition of a second antimicrobial agent should be considered.

Temafloxacin has been compared with ciprofloxacin in three separate clinical studies.[72-74] In these trials, patients received 7- to 28-day courses of either temafloxacin, 600 mg p.o. twice daily, or ciprofloxacin, 750 mg (as the hydrochloride salt) p.o. twice daily. The overall response rate (cure plus improvement) in the temafloxacin group was 97.6%; in the ciprofloxacin group it was 100%. Bacterial eradication rates were similar in both treatment groups. Thus, temafloxacin and ciprofloxacin administered twice daily were equally effective in the treatment of skin and skin-structure infections.

Urinary-Tract Infections. In general, the fluoroquinolones are well suited for the treatment of urinary-tract infections (UTIs). These agents achieve high concentrations in the urine and are active against most of the common bacterial pathogens. Lomefloxacin has been evaluated in both complicated and uncomplicated UTIs in comparison with reference fluoroquinolones.

In the treatment of uncomplicated UTIs, lomefloxacin has been compared with norfloxacin and trimethoprim–sulfamethoxazole. In one trial, three- and seven-day therapy with once-daily lomefloxacin was compared with a seven-day course of norfloxacin administered twice daily.[75] The three regimens were evaluated in 475 patients, with approximately equal numbers in each treatment group. Clinical cure and bacteriological eradication rates were similar in both seven-day treatment groups. The three-day lomefloxacin treatment resulted in lower eradication and cure rates than the seven-day regimens.

A second study compared a 7- to 10-day course of once-daily lomefloxacin with twice-daily norfloxacin.[76] Both agents achieved clinical cure rates greater than 90% and eradication rates exceeding 95%. Thus, lomefloxacin is effective in the treatment of uncomplicated UTIs, although the three-day regimen is somewhat less efficacious. Another study, involving 254 patients, compared trimethoprim–sulfamethoxazole administered twice daily for 7–10 days with lomefloxacin (400 mg p.o. once daily).[77] Both agents achieved similar clinical success rates (>98%) and bacteriologic eradication (>95%) at five to nine days after therapy.

In the therapy of complicated or recurrent UTIs in male and female patients, once-daily lomefloxacin 400 mg was compared with twice-daily ciprofloxacin 500 mg (as the hydrochloride salt).[78] Lomefloxacin and ciprofloxacin achieved clinical response rates of 98.6% and 95.7%, respectively. Eradication of the causative organism occurred in 97.2% of the lomefloxacin group and 95.7% of the ciprofloxacin group. Thus, the two agents seem to be equally effective in the treatment of complicated or recurrent UTIs.

Temafloxacin has been evaluated in clinical studies of complicated and uncomplicated UTIs compared with reference agents. These therapies included trimethoprim–sulfamethoxazole (160 mg and 800 mg), ciprofloxacin 250 mg (as the hydrochloride salt), and norfloxacin 400 mg. In a comparative trial with norfloxacin, both agents were administered twice daily for 10–14 days to male and female patients (mostly females) with complicated UTIs.[79] Of the 279 patients enrolled, 110 were unevaluable for reasons including lack of identifiable pathogen and missed examinations. Among patients receiving temafloxacin, 74% were cured and an additional 22% were classified as improved. In the norfloxacin group, 87% were cured and another 11% were improved. Bacterial eradication rates exceeded 95% in both treatment groups, with *Escherichia coli* being the most prevalent pathogen. Thus, temafloxacin 400 mg twice daily was as effective as norfloxacin in the treatment of complicated UTIs.

In the treatment of uncomplicated UTIs, temafloxacin 400 mg once daily for seven days exhibited a 93% cure rate, as compared with trimethoprim–sulfamethoxazole twice daily for 10 days, which exhibited a 95% cure rate.[80] Clinical improvement was noted in an additional 5% in each treatment group. Bacterial eradication was seen in 100% of the patients receiving temafloxacin and 97% of those receiving trimethoprim–sulfamethoxazole. Thus, the two regimens were equally effective. Further study has indicated that temafloxacin 400 mg given once daily for three days is as effective as ciprofloxacin 250 mg (as the hydrochloride salt) administered twice daily for seven days.[81] Both agents produced clinical cure rates over 90% at five to nine days after therapy, with bacteriological eradication seen in 97% of the patients receiving temafloxacin and 96% of those receiving ciprofloxacin.

Urinary-Tract Surgical Prophylaxis. Almost all urologists use perioperative antimicrobial prophylaxis in transurethral surgery, and many continue the antimicrobial agent postoperatively for three to four days, until the Foley catheter is removed. Controlled studies have demonstrated the efficacy of prophylaxis for procedures involving penetration through the urethra, such as prostate biopsy and transurethral surgery.[82] A preoperative urine culture should be obtained and, if the results are positive, treatment should be maintained for 10–14 days. Antimicrobial prophylaxis is not necessary in simple cystoscopy or bladder catheterization, in which the risk of infection is minimal.[82]

Lomefloxacin is well suited for prophylaxis because of its extended terminal elimination half-life, excellent activity against Enterobacteriaceae, and good oral bioavailability. A single 400-mg dose of lomefloxacin will maintain adequate concentrations in the urine for at least 48 hours.[35] Lomefloxacin given as a single 400-mg oral dose two to six hours preoperatively was compared with a single 1.5-g intravenous dose of cefuroxime administered one to three hours preoperatively.[83] Five days after surgery, UTIs occurred in 11.1% of the 27 evaluable patients receiving lomefloxacin and 11.5% of the 26 evaluable patients receiving cefuroxime. These findings indicate that lomefloxacin administered orally is equivalent to cefuroxime administered intravenously.

Lomefloxacin has also been compared with cefotaxime (1 g as the sodium salt i.v. or i.m. given 30–90 minutes before surgery) in two randomized investigations.[84] Of the 413 evaluable patients, 207 received lomefloxacin and 206 received cefotaxime. Most of the unevaluable patients either had missed cultures or received concomitant antimicrobials. Lomefloxacin was more effective ($p = 0.047$) in preventing postsurgical infections than cefotaxime, with overall success rates of 98.6% in the lomefloxacin group and 95.1% in the cefotaxime group.

Bacterial Prostatitis. Temafloxacin, like all quinolones, is well suited for the treatment of chronic bacterial prostatitis (CBP) because it attains adequate tissue concentrations in the uninflamed prostate; failure to do so has been a problem with other therapies, such as trimethoprim–sulfamethoxazole.[85]

Recently, temafloxacin was administered at a dosage of 400 mg twice daily for 28 days to 112 patients with CBP.[86] Of the 81 evaluable patients examined five to nine days after their course of therapy, 70.4% were cured and 21% displayed clinical improvement. One month after treatment, the total clinical success rate was 86% (cure plus improvement). Of 71 patients who could be evaluated microbiologically, 92% showed eradication of the pretreatment pathogens at 30 days. Based on these findings, temafloxacin appears to be a useful agent for the treatment of CBP. Similar response rates were found in another study,[87] in which temafloxacin was evaluated in 61 patients diagnosed with CBP, with 90% of the clinically and bacteriologically evaluable patients cured five to nine days after treatment.

Because of the nature of CBP infections, response to antimicrobial therapy is difficult to assess with follow-up periods of less than one year.[88] While the currently available results are promising, further study should be done to assess long-term efficacy.

Sexually Transmitted Diseases. The fluoroquinolones appear to be effective in the treatment of most gonococcal infections. They all possess favorable pharmacokinetic profiles that make them good alternatives to currently accepted therapies. Temafloxacin is no exception, with activity against *N. gonorrhoeae* comparable to that of most other fluoroquinolones. In addition, temafloxacin has good activity against *C. trachomatis*, currently the leading cause of sexually transmitted bacterial diseases in the United States, whereas other agents display only moderate-to-poor activity (with the exception of ofloxacin).[89,90]

Temafloxacin as a single 200- or 400-mg oral dose has been evaluated in the treatment of uncomplicated gonococcal urethritis and cervicitis compared with 250 mg of intramuscular ceftriaxone (as the sodium salt).[91] Of the 253 evaluable patients, 39 received 200 mg of temafloxacin, 102 received 400 mg of temafloxacin, and 112 received ceftriaxone. Temafloxacin produced cures in 97.4% of the subjects who received 200 mg and 92.2% of those who received 400 mg. The ceftriaxone group exhibited a cure rate of 94.6%. Most of the unevaluable patients had no identifiable baseline pathogen, missed a culture, or were noncompliant. Thus, temafloxacin appears to be a suitable single-dose agent for gonococcal cervicitis and urethritis.

Temafloxacin has also been studied in the treatment of nongonococcal urethritis and cervicitis in comparison with doxycycline.[92] Patients received either temafloxacin 400 mg twice daily or doxycycline 100 mg twice daily, for seven days. Cure rates at 21 to 28 days after therapy were significantly higher in the temafloxacin group than in the doxycycline group (89% and 69%, respectively, $p = 0.05$). While both agents were equally effective in eradicating *C. trachomatis*, temafloxacin showed significantly greater activity against *M. hominis*, with 90% eradication in the temafloxacin group and 33% in the doxycycline group ($p = 0.002$). Thus, temafloxacin is an excellent alternative to doxycycline, the current standard, for the treatment of nongonococcal urethritis and cervicitis. Neither temafloxacin nor doxycycline should be used to treat chlamydial genital infections in pregnant women; erythromycin is most commonly used in such cases.

Safety

Safety data regarding the use of lomefloxacin have been analyzed in 2869 patients receiving the antibiotic during clinical trials.[93] Adverse events noted in clinical and pharmacokinetic evaluations have included nausea (3.7%), headache (3.2%), photosensitivity (2.4%), dizziness (2.3%), and diarrhea (1.4%). Most of these adverse events were considered mild to moderate, and their overall frequency was similar to that of other antimicrobials being studied. The number of subjects withdrawn from studies because of adverse effects was comparable to those with other fluoroquinolones.

The adverse events observed with temafloxacin during Phase I–III studies have been summarized.[94] Temafloxacin was administered to 572 patients in Phase I trials and to 2602 patients in Phase II and III studies. Adverse events noted during Phase I studies involving multiple dosing most frequently included headache (10.9%), dizziness (5.5%), nausea (4.0%), diarrhea (3.5%), dyspepsia (1.0%), and somnolence (0.5%). In general, the occurrence of adverse events was dose dependent, with a 29.2% frequency with 400 mg and a 45.8% frequency with 800 mg. The frequency of headaches in these trials was significantly higher in the placebo group (17.7%) than in the temafloxacin group. Headaches in Phase I clinical trials were commonly caused by caffeine abstinence, which was required in early protocols.

In Phase II and III studies, temafloxacin was compared with both quinolones and nonquinolones to examine its comparative efficacy in various infections.[94] The total frequency of adverse events for temafloxacin was 31.5%, compared with 30.4% in the quinolone comparison group and 29.4% in the nonquinolone group. Adverse effects were reported much more frequently in the trials that used patient diary cards (41.5%) than in those that did not (23.5%). Treatment was halted prematurely in 4.1% of the study subjects receiving temafloxacin; this was not significantly different from the percentage in other study groups. Most adverse effects in all three treatment groups were gastrointestinal. Gastrointestinal events were associated with higher dosages and tended to occur more frequently in subjects with decreased renal function (creatinine clearance, <70 mL/min).[94]

Premarketing studies, which involved approximately 5000 subjects,[95] had shown temafloxacin to be well tolerated. However, spontaneous postmarketing reports of serious adverse reactions (including three deaths) in 50 patients[95] followed use of the drug by approximately 300,000 patients worldwide (Newman J, Abbott Laboratories. Personal communication. 1992 Jun 8). These adverse reactions were considered severe, appeared to be caused by temafloxacin, and had not been discovered in premarketing trials; their exact nature had not been disclosed at the time of this writing.

The limitations of spontaneous reporting—false positive and false negative drug–event associations, underreporting by the health-care community, and failure to identify the populations at risk—prevent accurate estimation of the actual frequency of severe adverse effects.[96] Nevertheless, the temafloxacin experience has confirmed that postmarketing surveillance can reveal adverse reactions that are not apparent during premarketing trials.

Drug Interactions

The fluoroquinolones have been shown to interact with a number of widely used drugs. These include the methylxanthines, antacids, cimetidine, nonsteroidal anti-inflammatory drugs (NSAIDs),[97,98] and possibly warfarin.[99] Of these interactions, the most extensively studied has been that involving theophylline and earlier fluoroquinolones, such as ciprofloxacin and enoxacin.[97,100,101] It has been suggested that the extent of this interaction is related to the relative proportion of the fluoroquinolone that is converted to an oxometabolite; however, this metabolite is not directly responsible for the metabolic inhibition.[101,102] To date, neither lomefloxacin nor temafloxacin has been shown to inhibit theophylline metabolism to any significant degree.[103-107] This holds true for caffeine as well.[108,109]

Multivalent cations may lead to decreased absorption of fluoroquinolones. This interaction is well documented and has been shown to occur with all fluoroquinolones, including lomefloxacin and temafloxacin.[110] Ciprofloxacin and enoxacin have also been shown to interact with dairy products when given alone, not with meals.[111,112] However, this should not be extrapolated to the newer agents, because this interaction has not been examined with lomefloxacin and temafloxacin. Both lomefloxacin and temafloxacin have been shown not to interact with food.[45,48]

Fluoroquinolones have also been shown to inhibit binding of γ-aminobutyric acid (GABA) in the central nervous system, which may lead to increased excitation and possible seizures.[113] When lomefloxacin was administered with NSAIDs, particularly fenbufen, GABA-binding inhibition was potentiated, causing seizures in laboratory animals.[114] Temafloxacin has not exhibited this increase in GABA inhibition when combined with NSAIDs.[115] Only enoxacin in combination with fenbufen has elicited seizures in humans.[116]

Sporadic anecdotal reports have appeared in the literature concerning interactions between some fluoroquinolones, such as ciprofloxacin, ofloxacin, and norfloxacin in combination with warfarin.[117] This suspected interaction has yet to be proved in a controlled clinical investigation.[117-119] Temafloxacin was shown not to alter warfarin's anticoagulant effect in healthy volunteers.[120]

A drug interaction has recently become apparent between certain fluoroquinolones and cimetidine. Coadministration of cimetidine was shown to decrease the total clearance of temafloxacin by 19%, compared with baseline.[121] This interaction appears to be the result of competition for active tubular secretion within the kidney. While the extent of this interaction is low, it may become significant in patients with pre-existing renal disease.

Administration of crushed temafloxacin through a nasogastric tube, with and without enteral feeding, has been examined in healthy adult volunteers.[122] When compared with a reference oral dose (intact tablet) the enteral feedings had no significant effect on the relative bioavailability of temafloxacin.

Dosage and Administration

Lomefloxacin is administered as a single oral 400-mg dose daily for 10 days when treating simple cystitis or acute bacterial exacerbations in chronic bronchitis.[11] In complicated UTIs, treatment should be maintained for 14 days. In transurethral surgical procedures in which prophylaxis is recommended, lomefloxacin may be given as a single 400-mg oral dose two to six hours before the procedure.

In the treatment of pneumonia or acute bacterial exacerbations in chronic bronchitis, temafloxacin was given twice daily as a 600-mg oral dose for 10–14 days, and in the treatment of skin and skin-structure infections it was given for 7–14 days.[12] In the treatment of complicated UTIs and bacterial prostatitis, the dosage was 400 mg twice daily; it was 400 mg once daily for three days in uncomplicated UTIs. It was recommended that treatment for complicated UTIs be given for 10–14 days and treatment for bacterial prostatitis be maintained for 28–31 days.

Because the elimination of both agents depends heavily on renal function, dosages must be reduced in renal insufficiency accordingly. Lomefloxacin dosage should be decreased to 200 mg once daily following a 400-mg loading dose when the creatinine clearance (CL_{cr}) is <40 mL/min/1.73 sq m but greater than 10 mL/min/1.73 sq m.[11] Recommendations for temafloxacin dosing in patients with reduced renal function followed a stepwise approach based on initial dosage.[12] Patients who received 400 mg once daily required no adjustment while the CL_{cr} remained >10 mL/min. Individuals requiring 400 mg twice daily warranted a dosage reduction when their CL_{cr} ranged between 10–40 mL/min. Finally, patients requiring 600 mg twice daily were given 400 mg twice daily if their CL_{cr} fell between 40 and 80 mL/min or 600 mg once daily if between 10 and 40 mL/min.

Cost

The average wholesale price for lomefloxacin is $107.28 for 20 400-mg tablets (Campbell University Drug Information Center. Personal communication. 1992 Apr). The average wholesale price for temafloxacin was $130.63 for 50 400-mg tablets and $143.75 for 50 600-mg tablets. Based on these prices, the cost of a 10-day course of lomefloxacin 400 mg once daily would be $53.64. The cost of a 10-day course of temafloxacin 600 mg twice daily would have been $57.50.

Instructions to the Patient

Like all fluoroquinolones, lomefloxacin should not be administered concurrently with agents that contain divalent cations.[11,12] Antacids, iron, multivitamins with minerals, and sucralfate are best avoided, but if necessary, they should be taken at least two hours before or two hours after the fluoroquinolone. Lomefloxacin may be administered without regard to meals, as food does not significantly alter its absorption.

Patients should be instructed to drink fluids liberally and to avoid excess exposure to sunlight while receiving lomefloxacin. It may also cause lightheadedness or dizziness in certain individuals; thus, patients should be cautioned to determine how this agent affects their ability to operate an automobile or heavy machinery.

No fluoroquinolone should be administered to pregnant women or to pediatric patients, because their safety in these patient populations has not been established. As with all antimicrobials, patients should be advised to contact their physician if a skin rash or other allergic reaction develops after the first dose.

Instructions regarding temafloxacin would have been essentially identical to those for lomefloxacin.

FDA-Approved Labeling

Lomefloxacin's FDA-approved labeling states that the drug is indicated for the treatment of acute bacterial exacerbations in chronic bronchitis caused by *H. influenzae* or *M. catarrhalis*.[11] It should not be used when *Strep. pneumoniae* is suspected or if a sputum Gram's stain displays a predominance of gram-positive organisms. Lomefloxacin is also indicated for the treatment of uncomplicated UTIs caused by *E. coli*, *K. pneumoniae*, *P. mirabilis*, or *Staph. saprophyticus* and for complicated infections due to *E. coli*, *K. pneumoniae*, *P. mirabilis*, *Ps. aeruginosa*, *Citrobacter diversus*, or *Enterobacter cloacae*. Lomefloxacin is the only fluoroquinolone that is indicated for prophylaxis before transurethral surgical procedures in which infection is likely to occur.

Before its recall, temafloxacin's FDA-approved labeling stated that the drug was indicated for treatment of (1) infections of the lower respiratory tract, including acute bacterial exacerbations in chronic bronchitis caused by *H. influenzae*, *M. catarrhalis*, or *Strep. pneumoniae* and pneumonia due to *H. influenzae* or *Strep. pneumoniae*; (2) uncomplicated skin and skin-structure infections caused by *Acinetobacter calcoaceticus*, *E. coli*, *Ps. aeruginosa*, *Staph. aureus*, or *Strep. pyogenes*; (3) uncomplicated UTIs caused by *E. coli*, *P. mirabilis*, or *Staph. epidermidis*; (4) complicated infections due to *E. coli* or *K. pneumoniae*; and (5) bacterial prostatitis caused by *Enterococcus faecalis*, *E. coli*, or *P. mirabilis*.[12]

Formulary Recommendation

Lomefloxacin's advantages over other quinolones make it an attractive formulary addition. Its long terminal elimination half-life allows once-daily dosing, which will provide potential cost savings and possibly improve patient compliance when administered in the outpatient setting. Lomefloxacin may be administered safely to individuals receiving concomitant theophylline therapy. Also, this agent is the only fluoroquinolone that is indicated for prophylaxis before transurethral surgery, which will provide a substantial cost savings over intravenous regimens.

If temafloxacin were to become available again, its safety would have to be considered carefully before formulary recommendations could be made.

Conclusion

Lomefloxacin is a new oral fluoroquinolone that is indicated for the treatment of various bacterial infections. Temafloxacin, another new fluoroquinolone, appeared to have some favorable characteristics but has been withdrawn from the market.

---

[a]Campbell University Drug Information Center. Personal communication. 1992 Apr.

References

1. Percival A. Impact of chemical structure on quinolone potency, spectrum and side effects. *J Antimicrob Chemother*. 1991; 28(Suppl C):1-8.
2. Hirose T, Okezaki E, Kato H et al. In vitro and in vivo activity of ny-198, a new difluorinated quinolone. *Antimicrob Agents Chemother*. 1987; 31:854-9.
3. Hardy D, Swanson RN, Hensey DM et al. Comparative antibacterial activities of temafloxacin hydrochloride (A-62254) and two reference fluoroquinolones. *Antimicrob Agents Chemother*. 1987; 31:1768-74.
4. Sanders CC. Microbiology of fluoroquinolones. In: Sanders WE, Sanders CC, eds. Fluoroquinolones in the treatment of infectious diseases. Glenview, IL: Physicians and Scientists; 1990:1-27.
5. Shen LL, Pernet AG. Mechanism of inhibition of DNA gyrase by analogues of nalidixic acid: the target of the drugs is DNA. *Proc Natl Acad Sci USA*. 1985; 82:307-11.
6. Leigh DA, Tait S, Walsh B. Antibacterial activity of lomefloxacin. *J Antimicrob Chemother*. 1991; 27:589-98.
7. Chin N, Novelli A, Neu HC. In vitro activity of lomefloxacin (SC-47111; NY-198), a difluoroquinolone 3-carboxylic acid, compared with those of other quinolones. *Antimicrob Agents Chemother*. 1988; 32:656-62.
8. Chin N, Figueredo VM, Novelli A et al. In vitro activity of temafloxacin, a new difluoroquinolone antimicrobial agent. *Eur J Clin Microb Infect Dis*. 1988; 7:58-63.
9. Nakanishi N, Inour M, Inoue K et al. In vitro activity of

temafloxacin hydrochloride (TA-167 or A-62254), a new fluorinated 4-quinolone. *Chemotherapy*. 1990; 36:345-55.
10. Nye K, Shi YG, Andrews JM et al. The in-vitro activity, pharmacokinetics and tissue penetration of temafloxacin. *J Antimicrob Chemother*. 1989; 24:415-24.
11. Searle Laboratories. Maxaquin package insert. Skokie, IL; 1992 Mar.
12. Abbott Laboratories. Omniflox package insert. North Chicago, IL; 1992 Feb.
13. Simor AE, Fuller SA, Low DE. Comparative in vitro activities of sparfloxacin (CI-978; AT-4140) and other antimicrobial agents against staphylococci, enterococci, and respiratory tract pathogens. *Antimicrob Agents Chemother*. 1990; 34:2283-6.
14. Mazzulli T, Simor AE, Jaeger R et al. Comparative in vitro activities of several new fluoroquinolones and β-lactam antimicrobial agents against community isolates of *Streptococcus pneumoniae*. *Antimicrob Agents Chemother*. 1990; 34:467-9.
15. Kenny GE, Cartwright FD. Susceptibility of *Mycoplasma pneumoniae* to several new quinolones, tetracycline, and erythromycin. *Antimicrob Agents Chemother*. 1991; 35:587-9.
16. Hoppe JE, Simon CG. In vitro susceptibilities of *Bordetella pertusis* and *Bordetella parapertusis* to seven fluoroquinolones. *Antimicrob Agents Chemother*. 1990; 34:2287-8.
17. Waites KB, Cassell GH, Canupp KC et al. In vitro susceptibilities of mycoplasmas and ureaplasmas to new macrolides and fluoroquinolones. *Antimicrob Agents Chemother*. 1988; 32:1500-2.
18. Gorzynski EA, Gutman SI, Allen W. Comparative antimycobacterial activities of difloxacin, temafloxacin, enoxacin, pefloxacin, reference quinolones, and a new macrolide, clarithromycin. *Antimicrob Agents Chemother*. 1989; 33:591-2.
19. Talbot H, Romanowski B. In vitro activities of lomefloxacin, tetracycline, penicillin, spectinomycin, and ceftriaxone against *Neisseria gonorrhoeae* and *Chlamydia trachomatis*. *Antimicrob Agents Chemother*. 1989; 33:2049-51.
20. Kenny GE, Hooton TM, Roberts MC et al. Susceptibilities of genital mycoplasmas to the newer quinolones as determined by the agar dilution method. *Antimicrob Agents Chemother*. 1989; 33:103-7.
21. Barry AL, Jones RN. In-vitro activities of temafloxacin, tosufloxacin (A-61827), and five other fluoroquinolone agents. *J Antimicrob Chemother*. 1989; 23:527-35.
22. Segreti J, Kessler HA, Kapell KS et al. In vitro activities of temafloxacin (A-62254) and four other antibiotics against *Chlamydia trachomatis*. *Antimicrob Agents Chemother*. 1989; 33:118-9.
23. Segreti J, Nelson JA, Goodman LJ et al. In vitro activities of lomefloxacin and temafloxacin against pathogens causing diarrhea. *Antimicrob Agents Chemother*. 1989; 33:1385-7.
24. Hardy DJ, Hansen CW, Hensey DM et al. Susceptibility of *Campylobacter pylori* to macrolides and fluoroquinolones. *J Antimicrob Chemother*. 1988; 22:631-6.
25. Simor AE, Ferro S, Low DE. Comparative in vitro activities of six new fluoroquinolones and other oral antimicrobial agents against *Campylobacter pylori*. *Antimicrob Agents Chemother*. 1989; 33:108-9.
26. Wexler HM, Molitoris E, Finegold SM. In vitro activities of three of the newer quinolones against anaerobic bacteria. *Antimicrob Agents Chemother*. 1992; 36:239-43.
27. Finegold SM, Molitoris E, Reeves D et al. In-vitro activity of temafloxacin against anaerobic bacteria: a comparative study. *J Antimicrob Chemother*. 1991; 28(Suppl C):25-30.
28. Appelbaum PC. Mechanisms and frequency of resistance to temafloxacin. *Am J Med*. 1991; 91(Suppl 6A):27S-30S.
29. Sonstein SA. Mode of action of quinolones: antibacterial aspects. In: Siporin C, Heifetz CL, Domagala JM, eds. The new generation of quinolones. New York: Marcel Dekker; 1990.
30. Kaatz GW, Sep SM, Ruble CA. Mechanisms of fluoroquinolone resistance in *Staphylococcus aureus*. *J Infect Dis*. 1991; 163:1080-6.
31. Ball P. Emergent resistance to ciprofloxacin amongst *Pseudomonas aeruginosa* and *Staphylococcus aureus*: clinical significance and therapeutic approaches. *J Antimicrob Chemother*. 1990; 26(Suppl F):165-79.
32. Okezaki E, Makino E, Ohmochi K et al. Disposition and metabolism of NY-198. II. HPLC and bioassay studies of absorption and excretion in the dog. *Chemotherapy*. 1988; 36(Suppl 2):138-43.
33. Kovarik JM, DeHond JAPM, Hoepelman IM et al. Intraprostatic distribution of lomefloxacin following multiple-dose administration. *Antimicrob Agents Chemother*. 1990; 34:2398-2401.
34. Baldwin DR, Honeybourne D, Andrews JM et al. Concentrations of oral lomefloxacin in serum and bronchial mucosa. *Antimicrob Agents Chemother*. 1990; 34:1017-9.
35. Stone JW, Andrews JM, Ashby JP et al. Pharmacokinetics and tissue penetration of orally administered lomefloxacin. *Antimicrob Agents Chemother*. 1988; 32:1508-10.
36. Granneman GR, Senello LT. High-performance liquid chromatographic procedures for the determination of difloxacin and its metabolites in biological matrices. *J Chromatogr*. 1987; 413:199-206.
37. Granneman GR, Varga LL. High-performance liquid chromatographic procedures for the determination of temafloxacin in biological matrices. *J Chromatogr*. 1991; 568:197-206.
38. Mahr G, Granneman GR, Sorgel F. Hepatobiliary elimination of temafloxacin. *Clin Pharmacokinet*. 1992; 22(Suppl 1):33-42.
39. Mant TGK. Multiple-dose pharmacokinetics of lomefloxacin: rationale for once-a-day dosing. *Am J Med*. 1992; 92(Suppl 4A):26S-32S.
40. Granneman GR. Pharmacokinetics of temafloxacin after multiple oral administration. *Clin Pharmacokinet*. 1992; 22(Suppl 1):14-23.
41. Granneman GR, Braeckman R, Kraut J et al. Temafloxacin pharmacokinetics in subjects with normal and impaired renal function. *Antimicrob Agents Chemother*. 1991; 35:2345-51.
42. Nix DE, DeVito JM. Ciprofloxacin and norfloxacin, two fluoroquinolone antimicrobials. *Clin Pharm*. 1987; 6:105-17.
43. Sorgel F, Naber KG, Stephan U et al. Pharmakokinetik und analytik von gyrase-hemmern. *Fortschr Antimikrob Antineoplast Chemother*. 1987; 6-10:1907-61.
44. Morrison PJ, Mant TGK, Norman GT et al. Pharmacokinetics and tolerance of lomefloxacin after sequentially increasing oral doses. *Antimicrob Agents Chemother*. 1988; 32:1503-7.
45. Hooper WD, Dickinson RG, Eadie MJ. Effect of food on absorption of lomefloxacin. *Antimicrob Agents Chemother*. 1990; 34:1797-9.
46. Granneman R, Braeckman R, Carpentier P et al. Pharmacokinetics of temafloxacin after single intravenous 100, 200, 400, 600, and 800 mg doses. Paper presented at 17th International Congress of Chemotherapy. Berlin, Germany: 1991.
47. Granneman GR, Carpentier P, Morrison PJ et al. Pharmacokinetics of temafloxacin in humans after single oral doses. *Antimicrob Agents Chemother*. 1991; 35:436-41.
48. Granneman GR, Mukherjee D. The effect of food on the bioavailability of temafloxacin: a review of 3 studies. *Clin Pharmacokinet*. 1992; 22(Suppl 1):48-56.
49. Sorgel F, Jaehde U, Naber K et al. Pharmacokinetic disposition of quinolones in human body fluids and tissues. *Clin Pharmacokinet*. 1989; 16(Suppl 1):5-24.
50. Leroy A, Fillastre JP, Humbert G. Lomefloxacin pharmacokinetics in subjects with normal and impaired renal function. *Antimicrob Agents Chemother*. 1990; 34:17-20.
51. Wise R, Baldwin DR, Andrews JM et al. Comparative pharmacokinetic disposition of fluoroquinolones in the lung. *J Antimicrob Chemother*. 1991; 28(Suppl C):65-71.
52. Fornara P, Schollmayer E, Seelman R et al. Penetration of temafloxacin into prostatic tissue. Paper presented at 3rd International Symposium on New Quinolones. Vancouver, British Columbia: 1990 Jul 12-14.
53. Sunder-Plassman L, Refior HJ, Seelman R et al. Penetration of temafloxacin into bone tissue. Paper presented at 3rd

International Symposium on New Quinolones. Vancouver, British Columbia: 1990 Jul 12-14.

54. Kastenbauer E, Luckhaupt H, Muth P et al. The penetration of temafloxacin into tonsils. Paper presented at 3rd International Symposium on New Quinolones. Vancouver, British Columbia: 1990 Jul 12-14.
55. Sorgel F. Penetration of temafloxacin into body tissues and fluids. *Clin Pharmacokinet*. 1992; 22(Suppl 1):57-63.
56. Seelman R, Sorgel F, Granneman R et al. Pharmacokinetics of temafloxacin in patients with liver impairment. Paper presented at 17th International Congress of Chemotherapy. Berlin, Germany: 1991.
57. Sorgel F, Naber KG, Jaehde U et al. Gastrointestinal secretion of ciprofloxacin. *Am J Med*. 1989; 87(Suppl 5A):62S-5S.
58. Sorgel F, Naber KG, Mahr G et al. Transintestinal elimination of ofloxacin. Paper presented at 17th International Congress of Chemotherapy. Berlin, Germany: 1991.
59. Blum RA, Schultz RW, Schentag JJ. Pharmacokinetics of lomefloxacin in renally compromised patients. *Antimicrob Agents Chemother*. 1990; 34:2364-8.
60. Pernet AG. Temafloxacin: a safe antibiotic for the elderly, patients with comorbidities, and other special populations. *Am J Med*. 1991; 91(Suppl 6A):162S-5S.
61. Schentag JJ, Goss TF. Quinolone pharmacokinetics in the elderly. *Am J Med*. 1991; 92(Suppl 4A):33S-7S.
62. Kemper P, Köhler D. A double-blind study of two dosage regimens of lomefloxacin in bacteriologically proven exacerbations of chronic bronchitis of gram-negative etiology. *Am J Med*. 1992; 92(Suppl 4A):98S-102S.
63. Saenz C. Lomefloxacin (LOM) vs. amoxicillin (AMOX) in treatment of acute exacerbations of chronic bronchitis: Latin America. Paper presented at 30th Interscience Conference on Antimicrobial Agents and Chemotherapy. Atlanta, GA: 1990 Oct 24.
64. Grassi C, Albera C, Pozzi E. Lomefloxacin versus amoxicillin in the treatment of acute exacerbations of chronic bronchitis: an Italian multicenter study. *Am J Med*. 1992; 92(Suppl 4A):103S-7S.
65. Kandziora J, Zaltenbach G. Lomefloxacin (LOM) vs. amoxicillin (AMOX) in the treatment of acute exacerbations of chronic bronchitis: German experience. Paper presented at 30th Interscience Conference on Antimicrobial Agents and Chemotherapy. Atlanta, GA: 1990 Oct 24.
66. Russell D. Lomefloxacin (LOM) vs. amoxicillin (AMOX) in treatment of acute exacerbations of chronic bronchitis: United Kingdom. Paper presented at 30th Interscience Conference on Antimicrobial Agents and Chemotherapy. Atlanta, GA: 1990 Oct 24.
67. Gottfried MH, Ellison WT. Safety and efficacy of lomefloxacin versus cefaclor in the treatment of acute exacerbations of chronic bronchitis. *Am J Med*. 1992; 92(Suppl 4A):108S-13S.
68. Ball P. The role of temafloxacin in the community setting: an overview. *J Antimicrob Chemotherapy*. 1991; 28(Suppl C):121-30.
69. Carbon C, Leophonte P, Petitpretz P et al. Efficacy and safety of temafloxacin versus those of amoxicillin in hospitalized adults with community-acquired pneumonia. *Antimicrob Agents Chemother*. 1992; 36:833-839.
70. Vogel F, Lode H. The use of oral temafloxacin compared with a parenteral cephalosporin in hospitalized patients with pneumonia. *J Antimicrob Chemother*. 1991; 28(Suppl C):81-6.
71. Neldner KH. Double-blind randomized study of oral temafloxacin and cefadroxil in patients with mild to moderate severe bacterial skin infections. *Am J Med*. 1991; 91(Suppl 6A):111S-4S.
72. Parish L. Temafloxacin compared to ciprofloxacin in the treatment of mild-to-severe bacterial skin or skin structure infections. Paper presented at 3rd International Symposium on New Quinolones. Vancouver, British Columbia: 1990 Jul 12-14.
73. Kampfer M. Temafloxacin versus ciprofloxacin for the treatment of skin or skin structure infection. Paper presented at 3rd International Symposium on New Quinolones. Vancouver, British Columbia: 1990 Jul 12-14.
74. Pein F, Craft J. Temafloxacin 600 mg bid compared to ciprofloxacin 750 mg bid in the treatment of moderate-to-severe bacterial skin infections. Paper presented at 3rd International Symposium on New Quinolones. Vancouver, British Columbia: 1990 Jul 12-14.
75. Forsgren A, Hansson C, Neringer R et al. Lomefloxacin vs. norfloxacin in the treatment of patients with uncomplicated urinary tract infections: three vs. seven day therapy. Paper presented at 3rd International Symposium on New Quinolones. Vancouver, British Columbia: 1990 Jul 12-14.
76. Iravani A. A multicenter comparison of the safety and efficacy of lomefloxacin and norfloxacin in the treatment of uncomplicated urinary tract infection (UTI). Paper presented at 3rd International Symposium on New Quinolones. Vancouver, British Columbia: 1990 Jul 12-14.
77. Andrade-Villanueva J, Flores-Gaxiola A, Lopez-Guillen P et al. Comparison of the safety and efficacy of lomefloxacin and trimethoprim/sulfamethoxazole in the treatment of uncomplicated urinary tract infections: results from a multicenter study. *Am J Med*. 1992; 92(Suppl 4A):71S-4S.
78. Cox CE. A comparison of the safety and efficacy of lomefloxacin and ciprofloxacin in the treatment of complicated or recurrent urinary tract infections. *Am J Med*. 1992; 92(Suppl 4A):82S-6S.
79. Cox CE. Oral temafloxacin compared to norfloxacin for the treatment of complicated urinary tract infections. *Am J Med*. 1991; 91(Suppl 6A):129S-33S.
80. Iravani A. Comparative, double-blind, prospective, multicenter trial of temafloxacin versus trimethoprim–sulfamethoxazole in uncomplicated urinary tract infections in women. *Antimicrob Agents Chemother*. 1991; 35:1777-81.
81. Stein GE, Philip E. Comparison of three-day temafloxacin with seven-day ciprofloxacin treatment of urinary tract infections in women. *J Fam Pract*. 1992; 34:180-4.
82. Amin M. Antibacterial prophylaxis in urology: a review. *Am J Med*. 1992; 92(Suppl 4A):114S-7S.
83. Charton M, Mombet A, Gattegno B. Urinary tract infection prophylaxis in transurethral surgery: oral lomefloxacin versus parenteral cefuroxime. *Am J Med*. 1992; 92(Suppl 4A):118S-20S.
84. Klimberg IW, Childs SJ, Madore RJ et al. A multicenter comparison of oral lomefloxacin versus parenteral cefotaxime as prophylactic agents in transurethral surgery. *Am J Med*. 1992; 92(Suppl 4A):121S-5S.
85. Meares EM. Prostatitis syndromes: new perspectives about old woes. *J Urol*. 1980: 123;141-7.
86. Cox CE, Childs SJ. Treatment of chronic bacterial prostatitis with temafloxacin. *Am J Med*. 1991; 91(Suppl 6A):134S-9S.
87. Naber KG, Boerema JBJ, Bischoff W et al. An assessment of temafloxacin in the treatment of chronic bacterial prostatitis. *J Antimicrob Chemother*. 1991; 28(Suppl C):87-96.
88. Pfau A. Prostatitis, a continuing enigma. *Urol Clin N Amer*. 1986; 13:695-715.
89. Mogabgab WJ. Recent developments in the treatment of sexually transmitted diseases. *Am J Med*. 1991; 91(Suppl 6A):140S-4S.
90. Batterger BE, Jones RB, White A. Efficacy and safety of ofloxacin in the treatment of nongonococcal sexually transmitted disease. *Am J Med*. 1989; 87(Suppl 6C):75S-7S.
91. Mogabgab WJ. Single-dose oral temafloxacin versus parenteral ceftriaxone in the treatment of gonococcal urethritis/cervicitis. *Am J Med*. 1991; 91(Suppl 6A):145S-9S.
92. McCarty J, Rodrigeuz M, Segreti J et al. Temafloxacin versus doxycycline in the treatment of non-gonococcal urethritis or cervicitis. Paper presented at 3rd International Symposium on New Quinolones. Vancouver, British Columbia: 1990 Jul.
93. Rizk E. The U.S. clinical experience with lomefloxacin, a new once-daily fluoroquinolone. *Am J Med*. 1992; 92(Suppl 4A):130S-5S.

94. Norby SR, Pernet AG. Assessment of adverse events during drug development: experience with temafloxacin. *J Antimicrob Chemother*. 1991; 20(Suppl C):111-9.
95. Burton TM. Adverse patient reactions force Abbott to pull new antibiotic from market. *Wall St J*. 1992; 219(Jun 8):B8.
96. Strom BL, Tugwell P. Pharmacoepidemiology: current status, prospects, and problems. *Ann Intern Med*. 1990; 113:179-81. Letter.
97. Janknegt R. Drug interactions with quinolones. *J Antimicrob Chemother*. 1990; 26(Suppl D):7-29.
98. Hori S, Shimada J, Saito A et al. Comparison of the inhibitory effects of new quinolones on gaba receptor binding in the presence of antiinflammatory drugs. *Rev Infect Dis*. 1989; 11(Suppl 5):S1397-8.
99. Jolson HM, Tanner LA, Green L et al. Adverse reaction reporting of interaction between warfarin and fluoroquinolones. *Arch Intern Med*. 1991; 151:1003-4.
100. Edwards DJ, Bowles SK, Svensson CK et al. Inhibition of drug metabolism by quinolone antibiotics. *Clin Pharmacokinet*. 1988; 15:194-204.
101. Rogge MC, Solomon WR, Sedman AJ et al. The theophylline–enoxacin interaction: i. Effect of enoxacin dose size on theophylline disposition. *Clin Pharmacol Ther*. 1988; 44:579-87.
102. Edwards DJ, Waite NM, Svesson CK. Effect of enoxacin and 4-oxo-enoxacin on antipyrine disposition in the rat. *Drug Metabol Dispos*. 1988; 16:653-4.
103. Nix DE, Norman A, Schentag JJ. Effect of lomefloxacin on theophylline pharmacokinetics. *Antimicrob Agents Chemother*. 1989; 33:1006-8.
104. LeBel M, Vallee F, St-Laurent M. Influence of lomefloxacin on the pharmacokinetics of theophylline. *Antimicrob Agents Chemother*. 1990; 34:1254-6.
105. Wijnands GJA, Cornel JH, Martea M et al. The effect of multiple-dose oral lomefloxacin on theophylline metabolism in man. *Chest*. 1990; 98:1440-4.
106. Sorgel F, Mahr G, Granneman R et al. Effects of two quinolone antibacterials, temafloxacin and enoxacin, on theophylline pharmacokinetics. *Clin Pharmacokinet*. 1992; 22(Suppl C):65-74.
107. Ruff F, Santais MC, Callens E et al. Effect of temafloxacin on the pharmacokinetics of theophylline. *Am J Med*. 1991; 91(Suppl 6A):76S-80S.
108. Harder S, Staib AH, Beer C et al. 4-Quinolones inhibit biotransformation of caffeine. *Eur J Clin Pharmacol*. 1988; 35:651-6.
109. Mahr G, Sorgel F, Granneman R et al. Effects of temafloxacin and ciprofloxacin on the pharmacokinetics of caffeine. *Clin Pharmacokinet*. 1992; 22(Suppl 1):90-7.
110. Granneman GR, Stephan U, Birner B et al. Effect of antacid medication on the pharmacokinetics of temafloxacin. *Clin Pharmacokinet*. 1992; 22(Suppl 1):83-9.
111. Neuvonen PJ, Kivistö KT, Lehto P. Interference of dairy products with the absorption of ciprofloxacin. *Clin Pharmacol Ther*. 1991; 50:498-502.
112. Kivistö KT, Ojala-Karlsson P, Neuvonen PJ. Inhibition of norfloxacin absorption by dairy products. *Antimicrob Agents Chemother*. 1992; 36:489-91.
113. Tsuji A, Sato H, Kume Y et al. Inhibitory effects of quinolone antibacterial agents on gamma-aminobutyric acid binding to receptor sites in rat brain membranes. *Antimicrob Agents Chemother*. 1988; 32:190-4.
114. Christ W, Gindler K, Gruene W et al. Interactions of quinolones with opioids and fenbufen, a nonsteroidal antiinflammatory drug: involvement of dopaminergic neurotransmission. *Rev Infect Dis*. 1989; 11(Suppl 5):S1393-4.
115. Giardinia WJ. Assessment of temafloxacin neurotoxicity in rodents. *Am J Med*. 1990; 91(Suppl 6A):42S-4S.
116. Morikawa K, Nagata O, Kubo S et al. Unusual CNS toxic action of new quinolones. Paper presented at 27th Interscience Conference on Antimicrobial Agents and Chemotherapy. New York, NY: 1987 Oct 5.
117. Toon S, Hopkins KJ, Garstang FM et al. Enoxacin–warfarin interaction: pharmacokinetic and stereochemical aspects. *Clin Pharmacol Ther*. 1987; 42:33-41.
118. Rocci ML, Vlasses PH, Distlerath LM et al. Norfloxacin does not alter warfarin's disposition or anticoagulant effect. *J Clin Pharmacol*. 1990; 30:728-32.
119. Rindone JP, Keuey CL, Jones WN et al. Hypoprothrombinemic effect of warfarin not influenced by ciprofloxacin. *Clin Pharm*. 1991; 10:136-8.
120. Millar E, Coles S, Wyld P et al. Temafloxacin does not potentiate the anticoagulant effect of warfarin in healthy subjects. *Clin Pharmacokinet*. 1992; 22(Suppl 1):102-6.
121. Sorgel F, Granneman GR, Stephan U et al. Effect of cimetidine on the pharmacokinetics of temafloxacin. *Clin Pharmacokinet*. 1992; 22(Suppl 1):75-82.
122. Lubowski TJ, Nightingale CH, Sweeney K et al. The relative bioavailability of temafloxacin administered through a nasogastric tube with and without enteral feeding. *Clin Pharmacokinet*. 1992; 22(Suppl 1):43-7.

Tuberculosis Morbidity in the United States

The number of tuberculosis cases reported to CDC has been increasing since 1988, after a long historic decline. In 1990, 25,701 cases were reported, an increase of 9.4% over the 1989 figure and the largest annual increase since 1953. From 1985 to 1990, reported cases increased by 15.8%. Disproportionately greater increases in reported cases occurred among Hispanics, non-Hispanic blacks, and Asians/Pacific Islanders. In contrast, decreases were observed among non-Hispanic whites and American Indians/Alaskan Natives. By age, the largest increase in reported cases occurred in the 25- to 44-year age group; this increase may be largely attributable to rising numbers of tuberculosis cases among persons with human immunodeficiency virus infection or acquired immunodeficiency syndrome. Notable increases also occurred among children. The proportion of cases among foreign-born persons has risen steadily, from 21.6% in 1986 to 24.4% in 1990.

—Jereb JA, Kelly GD, Dooley SW Jr et al. Tuberculosis morbidity in the United States: final data, 1990. *MMWR*. 1991; 40(SS-3):23-7.

Therapy Review

Treatment of adult acute leukemia

Dayna L. McCauley

Abstract: The epidemiology, etiology, pathophysiology, classification, and clinical appearance of adult acute leukemia are reviewed, and treatment strategies are discussed.

Some 18,000 Americans die of leukemia each year, with acute leukemia accounting for half of these deaths. The etiology of acute leukemia is unknown, but current theories propose that the disease is caused by environmental factors acting on a genetically susceptible host. Acute leukemia occurs when a single hematopoietic precursor cell undergoes neoplastic transformation; autonomous proliferation of the leukemia clone continues until the patient dies of infection or bleeding. Acute leukemias are broadly classified as myelogenous and lymphocytic on the basis of cell lineage. Signs and symptoms are related to infiltration of the bone marrow by leukemic cells and the resultant failure of normal hematopoiesis. Therapy for acute myelogenous leukemia includes remission induction and consolidation with an array of antineoplastic agents. Allogeneic or autologous bone marrow transplantation is the therapy of choice for eligible patients in the first complete remission. Neither low-dose maintenance therapy nor prophylaxis for CNS involvement is indicated. Therapy for acute lymphocytic leukemia includes induction, consolidation, maintenance, and CNS prophylaxis. Allogeneic bone marrow transplantation should be reserved for standard-risk patients in second or subsequent complete remission and for high-risk patients in first remission.

Intensive combination chemotherapy and bone marrow transplantation have improved the outlook for many adult patients with acute leukemia.

Index terms: Antineoplastic agents; Epidemiology; Leukemia; Transplantation
Clin Pharm. 1992; 11:767-96

Leukemias are malignant neoplasms arising from blood-forming units in the bone marrow. They are characterized by the autonomous proliferation and accumulation of immature or dysfunctional blood cells, with resultant failure of normal hematopoiesis.[1] Leukemias are classified as myeloid or lymphoid depending on the predominant cell type and as acute or chronic depending on the survival time after diagnosis.[2] Historically, a diagnosis of acute leukemia conferred a dismal prognosis and carried an anticipated life expectancy of only weeks to a few months. However, with advances in intensive combination chemotherapy and bone marrow transplantation, acute leukemia is now potentially curable.

This paper reviews the epidemiology, etiology, pathophysiology, classification, clinical presentation, diagnosis, prognostic features, and treatment of acute myelogenous and lymphocytic leukemias in adults. A rationale for the approach to treatment is provided and new drug therapies are discussed.

Epidemiology and Prevalence

Approximately 26,000 cases of leukemia occur in the United States annually; these cases account for 7–8% of all new cancer cases reported.[3] Approximately 18,000 Americans die of leukemia each year, with acute leukemia accounting for 50% of these deaths. All types of leukemia are more common in men than women; the male-to-female ratio is 3:2 for acute leukemia. Although the overall frequencies of acute lymphoblastic leukemia (ALL) and acute myelogenous leukemia (AML) in the United States are approximately equal, there are marked differences in their distribution by age.[1-3] Childhood leukemias are primarily lymphoid in origin, with ALL accounting for 80–85%

Dayna L. McCauley, Pharm.D., is Clinical Pharmacist, Adult Hematology and Oncology Ambulatory Care Clinic, University of Michigan Medical Center, Ann Arbor.

Address reprint requests to Dr. McCauley at Pharmacy Administration, UHB2D 301, Box 0008, University of Michigan Hospitals, 1500 E. Medical Center Drive, Ann Arbor, MI 48109-0008.

This is **article 680-204-9223** in the **ASHP Continuing Education System;** it qualifies for 2.0 hours of continuing-education credit. See page 812 for learning objectives and test questions.

The assistance of Michael L. Pearl, M.D., is acknowledged.

of all acute leukemias between the ages of 2 and 10 years. In adults the ratios are reversed: AML accounts for 80–85% of all acute leukemias and ALL the remaining 15–20%.[1,2]

Etiology

The exact cause of acute leukemia is unknown, although several factors are known to influence the frequency of the disease. Current theories propose that acute leukemias result from environmental factors acting on a genetically susceptible individual.

Ionizing Radiation. Large doses of ionizing radiation are clearly associated with an increased incidence of acute and chronic myeloid leukemias. In survivors of atomic bombings, the risk of acute leukemia was directly proportional to the total body exposure to radiation and inversely proportional to the distance from the hypocenter.[4,5] The high incidence of leukemia in pioneering radiologists and in patients treated with large doses of radiation confirms the role of radiation in leukemogenesis.[6,7] In contrast, the relationship between small amounts of radiation and leukemia is unknown, and whether a threshold dose exists, below which there is no attendant risk of leukemia, remains controversial. No data suggest that exposure to the doses of radiation currrently used in diagnostic procedures or emitted by video display terminals is associated with an increased incidence of leukemia.

Chemical Agents. Chemicals or drugs that injure bone marrow are associated with development of leukemia. Benzene is the best-known chemical carcinogen; data describing its role in the development of hematologic neoplasms were reviewed by Cronkite.[8] The drugs most commonly implicated in the development of leukemia are the antineoplastic agents, particularly alkylating agents such as chlorambucil, busulfan, nitrogen mustard, and melphalan. Secondary leukemia has been described in patients treated for Hodgkin's disease,[9,10] non-Hodgkin's lymphomas,[11] multiple myeloma,[12] ovarian cancer,[13] and other cancers.[1] Secondary leukemias caused by alkylating agents may be acute or chronic, are predominantly of myeloid origin, are preceded by a preleukemic or myelodysplastic phase, respond poorly to therapy, and confer a poor prognosis.[10,11] Chloramphenicol and phenylbutazone, drugs associated with marrow aplasia, have also been implicated in acute leukemia.[12]

Viruses. The role of viruses in the etiology of human leukemia is unclear. The Epstein-Barr virus, a DNA virus, has been implicated as a causative agent in Burkitt's lymphoma, and type C RNA viruses have been associated with leukemia in animals.[14] The only viruses implicated in human leukemia have been type C RNA viruses (retroviruses) that produce viral DNA from an RNA template with reverse transcriptase. While type C viral particles and reverse transcriptase have been identified in human leukemia cells,[1,2] there are no conclusive data linking these viruses to human leukemia. Research into a viral cause of human leukemia is focusing on the human T-cell lymphotropic viruses (HTLV), of which only HTLV type 1 has been shown to be associated with adult T-cell malignancies.[14]

Hereditary Factors. In general, acute leukemia is not a hereditary disease. However, an increased incidence of acute leukemia has been identified among identical twins of persons with leukemia; the chance of acute leukemia developing in the identical twin of a patient with this disease is approximately 20%.[2] The risk of leukemia developing in the fraternal twin of someone with leukemia is slightly higher than in age-matched controls but not as high as for identical twins. The difference is most likely accounted for by the fact that identical twins share identical genetic material, including chromosomal abnormalities that may predispose them to leukemia. Children with Down's syndrome have a 20-fold higher risk of developing acute leukemia than children without this defect. Other congenital diseases associated with an increased incidence of leukemia include Fanconi's anemia, congenital sex-linked agammaglobulinemia, and Wiskott-Aldrich, Klinefelter's, and Bloom's syndromes.[2] The genetic defects in these diseases vary, but all are characterized by a chromosomal abnormality or instability that seems to favor the development of hematologic neoplasms.

Antecedent Hematopoietic Disorders. Other nonmalignant syndromes caused by abnormal stem-cell function may precede the development of acute leukemia. The myelodysplastic syndromes are a heterogeneous group of disorders characterized by refractory anemia and impaired hematologic function. Transformation to AML occurs in 10–75% of patients with a myelodysplastic syndrome.[15] In contrast, a myelodysplastic syndrome or preleukemia does not precede ALL.

Pathophysiology

Normal Hematopoiesis. Hematopoiesis is the formation and development of blood cells from the bone marrow. This process is highly structured and complex and begins with a single pluripotent stem-cell population (Figure 1). Stem cells, which are normally quiescent, self-replicate or differentiate when stimulated into committed stem-cell populations of myeloid (bone marrow) or lymphoid origin. Stimuli include stress, infection, bleeding, bone marrow depletion, and hematopoietic growth factors.

Hematopoietic growth factors are glycoprotein hormones secreted by stromal bone marrow cells or accessory cells of the immune system. These factors regulate hematopoietic cells in a hierarchical fashion. For example, the pluripotent and multilineage hematopoietic growth factors (interleukin-1, interleukin-6, interleukin-3, c-*kit* ligand) work in concert with lineage-restricted growth factors (erythropoietin, granulocyte colony-stimulating factor, macrophage colony-stimulating factor, thrombopoietin) to aug-

Figure 1. Normal hematopoiesis. Adapted, with permission, from Cline MJ, Golde DW. *Blood.* 1979; 53:157-65.

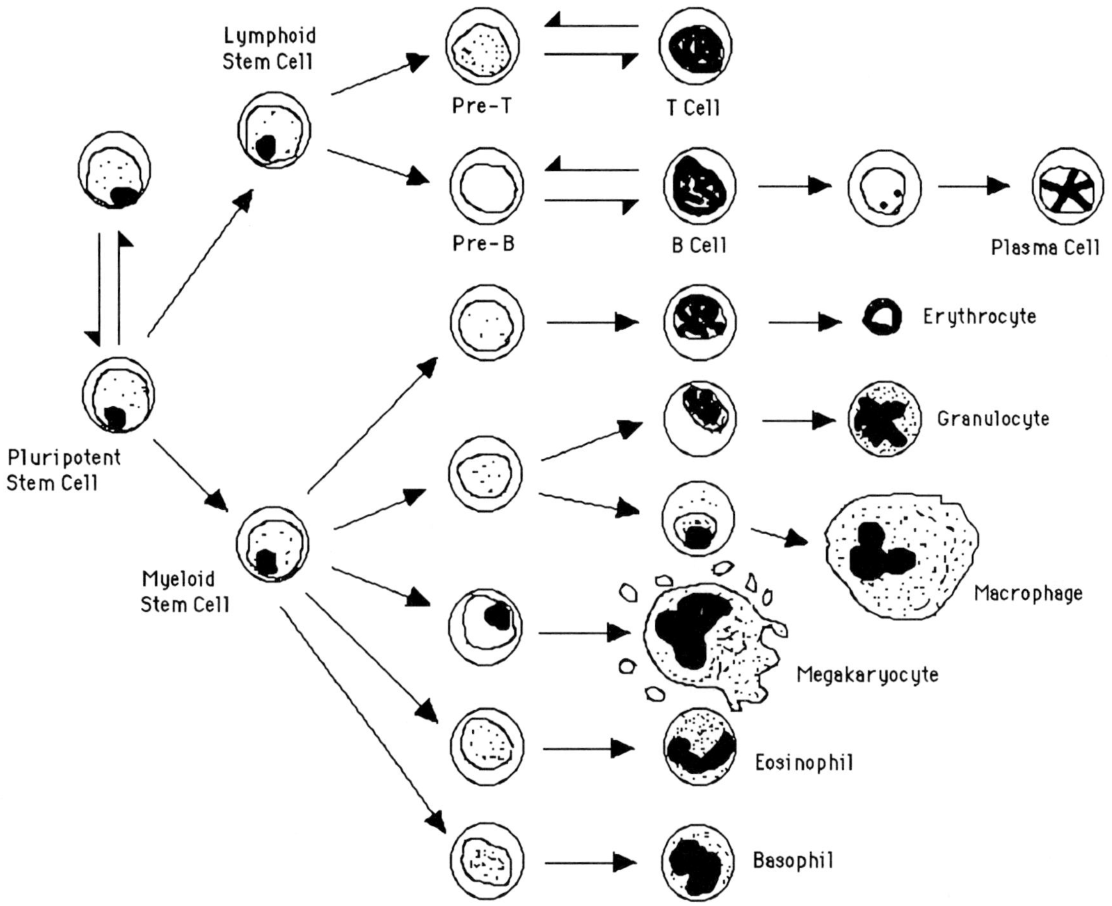

ment the proliferation, differentiation, maturation, and function of blood cells. As differentiation and maturation occur, the capacity for self-renewal is lost. Ultimately, highly specialized nondividing mature cells are formed.

When mature cells reach the end of their life cycle, they must be replaced by immature progenitor cells. A continuous supply of hematopoietic precursors is ensured by a delicate balance between the differentiation and self-renewal potentials of pluripotent stem cells. The capacity to differentiate ensures a supply of immature progenitor cells. The capacity for self-renewal ensures an unlimited hematopoietic reserve.

Leukemogenesis. Acute leukemia occurs when a single hematopoietic precursor cell undergoes neoplastic transformation, escapes the host's normal defenses, and begins to proliferate autonomously. Leukemia is characterized by an arrest of maturation along committed stem-cell lines. The leukemic transformation codes for cells that are genetically incapable of terminal differentiation and maturation. The type of leukemia that will be expressed is determined by the level of arrest of maturation. For example, if the defect occurs along the myeloid cell line at the level of the promyelocyte, promyelocytic leukemia will result. Because these cells fail to undergo terminal differentiation, they retain their stem-cell capabilities. The persistent stem-cell capabilities contribute to the clonal nature of leukemia, resulting in the persistent generation of immature dysfunctional cells identical to the leukemic clone. Lack of response to normal hematopoietic regulatory mechanisms bestows an additional survival advantage on leukemic cells. The culmination of these events is the autonomous proliferation of the leukemic clone that continues until the patient dies of bleeding or infection.

Classification

Acute leukemias are broadly classified as myelogenous (nonlymphocytic) and lymphocytic on the basis of cell lineage. Leukemias are further subdivided on the basis of morphologic, immunologic, and biochemical criteria. These classifications have been proposed in an attempt to define prognostic features, responses to chemotherapy, and outcomes.

Morphologic Classification. The morphologic classification of acute leukemia proposed by the French–

American–British (FAB) Cooperative Group in 1976 remains widely used today.[16] According to the FAB classification system, ALL is divided into three subgroups (L1, L2, and L3), depending on such criteria as cell size, chromatin content, nuclear shape, and the presence of nucleoli and cytoplasmic basophilia.[16,17] In childhood ALL, L1 morphology predominates; in adult ALL, L2 morphology is most commonly seen. L3 morphology, the type seen in Burkitt's lymphoma, is rare in both children and adults. Six subtypes were originally defined for leukemias of myeloid origin (M1–M6), depending on the direction of differentiation and degree of maturation along the various myeloid cell lines.[16,17] This nomenclature has been updated to include megakaryocytic leukemia (M7).[18]

Immunologic Classification. Acute leukemias, particularly ALL, may also be classified according to their immune features. In this classification system lymphoid cells are classified as common, T-cell, B-cell, or null-cell phenotypes, depending on the presence or absence of specific surface or cytoplasmic immunoglobulins. The distribution of phenotypes varies with age. In children, common-type ALL is the predominant phenotype, accounting for approximately 75% of all cases. However, in adults the distribution is approximately 50% common-type, 20% T-cell, and 20% null-cell, with B-cell ALL constituting <10% of all cases.[19] Monoclonal antibodies to granulocyte, monocyte, and erythrocyte cell lines are being used in an attempt to aid in the subclassification of myeloid leukemias. However, their clinical utility is limited by a lack of specificity.[20,21]

Biochemical Classification. Specific cell stains are useful in differentiating between lymphoid and myeloid leukemias. The best example of the application of these biochemical markers is the reddish purple staining of needle-like cytoplasmic inclusions with Wright's and Giemsa stains. These inclusions, called Auer rods, are present in the cytoplasm of myeloblasts, myelocytes, and monoblasts. Their presence is considered pathognomonic for AML. Peroxidase and Sudan Black are also useful in diagnosing myeloid leukemias. These stains detect myeloperoxidase and intracellular lipids, substances found in abundance in granulocyte, basophil, and eosinophil cell lines and absent or very sparse in lymphoid cell lines. The periodic acid-Schiff stain detects cytoplasmic glycogen and is useful primarily for confirming the diagnosis of erythroid or lymphoid leukemia. Terminal-deoxynucleotidyl-transferase is an intracellular enzyme whose presence strongly supports a diagnosis of ALL.

Clinical Presentation

The signs and symptoms of acute leukemia are related to the infiltration of the bone marrow by leukemic cells and the resultant failure of normal hematopoiesis. Infiltration of other organs by leukemic cells may also contribute to the clinical presentation.

AML. The symptoms of AML arise abruptly. Spontaneous bruising, abnormal bleeding and severe fatigue, and fever and infection are common and are related to progressive thrombocytopenia, anemia, and neutropenia, respectively.[22] Because of the abrupt onset of this illness, severe weight loss and cancer cachexia are uncommon. Physical examination often reveals pallor and petechiae. Lymphadenopathy and splenomegaly are uncommon. Gingival hyperplasia or skin lesions are seen frequently in patients with monocytic myeloid leukemia (FAB classification M5) because of the propensity for monocytes to accumulate in tissues. Laboratory examination reveals a normochromic, normocytic anemia, thrombocytopenia, and variable effects on white blood cell (WBC) counts. WBC counts are equally likely to be high, normal, or low, and leukemic blasts are almost always present in the peripheral smear. Owing to increased cell turnover, serum lactate dehydrogenase (LDH), alkaline phosphatase, and uric acid concentrations are usually elevated. Overt central nervous system (CNS) involvement is uncommon at diagnosis. However, patients with hyperleukocytosis (WBC count >100,000/cu mm) or myelomonocytic leukemia (FAB classification M4) are at higher risk for developing CNS disease. Bleeding and evidence of disseminated intravascular coagulation can occur in any of the FAB subtypes and are common manifestations at diagnosis in the promyelocytic subtype (M3).

ALL. The signs and symptoms of ALL are more insidious than those of AML. A history of generalized fatigue, headache, weight loss, and bone pain for several weeks is common. Lymphadenopathy and splenomegaly are noted in almost all patients.[22] A mediastinal mass may be seen in chest roentgenograms, particularly in T-cell ALL. Laboratory tests show mild to moderate anemia and thrombocytopenia in less than one third of patients. The total WBC count is elevated in almost all patients, and lymphoblasts are present in the peripheral smear. Serum LDH and uric acid concentrations are elevated in almost every patient; the degree of elevation is positively correlated with the leukemic cell burden in the bone marrow. Leukemic meningitis occurs more frequently in ALL than AML and may be present in up to 10% of adults at diagnosis. Disseminated intravascular coagulation is not seen in ALL.

Prognostic Features

AML. Few clinical features correlate with prognosis in AML. The most important indicators of outcome are the duration of the first remission and the cytogenetic profile. Patients whose first remission lasts less than six months and patients who do not achieve an initial complete remission have a very poor prognosis.[23-27] Chromosomal abnormalities are present in more than 90% of patients with AML, disappear during treatment, and reappear upon relapse. Examples of nonrandom chromosomal abnormalities that are associated with a good prognosis are inversion of chromosome 16 and translocations involving chromosomes 8 and 21.[1,25,26] Translocations involving chromosomes 15 and 17, commonly found in acute promyelocytic leukemia, suggest an intermediate prognosis. Abnormalities in chromosome 5 or 7 are commonly associated with therapy-related myeloid malignancies and are associated with a dismal prognosis. Older patients and patients with a history of myelodysplasia also respond poorly to therapy and have a poor prognosis. There is no difference in outcome based on the FAB classification in myeloid leukemia.[28,29]

ALL. The prognostic relevance of various immunologic, morphologic, and clinical features of adult ALL has been reviewed.[19] In general, L3 morphology is associated with short remissions and a poor prognosis. T-cell ALL in adults, unlike that in children, is associated with a favorable outcome.[30] Another feature associated with a poor prognosis in adults with ALL is a high WBC count (at least 25,000–35,000/cu mm).[31,32] Patients who achieve remission within four weeks have a significantly better prognosis than those whose remissions are achieved after a longer period.[32] Examination of the cytogenetic profile is gaining favor as a means of assigning risk categories for patients with ALL. Chromosomal abnormalities associated with a poor prognosis include translocations involving chromosomes 9 and 22 (the Philadelphia chromosome), 4 and 11, and 8 and 14.[19,33] Hyperploidy, the presence of more than 50 chromosomes in the leukemic cells, suggests a favorable prognosis for both adults and children.[19,33]

Diagnosis

A complete diagnostic workup, including a detailed personal and family medical history and a thorough physical examination, is essential before therapy begins. The medical history should seek to uncover any known prior exposure to chemical toxins or radiation. The physical examination should focus on node-bearing sites, temperature, and potential sites of infection including the oropharynx and gingivae, lungs, perianal area, skin, and axillae. Height, weight, and body surface area should be determined. Laboratory studies should include a complete blood count with differential; determination of serum electrolyte, uric acid, blood urea nitrogen, creatinine, and liver enzyme concentrations; urinalysis; and a coagulation profile. A transfusion workup to determine blood type, cytomegalovirus serology, and human leukocyte antigen typing should be performed on both the patient and family members.

Other necessary tests include a baseline chest roentgenogram and electrocardiogram. A bone marrow biopsy is necessary to determine marrow cellularity; adequate bone marrow aspirates are necessary to determine cell morphology, immunophenotyping, biochemical staining characteristics, and cytogenetic profile. A lumbar puncture should be performed on all patients with ALL and in AML-afflicted patients with FAB classification M4. To avoid intracerebral hemorrhage, lumbar punctures should be performed only on patients with platelet counts greater than 50,000/cu mm. In addition, to avoid the risk of leukemic contamination in the CNS, the lumbar puncture should be delayed until peripheral blast cells have been cleared by therapy. An exception is patients who have overt signs of leukemic meningitis. A lumbar puncture is required in all these patients in order to institute intrathecal chemotherapy.

Treatment Strategies in Adult Acute Leukemia

General Principles. Leukemias are blood-borne tumors that rarely appear as solitary masses of malignant cells. Consequently, surgery and radiation are not commonly used in treatment. Because acute leukemia is characterized by a high growth fraction and rapid doubling, it is sensitive to treatment with antineoplastic agents. Indeed, cytoreduction with antineoplastic agents, particularly antimetabolites such as methotrexate and cytarabine, remains the cornerstone of therapy.

Approximately 10^{11}–10^{12} leukemic cells are typically present at diagnosis. Therefore, when antitumor therapy reduces the tumor burden by 99.9%, as many as 10^9 malignant cells may still be present. An important concept in understanding the rationale behind antileukemic strategies is that complete remission does not mean absence of tumor cells but absence of clinically detectable disease. Therefore, the goals of antileukemic therapy are (1) to reduce the leukemic tumor burden to a level that allows the restoration of normal hematopoietic function and (2) to prevent relapse due to regrowth of the leukemic clone. These goals are accomplished by the administration of combinations of antineoplastic agents in several distinct phases. Combinations of drugs with different mechanisms of action and toxicity profiles are used in an attempt to minimize nonhematologic toxicity, produce additive or synergistic antileukemic effects, and prevent tumor resistance from developing.

In leukemia nomenclature, remission-induction therapy refers to an initial course of antineoplastic agents given to rapidly reduce the tumor burden in order to achieve complete remission. The definition of complete remission varies with the investigator but is usually defined as less than 5% leukemic blast cells in the bone marrow and normalization of peripheral blood counts, including hemoglobin concentration, hematocrit, granulocytes, and platelets. A bone marrow biopsy is usually performed at the nadir following a course of antileukemic therapy; if bone marrow cellularity is greater than 5%, another course of therapy is administered, and the biopsy is repeated until marrow aplasia is achieved.

Consolidation therapy refers to the administration of antineoplastic agents shortly after the induction of remission (usually four to six weeks after the achievement of complete remission). Drugs used in consolidation regimens may be the same as those given in the induction phase or may be different drugs that are non-cross-resistant. Intensification therapy refers to antineoplastic agents given after the induction of remission; the same drugs are used as in the induction phase but at higher dosages. Intensification therapy may also be given intermittently during consolidation therapy. Maintenance therapy refers to the daily or weekly administration of low doses of antineoplastics.

Supportive Care. Because of the severity of the illness, patients with a diagnosis of acute leukemia should be transferred immediately to a tertiary-care center with appropriate supportive-care facilities and a team of physicians, pharmacists, and nurses experienced in managing patients with acute leukemia. Preferably, treatment should begin within 48 hours of diagnosis.

Hemorrhage or infection, if present at diagnosis, should be treated before antineoplastic therapy is begun. Because the risk of acute tumor lysis syndrome is high, patients should receive allopurinol prophylactically beginning 24 hours before antineoplastic agents are first given and continuing until induction therapy is complete. Blood products should be administered as necessary throughout treatment to prevent severe anemia or fatal hemorrhage. Placement of a central venous catheter is recommended before the start of therapy. Parenteral nutrition may be necessary if oral mucositis is severe.

Adequate prophylaxis of infection is vital to the successful treatment of acute leukemia. Because the oropharynx is a common site of infection, mouth rinses with chlorhexidine and sodium bicarbonate and the use of soft-bristle toothbrushes are recommended for all patients. Atypical fungal, viral, and protozoan infections are common in patients with ALL. Prophylaxis with oral trimethoprim–sulfamethoxazole and acyclovir is recommended to prevent *Pneumocystis carinii* pneumonia and herpes simplex virus infection, respectively. Oral candidiasis can be prevented with clotrimazole troches, oral nystatin, ketoconazole, or fluconazole. Severe, prolonged neutropenia occurs after therapy for AML and, less commonly, for ALL. During this time, the patient is at risk for death due to infection by gram-negative bacteria or fungi. Empirical therapy with antimicrobials with a broad gram-negative spectrum should be initiated at the first temperature greater than 38.5 °C and a neutrophil count less than 500/cu mm. Systemic antifungal therapy with amphotericin B or fluconazole is often necessary in neutropenic patients whose fevers do not respond to broad-spectrum antimicrobials.

Treatment of Acute Myelogenous Leukemia

The natural history of AML is exceedingly grim. Without therapy, patients with AML die of infection or bleeding in a median time of six weeks. A major obstacle to the successful treatment of AML is the lack of specificity exhibited by the drugs used in treating this disease. Because normal hematopoietic precursors are sensitive to destruction by antineoplastic agents, it is impossible to completely eradicate leukemic clones of myeloid origin without simultaneously eradicating a portion of the normal stem-cell pool. Consequently, therapy for AML causes severe aplasia and pancytopenia that lasts for a minimum of three weeks.

Remission Induction. *Cytarabine and Daunorubicin Hydrochloride.* Single-agent therapy is rarely sufficient to induce the bone marrow aplasia necessary to eradicate the leukemic clone and hence has no place in modern induction therapy. Many uncontrolled studies and a few randomized trials have been conducted in the past 20 years in an attempt to determine the best remission-induction regimen. For all the drug combinations studied, the cornerstone of therapy remains cytarabine and daunorubicin hydrochloride.

Cytarabine is a synthetic pyrimidine analogue. The parent compound is a prodrug that is rapidly deaminated in the plasma to the inactive metabolite uracil arabinoside. Uptake of cytarabine into target cells and conversion by intracellular deoxycytidine kinases to the active metabolite, cytidine triphosphate, is a prerequisite for antileukemic activity. Cytidine triphosphate is a potent inhibitor of DNA polymerase that exerts its cytotoxic effects only on actively dividing cells and thus is cell-cycle specific.

Daunorubicin is a naturally occurring anthracycline antibiotic that intercalates between base pairs of the DNA double helix, interfering with DNA activity and inhibiting DNA-dependent DNA and RNA polymerases. This agent also blocks DNA repair mechanisms and produces DNA strand scission. Daunorubicin is not cell-cycle specific, being cytotoxic to both dividing and nondividing cells.

The superior activity of this combination of drugs was documented in a pioneering study by Gale and Cline,[34] who administered "TAD" (thioguanine 100 mg/sq m orally every 12 hours for seven days, cytarabine 100 mg/sq m intravenously for seven days, and daunorubicin 60 mg/sq m [as the hydrochloride salt] intravenously daily for three days) to 28 patients with newly diagnosed AML. These authors reported a complete remission rate of 80% and a median duration of remission of 9.3 months. In the same year, Rees et al.[35] reported a complete remission rate of 85% and a median duration of remission of 12 months in 20 patients given the "DAT" regimen (daunorubicin 50 mg/sq m [as the hydrochloride salt] intravenously [one dose], cytarabine 100 mg/sq m intravenously or subcutaneously every 12 hours for five days, and thioguanine 100 mg/sq m orally every 12 hours for five days). Cassileth and Katz[36] reported a complete remission rate of 67% and a median duration of remission of 12 months in 21 patients given the "3 + 7" regimen (daunorubicin 45 mg/sq m [as the hydrochloride salt] intravenously for three days and cytarabine 100 mg/

sq m by continuous intravenous infusion for seven days).

These provocative early results paved the way for other investigators to examine the effectiveness of the regimens in prospective open and randomized multicenter trials (Table 1). Several factors make direct comparisons among these studies difficult. First, the definition of complete remission was not standardized. Second, patient-selection criteria varied. Third, the life expectancy of patients with acute leukemia has increased in the past decade regardless of the treatment protocol used, reflecting improved blood product support and antimicrobial therapy for febrile neutropenic episodes. Nonetheless, the salient results of these large multicenter trials will be described here.

Approximately two thirds of the patients treated for AML achieved complete remission.[37-49] Of note, however, is the failure of the multicenter trials to reproduce the high remission rates originally reported.[34,35] This probably reflects the patient-selection bias inherent in single-institution studies conducted in small numbers of patients. The addition of prednisone, vincristine sulfate, or thioguanine did not increase the rate of complete remission[38,42,43,49-51]; consequently, these drugs have been dropped from current treatment protocols. None of the variations proposed proved to be more effective than the combination of daunorubicin hydrochloride and cytarabine.[43,47]

The administration of cytarabine by continuous infusion or by intermittent bolus injection produced comparable results.[45] Although the plasma half-life of cytarabine is short (two hours), the half-life of the active metabolite, cytidine triphosphate, is approximately six hours, making an every-12-hour regimen acceptable. Giving cytarabine for seven days appeared to maximize the therapeutic effects while minimizing toxicity.[43,45] The administration of daunorubicin hydrochloride at the beginning (days 1–3) or end (days 5–7) of the cytarabine infusion did not influence efficacy or toxicity.[52]

In most[38,40-47,50,53] but not all[34-37] of these studies of remission induction, age was inversely associated with a response to therapy. Complete remission rates higher than 30–40% were rarely reported in patients older than 50 years. This age-related difference in the ability to achieve complete remission is due to a high rate of mortality from nonhematologic toxicity during induction therapy in the elderly. In young patients, failure to achieve complete remission is usually due to the persistence of resistant leukemia.

Although daunorubicin hydrochloride and doxorubicin have been found to be equally efficacious,[39,42,49,53] daunorubicin has replaced doxorubicin as the anthracycline of choice because of a lower incidence of mucositis and necrotizing colitis.[39] No significant differences in response among FAB classifications have been reported.[37,44,46,49]

Other Agents for Inducing Remission. Two newer agents have been evaluated for inducing remission in AML. Idarubicin (4-demethoxydaunorubicin) is a synthetic daunorubicin analogue that lacks a methoxy group at position 4 in the chromophore ring of the parent compound. Mitoxantrone is an anthracenedione that is structurally related to daunorubicin but lacks the sugar moiety on the A ring of the anthracycline molecule. Both agents have shown considerable antileukemic activity.

Four randomized trials have compared either idarubicin hydrochloride plus cytarabine or mitoxantrone plus cytarabine with daunorubicin plus cytarabine (Table 2).[54-57] The most informative study evaluating the role of idarubicin in the treatment of AML was conducted by Wiernik et al.,[55] who randomly assigned 214 newly diagnosed patients of all ages and risk categories to receive idarubicin hydrochloride or daunorubicin hydrochloride in conjunction with cytarabine. There was no significant difference in the rates of complete remission when patients of all ages were considered. However, among patients less than 50 years of age, complete remission was more frequent in those given idarubicin hydrochloride than in those who received daunorubicin hydrochloride (88% versus 70%, $p = 0.035$). In addition, more patients with hyperleukocytosis (WBC count >50,000/cu mm) achieved complete remission when treated with idarubicin hydrochloride than when treated with daunorubicin hydrochloride (68% versus 32%, $p = 0.019$). Duration of remission and overall survival time were also significantly longer in patients treated with idarubicin hydrochloride (9.4 versus 8.4 months, $p = 0.021$, and 12.9 versus 8.7 months, $p = 0.038$, respectively). Berman et al.[54] reported similar results in a smaller, single-institution study. Arlin et al.[57] compared mitoxantrone with a standard 3 + 7 regimen in a multicenter trial. There was no difference in complete remission rates between mitoxantrone-treated patients and daunorubicin-treated patients when all age categories were considered. Neither the duration of remission nor survival time was different between the two groups.

These four trials[54-57] suggest that neither idarubicin nor mitoxantrone is less toxic than daunorubicin. Specific conclusions about the cardiotoxic potential of these analogues relative to that of daunorubicin are difficult to draw. Information on factors known to influence the development of anthracycline-induced cardiotoxicity, such as pre-existing heart disease and prior irradiation of the chest wall,[58] was not provided in these trials. Furthermore, the cumulative doses of all three agents were low, and left ventricular function was assessed only sporadically by appropriate tests, such as radionuclide scans.

These data suggest that idarubicin hydrochloride may represent a true therapeutic advance in young patients and patients with hyperleukocytosis who are newly diagnosed with AML. Indeed, the Southwest Oncology Group and the Eastern Cooperative Oncology Group are now using idarubicin hydrochloride in conjunction with cytarabine for first-line therapy in a new intergroup study evaluating postremission thera-

Table 1.
Representative Regimens for Remission Induction in Acute Myelogenous Leukemia

Reference	Study Design	No. Subjects	Regimen[a]	% Complete Remission
37	Open[b]	107	Ara-C 100 mg/sq m q 12 hr for 7 days plus DNR 60 mg/sq m/day for 3 days plus TG 100 mg/sq m p.o. q 12 hr for 7 days	76
38	Open	139	Ara-C 100 mg/sq m q 12 hr for 7 days plus DNR 70 mg/sq m/day for 3 days plus TG 100 mg/sq m p.o. q 12 hr for 7 days plus PRED 40 mg/sq m/day p.o. for 7 days plus VCR 1 mg/sq m on days 1 and 7	60
39	Randomized	653	Ara-C 100 mg/sq m/day c.i. for 7 days plus DNR 45 mg/sq m/day for 3 days	58[c]
			or	
			Ara-C 100 mg/sq m/day c.i. for 7 days plus DNR 30 mg/sq m/day for 3 days	55
			or	
			Ara-C 100 mg/sq m/day c.i. for 7 days plus DOX 30 mg/sq m/day for 3 days	50
40	Open	576	Ara-C 100 mg/sq m/day c.i. for 2 days, then 100 mg/sq m q 12 hr for 7 days, plus DNR 60 mg/sq m/day for 3 days plus TG 200 mg/sq m/day p.o. for 7 days	65
41	Open	1127	Ara-C 100 mg/sq m q 12 hr for 5 days plus DNR 50 mg/sq m/day for 1 day plus TG 100 mg/sq m p.o. q 12 hr for 5 days	67
42	Open	295	Ara-C 80 mg/sq m q 12 hr for 6 days plus DOX 50 mg/sq m on day 1 plus VCR 1 mg/sq m on day 1	64
43	Randomized	668	Ara-C 100 mg/sq m/day c.i. for 7 days plus DNR 45 mg/sq m/day for 3 days	53[c]
			or	
			Ara-C 100 mg/sq m/day c.i. for 10 days plus DNR 45 mg/sq m/day for 3 days	57
			or	
			Ara-C 100 mg/sq m/day c.i. for 7 days plus DNR 45 mg/sq m/day for 3 days plus TG 100 mg/sq m p.o. q 12 hr for 7 days	57
44	Open	191	Ara-C 200 mg/sq m/day c.i. for 5 days plus DNR 60 mg/sq m/day for 3 days plus TG 100 mg/sq m p.o. q 12 hr for 5 days	66
45	Randomized	352	Ara-C 100 mg/sq m/day c.i. for 7 days plus DNR 45 mg/sq m/day for 3 days	55[d]
			or	
			Ara-C 100 mg/sq m q 12 hr for 7 days plus DNR 45 mg/sq m/day for 3 days	46
			or	
			Ara-C 100 mg/sq m/day c.i. for 5 days plus DNR 45 mg/sq m/day for 2 days	39
			or	
			Ara-C 100 mg/sq m q 12 hr for 5 days plus DNR 45 mg/sq m/day for 2 days	29
46	Open	283	Ara-C 200 mg/sq m/day c.i. for 5 days plus DNR 60 mg/sq m/day for 3 days plus TG 100 mg/sq m p.o. q 12 hr for 5 days	65
47	Randomized	264	Ara-C 100 mg/sq m/day c.i. for 7 days plus DNR 50 mg/sq m/day for 3 days	56[e]
			or	
			Ara-C 100 mg/sq m/day c.i. for 7 days plus DNR 50 mg/sq m/day for 3 days plus ETOP 75 mg/sq m/day for 7 days	59
48	Open	508	Ara-C 100 mg/sq m/day c.i. for 7 days plus DNR 45 mg/sq m/day for 3 days	66

[a]All regimens involve the intravenous route of administration unless otherwise specified. Ara-C = cytarabine, DNR = daunorubicin (as the hydrochloride salt), TG = thioguanine, PRED = prednisone, VCR = vincristine sulfate, c.i. = continuous infusion, DOX = doxorubicin, ETOP = etoposide.
[b]Denotes open, consecutive enrollment.
[c]No significant differences in complete remission rates among the treatments.
[d]Significant difference in complete remission rates for the 7 + 3 regimens compared with the 5 + 2 regimens by multivariate analysis ($p < 0.01$).
[e]Significant difference in complete remission rates ($p = 0.01$).

Table 2.
Randomized Trials Comparing Idarubicin Hydrochloride or Mitoxantrone with Daunorubicin Hydrochloride plus Cytarabine for Remission Induction in Adult Acute Myelogenous Leukemia

Reference	No. Subjects	Regimen[a]	% Complete Remission	*p*
54	120	Ara-C 200 mg/sq m/day c.i. for 5 days plus DNR 50 mg/sq m/day for 3 days	58	0.005
		or		
		Ara-C 200 mg/sq m/day c.i. for 5 days plus IDA 12 mg/sq m/day for 3 days	80	
55	214	Ara-C 100 mg/sq m/day c.i. for 7 days plus DNR 45 mg/sq m/day for 3 days	59	0.08
		or		
		Ara-C 100 mg/sq m/day c.i. for 7 days plus IDA 13 mg/sq m/day for 3 days	70	
56	85	Ara-C 100 mg/sq m/day c.i. for 7 days plus DNR 45 mg/sq m/day for 3 days	57	0.09
		or		
		Ara-C 100 mg/sq m/day c.i. for 7 days plus IDA 12 mg/sq m/day for 3 days	74	
57	200	Ara-C 100 mg/sq m/day c.i. for 7 days plus DNR 45 mg/sq m/day for 3 days	53	0.15
		or		
		Ara-C 100 mg/sq m/day c.i. for 7 days plus MIT 12 mg/sq m/day for 3 days	63	

[a]All regimens involve the intravenous route of administration unless otherwise specified. Ara-C = cytarabine, c.i. = continuous infusion, DNR = daunorubicin (as the hydrochloride salt), IDA = idarubicin hydrochloride, MIT = mitoxantrone.

py in patients with AML. From currently available data, mitoxantrone does not appear to offer any advantage over daunorubicin hydrochloride as a first-line therapy in the induction of remission.

Hyperleukocytosis. A few patients with AML have a very high WBC count (>100,000/cu mm). While hyperleukocytosis is less of a concern in other types of leukemia (e.g., chronic lymphocytic leukemia), it is frequently an emergency in patients with AML. Leukemic myeloblasts are large and, when present in very high numbers, are prone to occluding the microcirculation of the lungs, CNS, and other organs.[59] In addition, instituting cytotoxic chemotherapy without first reducing the leukemic tumor burden can precipitate acute tumor lysis syndrome and fatal hemorrhage.[59,60] Thus, techniques to lower the WBC count are advocated before cytotoxic chemotherapy is begun.

Therapy for hyperleukocytosis is controversial. There are no clear guidelines based on the WBC count or clinical condition. Rapidly lowering the WBC count by leukapheresis or chemotherapy is advocated by some investigators. Multiple pheresis procedures have been used successfully to lower the WBC count by 20–60%.[59,60] Oral hydroxyurea 2–3 g every six hours is an alternative therapy, albeit a much slower one. If a patient has altered mentation and hyperleukocytosis, some investigators advocate emergently irradiating the cranium; others have questioned the use of this procedure.[61] Once the WBC count is lowered to a level deemed safe by the treating physician, induction therapy is initiated.

The clinical outcome for patients with hyperleukocytosis is worse than that of patients with lower initial WBC counts. Induction therapy is complicated by a high mortality rate, particularly in patients with pulmonary leukostasis, hepatomegaly, hyperbilirubinemia, and hypofibrinogenemia.[62] For patients who survive induction therapy, survival time is short.[60]

Postremission Therapy. Advances in remission-induction therapy have resulted in complete remission in approximately two thirds of all patients after the administration of one or two courses of cytarabine and daunorubicin hydrochloride at standard dosages. Despite the improvement in the initial response rate, most patients ultimately relapse and die of their disease. Long-term disease-free survival rates rarely exceed 20%.[40-43,45,46,63] Since long-term survival is positively correlated with the duration of the first remission, the challenge in treating patients with AML is to extend this initial remission. Postremission strategies include the sequential administration of combinations of antineoplastic agents in maintenance, consolidation, or intensification programs or consolidation with allogeneic or autologous bone marrow transplantation.

Antineoplastic Drug Therapy. The relative merits of consolidation with or without maintenance therapy (Table 3) and of maintenance therapy alone (Table 4) have been evaluated in randomized multicenter trials. Postremission therapy improved survival, compared with patients receiving no further therapy.[44,65] However, differences in study design make it difficult to assess the impact of the maintenance or consolidation component.

The value of maintenance therapy after the induction of remission in AML is controversial. Although

Table 3.
Randomized Trials Evaluating Postremission Consolidation Therapy with or without Maintenance Therapy in Adult Acute Myelogenous Leukemia

Reference	No. Subjects	Consolidation Regimen[a]	Maintenance Regimen[a]	Median Duration of Remission (mo)	Median Survival Time (mo)
40	145	Ara-C 100 mg/sq m/day c.i. for 2 days, then 100 mg/sq m q 12 hr for 5 days plus DNR 60 mg/sq m/day for 3 days plus TG 200 mg/sq m/day p.o. for 7 days	Ara-C 100 mg/sq m s.c. q 12 hr for 5 days plus DNR 45 mg/sq m/day for 2 days (cycle 1) Ara-C 100 mg/sq m s.c. q 12 hr for 5 days plus TG 200 mg/sq m/day p.o. for 5 days (cycles 2 and 4) Ara-C 100 mg/sq m s.c. q 12 hr for 5 days plus CTX 1000 mg/sq m for 1 dose (cycle 3) Alternate cycles 1–4 every month for 3 yr	13[b]	...[c]
		or			
		Consolidation as above	No further therapy	8	...
46	146	DNR 45 mg/sq m/day for 2 days plus Ara-C 100 mg/sq m q 12 hr for 5 days plus TG 100 mg/sq m p.o. q 12 hr for 5 days; repeat twice	TG 40 mg/sq m p.o. q 12 hr for 4 days per week plus Ara-C 60 mg/sq m s.c. once weekly; repeat every week for 2 yr	10[d]	18[e]
		or			
		No consolidation	TG and Ara-C given as above for 2 yr	8.5	21
48	335	AZA 150 mg/sq m/day c.i. for 5 days; repeat three times	Ara-C 100 mg/sq m c.i. for 5 days plus DNR 45 mg/sq m/day for 2 days; repeat every 13 wk for 1 yr	17.4[f]	29[e]
		or	or		
		AZA 150 mg/sq m/day c.i. for 5 days plus DTG 300 mg/sq m/day for 3 days; repeat three times	BCG 0.25 mL 2 times per week for 4 weeks, then once a month for 1 yr	9.4	21
		or	or		
		Ara-C 100 mg/sq m q 12 hr for 5 days plus TG 100 mg/sq m p.o. q 12 hr for 5 days plus DNR 10 mg/sq m/day for 5 days; repeat three times	Ara-C plus DNR plus BCG (dosages as above); repeat for 1 yr	9.5	21
63	248	Ara-C 200 mg/sq m/day for 7 days plus DNR 45 mg/sq m for 1 dose plus VCR 1 mg/sq m for 1 dose	Ara-C 100 mg/sq m s.c. q 12 hr for 5 days plus DNR 45 mg/sq m for 1 dose plus VCR 1 mg/sq m for 1 dose; repeat for 6 courses	...	12[e,g]
			or		
			AMSA 150 mg/sq m for 1 dose plus Ara-C 3 g/sq m[h] q 12 hr for 2 days, alternating with AMSA 150 mg/sq m for 1 dose plus AZA 150 mg/sq m/day for 3 days; repeat for 6 courses in all (3 each)		
64	74	Ara-C 100 mg/sq m/day c.i. for 7 days plus DNR 45 mg/sq m/day for 3 days plus VCR 0.8 mg/sq m for 1 dose (cycles 1, 3, and 4)	Ara-C 100 mg/sq m s.c. q 12 hr for 5 days plus TG 100 mg/sq m p.o. q 12 hr for 5 days (cycle 1)	18[d]	30[e]
		Ara-C 100 mg/sq m/day c.i. for 5 days plus DNR 45 mg/sq m/day for 2 days plus VCR 0.8 mg/sq m for 1 dose (cycle 2)	Ara-C 100 mg/sq m s.c. q 12 hr for 5 days plus PRED 40 mg/sq m/day p.o. for 5 days plus VCR 0.8 mg/sq m for 1 dose (cycle 2); alternate cycles 1 and 2 every 8 wk for 2 yr	...	...
			or		
			No maintenance therapy	18	30

[a]All regimens involve the intravenous route of administration unless otherwise specified. DNR = daunorubicin (as the hydrochloride salt), Ara-C = cytarabine, TG = thioguanine, c.i. = continuous infusion, CTX = cyclophosphamide, AZA = azacitidine, DTG = β-deoxythioguanosine, BCG = bacillus Calmette-Guérin, VCR = vincristine sulfate, AMSA = amsacrine, PRED = prednisone.

[b]Significant difference in median duration of remission ($p = 0.003$).

[c]Information was not reported.

[d]No significant difference in median duration of remission.

[e]No significant difference(s) in median survival time.

[f]Significant differences in median duration of remission produced by consolidation therapy followed by maintenance therapy with Ara-C plus DNR versus BCG alone ($p = 0.01$) and with Ara-C plus DNR versus Ara-C plus DNR plus BCG ($p = 0.02$).

[g]Disease-free survival.

[h]Defined as high-dose cytarabine.

Table 4.
Randomized Trials Evaluating Postremission Maintenance Therapy in Adult Acute Myelogenous Leukemia

Reference	No. Patients	Maintenance Regimen[a]	Median Duration of Remission (mo)	Median Survival Time (mo)
42	158	MP 70 mg/sq m/day p.o. days 1–14 plus MTX 15 mg/sq m i.m. twice weekly days 15–28; DNR 35 mg/sq m for 1 dose plus VCR 1 mg/sq m for 1 dose; repeat cycle every month for 2 yr	. . .[b]	22[c]
		or		
		MP, MTX, DNR, and VCR given as above plus stanozolol 0.15 mg/kg/day p.o.; repeat for 2 yr	. . .	22
		or		
		TG 70 mg/sq m p.o. 4 days per week plus Ara-C 80 mg/sq m s.c. once weekly; repeat for 2 yr	. . .	22
		or		
		TG and Ara-C given as above plus *Vibrio cholerae* neuraminidase; repeat for 2 yr	. . .	22
43	151	Ara-C 100 mg/sq m q 12 hr for 5 days plus TG 100 mg/sq m p.o. q 12 hr for 5 days (cycle 1) Ara-C 100 mg/sq m s.c. q 12 hr for 5 days plus PRED 40 mg/sq m/day p.o. for 5 days plus VCR 2 mg/sq m (maximum, 2 mg) for 1 dose (cycles 2 and 4) Ara-C 100 mg/sq m s.c. q 12 hr for 5 days plus DNR 45 mg/sq m/day for 2 days (cycle 3) Maintenance as above for 8 mo	11.3[d]	. . .[b]
		or		
		Maintenance as above for 3 yr	17.5	23
44	51	Ara-C 60 mg/sq m s.c. once weekly plus TG 40 mg/sq m p.o. q 12 hr for 4 days per week; repeat for 2 yr	8.1[e]	16.1[c]
		or		
		No therapy	4.1	12.7
45	125	Ara-C 100 mg/sq m q 12 hr for 5 days plus TG 100 mg/sq m p.o. q 12 hr for 5 days (cycle 1) Ara-C 100 mg/sq m q 12 hr for 5 days plus CTX 1000 mg/sq m for 1 dose (cycle 2) Ara-C 100 mg/sq m q 12 hr for 5 days plus CCNU 75 mg/sq m p.o. for 1 dose (cycle 3) Ara-C 100 mg/sq m q 12 hr for 5 days plus DNR 45 mg/sq m/day for 2 days (cycle 4) Alternate cycles 1–4 every month for 2 yr	8[f]	15[g]
		or		
		Therapy given as above except Ara-C administered s.c.	18	26

[a]All regimens involve the intravenous route of administration unless otherwise specified. Ara-C = cytarabine; TG = thioguanine, PRED = prednisone, VCR = vincristine sulfate, DNR = daunorubicin (as the hydrochloride salt), MP = mercaptopurine, MTX = methotrexate (as the sodium salt), CTX = cyclophosphamide, CCNU = lomustine.
[b]Information was not reported.
[c]No significant differences in median survival time.
[d]No significant difference in median duration of remission.
[e]Significant difference in median duration of remission ($p = 0.002$).
[f]Significant difference in median duration of remission ($p = 0.05$).
[g]Significant difference in median survival time ($p = 0.02$).

some investigators have extended the duration of remission beyond 12 months with maintenance therapy alone,[43,45] most have not been able to establish a role for low-dose maintenance therapy.[42,65,66] Maintenance therapy after consolidation did not prolong remission in the majority of studies.[41,46,63,64,67] Since the most aggressive myeloablative therapies fail to achieve initial remission in 20–40% of patients, it is unlikely that low-dose daily or weekly therapy will greatly affect the duration of complete remission.

It is not easy to define the best consolidation regimen by looking at the results of the randomized multicenter trials (Table 3). Repeated courses of consolidation therapy with the same drugs at dosages equivalent to or less than those used during remission induction extended the duration of remission in some[40,41,64] but not all[46,63] of the studies. One study suggests an advantage to using drugs in consolidation therapy that are non-cross-resistant with the drugs used during induction.[48] Despite the various drugs and combinations used, there has been no real progress in improving long-term disease-free suvival.

Data from small open trials suggest that increasing the intensity and duration of consolidation therapy improves survival.[68-70] The most provocative data supporting the use of intensified postremission chemotherapy comes from open nonrandomized trials in which high-dose cytarabine was given (2–3 g/sq m every 12 hours for 4–12 doses) alone or in combination with an anthracycline. Median durations of remission reported in these studies ranged from 12 to 31 months, and disease-free survival rates of 26–51% at three years were reported.[71-77] The improvement in survival was especially prominent in younger patients.[73,77] Although the authors of the pilot study of high-dose cytarabine[75] have been criticized for using highly selected younger patients, improvement in the disease-free survival rate to 45% at three years was reported in a subsequent large study that included non-age-selected patients up to 70 years old.[73]

The value of high-dose cytarabine consolidation therapy has also been evaluated prospectively. After providing standard induction therapy with a usual dose of cytarabine (100 mg/sq m per dose or per day), daunorubicin hydrochloride, and thioguanine, Champlin et al.[77] compared consolidation with high-dose cytarabine plus daunorubicin hydrochloride against alternating cycles of azacitidine plus doxorubicin and TAD. The five-year disease-free survival rate was 32% among the patients who received high-dose cytarabine, compared with 20% among those given azacitidine (p = 0.03). This finding suggests that consolidation with high-dose cytarabine-containing regimens may be more effective than consolidation with non-cross-resistant drugs, even in patients treated with cytarabine during remission induction. These data also strongly suggest that the cytoreduction observed with cytarabine is dose related. These results have prompted investigators to hypothesize that high-dose cytarabine administered as first-line therapy in previously untreated patients with AML may increase the percentage of patients attaining complete remission and extend the initial remission.[78]

While the value of aggressive postremission therapy with high-dose cytarabine cannot be underestimated, it must be noted that the associated rates of morbidity and mortality are alarmingly high. The incidence of death from toxicity during therapy with high-dose cytarabine has ranged from 3% to 22%.[72-75] Toxic effects unique to high-dose cytarabine include chemical conjunctivitis, hepatotoxicity, toxic epidermal necrolysis, and cerebellar neurotoxicity.[79] Furthermore, patients must withstand profound aplasia lasting a median of 30 days, during which they are at high risk for bacterial and fungal infections. The benefits of these intensive regimens must be weighed carefully against the risks, with the most aggressive treatment being reserved for younger patients, patients with excellent performance status before therapy, and those who have recovered fully from the toxicities incurred during induction therapy.

Bone Marrow Transplantation. The advent of bone marrow transplantation has improved the outlook for some patients with AML. Briefly, bone marrow transplantation involves ablation of the diseased marrow with chemotherapy or radiation or both. Rescue is achieved by infusing allogeneic, syngeneic, or autologous marrow. Allogeneic marrow is obtained from a donor, usually a sibling, who is matched for the major human histocompatibility antigen. Syngeneic marrow is obtained from an identical twin (the best immunologic match possible). Autologous marrow is marrow obtained from the patient during hematologic remission. Prevention of graft-versus-host disease with immunosuppressive therapy is necessary after allogeneic and, to a lesser degree, syngeneic marrow infusion. For a detailed discussion of the immunobiology and techniques involved in bone marrow transplantation, the reader is referred elsewhere.[80-85]

Allogeneic bone marrow transplantation was initially restricted to patients with multiply relapsed and refractory leukemia.[80,81,85] A small number of these patients were cured of an otherwise fatal disease, encouraging investigators to explore this technique for patients in first remission. The authors of several uncontrolled studies reported long-term disease-free survival rates of 44–70% in patients with AML in first remission.[82,85,86] Most prospectively randomized trials comparing allogeneic bone marrow transplantation with postremission chemotherapy in patients with AML in first complete remission showed better survival rates in the patients given transplants.[87,88] In 1980 Powles et al.[87] reported a 64% survival rate at three years in 22 patients undergoing allogeneic bone marrow transplantation in first remission, compared with 29% in 28 patients receiving postremission chemotherapy. Four years later, in a randomized study Appelbaum et al.[88] compared 33 patients given allogeneic bone marrow transplants with 46 patients given two courses of consolidation therapy followed by maintenance therapy. At a median follow-up time of three years there was a significant survival advantage for the patients who received bone marrow transplants (49% versus 20%, $p < 0.0001$). In both of these studies, the survival advantage conferred by transplantation was maintained at five years.[89,90] In contrast, Champlin et al.[91] did not see a significant survival advantage in 23 patients given allogeneic bone marrow transplantation during the first complete remission over 44 patients given intensive consolidation therapy with alternating cycles of azacitidine plus doxorubicin and TAD (40% versus 27% survival at four years, $p > 0.04$). These authors cited small patient numbers and a high transplant-related mortality rate as factors contributing to the lack of significant differences between the two groups.

Despite small patient numbers, differences in the induction and consolidation regimens used, and variations in the criteria used to select patients for bone marrow transplantation, three findings are consistent in these and other studies. First, the rate of leukemic relapse in patients who undergo allogeneic bone marrow transplantation is significantly lower than in patients receiving antineoplastic agents. This effect of transplantation may be due to immunocompetent cytotoxic T cells in the donor marrow eradicating residual host leukemia cells through antigen recognition (i.e., the graft-versus-leukemia effect).[83,84,92,93] Second, a higher incidence of early mortality (defined as death within the first six months of complete remission) is noted in transplant patients.[88,91] This increased early mortality is caused by procedure-related complications, such as interstitial pneumonia, infection, and graft-versus-host disease.[84,92] Third, in allogeneic bone marrow transplant patients, survival is negatively correlated with age.[86,88,91,94] In a review of 363 patients given allogeneic transplants for AML at the Fred Hutchinson Cancer Research Center, the five-year disease-free survival rate was 60% for patients who were younger than 20 years at the time of the procedure, compared with 40% for patients who were older than 20 ($p < 0.0001$).[92] For patients 35–50 years of age, five-year survival was comparable to that in chemotherapy-treated patients. Because of these age-related differences in mortality, most centers exclude patients older than 50 years from their allogeneic transplant protocols. The age factor has implications for the practical application of this procedure in a population of patients whose mean age at diagnosis is 50 years. The limited availability of matched siblings and matched unrelated donors further restricts the broad application of this therapy.

The use of autologous marrow for rescue after ablative chemotherapy is a new transplantation strategy designed to circumvent the age and donor limitations inherent in allogeneic programs. While this technique would greatly increase the number of patients eligible for this potentially curative therapy, there is a risk of microscopic leukemic contamination of the harvested marrow, as well as loss of the beneficial graft-versus-leukemia effect. McMillan et al.[95] evaluated the efficacy of autologous bone marrow transplantation in 82 adult patients (age, 16–57 years) with AML in first remission. Twenty-five patients received a second autologous bone marrow transplant within a median of 90 days after the first autograft. At a median follow-up time of 31 months, the researchers projected the five-year disease-free survival rate to be 48% for all 82 patients and 67% for the 25 patients who underwent double autologous bone marrow transplantation. The procedure had a mortality rate of 6% and was associated with severe bone marrow suppression and infection. Twenty-seven (33%) of the patients relapsed. Although the follow-up time was short, the authors noted that all the relapses occurred within 26 months. Others have reported similar findings. Gorin et al.,[96] in a survey of 424 patients with AML in first complete remission, reported a disease-free survival rate of 36% seven years after autologous transplantation. While these are pooled results from centers that used different selection criteria and conditioning regimens, it seems that autografts may indeed result in extended remissions.

The comparative merits of autologous bone marrow transplantation, allogeneic bone marrow transplantation, and chemotherapy have been evaluated prospectively. Lowenberg et al.[97] evaluated 117 consecutive patients undergoing therapy for AML. Of 90 patients who achieved complete remission, 32 and 23 had received autologous and allogeneic marrow, respectively. Three years after the procedure, survival rates were 37% and 66% and actuarial rates of relapse were 60% and 34% for the autograft and allograft recipients, respectively. Of 37 patients who received only consolidation therapy, only 10% were alive at three years. Reiffers et al.[98] reported disease-free survival rates at 32 months of 66%, 41%, and 16% and actuarial rates of relapse of 18%, 50%, and 83% in 20, 12, and 20 patients receiving allogeneic marrow, autologous marrow, or no transplant, respectively. The number of patients was small in both studies, and various remission-induction and consolidation protocols were used that might influence interpretation of the results. Nonetheless, both research groups concluded that allogeneic bone marrow transplantation is associated with a higher survival rate than autologous transplantation.

Thus, bone marrow transplantation offers the potential for a cure in patients with AML. For young patients with matched sibling donors, allogeneic bone marrow transplantation is currently the therapy of choice. The future availability of unrelated matched donors through national bone marrow registries may increase the number of patients who can be treated with this approach. Autologous transplantation is essentially ablative consolidation therapy followed by hematologic rescue with host marrow. Initial results from recent studies of autologous transplantation are provocative. Low transplant-related mortality and a lack of age- or donor-related limitations are attractive considerations. A reduced incidence of leukemic relapse and improved survival have been noted in patients who received autologous marrow transplants, compared with consolidation chemotherapy alone. Currently, the relapse rates after autologous transplantation are higher than those after allogeneic transplantation, presumably because of loss of the graft-versus-leukemia effect. The identification of successful techniques for purging autologous marrow of residual leukemia cells in vitro may improve these results. Until then, autologous bone marrow transplantation should be used as consolidation therapy for patients with AML in first complete remission who do not have an available allogeneic donor.

Therapy for Relapsed or Refractory AML. Despite advances in the induction of remission in AML, the long-term prognosis remains poor for patients who are not eligible to receive bone marrow transplants. Ultimately, 80–85% of all patients will relapse within two years of diagnosis and die of their disease.[1,40-43,45,46,63] Once a patient has relapsed, cure by conventional chemotherapy alone is rarely possible. Second remissions are more difficult to achieve and are briefer. The median survival time after relapse is six months.

The treatment of relapsed or refractory AML is complicated by features unique to the pathogenesis of these diseases. Relapse may occur as a result of the proliferation of subpopulations of resistant cells or because the dosages of antineoplastics have been subtherapeutic. It is usually impossible to elucidate the causes of relapse in individual patients. Refractory AML is inherently drug insensitive. Treatment strategies for relapsed or refractory disease are designed to circumvent natural or acquired resistance mechanisms and include single-agent or combination chemotherapy that is dose intensified or non-cross-resistant with agents used during induction and bone marrow transplantation.

Antineoplastic Drug Therapy. The results of representative studies of single-agent and combination regimens used in the treatment of relapsed or refractory AML are summarized in Tables 5 and 6, respectively. No single agent or combination regimen emerges as the most reproducibly effective therapy for relapsed or refractory disease. Response rates vary widely among the studies, including those with identical regimens. Many studies were Phase I or II trials in which small sample sizes and differences in study design complicate interpretation. Despite many discrepancies, some of the observations are noteworthy.

Chemotherapy is more active in relapsed than refractory AML. Whether single-agent or combination therapy is administered, complete remission rates are higher for patients in relapse than for patients with refractory AML. High-dose cytarabine is the most active single agent and is a component of the most active combination therapies. High-dose cytarabine induces complete remission in patients who fail to respond to or relapse with standard-dose cytarabine.[79,99-102] In addition, high-dose cytarabine is effective in therapy-related (secondary) AML, which is notoriously resistant to chemotherapy.[142]

Mitoxantrone, amsacrine, or idarubicin hydrochloride is effective in patients who are pretreated with an anthracycline.[102,104,105,107,111,114-118] All three of these agents show a lack of cross-resistance by producing complete remissions in patients who fail to respond to anthracycline therapy. Although results obtained with azacitidine are comparable to those for other agents, its poor stability and investigational status make it inferior from a practical standpoint.[108] Newer agents with comparable activity will make azacitidine obsolete.

The median duration of second remission is five months and is independent of the type of chemotherapy received. Most studies showing longer second remissions were conducted in highly selected patients with a favorable prognosis.[123,134]

Although response rates are comparable among combination regimens, differences in toxicity profiles make some regimens more attractive than others. The addition of an anthracycline to high-dose cytarabine appears to improve response, with no additional toxicity.[125] Herzig et al.[125] compared 34 patients given high-dose cytarabine alone with 44 patients given a combination of high-dose cytarabine and daunorubicin hydrochloride or doxorubicin. Although no significant difference in complete remission rates was noted when patients with relapsed and refractory disease were evaluated together (47% versus 59% for the high-dose cytarabine group and the high-dose cytarabine plus anthracycline group, respectively), a significant difference was noted for patients with refractory disease only (20% versus 56% for the high-dose cytarabine group and the high-dose cytarabine plus anthracycline group, respectively, $p = 0.02$). No significant difference in toxicity was noted between the two groups. The addition of mitoxantrone, idarubicin hydrochloride, or amsacrine to high-dose cytarabine also did not appear to enhance toxicity. Although studies of high-dose cytarabine in combination with mitoxantrone[122] or with amsacrine[127] showed treatment-related mortality rates of 25% and 28%, high-dose cytarabine was most likely the offending agent. When these same agents were used with lower doses of cytarabine, treatment-related mortality was diminished. Although amsacrine and etoposide have been investigated in combination, severe gastrointestinal toxicity precludes clinical utility.[137-139]

Role of High-Dose Cytarabine. As discussed, high-dose cytarabine is the most effective single agent for relapsed or refractory AML. The rationale for using high-dose cytarabine is to overcome the cellular resistance that can occur at standard dosages. The mechanisms of resistance to cytarabine may involve decreased uptake of the drug into leukemic cells, intrinsic variations in the intracellular rate of phosphorylation to cytidine triphosphate, or increased catabolism to arabinosyl uracil.[143,144] Whatever the mechanism, clinical and pharmacokinetic data indicate that the response to therapy is positively correlat-

Table 5.
Single-Agent Therapy for Relapsed or Refractory Adult Acute Myelogenous Leukemia

Drug	Dosage[a]	% Complete Remission	Median Duration of Remission (mo)	References
Cytarabine	3 g/sq m[b] q 12 hr for 6 days	12–70	3–5	79, 99–103
Amsacrine	120 mg/sq m/day for 5 days	8–28	1–3	104–107
Azacitidine	150–400 mg/sq m/day for 5 days	20–33	2–6	108–110
Mitoxantrone	12 mg/sq m/day for 5 days	31–56	3–10	111–115
Idarubicin hydrochloride	7–15 mg/sq m/day for 3–5 days	17–22	2	116–118

[a]All dosages are intravenous unless otherwise specified.
[b]Defined as high-dose cytarabine.

Table 6.
Representative Combination Regimens for the Treatment of Relapsed or Refractory Adult Acute Myelogenous Leukemia

Reference	No. Subjects	Regimen[a]	% Complete Remission	Median Duration of Remission (mo)
Cytarabine plus Mitoxantrone				
119	38	Ara-C 1 g/sq m q 12 hr for 3 days plus MIT 10–12 mg/sq m/day for 5 days	47	10
120	36	Ara-C 1 g/sq m over 6 hr daily for 6 days plus MIT 6 mg/sq m over 3 hr (after Ara-C) daily for 6 days	67	5
121	9	Ara-C 2 g/sq m[b] q 12 hr for 4 days plus MIT 12 mg/sq m/day c.i. for 2 days	44	6
122	40	Ara-C 3 g/sq m[b] q 12 hr for 4 days plus MIT 12 mg/sq m/day for 3 days	53	4.5
123	26	Ara-C 3 g/sq m/day[b] for 5 days plus MIT 7 mg/sq m/day for 5 days	58	12
124	49	Ara-C 100 mg/sq m/day c.i. for 7 days plus MIT 10 mg/sq m/day for 3 days	45	8
Cytarabine plus Doxorubicin or Daunorubicin Hydrochloride				
125	44	Ara-C 3 g/sq m[b] q 12 hr for 6 days plus DOX 20 mg/sq m/day for 3 days or DNR 30 mg/sq m/day for 3 days	59	5
126	37	Ara-C 45 mg/kg c.i. over 72 hr on days 1–3 and 8–10 plus DNR 1 mg/kg/day for 3 days	56	7
Cytarabine plus Amsacrine				
127	40	Ara-C 3 g/sq m[b] q 12 hr for 6 days plus AMSA 75–100 mg/sq m/day for 3 days	70	6
128	22	Ara-C 3 g/sq m[b] q 12 hr for 6 days plus AMSA 75 mg/sq m/day for 3 days	36	5
129	27	Ara-C 3 g/sq m[b] over 3 hr daily for 5 days plus AMSA 200 mg/sq m/day for 3 days	52	. . .[c]
130	34	Ara-C 1 g/sq m q 12 hr for 6 days plus AMSA 120 mg/sq m/day for 3 days	68	4.5
Cytarabine plus Idarubicin Hydrochloride				
131	35	Ara-C 1 g/sq m q 12 hr for 3 days plus IDA 8 mg/sq m/day for 5 days	60	4.5
132	10	Ara-C 600 mg/sq m q 12 hr for 6 days plus IDA 12 mg/sq m/day for 3 days	70	3
133	7	Ara-C 2 g/sq m[b] over 3 hr daily for 3 days plus IDA 12 mg/sq m/day for 3 days	57	2–3
134	16	Ara-C 120 mg/sq m q 12 hr for 7 days plus IDA 12 mg/sq m/day for 3 days	56	11
Cytarabine plus Etoposide				
135	21	Ara-C 3 g/sq m[b] q 12 hr for 6 days plus ETOP 100 mg/sq m/day for 5 days	52	4.6
136	9	Ara-C 500 mg/sq m q 12 hr for 12 doses plus ETOP 200 mg/sq m q 12 hr for 12 doses	33	. . .
Amsacrine plus Etoposide				
137	17	AMSA 100 mg/sq m/day for 5 days plus ETOP 100 mg/sq m/day for 5 days	19	. . .
138	20	AMSA 210 mg/sq m/day for 3 days plus ETOP 100 mg/sq m over 1 hr daily for 5 days followed by 110, 200, or 230 mg/sq m c.i. over 23 hr daily for 5 days	0	. . .
139	38	AMSA 120 mg/sq m/day for 5 days plus ETOP 80 mg/sq m/day c.i. for 5 days plus vinblastine sulfate 6 mg/sq m for 1 dose in 27 pts.	47	2
Cytarabine plus Mitoxantrone plus Etoposide				
140	72	Ara-C 500 mg/sq m/day c.i. for 3 days (days 1–3 and 8–10) plus MIT 12 mg/sq m for 3 days (days 1–3) plus ETOP 200 mg/sq m/day c.i. for 3 days (days 8–10)	61	6
141	32	Ara-C 1 g/sq m over 6 hr for 6 days plus MIT 6 mg/sq m/day for 6 days plus ETOP 80 mg/sq m/day for 6 days	66	4

[a]All regimens involve the intravenous route of administration unless otherwise specified. Ara-C = cytarabine, MIT = mitoxantrone, c.i. = continuous infusion, DOX = doxorubicin, DNR = daunorubicin (as the hydrochloride salt), AMSA = amsacrine, IDA = idarubicin hydrochloride, ETOP = etoposide.
[b]Defined as high-dose cytarabine.
[c]Information was not reported.

ed with the intracellular concentration of cytidine triphosphate.[143,145,146] Kantarjian et al.[145] evaluated the intracellular pharmacokinetics of cytarabine in 41 patients with refractory acute leukemia who were given high-dose cytarabine (3 g/sq m intravenously every 12 hours for 12 doses). Eight (44%) of 18 patients with a median trough intracellular cytidine triphosphate concentration greater than 75 μM achieved complete remission, compared with 3 (13%) of 23 patients whose median trough cytidine triphosphate concentration was less than 75 μM. These results were significantly different when patients dying from early causes or aplasia were excluded (complete remission in 8 of 12 [67%] and 3 of 19 [16%] patients with concentrations greater and less than 75 μM, respectively, $p = 0.01$).

While these results are provocative from a pharmacokinetic point of view, they are not widely applicable from a practical one. Assays measuring intracellular concentrations of cytidine triphosphate are tedious and are not readily available. In contrast, assays for measuring the parent compound in plasma are readily available. However, because of large interpatient variations in the distribution and metabolism of cytarabine within leukemic cells,[143,144] there is little correlation between a given plasma cytarabine concentration and the intracellular concentration of an active metabolite[144,147] or the response to therapy.[148] It appears that pharmacokinetic information based on plasma cytarabine concentrations is not currently useful for optimizing therapy for individual patients.

Although cytarabine has been used in intensified dosages for over a decade, the optimum high-dose regimen has not been well defined. In the most widely used regimens, 3 g/sq m is given intravenously every 12 hours for 12 doses.[79] Increasing the dose above 3 g/sq m or the number of doses beyond 12 results in an unacceptably high incidence of neurological and gastrointestinal toxicity, respectively.[79] However, pharmacokinetic data suggest that dosages this large may not be necessary. The intracellular rate of phosphorylation to cytidine triphosphate is nonlinear, and enzyme saturation occurs at plasma cytarabine concentrations of 3–10 μM.[149] Plasma concentrations after the infusion of cytarabine 2–3 g/sq m over two hours are 10 times higher than those necessary to saturate the intracellular phosphorylation enzymes.[150,151] Plunkett et al.[152] proposes that dosages of cytarabine designed to keep the plasma concentration at 7 μM (200–250 mg/sq m/hr) would optimize efficacy and minimize toxicity. Data for small numbers of patients with relapsed AML suggest that 500–1000 mg/sq m every 12 hours for 12 doses produces response rates that are comparable to those produced by 3 g/sq m.[153,154] Doses smaller than 3 g/sq m do not produce responses in patients with refractory AML.[153] Further investigation into the pharmacokinetics and pharmacodynamics of cytarabine is warranted.

Prognostic Features. To improve the management of patients in relapse, investigators have searched for variables with prognostic relevance to response and survival. Several large retrospective analyses demonstrate that the duration of the initial remission is positively correlated with response to therapy. In one such study, 19% of patients achieved complete remission after reinduction therapy when the initial remission lasted less than 12 months, compared with 60% of patients when the first remission lasted more than 12 months ($p < 0.01$).[23] These results have been substantiated by other investigators.[24-27] Another factor strongly associated with response to therapy is a favorable cytogenetic profile (translocations involving chromosomes 15 and 17 or 8 and 21, or inversion of chromosome 16).[23,25,26] On the basis of this information, standardized definitions of refractory and relapsed disease have been proposed.[27] Future trials should incorporate these definitions.

Role of Bone Marrow Transplantation. Allogeneic bone marrow transplantation was originally introduced for use in patients with relapsed or refractory leukemia and still plays an important role in this population. Although the results for patients in second remission or subsequent remissions are inferior to those obtained during first remission, bone marrow transplantation remains the only option for curative therapy once relapse has occurred.

Long-term disease-free survival can be achieved with allogeneic bone marrow transplantation applied immediately after a second complete remission is induced with salvage chemotherapy. In a retrospective review of 363 patients who underwent allogeneic bone marrow transplantation, Clift et al.[92] reported a five-year disease-free survival rate of 28% for 49 patients who were in second complete remission at the time of the procedure. Other investigators have reported disease-free survival rates as high as 64% at two years in similar but smaller groups.[86,94] Achievement of a second complete remission may not even be necessary. A 30% five-year disease-free survival rate was observed in 54 patients who underwent allogeneic bone marrow transplantation during early first relapse (bone marrow blast-cell fraction, <50%).[92] Santos et al.[86] reported a similar finding. An advantage of this strategy is improving performance status at the time of transplantation by avoiding the rigors and complications of prior salvage chemotherapy. An obvious disadvantage is the need to detect relapse at an early stage and begin the procedure promptly.

Survival is unlikely in patients with multiply relapsed or resistant AML, despite the use of allogeneic bone marrow transplantation. Disease-free survival rates in this patient population range from 0% to 12%.[85,86,94] As expected, leukemic relapse is common, despite the use of myeloablative drug and radiation therapies. Relapse is the leading cause of death and occurs in 38–56% of patients.[85,86,94]

Few studies have been published on the use of autologous bone marrow transplantation in patients in second or subsequent relapse. This treatment modality is attractive because there are no age or donor limitations; however, attainment of a second or subsequent complete remission is necessary in order to harvest donor marrow, and the risk of leukemic relapse is substantial. Analysis of pooled results for patients who received autologous bone marrow transplants during second complete remission showed disease-free survival rates of 30% in 136 low-risk patients at four years and 28% in 14 high-risk patients at seven months.[96] In contrast, the results obtained when autologous transplantation is applied during relapse are abysmal. Remission durations of three to five months and less than 10% survival at one year were reported for the few patients who underwent autologous bone marrow transplantation at the time of relapse and who were refractory to conventional chemotherapy.[155-157]

CNS Leukemia. Leukemic cells may spread hematogenously to the CNS and become foci for primary disease or relapse. CNS involvement in adult AML is uncommon at diagnosis; during the course of the disease it occurs in 0.5–11% of patients.[158] Intrathecal chemotherapy does not decrease the incidence of CNS disease, delay systemic relapse, or improve survival in adults with AML.[41] Therefore, empirical prophylaxis with intrathecal chemotherapy is usually not recommended.[41,159]

There are three treatment options for patients with documented CNS leukemia: intrathecal chemotherapy, cranial irradiation, and high-dose systemic chemotherapy that achieves cytotoxic drug levels in the cerebrospinal fluid.

Intrathecal Chemotherapy. Methotrexate sodium and cytarabine are two commonly used intrathecal agents. Clinical experience suggests that the dosage of intrathecal methotrexate sodium should be based on age and not on body surface area.[160] The volume of the CNS compartment does not correlate with body surface area and reaches 85–90% of the maximum value by the age of three years; hence, dosing intrathecal methotrexate on the basis of body surface area alone may underdose infants and overdose adults.[160] The recommended adult dose of intrathecal methotrexate is 12 mg.[160] The number of doses and the dosage interval vary with the extent of CNS disease and the presence of CNS toxicity. Methotrexate appears in the systemic circulation after it is cleared from the cerebrospinal fluid. Although the risk of systemic toxicity is low, the use of low-dose oral leucovorin calcium is recommended.

Cytarabine is effective for the treatment of CNS leukemia and exhibits sustained activity in the cerebrospinal fluid because of low concentrations of cytidine deaminase in this compartment.[150,151] The adult dosage of intrathecal cytarabine is not well established. Published recommendations range from 20 to 100 mg/sq m given every two to five days until the cerebrospinal fluid has cleared.[158,159,161] Paraplegia was reported in one patient given 100 mg/sq m/day intrathecally for five days.[161] Experience with intrathecal methotrexate sodium suggests that dosing of intrathecal cytarabine should be based on age and not body surface area.

Cranial Irradiation. Cranial irradiation is an option when intrathecal chemotherapy has failed, but data on the use of cranial irradiation in adults with AML are scarce. Most data on the use of cranial irradiation in leukemia are derived from children or adults with ALL, and the reported dosage of radiation varies. A typical regimen is 2400 rad given in 12 fractions over three weeks.[159]

High-Dose Systemic Chemotherapy. Cytarabine in doses of 2–3 g/sq m achieves concentrations in cerebrospinal fluid that are 10–15% of the concomitant plasma concentrations.[151] Cerebrospinal fluid cytarabine concentrations of 10–15 μM have been reported[151]—substantially higher than the proposed minimum effective concentration of 0.2 μM.[150] Standard-dose cytarabine does not produce measurable concentrations in cerebrospinal fluid[151] and therefore is not useful for treating documented CNS disease. High-dose cytarabine has been used successfully to treat CNS leukemia[148,162,163] and is potentially the therapy of choice for patients with combined CNS and bone marrow disease. The increasing use of high-dose cytarabine as first-line or consolidation therapy may partially explain the low frequency of CNS disease in adults with AML.

Differentiation Therapy. Acute leukemia represents an imbalance between incomplete cell differentiation and maturation and autonomous proliferation of neoplastic cells. Traditional therapies are directed toward suppressing proliferation. A novel approach to the treatment of AML involves administering drugs that circumvent the arrest in cell maturation and induce differentiation and terminal cell division. Drugs that have shown promise are low-dose cytarabine, tretinoin (all-*trans*-retinoic acid), and sargramostim (recombinant granulocyte–macrophage colony-stimulating factor).

Low-Dose Cytarabine. Cytarabine was the first agent explored for the ability to stimulate differentiation of myelogenous leukemia cells. In contrast to traditional and high doses of cytarabine, which are clearly cytotoxic, low doses have been shown to induce differentiation of myeloid leukemia cells in vitro.[164] In vivo, complete remission (bone marrow blast-cell fraction <5% and normalization of peripheral blood cell counts) has been noted to occur in the absence of the marrow aplasia characteristic of high-dose therapy[165-167] and to be more frequent in patients whose initial bone marrow cellularity is low.[168] These results suggest that the mechanism of action is stimulation of differentiation to normal myeloid elements.

Most studies of low-dose cytarabine have been conducted in elderly patients, for whom minimally toxic alternatives to standard chemotherapy are desirable. Pooled data from small studies indicate that complete remission can be attained in 43% of elderly patients (age, >65 years) by giving 10 mg/sq m subcutaneously every 12 hours for 15–21 days.[165,166] Tilly et al.[167] randomly assigned 87 previously untreated elderly patients to receive cytarabine 10 mg/sq m subcutaneously every 12 hours for 21 days or intensive chemotherapy with rubidazone (an anthracycline analogue) 100 mg/sq m intravenously for four days plus cytarabine 200 mg/sq m given by continuous intravenous infusion for seven days, followed by intensive maintenance therapy. Significantly more patients given intensive chemotherapy achieved complete remission (52% versus 32%, $p = 0.001$), and significantly more patients failed to respond to therapy with cytarabine alone (36% versus 15%, $p = 0.001$). However, the rate of early death was significantly higher in the intensive chemotherapy group (31% versus 10%, $p < 0.01$). Despite the higher remission rate in the patients given intensive therapy, the median duration of remission and median survival time were not significantly different between the two groups. In addition, there was no significant difference in survival time for patients achieving complete or partial remission between the low-dose cytarabine group (8.3 months) and the intensive chemotherapy group (10.5 months). Complete remission has also been achieved in patients with secondary AML[166,168] and in patients with relapsed or refractory AML.[166] Decreased red blood cell and platelet transfusion requirements and the ability to use an outpatient setting for treatment are advantages that can improve the quality of life. Thus, low-dose cytarabine therapy is an effective alternative for elderly patients.

Tretinoin. Tretinoin, a major endogenous metabolite of vitamin A, can induce differentiation and terminal cell division in myeloid leukemia cells in vitro.[169-172] Clinically, oral tretinoin has induced complete remission in 64–100% of previously untreated or relapsed patients with acute promyelocytic leukemia (APL).[169,170,173] Patients with other FAB classifications of acute leukemia failed to respond. The chromosomal translocation that characterizes APL (chromosomes 15 and 17) is believed to be the link to the response to tretinoin. The gene that codes for retinoic acid-receptor α is located on chromosome 17, near the translocation break point. Abnormal receptor expression occurs in APL, leading to faulty differentiation of myeloid leukemia cells. Although the exact mechanism of action is unknown, tretinoin may induce myeloid leukemia cells to differentiate by stimulating retinoic acid-receptor α.[169]

Oral dosages of tretinoin range from 45 to 100 mg/sq m/day for 40–90 days.[169,170] Response occurs in approximately 40 days and is characterized by normal or hypercellular marrow aspirates full of mature cells lacking chromosomal abnormalities. Of special interest is the absence of the disseminated intravascular coagulation that is often seen in APL after cytotoxic chemotherapy. Toxicity after tretinoin therapy is tolerable and includes dry mucous membranes, headache, and bone pain. A worldwide study comparing tretinoin with standard-dose cytarabine and daunorubicin hydrochloride for the induction of remission in APL has been launched. The agent's role in the maintenance of remission after consolidation chemotherapy will also be evaluated in this trial.

Sargramostim. Sargramostim is a recombinant glycoprotein hormone that promotes the formation, maturation, and survival of committed myeloid stem cells.[174,175] In addition, this growth factor enhances the function of more mature cells.[174,175] Demonstration of granulocyte–macrophage colony-stimulating factor receptors on malignant myeloid cells in vitro has discouraged the use of sargramostim in patients with myeloid malignancies. Recently, however, the differentiation-promoting properties of sargramostim have been exploited for therapeutic benefit. Limited data in patients with AML suggest that sargramostim 125–250 µg/sq m/day given by continuous intravenous infusion for two to seven days before remission induction with cytarabine and daunorubicin hydrochloride increases the percentage of cells entering the synthesis (S_1) phase and thus their sensitivity to the cytotoxic effects of cell cycle-specific agents.[176-178] Toxicities reported have been mild at these dosages, with fever and weight gain predominating. Because the percentage of blast cells can increase rapidly under the influence of growth factor, some investigators suggest that sargramostim not be given for patients with high initial WBC counts (>30,000/cu mm).[176] The use of cytotoxic chemotherapy under these conditions can cause massive tumor lysis syndrome and should be avoided.

The use of sargramostim as a differentiation-promoting agent is in its infancy. More experience and larger trials will help define the role of this novel approach in the treatment of AML.

Treatment of Acute Lymphocytic Leukemia

Treatment strategies for ALL are quite different from those for AML. Therapy for ALL is divided into remission induction, consolidation, maintenance, and CNS prophylaxis. A program including all these phases requires two to three years. Many of the drugs used successfully to treat ALL are selectively cytotoxic for lymphocytes; therefore, adequate antileukemic effects can be achieved while sparing normal hematopoietic function. Because bone marrow suppression can be mild, particularly during the maintenance phase, many patients are successfully managed in outpatient programs.

Remission Induction. Multiple-drug therapy is necessary to induce remission in adults with ALL. Defining an optimum remission-induction regimen for adults has been hindered by a paucity of research data. Many of the treatment strategies for adults have been extrapolated from the results of childhood ALL treatment protocols. However, differences in prognostic variables and age-related differences in responses to chemotherapy make direct comparisons between adults and children invalid. In addition, few randomized trials have addressed induction therapy in adults. The open, consecutive trials that have been conducted included small numbers of patients and failed to standardize entry criteria. Nonetheless, some of the findings deserve to be highlighted.

Combination therapy with three or more drugs is necessary to produce satisfactory results in adults.[31,179,180] Vincristine sulfate and prednisone, two selectively lymphotoxic agents, produce complete remission in about 90% of children with previously untreated ALL.[181,182] Although these two drugs are the cornerstone of remission-induction protocols in adults, the rate of complete remission after induction therapy with these two drugs alone rarely exceeds 40%.[183-185] A higher proportion of cases of Philadelphia chromosome-positive ALL in adults than in children is proposed as an explanation for the poor response to two-drug therapy.[186] Philadelphia chromosome-positive ALL is notoriously unresponsive to chemotherapy and carries a poor prognosis. Drugs added to the vincristine sulfate plus prednisone regimen in adults over the past decade include asparaginase,[30,31,187-190] daunorubicin hydrochloride,[30,31,180,188,189] doxorubicin,[25,190-194] methotrexate,[179] cyclophosphamide,[32] mercaptopurine,[30] and cytarabine.[30]

Of all the drugs used in combination with vincristine sulfate and prednisone, an anthracycline is the most beneficial. Gottlieb et al.[188] prospectively compared induction with vincristine sulfate, prednisone, and asparaginase with an identical regimen including daunorubicin hydrochloride in 177 previously untreated adults with ALL. Complete remission was achieved in 47% and 83% of the patients who received the three- and four-drug combinations, respectively ($p = 0.003$). Although severe (<1000 cells/cu mm) or life-threatening (<500 cells/cu mm) granulocytopenia was more frequent in the anthracycline-treated patients, the incidence of infection or bleeding was not significantly different between the two groups. The results of smaller nonrandomized trials confirmed the beneficial effects of an anthracycline addition for remission induction and suggested that doxorubicin hydrochloride and daunorubicin are equally effective additions.[30,31,180,187,189-194]

The contribution by drugs other than vincristine, prednisone, and anthracyclines to remission induction in these studies is unclear. Asparaginase is very active against ALL and is theoretically advantageous because of its marrow-sparing effects. However, the addition of asparaginase to combination therapy with vincristine, prednisone, and an anthracycline did not improve response in two studies.[30-31] Other studies also failed to show any additional benefit with asparaginase.[30,31,187,190] Similarly, methotrexate,[179] cyclophosphamide,[30] cytarabine,[30] and mercaptopurine[30] did not appear to provide any additional benefit.

Complete remission rates for combination therapy with three or more drugs range from 68% to 94%,[30,31,179-194] although investigators reporting the highest remission rates usually excluded high-risk patients.[189] In all the trials, advanced age was adversely associated with the ability to achieve complete remission.[31,32,187,188,193-195] A high initial WBC count and documented CNS disease at diagnosis were also adversely associated with the ability to achieve complete remission.[31,32]

Therefore, on the basis of available data, combination therapy with vincristine sulfate, prednisone, and an anthracycline is recommended for inducing remission in adults with ALL. The L10M protocol developed at the Memorial Sloan-Kettering Cancer Institute is depicted in Table 7. This regimen represents the most commonly used drugs and dosages for remission induction, consolidation, and maintenance in adult ALL.

Postremission Therapy. Effective postremission therapy is necessary to extend remission and improve survival; intensified induction therapy alone does not influence the duration of remission or survival.[188] However, as with induction therapy, most well-designed clinical trials evaluating postremission therapy were conducted in children. Strategies used in children are often insufficient to improve survival in adults.[31,187] Furthermore, the studies that have been completed in adults had small numbers of patients and inadequate follow-up and were neither randomized nor controlled.

Despite these limitations, a general treatment philosophy has evolved. Evidence from uncontrolled studies indicates that, unlike low-dose maintenance therapy,[31,187] intensified postremission therapy improves outcome.[30-32,189,192,194] Consequently, adult protocols include consolidation and maintenance phases incorporating alternating cycles of drugs with different mechanisms of action and nonhematologic toxicities. This strategy is designed to provide maximum antileukemic activity while minimizing toxicity and preventing the development of drug resistance. The optimum duration of postremission therapy is unknown. The benefits of continuing antileukemic therapy must be weighed against the risks of persistent immunosuppression. In most programs therapy continues for two to three years.[31,32,180,188,189,192]

The two most active drugs for maintaining remission are methotrexate sodium and mercaptopurine. These two drugs are part of all current postremission protocols. Other drugs used for maintaining remission include cytarabine, asparaginase, prednisone, cyclophosphamide, anthracyclines, vincristine sulfate, dactinomycin, and carmustine.[30-32,179-194] Dosages and the duration of therapy vary. Table 7 depicts a representative postremission program. Since postremission therapy is usally continued for at least two years, cumulative toxicity is a concern. Anthracycline-induced cardiomyopathy or severe vincristine-induced peripheral neuropathy can necessitate premature discontinuation of therapy.

Median durations of remission reported over the past 10 years range from 15 months to more than 48 months.[30-32,179-194] In a limited number of trials with adequate follow-up, five-year disease-free survival rates of 17–32% have been reported.[179,187] Although

Table 7.
Representative Combination Chemotherapy Program for Adult Acute Lymphoblastic Leukemia[a]

Therapy	Regimen[b]
Remission induction (days 1–36)	VCR[c] 2 mg/sq m on days 1, 8, 15, 22, and 29; PRED 60 mg/sq m p.o. on days 1–36, then taper over 7 days and discontinue; DOX 20 mg/sq m on days 17–19; and DOX 30 mg/sq m plus CTX 600 mg/sq m on day 36
Central nervous system prophylaxis	MTX 6 mg/sq m i.t. on days 3, 5, 15, 17, 34, and 36
Consolidation (days 1–110)	MTX 15 mg/sq m/day for 5 days plus Ara-C 200 mg/sq m/day c.i. for 5 days beginning on days 1, 36, and 71, alternating with TG 120 mg/sq m p.o. q 12 hr for 6 days plus Ara-C 150 mg/sq m q 12 hr for 6 days beginning on days 15, 50, and 85, VCR 1.4 mg/sq m on days 50 and 57, PRED 60 mg/sq m/day p.o. on days 50–57, ASP 60,000 IU/sq m 3 times per week for 6 doses beginning on day 99, CTX 1200 mg/sq m on day 110, and MTX 6 mg/sq m i.t. on days 15, 17, 57, and 59
Maintenance (repeat cycle every 21 wk for 36 mo)	VCR 1 mg/sq m on days 1, 8, 78, and 85; PRED 90 mg/sq m/day p.o. for 7 days beginning on days 1 and 78; DOX 20 mg/sq m on days 15–17; MP 90 mg/sq m/day p.o. on days 36–65 and 106–134; MTX 20 mg/sq m on days 43, 50, 57, 64, 113, 120, 127, and 134; dactinomycin 1000 μg/sq m on days 71 and 147; CTX 800 mg/sq m on day 91; BCNU 80 mg/sq m on day 91; and MTX 6 mg/sq m i.t. on days 36, 38, 106, and 108

[a]Adapted from reference 192, with permission.
[b]All regimens involve the intravenous route of administration unless otherwise specified. VCR = vincristine sulfate, PRED = prednisone, DOX = doxorubicin hydrochloride, CTX = cyclophosphamide, MTX = methotrexate (as the sodium salt), i.t. = intrathecally, Ara-C = cytarabine, c.i. = continuous infusion, TG = thioguanine, ASP = asparaginase, MP = mercaptopurine, BCNU = carmustine.
[c]Total dose not to exceed 4 mg for patients less than 60 years of age or 2.5 mg for patients over 60 years of age.

single-institution studies have yielded better results for remission duration and survival,[32,180,189-191] most have excluded older patients or patients with phenotypes carrying a poor prognosis, such as null-cell or Philadelphia chromosome-positive ALL. Results obtained in these trials are therefore not applicable to high-risk patients.

Several factors have been analyzed for their prognostic bearing on the duration of complete remission and survival and help to further define standard-risk and high-risk patient groups. T-cell and common-type ALL, age less than 35 years, a WBC count below 35,000/cu mm on admission, and early response to chemotherapy are associated with longer remission duration and longer survival.[30-32,188,190,194,195] In contrast, patients with null-cell or B-cell ALL, age more than 35 years, a high initial WBC count, or delayed response to chemotherapy have a dismal prognosis.[30-32,187,188,190,194] The use of standard definitions of high-risk patients in national clinical trials will assist in making comparisons among studies and in determining the best therapy for adult patients with ALL. Until then, no currently used postremission therapy can be recommended as a standard of care for all patients.

Prophylaxis and Treatment of CNS Involvement. Meningeal invasion by leukemic cells is common in ALL. Although documented CNS disease at diagnosis occurs in less than 10% of adults,[31,188,189] up to 40% of adults will ultimately relapse at this site without adequate prophylaxis.[179,196] Longer median survival or better migratory prowess of lymphocytes compared with myelocytes may partially explain the higher incidence of CNS involvement in ALL than AML. Findings associated with CNS disease at diagnosis are a high WBC count,[31] B-cell morphology,[31,197] and a high serum LDH concentration (>600 units/L).[197] These findings indicate a large tumor burden, are adversely associated with the ability to achieve complete remission, and confer a poor prognosis.[31,197]

The value of prophylaxis of CNS leukemia in children has been clearly shown in randomized controlled trials.[198,199] Consequently, all adult protocols incorporate such prophylaxis. One randomized trial showed that prophylaxis of CNS involvement in adults is warranted. Omura et al.[179] randomly assigned 99 adults with previously untreated ALL to receive intrathecal methotrexate sodium plus cranial irradiation or no prophylaxis. Time to relapse at a CNS site was 26 months in the patients who received prophylactic therapy, compared with 19 months in those who did not ($p = 0.008$). There was no difference in time to bone-marrow relapse or survival between the two groups. Retrospective studies have confirmed these observations.[31,200]

Combination therapy with intrathecal methotrexate sodium and cranial irradiation is the most commonly used prophylactic regimen in adults.[30,179,180,187-191,193-200] Prophylactic therapy is initiated after complete remission is attained and is given along with consolidation or maintenance therapy. Methotrexate dosages vary from 6 to 12 mg/sq m (as the sodium salt) twice weekly for four to six doses. Most investigators limit the total dose of methotrexate in adults to 12 or 15 mg (as the sodium salt).[160] Methotrexate is effective when administered intrathecally or via an Ommaya reservoir, an indwelling intraventricular device.[201] Some investigators recommend the intraventricular route for ease of administration if prophylactic therapy is prolonged.[202] If the intraventricular route is used, single doses should not exceed 6 mg.[203] Cranial irradiation most commonly consists of 2400 Gy administered in divided doses over two to three weeks. With combined-modality therapy, relapse of disease at a CNS site occurs in 3–13% of adults.[179,180,187,189,193]

CNS disease prophylaxis with these regimens has been associated with substantial toxicities in children, including paraplegia, seizures, leukoencephalopathy, bone marrow suppression, impaired cognitive function, and death.[204-207] Adverse effects occur in 10–20% of adult patients and are comparatively mild. They include transient paraplegia, headache, arachnoiditis, meningismus, somnolence syndrome, and Ommaya reservoir-associated infection.[179,189,201] Whether therapy is actually better tolerated in adults or adverse effects simply are reported less frequently is unknown.

To avoid the toxicities associated with combined-modality therapy, other approaches to prophylaxis have been explored. Schauer et al.[32] evaluated the efficacy of methotrexate sodium without the addition of cranial irradiation. Seventy-two patients received intrathecal or intraventricular methotrexate 6.25 mg/sq m (as the sodium salt) two times per week during induction, consolidation, and maintenance therapy over three years. Relapse in the CNS occurred in 3% of the patients. Transient meningismus and Ommaya reservoir-related infection were the most common toxicities, occurring in less than 10% of the patients. Other investigators have reported similar results with intrathecal methotrexate sodium alone.[192,200]

Incorporating high-dose chemotherapy capable of achieving cytotoxic drug levels in the CNS into the remission-induction or consolidation phase is another way to circumvent the use of more toxic prophylactic measures. High-dose methotrexate sodium and high-dose cytarabine have been used for this purpose. Esterhay et al.[195] used high-dose methotrexate (100–300 mg/kg/dose [as the sodium salt] given monthly for 12 months) as consolidation therapy in 38 previously untreated adults with ALL. Relapse in the CNS occurred in 8.3% of the patients. Methotrexate concentrations in the cerebrospinal fluid were 10^{-7}–10^{-4} M. Specific CNS toxicities were not described. Systemic toxicities were mild and included reversible bone marrow suppression and stomatitis. In a study by Kantarjian et al.,[194] systemic high-dose cytarabine (2 g/sq m every 12 hours for 12 doses) and methotrexate (200–800 mg/sq m [as the sodium salt]) incorporated into multidrug consolidation and maintenance programs were also effective in reducing the incidence of CNS relapse. The incidence of CNS relapse was 11%—similar to results obtained with intrathecal chemotherapy and irradiation. Toxicities specifically related to each of these two drugs are difficult to assess, as both were incorporated into the treatment regimens.

The results of these studies suggest that the value of cranial irradiation should be reassessed. Prolonged therapy with intrathecal methotrexate sodium or high-dose systemic therapy is as effective as combination therapy with intrathecal methotrexate sodium and radiation. Furthermore, radiation is immunosuppressive and places the patient at risk for marrow relapse or infection. High-dose systemic therapy has the added advantage of providing systemic antileukemic effects while simultaneously exerting a prophylactic effect in the CNS and other sanctuary sites. Randomized trials with long-term follow-up comparing systemic high-dose chemotherapy against standard therapy with intrathecal methotrexate sodium and cranial irradiation are needed to clarify the risks and benefits of these treatment options.

Not many studies have explored treatment for established CNS leukemia in adults. Some investigators reinstitute intrathecal methotrexate sodium therapy and cranial irradiation at dosages equivalent to those used for prophylaxis,[179] while others advocate increasing the radiation dose to 27 Gy[189] or 30 Gy.[30] Still other approaches are giving weekly intrathecal methotrexate sodium until the cerebrospinal fluid is clear of leukemic cells[188] or alternating intrathecal methotrexate sodium with intrathecal cytarabine.[201] When prolonged therapy with intrathecal methotrexate sodium is begun, cerebrospinal fluid methotrexate concentrations should be monitored carefully. Leukemic infiltration of the CNS can impede methotrexate elimination, resulting in elevated cerebrospinal fluid methotrexate concentrations and clinically significant neurotoxicity.[160,208,209] Maintenance of cerebrospinal fluid methotrexate concentrations in excess of 10^{-8} M for prolonged periods is associated with increased toxicity.[208] If concentrations exceed this value, further therapy should be withheld until they decline to an appropriately nontoxic value. Although remissions of CNS leukemia can be achieved, bone marrow relapse is usually imminent and survival time short.

Therapy for Relapsed or Refractory ALL. Ultimately, the majority of adults with ALL relapse and die of their disease. Although second remissions can be achieved in approximately 50% of patients, second and subsequent remissions are always shorter than the initial remission.[24,210] Patients with a long initial remission and patients who relapse after completing maintenance therapy, rather than during it, are more likely to achieve second complete remissions.[24,210] Median survival time after relapse is less than one year.[24]

Single-agent and combination therapies used in adults with ALL are detailed in Tables 8 and 9. As in AML, single-agent therapy is rarely useful in ALL. Combination therapy with non-cross-resistant agents is given in an attempt to overcome natural or acquired resistance. High-dose cytarabine, administered as a single agent[100] or in combination with an anthracycline analogue such as idarubicin,[132,133] mitoxantrone,[121,213,214] or amsacrine,[129,212,215,216] is one of the most effective drugs for treating relapsed or refractory ALL. By the time most patients relapse, they have been heavily treated with anthracyclines throughout the induction and postremission regimens. Therefore, the

Table 8.
Single-Agent Therapy for Relapsed or Refractory Adult Acute Lymphoblastic Leukemia

Drug	Dosage[a]	% Complete Remission	Median Duration of Remission (mo)	References
Cytarabine	3 g/sq m[b] q 12 hr for 2–6 days	27–33	10	79, 100
Mitoxantrone	8–20 mg/sq m/day for 5 days	20–40	1–10	111, 115, 211
Amsacrine	120 mg/sq m/day for 5 days	6–27	2	104, 105, 107, 212
Idarubicin hydrochloride	8–15 mg/sq m/day for 3 days	30	2	116, 117

[a]All dosages are intravenous unless otherwise specified.
[b]Defined as high-dose cytarabine.

Table 9.
Combination Therapy for Relapsed or Refractory Adult Acute Lymphoblastic Leukemia

Reference	No. Subjects	Regimen[a]	% Complete Remission	Median Duration of Remission (mo)
High-dose Cytarabine plus Mitoxantrone				
121	20	Ara-C 2 g/sq m q 12 hr for 4 days plus MIT 12 mg/sq m/day c.i. for 2 days	80	5
213	25	Ara-C 3 g/sq m q 12 hr for 3 days plus MIT 5 mg/sq m/day for 5 days	36	2
214	24	Ara-C 3 g/sq m q 12 hr for 1–4 days plus MIT 10 mg/sq m/day for 4 days	50	3.5
Cytarabine plus Idarubicin Hydrochloride				
133	13	Ara-C 2 g/sq m[b] over 3 hr daily for 3 days plus IDA 12 mg/sq m/day for 3 days	54	4
132	6	Ara-C 600 mg/sq m q 12 hr for 6 days plus IDA 12 mg/sq m/day for 3 days	83	3
Cytarabine plus Amsacrine				
129	13	Ara-C 3 g/sq m[b] over 3 hr daily for 5 days plus AMSA 200 mg/sq m/day for 3 days	67	. . .[c]
215	14	Ara-C 3 g/sq m[b] q 12 hr for 2 days plus AMSA 90–120 mg/sq m/day for 5 days	21	7
212	13	Ara-C 200 mg/sq m/day c.i. for 5 days plus AMSA 120–185 mg/sq m/day for 5 days	23	. . .
216	36	Ara-C 3 g/sq m[b] over 3 hr daily for 5 days	75	4
Cytarabine plus Teniposide				
217	19	Ara-C 300 mg/sq m 2 times per week for 4 wk plus TEN 165 mg/sq m 2 times per week for 4 wk	42	2
218	5	Ara-C 3 g/sq m[b] q 12 hr for 6 days plus TEN 100 mg/sq m on days 7 and 14	60	1–8
Vincristine Sulfate plus Doxorubicin plus Dexamethasone				
219	64	VCR 0.4 mg/sq m/day c.i. for 4 days plus DOX 12 mg/sq m/day c.i. for 4 days plus DEX 40 mg/day on days 1–4, 9–12, and 17–20 plus CTX 1 g/sq m on day 24	39	7
Methotrexate Sodium plus Asparaginase				
220	17	MTX 60 mg/sq m for 1 dose plus ASP 10,000 U/sq m 24 hr after MTX; repeat every week and increase MTX dosage by 50% with each course	58	2
221	38	VCR 2 mg on days 1, 10, and 20 plus PRED 40 mg/sq m/day plus MTX 125 mg/sq m on days 10, 20, and 30 plus ASP 6000 U/sq m on days 1, 11, 21, and 31; increase MTX dosage by 50 mg/sq m with each course	25	5
222	37	MTX 50–80 mg/sq m on day 1 plus ASP 20,000–40,000 U/sq m 3 hr after the MTX; repeat sequence every 7–14 days and increase MTX dosage by 40 mg/sq m per course as tolerated	58	4

[a]All regimens involve the intravenous route of administration unless otherwise specified. Ara-C = cytarabine, c.i. = continuous infusion, MIT = mitoxantrone, IDA = idarubicin hydrochloride, AMSA = amsacrine, TEN = teniposide, DOX = doxorubicin, DEX = dexamethasone, CTX = cyclophosphamide, MTX = methotrexate (as the sodium salt), ASP = asparaginase, VCR = vincristine sulfate, PRED = prednisone.
[b]Defined as high-dose cytarabine.
[c]Information was not reported.

addition of a second agent with non-cross-resistant activity is necessary to improve response. Thus, idarubicin hydrochloride, mitoxantrone, and amsacrine play an important role in the treatment of relapsed or refractory ALL.

Two drugs unique to the antineoplastic armamentarium for relapsed and refractory ALL are teniposide and moderate- to high-dose methotrexate. Teniposide is a podophyllotoxin derivative that has shown substantial activity in combination with cytarabine for treating high-risk ALL in children.[223,224] Limited data for adults suggest that this combination is effective in inducing second or subsequent remissions of short duration.[217,218] Myelosuppression and gastrointestinal toxicity are dose-limiting effects of teniposide. A pharmacodynamic relationship between dosage and response has been observed in children.[225] Thus far there are no comparable data for adults.

Moderate- and high-dose methotrexate regimens are increasingly being used to extend complete remission in children.[226,227] Although there is no standard definition of high-dose methotrexate, this term usually refers to doses that produce measurable plasma methotrexate concentrations in excess of 10^{-8} or 10^{-7} M for longer than 48 hours. Close pharmacokinetic monitoring is necessary, as these concentrations have been associated with toxicity.[228] Evans et al.[227] described a pharmacodynamic relationship between plasma methotrexate concentration and response to therapy in children with ALL. In this seminal study, children with plasma methotrexate concentrations less than 16×10^{-6} M were three times more likely to relapse at any site and seven times more likely to relapse in the bone marrow than children whose plasma methotrexate concentrations were greater than 16×10^{-6} M. Although this information is often used in clinical practice to improve therapy in adults, no adult studies have been published.

Adenosine deaminase is present in high concentrations in lymphocytes, in particular thymus-derived lymphocytes. This enzyme is necessary to produce deoxynucleotides required in DNA synthesis. Pentostatin is an agent derived from *Streptomyces antibioticus* that exerts selective lymphocytic activity by inhibiting adenosine deaminase.[229,230] Pentostatin recently received FDA-approved labeling for use in the treatment of hairy cell leukemia. Although not bearing approved labeling for other uses, pentostatin has been used successfully to treat a limited number of patients with relapsed or refractory ALL. Responses are seen only in subsets of patients with T-cell ALL.[230-233] Evaluations of this unique drug in combination with traditional therapies are eagerly awaited.

Role of Bone Marrow Transplantation. The role of bone marrow transplantation in the treatment of adult ALL is ill-defined. Reasonable response rates with chemotherapy alone and cumulative toxicity during prolonged chemotherapy are two reasons why many hematologists are reluctant to recommend bone marrow transplantation for adults with ALL.

Allogeneic bone marrow transplantation was originally reserved for patients with refractory leukemia or multiple relapses.[85] In these early studies it was clear that survival time after allogeneic transplantation for ALL was greater when the procedure was performed during remission than when it was done after relapse.[85,234] In one study,[235] 27% of patients with ALL who received transplants during remission remained in continuous complete remission at five years, compared with 15% of patients who underwent the procedure after relapse ($p = 0.02$). There is little agreement, however, on whether transplantation should be performed during the first remission or a subsequent one. Because intensive combination chemotherapy alone can produce long-term disease-free survival in many patients,[30,189] some investigators advocate withholding allogeneic bone marrow transplantation until a second complete remission has been achieved.[234,236,237] While this may be appropriate therapy for standard-risk patients, evidence suggests that high-risk adults should undergo allogeneic bone marrow transplantation during the first complete remission. In a retrospective review of 444 patients with one or more high-risk features, Herzig et al.[238] found that the disease-free survival rate and the relapse rate at four years were significantly better for patients undergoing allogeneic bone marrow transplantation during the first remission than for patients receiving transplants during a second remission (survival rate, 45% versus 22%, $p < 0.0002$, and relapse rate, 26% versus 56%, $p < 0.0001$). High risk was defined as an age of less than 2 years or more than 16 years, an initial WBC count above 50,000/cu mm, CNS involvement, B-cell ALL, an L3 morphology, and unfavorable chromosomal abnormalities. Authors of smaller studies with similar risk criteria reported comparable results at shorter follow-up times.[239,240] In a study of 10 patients with Philadelphia chromosome-positive ALL who received allogeneic transplants during a second or subsequent relapse, six patients experienced remission lasting a median of 19 months, suggesting that bone marrow transplantation may be the therapy of choice in such patients.[241]

No prospective randomized trials have been conducted to compare combination chemotherapy with allogeneic bone marrow transplantation in adults with ALL. Data from uncontrolled studies and historical controls suggest that disease-free survival is longer after allogeneic bone marrow transplantation performed during first or second remission than after chemotherapy alone.[236,242]

Autologous bone marrow transplantation has also been explored in patients with ALL. Kersey et al.[243] compared autologous with allogeneic bone marrow transplantation for the treatment of high-risk and refractory ALL in adults and children. Forty-six patients underwent allogeneic transplantation and 45 received autologous transplants after being conditioned with cyclophosphamide and total-body irradiation with or without cytarabine. Compared with allogeneic marrow recipients, autologous marrow recipients had a shorter median time to engraftment (24 versus 31 days, $p = 0.008$), a shorter hospital stay (41 versus 51 days, $p = 0.004$), and a lower incidence of procedure-related death (4% versus 26%, $p < 0.01$). Leukemic relapse was the most common cause of treatment failure and occurred more often in autologous marrow recipients (79%) and in allogeneic marrow recipients who did not develop graft-versus-host disease (75%) than in the allogeneic group that did develop graft-versus-host disease (37%, $p = 0.03$). Long-term disease-free survival rates were not different between the autologous and allogeneic marrow recipients (20% versus 27%). Similar relapse and survival rates after autologous bone marrow transplantation were reported in two small uncontrolled studies.[242,244]

As in patients with AML, leukemic relapse remains the greatest obstacle to successful treatment of ALL after rescue therapy with autologous marrow. In an effort to reduce the number of malignant lymphoblasts, some investigators advocate purging autologous marrow in vitro with monoclonal antibodies,[243,245] immunotoxins,[246] or antileukemic antineoplastics.[247] It is unclear whether marrow purging decreases the incidence of leukemic relapse; no prospective trials have been conducted. Many of the techniques used for purging are nonselective for lymphocytes and simultaneously deplete normal hematopoietic precursors, resulting in delayed engraftment. The use of sargramostim may accelerate engraftment. Sargramostim can be safely administered to patients with lymphoid malignancies and accelerates the engraftment of purged autografts as long as a sufficient number of hematopoietic precursor cells are infused.[248]

On the basis of the data available, allogeneic bone marrow transplantation is recommended for standard-risk patients in second or subsequent remission and for high-risk patients in first or subsequent remission. Autologous marrow transplantation is an alternative for high-risk patients in first remission who do not have a donor. The value of autologous transplantation for patients in second or subsequent relapse is unknown; for these patients the procedure should be considered experimental at best.

Conclusion

There has been substantial progress in the treatment of adult acute leukemia. The cornerstone of therapy for both AML and ALL remains intensive combination chemotherapy. Bone marrow transplantation has changed the outlook for some patients and offers the potential of a cure in young and otherwise healthy patients; however, much research is needed to decrease the frequency and severity of complications. Differentiation therapy with tretinoin, sargramostim, or low-dose cytarabine offers a less toxic alternative to intensive chemotherapy. New drug entities such as idarubicin hydrochloride and pentostatin are other important additions to the antileukemic armamentarium. Future advances may depend on identifying which patients will benefit most from specific treatments.

References

1. Jandl JH. Hematopoietic malignancies. In: Blood: textbook of hematology. Boston: Little, Brown; 1987:589-629.
2. Clarkson B. The acute leukemias. In: Petersdorf RG, Adams RD, Braunwald E et al., eds. Harrison's principles of internal medicine. 10th ed. New York: McGraw-Hill; 1983:798-807.
3. American Cancer Society. American Cancer Society facts and figures. New York: American Cancer Society; 1989.
4. Ishimaru T, Hoshino R, Ichimaru M et al. Leukemia in atomic bomb survivors, Hiroshima and Nagasaki, 1 October 1950–30 September 1966. *Radiat Res*. 1971; 45:216-33.
5. Bizzozero OJ, Johnson KG, Ciocco A. Radiation-related leukemia in Hiroshima and Nagasaki, 1946–1964. *N Engl J Med*. 1966; 274:1095-101.
6. March HC. Leukemia in radiologists, ten years later. *Am J Med Sci*. 1961; 242:137-48.
7. Court-Brown WM, Doll R. Leukemia and aplastic anemia in patients irradiated for ankylosing spondylitis. London: Her Majesty's Stationery Office, 1957; British Medical Research Report no. 295.
8. Cronkite EP. Chemical leukemogenesis: benzene as a model. *Semin Hematol*. 1987; 24:2-11.
9. Pedersen-Bjergaard J, Larsen SO. Incidence of acute nonlymphocytic leukemia, preleukemia, and acute myeloproliferative syndrome up to 10 years after treatment of Hodgkin's disease. *N Engl J Med*. 1982; 307:965-71.
10. Casciota DA, Scott JL. Acute leukemia following prolonged cytotoxic agent therapy. *Medicine*. 1979; 58:32-45.
11. Fougar K, McKenna RW, Bloomfield CD et al. Therapy-related leukemia, a panmyelosis. *Cancer*. 1979; 43:1285-96.
12. Bloomfield CD, Brunning RD. Acute leukemia as a terminal event in nonleukemic hematopoietic disorders. *Semin Oncol*. 1976; 3(3):297-314.
13. Greene MH, Boice JD, Greer BE et al. Acute nonlymphocytic leukemia after therapy with alkylating agents for ovarian cancer: a study of five randomized trials. *N Engl J Med*. 1982; 307:1416-21.
14. Gallo RC, Wong-Staal F. Retroviruses as etiologic agents of some animal and human leukemias and lymphomas and as tools for elucidating the molecular mechanism of leukemogenesis. *Blood*. 1982; 60:545-57.
15. Cheson BD. The myelodysplastic syndromes: current approaches to therapy. *Ann Intern Med*. 1990; 112:932-41.
16. Bennett JM, Catovsky D, Daniel M-T et al. Proposals for the classification of the acute leukaemias: French–American–British (FAB) Cooperative Group. *Br J Haematol*. 1976; 33:451-8.
17. Gralnick HR, Galton DAG, Catovsky D et al. Classification of acute leukemia. *Ann Intern Med*. 1977; 87:740-53.
18. Bennet JM, Catovsky D, Daniel M-T et al. Criteria for the diagnosis of acute leukemia of megakaryocyte lineage (M7): a report of the French–American–British Cooperative Group. *Ann Intern Med*. 1985; 103:460-2.
19. Hoelzer D, Gale RP. Acute lymphoblastic leukemia in adults: recent progress, future directions. *Semin Hematol*. 1987; 24:27-39.
20. Ball ED, Fanger MW. The expression of myeloid-specific antigens on myeloid leukemia cells: correlation with leukemia subclasses and implications for normal myeloid differentiation. *Blood*. 1983; 61:456-63.
21. Drexler HG. Classification of AML—comparison of FAB and immunophenotyping. *Leukemia*. 1987; 1:697-705.
22. Burns CP, Armitage JO, Frey AL. Analysis of the presenting features of adult acute leukemia: the French–American–British classification. *Cancer*. 1981; 47:2460-9.
23. Hoelzer D, Thiel E, Loffler H et al. Intensified therapy in acute lymphoblastic and acute undifferentiated leukemia in adults. *Blood*. 1984; 64:38-47.
24. Baccarani M, Corbelli G, Amadori S et al. Adolescent and adult acute lymphoblastic leukemia: prognostic features and outcome of therapy: a study of 293 patients. *Blood*. 1982; 60:677-84.
25. Schauer P, Arlin ZA, Mertelsmann R et al. Treatment of acute lymphoblastic leukemia in adults: results of the L-10 and L-10M protocols. *J Clin Oncol*. 1983; 1:462-70.
26. Look AT. The emerging genetics of acute lymphoblastic leukemia: clinical and biologic implications. *Semin Oncol*. 1985; 12:92-104.
27. Keating MJ, Kantarjian H, Smith TL et al. Response to salvage therapy and survival after relapse in acute myelogenous leukemia. *J Clin Oncol*. 1989; 7:1071-80.

28. Smits P, Schoosts L, de Pauw BE et al. Prognostic factors in adult patients with acute leukemia at first relapse. *Cancer.* 1987; 59:1631-4.
29. Estey E, Plunkett W, Dixon M et al. Variables predicting response to high dose cytosine arabinoside therapy in patients with refractory acute leukemia. *Leukemia.* 1987; 1:580-83.
30. Kantarjian HM, Keating MJ, Walters RS et al. The characteristics and outcome of patients with late relapse acute myelogenous leukemia. *J Clin Oncol.* 1988; 6:232-8.
31. Hiddemann W, Martin WR, Sauerland CM et al. Definition of refractoriness against conventional chemotherapy in acute myeloid leukemia: a proposal based on the results of retreatment by thioguanine, cytosine arabinoside, and daunorubicin (TAD 9) in 150 patients with relapse after standardized first line therapy. *Leukemia.* 1990; 4:184-8.
32. Mertelsmann R, Thaler T, To L. Morphological classification, response to therapy, and survival in 263 adult patients with acute nonlymphoblastic leukemia. *Blood.* 1980; 56:773-81.
33. Bennett JM, Begg CB. Eastern Cooperative Oncology Group study of the cytochemistry of adult acute myeloid leukemia by correlation of subtypes with response and survival. *Cancer Res.* 1981; 41:4833-7.
34. Gale PG, Cline MJ. High remission-induction rate in acute myeloid leukemia. *Lancet.* 1977; 1:497-9.
35. Rees JKH, Sandler RM, Challener J et al. Treatment of acute myeloid leukaemia with a triple cytotoxic regime: DAT. *Br J Cancer.* 1977; 36:770-6.
36. Cassileth PA, Katz ME. Chemotherapy for adult acute nonlymphocytic leukemia with daunorubicin and cytosine arabinoside. *Cancer Treat Rep.* 1977; 61:1441-5.
37. Foon KA, Zighelboim J, Yale C et al. Intensive chemotherapy is the treatment of choice for elderly patients with acute myelogenous leukemia. *Blood.* 1981; 58:467-70.
38. Glucksberg H, Cheever MA, Farewell VT et al. High-dose combination chemotherapy for acute nonlymphoblastic leukemia in adults. *Cancer.* 1981; 48:1073-81.
39. Yates J, Glidewell O, Wiernik P et al. Cytosine arabinoside with daunorubicin or adriamycin for therapy of acute myelocytic leukemia: a CALGB study. *Blood.* 1982; 60:454-62.
40. Buchner T, Urbanitz D, Hiddemann W et al. Intensified induction and consolidation with or without maintenance chemotherapy for acute myeloid leukemia (AML): two multicenter studies of the German AML Cooperative Group. *J Clin Oncol.* 1985; 3:1583-9.
41. Rees JKH, Gray RG, Swirsky D et al. Principal results of the Medical Research Council's 8th acute myeloid leukaemia trial. *Lancet.* 1986; 2:1236-41.
42. Hayat M, Jehn U, Willemze R et al. A randomized comparison of maintenance treatment with androgens, immunotherapy, and chemotherapy in adult acute myelogenous leukemia: a Leukemia–Lymphoma Group trial of the EORTC. *Cancer.* 1986; 58:617-23.
43. Preisler H, Davis RB, Kirshner J et al. Comparison of three remission induction regimens and two postinduction strategies for the treatment of acute nonlymphocytic leukemia: a Cancer and Leukemia Group B study. *Blood.* 1987; 69:1441-9.
44. Cassileth PA, Harrington DP, Hines JD et al. Maintenance chemotherapy prolongs remission duration in adult acute nonlymphocytic leukemia. *J Clin Oncol.* 1988; 6:583-7.
45. Rai KR, Holland JF, Glidewell OJ et al. Treatment of acute myelocytic leukemia: a study by Cancer and Leukemia Group B. *Blood.* 1981; 58:1203-12.
46. Cassileth PA, Begg CB, Bennett JM et al. A randomized study of the efficacy of consolidation therapy in adult acute nonlymphocytic leukemia. *Blood.* 1984; 63:843-7.
47. Bishop JF, Lowenthal RM, Joshua D et al. Etoposide in acute nonlymphocytic leukemia. *Blood.* 1990; 75:27-32.
48. Vogler WR, Winton EF, Gordon DS et al. A randomized comparison of postremission therapy in acute myelogenous leukemia: a Southeastern Cancer Study Group trial. *Blood.* 1984; 63:1039-45.
49. Keating MJ, Smith TL, McCredie KB et al. A four-year experience with anthracycline, cytosine arabinoside, vincristine and prednisone combination chemotherapy in 325 adults with acute leukemia. *Cancer.* 1981; 47:2779-88.
50. Glucksberg H, Buckner CD, Fefer A et al. Combination chemotherapy for acute nonlymphoblastic leukemia in adults. *Cancer Chemother Rep Part 1.* 1975; 59:1131-7.
51. Peterson BA, Bloomfield CD, Bosl GJ et al. Intensive five-drug combination chemotherapy for adult acute non-lymphocytic leukemia. *Cancer.* 1980; 46:663-8.
52. Archimbaud E, Fiere D, Treille-Ritouet D et al. Influence of daunorubicin and cytarabine sequencing on the outcome of therapy in acute myelogenous leukemia: a randomized trial. *Cancer Treat Rep.* 1987; 71:571-4.
53. Preisler HD, Rustum Y, Henderson ES et al. Treatment of acute nonlymphocytic leukemia: use of anthracycline–cytosine arabinoside induction therapy and comparison of two maintenance regimens. *Blood.* 1979; 53:455-64.
54. Berman E, Heller G, Santorsa J et al. Results of a randomized trial comparing idarubicin and cytosine arabinoside with daunorubicin and cytosine arabinoside in adult patients with newly diagnosed acute myelogenous leukemia. *Blood.* 1991; 77:1666-74.
55. Wiernik PH, Banks PLC, Case DC et al. Cytarabine plus idarubicin or daunorubicin as induction and consolidation therapy for previously untreated adult patients with acute myeloid leukemia. *Blood.* 1992; 79:1-8.
56. Vogler WR, Velez-Garcia E, Omura G et al. A Phase III trial comparing daunorubicin or idarubicin combined with cytosine arabinoside in acute myelogenous leukemia. *Semin Oncol.* 1989; 16(1 Suppl 2):21-4.
57. Arlin Z, Case DC Jr, Moore J et al. Randomized multicenter trial of cytosine arabinoside with mitoxantrone or daunorubicin in previously untreated adult patients with acute nonlymphocytic leukemia (ANLL). *Leukemia.* 1990; 4:177-83.
58. Von Hoff DD, Layard MW, Basa P et al. Risk factors for doxorubicin-induced congestive heart failure. *Ann Intern Med.* 1979; 91:710-7.
59. Lichtman MA, Rowe JM. Hyperleukocytic leukemias: rheological, clinical, and therapeutic considerations. *Blood.* 1982; 60:279-83.
60. Dutcher JP, Schiffer CA, Wiernik PH. Hyperleukocytosis in adult acute nonlymphocytic leukemia: impact on remission rate and duration, and survival. *J Clin Oncol.* 1987; 5:1364-72.
61. Maurer HS, Steinherz PG, Gaynon PS et al. The effect of initial management of hyperleukocytosis on early complications and outcome of children with acute lymphoblastic leukemia. *J Clin Oncol.* 1988; 6:1425-32.
62. Ventura GJ, Hester JP, Smith TL et al. Acute myeloblastic leukemia with hyperleukocytosis: risk factors for early mortality in induction. *Am J Hematol.* 1988; 27:34-7.
63. Zittoun R, Jehn U, Fiere D et al. Alternating v repeated postremission treatment in adult acute myelogenous leukemia: a randomized Phase III study (AML6) of the EORTC Leukemia Cooperative Group. *Blood.* 1989; 73:896-906.
64. Sauter C, Fopp M, Imbach P et al. Acute myelogenous leukaemia: maintenance chemotherapy after early consolidation treatment does not prolong survival. *Lancet.* 1984; 1:379-82.
65. Marcus RE, Catovsky D, Goldman JM et al. Maintenance and consolidation therapy in AML. *Lancet.* 1984; 1:686-7.
66. Jacobs P, Dubovsky DW, Wood L. In adult acute nonlymphoblastic leukaemia extended maintenance chemotherapy has no benefit. *Am J Hematol.* 1984; 16:255-65.
67. Petti MC, Broccia G, Caronia F et al. Therapy of acute myelogenous leukemia in adults. *Hamatol Bluttransfus.* 1990; 33:249-53.
68. Mayer RJ, Weinstein HJ, Coral FS et al. The role of intensive postinduction chemotherapy in the management of patients with acute myelogenous leukemia. *Cancer Treat Rep.* 1982; 66:1455-62.
69. Preisler HD, Brecher M, Browman G et al. The treatment of acute myelocytic leukemia in patients 30 years of age and

younger. *Am J Hematol*. 1982; 13:189-98.
70. Weinstein HJ, Mayer RJ, Rosenthal DS et al. Treatment of acute myelogenous leukemia in children and adults. *N Engl J Med*. 1980; 303:473-8.
71. Kurrle E, Ehninger G, Fackler-Schwalbe E et al. Consolidation therapy with high-dose cytosine arabinoside: experiences of a prospective study in acute myeloid leukemia. *Hamatol Bluttransfus*. 1990; 33:255-61.
72. Cassileth PA, Begg CB, Silber R. Prolonged unmaintained remission after intensive consolidation therapy in adult acute nonlymphocytic leukemia. *Cancer Treat Rep*. 1987; 71:137-40.
73. Preisler HD, Raza A, Early A et al. Intensive remission consolidation therapy in the treatment of acute nonlymphocytic leukemia. *J Clin Oncol*. 1987; 5:722-30.
74. Tallman MS, Appelbaum FR, Amos D et al. Evaluation of intensive postremission chemotherapy for adults with acute nonlymphocytic leukemia using high-dose cytosine arabinoside with L-asparaginase and amsacrine with etoposide. *J Clin Oncol*. 1987; 5:918-26.
75. Wolff SN, Marion J, Stein RS et al. High-dose cytosine arabinoside and daunorubicin as consolidation therapy for acute nonlymphocytic leukemia in first remission: a pilot study. *Blood*. 1985; 65:1407-11.
76. Champlin R, Ho W, Winston D et al. Treatment of adults with acute myelogenous leukemia: prospective evaluation of high-dose cytarabine in consolidation chemotherapy and with bone marrow transplantation. *Semin Oncol*. 1987; 14(2 Suppl 1):1-6.
77. Champlin R, Gajewski J, Nimer S et al. Postremission chemotherapy for adults with acute myelogenous leukemia: improved survival with high-dose cytarabine and daunorubicin consolidation treatment. *J Clin Oncol*. 1990; 8:1199-206.
78. Lazarus HM, Vogler RW, Burns CP et al. High-dose cytosine arabinoside and daunorubicin as primary therapy in elderly patients with acute myelogenous leukemia. A Phase I–II study of the Southeastern Cancer Study Group. *Cancer*. 1989; 63:1055-9.
79. Herzig RH, Wolff SN, Lazarus HM et al. High-dose cytosine arabinoside therapy for refractory leukemia. *Blood*. 1983; 62:361-9.
80. Thomas ED, Storb R, Clift RA et al. Bone marrow transplantation. Part 1. *N Engl J Med*. 1975; 292:832-43.
81. Thomas ED, Storb R, Clift RA et al. Bone marrow transplantation. Part 2. *N Engl J Med*. 1975; 292:895-902.
82. Thomas ED, Clift RA, Buckner CD. Marrow transplantation for patients with acute nonlymphoblastic leukemia who achieve a first remission. *Cancer Treat Rep*. 1982; 66:1463-6.
83. Storb R, Buckner CD, Clift RA et al. Marrow grafting for acute leukemia: results and future treatment strategies. *Hamatol Bluttransfus*. 1990; 33:629-35.
84. Champlin RE, Gale RP. Role of bone marrow transplantation in the treatment of hematologic malignancies and solid tumors: critical review of syngeneic, autologous and allogeneic transplants. *Cancer Treat Rep*. 1984; 68:145-59.
85. Thomas ED, Buckner CD, Banaji M et al. One hundred patients with acute leukemia treated by chemotherapy, total body irradiation, and allogeneic marrow transplantation. *Blood*. 1977; 49:511-33.
86. Santos GW, Tutxchka PJ, Brookmeyer R et al. Marrow transplantation for acute nonlymphocytic leukemia after treatment with busulfan and cyclophosphamide. *N Engl J Med*. 1983; 309:1347-53.
87. Powles RL, Clink HM, Bandini G et al. The place of bone-marrow transplantation in acute myelogenous leukaemia. *Lancet*. 1980; 1:1047-50.
88. Appelbaum FR, Dahlberg S, Thomas ED et al. Bone marrow transplantation or chemotherapy after remission induction in adults with acute nonlymphoblastic leukemia. *Ann Intern Med*. 1984; 101:581-8.
89. Appelbaum FR, Fisher LD, Thomas ED. Chemotherapy v marrow transplantation for adults with acute nonlymphocytic leukemia: a five-year follow-up. *Blood*. 1988; 72:179-84.
90. Powles RL, Watson JG, Morgenstern GR et al. Bone marrow transplantation in leukaemia remission. *Lancet*. 1982; 1:336-7.
91. Champlin RE, Ho WG, Gale RP et al. Treatment of acute myelogenous leukemia: a prospective controlled trial of bone marrow transplantation versus consolidation chemotherapy. *Ann Intern Med*. 1985; 102:285-91.
92. Clift RA, Buckner CD, Thomas ED et al. The treatment of acute non-lymphoblastic leukemia by allogeneic marrow transplantation. *Bone Marrow Transplant*. 1987; 2:243-58.
93. Butturini A, Bortin MM, Gale RP. Graft-versus-leukemia following bone marrow transplantation. *Bone Marrow Transplant*. 1987; 2:233-42.
94. Dinsmore R, Kirkpatrick D, Flomenberg N et al. Allogeneic bone marrow transplantation for patients with acute nonlymphocytic leukemia. *Blood*. 1984; 63:649-56.
95. McMillan AK, Goldstone AH, Linch DC et al. High-dose chemotherapy and autologous bone marrow transplantation in acute myeloid leukemia. *Blood*. 1990; 76:480-8.
96. Gorin NC, Aegerter P, Auvert B. Autologous bone marrow transplantation for acute leukemia in remission: an analysis of 1322 cases. *Hamatol Bluttransfus*. 1990; 33:660-6.
97. Lowenberg B, Verdonck LJ, Dekker AW et al. Autologous bone marrow transplantation in acute myeloid leukemia in first remission: results of a Dutch prospective study. *J Clin Oncol*. 1990; 8:287-94.
98. Reiffers J, Gaspard MH, Maraninchi D et al. Comparison of allogeneic or autologous bone marrow transplantation and chemotherapy in patients with acute myeloid leukaemia in first remission: a prospective controlled trial. *Br J Haematol*. 1989; 72:57-63.
99. Cantin G, Brennan JK. High-dose cytosine arabinoside for acute nonlymphocytic leukemia. *Am J Hematol*. 1984; 16:59-66.
100. Kantarjian HM, Estey EH, Plunkett W et al. Phase I–II clinical and pharmacologic studies of high-dose cytosine arabinoside in refractory leukemia. *Am J Med*. 1986; 81:387-94.
101. Takaku F, Urabe A, Mizoguchi H et al. High-dose cytosine arabinoside in the treatment of resistant leukemia. *Semin Oncol*. 1985; 12(Suppl 3):144-9.
102. Vogler WR, Preisler HD, Winton EF et al. Randomized trial of high-dose cytarabine versus amsacrine in acute myelogenous leukemia in relapse: a leukemia intergroup study. *Cancer Treat Rep*. 1986; 70:455-9.
103. Willemze R, Zwaan FE, Colpin G et al. High dose cytosine arabinoside in the management of refractory acute leukaemia. *Scand J Haematol*. 1982; 29:141-6.
104. Estey EH, Keating MJ, Smith TL et al. Prediction of complete remission in patients with refractory acute leukemia treated with AMSA. *J Clin Oncol*. 1984; 2:102-6.
105. Legha SS, Keating MJ, McCredie KB et al. Evaluation of AMSA in previously treated patients with acute leukemia: results of therapy in 109 adults. *Blood*. 1982; 60:484-90.
106. Omura GA, Winton EF, Vogler WR et al. Phase II study of amsacrine gluconate in refractory leukemia. *Cancer Treat Rep*. 1983; 67:1131-2.
107. Winton EF, Hearn EB, Vogler WR et al. Amsacrine in refractory adult acute leukemia: a pilot study of the Southeastern Cancer Study Group. *Cancer Treat Rep*. 1983; 67:977-80.
108. Von Hoff DD, Slavik M, Muggia FM. 5-Azacytidine: a new anticancer drug with effectiveness in acute myelogenous leukemia. *Ann Intern Med*. 1976; 85:237-45.
109. Larson RA, Sweet DL, Golomb HM et al. Response to 5-azacytidine in patients with refractory acute nonlymphocytic leukemia and association with chromosome findings. *Cancer*. 1982; 49:2222-5.
110. Vogler WR, Miller DS, Keller JW. 5-Azacytidine (NCS 102816): a new drug for the treatment of myeloblastic leukemią. *Blood*. 1976; 48:331-7.
111. Vorobiof DA, Falkson G, Coccia-Portugal MA et al. Mitoxantrone in the treatment of acute leukemia. *Invest New Drugs*. 1987; 5:383-8.
112. Kaminer LS, Choi KE, Daley KM. Continuous infusion mi-

toxantrone in relapsed acute non-lymphocytic leukemia. *Cancer*. 1990; 65:2619-23.

113. Moore JO, Olsen GA. Mitoxantrone in the treatment of relapsed and refractory acute leukemia. *Semin Oncol*. 1984; 11(Suppl 1):41-6.
114. Larson RA, Daly KM, Choi KE. A clinical and pharmacokinetic study of mitoxantrone in acute nonlymphocytic leukemia. *J Clin Oncol*. 1987; 5:391-7.
115. Bezwoda WR, Bernasconi C, Hutchinson RM et al. Mitoxantrone for refractory and relapsed acute leukemia. *Cancer*. 1990; 66:418-22.
116. Carella AM, Santini G, Martinengo M et al. 4-Demethoxydaunorubicin (idarubicin) in refractory or relapsed acute leukemias. *Cancer*. 1985; 55:1452-4.
117. Daghestani AN, Arlin ZA, Leyland-Jones et al. Phase I and II clinical and pharmacological study of 4-demethoxydaunorubicin (idarubicin) in adult patients with acute leukemia. *Cancer Res*. 1985; 45:1408-12.
118. Harousseau JL, Hurteloup P, Reiffers J et al. Idarubicin in the treatment of relapsed and refractory acute myeloid leukemia. *Cancer Treat Rep*. 1987; 71:991-2.
119. Brito-Babapulle F, Catovsky D, Slocombe G et al. Phase II study of mitoxantrone and cytarabine in acute myeloid leukemia. *Cancer Treat Rep*. 1987; 71:161-3.
120. Amadori S, Meloni G, Petti MC et al. Phase II trial of intermediate dose Ara-C (IDAC) with sequential mitoxantrone (MITOX) in acute myelogenous leukemia. *Leukemia*. 1989; 3:112-4.
121. Lejeune C, Tubiana N, Gastaut JA et al. High-dose cytosine arabinoside and mitoxantrone in previously treated acute leukemia patients. *Eur J Haematol*. 1990; 44:240-3.
122. Hiddemann W, Kreutzmann H, Straif K et al. High-dose cytosine arabinoside and mitoxantrone: a highly effective regimen in refractory acute myeloid leukemia. *Blood*. 1987; 69:744-9.
123. Martiat P, Ghilain JM, Ferrant A et al. High-dose cytosine arabinoside and amsacrine or mitoxantrone in relapsed and refractory acute myeloid leukaemia: a prospective randomized trial. *Eur J Haematol*. 1990; 45:164-7.
124. Paciucci PA, Dutcher JP, Cuttner J et al. Mitoxantrone and Ara-C in previously treated patients with acute myelogenous leukemia. *Leukemia*. 1987; 1:565-7.
125. Herzig RH, Lazarus HM, Wolff SN et al. High-dose cytosine arabinoside therapy with and without anthracycline antibiotics for remission reinduction of acute nonlymphoblastic leukemia. *J Clin Oncol*. 1985; 3:992-7.
126. Fiere D, Campos L, Van HV et al. Intensive timed chemotherapy protocol for 37 resistant or relapsing acute myeloid leukemias. *Cancer Treat Rep*. 1986; 70:285-6.
127. Hines JD, Oken MM, Mazza JJ et al. High-dose cytosine arabinoside and m-AMSA is effective therapy in relapsed acute nonlymphocytic leukemia. *J Clin Oncol*. 1984; 2:545-9.
128. Decker RW, Ho WG, Champlin RE et al. Phase II study of amsacrine and high-dose cytarabine for resistant acute myelogenous leukemia. *Cancer Treat Rep*. 1987; 71:881-2.
129. Arlin ZA, Ahmed T, Mittelman A et al. A new regimen of amsacrine with high-dose cytarabine is safe and effective therapy for acute leukemia. *J Clin Oncol*. 1987; 5:371-5.
130. Jehn U, Heinemann V. Intermediate-dose Ara-C/m-AMSA for remission induction and high-dose Ara-C/m-AMSA for intensive consolidation in relapsed and refractory adult acute myelogenous leukemia. *Hamatol Bluttransfus*. 1990; 33:333-5.
131. Harousseau JL, Reiffers J, Hurteloup P et al. Treatment of relapsed acute myeloid leukemia with idarubicin and intermediate-dose cytarabine. *J Clin Oncol*. 1989; 7:45-9.
132. Leone G, Pagano L, Marra R et al. Idarubicin combined with intermediate-dose cytosine arabinoside in the treatment of refractory acute leukemia. *Haematologia*. 1989; 74:57-61.
133. Carella AM, Pungolino E, Piatti G et al. Idarubicin in combination with intermediate-dose cytarabine in the treatment of refractory or relapsed acute leukemias. *Eur J Haematol*. 1989; 43:309-13.
134. Lambertenghi-Deliliers G, Maiolo AT, Annaloro C et al. Idarubicin in sequential combination with cytosine arabinoside in the treatment of relapsed and refractory patients with acute non-lymphoblastic leukemia. *Eur J Cancer Clin Oncol*. 1987; 23:1041-5.
135. Freund M, Link H, Diedrich H et al. High dose Ara-C and etoposide in the treatment of refractory or relapsing acute leukemia. *Blut*. 1987; 55:215. Abstract.
136. Chan HY, Meyers FJ, Lewis JP et al. High-dose VP-16 with intermediate-dose cytosine arabinoside in the treatment of relapsed acute nonlymphocytic leukemia. *Cancer Chemother Pharmacol*. 1987; 20:265-6.
137. Abrams RA, Hanson G, Hansen RM et al. Phase II study of combination chemotherapy with etoposide and amsacrine in relapsed adult leukemia. *Cancer Treat Rep*. 1986; 70:535.
138. Hiddemann W, Urbanitz D, Preusser P et al. Treatment of refractory acute myeloid leukemia with m-AMSA and VP-16-213 in combination. Results of a clinical Phase I/II study. *Hematol Oncol*. 1989; 7:267-73.
139. Tschopp L, Von Fliedner VE, Sauter C et al. Efficacy and clinical cross-resistance of a new combination therapy (AMSA/VP-16) in previously treated patients with acute nonlymphocytic leukemia. *J Clin Oncol*. 1986; 4:318-24.
140. Archimbaud E, Leblond V, Michallet M et al. Intensive sequential chemotherapy with mitoxantrone and continuous infusion etoposide and cytarabine for previously treated acute myelogenous leukemia. *Blood*. 1991; 77:1894-900.
141. Amadori S, Arcese W, Isacchi G et al. Mitoxantrone, etoposide, and intermediate-dose cytarabine: an effective and tolerable regimen for the treatment of refractory acute myeloid leukemia. *J Clin Oncol*. 1991; 9:1210-4.
142. Preisler HD, Early AP, Raza A et al. Therapy of secondary acute nonlymphocytic leukemia with cytarabine. *N Engl J Med*. 1983; 308:21-3.
143. Rustum YM, Preisler HD. Correlation between leukemic cell retention of 1-β-D-arabinofuranosylcytosine 5'-triphosphate and response to therapy. *Cancer Res*. 1979; 39:42-9.
144. Riva CM, Rustum YM, Preisler HD. Pharmacokinetics and cellular determinants of response to 1-β-arabinofuranosylcytosine (Ara-C). *Semin Oncol*. 1985; 12(Suppl 3):1-8.
145. Kantarjian HM, Estey EH, Plunkett W et al. Phase I–II clinical and pharmacologic studies of high-dose cytosine arabinoside in refractory leukemia. *Am J Med*. 1986; 81:387-94.
146. Chou TC, Arlin Z, Clarkson BD et al. Metabolism of 1-β-D-arabinofuranosylcytosine in human leukemic cells. *Cancer Res*. 1977; 37:3561-70.
147. Liliemark JO, Plunkett W, Dixon DO. Relationship of 1-β-D-arabinofuranosylcytosine in plasma to 1-β-D-arabinofuranosylcytosine 5'-triphosphate levels in leukemic cells during treatment with high dose 1-β-D-arabinofuranosylcytosine. *Cancer Res*. 1985; 45:5952-7.
148. Early AP, Preisler HD, Slocum H et al. A pilot study of high-dose 1-β-D-arabinofuranosylcytosine for acute leukemia and refractory lymphoma: clinical response and pharmacology. *Cancer Res*. 1982; 42:1587-94.
149. Plunkett W, Liliemark JO, Adams TM et al. Saturation of 1-β-D-arabinofuranosylcytosine 5'-triphosphate accumulation in leukemic cells during high dose 1-β-D- arabinofuranosylcytosine therapy. *Cancer Res*. 1987; 47:3005-11.
150. Ho DHW, Frei E. Clinical pharmacology of 1-β-D-arabinofuranosylcytosine. *Clin Pharmacol Ther*. 1971; 12:944-54.
151. Breithaupt H, Pralle H, Eckhardt T et al. Clinical results and pharmacokinetics of high-dose cytosine arabinoside (HD ARA-C). *Cancer*. 1982; 50:1248-57.
152. Plunkett W, Liliemark JO, Estey E et al. Saturation of ara-CTP accumulation during high-dose ara-C therapy: pharmacologic rationale for intermediate-dose ara-C. *Semin Oncol*. 1987; 14(Suppl 1):159-66.
153. Willemze R, Fibbe WE, Zwaan FE. Experience with intermediate and high-dose cytosine arabinoside in relapsed and refractory acute leukaemia. *Neth J Med*. 1983; 26:215-9.
154. Van Prooijen HC, Dekker AW, Punt K. The use of intermediate dose cytosine arabinoside (ID Ara-C) in the treatment of

acute non-lymphocytic leukaemia in relapse. *Br J Haematol.* 1984; 57:291-9.
155. Gorin NC, David R, Stachowiak J et al. High dose chemotherapy and autologous bone marrow transplantation in acute leukemias, malignant lymphomas and solid tumors: a study of 23 patients. *Eur J Cancer.* 1981; 17:557-68.
156. Zander AR, Dicke KA, Vellekoop et al. Autografting in acute leukemia. In: Gale RP, ed. Recent advances in bone marrow transplantation. New York: Liss; 1983:659-78.
157. Herzig GP, Phillips GL, Mill W et al. Treatment of hematologic malignancy with cyclophosphamide (CY), total body irradiation (TBI) and autologous bone marrow transplantation (BMTX). *Blood.* 1978; 52(Suppl 1):253. Abstract.
158. Stewart DJ, Keating MJ, McCredie KB et al. Natural history of central nervous system acute leukemia in adults. *Cancer.* 1981; 47:184-96.
159. Foon KA, Gale RP. Controversies in the therapy of acute myelogenous leukemia. *Am J Med.* 1982; 72:963-79.
160. Bleyer WA. Clinical pharmacology of intrathecal methotrexate. II. An improved dosage regimen derived from age-related pharmacokinetics. *Cancer Treat Rep.* 1977; 61:1419-25.
161. Wolff L, Zighelboim J, Gale RP. Paraplegia following intrathecal cytosine arabinoside. *Cancer.* 1979; 43:83-5.
162. Frick J, Ritch PS, Hansen RM et al. Successful treatment of meningeal leukemia using systemic high-dose cytosine arabinoside. *J Clin Oncol.* 1984; 2:365-8.
163. Morra E, Lazzarino M, Alessandrino EP et al. Central nervous system (CNS) leukemia: the role of high dose cytarabine (HDAra-C). *Bone Marrow Transplant.* 1989; 4(1):101-3.
164. Sachs L. The differentiation of myeloid leukemia cells: new possibilities for therapy. *Br J Haematol.* 1979; 40:509-17.
165. Castaigne S, Daniel MT, Tilly H et al. Does treatment with Ara-C in low dosage cause differentiation of leukemic cells? *Blood.* 1983; 62:85-6.
166. Shtalrid M, Lotem J, Sachs L et al. Review of clinical and haematological response to low dose cytosine arabinoside in acute myeloid leukaemia. *Eur J Haematol.* 1987; 38:3-11.
167. Tilly H, Castaigne S, Bordessoule D et al. Low-dose cytarabine versus intensive chemotherapy in the treatment of acute nonlymphocytic leukemia in the elderly. *J Clin Oncol.* 1990; 8:272-9.
168. Tilly H, Castaigne S, Bordessaule D et al. Low-dose cytosine arabinoside treatment for acute nonlymphocytic leukemia in elderly patients. *Cancer.* 1985; 55:1633-6.
169. Warrell RP, Frankel SR, Miller WH et al. Differentiation therapy of acute promyelocytic leukemia with tretinoin (all-*trans*-retinoic acid). *N Engl J Med.* 1991; 324:1385-93.
170. Meng-er H, Yu-chen Y, Shu-rong C et al. Use of all-*trans*-retinoic acid in the treatment of acute promyelocytic leukemia. *Blood.* 1988; 72:567-72.
171. Castaigne S, Chomienne C, Daniel MT et al. All-*trans*-retinoic acid as a differentiation therapy for acute promyelocytic leukemia. I. Clinical results. *Blood.* 1990; 76:1704-9.
172. Chomienne C, Ballerini P, Balitrand N et al. All-*trans*-retinoic acid in acute promyelocytic leukemias. II. In vitro studies: structure–function relationship. *Blood.* 1990; 76:1710-7.
173. Degos L, Chomienne C, Daniel MT et al. Treatment of first relapse in acute promyelocytic leukaemia with all-*trans*-retinoic acid. *Lancet.* 1990; 336:1440-1.
174. Groopman JE, Molina JM, Scadden DT. Hematopoeitic growth factors. Biology and clinical applications. *N Engl J Med.* 1989; 321:1449-59.
175. Metcalf D. The granulocyte–macrophage colony-stimulating factors. *Science.* 1985; 229:16-22.
176. Bettelheim P, Valent P, Andreeff M et al. Recombinant human granulocyte–macrophage colony-stimulating factor in combination with standard induction chemotherapy in de novo acute myeloid leukemia. *Blood.* 1991; 77:700-11.
177. Estey E, Kantarjian H, Keating M et al. Use of GM-CSF prior to chemotherapy of AML: effects on circulating blast count, thymidine incorporation and ARA-CTP formation. *Blood.* 1990; 76(Suppl 1):142. Abstract.
178. Tafuri A, Estey E, Valent P et al. Cell kinetic effects in vivo of rhGM-CSF as pre-induction treatment in acute myeloblastic leukemia. *Blood.* 1990; 76(Suppl 1):168. Abstract.
179. Omura GS, Moffitt S, Vogler WR et al. Combination chemotherapy of adult acute lymphoblastic leukemia with randomized central nervous system prophylaxis. *Blood.* 1980; 55:199-204.
180. Blacklock HA, Matthews FRD, Buchanan JG et al. Improved survival from acute lymphoblastic leukemia in adolescents and adults. *Cancer.* 1981; 48:1931-5.
181. Hardisty RM, McElwain TJ, Darby CW. Vincristine and prednisone for the induction of remissions in acute childhood leukemia. *Br Med J.* 1969; 2:662-5.
182. George P, Hernandez K, Hustu O et al. A study of "total therapy" of acute lymphocytic leukemia in children. *J Pediatr.* 1968; 72:399-408.
183. Willemze R, Hillen H, Hartgrink-Groeneveld CA et al. Treatment of acute lymphoblastic leukemia in adolescents and adults: a retrospective study of 41 patients (1970–1973). *Blood.* 1975; 46:823-34.
184. Hess CE, Zirkle JW. Results of induction therapy with vincristine and prednisone alone in adult acute lymphoblastic leukemia: report of 43 patients and a review of the literature. *Am J Hematol.* 1982; 13:63-71.
185. Amadori S, Montuoro A, Meloni G et al. Combination chemotherapy for acute lymphocytic leukemia in adults: results of a retrospective study in 82 patients. *Am J Hematol.* 1980; 8:175-83.
186. Bloomfield CD, Lindquist LL, Arthur D et al. Chromosomal abnormalities in acute lymphoblastic leukemia. *Cancer Res.* 1981; 41:4838-43.
187. Henderson ES, Scharlau C, Cooper MR et al. Combination chemotherapy and radiotherapy for acute lymphocytic leukemia in adults: results of CALGB protocol 7113. *Leukemia Res.* 1979; 3:395-407.
188. Gottlieb AJ, Weinberg V, Ellison RR et al. Efficacy of daunorubicin in the therapy of adult acute lymphocytic leukemia: a prospective randomized trial by Cancer and Leukemia Group B. *Blood.* 1984; 64:267-74.
189. Linker CA, Levitt LJ, O'Donnell M et al. Improved results of treatment of adult acute lymphoblastic leukemia. *Blood.* 1987; 69:1242-8.
190. Smedmyr B, Killander A, Simonsson B et al. Aggressive treatment improves survival in adult acute lymphoblastic leukemia. *Eur J Haematol.* 1988; 41:478-81.
191. Stein RS, Flexner JM, Collins R. Effective multidrug, multimodality consolidation therapy of adult acute lymphocytic leukemia: a preliminary report. *Cancer.* 1982; 49:846-9.
192. Hussein KK, Dahlberg S, Head D et al. Treatment of acute lymphoblastic leukemia in adults with intensive induction, consolidation, and maintenance chemotherapy. *Blood.* 1989; 73:57-63.
193. Radford JE, Burns CP, Jones MP et al. Adult acute lymphoblastic leukemia: results of the Iowa HOP-L protocol. *J Clin Oncol.* 1989; 7:58-66.
194. Kantarjian HM, Walters RS, Keating MJ et al. Results of the vincristine, doxorubicin, and dexamethasone regimen in adults with standard- and high-risk acute lymphocytic leukemia. *J Clin Oncol.* 1990; 8:994-1004.
195. Esterhay RJ, Wiernik PH, Grove WR et al. Moderate dose methotrexate, vincristine, asparaginase, and dexamethasone for treatment of adult acute lymphocytic leukemia. *Blood.* 1982; 59:334-45.
196. Omura GA, Raney M. Long-term survival in adult acute lymphoblastic leukemia: follow-up of a Southeastern Cancer Study Group trial. *J Clin Oncol.* 1985; 3:1053-8.
197. Kantarjian HM, Walters RS, Smith TL et al. Identification of risk groups for development of central nervous system leukemia in adults with acute lymphocytic leukemia. *Blood.* 1988; 72:1784-9.
198. Sullivan MP, Chen T, Dyment PG et al. Equivalence of intrathecal chemotherapy and radiotherapy as central nervous system prophylaxis in children with acute lymphatic

leukemia: a Pediatric Oncology Group study. *Blood.* 1982; 60:948-58.
199. Daniel M, Green DM, Freeman AI et al. Comparison of three methods of central nervous system prophylaxis in childhood acute lymphoblastic leukemia. *Lancet.* 1986; 2:1398.
200. Willemze R, Drenthe-Schonk AM, van Rossum J et al. Treatment of acute lymphoblastic leukaemia in adolescents and adults. *Scand J Haematol.* 1980; 24:421-6.
201. Haaxma-Reiche H, Daenen S. Acute lymphoblastic leukemia in adults: results of intraventricular maintenance chemotherapy for central nervous system prophylaxis and treatment. *Eur J Cancer Clin Oncol.* 1988; 24:615-20.
202. Shapiro WR, Young DF, Mehta BM. Methotrexate: distribution in cerebrospinal fluid after intravenous, ventricular and lumbar injections. *N Engl J Med.* 1975; 293:161-6.
203. Strother DR, Glynn-Barnhart A, Kovnar E et al. Variability in the disposition of intraventricular methotrexate: a proposal for rational dosing. *J Clin Oncol.* 1989; 7:1741-7.
204. Luddy RE, Gilman PA. Paraplegia following intrathecal methotrexate. *J Pediatr.* 1973; 83:988-92.
205. McIntosh S, Aspnes GT. Encephalopathy following CNS prophylaxis in childhood lymphoblastic leukemia. *Pediatrics.* 1973; 52:612-5.
206. Back EH. Death after intrathecal methotrexate. *Lancet.* 1969; 2:1005. Letter.
207. Peylan-Ramu N, Poplack DG, Pizzo PA et al. Abnormal CT scans of the brain in asymptomatic children with acute lymphocytic leukemia after prophylactic treatment of the central nervous system with radiation and intrathecal chemotherapy. *N Engl J Med.* 1978; 298:815-8.
208. Bleyer WA, Drake JC, Chabner BA. Neurotoxicity and elevated cerebrospinal fluid methotrexate concentration in meningeal leukemia. *N Engl J Med.* 1973; 289:770-3.
209. Duffner PK, Cohen ME, Brecher ML et al. CT abnormalities and altered methotrexate clearance in children with CNS leukemia. *Neurology.* 1984; 34:229-33.
210. Woodruff RK, Lister TA, Paxton AM et al. Combination chemotherapy for hematologic relapse in adult acute lymphoblastic leukemia (ALL). *Am J Hematol.* 1978; 4:173-7.
211. Pacciucci PA, Ohnuma T, Cuttner J et al. Mitoxantrone in patients with acute leukemia in relapse. *Cancer Res.* 1983; 43:3919-22.
212. Arlin ZA, Fanucchi MP, Gee TS et al. Treatment of refractory adult lymphoblastic leukemia (ALL) with 4'-(9-acridinylamino)methanesulfon-*m*-anisidide (AMSA). *Blood.* 1982; 60:1224-6.
213. Kantarjian HM, Waters RL, Keating MJ et al. Mitoxantrone and high-dose cytosine arabinoside for the treatment of refractory acute lymphocytic leukemia. *Cancer.* 1990; 65:5-8.
214. Hiddemann W, Buchner T, Heil G et al. Treatment of refractory acute lymphoblastic leukemia in adults with high dose cytosine arabinoside and mitoxantrone (HAM). *Leukemia.* 1990; 4:637-40.
215. Zittoun R, Bury J, Stryckmaus P et al. Amsacrine with high-dose cytarabine in acute leukemia. *Cancer Treat Rep.* 1985; 69:1447-8.
216. Arlin ZA, Feldman E, Kempin S et al. Amsacrine with high-dose cytarabine is highly effective therapy for refractory and relapsed acute lymphoblastic leukemia in adults. *Blood.* 1988; 72:433-5.
217. Sanz GF, Sanz MA, Rafecas FJ et al. Teniposide and cytarabine combination chemotherapy in the treatment of relapsed adolescent and adult acute lymphoblastic leukemia. *Cancer Treat Rep.* 1986; 70:1321-3.
218. Larson RA, Gaynor ER, Shepard KV et al. High-dose Ara-C plus VM-26 in adult acute lymphoblastic leukemia. *Eur J Cancer Clin Oncol.* 1985; 21:1261-3.
219. Kantarjian HM, Walters RS, Keating MJ et al. Experience with vincristine, doxorubicin and dexamethasone (VAD) chemotherapy in adults with refractory acute lymphocytic leukemia. *Cancer.* 1989; 64:16-22.
220. Amadori S, Tribalto M, Pacilli L et al. Sequential combination of methotrexate and L-asparaginase in the treatment of refractory acute leukemia. *Cancer Treat Rep.* 1980; 64:939-42.
221. Terebelo HR, Anderson K, Wiernik PH et al. Therapy of refractory adult acute lymphoblastic leukemia with vincristine and prednisone plus tandem methotrexate and L-asparaginase. Results of a Cancer and Leukemia Group B study. *Am J Clin Oncol.* 1986; 9:411-5.
222. Yap BS, McCredie KB, Keating MJ et al. Asparaginase and methotrexate combination chemotherapy in relapsed acute lymphoblastic leukemia in adults. *Cancer Treat Rep.* 1981; 65(Suppl 1):83-7.
223. Rivera G, Aur RJ, Dahl GV et al. Combined VM-26 and cytosine arabinoside in treatment of refractory childhood lymphocytic leukemia. *Cancer.* 1980; 45:1284-8.
224. Rivera G, Dahl GV, Bowman WP et al. VM-26 and cytosine arabinoside combination chemotherapy for initial induction failures in childhood lymphocytic leukemia. *Cancer.* 1980; 46:1727-30.
225. Rodman JH, Abromowitch M, Sinkule JA et al. Clinical pharmacodynamics of continuous infusion teniposide: systemic exposure as a determinant of response in a Phase I trial. *J Clin Oncol.* 1987; 7:1007-14.
226. Borsi JD, Moe PJ. Systemic clearance of methotrexate in the prognosis of acute lymphoblastic leukemia in children. *Cancer.* 1987; 60:3020-4.
227. Evans WE, Crom WR, Abromowitch M et al. Clinical pharmacodynamics of high-dose methotrexate in acute lymphocytic leukemia. *N Engl J Med.* 1986; 314:471-7.
228. Stoller RG, Hande KR, Jacobs SA et al. Use of plasma pharmacokinetics to predict and prevent methotrexate toxicity. *N Engl J Med.* 1977; 297:630-4.
229. O'Dwyer PJ, Wagner B, Leyland-Jones B et al. 2'-Deoxycoformycin (pentostatin) for lymphoid malignancies: rational development of an active new drug. *Ann Intern Med.* 1988; 108:733-43.
230. Prentice HG, Lee N, Blocklock H et al. Therapeutic selectivity of and prediction of response to 2'-deoxycoformycin in acute leukaemia. *Lancet.* 1981; 2:1250-4.
231. Smyth JF, Paine RM, Jackman AL et al. The clinical pharmacology of the adenosine deaminase inhibitor 2'-deoxycoformycin. *Cancer Chemother Pharmacol.* 1980; 5:93-101.
232. Ho AD, Thaler J, Willemze R et al. Pentostatin (2'-deoxycoformycin) for the treatment of lymphoid neoplasms. *Cancer Treat Rev.* 1990; 17:213-5.
233. Poplack DG, Sallan SE, Rivera G et al. Phase I study of 2'-deoxycoformycin in acute lymphoblastic leukemia. *Cancer Res.* 1981; 41:3343-6.
234. Thomas ED, Sanders JE, Flournoy N et al. Marrow transplantation for patients with acute lymphoblastic leukemia in remission. *Blood.* 1979; 54:468-76.
235. Thomas ED, Sanders JE, Flournoy N et al. Marrow transplantation for patients with acute lymphoblastic leukemia: a long-term follow-up. *Blood.* 1983; 62:1139-41.
236. Woods WG, Nesbit ME, Ramsay NKC et al. Intensive therapy followed by bone marrow transplantation for patients with acute lymphocytic leukemia in second or subsequent remission: determination of prognostic factors. *Blood.* 1983; 61:1182-9.
237. Dinsmore R, Kirkpatrick D, Flomenberg N et al. Allogeneic bone marrow transplantation for patients with acute lymphoblastic leukemia. *Blood.* 1983; 62:381-8.
238. Herzig HH, Barrett AJ, Gluckman E et al. Bone-marrow transplantation in high-risk acute lymphoblastic leukaemia in first and second remission. *Lancet.* 1987; 1:786-9.
239. Weisdorf DJ, Nesbit ME, Ramsay NKC et al. Allogeneic bone marrow transplantation for acute lymphoblastic leukemia in remission: prolonged survival associated with acute graft-versus-host disease. *J Clin Oncol.* 1987; 5:1348-55.
240. Blume KG, Forman SJ, Snyder DS et al. Allogeneic bone marrow transplantation for acute lymphoblastic leukemia during first complete remission. *Transplantation.* 1987; 43:389-92.
241. Forman SJ, O'Donnell MR, Nademanee AP et al. Bone marrow transplantation for patients with Philadelphia chromo-

some-positive acute lymphoblastic leukemia. *Blood*. 1987; 70:587-8.

242. Proctor SJ, Hamilton PJ, Taylor P et al. A comparative study of combination chemotherapy versus marrow transplant in first remission in adult acute lymphoblastic leukaemia. *Br J Haematol*. 1988; 69:35-9.
243. Kersey JH, Weisdorf D, Nesbit ME et al. Comparison of autologous and allogeneic bone marrow transplantation for treatment of high-risk refractory acute lymphoblastic leukemia. *N Engl J Med*. 1987; 317:461-7.
244. Ramsay N, LeBien T, Nesbit M et al. Autologous bone marrow transplantation for patients with acute lymphoblastic leukemia in second or subsequent remission: results of bone marrow treated with monoclonal antibodies BA-1, BA-2, and BA-3 plus complement. *Blood*. 1985; 66:508-13.
245. Ritz J, Bast RC, Clavell LA et al. Autologous bone-marrow transplantation in CALLA-positive acute lymphoblastic leukaemia after in-vitro treatment with J5 monoclonal antibody and complement. *Lancet*. 1982; 2:60-3.
246. Muirhead M, Martin PJ, Torok-Storb B et al. Use of an antibody–ricin-A-chain conjugate to delete neoplastic B cells from human bone marrow. *Blood*. 1983; 62:327-32.
247. Kaizer H, Stuart RK, Brookmeyer R et al. Autologous bone marrow transplantation in acute leukemia: a Phase I study of in vitro treatment of marrow with 4-hydroperoxycyclophosphamide to purge tumor cells. *Blood*. 1985; 65:1504-10.
248. Blazer BR, Kersey JH, McGlave PB et al. In vivo administration of recombinant human granulocyte/macrophage colony-stimulating factor in acute lymphoblastic leukemia patients receiving purged autografts. *Blood*. 1989; 73:849-57.

Commentary

White clot syndrome and thrombocytopenia: Reasons to abandon heparin i.v. lock flush solution

JAMES C. GARRELTS

Clin Pharm. 1992; 11:797-9

The choice of heparin or 0.9% sodium chloride solution (saline) as a flush solution for maintaining patency of indwelling intermittent-injection devices has been controversial since Epperson[1] first showed saline to be equivalent to heparin in 1984. Many letters and editorials have been written in an attempt to solidify opinion behind one flush solution or the other.[2-9] Some authors have argued against switching to saline for the sole purpose of saving money.[2,4,5] Others have warned that adoption of saline as an institution's flush solution may increase liability if an adverse outcome occurs, especially since heparin has been considered the national standard of practice.[2,5] However, as shown by a recently described law case, the use of heparin to flush i.v. locks actually increases an institution's liability.[10] I agree that cost should be considered only if all other things are equal. I also believe that safety and liability problems need to be addressed.

Efficacy. To understand how heparin became the national standard, it is necessary to review the early supporting literature. Most people may be surprised to learn that the "gold standard" study supporting heparin use was conducted in eight beagles. Hanson and coworkers[11] instilled into peripheral i.v. locks 0.3 mL of saline containing heparin sodium at concentrations of 0, 1, 3, 10, and 30 units/mL. They then drew blood into the lock and allowed it to sit for four hours, at which time they checked for patency. Although they provided no specific data, the authors stated that only the solutions containing heparin sodium 10 and 30 units/mL prevented clotting. The investigators then conducted an open study of heparin sodium 10 units/mL in 10 healthy volunteers. Saline was not tested in this part of the study. As expected, heparin prevented clot formation.

Neither part of the study by Hansen et al. reflects the way peripheral i.v. locks are used in practice today. Currently, i.v. locks are used for administering fluids and medications. When fluids and medications are administered, blood does not enter the i.v. lock. Therefore, stasis and clotting within the lock would not be expected to occur, and heparin should not be necessary. On the other hand, when an i.v. lock is used to obtain blood samples, it seems prudent to flush it with heparin afterward. Holford and colleagues[12] reported that heparin is more effective than saline when frequent blood samples are drawn from subjects participating in pharmacokinetic studies.

Many investigators have compared the efficacy of heparin with that of saline in maintaining patency of i.v. locks under usual clinical conditions.[1,13-23] In these studies the i.v. locks were usually changed every 48 to 72 hours, even if they were still functioning well. With one exception,[21] saline produced patency rates equivalent to those of both heparin sodium 10 units/mL and heparin sodium 100 units/mL; phlebitis also occurred with equal frequency. While fibrin strands at the catheter tip have been noted more frequently in patients receiving saline, they have not been of clinical significance.[13] Weber[24] has provided a detailed review of these studies. A meta-analysis involving nearly 3500 patients also supported the equivalence of saline in terms of patency, the incidence of phlebitis, and the time that i.v. locks function.[25] These studies would seem to have laid to rest the issue of whether saline is as effective as heparin as an i.v. lock flush solution in adult patients. The remaining question, then, concerns safety.

Safety. Bleeding is the most common complication of heparin therapy. While bleeding is unlikely to occur with the small doses of heparin sodium used to flush indwelling i.v. locks (usually 10 to 100 units/mL), it can occur when the patient receives multiple flushes. Passannante and Macik[26] described a patient who developed postoperative bleeding and hypotension after receiving multiple i.v. lock flushes with heparin in the perioperative period. Upon surgical re-exploration,

JAMES C. GARRELTS, PHARM.D., is Assistant Director of Pharmacy (Clinical), St. Francis Regional Medical Center, and Adjunct Associate Professor of Medicine, University of Kansas School of Medicine, Wichita.

Address reprint requests to Dr. Garrelts at the Department of Pharmacy, St. Francis Regional Medical Center, 929 North St. Francis Street, Wichita, KS 67214-3882.

The contributions of Dale F. Smith, Jr., M.S., (manuscript review) and Vannessa Petersen (manuscript preparation) are acknowledged.

1500 mL of blood was found in the peritoneal cavity.

Other potential complications, even with the small doses of heparin used to flush i.v. locks, are thrombocytopenia and paradoxical thromboembolism (white clot syndrome).[27-33] Small doses of heparin can change the platelet membrane such that the platelet becomes recognized as a foreign substance by the immune system. Rhodes and colleagues[33] showed that an immunoglobulin G-dependent antibody binds to the modified platelet, causing aggregation. Extensive platelet aggregation produces thrombocytopenia and sometimes the paradoxical formation of clots consisting of aggregated platelets (white clots). Thrombocytopenia usually begins several days after the patient has begun heparin treatments. Clinical manifestations of white clot syndrome include unexplained pain, a cold extremity, and apparent resistance to the effects of heparin.[34, 35] Obstruction of blood flow by the white clot may produce upper or lower limb ischemia, myocardial infarction, or a cerebrovascular accident. Less commonly reported complications include skin necrosis, mesenteric thrombosis, renal artery thrombosis, adrenal thrombosis, and spinal artery thrombosis.[35] The frequency of morbidity (e.g., loss of limb, renal failure) and mortality is often high, especially when the cause of the problem goes unrecognized for some time.

Some might question whether i.v. lock flushes with heparin can cause such severe adverse consequences. At least 11 patients have been reported to have developed thrombocytopenia or white clot syndrome or both after heparin flushes.[27-32] Heeger and Backstrom[31] described a patient whose platelet count fell from 541,000/cu mm to 50,000/cu mm while receiving heparin flushes (<500 units of heparin sodium per day). Laster et al.[32] described a patient who developed thrombocytopenia and died of a massive lower intestinal hemorrhage while continuing to receive heparin flushes. Rizzoni and colleagues[30] reported a case of heparin-induced pulmonary embolus in which the platelet count was as low as 2000/cu mm. Clots were found in the right external iliac vein and the origin of the right renal vein. Despite multiple transfusions of platelets, the platelet count did not begin to rise until five days after the heparin flushes had been discontinued. Finally, Doty and coworkers[28] described two patients who developed thrombocytopenia after heparin flushes. Both patients experienced acute neurological deterioration secondary to epidural hematomas occurring at the site of surgery for tumor removal. The course of one of these patients was further complicated by recurrent gastrointestinal hemorrhage. The severity of these cases should leave little doubt about the dangers associated with using heparin flushes.

What are the frequencies of heparin-induced thrombocytopenia and paradoxical thromboembolism? How often do these reactions go unrecognized and produce morbidity or mortality? How often does the physician not even realize that his or her patient is receiving heparin during i.v. lock flushes? The answers to many of these questions are unknown. Warkenton and Kelton[34] analyzed data from prospective studies of 1500 patients receiving therapeutic dosages of heparin. They found the incidence of heparin-induced thrombocytopenia to be 5.5% for beef lung heparin and 1% for heparin from porcine intestine; probable or possible paradoxical thromboembolism occurred in 1.7% and 0.3% of these patients, respectively. These figures indicate that white clot syndrome occurs in up to 30% of patients who develop heparin-induced thrombocytopenia. Similarly, Laster et al.[32] reported that 38 (22.5%) of 169 patients who developed heparin-induced thrombocytopenia in a three-year period developed clinically important bleeding or thromboembolic complications.

Conclusion. The risks associated with using heparin to flush indwelling intermittent-injection devices are much greater than those associated with using 0.9% sodium chloride solution. Both flush solutions are equally effective in maintaining patency under usual clinical circumstances; the exception is when blood is drawn and allowed to remain in the catheter. The issue of cost need not even be raised. Our responsibility as pharmacists mandates the use of saline as the preferred i.v. lock flush solution. I encourage ASHP and other national pharmacy organizations to adopt policies recommending saline as the standard solution for this use. I encourage practicing pharmacists to make saline the flush solution of choice at their institutions.

References

1. Epperson EL. Efficacy of 0.9% sodium chloride injection with and without heparin for maintaining indwelling intermittent injection sites. *Clin Pharm.* 1984; 3:626-9.
2. Habeger B, VanDyke DS. Maintaining i.v. catheter patency: can saline replace heparin as agent of choice? *Hosp Formul.* 1991; 26:230. Letter.
3. Dean T, Ridley P. Use of 0.9% sodium chloride without heparin for maintaining indwelling intermittent injection sites. *Clin Pharm.* 1985; 4:488. Letter.
4. Ferraro JM, Guanci RF, Stoneburner RJ. Use of 0.9% sodium chloride injection without heparin for maintaining indwelling intermittent injection sites. *Clin Pharm.* 1985; 4:488-9. Letter.
5. Cole MG. Flushing heparin locks: is saline flushing really cost-effective? *J Intraven Nurs.* 1989; 12(Suppl):S23-9.
6. Rushaidat R. What concentration of heparin is optimal for flushing heparin-locks? *US Pharm.* 1986; 11:16. Letter.
7. Crabbe SJ. Flushing heparin locks. *Hosp Ther.* 1990; Feb:165-6. Letter.
8. Todd MW, Montanez EJ. What are the advantages and disadvantages of using heparin versus a saline flush for maintaining i.v. catheter patency? *Hosp Formul.* 1990; 25:1185-6. Letter.
9. Hook ML, Ose P. Heparin versus normal saline. *J Intraven Nurs.* 1990; 13:150. Letter.
10. Brushwood DB. Hospital liable for allergic reaction to heparin used in needle flush. *Am J Hosp Pharm.* 1992; 49:1491-2.
11. Hanson RL, Grant AM, Majors KR. Heparin-lock maintenance with 10 units of sodium heparin in one milliliter of normal saline solution. *Surg Gynecol Obstet.* 1976; 142:373-6.
12. Holford NHG, Vozeh S, Coates P et al. More on heparin lock. *N Engl J Med.* 1977; 296:1300. Letter.
13. Garrelts JC, LaRocca J, Ast D et al. Comparison of heparin and 0.9% sodium chloride injection in the maintenance of indwelling intermittent i.v. devices. *Clin Pharm.* 1989; 8:34-9.

14. Hamilton RA, Plis JM, Clay C et al. Heparin sodium versus 0.9% sodium chloride injection for maintaining patency of indwelling intermittent infusion devices. *Clin Pharm.* 1988; 7:439-43.
15. Shaw P, Baker D. Flushing solutions for indwelling intravenous catheters. *Pharm J.* 1988; 241:122-3.
16. Barrett PJ, Lester RL. Heparin versus saline flushing solutions in a small community hospital. *Hosp Pharm.* 1990; 25:115-8.
17. Miracle V, Fangman B, Kayrouz P et al. Normal saline versus heparin lock flush solution: one institution's findings. *Ky Nurse.* 1989; 37:5-7.
18. Lombardi TP, Gundersen B, Zammett LO et al. Efficacy of 0.9% sodium chloride injection with or without heparin sodium for maintaining patency of intravenous catheters in children. *Clin Pharm.* 1988; 7:832-6.
19. Donham JA, Denning V. Heparin versus saline in maintaining patency of intermittent infusion devices: pilot study. *Kans Nurse.* 1987; 62:6-7.
20. Dunn DL, Lenihan SF. The case for the saline flush. *Am J Nurs.* 1987; 87:798-9.
21. Cyganski JM, Donahue JM, Heaton JS. The case for the heparin flush. *Am J Nurs.* 1987; 87:796-7.
22. Shearer J. Normal saline flush versus dilute heparin flush. *NITA.* 1987; 10:425-7.
23. Ashton J, Gibson V, Summers S. Effect of heparin versus saline solution on intermittent infusion device irrigation. *Heart Lung.* 1990; 19:608-12.
24. Weber DR. Is heparin really necessary in the lock and, if so, how much? *DICP Ann Pharmacother.* 1991; 25:399-406.
25. Goode CJ, Titler M, Rakel B et al. A meta-analysis of effects of heparin flush and saline flush: quality and cost implications. *Nurs Res.* 1991; 40:324-30.
26. Passannante A, Macik BG. Case report: the heparin flush syndrome: a cause of iatrogenic hemorrhage. *Am J Med Sci.* 1988; 296:71-3.
27. Cines DB, Tomaski A, Tannenbaum S. Immune endothelial-cell injury in heparin-associated thrombocytopenia. *N Engl J Med.* 1987; 316:581-9.
28. Doty JR, Alving BM, McDonnell DE et al. Heparin-associated thrombocytopenia in the neurosurgical patient. *Neurosurgery.* 1986; 19:69-72.
29. Kappa JR, Fisher CA, Berkowitz HD et al. Heparin-induced platelet activation in sixteen surgical patients: diagnosis and management. *J Vasc Surg.* 1987; 5:101-9.
30. Rizzoni WE, Miller K, Rick M et al. Heparin-induced thrombocytopenia and thromboembolism in the post-operative period. *Surgery.* 1988; 103:470-6.
31. Heeger PS, Backstrom JT. Heparin flushes and thrombocytopenia. *Ann Intern Med.* 1986; 105:143. Letter.
32. Laster J, Cikrit D, Walker N et al. The heparin-induced thrombocytopenia syndrome: an update. *Surgery.* 1987; 102:763-70.
33. Rhodes GR, Dixon RH, Silver D. Heparin-induced thrombocytopenia with thrombotic and hemorrhagic manifestations. *Surg Gynecol Obstet.* 1973; 136:409-16.
34. Warkenton TE, Kelton JG. Heparin and platelets. *Hematol Oncol Clin N Am.* 1990; 4:243-64.
35. Becker PS, Miller VT. Heparin-induced thrombocytopenia. *Stroke.* 1989; 20:1449-59.

Grand Rounds

Dapsone-induced methemoglobinemia and hemolytic anemia

Brian L. Erstad

Abstract: The treatment of two common adverse effects of dapsone (methemoglobinemia and hemolytic anemia) is discussed, and a case of acute dapsone intoxication is described.

A pregnant 29-year-old woman was admitted to an emergency room three hours after ingesting 50 tablets of dapsone (100 mg each) and six alcoholic drinks. One hour after admission 50 g of activated charcoal was given p.o., and 65 mg of methylene blue was given i.v. The patient was found to have a methemoglobin concentration of 25.1%. Arterial blood gases while the patient was breathing 4 L/min of oxygen by nasal cannula were Po_2, 136 mm Hg (72.1% saturation); Pco_2, 28.9 mm Hg; bicarbonate content, 18.9 mmol/L; and pH, 7.42. Oxygen therapy was changed to 100% oxygen by face mask, 50 g of activated charcoal in sorbitol was administered p.o., and another 65 mg of methylene blue was given i.v. Two more 50-g doses of activated charcoal in sorbitol were given (18.5 and 22 hours after dapsone ingestion). Methylene blue 130 mg was given 14 hours after dapsone ingestion, and 65 mg was given 21, 36, and 55.5 hours after ingestion. Methemoglobin concentrations never rose above 20% after the sixth dose of methylene blue. On hospital days 2 and 3, laboratory values were consistent with a diagnosis of hemolytic anemia; the patient received two units of packed red blood cells. The hematocrit decreased over the next three days to 23.9%, and the patient received four units of packed red blood cells. On day 8 oxygen therapy was changed to oxygen 2 L/min by nasal cannula, and on day 10 the patient was breathing room air.

Oral doses of activated charcoal have been used to treat acute dapsone poisoning. Methylene blue acts as a cofactor for the nicotinamide adenine dinucleotide phosphate system to convert methemoglobin to hemoglobin. Methylene blue, however, sometimes aggravates the adverse effects of dapsone, particularly in patients with glucose 6-phosphate dehydrogenase deficiency. Total methylene blue dosages exceeding 4 mg/kg are more likely to aggravate the methemoglobinemia and possibly cause or aggravate an acute hemolytic state.

Most cases of dapsone-induced methemoglobinemia and hemolysis resolve when the offending drug is discontinued. When methylene blue is required for symptomatic patients with an elevated methemoglobin concentration (more than 30%), careful monitoring of drug dosage and clinical progress is indicated.

Index terms: Anemia; Antidotes; Charcoal activated; Dapsone; Dosage; Methemoglobinemia; Methylene blue; Poisoning; Toxicity
Clin Pharm. 1992; 11:800-5

Dapsone is a drug of choice for treating leprosy and dermatitis herpetiformis, but more recent investigational uses (e.g., treatment of *Pneumocystis carinii* pneumonia[1]) have required an increasing number of clinicians to be aware of the potential toxicities of the drug. The case of a patient who attempted suicide with dapsone will be described. The case report will be followed by a discussion of the treatment of two common, dose-related adverse effects of dapsone: methemoglobinemia and hemolytic anemia.

Case Report

A 29-year-old, pregnant white woman (67 kg) arrived in a local emergency room three hours after reportedly ingesting 50 tablets of dapsone (100 mg each) in a suicide attempt. Six alcoholic drinks also were reported to have been consumed around the time of the dapsone ingestion. The patient had no signs or symptoms of toxicity other than cyanosis, which was especially prominent on mucosal surfaces. The patient had a history of dermatitis herpetiformis, for which the dapsone had been pre-

Brian L. Erstad, Pharm.D., is Assistant Professor, Department of Pharmacy Practice, College of Pharmacy, The University of Arizona, Tucson, AZ 85721.

This is **article 680-204-9220** in the **ASHP Continuing Education System**; it qualifies for 1.0 hour of continuing-education credit. See page 811 for learning objectives and test questions.

scribed. The patient also had a history of depression and gluten hypersensitivity, and she recently had had episodes of vaginal bleeding. Blood methemoglobin (normal, <1%) and ethanol (normal, <2.2 mmol/L) concentrations obtained one-half hour after admission were 21.7% and 33 mmol/L (150 mg/dL), respectively. Arterial blood gases while the patient was breathing room air were Po_2 61.8 mm Hg (93.2% saturation); Pco_2, 26 mm Hg; bicarbonate content, 18.5 mmol/L; and pH, 7.46. One hour after admission, activated charcoal 50 g p.o. and methylene blue 65 mg i.v. were given. The next methemoglobin concentration obtained approximately one-half hour after the injection of methylene blue was 10.1%.

Five and one-half hours after the ingestion of dapsone, the patient was transferred to our facility, where her methemoglobin concentration was found to be 25.1%. The patient had shortness of breath at this time. Arterial blood gases while the patient was breathing 4 L/min of oxygen by nasal cannula were Po_2, 136 mm Hg (72.1% saturation); Pco_2, 28.9 mm Hg; bicarbonate content, 18.9 mmol/L; and pH, 7.42. The patient was given 100% oxygen to breathe by face mask. A laboratory workup that included renal and liver function tests revealed no abnormalities other than a serum carbon dioxide content of 18.3 mmol/L. At this time activated charcoal 50 g in sorbitol was administered p.o., and another 65 mg of methylene blue was given i.v. Two additional doses of activated charcoal 50 g in sorbitol were given 18.5 and 22 hours after dapsone ingestion. The patient had small amounts of emesis after receiving the charcoal, and she subsequently refused to continue taking the charcoal. A methemoglobin concentration determined 14 hours after the ingestion was 43.2%, and methylene blue 130 mg i.v. was given. The next methemoglobin concentration at 16.5 hours after ingestion was 15.9%. Additional i.v. doses of methylene blue (65 mg each) were given at 21, 36, and 55.5 hours after dapsone ingestion in response to methemoglobin concentrations of approximately 30%, and subsequent methemoglobin concentrations were approximately 16%. Methemoglobin concentrations never rose above 20% after the sixth and final dose of methylene blue. The total dose of methylene blue was approximately 7 mg/kg.

On hospital day 2 a complete blood count revealed a hematocrit of 29.8% (normal, 37–47%), and the patient received two units of packed red blood cells. The laboratory did not mention whether the patient's blood was chocolate-brown in color or whether there was Heinz body formation in red blood cells. On hospital day 3, the following laboratory measurements were obtained: hematocrit, 31.9%; total serum bilirubin concentration, 37.6 μmol/L (2.2 mg/dL); direct serum bilirubin concentration, 8.55 μmol/L (0.5 mg/dL); haptoglobin, <0.05 g/L (normal, 0.4–1.7 g/L); and corrected reticulocyte count, 1.7% (normal, 0.5–1.5%). These results were consistent with a diagnosis of hemolytic anemia. The hematocrit decreased over the following three days to a low of 23.9% on hospital day 6, at which time the patient received four units of packed red blood cells. Serum lactate dehydrogenase measurements, which were first obtained on hospital day 6, were also elevated. Laboratory findings relevant to the patient's hemolytic state are provided in Table 1.

On hospital day 4, the patient complained of abdominal pain, and physical examination revealed splenomegaly. Ultrasonography of the spleen demonstrated enlargement, but no infarct or hemorrhage. The splenomegaly and pain gradually resolved over the ensuing two weeks.

On hospital day 6, therapy with hydrocortisone (100 mg i.v. [as the sodium succinate ester] every six hours) was started in an attempt to decrease the continued hemolysis. Steroid therapy was changed the following day to oral prednisone (100 mg/day), which was then tapered off over the next few days. On day 8 the patient's oxygen therapy was changed to 2 L/min of oxygen by nasal cannula, and on day 10 she was breathing room air.

Papers in the Grand Rounds *section are patient case reports and literature review combined in a way that gives them high educational value. The papers lead off with a well-documented case report of an unusual drug experience (e.g., adverse drug reaction or other unexpected drug response, experimental use of a drug). The case generally deals with a difficult therapeutic problem or dilemma that is commonly encountered but may be overlooked or misunderstood. (Esoteric or rare occurrences of minor importance do not make good* Grand Rounds *material.) A literature review puts the case in perspective with previously reported similar cases and alternative treatments. The review is integrated with related discussion of the case being reported.*

CP *readers are encouraged to use* Grand Rounds *for educational group discussions. For this purpose, discussion questions are printed at the end of* Grand Rounds *papers.*

Table 1.
Laboratory Findings Associated with Dapsone Intoxication

Variable[a] (Normal Range)	Day of Hospitalization 1	2	3	4	5	6	7	8	9	10	11	12
HCT (37–47%)	NA[b]	29.8[c]	31.9	28.2	28.1	23.9[c]	27.9	26.8[c]	24.4[c]	30.9	33.3	34.6
TB (0.2–1.2 mg/dL)	0.3	NA	2.2	NA	NA	3.6	4.3	4.1	1.7	1.1	0.8	0.7
DB (0.0–0.4 mg/dL)	NA	NA	0.5	NA	NA	0.6	0.6	0.6	0.4	0.3	0.2	0.1
LDH (95–175 IU/L)	NA	NA	NA	NA	NA	340	405	436	345	338	282	233
Retic (0.5–1.5%)	NA	NA	1.7	NA	NA	NA	3.3	4.2	2.1	2.4	4.3	NA

[a]HCT = hematocrit; TB = serum total bilirubin concentration; DB = serum direct bilirubin concentration; LDH = serum lactate dehydrogenase concentration; Retic = reticulocyte count (corrected).
[b]NA = not available.
[c]Packed red blood cells given.

Discussion

As in this case, most reports of dapsone toxicity have involved patients who had ingested the drug over a short time.[2] This case was also similar to other poisonings in that other drugs or toxins were involved (e.g., alcohol). The increased use of dapsone for diseases other than leprosy and dermatitis herpetiformis could lead to an increasing number of patient admissions for toxic ingestions. Patients who are anemic or hypoxemic would be less likely to tolerate the hematologic adverse effects related to dapsone, and they could become symptomatic after the administration of usual dosages of dapsone.

Nonhematologic complications have occurred after dapsone administration. Permanent retinal damage was observed in one patient who took 7.5 g of dapsone in a suicide attempt.[3] Another patient died from what appeared to be a severe hypersensitivity reaction to dapsone.[4] Such reactions appear to be uncommon and will not be discussed here.

One of the first reported cases of dapsone toxicity occurred in a child who swallowed a paste containing dapsone that was intended for veterinary use only.[5] Because the author did not find evidence of methemoglobinemia, methylene blue was withheld. The child died from what the author thought was either dapsone-induced anemia or a toxic effect of dapsone on the central nervous system. Compared with other reports of dapsone poisoning, this case is atypical in two ways: methylene blue was not administered, and the patient died.

Hematologic Effects of Dapsone. The primary adverse effects of dapsone are dose-related methemoglobinemia and hemolysis.[6] Both of these toxicities occurred in the patient described here. These adverse effects are thought to be due to hydroxyl metabolites of dapsone—in particular, dapsone monohydroxylamine.[7,8]

There are three systems in erythrocytes that keep methemoglobin levels low. The most important system under normal circumstances involves reduced nicotinamide adenine dinucleotide (NADH), which converts methemoglobin to hemoglobin when adequate amounts of the enzyme NADH-methemoglobin reductase are available.[9] The second system, which can potentially convert methemoglobin to hemoglobin, consists of (1) reduced nicotinamide adenine dinucleotide phosphate (NADPH) formed by the hexose monophosphate shunt pathway, (2) the enzyme NADPH-methemoglobin reductase, and (3) a cofactor. Although this system is unimportant under normal clinical conditions, it is notable when methylene blue is being administered for methemoglobinemia.[10]

The third system uses NADPH to convert oxidized glutathione to reduced glutathione. Reduced glutathione prevents various oxidizing agents from converting hemoglobin to methemoglobin. This system plays a minor role in limiting methemoglobinemia, but it is necessary for the detoxification of intracellular oxidants (including drugs such as dapsone) that may cause Heinz body hemolytic anemias.[9] Heinz bodies are thought to represent degradation of hemoglobin in red blood cells, and affected cells appear to have reduced survival.[11,12] It has been reported that the percentage of red cells having Heinz bodies may correlate with the risk of hemolytic anemia. When fewer than 20% of red cells have Heinz bodies, the risk of frank hemolytic anemia is low.[11]

Most patients experiencing dapsone-related methemoglobinemia are asymptomatic until approximately 30% of hemoglobin is present as methemoglobin, although lower levels are associated with cyanosis. Initial signs and symptoms of toxicity include fatigue, headache, and tachycardia, with higher levels of methemoglobin leading to dyspnea, coma, and bradycardia.[9] As mentioned previously, individuals with preexisting anemia, hypoxemia, or both may be susceptible to adverse effects at lower methemoglobin levels.

Cases of dapsone ingestion in which hemolytic anemia is not reported are more the exception than the rule. One such case involved an 18-month-old child who had ingested a single 100-mg dapsone tablet.[13] The initial peak methemoglobin concentration was 27%. The patient was given a single i.v. dose of methylene blue and multiple doses of activated charcoal. This patient was discharged after four days of hospitalization with no mention of decreased hemoglobin or of Heinz body formation.

Laboratory testing for suspected dapsone toxicity should include reticulocyte and complete blood counts, methemoglobin levels, arterial blood gas measurements, and visual examination of blood for the chocolate-brown color often seen with methemoglobinemia. The laboratory may not routinely note the color of blood or the presence of Heinz bodies, but such information should be actively sought. Arterial blood gases should be interpreted with caution because, in some institutions, oxygen saturation may be calculated rather than measured from oxygen tension. Calculated oxygen saturation may be normal, despite clinically important methemoglobinemia.[14] This is a likely explanation for the discrepancy between the methemoglobin concentration (21.7%) and the oxygen saturation (92.3%) recorded by the institution that initially treated the patient described in this report. Our hospital uses a co-oximeter to measure oxyhemoglobin as a fraction of total hemoglobin; thus, the patient had low oxygen saturation (72.1%), as would be expected considering the increased percentage of methemoglobin. Pulse oximetry monitoring common to intensive-care units may be misleading or inaccurate in a patient with methemoglobinemia; methylene blue administration may also affect oximetric determinations.[15]

Treatment. Pharmacokinetic properties of dapsone that are important treatment considerations include its prolonged half-life (14–83 hours for dapsone and its main metabolite), marked protein binding (70–90% for dapsone and close to 100% for its main metabolite), large volume of distribution (1.5 L/kg), and enterohepatic circulation.[16] Suggested treatments of dapsone toxicity are based largely on isolated case reports demonstrating changes in various pharmacokinetic values such as half-life. The reports and conclusions should be interpreted with caution.

Activated Charcoal. Single oral doses of activated charcoal are frequently recommended for the acutely poisoned patient and cause infrequent adverse effects when the poisoned patient is conscious.[17] There is a paucity of pharmacokinetic or outcome information documenting the efficacy of single doses of charcoal for dapsone intoxication. Some investigators have suggested that multiple doses of activated charcoal may be useful for acute dapsone poisoning because they interrupt enterohepatic circulation.[13,18] Repeated doses of charcoal resulted in decreases in the elimination half-life of both dapsone (mean ± S.E. half-life without charcoal, 77 ± 23 hours; with charcoal, 12.7 ± 0.7 hours) and the metabolite monoacetyldapsone (mean ± S.E. half-life without charcoal, 51 ± 10 hours; with charcoal, 13.3 ± 1.0 hours) in three dapsone-intoxicated patients. However, activated charcoal is not innocuous, and multiple doses of charcoal may be associated with an increased risk of aspiration. The emesis experienced by the patient described in this report not only raised concern about aspiration but also demonstrated the problems in achieving compliance with the administration of charcoal.

Invasive Therapy. Other, more invasive, maneuvers have been used to treat dapsone poisoning. Charcoal hemoperfusion was used to hasten the removal of dapsone and its metabolites in one patient.[19] The half-life of dapsone during the charcoal hemoperfusion was approximately 90 minutes, which resulted in clinical improvement of the patient. But complications related to hemoperfusion (e.g., hypotension) generally limit its use to patients in whom activated charcoal cannot be used.[2,19] Plasma exchange and dialysis also have been investigated for dapsone intoxication, but the pharmacokinetic properties of dapsone (large volume of distribution and extensive protein binding) and complications related to the procedures have limited their effectiveness.[19-21]

Methylene Blue. Methylene blue has been advocated for the treatment of methemoglobinemia (such as that seen with dapsone toxicity) since the first reports of dapsone poisoning appeared in the literature.[22] Methylene blue acts as a cofactor for the NADPH system to convert methemoglobin to hemoglobin. Methylene blue is reduced to leukomethylene blue by NADPH, and leukomethylene blue subsequently reduces methemoglobin to hemoglobin.[9] But methylene blue does not always alleviate dapsone toxicity and may actually aggravate some of the adverse effects of dapsone; that may have occurred in the patient described in this report.

Methylene blue is particularly likely to aggravate the adverse effects of dapsone in patients with glucose 6-phosphate dehydrogenase deficiency. Glucose 6-phosphate dehydrogenase is the enzyme that catalyzes the reaction that results in the formation of NADPH. When NADPH is decreased, the formation of reduced glutathione is decreased. Reduced glutathione prevents Heinz body hemolytic anemia by reducing intracellular oxidants.[9] The patient described in this report was not tested for glucose 6-phosphate dehydrogenase deficiency.

In 1974 Goldstein[23] described the case of a patient with systemic lupus erythematosus who had ingested an unknown quantity of dapsone after a cerebrovascular accident. In contrast to many of the previously reported cases of dapsone poisoning, the clinical course of this patient, including relevant laboratory data, was described in detail. On presentation the patient was found to have the following laboratory values: methemoglobin, 36%; hematocrit, 37%; red cell reduced glutathione, 4.48 μmol per gram of hemoglobin; and Heinz bodies in 50% of red cells. After three days with little change in the methemoglobin levels and a decreasing hematocrit (29%), a single dose of methylene blue was given. Although the methylene blue led to an immediate decrease in the methemoglobin levels, there were also decreases in reduced glutathione and the hematocrit. The reticulocyte count markedly increased (peak of 33%), and almost all red cells were noted to have Heinz bodies. The patient eventually recovered, and all laboratory values returned to normal. Glucose 6-phosphate dehydrogenase activity was not impaired in this patient.

Two separate in vitro trials were then performed to try to reproduce the hematologic changes observed in the patient.[23] In the first trial sodium nitrite was added to normal red cells to artificially elevate the methemoglobin levels, and an azoester was used to oxidize the reduced glutathione of the cells. Methemoglobin and glutathione levels were then determined before the addition of methylene blue. The ability of the methylene blue to decrease the methemoglobin level was inhibited in direct proportion to the decrease in reduced glutathione. In the second experiment with methemoglobinemic red cells and subsequent oxidation of reduced glutathione in these cells, methylene blue was found to inhibit the conversion of oxidized glutathione back to its reduced form.

It was postulated that the patient probably had substantial stimulation of the hexose monophosphate shunt pathway to form the NADPH needed for production of reduced glutathione.[23] NADPH also was needed to reduce methylene blue to leukomethylene blue, in order to convert methemoglobin to hemoglobin. This competition for NADPH may have resulted in methemoglobin being reduced at the expense of increasing the Heinz body hemolytic anemia because of a relative lack of reduced glutathione.

Aggravation of hemolytic anemia also occurred when methylene blue was used for nitrate- and aniline-induced methemoglobinemia.[24,25] In nitrate poisoning, hemolytic anemia is not thought to occur because of toxic ingestion; thus, methylene blue is implicated as the inciting agent.[26]

The usual recommended dose of methylene blue for methemoglobinemia is 1–2 mg/kg, which can be repeated in approximately one hour if a suboptimal response is noted.[27] Intravenous infusions of methylene blue also have been used (0.1–0.15 mg/kg/hr), although an initial loading dose is still recommended.[2] The response to methylene blue is determined by the resolution of the signs and symptoms of methemoglobinemia (e.g., hypoxia). Elimination of cyanosis should not be used as an endpoint because resolution of cyanosis may lag behind symptomatic relief.[9] Additionally, methylene blue may cause a bluish discoloration of the skin that could be confused with cyanosis.

There is little reason to aggressively treat most patients with mild methemoglobinemia, which is usually seen when methemoglobin concentrations are lower than 30%.[28] Supportive care and the administration of oxygen are all that are needed for most ingestions that cause methemoglobinemia. If methylene blue is deemed necessary after supportive measures have failed, care should be taken when adequate doses of the drug fail to substantially decrease the methemoglobin levels. Total methylene blue dosages exceeding 4 mg/kg are more likely to aggravate the methemoglobinemia and possibly cause or aggravate an acute hemolytic state.

Failure to respond to usual doses of methylene blue or aggravation of a preexisting hemolytic anemia by methylene blue may require that additional testing be done. Lambert et al.[29] reported the case of a man who had ingested 3 g of dapsone, which resulted in a methemoglobin concentration of 41.5%. The patient also developed sulfhemoglobinemia. Sulfhemoglobinemia is caused by many of the same drugs that cause methemoglobinemia. It is not a common disorder, which is fortunate because there is no way to readily reverse its toxicity.[10] Multiple doses of methylene blue were given, and the patient developed hemolytic anemia, which was still present 20 days after the ingestion.[29]

Other uncommon causes of methylene blue treatment failure or toxicity include associated glucose 6-phosphate dehydrogenase deficiency and congenital methemoglobinemias.[30,31] Although problems such as sulfhemoglobinemia are not readily reversible, they must be differentiated from situations in which additional doses of methylene blue might be indicated.[10] For example, the long half-life of dapsone may require that multiple doses of methylene blue be administered to an intoxicated patient who remains symptomatic, although this may increase the risk of methylene blue toxicity (e.g., aggravation of hemolytic anemia).

Other Possible Treatments. Various treatments other than methylene blue have been suggested for management of dapsone-induced hematologic effects. Some of the suggested treatments, such as administration of ascorbic acid, would seem to have theoretical benefits because they reduce methemoglobin to hemoglobin in the presence of reduced glutathione,[10] but clinical trials demonstrating efficacy are lacking.[32] Cimetidine has been used to decrease the formation of toxic metabolites of dapsone by inhibiting hepatic cytochrome P-450 activity. The P-450 system is responsible for the formation of the hydroxyl metabolite of dapsone, which appears to be responsible for the hematologic problems. Cimetidine's actions may prove useful in patients who must receive dapsone but have congenital methemoglobinemia or glucose 6-phosphate dehydrogenase deficiency.[33] Cimetidine has not been investigated as a treatment for acute dapsone intoxication.

Attempts to offset the hemolysis associated with dapsone and methylene blue have been largely unsuccessful. Vitamin E has antioxidant effects that could potentially decrease the hemolysis associated with the oxidizing actions of various chemicals, including active metabolites of dapsone. However, vitamin E was found to be ineffective in decreasing the hemolytic toxicity of usual therapeutic doses of dapsone (100 mg/day).[34] Similarly, the use of corticosteroids for alleviating the hemolytic process associated with dapsone and methylene blue is unsupported. Corticosteroids were administered to the patient described in this report on the assumption that the hemolysis was antibody mediated, but there is no evidence that this occurs in dapsone intoxication.[26]

Conclusion

Most cases of dapsone-induced methemoglobinemia and hemolysis resolve when the offending drug is discontinued. When methylene blue is required for symptomatic patients with elevated methemoglobin concentrations (more than 30%), careful monitoring of drug dosage and clinical progress is indicated.

Discussion Questions

1. What are the three erythrocyte mechanisms that keep the methemoglobin concentration low?
2. Describe the laboratory findings and clinical presentation associated with dapsone-induced hematologic abnormalities.
3. What are the effects of methylene blue on dapsone-induced hematologic abnormalities?
4. What dosage regimen would you recommend for methylene blue for the treatment of dapsone-induced methemoglobinemia?
5. Which two drugs other than methylene blue may have a theoretical role in the treatment of dapsone-induced hematologic effects?

References

1. Mills J, Leoung G, Medina I et al. Dapsone treatment of *Pneumocystis carinii* pneumonia in the acquired immunodeficiency syndrome. *Antimicrob Agents Chemother.* 1988; 32:1057-60.
2. Dawson AH, Whyte IM. Management of dapsone poisoning complicated by methaemoglobinaemia. *Med Toxicol Adverse Drug Exp.* 1989; 4:387-92.
3. Kenner DJ, Holt K, Agnello R et al. Permanent retinal damage following massive dapsone overdosage. *Br J Ophthalmol.* 1980; 64:741-4.

4. Frey HM, Gershon AA, Borkowsky W et al. Fatal reaction to dapsone during treatment of leprosy. *Ann Intern Med.* 1981; 94:777-9.
5. Davies R. Fatal poisoning with udolac. *Lancet.* 1950; 1:905-6.
6. Hjelm M, de Verdier CH. Biochemical effects of aromatic amines: I. Methaemoglobinaemia, haemolysis and Heinz-body formation induced by 4,4'-diaminodiphenylsulphone. *Biochem Pharmacol.* 1965; 14: 1119-28.
7. Glader BE, Conrad ME. Hemolysis of diphenylsulfones: comparative effects of DDS and hydroxylamine-DDS. *J Lab Clin Med.* 1973; 81:267-72.
8. Grossman SJ, Jollow DJ. Role of dapsone hydroxylamine in dapsone-induced hemolytic anemia. *J Pharmacol Exp Ther* 1988; 244:118-25.
9. Curry S. Methemoglobinemia. *Ann Emerg Med.* 1982; 11:214-21.
10. Goldfrank LR, Price D, Kirstein RH. Nitroglycerin (methemoglobinemia). In: Goldfrank LR, Weisman RS, Flomenbaum NE et al., eds. Goldfrank's toxicologic emergencies. 4th ed. Norwalk, CT: Appleton and Lange; 1990:391-6.
11. Smith RS, Alexander S. Heinz-body anaemia due to dapsone. *Br Med J.* 1959; 1:625-7.
12. Mayer K, Ley AB. Hemolysis of red cells due to sulfone. *Ann Intern Med.* 1970; 72:711-14.
13. Reigart JR, Trammel HL, Lindsey JM. Repetitive doses of activated charcoal in dapsone poisoning in a child. *J Toxicol Clin Toxicol.* 1982-3; 19:1061-6.
14. Linakis JG, Shannon M, Woolf A et al. Recurrent methemoglobinemia after acute dapsone intoxication in a child. *J Emerg Med.* 1989; 7:477-80.
15. Schnapp LM, Cohen NH. Pulse oximetry: uses and abuses. *Chest.* 1990; 98:1244-50.
16. Zuidema J, Hilbers-Modderman ESM, Merkus FWHM. Clinical pharmacokinetics of dapsone. *Clin Pharmacokinet.* 1986; 11:299-315.
17. Albertson TE, Derlet RW, Foulke GE et al. Superiority of activated charcoal alone compared with ipecac and activated charcoal in the treatment of acute toxic ingestions. *Ann Emerg Med.* 1989; 18:56-9.
18. Neuvonen PJ, Elonen E, Haapanen EJ. Acute dapsone intoxication: clinical findings and effect of oral charcoal and haemodialysis on dapsone elimination. *Acta Med Scand.* 1983; 214:215-20.
19. Endre ZH, Charlesworth JA, MacDonald GJ et al. Successful treatment of acute dapsone intoxication using charcoal hemoperfusion. *Aust N Z J Med.* 1983; 13:509-12.
20. Berlin G, Brodin B, Hilden J et al. Acute dapsone intoxication: a case treated with continuous infusion of methylene blue, forced diuresis and plasma exchange. *Clin Toxicol.* 1984-5; 22:537-48.
21. Stanfield JP. A case of acute poisoning with dapsone. *J Trop Med Hyg.* 1963; 66:292-5.
22. Cooke TJL. Dapsone poisoning. *Med J Aust.* 1970; 1:1158-9.
23. Goldstein BD. Exacerbation of dapsone-induced Heinz body hemolytic anemia following treatment with methylene blue. *Am J Med Sci.* 1974; 267:291-7.
24. Goluboff N, Wheaton R. Methylene blue induced cyanosis and acute hemolytic anemia complicating the treatment of methemoglobinemia. *J Pediatr.* 1961; 58:86-9.
25. Harvey JW, Keitt AS. Studies of the efficacy and potential hazards of methylene blue therapy in aniline-induced methaemoglobinaemia. *Br J Haematol.* 1983; 54:29-41.
26. Arena JM, Drew RH. Poisoning: toxicology, symptoms, treatments. 5th ed. Springfield, IL: Charles C Thomas; 1986:454-680.
27. Harris JC, Rumack BH, Peterson RG et al. Methemoglobinemia resulting from absorption of nitrates. *JAMA.* 1979; 242:2869-71.
28. Woodhouse KW, Henderson DB, Charlton B et al. Acute dapsone poisoning: clinical features and pharmacokinetic studies. *Hum Toxicol.* 1983; 3:507-10.
29. Lambert M, Sonnet J, Mahieu P et al. Delayed sulfhemoglobinemia after acute dapsone intoxication. *J Toxicol Clin Toxicol.* 1982; 19:45-50.
30. Hall AH, Kulig KW, Rumack BH. Drug- and chemical-induced methaemoglobinaemia. *Med Toxicol.* 1986; 1:253-60.
31. Rosen PJ, Johnson C, McGehee WG. Failure of methylene blue treatment in toxic methemoglobinemia. *Ann Intern Med.* 1971; 75:83-6.
32. Bolyai JZ, Smith RP, Gray CT. Ascorbic acid and chemically induced methemoglobinemias. *Toxicol Appl Pharmacol.* 1972; 21:176-85.
33. Coleman MD, Scott AK, Breckenridge AM et al. The use of cimetidine as a selective inhibitor of dapsone *N*-hydroxylation in man. *Br J Clin Pharmacol.* 1980; 30:761-7.
34. Kelly JW, Scott J, Sandland M et al. Vitamin E and dapsone-induced hemolysis. *Arch Dermatol.* 1984; 120:1582-4.

“

Outbreaks of Drug-Resistant Tuberculosis

In the past two years, at least six outbreaks of tuberculosis resistant to multiple drugs have been investigated by the CDC. About 200 cases of drug-resistant disease have been identified. . . .

Although to date large outbreaks of drug-resistant tuberculosis have been reported only in Florida and New York, a CDC survey for the first quarter of 1991 found *M. tuberculosis* isolates resistant to isoniazid and rifampin in 11 other states. Drug-resistant tuberculosis among HIV-infected patients has also been reported from outside the United States, and given the high rates of drug resistance in many developing countries, further global spread of drug-resistant tuberculosis is a very real source of concern.

—Jereb JA, Kelly GD, Dooley SW Jr et al. Tuberculosis morbidity in the United States: final data, 1990. *MMWR.* 1991; 40(SS-3):23-7.

”

Drug Experience

Straightforward reports of unusual drug experiences are included in this section. These may be confirmations of previously reported drug experiences or brief apparent first reports. While selected references may be cited, the purpose of a Drug Experience *report is not to present an extensive review of the literature.*

A related section, Grand Rounds, *includes papers that are well-documented patient case reports with a thorough review of the important literature to help put the case in perspective.*

Apparent potentiation of warfarin activity by tetracycline

ERICA A. DANOS

Clin Pharm. 1992; 11:806-8

Several antimicrobial agents have been reported to enhance the effect of oral anticoagulants. Trimethoprim–sulfamethoxazole[1,2] and erythromycin,[3] for example, may prolong the prothrombin time (PT) in patients receiving warfarin. This report describes an apparent interaction between tetracycline and warfarin.

Case Report. On January 8, 1991, a 50-year-old Hispanic man came to the vascular surgery clinic for monitoring and possible adjustment of his warfarin therapy. Although he had no external signs of bleeding, he had an International Normalized Ratio (INR) of 7.66 and was admitted to the hospital.

The patient had had "blue toe syndrome" caused by multiple peripheral emboli and had undergone left transmetatarsal amputation and left femoral–popliteal bypass grafting six months earlier (July 1990). Since then, he had received warfarin (Coumadin, DuPont) to maintain graft patency. (The brand of warfarin did not change during therapy.) Coagulation studies had revealed hypercoagulable platelets but no other hemostatic disorders.

The patient had type II diabetes mellitus, for which he had been treated with glyburide. He lost 12 kg through dieting and had several episodes of hypoglycemia. Glyburide therapy was then discontinued, and the diabetes was considered controlled by diet.

The patient described himself as active and denied past or present use of tobacco, illicit drugs, or alcohol. He used an alarm clock to help himself take his medications at the same time every day.

The warfarin sodium dosage had been 5 mg and 7.5 mg orally on alternate nights for four months before admission (Table 1). The patient's only other medication was dipyridamole 25 mg orally three times daily, which he had also been taking since the bypass operation. Warfarin therapy had been adjusted to keep the INR between 2.0 and 3.0. On October 30, 1990, 10 weeks before admission, the INR was approximately 2.2.

On November 27, 1990, six weeks before admission, the patient began taking tetracycline hydrochloride 250 mg (Achromycin, Lederle) orally four times daily for chronic blepharitis. (The brand of tetracycline did not change during therapy.) The INR on that day was within the desired range. Clinicians in the vascular surgery clinic were unaware of the addition of tetracycline therapy, and the next clinic visit was scheduled for January 8, 1991. It was at this clinic visit that the PT and INR were found to be supratherapeutic, and the patient was admitted to the hospital.

During hospitalization, anticoagulant therapy was withheld for three nights, and the INR fell to 2.70. Therapy was restarted at a warfarin sodium dosage of 2.5 mg and 5 mg orally on alternate nights, and the patient was discharged.

The patient's ophthalmologist was informed of the possible interaction between tetracycline and warfarin but declined to alter his choice of antimicrobials. Over the next several months, changes in the INR generally paralleled changes in the tetracycline dosage; as the dosage of tetracycline decreased, so did the INR (Table 1). The warfarin dosage was adjusted periodically in response to changes in the INR. After discontinuation of tetracycline therapy (one year after admission), the INR remained stable while the patient took a consistent dosage of warfarin.

Discussion. Standard drug-interaction references suggest a tentative association between the concurrent use of warfarin and tetracycline and the augmentation

ERICA A. DANOS, PHARM.D., BCPS, is Clinical Assistant Professor, Department of Pharmacy Practice, University of Illinois–Chicago, College of Pharmacy M/C 886, 833 South Wood Street, Chicago, IL 60612, and Pharmacotherapist, General Medicine Clinic and Combined Medicine/Pediatric Clinic, University of Illinois Hospital and Clinics, Chicago.

Table 1.
Effect of Warfarin and Tetracycline Therapy on Measurements of Anticoagulation[a]

Date	Change in Warfarin Sodium Therapy	Change in Tetracycline Hydrochloride Therapy	PT (sec)	INR
4 Sep 1990	None[b]	...	18.4	2.0[c]
30 Oct 1990	None	...	19.7	2.2[d]
27 Nov 1990	None	Started 250 mg q.i.d.	20.2	2.59
8 Jan 1991	Withheld for 3 nights	None	36.5	7.66
10 Jan 1991	...	None	20.6	2.70
11 Jan 1991	Started alternating 2.5 and 5 mg nightly	None	...	...
15 Jan 1991	None	None	17.6	2.02
25 Jan 1991	None	None	21.7	2.95
1 Feb 1991	None	Decr. to 250 mg t.i.d.	22.1	3.06
8 Feb 1991	None	None	18.1	2.10
11 Mar 1991	None	None	18.2	2.13
22 Mar 1991	None	Decr. to 250 mg b.i.d.	...	...
29 Mar 1991	Incr. to 5 mg nightly	None	16.9	1.86
4 Apr 1991	None	None	22.1	3.05
1 May 1991	None	Decr. to 250 mg daily	...	...
10 May 1991	Withheld for 2 nights	None[e]	27.9	4.67
12 May 1991	Started 3.75 mg nightly	None	...	...
24 May 1991	None	Incr. to 250 mg b.i.d.	16.4	1.76
24 Jun 1991	None	Decr. to 250 mg daily	17.2	1.93
13 Aug 1991	None	None	19.3	2.31
30 Aug 1991	None	None	18.6	2.23
8 Nov 1991	None	None	18.1	2.03
10 Jan 1992	None	Discontinued	...	...
24 Jan 1992	Incr. to 5 mg nightly	...	16.5	1.78
28 Jan 1992	None	...	18.9	2.31
20 Feb 1992	None	...	19.1	2.25
17 Apr 1992	None	...	18.5	2.13

[a]All doses of warfarin and tetracycline were oral. PT = prothrombin time, INR = International Normalized Ratio (INR = $[\text{patient's PT/control PT}]^{ISI}$, where ISI = International Sensitivity Index).

[b]Nightly warfarin sodium dosage until 8 Jan 1991 was 5 mg alternating with 7.5 mg.

[c]Estimate based on an ISI of 1.83 and an average institutional control PT of 12.7 sec. The actual control PT was not available for this day. Because control PTs during this period ranged from 11.4 to 14.0 sec, the actual INR could have ranged from 1.65 to 2.40.

[d]Estimate. Actual INR could have ranged from 1.87 to 2.72.

[e]Although the dosage was supposed to have been 250 mg daily, the patient revealed that he had again started to take 250 mg twice daily. He reduced the dosage to 250 mg daily after this clinic visit.

of warfarin's anticoagulant effect.[4-7] These references cite a report of a woman whose PTs had been stable and in the desired range during 15 months of warfarin therapy.[8] She developed a PT of 51 seconds, menorrhagia, and a severe drop in hematocrit and hemoglobin concentration after a 10-day course of oral doxycycline therapy.

Searcy et al.[9] studied the effects of tetracycline on blood clotting in 25 patients who were receiving the drug intravenously for a variety of infections. When measured by Quick's method, prothrombin activity varied greatly, but when measured by the modified one-stage procedure (which is generally considered to be more accurate), prothrombin activity was essentially normal. The report is difficult to interpret because it provides relatively few data. However, the lack of substantial changes in prothrombin activity may suggest that tetracycline, by itself, does not affect hemostasis.

Magid[10] reported that chlortetracycline, alone and in combination with other antimicrobials, may increase the hypoprothrombinemic effects of oral anticoagulants. In another report, the combination of nystatin and tetracycline was implicated as a cause of bleeding in two patients who had been clinically stable while taking warfarin.[11]

The previous literature and the current case suggest that tetracycline can indeed enhance the hypoprothrombinemic effect of warfarin. The INR in this case appeared to change in response to changes in tetracycline dosage. Except for one instance, when the wrong tetracycline dosage was taken, the patient seemed to be extremely compliant with his medication regimen. His self-reports, medication-refill records, and clinic-appointment attendance all suggested good compliance. Changes in liver function may have influenced the degree of anticoagulation, but liver function was not monitored during therapy.

Tetracycline is used fairly commonly, so the lack of a well-documented interaction between it and warfarin is conspicuous. Although long-term tetracycline therapy may sometimes be indicated, patients generally receive tetracycline for a relatively short time (i.e., 7–10 days). Even if the PT increased during short-term tetracycline therapy, this change might not be detected.

Drug-interaction references generally classify the likelihood of a tetracycline–warfarin interaction as "possible" or "unlikely." It would seem prudent to revise the classification to "suspected" or "probable." This change would alert clinicians to this potentially serious interaction.

Conclusion. Oral tetracycline appeared to increase the INR in a patient taking warfarin.

References

1. Reilly RA, Motley CH. Racemic warfarin and trimethoprim–sulfamethoxazole interaction in humans. *Ann Intern Med*. 1979; 91:34-6.
2. Reilly RA. Stereoselective interaction of trimethoprim–sulfamethoxazole with the separated enantiomorphs of racemic warfarin in man. *N Engl J Med*. 1980; 302:33-5.
3. Weibert RT, Lorentz SM, Townsend RJ et al. Effect of erythromycin in patients receiving long-term warfarin therapy. *Clin Pharm*. 1989; 8:210-4.
4. Tatro DS, ed.: Drug interaction facts. St. Louis, MO: Lippincott; 1992.
5. Hansten PD, Horn JR, eds. Drug interactions and updates. Malvern, PA: Lea & Febiger; 1990.
6. Anon. Drug–drug interaction report: warfarin and tetracycline (drug consult). In: Gelman DR, Rumack BH, eds. DRUGDEX information system. Denver, CO: Micromedex; 1989.
7. Zucchero FJ, Hogum MJ, eds. Evaluation of drug interactions. St. Louis, MO: Professional Drug Systems; 1990.
8. Westfall LK, Mintzer DL, Wiser TH. Potentiation of warfarin by tetracycline. *Am J Hosp Pharm*. 1980; 37:1620,1625. Letter.
9. Searcy RL, Sims NM, Foreman JA et al. Evaluation of blood clotting mechanisms in tetracycline-treated patients. *Antimicrob Agents Chemother*. 1964; 4:179-83.
10. Magid E. Tolerance to anticoagulants during antibiotic therapy. *Scand J Clin Lab Invest*. 1962; 14:565-6.
11. O'Donnell D. Antibiotic-induced potentiation of oral anticoagulants. *Med J Aust*. 1989; 150:163-4.

DUE Criteria

The DUE Criteria *section of* Clinical Pharmacy *features model drug-use evaluation criteria that may be employed as a component of a comprehensive quality assurance program. The criteria sets are presented in the format used in the ASHP book* Criteria for Drug Use Evaluation. *Some of the criteria sets will have been originally published in that book; others will be presented here for the first time and published in future volumes of the ASHP book. The practitioners who developed a criteria set are acknowledged.*

In selecting drug products for coverage in DUE Criteria, *priority is given to products that have been recently marketed, those that are frequently prescribed, those that have high potential risk associated with their use, and those that are expensive. When feasible, a criteria set will be linked with a Drug Review that appears in the same issue.*

These criteria sets are a starting point for the development of DUE criteria for a specific practice setting. Readers are encouraged to modify the model criteria to fit their own circumstances.

Criteria for use of amphotericin B bladder irrigation in adult inpatients[a]

Element	Standard 100%	Standard 0%	Exception	Sources of Information
Justification for Use				
1. Urine culture positive for yeast when collected by midstream clean-catch method[1] or straight catheterization,[1] or urine culture positive for >10,000 colony-forming units/mL when collected by another method[2,3] and	X		1A. None	1. Laboratory reports
2. Clinical course includes one or more of the following: a. Symptoms of urinary tract infection (UTI) (e.g., urinary frequency, dysuria, fever, and lower-abdominal discomfort)[1,3] b. Pyuria[4] c. Predisposing risk factor for candidal UTI that cannot be adequately corrected or eliminated (e.g., structural abnormality, diabetes, and antibiotic or immunosuppressive therapy)[1,2] d. Repeat urine culture positive for yeast >3 days after initial positive culture[1,2]	X		2A. None	2. History and physical (H&P), progress notes, laboratory reports, medication administration record (MAR), nursing notes, nursing flow sheets
Critical (Process) Indicators				
3. Bladder irrigation not sole antifungal therapy for patient with ureteral obstruction caused by fungus ball or with systemic fungal infection[2]	X		3A. None	3. H&P, physician orders, progress notes, laboratory reports, MAR, radiology reports
4. Temperature monitored at least every 8 hr until normal	X		4A. Temperature monitored daily in patient with normal temperature initially	4. Physician orders, progress notes, nursing notes, nursing flow sheets 4A. H&P, progress notes, nursing flow sheets

Prepared by Patricia A. Montgomery, Pharm.D., Clinical Pharmacist and Clinical Assistant Professor; Patricia S. Woster, Pharm.D., Clinical Pharmacist and Clinical Assistant Professor; and Pamala A. Jacobson, Pharm.D., Clinical Pharmacist and Clinical Assistant Professor, Department of Pharmacy Services, University of Michigan Medical Center and College of Pharmacy, Ann Arbor, MI.

Element	Standard 100%	Standard 0%	Exception	Sources of Information
5. Amphotericin B 10–50 mg in 1 L of sterile water for irrigation infused continuously over 24 hr[2-5] or 100–200 mL of amphotericin B 37.5–50 mg/L[6-8] in sterile water for irrigation[4] instilled every 3–12 hr with tubing clamped for at least 30 min after dose[6-8]	X		5A. None	5. Physician orders, pharmacy i.v. admixture preparation records, progress notes, MAR, nursing notes
6. Duration of therapy five to seven days[5,6]	X		6A. Patient requalifies for therapy as defined under justification for use (systemic fungal infection ruled out)	6. Physician orders, progress notes, MAR 6A. Progress notes, laboratory reports, nursing notes, nursing flow sheets
Outcome Measure				
7. Follow-up urine culture negative >24 hr after end of treatment[5]	X		7A. None	7. Progress notes, laboratory reports, MAR

[a]Criteria address justification for use (indications), critical (process) indicators, complications of therapy, and patient outcome. Each criterion consists of an element, a standard, exceptions to the standard, and sources of information. The element is the minimum level of evidence needed to show that patient care was optimal. The standard defines the deviation from an element that is acceptable. If no deviation is acceptable, the standard is 100%. Exceptions are identified by the number assigned to the element or exception (e.g., 4,4A).

References

1. Michigan S. Genitourinary fungal infection. *J Urol.* 1976; 116:390-7.
2. Fisher JF, Chew WH, Shadomy S et al. Urinary tract infections due to *Candida albicans. Rev Infect Dis.* 1982; 4:1107-18.
3. Wise GJ, Goldberg P, Kozinn PJ. Genitourinary candidiasis: diagnosis and treatment. *J Urol.* 1976; 116:778-80.
4. Wise GJ, Wainstein S, Goldberg P et al. Candidal cystitis. Management by continuous bladder irrigation with amphotericin B. *JAMA.* 1973; 224:1636-7.
5. Wise GJ, Kozinn PJ, Goldberg P. Amphotericin B as a urologic irrigant in the management of noninvasive candiduria. *J Urol.* 1982; 128:82-4.
6. Goldman HJ, Littman ML, Oppenheimer GD et al. Monilial cystitis—effective treatment with instillations of amphotericin B. *JAMA.* 1960; 174:359-62.
7. O'Connell CJ, Hardner GJ. Thrush of urinary bladder due to *Candida guilliermondii. NY State J Med.* 1973; 73:1685-6.
8. Cuetara MM, Mallo N, Dalet F. Amphotericin B lavage in the treatment of candidal cystitis. *Br J Urol.* 1972; 44:475-80.

Need for Aggressive Efforts To Control Tuberculosis

. . . Aggressive efforts must be made to identify and control the current outbreaks of drug-resistant tuberculosis and to prevent additional ones. For the emergence of drug-resistant strains to be controlled, the completion of therapy by all patients with tuberculosis must be ensured. Full implementation of the core program of tuberculosis prevention and control requires additional local, state, and federal efforts. We must also ensure the availability of tuberculosis drugs, more extensive and rapid drug-susceptibility testing, and the implementation of measures to prevent airborne spread, especially in settings where HIV-infected persons receive care. While continuing to do what we now know how to do, we must also intensify efforts to develop rapid diagnostic and drug-susceptibility tests and new drugs that can be effective and that require a shorter therapeutic course. We must also reevaluate the need for an effective tuberculosis vaccine.

—Jereb JA, Kelly GD, Dooley SW Jr et al. Tuberculosis morbidity in the United States: final data, 1990. *MMWR.* 1991; 40(SS-3):23-7.

Current Literature

Drug Reaction Alerts

Drug Reaction Alerts focuses primarily on serious, unlabeled reactions to new chemical entities. The citations are compiled monthly from International Pharmaceutical Abstracts, *which covers over 800 pharmacy and health-related journals worldwide. An address for reprints (when available) follows the name of the corresponding author in each citation.*

Pharmacists may use the FDA Adverse Reaction Report form that appears in the January and July issues of Clinical Pharmacy *for submitting reports of adverse drug reactions directly to FDA.*

Anabolic Agents

Montine TJ, Gaede JT (Duke University Medical Center, Durham, NC 27710). Massive pulmonary embolus and **anabolic steroid** abuse. *JAMA.* 1992. 267:2328-9. Case. (36-year-old man; abused anabolic steroids over unknown number of years; developed pulmonary embolism and died; examination at autopsy revealed large pulmonary embolus obstructing right and left pulmonary arteries and small, peripheral emboli and associated infarcts without evidence of cerebral or coronary infarcts)

Antibiotics

Morris JT, McAllister CK (Brook Army Medical Center, Fort Sam Houston, TX 78234-6200). **Cefotetan**-induced singultus. *Ann Intern Med.* 1992; 116:522-3. Case. (62-year-old man with osteomyelitis; received cefotetan 1 g twice daily by i.v. injection for four weeks; developed prolonged, recurrent hiccups; withdrawal of cefotetan for one day led to resolution of hiccups; positive rechallenge; complete withdrawal of cefotetan and therapy with oral antibiotic led to resolution of hiccups)

Anxiolytics, Sedatives, and Hypnotics

Ansseau M, Pitchot W, Hansenne M et al. (Moreno AG, Psychiatric Unit, University of Liège, CHU du Sart Tilman, B-4000 Liège, Belgium). Psychotic reactions to **zolpidem**. *Lancet.* 1992; 339:809. Cases. (two women, aged 26 and 27 years; received one tablet of zolpidem 10 mg; developed psychotic symptoms 20–30 minutes after receiving dose and developed amnesia of psychotic events)

Antineoplastic Agents

Tweedy CR (Nebraska Methodist Hospital, Omaha, NE 68114), Silverberg DA, Scott L. **Levamisole**-induced syndrome of inappropriate antidiuretic hormone. *N Engl J Med.* 1992; 326:1164. Case. (64-year-old man with stage B2 sigmoid colon carcinoma; received levamisole hydrochloride for two weeks; developed extreme dizziness, fatigue, one episode of near syncope, and orthostatic hypotension without edema or ascites; serum sodium concentration, 115 mM; concomitant fluorouracil and levothyroxine; therapy with 3% sodium chloride injection for three days led to serum sodium concentration of 129 mM; positive rechallenge; levamisole hydrochloride was discontinued)

Antivirals

De Jong MD (National AIDS Therapy Evaluation Center, Academy Medical Center, University of Amsterdam, 1105 AZ Amsterdam, Netherlands), Borleffs JC. **Didanosine** and heart failure. *Lancet.* 1992; 339:806-7. Cases. (three patients, aged 28–47 years, with AIDS; received didanosine; developed cardiac failure)

Benzodiazepines

Martí-Massó JF (Neurology Section, Hospital Ntra. Sra de Aránzazu, Paseo del Dr. Beguiristain s/n, Apdo. Correos 447, San Sebastián 20080, Spain), Lopez De Munain A, Lopez De Dicastillo G. Ataxia following gastric bleeding due to **omeprazole**–benzodiazepine interaction. *Ann Pharmacother.* 1992; 26:429-30. Cases. (two men, aged 66 and 75 years; 66-year-old man received **flurazepam** 60 mg/day and omeprazole 20 mg/day; 75-year-old man received **triazolam** 0.25 mg/day, **lorazepam** 1.5 mg/day, and omeprazole 20 mg/day; developed ataxia; withdrawal of benzodiazepine[s] led to improvement in gait)

Bronchodilators

Chin TW (Memorial Miller Children's Hospital, Long Beach Memorial Medical Center, 2801 Atlantic Avenue, Long Beach, CA 90801-1428), Nussbaum E. Detrimental effect of hypotonic **cromolyn sodium**. *J Pediatr.* 1992; 120:641-3. Study. (double-blind, placebo-controlled, crossover; 13 patients, aged 6–14 years, with asthma; received isotonic 1% cromolyn sodium solution in 0.9% sodium chloride solution, hypotonic 1% cromolyn sodium solution in distilled water, 0.9% sodium chloride solution with 1% lactose, or distilled water by nebulization; after treatment with hypotonic cromolyn sodium solution, midexpiratory flow rate between 25th and 75th percentile points was significantly less than after treatment with isotonic cromolyn sodium solution [$p < 0.05$])

Drug Abuse

Libby DM (Division of Pulmonary and Critical Care Medicine, 407 E. 70th Street, New York, NY 10021), Klein L, Altorki NK. Aspiration of the nasal septum: new complication of **cocaine** abuse. *Ann Intern Med.* 1992; 116:567-8. Case. (55-year-old man; abused cocaine by intranasal inhalation; aspirated nasal septum, which had ossified from chronic irritation; bone removed by using rigid bronchoscopy under general anesthesia; DNA probe confirmed bone as patient's bone)

Drug Interactions

Rex J (National Institutes of Health, Bethesda, MD 20892). **Itraconazole–digoxin** interaction. *Ann Intern Med.* 1992; 116:525. Case. (68-year-old man who received digoxin 0.25 mg/day as maintenance therapy to control atrial fibrillation; received itraconazole 400 mg/day for two weeks for fungal osteomyelitis; developed symptoms of digoxin toxicity and elevated serum digoxin concentration; withdrawal of digoxin and itraconazole led to resolution of symptoms and return of serum digoxin concentration to normal range; reinstitution of digox-

Continued on page 820

Current Literature *Continued from page 819*

in at 0.125 mg/day and of itraconazole at 400 mg/day did not lead to another incident)

Safferman AZ, Masiar SJ (Pilgrim Psychiatric Center, West Brentwood, NY 11717). Central nervous system toxicity after abrupt monoamine oxidase inhibitor switch: case report. *Ann Pharmacother*. 1992; 26:337-8. Case. (53-year-old woman who received **phenelzine** 15 mg/day; therapy with phenelzine replaced with **isocarboxazide** 10 mg/day; developed stuporous sensorium, hypertension, tachycardia tremor, and urinary retention within 48 hours; therapy with labetalol, haloperidol, and amitriptyline led to resolution of hypertension and of stuporous sensorium)

Heavy Metal Antagonists

Tenenbein M (Children's Hospital, 840 Sherbrook Street, Winnipeg, Manitoba R3A 1S1, Canada), Kowalski S, Sienko A et al. Pulmonary toxic effects of continuous desferrioxamine administration in acute iron poisoning. *Lancet*. 1992; 339:699-701. Cases. (three women and one man, aged 19–26 years, who were poisoned with 1.6–6.0 g of elemental iron and were without any known risk factors for developing adult respiratory distress syndrome [ARDS]; received **deferoxamine** 15 mg/kg/hr by continuous i.v. infusion for 65–92 hours [total dose, 57–120 g]; serum iron concentration was 77–111 μM 5–10 hours after iron ingestion [normal, 8–24 μM]; developed respiratory distress after receiving deferoxamine for 32–72 hours [24–120 g]; died 76–114 hours after iron ingestion; diagnosed with ARDS based on clinical and physiological criteria and examination at autopsy)

Hypotensive Agents

Lee ST (Taipei Municipal Chung Hsaio Hospital, Nankang, Taipei, Taiwan, Republic of China). Hyperprolactinemia, galactorrhea, and **atenolol**. *Ann Intern Med*. 1992; 116:522. Case. (38-year-old woman with hypertension; received atenolol 50 mg/day for 18 months; developed hyperprolactinemia and galactorrhea; serum prolactin concentration, 16.5 ng/mL; withdrawal of atenolol led to decrease of serum prolactin concentration to 15.6 ng/mL within two days and to 13.5 ng/mL in seven days, return of menstrual cycle to normal, and gradual cessation of galactorrhea; refused rechallenge)

Immunosuppressive Agents

Abramowicz D (Nephrology Department, Hôpital Erasme, 808 route de Lennik, B-1070 Brussels, Belgium), Pradier O, Marchant A et al. Induction of thromboses within renal grafts by high-dose prophylactic OKT3. *Lancet*. 1992; 339:777-8. Cases.(nine patients who received renal transplants; received **muromonab-CD3** 10 mg/day for two weeks as prophylaxis for graft rejection; developed intragraft thromboses in graft artery, graft vein, or glomerular capillaries with thrombotic microangiopathy; four hours after first muromonab-CD3 dose, plasma concentrations of prothrombin fragments 1 and 2 were greater than in transplant patients who received prophylaxis other than muromonab-CD3; failure of immunosuppressive therapy led to removal of graft)

Nozue T (Department of Pediatrics, Showa University Toyosu Hospital, Koto-ku, Toyosu, 4-1-18, Tokyo 135, Japan), Kobayashi A, Kodama T et al. Pathogenesis of **cyclosporine**-induced hypomagnesemia. *J Pediatr*. 1992; 120:638-40. Study. (case series; three girls and two boys, aged 5–18 years, with nephrosis; received cyclosporine at a mean dose of 5 mg/kg daily, adjusted to maintain whole blood cyclosporine concentration at 100–200 ng/mL; developed hypomagnesemia; serum magnesium concentration and urinary excretion of magnesium decreased, and magnesium concentration in mononuclear blood cells increased)

Continued on page 822

Continued from page 820

Pediatrics

Gourlay GK (Pain Management Unit, Flinders Medical Center, Bedford Park, South Australia 5042, Australia), Boas RA. Fatal outcome with use of rectal **morphine** for postoperative pain control in an infant. *Br Med J.* 1992; 304:766-7. Case. (7.5-month-old boy with postoperative pain; received morphine sulfate 4 mg every four hours as rectal suppository for five doses; experienced cardiac arrest three hours after fifth dose; serum morphine concentration was 0.094 μg/mL 1.5 hours after arrest and resuscitation; deteriorated without regaining consciousness, and died next day; review of patient's medical chart and discussion with nursing staff members indicated at least two doses probably were unnecessary but were administered becauses doses were scheduled)

Sympatholytic Agents

Bright RA (FDA Center for Devices and Radiological Health, HFZ-161, 5600 Fishers Lane, Rockville, MD 20857), Everitt DE. β-Blockers and depression: evidence against an association. *JAMA.* 1992; 267:1783-7. Study. (case–control; 4302 patients with depression and matched controls who were reported to New Jersey Medicaid Management Information System, July 1980–December 1983; case patients were more likely to have taken β blockers than control patients [odds ratio, 1.45; 95% confidence interval, 1.29–1.62], but this difference disappeared when confounding variables, such as benzodiazepine use, frequent outpatient visits, and frequent use of medications other than β blockers, were controlled; results did not vary by age, sex, race, nursing home status, or use of other selected medications)

Thrombolytic Agents

Urban P, Reynard C, Meier B (Center for Cardiology, Hôpital Cantonal University, 1205 Geneva, Switzerland). Thrombolysis and risk of intracranial bleeding. *Lancet.* 1992; 339:817. Study. (convenience sample; database with 358 patients who received **alteplase** 100 mg over three hours for myocardial infarction; mean age, 60 years; overall prevalence of stroke, 3.4%; stroke was secondary to intracranial hemorrhage in 10 patients)

Tocolytics

Lindenbaum C (University of Pennsylvania Medical Center, Department of Obstetrics and Gynecology, Division of Maternal–Fetal Medicine, 3400 Spruce Street, Philadelphia, PA 19104), Ludmir J, Teplick FB et al. Maternal glucose intolerance and the subcutaneous **terbutaline** pump. *Am J Obstet Gynecol.* 1992; 166:925-8. Study. (nonrandomized, controlled; 37 pregnant women who received individualized subcutaneous doses of terbutaline by pump, 54 pregnant women who received oral terbutaline 5 mg every four hours, and 634 control patients, none of whom had pregestational or gestational diabetes; after one-hour glucose tolerance test, gestational diabetes occurred in 6% of control patients, 5% of women using pump for subcutaneous terbutaline delivery, and 11% of women receiving oral terbutaline; of women who developed gestational diabetes, 8% of control patients required both insulin therapy and diet modification for glycemic control, compared with 100% of women using pump and 50% receiving oral terbutaline)

Toxicity

Clark RF (Department of Medical Toxicology, Good Samaritan Regional Medical Center, Phoenix Children's Hospital, Phoenix, AZ 85006). Crystalluria following **cephalexin** overdose. *Pediatrics.* 1992; 89:672-4. Case. (three-year-old boy with pharyngitis; accidentally ingested 2.5 g of cephalexin suspension prescribed for treatment of pharyngitis; developed hematuria and crystalluria; physical examination on admission, complete blood cell count, serum creatinine concentration, and blood urea nitrogen concentration were normal; therapy with oral fluids over next 24 hours led to resolution of hematuria and dysuria and normal follow-up examination on next day)

Vaccines

Benjamin CM, Chew GC, Silman AJ (Arthritis and Rheumatism Council Epidemiology Research Unit, Stopford Building, University of Manchester, Manchester M13 9PT, England). Joint and limb symptoms in children after immunization with **measles, mumps, and rubella vaccine**. *Br Med J.* 1992; 304:1075-8. Study. (nonrandomized, controlled; 1846 children who were immunized with measles, mumps, and rubella vaccine and 1075 children who were not yet immunized; during six-year period after immunization, immunized group had increased incidence of new episodes of joint and limb symptoms compared with nonimmunized children [relative risk, 1.6; 95% confidence interval, 1.2–2.1]; increased risk of first episodes of joint and limb symptoms in girls [relative risk, 3.5; 95% confidence interval, 1.1–12.2] but not in boys and in children aged <5 years [relative risk, 12.0; 95% confidence interval, 1.6–92.3] but not in older children; most episodes of joint and limb symptoms were self-limiting; three immunized children were referred to hospital for treatment of joint and limb symptoms)

Advertising Index

American Society of Hospital Pharmacists
AHFS Drug Information 92, 796
Basic Skills in Interpreting Laboratory Data, 799
The Elements of Quality in Pharmaceutical Care, 820
Handbook on Injectable Drugs, 7th Edition, 821
Medication Teaching Manual, 808
Amgen Inc.
Epogen, 748-749
Egleston Children's Hospital
Positions Available, 752
National Council on Patient Information and Education
Institutional, 814
Roche Laboratories, Division of Hoffmann-La Roche, Inc.
Rocephin, 745-746
SmithKline Beecham
Timentin, inside back cover, outside back cover
Wyeth-Ayerst Laboratories, Inc.
Ativan Injection, 816-818
Tubex, inside front cover

News

Finasteride approved for treatment of benign prostatic hyperplasia 825

Terfenadine and astemizole pose cardiovascular risks to certain patients, health professionals warned 825

News Briefs 829

Correction 829

Finasteride approved for treatment of benign prostatic hyperplasia

Finasteride (Proscar, Merck Sharp & Dohme) is the first drug to be approved by FDA for the treatment of symptomatic benign prostatic hyperplasia; marketing approval was granted in June.

Finasteride selectively inhibits 5α-reductase, which converts testosterone to 5α-dihydrotestosterone. Prostatic growth is mediated by 5α-dihydrotestosterone.

In one study, the mean bioavailability of finasteride given as a 5-mg tablet to healthy volunteers was 63%; the mean elimination half-life was six hours. The elimination half-life in elderly persons is about eight hours. Finasteride accumulates slowly in plasma when multiple doses are given; concentrations measured 17 days after the start of therapy were reported to be 47–54% higher than concentrations measured after the first dose. About 39% of a dose is excreted in the urine as metabolites and 57% is excreted in the feces.

Placebo-controlled trials involving some 1645 patients showed that finasteride decreased prostate size about 20% in patients treated for 12 months and increased urine flow and reduced symptoms in about 50% of patients. At least six months of therapy may be required to fully assess treatment effectiveness. Adverse effects reported by more than 2% of patients treated in 12-month controlled clinical trials include impotence (3.7%), decreased libido (3.3%), and decreased volume of ejaculate (2.8%).

Proscar is available as 5-mg tablets in unit-of-use bottles of 30 or 100 and unit dose packages of 100. The recommended daily dosage is 5 mg.

Terfenadine and astemizole pose cardiovascular risks to certain patients, health professionals warned

FDA and the manufacturers of terfenadine (Seldane, Marion Merrell Dow) and astemizole (Hismanal, Janssen Pharmaceutica) have warned health professionals that certain patients who use these antihistamines may be at risk of adverse cardiovascular events.

Rare cases of torsades de pointes, other ventricular arrhythmias, cardiac arrest, and death have been reported. In some cases, patients have complained of fainting, dizziness, or palpitations before arrhythmias were diagnosed. Several circumstances that contribute to high blood levels of the two antihistamines have been identified as risk factors. For terfenadine, risk factors include

Continued on page 829

OVERWHELMING

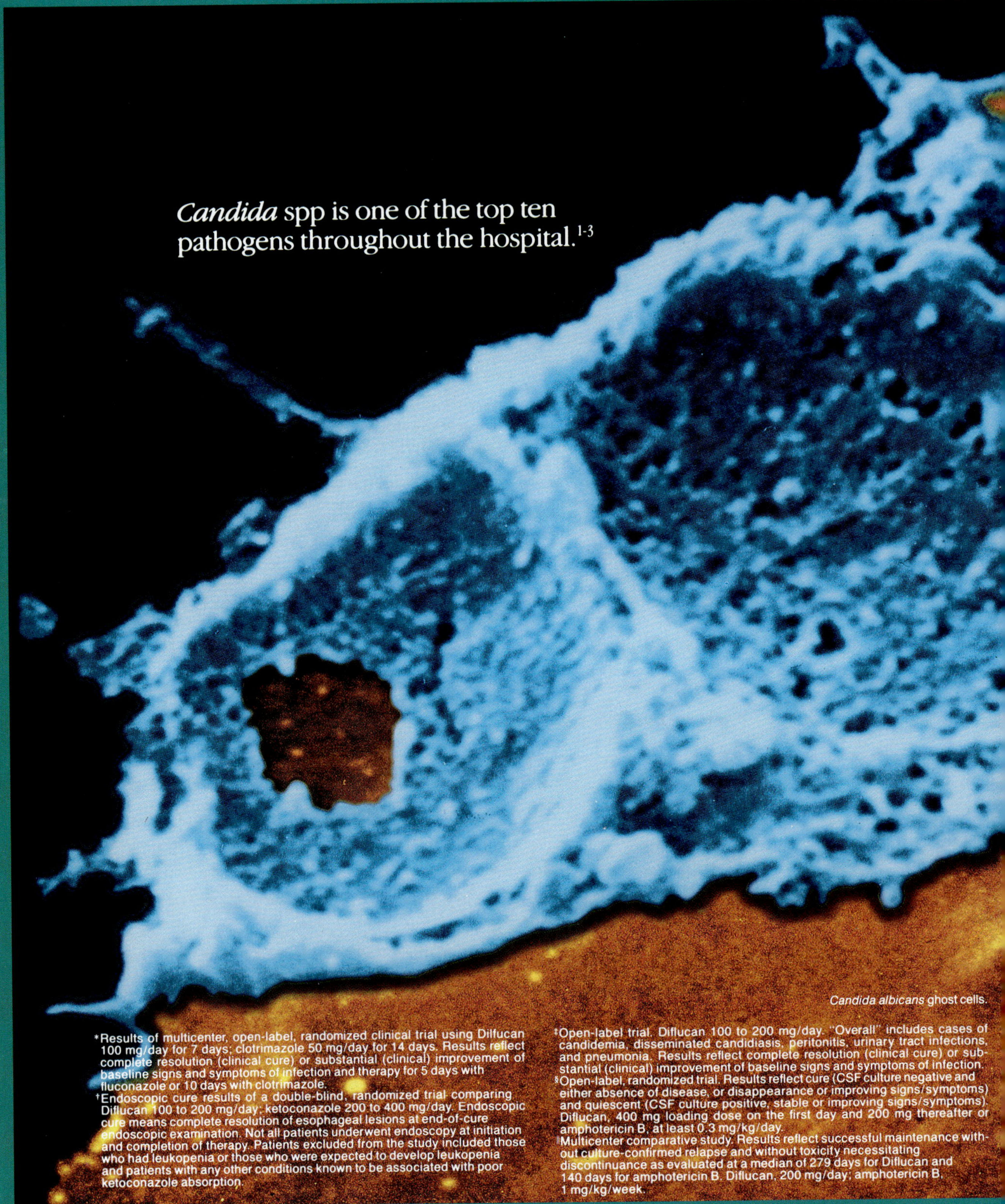

Candida albicans ghost cells.

*Results of multicenter, open-label, randomized clinical trial using Diflucan 100 mg/day for 7 days; clotrimazole 50 mg/day for 14 days. Results reflect complete resolution (clinical cure) or substantial (clinical) improvement of baseline signs and symptoms of infection and therapy for 5 days with fluconazole or 10 days with clotrimazole.

†Endoscopic cure results of a double-blind, randomized trial comparing Diflucan 100 to 200 mg/day; ketoconazole 200 to 400 mg/day. Endoscopic cure means complete resolution of esophageal lesions at end-of-cure endoscopic examination. Not all patients underwent endoscopy at initiation and completion of therapy. Patients excluded from the study included those who had leukopenia or those who were expected to develop leukopenia and patients with any other conditions known to be associated with poor ketoconazole absorption.

‡Open-label trial. Diflucan 100 to 200 mg/day. "Overall" includes cases of candidemia, disseminated candidiasis, peritonitis, urinary tract infections, and pneumonia. Results reflect complete resolution (clinical cure) or substantial (clinical) improvement of baseline signs and symptoms of infection.

§Open-label, randomized trial. Results reflect cure (CSF culture negative and either absence of disease, or disappearance or improving signs/symptoms) and quiescent (CSF culture positive, stable or improving signs/symptoms). Diflucan, 400 mg loading dose on the first day and 200 mg thereafter or amphotericin B, at least 0.3 mg/kg/day.

‖Multicenter comparative study. Results reflect successful maintenance without culture-confirmed relapse and without toxicity necessitating discontinuance as evaluated at a median of 279 days for Diflucan and 140 days for amphotericin B. Diflucan, 200 mg/day; amphotericin B, 1 mg/kg/week.

News *Continued from page 825*

concurrent use of ketoconazole or erythromycin, liver disease, and use of terfenadine at excessive dosages. A small number of patients who have developed arrhythmias have had no identifiable risk factors. Risk factors for astemizole include excessive dosage and liver disease. Most cases of cardiovascular toxicity with astemizole have occurred when the dosage was much higher than the recommended daily dosage of 10 mg; however, toxicity has occurred at daily dosages of 20 to 30 mg.

The product labeling for terfenadine now warns that the recommended dosage should not be exceeded and that terfenadine use is contraindicated in patients taking ketoconazole or erythromycin and in patients with significant hepatic dysfunction. If syncope occurs, terfenadine use should be promptly discontinued and the patient should be evaluated for arrhythmias.

Labeling for astemizole has also been revised; it contains a warning that patients with liver disorders should generally avoid use of this drug and warns against use of higher-than-recommended dosages. Use of dosages higher than 10 mg during the first few days of therapy is no longer recommended.

News Briefs

• Labeled indications for **recombinant interferon alfa-2b** (Intron A, Schering-Plough) have been expanded to include treatment of chronic hepatitis B.

• The Centers for Disease Control has updated its recommendations for the **prevention and control of influenza** (*MMWR*. 1992; 41(RR-9):1–17). The 1992–1993 vaccine differs from last year's vaccine; this year's vaccine contains A/Texas/36/91-like (H1N1), A/Beijing/353/89-like (H3N2), and B/Panama/45/90-like hemagglutinin antigens.

• To obtain a free, single copy of a report entitled **"Opportunities for Integration of Pharmacokinetics, Pharmacodynamics, and Toxicokinetics in Rational Drug Development,"** write to PD, PK, TK Report, American Association of Pharmaceutical Scientists, 1650 King Street, Alexandria, VA 22314-2747; the report was published in the June 1992 issue of *Pharmaceutical Research*.

• **"New Approaches to the Treatment of Headaches in Adults and Children,"** a symposium sponsored by The Cleveland Clinic Foundation, is now available on videotape; for more information, write to CME Video, 1916 Old Cuthbert Road, B-13, Cherry Hill, NJ 08034-1457, or call 800-284-8433 (fax, 800-284-5964).

• Free, single copies of a booklet entitled **"Answers to Your Questions about Urinary Tract Infections"** are available to consumers; the booklet may be obtained by writing to Bladder Health Council, c/o American Foundation for Urologic Disease, 300 West Pratt Street, Suite 401, Baltimore, MD 21201, or by calling 800-242-2383.

Correction

Table of contents (August 1992). On page 657, the first author of the Drug Review is Paul W. Jungnickel.

Therapy Consultation

The Therapy Consultation *section provides brief advice, in question-and-answer format, on how to handle specific drug-therapy problems. Readers are invited to submit questions, which will be referred to a consultant for an answer. The problems should not be highly specialized or unusual, nor should they be mundane. Questions are answered briefly, based largely on the judgment and personal experience of the consultant, although selected references may be cited to substantiate the consultant's advice.*

Assistance in identifying Therapy Consultation *topics is provided by the drug information centers at Medical College of Virginia Hospitals, Richmond; University of California Medical Center, San Diego; and University of Michigan Medical Center, Ann Arbor.*

Transdermal scopolamine for hyperemesis gravidarum

Question: A patient with hyperemesis gravidarum has not responded to any of the conventional treatments. Transdermal scopolamine has been suggested as an alternative. Are scopolamine patches effective for this indication and, perhaps more importantly, what are the effects on the fetus?

Answer: Hyperemesis gravidarum (HG) is a severe, intractable form of nausea and vomiting of pregnancy that most often develops early in pregnancy. It occurs in approximately 3.5 women per 1000 pregnancies.[1] Women diagnosed as having HG may lose ≥5% of their body weight, develop fluid and electrolyte problems, manifest ketonuria, and suffer from various nutritional deficits.[1,2] HG may resolve spontaneously, but in some cases the mother may develop neurologic, hepatic, or renal complications.[2]

The main therapeutic goal is to correct fluid and electrolyte imbalances and then begin nutritional support and antiemetic therapy if needed. Enteral nutrition may be successful in some women, while others require parenteral nutrition.[1-3] Antiemetics (e.g., metoclopramide, phenothiazines, and pyridoxine) have been used for treating HG, with varying results. No data are available that demonstrate the effectiveness of antiemetics for HG.[4] During the past 10 years, few articles have addressed drug therapy for HG. This may reflect the views of authors who believe that drugs have limited use in the treatment of HG.[4] Behavior modification and psychotherapy are also used.

The question has been raised as to whether scopolamine administered via a transdermal patch might be useful in decreasing HG symptoms in women who do not respond adequately to other antiemetics or another form of therapy. Scopolamine is available as a transdermal therapeutic system (Transderm Scop, Ciba Consumer Pharmaceuticals) for the prevention of nausea and vomiting that occurs with motion sickness. The product is not indicated for HG.

We searched the literature and contacted personnel at Ciba to determine if scopolamine, administered by any route, had been used to treat HG. We found only one reference that addressed maternal scopolamine use during pregnancy before term.[5] Information from the Collaborative Perinatal Project, in which 50,282 mother–child pairs were monitored, revealed 309 mother–child pairs exposed to scopolamine during the first trimester, with 881 exposures occurring any time during pregnancy. No fetal malformations were observed in the 309 exposures; however, this small number of exposures may not have been sufficient to demonstrate malformations. Furthermore, the project was performed before the transdermal scopolamine (TDS) patch was available; therefore, none of the scopolamine exposures occurred via the transdermal route. When mother–child pairs exposed to all parasympatholytic agents were grouped, a trend toward minor malformations was observed.[5]

Scopolamine has been studied at the time of delivery in pregnant women and their fetuses. Kanto et al.[6] determined the pharmacokinetics of scopolamine administered intramuscularly to six women undergoing elective cesarean section; they measured scopolamine concentrations in maternal venous (MV) blood, umbilical venous (UV) blood, and umbilical arterial (UA) blood in 15 maternal–fetal pairs. Peak maternal serum concentrations occurred within 10 minutes after administration, and mean ± S.D. elimination half-lives were calculated as 59 ± 23 min. No differences in scopolamine concentrations were noted among MV, UV, and UA blood samples. From these results, it appears that scopolamine administered intramuscularly is rapidly absorbed and readily

Continued on page 833

Continued from page 830

distributes to the placenta.[6]

Although there is no information on the use of transdermal scopolamine before delivery, the antiemetic effect of TDS in women who received epidural morphine analgesia for elective cesarean delivery has been studied in a randomized, double-blind study in which TDS was compared with placebo patches.[7] Women in the TDS and placebo groups were evaluated periodically for the first 24 hours after surgery and once thereafter for nausea, vomiting, retching, pain relief, and adverse effects. A significant decrease in nausea, vomiting, and retching was observed in the TDS group ($p = \leq 0.5$). Examination of data for specific intervals within the 24-hour period showed no significant difference between groups for nausea, vomiting, or retching during hours 0 to 2 or for vomiting or retching during the hours 6 to 8. Women in the TDS group needed fewer antiemetic doses. From the study results, it appears that TDS is effective for reducing nausea, vomiting, and retching associated with epidural morphine analgesia in women who undergo cesarean section.

Effects observed in fetuses whose mothers receive scopolamine during delivery include tachycardia, decreased heart rate decelerations, and decreased beat-to-beat variability.[8]

Yu et al.[9] studied possible scopolamine and chlorpromazine mutagenicity and teratogenicity by determining the frequency of chromosomal aberration and sister-chromatid exchange (SCE). This was done by adding scopolamine or chlorpromazine in various concentrations to healthy adult lymphocytes. The effects of these drugs on lymphocytes were compared with effects observed when lymphocytes were exposed to saline (normal control) or mitomycin (positive control). The effects of scopolamine on chromosomal aberration and SCE were significantly greater than for controls, but the investigators observed more chromosomal aberration and SCE damage with chlorpromazine than with scopolamine. For scopolamine doses equivalent to 1/50 and 1/10 of the lethal dose in 50% of mice (LD_{50}), incidences of malformations in mice were 3.8% and 8.2%, respectively. Incidences were 0% when a saline control was used and 28.6% when a cod liver oil control was used. Incidences for chlorpromazine were 38.5% and 42.7%. Malformations observed in scopolamine-treated mice included deformed limbs and short trunks; chlorpromazine caused additional types of deformities. The investigators believe that these teratogenicity studies should be repeated. They stated that scopolamine should be used cautiously in pregnant women, especially between weeks 3 and 6 of gestation, when organ formation occurs.

A variety of serious malformations, including limb deformities, buphthalmia, gastroschisis, and exencephaly were noted on the 12th day of incubation in hen embryos that were injected with 100-200 μg of scopolamine hydrobromide. Microphthalmia, buphthalmia, hydrocephaly, and exencephaly were noted in New Zealand rabbit fetuses whose mothers received scopolamine hydrobromide (473 μg/kg or 520 μg/kg in drinking water) on days 10–14 of gestation. No malformations were noted in the offspring of rabbits that received scopolamine hydrobromide 37–184 μg/kg i.m. every 12 hours during the same gestational time.[10]

Acetylcholine and choline concentrations were measured in the fetuses and placentas of rabbits exposed to scopolamine hydrobromide (100 μg/kg) between days 8 and 15 of gestation. This study was done because drugs that decrease acetylcholine, choline acetylase, and acetylcholinesterase may have ontogenetic effects. Scopolamine reduced choline but not acetylcholine concentrations.[11]

Information provided in the Transderm Scop package insert states that no teratogenic effects were noted in study rats but that a "marginal embryotoxic effect" was observed when pregnant rabbits had serum concentrations 100 times that achievable with Transderm Scop in humans.[12] Transderm Scop is classified as pregnancy category C because of its possible teratogenic potential in animals. We believe this classification is justified.

Since HG occurs early in pregnancy, maternal scopolamine use during the first trimester could place the fetus at risk if humans are susceptible to teratogenic or mutagenic effects of scopolamine. We believe more studies are needed to resolve this issue. Not only is more information needed on scopolamine, but more information is also needed on the treatment of HG.

1. Barclay BA. Experience with enteral nutrition in the treatment of hyperemesis gravidarum. *Nutr Clin Pract.* 1990; 5:153-5.
2. Levine MG, Esser D. Total parenteral nutrition for the treatment of severe hyperemesis gravidarum: maternal nutritional effects and fetal outcome. *Obstet Gynecol.* 1988; 72:102-7.
3. Wolk RA, Rayburn WF. Parenteral nutrition in obstetric patients. *Nutr Clin Pract.* 1990; 5:139-52.
4. Leathem AM. Safety and efficacy of antiemetics used to treat nausea and vomiting in pregnancy. *Clin Pharm.* 1986; 5:660-8.
5. Heinonen OP, Slone D, Shapiro S. Birth defects and drugs in pregnancy. Littleton, MA: Publishing Sciences Group; 1977.
6. Kanto J, Kentala E, Kaila T et al. Pharmacokinetics of scopolamine during caesarean section: relationship between serum concentration and effect. *Acta Anaesthesiol Scand.* 1989; 33:482-6.
7. Kotelko DM, Rottman RL, Wright WC et al. Transdermal scopolamine decreases nausea and vomiting following cesarean section in patients receiving epidural morphine. *Anesthesiology.* 1989; 71:675-8.
8. Briggs GG, Freeman RK, Yaffe SJ. Scopolamine. Drugs in pregnancy and lactation. 3rd ed. Baltimore: Williams & Wilkins; 1990:572.
9. Yu JF, Yang YS, Wang WY et al. Mutagenicity and teratogenicity of chlorpromazine and scopolamine. *Chin Med J (Peking).* 1988; 101:339-45.
10. McBride WG, Vardy PH, French J. Effects of scopolamine hydrobromide on the development of the chick and rabbit embryo. *Aust J Biol Sci.* 1982; 35:173-8.
11. McBride WG, Hicks LJ. Acetylcholine and choline levels in rabbit fetuses exposed to anticholinergics. *Int J Developmental Neuroscience.* 1987; 5:117-25.
12. Ciba Consumer Pharmaceuticals. Transderm Scop package insert. Edison, NJ: 1988 Feb.

ROSALIE SAGRAVES, PHARM.D., Professor of Pharmacy Practice
DOUGLAS C. ANDERSON, JR., PHARM.D., Pharmacotherapy Fellow in Adult Medicine

College of Pharmacy
University of Oklahoma Health Sciences Center
Oklahoma City, OK 73190

Drug Review

Recombinant interferon gamma for treatment of chronic granulomatous disease and other disorders

ANN M. BOLINGER AND MARY A. TAEUBEL

Abstract: The chemistry, biological activity, and pharmacokinetics of γ-interferon and recombinant interferon gamma are reviewed, and the agent's clinical efficacy, adverse effects, and dosage and administration for the treatment of chronic granulomatous disease (CGD) and other disorders are described.

Endogenous γ-interferon is a 166-amino-acid protein encoded by a single gene on chromosome 12. Recombinant human interferon gamma is purified from *Escherichia coli* as a monomer containing 139 amino acids. Gamma-interferon has antiviral, immunomodulatory, and antiproliferative activity. Serum concentrations of recombinant interferon gamma increase in proportion to the dose. Clearance after i.m. or s.c. administration fits a two-compartment model. The half-life is 3.5–7.5 hours, and bioavailability is 89%. Evidence that recombinant interferon gamma can enhance phagocytic oxidative metabolism led to its evaluation for use in the treatment of CGD. Clinical studies showed that the agent decreases the frequency of serious infections in patients with CGD. Recombinant interferon gamma has shown only limited success in the treatment of metastatic renal cell carcinoma (RCC), both as a single agent and in combination with recombinant interferon alfa. Similarly, although interferons appear to be able to change cytogenetic abnormalities in some patients with Philadelphia chromosome-positive chronic myelogenous leukemia, therapy with recombinant interferon gamma has led to minimal success. However, the agent has produced some encouraging results in atopic dermatitis. The adverse effects of recombinant interferon gamma in patients with CGD usually consist only of fever, chills, headache, and erythema. The recommended dosage in CGD-afflicted children whose body surface area is greater than 0.5 sq m is 50 μg/sq m given by s.c. injection three times a week for life.

Recombinant interferon gamma has given new hope to patients with CGD. Although the drug is very expensive, the cost may be offset by fewer hospitalizations to treat infection.

Index terms: Dosage; Drug administration; γ-Interferon; Granulomatous disease; Immunotherapy; Interferon gamma-1b; Pharmacokinetics; Toxicity
Clin Pharm. 1992; 11:834-50

Interferons are proteins that, along with interleukins, tumor necrosis factor, platelet-activating factor, and lymphotoxins, have been identified as factors involved in regulating the inflammatory response. Interferons were named after their discovery in 1957. During a study of viral interference, Isaacs and Lindenmann[1] identified a compound that induced cellular resistance to viral infection. In addition to inhibiting viral replication, interferons were found to be involved in the host defense system through activation of macrophages, leading to enhanced antimicrobial activity and augmented tumor-cell killing.

Interferons belong to a system of regulatory cytokines that become active participants in the host defense system during infection. Although initially it was believed that there was just one compound, it soon became clear that the interferons are a group of functionally and structurally related molecules. Three

ANN M. BOLINGER, PHARM.D., is Associate Professor of Clinical Pharmacy, Division of Clinical Pharmacy, School of Pharmacy, University of California, San Francisco, and Clinical Pharmacist in Pediatrics, University of California at San Francisco Medical Center, San Francisco. MARY A. TAEUBEL, PHARM.D., is Clinical Pharmacist in Pediatrics, Humana Hospital–Michael Reese, Chicago, IL, and Clinical Assistant Professor, Department of Pharmacy Practice, College of Pharmacy, University of Illinois at Chicago.

Address reprint requests to Dr. Bolinger at the School of Pharmacy, University of California, San Francisco, 521 Parnassus Avenue, Room C-152, Box 0622, San Francisco, CA 94143.

This is **article 680-204-9226** in the **ASHP Continuing Education System**; it qualifies for 1.0 hour of continuing-education credit. See page 892 for learning objectives and test questions.

classes of interferons have been described: α, β, and γ.[2] It is likely that other interferons exist, although they have yet to be identified.[3]

Alpha-interferon and β-interferon are described as type I, or classical, interferons, as they were the first interferons to be characterized; they are produced by leukocytes and fibroblasts, respectively.[4] Gamma-interferon was designated as the third type of interferon in 1965 and is described as a type II, or immune, interferon; it is produced by T lymphocytes and natural killer (NK) cells.[5] Whereas α-interferon and β-interferon are acid-stable compounds that are structurally related and genetically encoded on the same chromosome, γ-interferon is an acid-labile compound that is encoded on a different chromosome.[5] In addition, α-interferon and β-interferon exert biological activity by binding to the same cell-membrane receptor, while γ-interferon binds to a separate cell-surface receptor.[5,6]

Alpha-interferon and β-interferon increase expression of the class I major histocompatibility complex (MHC), enhance the activity of NK cells, interfere with viral replication, and decrease cell replication.[2,5,7] Not only does γ-interferon have the same biological activity as α-interferon and β-interferon, it can activate macrophages, increase expression of the class II MHC, and generate cytotoxic T lymphocytes.[7]

Investigators have distinguished two types of human γ-interferon receptors differing in molecular weight, acid stability, and the regulation of receptor expression.[8] These differences may be responsible for the various effects of γ-interferon on different types of cells. Epithelial cells, hematopoietic cell lines, and fibroblasts have all been found to have γ-interferon receptors.[6]

Recombinant DNA technology has made large amounts of purified interferons available for research, and many forms of γ-interferon are being investigated. Recombinant interferon gamma-1b is currently marketed in the United States by Genentech, Inc. (South San Francisco, CA), under the brand name Actimmune. It has received FDA-approved labeling for use in the treatment of chronic granulomatous disease (CGD) and has been granted orphan drug status because fewer than 200,000 people in the United States have this disease.

This article reviews the chemistry, biological activity, and pharmacokinetics of γ-interferon and recombinant interferon gamma and describes the clinical efficacy, adverse effects, and dosage and administration of recombinant interferon gamma for the treatment of CGD and other selected disorders.

Chemistry

Endogenous γ-interferon is a heterogeneous protein of 166 amino acids encoded by a single gene on chromosome 12.[9] Sodium dodecyl sulfate–polyacrylamide gel electrophoresis has shown that there are three separate monomeric forms of γ-interferon with molecular weights of 15,500, 20,000, and 25,000.[2] The different molecular weights can be explained by the extent of glycosylation. Natural γ-interferon under physiological conditions has been proposed to exist as a dimer with a molecular weight of 40,000–60,000.[2] Clusters of basic residues occur in the protein at positions 89–92 and 131–134 and are thought to be responsible for the loss of biological activity at low pH.[9]

Recombinant human interferon gamma is purified from *Escherichia coli* as a monomer containing 139 amino acids with a molecular weight of approximately 17,000. Protein variants of recombinant interferon gamma are identified by a number indicating the sequence at position 1 and a letter characterizing position 139. Recombinant interferon gamma-1b has hydrogen and methionine at position 1 and a hydroxyl group at position 139.[10] The activity of interferon gamma-1b is 3×10^7 units per milligram of protein, which is consistent with that of natural human γ-interferon.[2] A unit of activity is based on antiviral activity against encephalomyocarditis virus.

Biological Activity

Antiviral Activity. Interferons have a myriad of biological effects. All three classes of interferons are capable of inducing an antiviral state in host cells. Different steps of viral infection and replication are thought to be influenced by the antiviral state, including attachment, penetration, uncoating, transcription, assembly, and maturation. In addition, interferons inhibit viral translation through the induction and activation of two pathways, the 2,5-oligoadenylate synthetase pathway and the eukaryotic protein-synthesis initiation factor protein kinase phosphatase pathway.[11] Inducing 2,5-oligoadenylate synthetase leads to degradation of viral messenger RNA, while activation of protein-synthesis initiation factor inhibits viral translation.[12,13] While α-interferon and β-interferon are available as the host's first line of defense against certain viral infections, γ-interferon is produced only after T cells become sensitized to viral antigens. Gamma-interferon directly induces cellular resistance to cytomegalovirus, herpes simplex virus, and adenovirus in vitro, although the potential clinical value is unclear.[14-16] The major role of γ-interferon during viral infection appears to be activation of immune reactions rather than a direct antiviral effect.

Immunomodulation. Gamma-interferon must be present for the enhanced antimicrobial activity resulting from lymphokine-induced macrophage activation to occur.[17] Neutralization of γ-interferon with monoclonal antibody treatment prevents lymphokines from releasing hydrogen peroxide from macrophages, an activity associated with the activated state.[18] The ability of γ-interferon to regulate macrophage activation and boost antimicrobial activity appears to be particularly important in the elimination or inhibition of certain intracellular pathogens, including *Toxoplasma gondii*, *Leishmania donovani*, and *Chlamydia psittaci*.[19,20]

The induction of antigen processing and signaling by antigen-presenting cells may be another central function of γ-interferon.[21] The presence of γ-interferon rapidly increases class II MHC expression on the cell membranes of macrophages. The quantity of class II MHC on the macrophage cell membrane is crucial in enabling the cell to function as an antigen presenter. Gamma-interferon also enhances the release of interleukin-1, which is important in the activation of T cells.[21]

In addition to its role in stimulating cell-mediated responses, γ-interferon seems to participate in the regulation of humoral responses, although the latter role is not well understood. Investigators have found that γ-interferon can inhibit the proliferation and differentiation of normal and neoplastic B lymphocytes.[22] The inhibitory effect of γ-interferon appears to be responsible for the failure of some helper T-cell clones to stimulate B-cell maturation. Researchers have also demonstrated the ability of γ-interferon to inhibit the proliferation and stimulation of class II antigen expression and immunoglobulin E (IgE) secretion in B cells induced by B-cell stimulatory factor 1 (also known as interleukin-4).[23-25]

Gamma-interferon has a role in enhancing NK-cell activity. NK cells are effector cells derived from the bone marrow that exhibit spontaneous cytotoxicity without prior sensitization. NK cells act selectively against tumor cells and virus-infected cells and are therefore thought to be important in host defense. Gamma-interferon-mediated enhancement of NK-cell activity appears to depend on the NK-cell source and the nature of the target cell. Conversely, interferons can protect certain target cells (usually normal cells) against NK-cell activity. Thus, depending on the biological situation, γ-interferon may exhibit opposite effects on interactions of effectors and target cells.[25] Viruses, bacteria, mitogens, and cells can stimulate NK cells into making interferons. NK-cell production of γ-interferon provides an alternative route for macrophage activation in the presence of T-cell deficiency states.[25]

Effects on Tumor Cells. Interferons appear to have direct antiproliferative effects on tumor cells, as well as indirect effects through the activation of other mechanisms. The antiproliferative activities of interferons were first recognized in 1962.[26] Interferons decrease the growth and proliferation of both normal cells and tumor cells by prolonging the cell cycle. There are clear differences in sensitivity to the antiproliferative effect, which explains why some tumor cells may be very sensitive while others are resistant.[27] Although the role is not well defined, it is possible that interferon-induced 2,5-oligoadenylate synthetase and protein phosphokinase are involved in the actions of interferon on cell proliferation.[27] Other direct effects have been theorized, including an ability of interferons to reverse the phenotype of some malignant cells, possibly through an effect on oncogene expression.

Pharmacokinetics

Although information is limited, the pharmacokinetic properties of recombinant interferon gamma have been examined after intravenous, intramuscular, or subcutaneous administration in patients with a variety of malignancies. Concentrations in serum appear to increase proportionally with increasing doses. In a study by Kurzrock et al.,[28] 10 patients with metastatic cancer were given intramuscular and intravenous bolus doses of recombinant interferon gamma. The exposure time (concentration × time) after intramuscular injection increased from 1029 ng/mL · min for a dose of 100 μg/sq m to 24,640 ng/mL · min for a dose of 2500 μg/sq m. Exposure time after intravenous bolus doses ranged from 275 to 15,267 ng/mL · min for doses of 100 and 2500 μg/sq m, respectively.

Clearance of recombinant interferon gamma occurs rapidly after intravenous bolus administration and can be described by a one-compartment model.[28] The half-life has been reported to be 25–35 minutes, which is similar to the half-life of native γ-interferon.[28,29] After intramuscular or subcutaneous administration, absorption of interferon gamma is slow, with peak concentrations occurring within 6–13 hours.[17,30] Clearance after intramuscular or subcutaneous administration fits a two-compartment model; the half-life ranges from 3.5 to 7.5 hours.[30] Bioavailability after intramuscular or subcutaneous administration appears to be somewhat lower than after intravenous administration, with the manufacturer reporting 89% absorption of interferon gamma-1b given by these routes.[a]

It is not known whether the body metabolizes recombinant interferon gamma. Trace amounts have been detected in the urine of animals given an intravenous dose of 500 μg/kg. However, when an intravenous, intramuscular, or subcutaneous dose of 100 μg/sq m was given to healthy volunteers, recombinant interferon gamma could not be detected in the urine. No accumulation of the agent was observed after the administration of 100 μg/kg for 12 consecutive days in 38 healthy men.[a]

To date, pharmacokinetic studies in patients with CGD have not been reported.

Clinical Efficacy

Chronic Granulomatous Disease. *Description of the Disease.* When a phagocyte encounters opsonized bacteria or other acceptable stimuli, it activates a metabolic pathway that produces potent antimicrobial agents (Figure 1).[31,32] CGD is an uncommon inherited disorder in which there is a deficiency in phagocytic oxidative metabolism, or the respiratory burst. CGD was first described in 1957 in boys with recurrent bacterial infections and infiltration of several organs with granulomas; the patients died at a young age.[33,34] A decade later, it was discovered that CGD was related to a defect in bactericidal activity.

Figure 1. Metabolic pathway activated by phagocytosis. A microorganism interacts with the phagocytic-cell receptor, stimulating an enzyme complex affiliated with the plasma membrane of the phagocytic cell. The enzyme system moves oxygen (O_2) from the environment into the plasma membrane and reduces it to superoxide anion (O_2^-), which is then converted by superoxide dismutase to hydrogen peroxide (H_2O_2). Superoxide anion and hydrogen peroxide are then converted to a deadly combination of oxidizing radicals, such as hydroxyl radical (· OH), and oxidizing halogens, such as free chlorine (· Cl). The process has been labeled the respiratory burst, even though it is unrelated to cell respiration or energy generation. Adapted from reference 32, with permission.

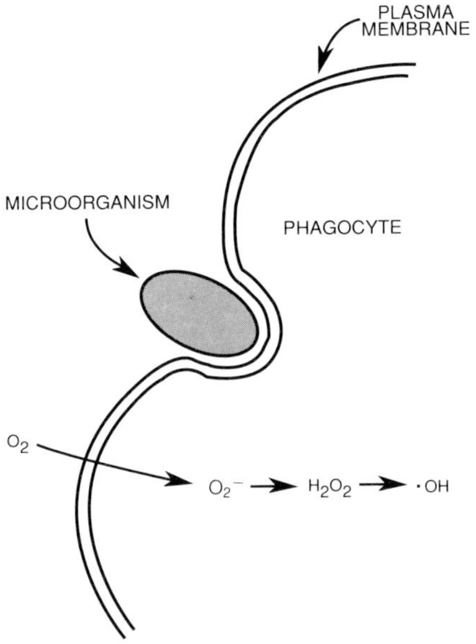

Neutrophils in patients with CGD showed normal chemotaxis, engulfment, and degranulation but failed to produce superoxide anion and other toxic metabolites necessary for host defense. During the 1970s, reduced nicotinamide adenine dinucleotide phosphate (NADPH) oxidase, the enzyme responsible for the respiratory burst, was defined.[34] Recently, there has been substantial progress in understanding the respiratory burst and the biology of CGD (Figure 2).[31-35] CGD is now recognized as a heterogeneous class of disorders characterized by defective phagocytic oxidative metabolism.

CGD is a rare disease; the prevalence is estimated to be 1 in 1 million.[35] Patients have many recurrent infections that are severe, lengthy, and hard to treat. The infections usually begin at an early age, and most patients are diagnosed in the first few years of life. Some patients have milder forms of CGD and are not diagnosed until adolescence or early adulthood.[34]

CGD may be inherited through X chromosome-linked transmission or an autosomal recessive gene. X chromosome-linked inheritance is responsible for about 60% of the cases. In families with X chromosome-linked CGD, the disease usually affects only men. Approximately 40% of cases are due to autosomal recessive inheritance. This form affects men and women with equal frequency.[31] A very small percentage of patients (less than 1%) have autosomal dominant inheritance.[35]

One method of classifying the various types of CGD is by determining the location of the defective component of the oxidase. The defect is broadly categorized as membrane bound or cytosolic and then is further classified by the specific component (Table 1).[33,36-44] Classic X chromosome-linked CGD is caused by a defect in the gp91-*phox* gene and is clinically manifested by an absence of detectable cytochrome *b*; the absence of gp91-*phox* appears to lead to a secondary absence of p22-*phox*.[33]

CGD is diagnosed by identifying an abnormality in NADPH oxidase. The respiratory burst can be evaluated through numerous measurements, including tests of oxygen consumption; the production of hydrogen peroxide, superoxide anion, hypoclorous acid, or oxidizing radicals; the release on exhalation of carbon dioxide labeled with carbon 14; and the chemiluminescence of phagocytes.[31,35] The most commonly used method is the nitroblue tetrazolium test. In this test, oxidative products reduce the water-soluble, yellow tetrazolium dye to an insoluble, deep-blue precipitate (formazan). Phagocytes from patients with CGD produce little or no superoxide anion; therefore little or no blue is seen. The inability of activated neutrophils to reduce tetrazolium dye is almost always diagnostic for CGD.[31]

Since the basic defect in CGD results in failure of the phagocyte to kill microorganisms, patients experience recurrent infections caused by catalase-positive bacteria (e.g., *Staphylococcus aureus*) or fungal organisms (e.g., *Aspergillus* species). Patients do not have trouble with common catalase-negative bacteria such as pneumococci or *Haemophilus influenzae*; these bacteria produce and excrete hydrogen peroxide, thereby providing the powerful oxidant that the phagocyte cannot produce.[45] Infections are usually seated in such areas as the skin, lungs, mucous membranes, and other environmental barriers that are constantly challenged by bacteria.[45]

Typically, infections in CGD consist of skin lesions, lymphadenitis, abscesses, respiratory-tract infections, and osteomyelitis.[31,33,35,45] Although skin infections are common, they are seldom life-threatening.[35] More serious infections involve the respiratory tract or abscess formation in the lungs or liver. Infections may develop anywhere, however, and have even been found in the conjunctivae, peritoneum, mediastinum, and urinary bladder.[31]

Other features of CGD are granulomatous lesions and obstructive complications. Granulomas can form in any organ system; the exact etiologic mechanism is unknown. It is possible that defective phagocytosis causes persistent inflammation.[45] Because CGD causes difficulty in eradicating microorganisms, they remain in the vacuoles of macrophages or neutrophils and lead to a chronic inflammatory state. Granulomas are formed as the body tries to wall off the areas of chronic infection.[33] The clinical appear-

Figure 2. Components of nicotinamide adenine dinucleotide phosphate (NADPH) oxidase and the metabolic abnormalities in chronic granulomatous disease (CGD). The glycolytic and hexose monophosphate pathways produce NADPH and stimulate NADPH oxidase, which catalyzes the one-electron (e^-) reduction of oxygen (O_2) to superoxide anion (O_2^-), oxidizing NADPH and producing hydrogen ion. NADPH oxidase is a multicomponent complex that, in resting cells, is separated between the plasma membrane and the cytoplasm. The membrane-associated components include a flavoprotein (flavin adenine dinucleotide [FAD]) and heterodimeric cytochrome b_{558}, which is composed of a 91-kDa glycoprotein (gp91-*phox*) and a 22-kDa peptide (p22-*phox*). The cytosol factors include a 47-kDa polypeptide (p47-*phox*), a 67-kDa polypeptide (p67-*phox*), and the NADPH-binding component (N). The cytosol factors, especially p47-*phox*, are required for activation of the respiratory burst. How the components of the oxidase are assembled and the exact function of each are not understood. FAD and cytochrome b_{558} pass electrons from NADPH to oxygen. X chromosome-linked CGD (X) involves a defect in gp91-*phox*; autosomal recessive CGD (AR) involves a defect in p22-*phox*, p47-*phox*, or p67-*phox*. PO_4 = phosphate. Adapted from reference 35, with permission.

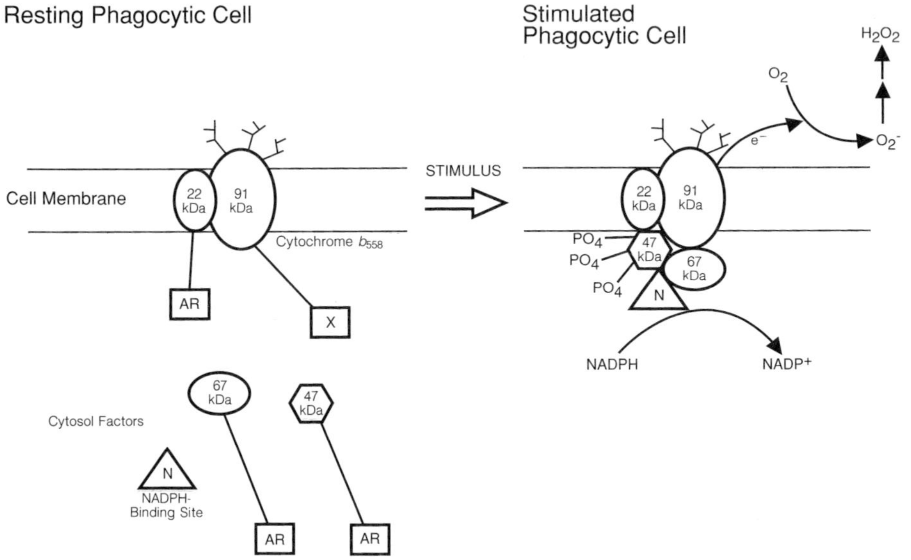

Table 1.
Classification of Types of Chronic Granulomatous Disease (CGD)

Cell Location, Defective Enzyme Component	Enzyme Defect	Inheritance[a]	Cytochrome b_{558} Spectrum[b]	Superoxide Anion Production	% CGD Cases
Membrane, gp91-*phox*	Absent	X	None	None	52
	Nonfunctional	X	Normal	None	3
	Partial deficiency	X	Low	Very low	2
	K_m defect[c]	X	Very low	Very low	<1
Membrane, p22-*phox*	Absent	AR	None	None	5
	Nonfunctional	AR	Normal	None	<1
Cytosol, p47-*phox*	Absent	AR	Normal	None	33
Cytosol, p67-*phox*	Absent	AR	Normal	None	5

[a]X = X chromosome-linked, AR = autosomal recessive.
[b]Amount of cytochrome b_{558} measured or present.
[c]Michaelis constant (K_m) for reduced nicotinamide adenine dinucleotide phosphate (NADPH) is altered.

ance usually involves a mass lesion or obstruction of the small intestine, esophagus, stomach, bladder, ureter, or other hollow organ.[32] Inflammatory changes in the lungs may lead to areas of focal necrosis, causing fibrosis and other lesions that result in decreased pulmonary function and possibly death.[31,33]

Another hallmark of CGD is an overactive reticuloendothelial system. One group of authors[45] observed hepatosplenomegaly and lymphadenopathy in more than 50% of patients.

The management of CGD has two primary goals: (1) to prevent and cure infections and (2) to manage the obstructive complications.[31] Aggressive supportive care continues to be the cornerstone of therapy.[32] The only cure is allogeneic bone marrow transplantation, but this treatment has complications and has brought only limited success.[33]

The standard treatment regimen for acute infections consists of high doses of appropriate antimicrobial agents administered for prolonged periods.[33] Abscesses should be treated with antimicrobial therapy, and prompt surgical drainage is necessary for both therapeutic and diagnostic reasons. However, caution should be used, as an increased risk of operative morbidity and mortality has been reported in patients with CGD.[33,45] Corticosteroids are contraindicated except in cases of invasive pulmonary disease and obstructive lesions of the genitourinary or gastrointestinal tract.[33,46-48]

Antimicrobial prophylaxis has changed the clinical course of CGD.[45,49-55] Although no prospective, controlled trials have been performed, clinical experience indicates that prophylactic antimicrobials (e.g., trimethoprim–sulfamethoxazole, dicloxacillin sodium) may result in fewer infections and improve the general well-being of patients with CGD.[56-58] Reports suggest that antimicrobial prophylaxis may increase the interval between life-threatening infections[56] or increase the length of infection-free periods.[45,57,59] While it appears that antimicrobial prophylaxis has potential benefits, some clinicians believe that it may contribute to an increased incidence of chronic complications and fungal infections.[45,46] Life-threatening infections remain a serious concern.

Uncontrolled Trials. Progress in understanding CGD has raised hopes for a cure or an ameliorative therapy. Pharmacologic correction of the defective phagocytes might be achieved by altering oxidative metabolism.[35] A 1983 study suggested that recombinant interferon gamma could enhance the respiratory burst in normal phagocytes.[60] As a result, in vitro and in vivo studies were performed to examine the effect of recombinant interferon gamma on phagocytes from patients with CGD.[39,61,62] The trials attempted to correlate the pattern of inheritance or the presence or absence of cytochrome *b* with an increase in superoxide anion production. All the trials evaluated superoxide anion production, while some also considered cytochrome *b* content and NADPH oxidase kinetics. In the in vitro studies (Table 2), phagocytes from patients with CGD were incubated with recombinant interferon gamma. Phagocytes from some of the patients responded with an increase in superoxide anion production. The trials showed that the patients most likely to respond to recombinant interferon gamma in vitro were patients with detectable cytochrome *b*. However, this finding was not all-inclusive, as some patients with X chromosome-linked CGD had a response and some patients with detectable cytochrome *b* did not respond.

For the most part, the in vivo responses (Table 3) paralleled the in vitro responses, although one patient whose phagocytes did not respond to in vitro therapy responded to in vivo administration of the drug. The trials suggest that in vitro testing of phagocytes might be useful in predicting increased superoxide anion production in vivo. This application is limited, however, since it does not exclude the possibility of an in vivo response. In addition, none of the trials examined the possible correlation between the in vivo effect of recombinant interferon gamma and the clinical outcome.

Controlled Trial. Since in vivo and in vitro studies indicated that recombinant interferon gamma can partially correct the metabolic defect in phagocytes of patients with CGD, a trial was designed to determine whether the agent could decrease the frequency and severity of infection and improve the chronic conditions and inflammation.[63] This study, the International Chronic Granulomatous Disease Cooperative Study, was a randomized, double-blind, placebo-controlled trial involving 128 patients from 13 centers in four countries. Patients were excluded for abnormal renal or hepatic function, active infection, severe heart disease, seizure disorders, or a life expectancy of less than three months. Women who were pregnant, breast feeding, or not practicing effective contraception were also excluded. Patients taking prophylactic antimicrobials could be enrolled. Patients taking corticosteroids could be enrolled only if they had been maintained on prednisone 10 mg/day or less for at least one month.

Patients were randomly enrolled and stratified according to the pattern of inheritance, use of prophylactic antimicrobials, use of corticosteroids, and location (United States or Europe). Sixty-three patients received recombinant interferon gamma and 65 patients received placebo (recombinant interferon gamma diluent) three times a week (on Monday, Wednesday, and Friday) for up to 12 months. Doses were based on body surface area (BSA). For a BSA greater than 0.5 sq m, the dose was 50 μg/sq m, and for a BSA less than 0.5 sq m, the dose was 1.5 μg/kg. The primary endpoint was the time from enrollment to the first serious infection, defined as an infection necessitating hospitalization and intravenous antimicrobial therapy. Quantitative estimates were used to evaluate the clinical conditions related to CGD and were made by using two scoring systems, a visual analogue scale to measure severity and a 7-point system to measure changes.

The two groups were comparable when they entered the study with respect to age, sex, pattern of inheritance of CGD, and use of prophylactic antimicrobials and corticosteroids. The median age was 15 years, but there were 37 patients less than nine years of age. The average duration of therapy was 8.9 months. Fifty-seven and 54 patients completed the study in the treatment and placebo groups, respectively. Six patients were removed from the treatment group and 11 patients from the placebo group because of adverse effects, accidental unblinding, or their request. Four patients were removed from the treatment group after reactions related to the agent: two patients for worsening constitutional symptoms, one patient for skin rash, and the remaining patient for worsening granulomatous colitis.

Of the 65 patients in the placebo group, 30 (46%) had a serious infection, compared with 14 (22%) of the 63 patients in the interferon gamma group (p = 0.0006). There was a 67% reduction in the relative risk of a serious infection during interferon gamma therapy. There were 56 serious infections in the placebo group and 20 serious infections in the treatment

Table 2.
In Vitro Trials of Recombinant Interferon Gamma for Treatment of Chronic Granulomatous Disease (CGD)

				Baseline		Response		
Ref.	Regimen	No. Patients	CGD Classification[a]	Cytochrome b_{558}	Superoxide Anion Production	Cytochrome b_{558}	Superoxide Anion Production	Comment
61	Granulocytes and monocytes incubated with 100 units/mL for 40 min to 4 hr	4	X	None	None	None	None	Patients who responded also had increased enzyme maximum velocity of NADPH[c] oxidase
		3	X	None[b]	Low	None	Increased	
		1	AR	Present	Low	Low	Low	
		1	AR	Present	None	None	None	
62	Monocytes cultured with 100 units/mL for 3 days	13	X	None	None	...[d]	Increased[e]	After treatment, superoxide anion production differed between group with cytochrome *b* and group without cytochrome *b* ($p < 0.01$)
		1	X	Present	None	...	None	
		1	AR	None	None	...	None	
		13	AR	Present	0[f], low[g]	...	Increased[f]	
		2	AD	Present	Low	...	Increased	

[a]X = X chromosome-linked, AR = autosomal recessive, AD = autosomal dominant.
[b]Low levels of cytochrome b_{558} were detected in two of these patients, according to Dinauer et al.[40]
[c]NADPH = reduced nicotinamide adenine dinucleotide phosphate.
[d]Information was not reported.
[e]Four patients.
[f]Twelve patients.
[g]One patient.

group ($p < 0.0001$). Interferon gamma was most effective in decreasing the frequency of adenitis, abscesses, cellulitis, and pulmonary infections. The placebo group had a total of 1493 hospital days, compared with 497 days for the treatment group; the average hospital stay for members of each group was 48 and 32 days, respectively. Patients under 10 years of age showed the greatest benefit.

With respect to chronic conditions associated with CGD, no significant benefit or detrimental effect of recombinant interferon gamma was identified. In contrast to previous reports,[39,61,62] there was no significant difference between the groups in superoxide anion production or bacterial killing.

In response to the results of the Cooperative Study, Mouy and colleagues[64] suggested that the clinical benefit of recombinant interferon gamma may be limited to patients with CGD who have an unusually high risk of infection. Their suggestion was based on data indicating that patients at centers in Paris and Zurich who were receiving only trimethoprim–sulfamethoxazole prophylaxis had a lower infection rate than did the placebo group in the Cooperative Study; Mouy et al.[64] reported an infection rate of 1.8 and 2.0 infections per 100 months for patients in each city, respectively. In comparison, the Cooperative Study showed the infection rate to be 9.7 per 100 months for the placebo group receiving prophylactic antimicrobials and 3.6 per 100 months for those receiving the combination of antimicrobial prophylaxis and recombinant interferon gamma. In addition, the decrease in the rate of serious infections reported in the Cooperative Study was not as dramatic for patients studied at the European centers.[64] It is unclear why infections were more frequent in patients in North America. A possible explanation is that diagnosis and treatment may differ between the two regions, influencing the primary endpoint of the time between enrollment and the first serious infection requiring intravenous antimicrobial therapy and hospitalization.[65]

Data from the Cooperative Study indicate that recombinant interferon gamma is safe and effective therapy for reducing the frequency of severe infections in patients with CGD. The results suggest that interferon gamma, either alone or in combination with prophylactic antimicrobials, should be used to help prevent infections in these patients. Although the study established an effective dose, dosage interval, and route of administration, additional trials must be done to determine the optimum dosage, and long-term follow-up is needed to evaluate the benefits and risks of extended therapy.

The Cooperative Study failed to show a correlation between the clinical benefit of recombinant interferon gamma and improvement in phagocytic function. The exact mechanisms by which recombinant interferon gamma improves host defenses in CGD remain elusive. The investigators proposed several mechanisms by which recombinant interferon gamma may bolster host defenses, including augmentation of oxygen-independent antimicrobial pathways of phagocytosis, improvement in the function of other components of the immune system such as T cells or B cells, failure to detect the changes in superoxide anion production, and generation of hydrogen peroxide in response to enhancement of the oxidase. Further study is necessary to characterize the effect of recombinant

Table 3.
In Vivo Trials of Recombinant Interferon Gamma for Treatment of Chronic Granulomatous Disease (CGD)

				Baseline		Response		
Ref.	Regimen	No. Patients	CGD Classification[a]	Cytochrome *b*558	Superoxide Anion Production	Cytochrome *b*558	Superoxide Anion Production	Comment
62	10 μg/sq m s.c. (test dose) followed 6 days later by 10 μg/sq m s.c. q.d. for 5 days	1	AR[b]	Present	None	Increased	Increased[c]	Presence of cytochrome *b*558 associated with augmented response. Enhanced bactericidal activity of monocytes and neutrophils against *Staphylococcus aureus*
	10 μg/sq m s.c. q.d. for 5 days	1	AD[b]	Present	Present	...[d]	Increased[e]	
	50 μg/sq m s.c. 3 days/wk for 2 wk	1	AR[b]	Present	Present	...	Increased[e]	
39	100 μg/sq m s.c. q.d. for 2 days	1	X classic[f]	None	None	Increased[g]	Increased[c]	Increased granulocyte microbial activity against *S. aureus* in all patients. Positive responses in vivo, even in patient without response in vitro
		2	X variant[b]	Present	Present	Increased[h]	Increased[c]	
		1	X variant[b]	None	Present	Increased[h]	Increased[c]	

[a]AR = autosomal recessive, AD = autosomal dominant, X = X chromosome-linked.
[b]Positive in vitro response to treatment with interferon gamma.
[c]By both monocytes and granulocytes.
[d]Information was not reported.
[e]Monocytes only.
[f]No in vitro response to treatment with interferon gamma.
[g]Increased to 30–50% of normal.
[h]Increased to approximately 10% of normal.

interferon gamma on the respiratory burst and other defense mechanisms.

Metastatic Renal Cell Carcinoma (RCC). Approximately 20,000 Americans are affected by RCC every year. Some 40–50% of patients have distant metastases at the time of diagnosis and will die of their disease.[66] The median survival time in patients with metastatic disease is 6–12 months; fewer than 10% survive two years.[66,67] Even among patients with no initial metastases, 50% experience tumor progression in subsequent years.[68] The only curative treatment for localized RCC is to completely remove the affected kidney, adrenal gland, and adjacent lymph nodes.[68] Metastatic RCC has been treated systemically with cytotoxic agents, radiation, and hormonal agents. Objective responses have been observed in 15–20% of patients after single-agent or combination chemotherapy, with vinblastine sulfate being the best single agent.[69,70]

Studies have suggested that human interferons and other biological response modifiers may show promise in the therapy of metastatic RCC. Recombinant interleukin-2 recently received FDA-approved labeling for use in metastatic RCC. Although studies have shown an overall response rate of 15%, therapy is associated with many adverse effects.[71] In general, patients with soft-tissue metastases, a limited metastatic burden, and good performance status appear to have a chance of responding to biological response modifiers, while patients with bone lesions, central nervous system metastases, and primary tumors rarely respond.[67] Of the human interferons, recombinant interferon alfa is the agent most widely used in treating metastatic RCC. Although dosages and schedules vary among studies of the use of recombinant interferon alfa in the treatment of RCC, the overall objective response rate is approximately 16.4%.[72,73]

Clinical experience with recombinant interferon gamma in the treatment of metastatic RCC is not as extensive. Recombinant interferon gamma has demonstrated activity against RCC in model systems. Studies of recombinant interferon gamma are complicated by differences in the source of the agent, route of administration, dosage, schedule, dose-modification strategy, and patient-selection and response criteria. Researchers have used intravenous, intramuscular, or subcutaneous administration continuously or intermittently, at high or low dosages or as an escalating dosage. Typically, a small number of patients with advanced tumor stages are enrolled in these studies.

In most trials, a complete response has been defined as the disappearance of all lesions for at least one month and a partial response as a 50% or greater reduction in the sum of the products of the diameters (length times width) of measurable lesions, with no existing lesion increasing in size or no new lesions developing. Stable disease refers to no progression or evidence of partial or complete remission. The objective response rate refers to the sum of the partial response rate and the complete response rate. In trials of recombinant interferon gamma only, the objective response rates have ranged from 0% to 32% (Table 4).[68,73-82] In two of the studies with the highest objective response rates, the dose of recombinant interferon gamma was 100 μg/sq m.[78,79] Several research groups have used combination therapy consisting of recombinant interferon gamma and escalating dosages of recombinant interferon alfa (Table 5).[66,67,76,83,84] From their reports, it is difficult to make any conclusions about the effectiveness of recombinant interferon gamma. In addition, the order in which the two agents are given may be important with respect to adverse effects and efficacy. Objective response rates in trials of the combination therapy have ranged from 0% to 28%.

Recombinant interferon gamma has shown limited success in the treatment of metastatic RCC, both as single-agent therapy and in combination with recombinant interferon alfa. Clinical experience has not yet defined the optimum dosage or the best agents to use in combination with recombinant interferon gamma.

Atopic Dermatitis (AD). AD is a chronically relapsing inflammatory skin disorder characterized by severe pruritus and frequent exacerbations.[85] The social and economic costs of this disorder are high and include missed school and work, the psychological impact of physical disfigurement, chronic use of medications, and frequent hospitalization for control of disease and infection. The primary cause of AD is unknown, although excessive IgE production in response to food and inhaled allergens is thought to play a role.[86] T cells from patients with AD have decreased production of γ-interferon[87] and appear to produce abnormally high levels of interleukin-4, which is important for IgE synthesis.[88]

Management of AD has emphasized symptomatic relief. Interferon gamma, through its ability to suppress IgE synthesis, may be an important new therapy. Boguniewicz et al.[89] reported on the use of recombinant interferon gamma in 22 patients with chronic, severe AD that was poorly responsive to other therapy. In the first phase of the study, 14 patients received three increasing doses of recombinant interferon gamma (10, 50, and 100 μg/sq m) administered as subcutaneous injections on five consecutive days per week, with a two-day rest period between each increase in the dose. In the second phase, eight patients received recombinant interferon gamma 50 μg/sq m/day for six weeks. Finally, one patient from phase 1 and all phase 2 patients continued to receive 50 μg/sq m three times weekly as maintenance therapy.

In phase 1, 10 of 12 patients receiving 10 μg/sq m and 9 of 12 patients receiving 100 μg/sq m showed inhibition of baseline de novo IgE synthesis by peripheral blood mononuclear cells. No decrease in serum IgE concentrations was noted; therefore it appeared that the inhibitory effects on IgE production by peripheral blood mononuclear cells represented only a partial inhibition of IgE synthesis. All dosages in phase 1 led to considerable decreases in the clinical severity of the disease; clinical severity worsened three days after the drug was discontinued. Patients in phase 2 had a progressive and substantial reduction in clinical severity during the six weeks of daily therapy. During the maintenance therapy, sustained clinical improvement occurred.

Reinhold et al.[90] reported on the use of recombinant interferon gamma in three patients with unremitting severe AD who had high serum IgE concentrations, high spontaneous production of IgE, and defective in vitro secretion of γ-interferon. Doses of 100 μg were administered subcutaneously for five days, followed by three doses per week for three weeks. The inflammatory condition improved within two weeks and had almost disappeared after four weeks. These patients were found to have decreased serum IgE concentrations, as well as a decrease in the spontaneous production of IgE in vitro.

It is difficult to make any conclusions about the clinical efficacy of recombinant interferon gamma in patients with AD on the basis of one small, uncontrolled trial and three case reports. However, the reduction in clinical severity in patients with severe AD receiving recombinant interferon gamma daily is encouraging. Placebo-controlled trials are warranted.

Lymphoproliferative Disorders. *Cutaneous T-cell Lymphoma (CTCL).* CTCL is an uncommon malignant lymphoproliferative disorder.[91] The clinical features include a premycotic stage with cutaneous eruptions that slowly progress to infiltrated plaques, eventually involving the lymph nodes and visceral organs. The leukemic phase of CTCL, known as Sézary syndrome, is characterized by generalized erythroderma, superficial lymphadenopathy, and splenomegaly. Patients have severe itching and atypical cells in the blood, lymph nodes, and cutaneous infiltrates.[92] Cures for both CTCL and Sézary syndrome have been extremely rare with conventional therapy. In 1986, patients with CTCL who were given recombinant interferon alfa were reported to have objective response rates of 29–85%, with the response lasting 3–36 months.[93] It was believed that recombinant interferon gamma, with its ability to activate macrophages and its antiproliferative effect, might provide additive or synergistic antitumor effects.[94]

Kaplan et al.[95] conducted a Phase II trial to evaluate the efficacy of recombinant interferon gamma in the treatment of CTCL. All 16 patients included in the trial had failed to respond to previous therapy with standard regimens of topical mechlorethamine hydrochloride, psoralen plus ultraviolet-A light, electron-beam irradiation, or antineoplastic drugs. Some patients had also received experimental treatment with recombinant interferon alfa, radioactively labeled monoclonal antibodies, or retinoids. The pa-

Table 4.
Selected Studies of Recombinant Interferon Gamma for Treatment of Metastatic Renal Cell Carcinoma

Ref.	Manufacturer	Regimen	No. Evaluable Patients	No. Complete Responses	No. Partial Responses	Objective Response Rate (%)	Duration of Response (mo)	Comment
68	Boehringer Ingelheim[a]	250 μg i.m. for 8 days given every 3–4 wk for up to 11 cycles	10	0	3	30	4–18	
73	Biogen[b]	Dosage escalated from 0.01 × 10^6 units/sq m to 75 × 10^6 units/sq m i.v. over 4 hr twice weekly	13	0	0	0	0	Phase I/II trial. Maximum tolerated dose was 75 × 10^6 units/sq m
74	Genentech	10–50 μg/sq m/day c.i.[c]	14	0	1	7	...[d]	
		250–1000 μg/sq m/day i.m.	16	0	1	6	...	
75	Shionogi[a]	8 × 10^6 to 12 × 10^6 units/sq m i.v. or i.m. daily for at least 4 wk	32	0	2	6	...	Japanese multicenter nonrandomized Phase II trial.
		40 × 10^6 units/sq m i.v. over 1 hr on days 1–5, 15–19, 29, 31, 33, 43, 45, 47	30	1	5	20	...	Intermittent therapy continued for >8 wk
76	Schering[a]	1 × 10^6 units/sq m s.c. three times weekly	21	...	...	5[e]	...	Patients prospectively randomized to receive interferon alfa or interferon gamma or a combination
77	Biogen[b]	Dosage escalated from 10 to 3000 μg/sq m i.v. over 2 hr or c.i. for 7 days every 3 wk	41	1	3	10	2–13+	Phase I/II trial. Schedule determined randomly
78	Genentech	10, 100, or 500 μg s.c. weekly followed by 100 μg s.c. weekly	20	2	4	30	6–24+	Open Phase I/II dosage finding trial
79	Biogen[b]	100 μg/sq m i.v. over 4 hr three times weekly every other week	22	2	5	32	11–45+	Prospective nonrandomized Phase II trial
		500 μg/sq m c.i. for 5 days every other week for stable or progressive disease	10	1	0	10	11–45+	
80	Genentech	100 μg/sq m/day i.v. over 4 hr 3 times weekly on alternate days every other week	32	0	1	3	...	Phase II trial
81	Schering[a]	0.25 × 10^6 units/sq m/day (100 μg/sq m/day) by i.v. c.i. for 5 days every 4 wk	24	0	0	0	...	Phase II trial. Twenty patients completed at least 2 cycles. Ten patients had stable disease
82	Toray/ Biogen[b]	6 × 10^6 to 12 × 10^6 units/sq m i.v. infusion daily for at least 14 days followed by i.m. therapy 6 days/wk	7	0	0	0	...	Five patients did not change, and two had progression of disease

[a]Information about the protein structure is not available.
[b]A 146-amino acid compound with a sequence of cysteine, tyrosine, and cystine at the amino terminus.
[c]c.i. = continuous infusion.
[d]Information was not reported.
[e]One patient had a response, but the report did not specify whether it was complete or partial.

Table 5.
Selected Studies of Combination Therapy with Recombinant Interferon Gamma and Recombinant Interferon Alfa for Treatment of Metastatic Renal Cell Cancer

Ref.	Manufacturer	Regimen: Interferon Gamma	Regimen: Interferon Alfa	No. Evaluable Patients	No. Complete Responses	No. Partial Responses	Objective Response Rate (%)	Duration of Response (mo)	Comment
66	Biogen[a]	30, 300, or 1000 μg/sq m i.v. for 5 days every 3 wk given 6 hr before interferon alfa	2.5×10^6 to 20×10^6 units/sq m s.c. in escalating doses	30	2	6	27	4–22+	Sequence of administration may play important role in decreasing adverse effects and increasing efficacy. Response not seen until after ≥2–7 mo
67	. . .[b]	100 μg/sq m s.c. twice weekly 100 μg/sq m s.c. twice weekly	Escalating dose 24 μg/sq m s.c. twice weekly	29 21	2 4	6 1	28 24	8–22+ . . .	In escalating-dose regimen, median time to response was 24–28 wk. In fixed-dose regimen, median time to response was 4–12 wk
76	Schering[c]	1×10^6 units/sq m s.c. three times weekly	2×10^6 units/sq m s.c. three times weekly	47	. . .	. . .	2[d]	. . .	Patients prospectively randomized to receive therapy with interferon alfa or interferon gamma or a combination
83	Genentech	2×10^6 units/sq m i.m. q.d. 2×10^5 units/sq m i.m. q.d. 5×10^6 units/sq m q.d. for 1 wk, repeat every 3 wk	2×10^6 units/sq m i.m. q.d. 2×10^6 units/sq m i.m. q.d. 10×10^6 units/sq m weekly for 3 wk	10 25 13	0 0 0	0 4 1	0 16 8	. . . 4–10 . . .	Second regimen was best tolerated. In first and second regimens, drugs were given simultaneously. In third regimen, interferon gamma was given, then interferon alfa was given, followed by 1 wk of rest
84	Genentech	100 μg/sq m s.c. twice weekly	6 μg/sq m s.c. twice weekly and increased by 6 μg/sq m/wk until maximally tolerated	31	2	6	26	8–35+	Cannot make any conclusions about interferon gamma

[a]A 146-amino acid compound with a sequence of cysteine and tyrosine at the amino terminus.
[b]Information was not reported.
[c]Information about the protein structure is not available.
[d]One patient had a response; it was not specified whether it was complete or partial.

tients received eight weeks of recombinant interferon gamma therapy starting at 250 μg/sq m/day for one week, which, if tolerated, was increased to 500 μg/sq m/day for the remaining seven weeks. None of the patients had a complete response, although favorable responses were noted in 11 patients. Five patients (31%) had a partial response (a 50% reduction in the size of measurable lesions lasting 3–32 months). Six patients (38%) had either a mixed response (some lesions regressing, others progressing, new lesions) or a minor response (less than a 50% reduction in lesion size). Six patients with stage IV disease at the beginning of the trial died of progressive disease despite the therapy. The small number of patients evaluated prevented an examination of a possible correlation between the response to recombinant interferon gamma and (1) prior therapy, (2) the dosage of recombinant interferon gamma, and (3) the stage of the disease. Although it is difficult to form conclusions because of the small sample size, future trials may establish a role for recombinant interferon gamma in combination with antineoplastic agents or other biologics in the treatment of CTCL.

Chronic Myelogenous Leukemia (CML). CML, another proliferative disorder, has a chronic phase lasting about three years followed by an acceleration to lymphoid or myeloid blast-cell transformation that is fatal within three to six months. Approximately 90% of patients with CML have cytogenetic abnormalities identified by the presence of the Philadelphia chromosome, a translocation of material from chromosome 22 to another chromosome, usually chromosome 9.[96] Treatment options in CML are aimed at early control of the chronic phase in the hope that intensive chemotherapy and irradiation may lead to a clinical and cytogenetic cure. Although the chronic phase of the disease can be controlled, the Philadelphia chromosome continues to be present in metaphase cells in the majority of patients, and the disease is almost invariably fatal.

Interferons were considered for use in the treatment of CML after they showed an ability to suppress the formation of both leukemic and normal cells in vitro.[97] Hematologic and cytogenetic improvement in Philadelphia chromosome-positive patients has been achieved after 12–78 months of therapy with recombinant interferon alfa; a 76% rate of complete remission and a 30% cytogenetic response rate were reported.[98] These encouraging results prompted an evaluation of recombinant interferon gamma.

Kurzrock et al.[99] evaluated 26 patients with Philadelphia chromosome-positive benign-phase CML who received intramuscular recombinant interferon gamma 250–500 μg/sq m/day for six weeks. Patients with complete or partial remission or having hematologic improvement continued therapy. A complete response was defined as a normalization of white blood cell (WBC) and platelet counts and an absence of the clinical signs and symptoms of CML. A partial response was defined as a 50% reduction in WBC counts or normalization of WBC counts but persistent splenomegaly. Although 16 patients had no response, 6 (23%) had a complete response and 4 (15%) had a partial response. None of the patients developed blast-cell crisis while receiving therapy. Cytogenetic improvement, with the return of normal diploid metaphases in the bone marrow, was reported in five of the patients with complete responses. The median duration of follow-up was only 7.5 months (range, 5–12 months).

In a study by Silver et al.,[100] 18 patients with Philadelphia chromosome-positive CML were treated with recombinant interferon gamma. Initially, the patients received 300 μg/sq m/week as a single intravenous bolus injection. If tolerated, the dosage was increased to a maximum of 1500 μg/sq m/day i.v. The median duration of treatment was 15 months, with most patients receiving 1500 μg/sq m three times a week. Progression of disease within three months of the start of therapy necessitated the removal of five patients from the trial. Of the remaining 13 patients, 4 (30%) had a complete response, 2 (15%) had a partial response, and 2 showed some improvement. Patients with a complete response were found to have normal blood counts and an absence of splenomegaly. A partial response was described as a 50% decrease in splenomegaly and only slight elevation in WBC and platelet counts. Some normal karyotypes were found in two of the four complete responders, although reversion to 100% Philadelphia chromosome-positive cells occurred after an average of 30 weeks. None of the patients developed blast-cell crisis during the study.

While the response rates were similar in both the Kurzrock et al. and the Silver et al. trials, it is difficult to make conclusions, since the investigators studied only a small number of patients and used different types of recombinant interferon gamma and different treatment regimens. Another factor that should be considered is the duration of therapy, which was relatively short in both studies. Information from the trials with recombinant interferon alfa suggest that prolonged treatment is necessary to achieve remission or cytologic changes.

Clinical experience with recombinant interferon gamma for the treatment of CML is limited. To date, the response rates reported for recombinant interferon gamma are lower than those seen with recombinant interferon alfa. Some patients failing to respond to recombinant interferon gamma have been reported to respond to recombinant interferon alfa, and the reverse has also been documented.[101,102] It appears unlikely that recombinant interferon gamma alone will have an important impact on CML.

The use of recombinant interferon gamma in combination therapy for CML has also been considered. Howard Ozer, M.D., Ph.D., designed a trial in which subcutaneous doses of recombinant interferon gamma 250 μg/sq m/day were alternated weekly with recombinant interferon alfa 25 μg/sq m/day in 100 patients with chronic-phase CML.[103] The hematologic response to the combination therapy was less than the response to recombinant interferon alfa alone. Toxicities during the periods of recombinant interferon gamma administration necessitated the removal of patients from the trial and may have been responsible for the weaker response to the combination therapy.

The ability of interferons to reverse the cytogenetic abnormalities in some patients with Philadelphia chromosome-positive CML is a breakthrough. Additional trials are needed, however, to help establish a role, either additive or synergistic, for recombinant interferon gamma used with other biological response modifiers or antineoplastic agents in the treatment of CML.

Adverse Effects

Adverse effects associated with recombinant interferon gamma primarily involve constitutional symptoms, although a variety of other adverse effects have also been reported. For the most part, subcutaneous recombinant interferon gamma appears to be well tolerated in patients with CGD (Table 6). No serious or life-threatening toxic effects have been directly attributed to the drug in this patient population. The International Chronic Granulomatous Disease Cooperative Study reported fever, chills, headache, and erythema to be the most common adverse effects.[63] The majority of reactions are mild and are ameliorated by giving concomitant acetaminophen. Administering the agent at bedtime results in fewer reactions.

Adverse effects have also been evaluated in patients with various malignancies (Table 6). In addition to constitutional symptoms, this population has been reported to have experienced occasional adverse effects involving the cardiovascular, gastrointestinal, renal, hematologic, pulmonary, and central nervous systems. The most common adverse effects are fever, chills, myalgias, arthralgias, headache, and fatigue. These flu-like symptoms are seen in nearly all patients receiving recombinant interferon gamma. They do not appear to be dose related, and tachyphylaxis is uncommon. Concomitant administration of acetaminophen or a nonsteroidal anti-inflammatory agent may help alleviate many of the symptoms. Night sweats are also reported frequently. Cardiovascular effects, including tachycardia and hypotension, have been reported rarely, although patients with underlying cardiac problems may be at a higher risk for toxicity.[104-106]

Gastrointestinal effects such as nausea, vomiting, stomatitis, and anorexia have been reported, as has weight loss.[104-108] Hepatotoxicity occurs in about 30% of patients; values for hepatic enzymes, usually aminotransferase, have been up to three times higher than baseline values.[105,106,108,109] The elevation in aminotransferase is rarely dose limiting and resolves two to four weeks after therapy is discontinued. In the Cooperative Study, elevations in hepatic enzyme values to less than three times normal concentrations were seen in 23% of the placebo group and 16% of the recombinant interferon gamma group.[63] Reversible hypertriglyceridemia has occurred, particularly in patients receiving long-term therapy.[109]

Renal toxicity has been reported and is usually manifested as proteinuria.[95,104,106,110] Acute renal failure occurred in a 12-year-old boy with acute lymphoblastic leukemia after he received recombinant interferon gamma 500 µg/sq m for 19 days.[111] Renal biopsy showed diffuse tubular damage and interstitial edema consistent with tubular necrosis. There was no evidence of immune-complex deposition. The child's renal function improved after recombinant interferon gamma was discontinued, although he did require short-term hemodialysis. Acute renal failure was also reported in a patient with metastatic RCC who was given both recombinant interferon alfa and interferon gamma.[83] Close monitoring of renal function with frequent urinalysis is recommended during recombinant interferon gamma therapy. If changes in renal

Table 6.
Adverse Reactions to Recombinant Interferon Gamma

	No. (%) Patients with Adverse Reaction			
			Metastatic Renal Cell Carcinoma	
Adverse Reaction	Chronic Granulomatous Disease ($n = 63$)[a]	Chronic Myelogenous Leukemia ($n = 30$)[b]	Low-Dose Regimen ($n = 14$)[c]	High-Dose Regimen ($n = 14$)[d]
Fever	33 (52)	30 (100)	14 (100)	14 (100)
Night sweats	...[e]	25 (83)	...	...
Headache	21 (33)	14 (47)	...	...
Rash	11 (18)	...	...	...
Chills	9 (14)	20 (67)	14 (100)	14 (100)
Erythema at injection site	9 (14)	...	...	...
Myalgia	4 (6)	20 (67)	...	...
Hypertriglyceridemia	...	22 (73)[f]	...	...
Hepatotoxicity	10 (16)[g]	10 (33)[g]	...	...
Neurotoxicity	...	1 (3)	...	...

[a]Interferon gamma 50 µg/sq m on Mondays, Wednesdays, and Fridays by s.c. injection. From reference 63.
[b]Interferon gamma 250–500 µg/sq m daily by i.m. injection. From reference 99.
[c]Interferon gamma 100 µg/sq m weekly by s.c. injection. From reference 78.
[d]Interferon gamma 500 µg/sq m weekly by s.c. injection. From reference 78.
[e]Information was not reported.
[f]Serum triglyceride concentrations were 1.5 times the baseline values.
[g]Serum hepatic enzyme concentrations were less than 3 times the baseline values.

function occur, the dosage should be decreased or therapy discontinued until renal function returns to normal.

A dose-dependent hematologic toxicity manifested as leukopenia, usually with granulocytopenia, has been reported in patients receiving recombinant interferon gamma dosages greater than 250 μg/sq m/day.[105-109,112,113] Reversible thrombocytopenia and anemia have been reported rarely,[104,106,112] and there has been one report of hemolytic anemia.[114]

Patients receiving recombinant interferon gamma at dosages greater than 250 μg/sq m/day have reported a variety of mild and reversible CNS effects, including dizziness, confusion, hallucinations, depression, and parkinsonian symptoms.[104-109,113] One patient with brain metastases developed seizures.[105]

Contraindications and Precautions

Recombinant interferon gamma-1b is purified from *E. coli*; therefore its use in patients with hypersensitivity to *E. coli* or *E. coli*-derived products is contraindicated.

Although adverse effects associated with recombinant interferon gamma are generally mild, special caution should be used in administering the drug to immunocompromised patients because reversible neutropenia has been reported when dosages equal or exceed 250 μg/sq m/day. Extra caution should also be used in initiating therapy in patients with seizure disorders or cardiac disease. Dosages of 250 μg/sq m/day or higher may exacerbate these conditions.

Little is known about the use of recombinant interferon gamma during pregnancy. Animal data suggest an increased risk of uterine bleeding, spontaneous abortion, and decreased neonatal viability with maternally toxic doses. Studies have not been performed in humans. Therefore, recombinant interferon gamma should be used during pregnancy only if absolutely necessary. It is not known if interferon gamma is excreted in breast milk. Because of the potential for adverse effects in the infant, women receiving recombinant interferon gamma should not breastfeed.

Although the efficacy and safety of recombinant interferon gamma have been evaluated in pediatric patients, data are not available for children less than one year of age.

Drug Interactions

Drug interactions involving recombinant interferon gamma have not been fully evaluated. It is possible that the agent could potentiate the toxicities of other myelosuppressive agents. Animal studies have shown inhibition of cytochrome P-450. Although the clinical significance of this effect in humans is not known, recombinant interferon gamma might decrease the hepatic metabolism of drugs that rely on this pathway for elimination.

Dosage and Administration

The current recommendations for dosages of recombinant interferon gamma-1b in the treatment of CGD are based on body weight or BSA. Children with a BSA greater than 0.5 sq m should receive 50 μg/sq m (1.5 million units/sq m) by subcutaneous injection three times a week. Children with a BSA less than or equal to 0.5 sq m should receive 1.5 μg/kg, again by subcutaneous injection three times weekly (e.g., on Monday, Wednesday, and Friday). To be successful, therapy must be continued for life.

The optimum dosages for patients with AD, metastatic RCC, or CML have not been established. In the larger trials for metastatic RCC, a dosage of 100 μg/sq m/day has been used and maintained as tolerated. In patients with Philadelphia chromosome-positive CML, the dosage schedule has typically included subcutaneous injections of 250–500 μg/sq m/day. Lower dosages (50–100 μg/sq m/day) have been used in the treatment of AD. Long-term therapy appears to be necessary to control all three disease states.

Patient Education

Since recombinant interferon gamma is given by subcutaneous injection, patients and their families should be instructed on proper storage, preparation, injection technique, and disposal of needles and syringes. Patients should be reminded that the drug must be stored in the refrigerator, not the freezer. If a vial is exposed to room temperature for longer than 12 hours, it must be discarded. Care should be taken not to shake the vials or subject them to excessive agitation.

Before use, vials of recombinant interferon gamma should be examined for particulate matter and discoloration. If possible, injections should be given into the right or left deltoid muscle or the anterior thigh. After administration, any unused portion should be discarded, and the syringe and needle should be disposed of in a puncture-resistant container. Patients who experience fever or headache should take acetaminophen. A dose of acetaminophen should be taken at least four hours before the injection, and additional doses should be taken at regular intervals for the next 24 hours. Administration of recombinant interferon gamma at bedtime may minimize some of the flu-like symptoms.

Availability, Cost, and Approved Labeling

The average wholesale price for a vial of recombinant interferon gamma-1b (Actimmnue, Genentech) is approximately $140, although packages of 12 vials are available for $1526 (approximately $127 per vial).[115] The cost of administering recombinant interferon gamma to a 28-kg, 1.0-sq m, 10-year-old child is approximately $380 per week or $19,800 per year; this cost does not include the pharmacist's fee or the cost of needles, syringes, and other supplies. Each 0.50 mL vial contains 100 μg (3 million units) of interferon gamma formulated in 20 mg of mannitol, 0.36 mg of sodium succinate, 0.05 mg of polysorbate 20, and sterile water for injection. Doses given to pediatric patients will frequently be less than the amount contained in a single vial. However, because of a lack of information on the drug's stability, the manufacturer states that each vial should be used only once.[116]

Recombinant interferon gamma-1b has orphan drug status and has FDA-approved labeling for use in the treatment of CGD. It is indicated for use in reducing the severity and frequency of serious infections associated with CGD. Clinical trials to evaluate its role in other disease states are under way.

Formulary Considerations

Recombinant interferon gamma represents an original form of therapy for the treatment of CGD and therefore should be granted formulary status. It is inevitable that recombinant interferon gamma will continue to be evaluated for use in other disease states, including malignancies and various primary immunodeficiency disorders. Because of cost considerations, it is important to establish specific criteria for the use of recombinant interferon gamma and other biological response modifiers.

Conclusion

Recombinant interferon gamma has given new hope to patients afflicted with chronic granulomatous disease. Although the agent does not provide a cure, it decreases the rate of serious infections and the need for hospitalization. The very high cost of recombinant interferon gamma may limit its use, although the cost may be offset by fewer hospitalizations. Another limiting factor is compliance; the drug must be injected three times a week for life.

It does not appear likely that recombinant interferon gamma alone will have an important role in the treatment of lymphoproliferative disorders and metastatic renal cell carcinoma, but its role in combination with other biological response modifiers or antineoplastic agents remains to be determined. The benefits of recombinant interferon gamma in the treatment of atopic dermatitis are encouraging.

---

[a]Buchanan J, Genentech, Inc. Personal communication. 1991 Sep 30.

References

1. Isaacs A, Lindenmann J. Virus interference: I. The interferon. *Proc R Soc Lond*. 1957; 147:258-67.
2. Pestka S, Langer JA, Zoon KC et al. Interferons and their actions. *Annu Rev Biochem*. 1987; 56:727-77.
3. Langer JA, Pestka S. Structure of interferons. *Pharmacol Ther*. 1985; 27:371-401.
4. Okita K, Kaneko T. The potential of interferons in malignant diseases. *Drugs*. 1990; 39:1-6.
5. Heremans H, Billiau A. The potential role of interferons and interferon antagonists in inflammatory disease. *Drugs*. 1989; 38:957-72.
6. Rubinstein M, Novick D, Fischer DG. The human interferon-gamma receptor system. *Immunol Rev*. 1987; 97:29-50.
7. Lewis DB, Wilson CB. Gamma-interferon: an immunoregulatory lymphokine with immunotherapeutic potential. *Pediatr Infect Dis J*. 1990; 9:642-51.
8. Fischer DG, Novick D, Orchansky P et al. Two molecular forms of the human interferon-gamma receptor: ligand binding, internalization and down-regulation. *J Biol Chem*. 1988; 263:2632-8.
9. DeMaeyer E, DeMaeyer-Guignard J, eds. Interferons and other regulatory cytokines. New York: Wiley; 1988:5-38.
10. Martindale: the extra pharmacopoeia. 29th ed. Reynolds JEF, ed. London: Pharmaceutical Press; 1989:696-9.
11. DeMaeyer E, DeMaeyer-Guignard J, eds. Interferons and other regulatory cytokines. New York: Wiley; 1988:114-33.
12. Verhaegen-Lewalle M, Kuwata T, Chang ZX et al. 2-5A synthetase activity induced by interferon alpha, beta, and gamma in human cell lines differing in their sensitivity to the anticellular and antiviral activities of these interferons. *Virology*. 1982; 117:245-54.
13. Samuel CE, Duncan R, Knutsen GS et al. Mechanism of interferon action: increased phosphorylation of protein synthesis initiation factor eIF-2a in interferon-treated, retrovirus-infected mouse l-929 fibroblasts in vitro and in vivo. *J Biol Chem*. 1984; 259:13451-7.
14. Yamamoto N, Shimokata K, Maeno K et al. Effect of recombinant human interferon gamma against human cytomegalovirus. *Arch Virol*. 1987; 94:323-9.
15. Mistchenko AS, Falcoff R. Recombinant human interferon gamma inhibits adenovirus multiplication in vitro. *J Gen Virol*. 1987; 68:941-4.
16. Scott GM. Clinical trials of interferons against viral diseases. In: Stringfellow DA, ed. Clinical application of interferons and their inducers. 2nd ed. New York: Dekker; 1986:149-96.
17. Murray HW. Interferon-gamma, the activated macrophage, and host defense against microbial challenge. *Ann Intern Med*. 1988; 108:595-608.
18. Nathan CF, Murray HW, Wiebe ME et al. Identification of interferon-gamma as the lymphokine that activates human macrophage oxidative metabolism and antimicrobial activity. *J Exp Med*. 1983; 158:670-89.
19. Murray HW, Rubin BY, Rothermel CD. Killing of intracellular *Leishmania donovani* by lymphokine-stimulated human mononuclear phagocytes: evidence that interferon-gamma is the activation factor. *J Clin Invest*. 1983; 72:1506-10.
20. Rothermel CD, Rubin BY, Murray HW. Gamma-interferon is the factor in lymphokine that activates human macrophages to inhibit intracellular *Chlamydia psittaci* replication. *J Immunol*. 1983; 131:2542-4.
21. Ijzermans JNM, Marquet RL. Interferon-gamma: a review. *Immunobiology*. 1989; 179:456-73.
22. Reynolds DS, Boom WH, Abbas AK. Inhibition of B lymphocyte activation by interferon-gamma. *J Immunol*. 1987; 139:767-73.
23. Rabin EM, Mond JJ, Ohara J et al. Interferon-gamma inhibits the action of B cell stimulatory factor (BSF)-1 on resting B cells. *J Immunol*. 1986; 137:1573-6.
24. Finkleman FD, Katona IM, Mosmann TR et al. IFN-gamma regulates the isotypes of Ig secreted during in vivo humoral immune responses. *J Immunol*. 1988; 140:122-7.
25. DeMaeyer E, DeMaeyer-Guignard J, eds. Interferons and other regulatory cytokines. New York: Wiley; 1988:221-73.
26. Paucker K, Cantel K, Henle W. Quantitative studies on viral interference in suspended L cells. *Virology*. 1962; 17:324-34.
27. DeMaeyer E, DeMaeyer-Guignard J, eds. Interferons and other regulatory cytokines. New York: Wiley; 1988:334-63.
28. Kurzrock R, Rosenblum MG, Sherwin SA et al. Pharmacokinetics, single dose tolerance, and biologic activity of recombinant gamma-interferon in cancer patients. *Cancer Res*.

1985; 45:2866-72.
29. Gutterman JU, Rosenblum MG, Rios AA et al. Pharmacokinetic study of partially pure gamma-interferon in cancer patients. *Cancer Res.* 1984; 44:4164-71.
30. Thompson JA, Cox WW, Lindgren CG et al. Subcutaneous recombinant gamma interferon in cancer patients: toxicity, pharmacokinetics, and immunomodulatory effects. *Cancer Immunol Immunother.* 1987; 25:47-53.
31. Bablor BM, Woodman RC. Chronic granulomatous disease. *Semin Hematol.* 1990; 27:247-59.
32. Johnston RB Jr. Resistance to infection: prospects for therapeutic manipulation. *Pediatr Res.* 1990; 27 (Suppl 6):S44-8.
33. Smith RM, Curnutte JT. Molecular basis of chronic granulomatous disease. *Blood.* 1991; 77:673-86.
34. Baehner RL. Chronic granulomatous disease of childhood: clinical, pathological, biochemical, molecular, and genetic aspects of the disease. *Pediatr Pathol.* 1990; 10:143-53.
35. Gallin JI, Malech HL. Update on chronic granulomatous disease of childhood: immunotherapy and potential for gene therapy. *JAMA.* 1990; 263:1533-7.
36. Curnutte JT. Classification of chronic granulomatous disease. *Hematol Oncol Clin North Am.* 1988; 2:241-52.
37. Dinauer MC, Curnutte JT, Rosen H et al. A missence mutation in the neutrophil cytochrome *b* heavy chain in cytochrome positive X-linked chronic granulomatous disease. *J Clin Invest.* 1989; 84:2012-6.
38. Bohler M-C, Seger RA, Mouy R et al. A study of 25 patients with chronic granulomatous disease: a new classification by correlating respiratory burst, cytochrome *b*, and flavoprotein. *J Clin Immunol.* 1986; 6:136-45.
39. Ezekowitz RAB, Dinauer MC, Jaffe HS et al. Partial correction of the phagocyte defect in patients with X-linked chronic granulomatous disease by subcutaneous interferon gamma. *N Engl J Med.* 1988; 319:146-51.
40. Dinauer MC, Pierce EA, Bruns GAP et al. Human neutrophil cytochrome-*b* light chain (p22-*phox*): gene structure, chromosome location, and mutations in cytochrome-negative autosomal recessive chronic granulomatous disease. *J Clin Invest.* 1990; 86:1729-37.
41. Dinauer MC, Muhlebach T, Erickson RW et al. A missence mutation of the p22-*phox* subunit of cytochrome *b* associated with a nonfunctional cytochrome *b* and chronic granulomatous disease. *Blood.* 1990; 76:179a. Abstract.
42. Clark RA, Malech HL, Gallin JI et al. Genetic variants of chronic granulomatous disease: prevalence of deficiencies of two cytosolic components of the NADPH oxidase system. *N Engl J Med.* 1989; 321:647-52.
43. Lomax KJ, Leto TL, Nunoi H et al. Recombinant 47-kilodalton cytosol factor restored NADPH oxidase in chronic granulomatous disease. *Science.* 1989; 245:409-12.
44. Leto TL, Lomax KJ, Volpp BD et al. Cloning of a 67-kD neutrophil oxidase factor with a similarity to a non-catalytic region of $p60^{c\text{-}src}$. *Science.* 1990; 248:727-30.
45. Forrest CB, Forehand JR, Axtell RA et al. Clinical features and current management of chronic granulomatous disease. *Hematol Oncol Clin North Am.* 1988; 2:253-66.
46. Gonzales LA, Hill HR. Advantages and disadvantages of antimicrobial prophylaxis in chronic granulomatous disease in childhood. *Pediatr Infect Dis J.* 1988; 7:83-5.
47. Quie PG, Belani KK. Corticosteroids for chronic granulomatous disease. *J Pediatr.* 1987; 111:393-4.
48. Chin TW, Stiehm ER, Falloon J et al. Corticosteroids in the treatment of obstructive lesions of chronic granulomatous disease. *J Pediatr.* 1987; 111:349-52.
49. Rubin RH, Swartz MN. Trimethoprim–sulfamethoxazole. *N Engl J Med.* 1980; 303:426-32.
50. Gmunder FK, Seger RA. Chronic granulomatous disease: mode of action of sulfamethoxazole/trimethoprim. *Pediatr Res.* 1981; 15:1533-7.
51. Johnston RB, Wilfert CM, Buckley RH et al. Enhanced bacteriocidal activity of phagocytes from patients with chronic granulomatous disease in the presence of sulfisoxasole. *Lancet.* 1975; 1:824-7.
52. Seger RA, Baumgartner S, Tiefenauer LX et al. Chronic granulomatous disease: effect of sulfamethoxazole/trimethoprim on neutrophil microbial function. *Helv Paediatr Acta.* 1981; 36:579-88.
53. Johnston RB, Reele BB, Misra HP et al. The role of superoxide anion generation in phagocytic bactericidal activity. *J Clin Invest.* 1975; 55:1357-72.
54. Curnutte JT, Whitten DM, Babior BM. Defective superoxide production by granulocytes from patients with chronic granulomatous disease. *N Engl J Med.* 1974; 290:593-7.
55. Stjernholm RL, Allen RC, Steele RH et al. Impaired chemiluminescence during phagocytosis of opsonized bacteria. *Infect Immun.* 1973; 7:313-4.
56. Gallin JI, Buescher ES, Seligmann BE et al. Recent advances in chronic granulomatous disease. *Ann Intern Med.* 1983; 99:657-74.
57. Mouy R, Fischer A, Vilmer E et al. Incidence, severity, and prevention of infections in chronic granulomatous disease. *J Pediatr.* 1989; 114:555-60.
58. Margolis DM, Melnick DA, Alling DW et al. Trimethoprim–sulfamethoxazole prophylaxis in the management of chronic granulomatous disease. *J Infect Dis.* 1990; 162:723-6.
59. Regelman W, Hays N, Quie PG. Chronic granulomatous disease: historical perspective and clinical experience at University of Minnesota Hospitals. In: Gallin JI, Fauci AS, eds. Advances in host defense mechanisms. Vol. 3. New York: Raven; 1983:3-24.
60. Nathan CF, Murray HW, Wiebe ME et al. Identification of interferon as the lymphokine that activates human macrophage oxidative metabolism and antimicrobial activity. *J Exp Med.* 1983; 158:670-89.
61. Ezekowitz RAB, Orkin SH, Newburger PE. Recombinant interferon gamma augments phagocyte superoxide production and X-chronic granulomatous disease gene expression in X-linked variant chronic granulomatous disease. *J Clin Invest.* 1987; 80:1009-16.
62. Sechler JMG, Malech HL, White CJ et al. Recombinant interferon-gamma reconstitutes defective phagocytic function in patients with chronic granulomatous disease of childhood. *Proc Natl Acad Sci.* 1988; 85:4874-8.
63. International Chronic Granulomatous Disease Cooperative Study Group. A controlled trial of interferon gamma to prevent infection in chronic granulomatous disease. *N Engl J Med.* 1991; 324:509-16.
64. Mouy R, Seger R, Veber F et al. Interferon gamma for chronic granulomatous disease. *N Engl J Med.* 1991; 325:1516. Letter.
65. Ezekowitz RAB. Interferon gamma for chronic granulomatous disease. *N Engl J Med.* 1991; 325:1516-7. Letter.
66. Ernstoff MS, Suresh N, Bahnson RR et al. A Phase IA trial of sequential administration of recombinant DNA-produced interferons: combination recombinant interferon gamma and recombinant interferon alfa in patients with metastatic renal cell carcinoma. *J Clin Oncol.* 1990; 8:1637-49.
67. Debruyne FMJ, Franssen MPH, Beniers AJMC et al. New prospects in the management of metastatic renal cell carcinoma: experimental and clinical data. *Prog Clin Biol Res.* 1990; 350:243-55.
68. Grups JW, Frohmuller HGW. Cyclic interferon gamma application in patients with renal cell carcinoma. *Prog Clin Biol Res.* 1990; 350:257-62.
69. Bell DR, Aroney RS, Fisher RJ et al. High-dose methotrexate with leucovorin rescue, vinblastine, and bleomycin with or without tamoxifen in metastatic renal cell carcinoma. *Cancer Treat Rep.* 1984; 68:587-90.
70. Rodriguez LH, Johnson DE. Clinical trial of cisplatin (NSC 119875) in metastatic renal cell carcinoma. *Urology.* 1987; 11:344-6.
71. Kintzel PE, Calis KA. Recombinant interleukin-2: a biological response modifier. *Clin Pharm.* 1991; 10:110-28.
72. Muss HB. The role of biologic response modifiers in meta-

static renal cell carcinoma. *Semin Oncol*. 1988; 15:30-4.
73. Rinehart JJ, Malspeis L, Young D et al. Phase I/II trial of human recombinant interferon gamma in renal cell carcinoma. *J Biol Response Mod*. 1986; 5:300-8.
74. Quesada JR, Kurzrock R, Sherwin SA et al. Phase II studies of recombinant human gamma in metastatic renal cell carcinoma. *J Biol Response Mod*. 1987; 6:20-7.
75. Recombinant Human Interferon Gamma (S-6810) Research Group on Renal Cell Carcinoma. Phase II study of recombinant human interferon gamma (S-6810): summary of two collaborative studies. *Cancer*. 1987; 60:929-33.
76. Foon K, Doroshow J, Bonnem E et al. A prospective randomized trial of alpha-2b-interferon/gamma-interferon or the combination in advanced metastatic renal cell carcinoma. *J Biol Response Mod*. 1988; 7:540-5.
77. Garnick MB, Reich SD, Maxwell B et al. Phase I/II study of recombinant interferon-gamma in advanced renal cell carcinoma. *J Urol*. 1988; 139:251-5.
78. Aulitzky W, Gastl G, Aulitzky WE et al. Successful treatment of metastatic renal cell carcinoma with a biologically active dose of recombinant interferon-gamma. *J Clin Oncol*. 1989; 7:1875-84.
79. Otto U, Schneider AW, Conrad S et al. Recombinant alpha-2 or gamma interferon in the treatment of metastatic renal cell carcinoma: results of two Phase II/III trials. *Prog Clin Biol Res*. 1990; 350:275-82.
80. Bruntsch U, de Mulder PHM, ten Bokkel Huinink WW et al. Phase II study of recombinant human interferon-gamma in metastatic renal cell carcinoma. *J Biol Response Mod*. 1990; 9:335-8.
81. Kuebler JP, Goodman PJ, Brown TD et al. Phase II study of continuous infusion recombinant gamma interferon in renal cell carcinoma. *Invest New Drugs*. 1990; 8:307-9.
82. Marmuo K, Murai M, Deguchi N et al. Immunologic effects of recombinant interferon-gamma in patients with renal cell carcinoma. *Keio J Med*. 1990; 39(2):97-101.
83. Quesada JR, Evans L, Saks SR et al. Recombinant interferon alpha and gamma in combination as treatment for metastatic renal cell carcinoma. *J Biol Response Mod*. 1988; 7:234-9.
84. De Mulder PHM, Debruyne FMJ, Franssen MPH et al. Phase I/II study of recombinant interferon-alpha and gamma in advanced progressive renal cell carcinoma. *Cancer Immunol Immunother*. 1990; 31:321-4.
85. Hanfin JM. Atopic dermatitis. *J Am Acad Dermatol*. 1982; 6:1-13.
86. Sampson HA. The role of food allergy and mediator release in atopic dermatitis. *J Allergy Clin Immunol*. 1988; 81:635-45.
87. Reinhold U, Pawelec G, Wehrmann W et al. Immunoglobulin E and immunoglobulin G subclass distribution in vivo and relationship to in vitro generation of interferon-gamma and neopterin in patients with severe atopic dermatitis. *Int Arch Allergy Appl Immunol*. 1988; 87:120-6.
88. Romagnani S, Del Prete G, Maggi E et al. Role of interleukins in induction and regulation of human IgE synthesis. *Clin Immunol Immunopathol*. 1989; 50:S13-23.
89. Boguniewicz M, Jaffe HS, Izu A et al. Recombinant gamma interferon treatment of patients with atopic dermatitis and elevated IgE levels. *Am J Med*. 1990; 88:365-70.
90. Reinhold U, Wehrmann W, Kukel S et al. Recombinant interferon-gamma in severe atopic dermatitis. *Lancet*. 1990; 335:1282. Letter.
91. Haynes BF, Metzgar RS, Minna JD et al. Phenotypic characterization of cutaneous T-cell lymphoma: use of monoclonal antibodies to compare with other malignant T cells. *N Engl J Med*. 1981; 304:1319-23.
92. Broder S, Edelson RL, Lutzner MA et al. The Sézary syndrome: a malignant proliferation of helper T cells. *J Clin Invest*. 1976; 58:1297-306.
93. Bunn PA, Ihde DC, Foon KA. The role of recombinant interferon alfa-2a in the therapy of cutaneous T-cell lymphomas. *Cancer*. 1986; 57:1689-95.
94. Rubin BY, Gupta SL. Differential efficacies of human type I and type II interferons as antiviral and antiproliferative agents. *Proc Natl Acad Sci U S A*. 1980; 77:5926-32.
95. Kaplan EH, Rosen ST, Norris DB et al. Phase II study of recombinant human interferon-gamma for treatment of cutaneous T-cell lymphoma. *J Natl Cancer Inst*. 1990; 82:208-12.
96. Canellos GP. Chronic leukemias. In: DeVita VT Jr, Hellmans S, Rosenberg SA, eds. Cancer: principles and practice of oncology. 2nd ed. Philadelphia: Lippincott; 1985:1739-52.
97. Kurzrock R, Gutterman JU, Kantarjian H et al. Therapy of chronic myelogenous leukemia with interferon. *Cancer Invest*. 1989; 7(1):83-91.
98. Talpaz M, Kantarjian H, Kurzrock R et al. Interferon-alpha produces sustained cytogenetic responses in chronic myelogenous leukemia. *Ann Intern Med*. 1991; 114:532-8.
99. Kurzrock R, Talpaz M, Kantarjian H et al. Therapy of chronic myelogenous leukemia with recombinant interferon-gamma. *Blood*. 1987; 70:943-7.
100. Silver RT, Benn P, Verma RS et al. Recombinant gamma-interferon has activity in chronic myeloid leukemia. *Am J Clin Oncol*. 1990; 13:49-54.
101. Silver RT, Coleman M, Benn P et al. Interferon alfa-2b has activity in treating chronic myeloid leukemia in recombinant interferon gamma failures. *Proc Am Soc Clin Oncol*. 1987; 6:587. Abstract.
102. Kantarjian HM, Talpaz M, Gutterman J. Biologic therapy of chronic myelogenous leukemia. *Oncology*. 1987; 1(Sep):35-40,48-9,52.
103. Silver RT. Interferon in the treatment of myeloproliferative disease. *Semin Hematol*. 1990; 27(Suppl 4):6-14.
104. Srikandan K, Garner P, Watkinson J et al. A toxicity study of recombinant interferon-gamma given by intravenous infusion to patients with advanced cancer. *Cancer Chemother Pharmacol*. 1986; 18:63-8.
105. Brown TD, Koeller J, Beougher K et al. A Phase I clinical trial of recombinant DNA gamma interferon. *J Clin Oncol*. 1987; 5:790-8.
106. Boman BM, Gagen MM, Bonnem E et al. Phase I study of recombinant gamma-interferon (rIFN-gamma). *J Biol Response Mod*. 1988; 7:438-46.
107. Ernstoff MS, Trautman T, Davis CA et al. A randomized Phase I/II study of continuous versus intermittent intravenous interferon gamma in patients with metastatic melanoma. *J Clin Oncol*. 1987; 5:1804-10.
108. Creagan ET, Schaid DJ, Ahmann DL et al. Recombinant interferons in the management of advanced malignant melanoma. *Am J Clin Oncol*. 1988; 11:652-9.
109. Kirkwood JM, Ernstoff MS. A clinical update: the role of interferon in the biotherapy of solid tumors. *Oncol Nurs Forum*. 1988; 15(Suppl):3-6.
110. Kurzrock R, Quesada JR, Talpaz M et al. Phase I study of multiple dose intramuscularly administered recombinant gamma interferon. *J Clin Oncol*. 1986; 4:1101-9.
111. Ault BH, Stapleton FB, Gaber L et al. Acute renal failure during therapy with recombinant human gamma interferon. *N Engl J Med*. 1988; 319:1397-400.
112. Cannon GW, Pincus SH, Emkey RD et al. Double-blind trial of recombinant gamma-interferon versus placebo in the treatment of rheumatoid arthritis. *Arthritis Rheum*. 1989; 843-4.
113. Di Bisceglie AM, Rustgi VK, Kassianides C et al. Therapy of chronic hepatitis B with recombinant human alpha and gamma interferon. *Hepatology*. 1990; 11:266-70.
114. Rabinowitz AP, Hu E, Watkins K et al. Hemolytic anemia in a cancer patient treated with recombinant interferon-gamma. *J Biol Response Mod*. 1990; 9:256-9.
115. American Druggist blue book. Edelstein E, ed. New York: Hearst; 1991.
116. Genentech, Inc. Actimmune package insert. South San Francisco, CA; 1990 Dec.

Therapy Review

Management of psychotropic-induced hyperprolactinemia

PATRICIA A. MARKEN, RADWAN F. HAYKAL, AND JOSEPH N. FISHER

Abstract: The effects of individual psychotropic medications on serum prolactin concentrations are described, and recommendations for dealing with adverse effects are provided.

Hyperprolactinemia can result in galactorrhea, amenorrhea, irregular menses, and anovulation; in men, impotence and azoospermia, with or without lactation and gynecomastia, can occur. Antipsychotics may block dopamine receptors in the pituitary prolactin-secreting cells and prevent dopamine-induced reduction of prolactin release. The magnitude of the increase in prolactin concentration correlates with the amount of antipsychotic drug given. The treatment of choice is reduction of the antipsychotic dosage or discontinuation of therapy. If adjustments to the antipsychotic dosage fail to resolve symptoms, the dopamine agonists bromocriptine and amantadine may be tried. Antidepressants may produce elevated serum prolactin concentrations, especially with long-term administration. However, the frequency of antidepressant-induced hyperprolactinemia is much lower than that seen with antipsychotics, and serious adverse clinical effects are uncommon. Other psychotropic drugs such as lithium, valproic acid, buspirone, carbamazepine, and benzodiazepines either are only rarely associated with symptomatic hyperprolactinemia or do not produce clinically important changes in prolactin concentrations.

Antipsychotic drugs are the psychotropic agents most likely to cause symptomatic hyperprolactinemia. Bromocriptine or amantadine may provide symptomatic relief if withdrawal or adjustment of the antipsychotic dosage does not eliminate the symptoms.

Index terms: Amantadine; Bromocriptine; Hyperprolactinemia; Prolactin inhibitors; Psychotherapeutic agents; Toxicity
Clin Pharm. 1992; 11:851-6

Prolactin was discovered in 1928; however, specific evidence of its existence in humans was not found until the early 1970s.[1] Prolactin secretion is affected by many medications and pathologic states. Many psychotropic drugs, especially those that alter dopaminergic function, have an important effect on serum prolactin concentrations. Although prolactin changes are not always clinically significant, patients can develop intolerable clinical manifestations that limit their ability to continue treatment with psychotropic drugs. Some effects may be distressing without being particularly uncomfortable. The amenorrhea associated with hyperprolactinemia, for example, may prevent a woman from realizing that she is pregnant. This paper reviews the regulation of prolactin, describes effects of individual psychotropic medications on prolactin, and provides recommendations for dealing with adverse effects.

Prolactin Physiology and Pathophysiology

Prolactin is a protein hormone synthesized and released by the anterior pituitary gland. Prolactin receptors have been found in humans in the mammary glands, liver, kidneys, brain, adrenal glands, ovaries, seminal vesicles, uterus, prostate, testes, and placen-

PATRICIA A. MARKEN, PHARM.D., is Assistant Professor of Pharmacy Practice and Psychiatry, Schools of Pharmacy and Psychiatry, University of Missouri-Kansas City, and Psychopharmacy Specialist, Western Missouri Mental Health Center, Kansas City. RADWAN F. HAYKAL, M.D., is Director, Mood Disorders Program, Charter Lakeside Hospital, Memphis, TN, and Clinical Associate Professor of Psychiatry, Department of Psychiatry, The University of Tennessee, Memphis. JOSEPH N. FISHER, M.D., is Professor of Medicine, Division of Endocrinology and Metabolism, Department of Medicine, The University of Tennessee, Memphis.

Address reprint requests to Dr. Marken at the University of Missouri-Kansas City, 2411 Holmes M3-C19, Kansas City, MO 64108.

 0278-2677/92/1001-0851$01.50.

ta.[2] Prolactin induces the synthesis and secretion of milk, suppresses gonadotropin secretion, and may stimulate testosterone synthesis.[3,4] Serum prolactin increases during sleep, peaks in the early morning, and declines immediately after awakening.[5] This variation should be considered when blood samples are collected for determination of serum prolactin concentration and when results of these determinations are interpreted. Basal concentrations vary considerably and range from 5 to 25 ng/mL in men and nonpregnant, nonlactating women.[6] Serum concentrations can rise during pregnancy to 200 ng/mL at term and to 300 ng/mL during nursing.[7]

The hypothalamus exerts tonic inhibitory control over prolactin release, mainly through the prolactin-inhibiting factor dopamine.[8] Dopaminergic neurons are located in the tuberoinfundibular tract of the hypothalamus and have corresponding receptors in the anterior pituitary gland.[9] Dopamine is released from the tuberoinfundibular tract and transported through the portal system to the prolactin-secreting cells (lactotrophs) of the anterior pituitary gland. Dopamine acts on lactotrophs to decrease prolactin release.

Prolactin-releasing factors, which include histamine, norepinephrine, opiates and opioids, estrogens, prostaglandins, protirelin (thyrotropin-releasing hormone), and cholecystokinin, act to increase serum prolactin concentrations.[8] Gamma-aminobutyric acid plays a dual role with respect to its effects on prolactin; it may be stimulatory at the central nervous system level and inhibitory in the anterior pituitary gland.[10] The effects of serotonin on prolactin regulation in humans are uncertain. Serotonin may act to increase prolactin concentrations by inhibiting dopamine[11] and by increasing the activity of prolactin-releasing factors.[12]

Hyperprolactinemia can result in galactorrhea, amenorrhea, irregular menses, and anovulation. In men, impotence and azoospermia, with or without lactation and gynecomastia, can occur.[5] Obesity and mild hirsutism can develop from the weak androgenic activity of prolactin.[5] Clinical symptoms may also be absent; galactorrhea may occur in as few as 20% of hyperprolactinemic women.[13] For galactorrhea to be manifested, prolactin concentrations must be elevated; the breast must have been prepared by normal amounts of insulin, growth hormone, glucocorticoids, estrogen, and progestin; and there must be an absolute or relative deficiency of estrogen.[5] If serum prolactin concentrations are greater than 60–100 ng/mL, amenorrhea will usually develop.[14]

The causes of hyperprolactinemia and its associated complications are numerous (Table 1). Assessment should include a pregnancy test in women who have child-bearing potential. A pituitary tumor will be present in 50–90% of nonpregnant, nonlactating patients with a basal serum prolactin concentration greater than 100–200 ng/mL.[15,16] A history of headache and visual changes may also indicate a pituitary tumor.[13] Gynecomastia can occur independently of elevated serum prolactin and may be a normal finding in newborn, adolescent, and elderly males.[17]

Antipsychotic Effects of Drugs

Patients with schizophrenia have normal serum prolactin concentrations when free of medication.[18] However, antipsychotics, the primary treatment for schizophrenia, have a profound effect on serum prolactin. Antipsychotics may block dopamine receptors in the pituitary lactotrophs and prevent dopamine-induced reduction of prolactin release.[19] Prolactin concentrations usually plateau within the first week after initiation of therapy with antipsychotics.[20] The magnitude of the increase in prolactin concentration correlates with the amount of antipsychotic drug given, up to a chlorpromazine dosage of 600 mg/day (or an equipotent dosage of another drug). Wide variations can exist, however.[19,21] Prolactin concentrations usually return to baseline within a few days after discontinuation of therapy with antipsychotics, although some patients continue to have elevated concentrations for up to three weeks.[22] Normalization of prolactin concentrations during continued antipsychotic treatment may also occur.[23-25] DeRivera et al.[26] found that 37.5% of men and 27% of women treated with antipsychotics for at least five years had normal prolactin concentrations. However, the morning serum prolactin concentration in a patient receiving long-term treatment with antipsychotics can exceed 5 to 10 times the normal concentration.[27]

The relationship between prolactin changes and antipsychotic therapy has been extensively investigated.

Table 1.
Potential Causes of Hyperprolactinemia[a]

Nonpathologic
Pregnancy
Nursing
Nipple stimulation
Coitus
Stress
Exercise
Neonatal state
Sleep
Pathologic
Prolactin-secreting pituitary tumors
Hypothalamic–pituitary stalk lesions
Hypothyroidism
Chronic renal failure
Severe liver disease
Drugs
Protirelin (thyrotropin-releasing hormone)
Antipsychotic agents
Opiates and opioids
Reserpine
Fenfluramine
Estrogens
Methyldopa
Metoclopramide
Amoxapine

[a]Adapted from references 8 and 13.

Attempts to predict antipsychotic response by assessing drug-induced prolactin changes have been unsuccessful because of great interindividual variability.[28] Attempts to correlate antipsychotic-induced changes in prolactin concentration with improvement in psychosis have also been inconclusive.[19-21] Use of elevated prolactin concentrations to evaluate medication compliance is not feasible because levels rise quickly, even after a single dose of an antipsychotic.[22]

The exact frequency of antipsychotic-induced hyperprolactinemia and the accompanying complications is not known. Galactorrhea has been reported in 0–80% of women receiving antipsychotics and has occurred at all dosages.[29,30] It has been reported as early as eight days after initiating therapy with antipsychotics.[30] Galactorrhea occurs more frequently in premenopausal than in postmenopausal women, possibly because of the positive influence of estrogen on prolactin release.[31] Antipsychotic-induced gynecomastia is rare.[30] Concern that chronically elevated prolactin concentrations could increase the likelihood of breast cancer has not been supported by several epidemiologic studies.[32] Nevertheless, therapy with antipsychotics is contraindicated in patients with hormone-dependent breast tumors.[33] Clozapine may differ from other antipsychotics with respect to its effects on serum prolactin. In several clinical trials involving clozapine, large increases in serum prolactin were absent, as were amenorrhea, galactorrhea, and inhibition of ejaculation.[18,34,35]

Treatment. The expected increase of prolactin concentrations in patients receiving antipsychotics should not be of concern unless complications develop. Patients who develop complications should be assessed for the other causes listed in Table 1. Reduction of the antipsychotic dosage or discontinuation of therapy is the treatment of choice. In fact, dosage reduction alone may alleviate symptoms. Dosage reductions must be individualized with consideration of both the risk of relapse and the severity of the adverse effects. Substituting another antipsychotic drug is unlikely to relieve symptoms, because most of these drugs block dopamine receptors.[30] Clozapine may be the exception; however, the potential for agranulocytosis makes automatic use of this agent too risky. Even though prolactin concentrations usually decrease within a few days after discontinuation of antipsychotic therapy,[20] breast symptoms may take three weeks to resolve.[30]

If adjustments to the antipsychotic dosage fail to resolve symptoms, the dopamine agonists bromocriptine and amantadine may be tried, although the data are somewhat limited. Bromocriptine acts by directly stimulating postsynaptic dopamine receptors, whereas amantadine probably acts by facilitating dopamine release from presynaptic neurons.[36]

Studies Involving Bromocriptine. Beaumont et al.[24] studied the efficacy of bromocriptine in treating antipsychotic-induced amenorrhea and galactorrhea in nine women who were otherwise gynecologically normal. Seven of the nine had irregular menses, and all had some degree of galactorrhea. Bromocriptine 2.5 mg (as the mesylate salt) twice a day was added to existing antipsychotic regimens. Galactorrhea, rated twice weekly for nine weeks, markedly decreased in the five patients in whom symptoms were most severe, although it did not completely resolve in any patient. Menses returned in only one patient. No important adverse effects were reported.

Matsuoka et al.[37] added bromocriptine 5–7.5 mg (as the mesylate salt) twice a day to the drug regimen of 16 patients with antipsychotic-induced amenorrhea, galactorrhea, or impotence. Menses returned in 7 of the 10 women, galactorrhea decreased substantially in 5 of 6 women, and testosterone concentration increased substantially in all 6 male patients. No worsening of psychotic symptoms was reported.

Cases reports also show that bromocriptine is effective in treating antipsychotic-induced amenorrhea and galactorrhea.[38,39] Bromocriptine 5–10 mg (as the mesylate salt) was given daily to two patients. Response occurred at 2 weeks in one patient[38] and at 24 weeks in the other.[39] Again, psychiatric adverse effects were minimal.

Bromocriptine 5–15 mg/day (as the mesylate salt) has been effective either when given alone or when antipsychotic therapy is continued.[24,37-39] Resolution of symptoms has occurred as soon as 15 days after the initiation of therapy with bromocriptine,[38] but 9 weeks of treatment was sometimes necessary to achieve a response.[24] When patients receive bromocriptine for a broad range of causes of hyperprolactinemia, the average time for the return of menses is 6–8 weeks, with a range of a few days to 24 weeks. Galactorrhea usually decreases by 75% after 7–12 weeks, although symptoms may never completely disappear. Tolerance does not seem to develop to the prolactin-reducing effects of bromocriptine.[36]

Studies Involving Amantadine. Amantadine has also improved symptoms of antipsychotic-induced hyperprolactinemia. Correa et al.[40] reported a significant decrease in serum prolactin in 9 of 10 patients receiving 200–300 mg of amantadine hydrochloride a day, although prolactin concentrations remained above normal. Therapy with antipsychotics was continued at prestudy doses in all patients. Gynecomastia resolved in four of six male subjects. Libido improved in 4 of 10 patients, breast tenderness decreased in 6 of 10 patients, and menses returned in all 3 amenorrheic women. An average weight loss of 8.2 pounds occurred during the three-week study. Seven of nine patients had a significant decrease in Brief Psychiatric Rating Scale (BPRS) scores after the addition of amantadine, whereas two worsened. BPRS scores, however, remained high (indicating relatively severe psychosis), with an average score after amantadine therapy of 35.6 on a scale of 18–146, and the clinical importance was minimal. No other adverse effects were reported.

Siever[41] administered amantadine hydrochloride 300 mg a day to 10 women and 1 man for 15 days. All five women experiencing galactorrhea improved after amantadine administration. Eight patients had serum prolactin concentrations assessed before and after treatment. Prolactin concentrations decreased significantly in six patients but remained above normal in all eight patients. BPRS scores showed no consistent changes, with only the severity of "unusual thought content" decreasing significantly.

Recommendations. Patients who develop hyperprolactinemia-induced complications and require continued treatment with antipsychotics present a therapeutic dilemma. If antipsychotic therapy is continued, symptoms are likely to return when dopamine agonists are withdrawn.[24,39] The literature does not contain specific recommendations for treating recurrent amenorrhea and galactorrhea in antipsychotic-dependent patients. Bromocriptine is indicated for short-term management of amenorrhea and galactorrhea caused by hyperprolactinemia.[36] However, in clinical practice, bromocriptine therapy is continued for many years.[14] Patients receiving therapy for longer than six months should be observed for pulmonary complications such as infiltrates, effusions, and pleural thickening.[36] The best approach may be minimizing dosages of antipsychotics and treating patients with short courses of dopamine agonists when symptoms become problematic.

Dopamine agonists can produce adverse effects, but studies and clinical experience with this patient population indicate few problems. Because more data are available for bromocriptine, it should be given first unless a specific contraindication, such as hypersensitivity to ergot alkaloids or peripheral vascular disease, exists. Bromocriptine most commonly causes nausea, headache, and dizziness. Adverse effects can be minimized by starting therapy with small, divided doses (e.g., 1.25 mg [as the mesylate salt] twice a day) and adjusting upward every few days until the desired daily dose (between 5 and 15 mg [as the mesylate salt]) is achieved. Coadministration with food will decrease stomach upset. The drug's transient hypotensive effect can be minimized if the first dose is taken while the patient is lying down and by avoiding rapid changes in posture. Women should be advised to use a nonhormonal contraceptive method during treatment, because bromocriptine can restore fertility.[36] Amantadine hydrochloride should be given at a dosage of 100 mg/day initially and raised weekly until a dosage of 200–300 mg/day has been achieved. Amantadine most commonly causes nausea, dizziness, and lightheadedness. Livedo reticularis, peripheral edema, anorexia, and constipation have also been reported.[41] Amantadine and bromocriptine should not be used together in patients receiving antipsychotic drugs.

Drug-induced psychiatric adverse effects are of special concern in patients taking antipsychotics. Confusion, hallucinations, delusions, nightmares, depression, and mania have occurred during bromocriptine therapy, especially at daily doses greater than 100 mg (as the mesylate salt).[36] The low dosages of bromocriptine used in patients with antipsychotic-induced hyperprolactinemia may account for the lack of psychiatric adverse effects. Amantadine can produce similar central nervous system adverse effects.[42] Even though improvement and worsening of BPRS scores have been reported with amantadine therapy, the data are insufficient to determine the clinical importance of these changes.

Effects of Antidepressants

Depression can affect serum prolactin in a variety of ways. Low,[43] normal,[44] and high prolactin concentrations[45] have been reported in depressed patients. A number of other abnormalities in neuroendocrine function, including decreased basal luteinizing-hormone concentrations,[46] decreased luteinizing-hormone response to gonadotropin-releasing hormone,[47] nonsuppression of cortisol after administration of dexamethasone,[48] and decreased thyrotropin response to protirelin,[49] can occur during a depressive episode.

Antidepressants may produce changes in serum prolactin concentrations through facilitation of serotonin activity. Other mechanisms may include inhibition of dopamine and norepinephrine reuptake in the synaptic cleft.[50] Some studies have demonstrated increased prolactin concentrations in healthy and depressed adults after short-term administration of tricyclic antidepressants, whereas others have shown no appreciable effect.[51,52] Long-term administration of antidepressants more consistently increases serum prolactin concentrations. However, the increases are small in comparison to those seen with antipsychotics and concentrations often do not exceed the upper limits of normal.[53]

The frequency of antidepressant-induced hyperprolactinemia is much lower than that seen with antipsychotics, and serious adverse clinical effects are uncommon.[54] Among antidepressants, amoxapine causes the most hyperprolactinemia, most likely because of its hydroxyl metabolite, which also exhibits antipsychotic properties.[55] There are case reports of imipramine,[56] amitriptyline,[57] maprotiline,[58] desipramine,[59] and clomipramine[59] causing hyperprolactinemia or galactorrhea. Fluoxetine can increase serum prolactin concentrations but rarely causes breast pain and galactorrhea.[60] In clinical trials of fluoxetine in 5920 patients, female lactation occurred in 0.07%, breast enlargement in 0.08%, and breast pain in 0.25% of patients (Beasley CM, Eli Lilly and Co. Personal communication. 1989 Feb 23).

Theoretically, bupropion hydrochloride can decrease serum prolactin concentrations because of its weak dopamine agonist properties.[53] Doses up to 200 mg have been found to have no effect on serum prolactin concentrations.[61,62] Othmer et al.,[63] in contrast, found a significant increase in menstrual disturbances after treatment with bupropion, but not with amitriptyline. However, serum prolactin concentrations were not reported. The frequency and importance of bupropion-induced changes in prolactin concentrations are yet to be clearly established.

Recommendations. Antidepressants do not usually produce serious prolactin-related adverse effects. Amenorrhea and galactorrhea should be treated with dosage reduction or withdrawal of the offending agent. If amoxapine is implicated, substituting another antidepressant should resolve the symptoms. Dopamine agonists have not been specifically evaluated in patients with antidepressant-induced amenorrhea and galactorrhea. They may be considered when symptoms continue despite dosage adjustments and trials with alternative agents. Because amenorrhea, galactorrhea, and gynecomastia are relatively rare complications of antidepressant therapy, other causes should always be investigated.

Effects of Other Psychotropic Drugs

Other psychotropic medications have limited effects on prolactin concentrations. Lithium produces important endocrine adverse effects, especially thyroid dysfunction. However, reports of lithium-induced changes in prolactin concentrations are conflicting. Joffe et al.[64] found that lithium elevated baseline concentrations of thyrotropin and prolactin and augmented the response of both to stimulation with protirelin in eight depressed patients. In contrast, other investigators have found unaltered baseline prolactin concentrations after lithium treatment.[65,66] Amenorrhea, galactorrhea, and gynecomastia should be considered to be very rare complications of lithium therapy, and occurrence of these disorders should prompt evaluation of other potential causes.

Valproic acid-induced enhancement of the activity of γ-aminobutyric acid has the potential to inhibit prolactin secretion.[67] Breast enlargement, galactorrhea, irregular menses, and amenorrhea secondary to valproic acid have occasionally been reported.[36]

Because of its effects on serotonin function, buspirone would be expected to cause hyperprolactinemia. Menstrual irregularities and galactorrhea have been reported; however, a causal relationship has yet to be established.[68] A review of the adverse-effect profile in 984 patients taking buspirone in clinical trials described all complications that occurred in more than 1% of the subjects. There were no reports of amenorrhea, galactorrhea, or gynecomastia in the review.[68]

Carbamazepine has been reported to augment the response of prolactin to arginine, although the clinical importance is uncertain.[69] Benzodiazepine-induced endocrine changes are uncommon and generally not clinically important.

Conclusion

Antipsychotic drugs are the psychotropic agents most likely to cause symptomatic hyperprolactinemia. If withdrawal or dosage adjustment of the offending antipsychotic drug does not successfully eliminate the symptoms of hyperprolactinemia, bromocriptine or amantadine may provide symptomatic relief.

References

1. Friesen H, Hwong P. Human prolactin. *Annu Rev Med.* 1973; 24:251-70.
2. Fluckiger E, Del Pozo E, Werder K. Prolactin: physiology, pharmacology and clinical findings. Berlin: Springer; 1982:1-64.
3. Thorner MO, Pogol AD, Evans WS et al. The effects of prolactin on gonadal function in man. In: McLeod RM, Scapagnini V, eds. Central and peripheral regulation of prolactin function. New York: Raven; 1980:271-82.
4. Rubin RT, Poland RE, Tower BB. Prolactin-related testosterone secretion in normal adult males. *J Clin Endocrinol Metab.* 1976; 42:112-6.
5. Martin JB, Reichlin S. Clinical neuroendocrinology. 2nd ed. Contemporary neurology series. Philadelphia: F. A. Davis; 1987.
6. Hororobin DF, Mtabaji JP, Karmali RA et al. Prolactin in mental illness. *Postgrad Med J.* 1976; 52:79-85.
7. Liddle GW, Liddle LA. Endocrinology. In: Smith LH, Their SO, eds. The biological principles of disease. Philadelphia: Saunders; 1981:653-754.
8. Hell K, Wernze H. Drug induced changes in prolactin secretion: clinical implications. *Med Toxicol.* 1988; 3:463-98.
9. Gudelsky GA. Tuberoinfundibular dopamine neurons and the regulation of prolactin secretion. *Psychoneuroendocrinology.* 1981; 6:3-16.
10. Cavagnini F, Benetti G, Invitti C et al. Effect of gamma amino butiric acid on growth hormone and prolactin secretion in man: influence of pimozide and domperidone. *J Clin Endocrinol Metab.* 1980; 51:789-92.
11. Pilotte NS, Porter JC. Dopamine in the hypophysial portal plasma and prolactin in systemic plasma of rats treated with 5-hydroxytryptomine. *Endocrinology.* 1981; 108:2137-41.
12. Clemens JA, Roush ME, Fuller RW. Evidence that serotonin neurons stimulate secretion of prolactin releasing factor. *Life Sci.* 1978; 22:2209-14.
13. Findling JW, Tyrrell JB. Anterior pituitary gland. In: Greenspan FS, ed. Basic and clinical endocrinology. 3rd ed. Los Altos, CA: Lange Medical Publications; 1991:103.
14. Friesen HG, Erzin C, Godden J et al., eds. Clinical endocrinology: a survey of current practice. New York: Appleton-Century-Crofts; 1977.
15. Watts NB, Keffer JH. Practical endocrine diagnosis. 3rd ed. Philadelphia: Lea & Febiger; 1982:11-27.
16. Tolis G, Somma M, vanCampenhout J et al. Prolactin secretion in 65 patients with galactorrhea. *Am J Obstet Gynecol.* 1974; 118:91-101.
17. Braunstein GD. The testes. In: Greenspan FS, Forshan PH, eds. Basic and clinical endocrinology. 2nd ed. Los Altos, CA: Lange Medical Publications; 1986:589-600.
18. Gruen PH, Sacher EJ, Langer G et al. Prolactin response to neuroleptics in normal and schizophrenic subjects. *Arch Gen Psychiatry.* 1978; 35:108-16.
19. Rubin RT, Hayes SE. The prolactin secretory response to neuroleptic drugs: mechanisms, applications and limitations. *Psychoneuroendocrinology.* 1980; 5:121-37.
20. Meltzer HY, Fang VS. The effects of neuroleptics on serum prolactin in schizophrenic patients. *Arch Gen Psychiatry.* 1976; 33:279-86.
21. Meltzer HY, Busch DA, Fang VS. Serum neuroleptic and prolactin levels in schizophrenic patients and clinical response. *Psychiatry Res.* 1983; 9:271-83.
22. Rubin RT. Prolactin in schizophrenia. In: Meltzer HY, ed. Psychopharmacology: the third generation of progress. New York: Raven; 1987:803-7.
23. Brown WA, Laughren T. Low serum prolactin and early relapse following neuroleptic withdrawal. *Am J Psychiatry.* 1981; 138:237-9.
24. Beaumont P, Bruwer J, Pimstone B et al. Brom-ergocryptine in

the treatment of phenothiazine-induced galactorrhea. *Br J Psychiatry*. 1975; 126: 285-8.
25. Laughren TP, Brown WA, Williams BW. Serum prolactin and clinical state during neuroleptic treatment and withdrawal. *Am J Psychiatry*. 1979; 136:108-10.
26. DeRivera JL, Ettigi P, Hontela S et al. Effect of acute and chronic neuroleptic therapy on serum prolactin levels in men and women of different age groups. *Clin Endocrinol*. 1976; 5:273-82.
27. Meltzer HY, Goode DJ, Fang VS. The effect of psychotropic drugs on endocrine function: I. Neuroleptics, precursors, and agonists. In: Lipton MD, DiMascio A, Killam KF, eds. Psychopharmacology, a generation of progress. New York: Raven; 1978:509-29.
28. Hayes SE, Rubin RT. Variability of prolactin release in response to intravenous and intramuscular haloperidol in normal adult males. *Psychopharmacology*. 1979; 61:17-24.
29. Shader R, DiMascio A. Psychotropic drug side effects: clinical and theoretical perspectives. Baltimore: Williams & Wilkins; 1970:63-85.
30. Perry PJ, Alexander B, Liskow BI. Psychotropic drug handbook. 5th ed. Cincinnati, OH: Harvey Whitney Books; 1988:3-43.
31. Apostolakis M, Kapetanakis S, Lazos G et al. In: Wolstenholm GEW, Knight J, eds. Lactogenic hormones. Edinburgh, Scotland: Churchill Livingstone; 1972:349-59.
32. Schyve PM, Smithline F, Meltzer H. Neuroleptic-induced prolactin level elevation and breast cancer. *Arch Gen Psychiatry*. 1978; 35:1291.
33. Simpson GM, Pi EH, Sramek JJ. Adverse effects of antipsychotic agents. *Drugs*. 1981; 21:138-51.
34. Meltzer HY, Goode DJ, Schyve PM et al. Effect of clozapine on human serum prolactin levels. *Am J Psychiatry*. 1979; 136:1550-5.
35. Kane JM, Cooper TB, Sacher EJ et al. Clozapine: plasma levels and prolactin response. *Psychopharmacology*. 1981; 73:184-7.
36. AHFS drug information 92. McEvoy GK, ed. Bromocriptine. Bethesda, MD: American Society of Hospital Pharmacists; 1992:2255-9.
37. Matsuoka I, Nakai T, Miyaki M et al. Effects of bromocriptine on neuroleptic-induced amenorrhea, galactorrhea and impotence. *Jpn J Psychiatry Neurol*. 1986; 40:639-46.
38. Varia IM, Cavenar JO, Taska RJ et al. Bromocriptine in the treatment of haloperidol-induced galactorrhea. *N C Med J*. 1982; 43:769-70.
39. Shenoy RS, Ettigi R, Johnson CH. Bromocriptine in the treatment of galactorrhea caused by haloperidol. A case study. *J Clin Psychopharmacol*. 1983; 3:187-8.
40. Correa N, Opler LA, Kay SR. Amantadine in the treatment of neuroendocrine side effects of neuroleptics. *J Clin Psychopharmacol*. 1987; 7:91-5.
41. Siever LJ. The effect of amantadine on prolactin levels and galactorrhea in neuroleptic-treated patients. *J Clin Psychopharmacol*. 1981; 1:2-7.
42. AHFS Drug Information 92. McEvoy GK, ed. Amantadine. Bethesda, MD: American Society of Hospital Pharmacists; 1992:2250-2.
43. Asnis GM, Nathan RS, Halbreich A et al. Prolactin changes in major depression. *Am J Psychiatry*. 1980; 137:1117-8.
44. Meltzer HY, Kolakowski T, Fang VS et al. Growth hormone and prolactin response to apomorphine in schizophrenia and the major affective disorders. *Arch Gen Psychiatry*. 1984; 41:512-9.
45. Mendlewicz J, Van Cauter E, Linkowski P. The 24-hour profile of prolactin in depression. *Life Sci*. 1980; 27:2015-24.
46. Altman N, Sachar EJ, Gruen PH et al. Reduced plasma LH concentration in post menopausal depressed women. *Psychosom Med*. 1976; 37:274-6.
47. Brambilla N, Smeraldi E, Sacchetti E et al. Deranged anterior pituitary responsiveness to hypothalamic hormones in depressed patients. *Arch Gen Psychiatry*. 1978; 35:1231-8.
48. Arana GW, Baldessarini RJ. Clinical use of the dexamethasone suppression test in psychiatry. In: Meltzer HY, ed. Psychopharmacology, the third generation of progress. New York: Raven; 1987:608-15.
49. Loosen PT, Prange AJ. Serum thyrotropin response to thyrotropin-releasing hormone in psychiatric patients: a review. *Am J Psychiatry*. 1982; 139:405-16.
50. Waldmier PC. Effects of antidepressant drugs on dopamine uptake and metabolism. *J Pharm Pharmacol*. 1982; 34:391-4.
51. Laakman G, Gugath M, Kuss HJ et al. Comparison of growth hormone and prolactin stimulation induced by clomipramine and desipramine in man in connection with clomipramine metabolism. *Psychopharmacology*. 1984; 82:62-7.
52. Jones RB, Luscombe DK, Groom GV. Plasma prolactin concentrations in normal subjects and depressive patients following oral clomipramine. *Postgrad Med J*. 1977; 53:166-71.
53. Meltzer HY, Gudelsky GA, Koenig J. Antipsychotics, tricyclic antidepressants and lithium. In: Nemeroff CB, Loosen PT, eds. Handbook of clinical psychoneuroendocrinology. New York: Guilford; 1987:266-92.
54. Blackwell B, Simon J. Antidepressant drugs. In: Dukes MNG, ed. Side effects of drugs annual 11. Amsterdam: Elsevier; 1987:12-23.
55. Hayes PE, Kristoff CA. Adverse reactions to five new antidepressants. *Clin Pharm*. 1986; 5:471-80.
56. Kleine J, Segal R, Pidrel-Warnek R. Galactorrhea due to imipramine. *N Engl J Med*. 1964; 271:510-2.
57. Liansky J, Fava GA, Buckman MT et al. Amitriptyline boosts plasma prolactin. *Psychopharmacology*. 1984; 84:331-5.
58. Perez OE, Henriques N. Galactorrhea associated with maprotalene HCl. *Am J Psychiatry*. 1983; 140:641. Letter.
59. Fowlie S, Burton J. Hyperprolactinemia and nonpuerperal lactation associated with clomipramine. *Scott Med J*. 1987; 32:52-3.
60. Meltor HY, Young M, Metz J et al. Extrapyramidal side effects and increased serum prolactin following fluoxetine, a new antidepressant. *J Neural Transm*. 1979; 45:165-75.
61. Whiteman PD, Peck AW, Fowlie ASE et al. Failure of bupropion to affect prolactin or growth hormone in man. *J Clin Psychiatry*. 1983; 44:209.
62. Laakmann G, Hoffmann N, Hofschuster E. The lack of effect of bupropion (Wellbutrin) on the secretion of growth hormone and prolactin in man. *Life Sci*. 1982; 30:1725-32.
63. Othmer E, Othmer SC, Stern WC et al. Long-term safety and efficacy of bupropion. *J Clin Psychiatry*. 1983; 44:153-6.
64. Joffe RT, Post RM, Ballenger R et al. The effects of lithium on neuroendocrine function in affectively ill patients. *Acta Psychiatr Scand*. 1986; 73:524-8.
65. Goodnick PJ, Meltzer HY. Effects of subchronic lithium treatment on apomorphine-induced change in prolactin and growth hormone secretion. *J Clin Psychopharmacol*. 1983; 4:239-43.
66. Tanimoto K, Maedak K, Yamaguchi N et al. Effect of lithium on prolactin response to thyrotropin-releasing hormone in patients with manic states. *Psychopharmacology*. 1981; 72:129-33.
67. Melis GB, Paoleth AM, Mais V. The effects of the gabaergic drug sodium valproate on prolactin secretion in normal and hyperprolactinemic subjects. *J Clin Endocrinol Metab*. 1982; 54:485-9.
68. Newton EJ, Marunycz JD, Alderdice MT et al. Review of the side effects profile of buspirone. *Am J Med*. 1986; 80(Suppl 3B):17-21.
69. Joffe RT, Post RM, Ballenger JC et al. Neuroendocrine effects of carbamazepine in patients with affective illness. *Epilepsia*. 1986; 27:156-60.

Therapy Update

Oral anticoagulant therapy in patients undergoing dental surgery

Robert T. Weibert

Abstract: The literature on dental surgery in patients receiving oral anticoagulants is reviewed, and methods of managing anticoagulant therapy to minimize the risk of complications are discussed.

Although blood loss during and after oral surgery in patients receiving oral anticoagulant drugs can be substantial, research indicates that most bleeding incidents are not serious and can be controlled by local measures. Studies of 241 anticoagulant-treated patients undergoing more than 500 dental extractions during the 1950s and 1960s showed that only 9 had postoperative bleeding. More recent studies indicate that continued anticoagulation can increase the frequency of prolonged bleeding and delay wound healing. An antifibrinolytic mouthwash containing tranexamic acid can effectively suppress postoperative bleeding. Gelatin sponges, oxidized cellulose, and microcrystalline collagen are other useful hemostatic agents. A reduction in the intensity of anticoagulation therapy has been recommended; the prothrombin time should be measured shortly before the procedure in such patients. In many patients the duration of subtherapeutic anticoagulation must be minimized to reduce the possibility of thromboembolism. An option for high-risk patients is to switch them to heparin. Each patient must be evaluated individually, and the level of risk of the dental procedure and the risk of thromboembolism should be taken into account.

In patients taking oral anticoagulants who must undergo dental surgery, careful control of the intensity of anticoagulation and improved methods of local hemostasis can minimize the risk of hemorrhagic complications and thromboembolism.

Index terms: Anticoagulants; Cellulose; Collagen; Gelatin; Hemorrhage; Hemostatics; Mouthwashes; Surgery; Toxicity; Tranexamic acid
Clin Pharm. 1992; 11:857-64

The management of oral anticoagulant therapy before dental procedures has been controversial for the past 40 years. Reports during the 1950s described profound bleeding resulting from dental extractions performed during anticoagulant therapy.[1,2] One patient developed a facial hematoma that interfered with vision, and another patient had a 50% decline in hemoglobin concentration.[1,2] Such reports led to a recommendation to discontinue anticoagulants before dental surgical procedures, including routine exodontia.[3] In 1954 Tulloch and Wright[4] had described prolonged bleeding from a dental extraction in one patient taking anticoagulants, while no complications occurred in 14 other patients in whom the prothrombin time (PT) was returned to near normal. Because cessation of anticoagulant therapy may increase the risk of thromboembolic complications, there have been recommendations to continue the therapy, decrease its intensity, or substitute heparin.

Methods of Monitoring Anticoagulation Therapy

An understanding of the differences in the measurement and reporting of the PT is needed to interpret information on oral anticoagulation therapy that has been reported over the past 40 years. While exact conversions are not possible, useful approximations of the relationships among results obtained with locally prepared thromboplastins, less sensitive commercial thromboplastins, and the thrombotest are helpful in interpreting the earlier reports.

The Quick PT test is the most widely used of several laboratory tests that measure the effect of oral anticoagulant therapy. To account for daily variations in instrumentation and testing procedures, the PT is reported as a ratio (PTR), which is the patient's PT divided by the laboratory's control PT. The PT test is performed by adding a mixture of thromboplastin and calcium to citrated plasma and is sensitive to three of

Robert T. Weibert, Pharm.D., is Clinical Professor, University of California San Francisco School of Pharmacy, and Anticoagulation Clinic Director, University of California San Diego Medical Center, 225 Dickinson Street, San Diego, CA 92103-8238.

 0278-2677/92/1001-0857$02.00.

The Therapy Update *section provides concise analytical reviews of narrowly defined, important topics in pharmacotherapy. Priority is given to articles that focus on new or emerging standards in drug therapy. Articles are not intended to be comprehensive reviews of drugs or of disease states and their treatment.*

the four vitamin K-dependent procoagulant clotting-factor proteins. Thromboplastin is an extract of tissue, usually brain; it contains tissue factor and phospholipid needed for factor VII to initiate coagulation by activating factors IX and X.

During the 1980s it was recognized that thromboplastins vary markedly in their responsiveness to the anticoagulant effects of warfarin, depending on their source and method of preparation.[5-11] In the 1950s and 1960s thromboplastin was prepared in local clinical laboratories, and these local reagents were more sensitive than the commercial rabbit brain thromboplastins that are now used.[8] With local thromboplastins, the early recommendation for a therapeutic range of anticoagulation was a PTR of 1.5 to 2.5.[8]

The International Committee on Thrombosis and Hemostasis and the International Committee for Standardization in Haematology have developed a calibration system based on the World Health Organization (WHO) international reference preparation (IRP) thromboplastin.[5] This system converts the observed PTR to an international normalized ratio (INR), which is the ratio that would be obtained by measuring the sample with the WHO IRP.[6-11] Commercial thromboplastins are compared with the IRP by a logarithmic plot. The international sensitivity index (ISI) is calculated from the slope of the orthogonal regression line. By definition, the IRP has an ISI of 1.0. The INR is calculated by raising the PTR to the power of the ISI of the specific thromboplastin ($INR = PTR^{ISI}$). The intent of this system is to reduce laboratory variations that can result in overanticoagulation if a low-sensitivity thromboplastin (high ISI) is used or underanticoagulation if a thromboplastin of greater sensitivity (low ISI) is used. Therapeutic guidelines involving the INR recommend an INR range of 2.0 to 3.0 for low-intensity anticoagulation and a range of 3.0 to 4.5 for conventional anticoagulation.[9]

The PT has also been reported as percent activity by calibrating PTs with serial dilutions of control plasma. In 1954 the American Heart Association recommended a therapeutic range of 17% to 23%.[7] Activity reported with this method was called prothrombin activity or prothrombin complex activity (PCA); the lower the percent PCA, the greater the anticoagulant effect. The thrombotest, which uses a weak bovine thromboplastin, is another method of measuring anticoagulation. This method has not changed in 35 years. Hirsch and Levine[8] estimated that a therapeutic thrombotest value of 7% to 10% is equivalent to a PTR of 1.5 to 1.7 determined with a less sensitive rabbit brain thromboplastin. The thrombotest range of 7% to 10% was also considered to be equivalent to the PTR therapeutic range of 1.5 to 2.5 measured with the early local thromboplastin preparations. These ranges are approximately equal to an INR of 2.75–3.75 (ISI = 2.5).

Blood Loss during Dental Surgery

Blood loss during and after dental surgery can be substantial. An early study described an average loss of 223 mL in patients not receiving anticoagulants.[12] Blood loss was greater in patients who had lengthy surgery and multiple tooth extractions. Postoperative bleeding from oral tissues can occur because of their highly vascular nature and the fibrinolytic activity of saliva and the oral mucosae.[13,14] In a more recent study of multiple dental extractions, less loss of blood—only 2.9 mL per tooth extracted—was reported.[15] Anticoagulant-treated patients with therapeutic prothrombin activity (14% to 28%) averaged 9.7 mL of blood loss per tooth. Total blood loss was three times greater in anticoagulant-treated patients (25.3 mL) than in control patients (8.6 mL). Two anticoagulant-treated patients with abnormally prolonged partial thromboplastin times (>100 seconds) had substantial blood loss (averaging 126 mL per patient and 46.5 mL per tooth). Other patients who were taking coumarin anticoagulants and did not have a prolonged partial thromboplastin time did not bleed more than the control patients.

Dental Extraction during Anticoagulation Therapy

Early Reports (1950s and 1960s). Askey and Cherry[16] described the extraction of 14 teeth in six patients. There was no unusual bleeding, despite continued dicumarol therapy and an average prothrombin activity of 28% (range, 14% to 51%). Shira et al.[17] performed 50 oral surgical procedures, including 41 extractions, on 18 anticoagulant-treated patients with PTRs of 2 to 2.5. The mean PT was 25.5 seconds (range, 17.4 to 50.7 seconds), the mean PTR was 2.17 (range, 1.48 to 4.31), and the mean prothrombin activity was 18.8% (range, 9.5% to 31%). Hemostatic techniques included the use of absorbable gelatin sponges, postoperative biting pressure for two hours, and ice packs applied intermittently for 24 hours. Only one patient required vitamin K treatment.

Behrman and Wright[18,19] reported on a series of 20 patients receiving anticoagulation therapy who underwent 45 dental procedures, including 36 extractions, without having any unusual or serious hemorrhage. The mean PT was 25.7 seconds (range, 17.6 to 37.3 seconds), and the mean PTR was 1.71 (range, 1.21 to 2.24). One patient developed minor oozing of blood after tooth extraction. The authors emphasized the importance of using constant pressure during surgery, multiple sutures placed under tension, absorbable gelatin placed in the tooth sockets, and heavy biting pressure immediately after surgery.

Kwapis[20] reported prolonged bleeding in 3 of 60 anticoagulant-treated patients after dental surgery. The bleeding was corrected with oral vitamin K_1. Kwapis's preferred method of surgical preparation was to reduce the PTR to the lower part of the therapeutic range of 1.5 to 2.0.

Frank et al.[21] reported no complications from 25 extractions in 11 patients. The average prothrombin activity was 23.4%. McIntyre[22] compared 106 anticoagulant-treated patients having thrombotest values of 7% to 15% with 106 control patients. All the patients underwent dental extractions, with an average of six teeth extracted per patient for the anticoagulant-treated group. The thrombotest value was adjusted to the upper end of the therapeutic range (less-intense anticoagulation). One patient in each group bled, with the test-group patient requiring vitamin K_1.

Waldrep and McKelvey[23] performed 76 procedures (60 extractions) on 20 patients who had an average prothrombin activity of 20.3%. Three patients had prolonged oozing, and all bleeding was stopped by local measures. The investigators concluded that the risk of hemorrhage was overemphasized and that most postoperative bleeding could be controlled by local measures or by a reduction in anticoagulation within the therapeutic range.

The seven reports described above represent more than 500 dental extractions in 241 patients. Postoperative bleeding occurred in nine patients (3.7%), and five of these patients were treated with vitamin K. The extractions were generally performed during "therapeutic anticoagulation" measured with the more sensitive locally prepared thromboplastins. The intensity of anticoagulation in these patients approximates conventional anticoagulation defined by current standards.

More Recent Reports (1980s). Anavi et al.[24] compared 15 patients whose anticoagulation treatment was continued during dental extraction with 15 patients whose treatment was interrupted for the surgery. No patient had uncontrollable bleeding, but there was oozing eight hours after surgery in seven anticoagulant-group patients (46%), compared with three control patients (20%). By 24 hours, bleeding had stopped in all the patients. The prothrombin activity averaged 27.5% (range, 19% to 36%) in patients continuing anticoagulation therapy and 52.3% (range, 38% to 70%) in patients interrupting anticoagulation. The authors concluded that extractions can be done safely in the presence of a prothrombin activity of 20% to 30%, which corresponds to lower-intensity anticoagulation.

Bailey and Fordyce[25] compared 25 anticoagulant-treated patients (average INR, 2.4; range, 1.2 to 4.3) with 25 age-matched controls. There were 156 teeth extracted in the experimental group and 227 teeth extracted in the control group. Postextraction bleeding was controlled with pressure packs, sutures, or oxidized methylcellulose and sutures. A numerical scoring system was used to categorize early and late bleeding. There was no difference between the groups in bleeding immediately after extraction. Late episodes of bleeding were classified as intermittent oozing (score = 1), continuous oozing (score = 2), or profuse bleeding (score = 3). Patients in the experimental group had more frequent late bleeding, more prolonged bleeding, and greater blood loss than the controls. Seven (28%) of the anticoagulant-treated patients developed profuse late bleeding; three of them required suturing. The total scores for late bleeding were 59 for the experimental patients and 31 for the control patients ($p = 0.057$). None of the controls had profuse late bleeding. No patient in either group had serious bleeding leading to trismus, upper airway obstruction, or hospitalization. While patients in the anticoagulant group had a greater tendency to bleed again one to five days postoperatively, all episodes were easily controlled by local measures. This trial did show increased bleeding in anticoagulant-treated patients with an average INR of 2.4.

These two studies indicate that continued anticoagulation, even at a relatively low intensity, can increase the frequency of prolonged bleeding after dental extractions. However, all the bleeding was controlled by local measures.

Routine Dental Procedures during Anticoagulation Therapy

Routine general dental treatment presents minimal risk of hemorrhage. These procedures include dental hygiene treatments, restorations, endodontics, prosthetics, minor periodontal therapy, and uncomplicated extractions. Rooney[26] successfully performed 85 dental procedures on patients with an average PTR of 1.7 (range, 1.1 to 2.2). Patients with a PTR greater than 2.5 were rescheduled. Although the type of thromboplastin used to measure the PT was not specified, the average PTR reported suggests that a less sensitive commercial rabbit brain thromboplastin was used. The dental procedures included subgingival restorations, prophylaxis by a dental hygienist, and closed curettage with periodontal packing. Three procedures resulted in intraoperative bleeding, which was controlled in the office. One patient had oozing for 24 hours that was controlled by pressure with a gauze pack. Rooney concluded that these procedures should be exempted from any routine reduction in the anticoagulant dosage. It was recommended, however, that patients schedule dental appointments on a day when the PT is to be routinely monitored to confirm that anticoagulation is not excessive and to avoid extra testing solely for dental purposes.

Benoliel et al.[27] described 490 general dental procedures performed on 30 patients with an average PTR of 2.0 (range, 1.3 to 2.5). One patient had bleeding 24 hours after surgery; the bleeding was controlled by local measures. The researchers recommended that routine dental treatment be performed without altering the PT when the PT is within the therapeutic range.

Antifibrinolytic Therapy

The fibrinolytic activity of saliva may contribute to excessive bleeding in dental surgery. Saliva contains activators of fibrinolysis but does not contain physiological inhibitors of fibrinolysis.

In a study by Sindet-Pedersen et al.,[28] an antifibrinolytic mouthwash reduced bleeding after oral surgery in patients receiving anticoagulation therapy. Therapeutic anticoagulation was defined as a thrombotest value of 5% to 12% or a prothrombin–proconvertin (factor VII) value of 10% to 20%. This corresponded to a PTR of 1.4 to 2.0 and an INR of 2.5 to 4.8. A 4.8% tranexamic acid mouthwash (10 mL) used four times daily for seven days decreased the number of bleeding episodes that could not be controlled by pressure with a gauze pack for 20 minutes. Eight of 20 patients who used a placebo mouthwash had postoperative bleeding (10 episodes), compared with only 1 patient in the tranexamic acid group. Bleeding episodes were treated with compression (one patient), locally applied tranexamic acid and compression (four), or local tranexamic acid and a local hemostatic agent (collagen or oxidized cellulose) (five). One patient required fresh frozen plasma. While the oral rinse with tranexamic acid did not completely suppress fibrinolysis for six hours, it did reduce fibrinolysis and bleeding complications. This suggests that local fibrinolysis is an important factor in postoperative bleeding in patients taking anticoagulants. This mouthwash must be compounded with injectable tranexamic acid, and the cost is substantial.

An animal study by Vinckier and Vermylen[29] provided information on the effect of anticoagulation on wound healing. After the extraction of a tooth, the blood clot that forms in the socket is held together by fibrin threads. Both thrombin and fibrin stimulate the growth of perivascular fibroblasts. The fibrin network also provides support for the migration of fibroblasts. Epithelium then grows over the developing connective tissue. Early disappearance of the fibrin clot leads to an empty socket, and delayed epithelialization occurs by ingrowth rather than overgrowth. The investigators measured wound healing in untreated and warfarin-treated rabbits after the extraction of four front teeth. The rate of wound healing was measured as the time necessary to complete epithelial closure, which was determined from color slides of the wounds. The wounds were stained with iodine, which stains granulation tissue but is not taken up by intact epithelium. In the untreated rabbits, most of the wounds were covered by day 5, and all the wounds were epithelialized by day 8. The PT was adjusted to 8% to 14% in the warfarin-treated rabbits by using thrombotest reagent and a calibration curve for rabbit plasma. The anticoagulant significantly delayed wound healing. The first wound closures occurred on day 8, and it took 15 days until all the wounds were covered. Because fibrin is continuously deposited in a wound and continuously removed by fibrinolysis, the effect of antifibrinolytic therapy was also investigated. Tranexamic acid impedes the proteolytic degradation of fibrin by preventing the attachment of plasminogen and plasmin. Tranexamic acid was given orally at a dosage of 100 mg/kg/day. Simultaneous oral administration of tranexamic acid to the warfarin-treated rabbits completely corrected the delayed healing. In warfarin-treated rabbits given apical packs of oxidized cellulose soaked in thrombin plus tranexamic acid, the first wounds closed on day 4, and all were covered by day 8. Antifibrinolytic therapy stabilizes the fibrin structure within the dental socket and accelerates wound healing. Antifibrinolytic therapy increases collagen synthesis and tensile strength in granulation tissue, presumably by preserving the fibrin matrix. However, socket packing alone does not facilitate wound healing and may increase the risk of infection. The quality of the fibrin network in the dental socket determines the rate of wound healing; oxidized cellulose is not an adequate substitute for fibrin. Vinckier and Vermylen produced normal wound healing in rabbits receiving warfarin by limiting packing to the apical third of the socket and administering oral tranexamic acid to impair fibrinolysis.

Local Hemostatic Agents

Local hemostatic agents assist in controlling bleeding after dental surgery. Absorbable hemostatic agents include gelatin sponges (Gelfoam, Upjohn), oxidized cellulose (Oxycel, Becton-Dickinson), oxidized regenerated cellulose (Surgicel, Johnson & Johnson), and microcrystalline collagen (Avitene, Alcon).[14] Topical thrombin powder or solution can control capillary and venous bleeding. Martinowitz et al.[30] performed 63 extractions in 40 patients who were undergoing anticoagulation therapy and had an average INR of 3.25 (range, 2.5 to 4.5). Local hemostasis was achieved by using thrombin-soaked gauze, a biologic adhesive (Beriplast, Behringwerke, Germany), a collagen fleece, and sutures. One patient developed a mild recurrence of bleeding. The biologic adhesive contained thrombin to convert fibrinogen to a fibrin clot, factor XIII to stabilize the clot, and aprotinin to slow fibrinolysis.

Reducing the Intensity of Anticoagulation

A reduction in the intensity of anticoagulation has also been recommended in patients undergoing dental surgery. In one study, oral anticoagulants were discontinued for one to two days until the PT activity returned to 50% of normal; this intensity of anticoagulation was maintained for 4 to 10 days postoperatively until healing was well established.[31] In 1987,[32] Mulligan described the response to anticoagulant withdrawal in 17 patients with a mean PTR of 1.93. The type of thromboplastin used was not specified. Warfarin was discontinued for two days (on 21 occasions in 11 patients), three days (15 occasions in 6 patients), or four to seven days (8 occasions in 7 patients). The mean PTRs were 1.38 (two days), 1.25 (three days), and 1.13 (four to seven days). The PTR was less than 1.5 after two days in 81% of the instances of warfarin withdrawal. No thromboembolic events occurred within six weeks after withdrawal. A return to a therapeutic PT took three to seven days after warfarin treatment was resumed. Mulligan recommended stopping warfarin for two days and measuring the PT on the morning of the day of the procedure. Dental surgery could proceed if the PTR was 1.5 to 2.0 or less.[32,33]

Yoshimura et al.[34] performed 23 extraction procedures in 16 patients with prosthetic heart valves. Warfarin was continued at the usual dosage (in 19 procedures), continued at a 60% lower dosage (1 procedure), stopped for two days (1 procedure), or stopped for one day (2 procedures). The PTR at surgery ranged from 1.1 to 2.0 and was ≤1.5 in 20 cases (the type of thromboplastin was not specified). None of the four procedures performed after a reduction in or withdrawal of warfarin resulted in postextraction bleeding. Bleeding occurred for 6 (32%) of the 19 procedures in which there was no change in anticoagulation therapy and for 5 (56%) of 9 cases in which three or more teeth were extracted during continued warfarin therapy. The authors suggested that it would be ideal to stop anticoagulation therapy two or three days before the extraction of a tooth.

Because of the prolonged elimination of warfarin and the delayed decrease in clotting factors, there is a delayed increase in the PT, and warfarin should be reinstituted quickly after dental surgery. For major nondental surgery, phytonadione is often given 24 to 36 hours beforehand to reverse the hypoprothrombinemia produced by oral anticoagulants.[35] However, the use of phytonadione to reverse anticoagulation before dental procedures has not been investigated and is not currently recommended.

Risk of Thromboembolism and Rebound Hypercoagulability

Early reports noted the danger of stopping anticoagulation therapy. Cosgriff[36] reported fatal cerebral emboli in a patient after dicumarol therapy was discontinued for 12 days for tooth extractions. This patient had rheumatic heart disease (mitral stenosis and insufficiency) and atrial fibrillation and had had two episodes of thromboembolism before starting anticoagulation therapy. Tulloch and Wright[4] reported a patient who developed cerebral and brachial emboli after dicumarol was stopped for eight days for extractions. The occurrence of thromboemboli after the abrupt discontinuation of anticoagulation therapy was postulated to be caused by a rebound hypercoagulable state.[37] Laboratory evidence supporting the existence of rebound hypercoagulability includes a temporary increase in factors VII and VIII after anticoagulants are stopped.[38] Harenberg et al.[39] found that discontinuation of oral anticoagulation therapy led to an increase in fibrinopeptide A that persisted 57 days later.

Sise et al.[37] speculated that the risk of rebound hypercoagulability was increased by abrupt withdrawal of anticoagulants, particularly after a bleeding episode. However, earlier studies comparing abrupt with gradual withdrawal did not show an increased rate of thromboembolic disease.[40-42] These studies supported the view that the risk of thrombosis is simply a return to the pre-existing level of risk. Michaels and Beamish[41] reported that abrupt removal of anticoagulants did not increase the rate of thromboembolism over that seen with gradual withdrawal. Michaels[43] subsequently reported that there was no clinically demonstrable risk of thromboembolism when anticoagulation therapy was discontinued because of hemorrhage. Physicians at the Mayo Clinic stopped anticoagulants for patients with cardiac valve prostheses who required other surgery (180 operations) and found no thromboembolic complications during the postoperative period.[44] Anticoagulants were usually stopped one to three days before surgery and restarted one to seven days after surgery.

In 1983, however, Hart and Coull[45] resurrected the possibility of rebound hypercoagulability by publishing a report on six patients who developed strokes four to seven days after discontinuing anticoagulation therapy.[45] The authors emphasized the fact that in patients with atrial fibrillation, the likelihood of a random stroke during a five-day interval is 1 in 1400. New evidence of a hypercoagulable state and increased risk of thromboembolism was obtained when warfarin was withdrawn from patients who had been receiving the drug prophylactically after myocardial infarction.[46] Of 47 patients, 9 developed thromboembolic complications within four weeks. The levels of factors VII and IX increased more rapidly than those of the anticoagulant proteins C and S after withdrawal of warfarin. This imbalance was greatest after one week. Increased plasma concentrations of fibrinopeptide A were further evidence of a hypercoagulable state.

The question over the risk of rebound hypercoagulability has not been definitively resolved. Withdrawal of oral anticoagulants for brief periods appears to be associated with low risk for most patients, and many patients occasionally miss doses and have subtherapeutic PTs without sustaining complications. However, it appears desirable to minimize the duration of subtherapeutic anticoagulation to reduce the possibility of hypercoagulability and thromboembolism.

The risk of thromboembolic complications must be evaluated for each patient receiving anticoagulation therapy who will undergo a dental procedure. For patients with a prosthetic heart valve, the risk of thromboembolism is related to the position and type of valve. A prosthesis in the aortic position is less thrombogenic (2% rate) than one in the mitral position (5%).[35] The design and hemodynamic performance of the St. Jude valve has reduced the risk of thromboembolism compared with earlier types of prosthetic heart valves.[47] Prophylaxis with a reduced dosage of warfarin to maintain the PTR at 1.5 can prevent thromboembolic complications in patients with the St. Jude valve.[47] Patients with a history of recurrent venous thromboembolic disease should be considered at high risk for thromboembolic complications when anticoagulation therapy is stopped, as should patients with atrial fibrillation and patients who have had myocardial infarction.[45,46]

Substituting Heparin for Oral Anticoagulants

Another recommendation for very high risk patients has been to switch them to heparin. Roser and Rosenbloom[48] administered intravenous heparin starting 24 hours after the discontinuation of a courmarin oral anticoagulant. When the PT returned to near normal, the heparin was stopped 12 to 24 hours before surgery. Oral anticoagulation therapy was resumed on the night of surgery. Heparin was resumed 12 to 24 hours after surgery and discontinued when the PT reached a therapeutic level.

Eckman et al.[49] examined the cost-effectiveness of hospitalizing patients with prosthetic heart valves for intravenous heparin infusions before and after noncardiac surgery. They reported that the marginal cost of prolonging hospitalization to administer heparin was prohibitively high because the rate of thromboembolic events is quite low and the period of increased risk is very short. For example, the marginal cost of giving intravenous heparin to a patient with a St. Jude valve in the aortic position (which carries a very low risk of thromboembolism) was $40,000 per quality-adjusted year of life gained. Clearly, the risks of hemorrhage from dental surgery do not warrant using the old technique of hospitalization to administer intravenous heparin. Hospitalization can be avoided by giving subcutaneous heparin in dosages sufficient to prolong the partial thromboplastin time to greater than 1.5 times control. Subcutaneous heparin is also inexpensive.

Summary of Approaches

Mulligan and Weitzel[33] classified dental procedures according to risk: Low-risk procedures included supragingival scaling, simple restorations, and local anesthetic injections in well-defined areas over bone; moderate-risk procedures were subgingival scaling, restorations with subgingival preparations, simple extractions, and regional injections of local anesthetics; and high-risk procedures were extensive surgeries. The authors suggested that in the cases of major hemorrhage that have been reported there is a possibility that the techniques of injection or surgery used may have contributed to the bleeding and that less traumatic techniques can reduce bleeding complications. They recommended no change in anticoagulation therapy for low-risk procedures. For moderate-risk procedures, Mulligan and Weitzel advised that the PT be verified; it should not exceed twice the control time. They suggested withholding warfarin for two days before a dental procedure, considering hospitalization for high-risk procedures, and returning patients to their usual anticoagulant dosage on either the evening of the day of the procedure or the next day.

The risk of serious hemorrhage due to dental surgery appears to be small. Both early and late bleeding can usually be controlled by local measures. Many patients have had dental extractions during anticoagulation therapy without complications. Adjusting the anticoagulation to a lower intensity (INR, 2.0 to 3.0) may further reduce the risk of serious hemorrhage. However, continuing anticoagulation therapy during dental extractions prolongs bleeding and can decrease wound healing. For extensive procedures, it is necessary to achieve near-normal hemostasis or to provide low-intensity anticoagulation therapy plus antifibrinolytic therapy; these approaches minimize bleeding, facilitate healing, and improve patient comfort.

The risk of thromboembolic complications is also small, although such complications can be catastrophic. Regulating the PT to the lowest therapeutic target level offers a reasonable compromise for minimizing postoperative oozing or bleeding while avoiding the risk associated with a complete reversal of anticoagulation. Patients should be carefully monitored to avoid prolonged periods of subtherapeutic anticoagulation.

Recommendations for Managing Oral Anticoagulation Therapy in Dental Surgery Patients

Low-Risk Procedures. For low-risk procedures, no changes are needed in patients with a therapeutic level of anticoagulation (INR, 2.0 to 4.5; PTR, 1.3 to 2.0). Routine dental work should be scheduled to take place shortly after a routine PT measurement.

Moderate-Risk Procedures. Warfarin dosages should be adjusted to achieve an INR of 2.0 to 3.0 (PTR, 1.3 to 1.5), with an INR of 2.5 set as a minimum in patients for whom the usual recommended level of anticoagulation is an INR of 3.0 to 4.5 (PTR, 1.5 to 2.0). For dental procedures with a relatively high risk of bleeding (e.g., tooth extractions), warfarin should be discontinued for 48 hours (two doses) before the procedure and reinstituted on the night of the day of surgery. The PT should be measured before surgery. Local hemostatics should be used to reduce postoperative bleeding.

Patients should be instructed to use external ice packs and biting pressure over gauze. They should avoid hot liquids, mouthwashes, hard foods, and aspirin and nonsteroidal anti-inflammatory drugs.

High-Risk Procedures. Dental procedures expected to cause substantial bleeding (multiple tooth extractions or other extensive surgeries) may require a return to normal hemostasis. This requires withholding warfarin for five days or longer. The PT should be measured before surgery to verify a return to near-normal hemostasis. The usual warfarin dosage should be resumed the night after surgery. Alternatively, patients undergoing multiple tooth extractions can discontinue warfarin therapy for 48 hours (two doses) and use a 5% tranexamic acid mouthwash. This approach avoids prolonged interruption of anticoagulation.

Long periods of inadequate anticoagulation may endanger patients considered to be at very high risk for thromboembolic complications. Warfarin should be discontinued and subcutaneous heparin should be started when the PT decreases to a subtherapeutic value. The heparin dosage should be adjusted to achieve an activated partial thromboplastin time of 1.5 to 2.0 times control midway between injection times. Heparin should be stopped for a minimum of 12 hours before surgery. Adjusted-dose subcutaneous heparin should be resumed 12 to 24 hours postoperatively and continued until the PT returns to the therapeutic range. The usual warfarin dosage should be resumed the night after the dental surgery or the following day.

Conclusion

In patients taking oral anticoagulants who must undergo dental surgery, careful control of the intensity of anticoagulation and improved methods of local hemostasis can minimize the risk of hemorrhagic complications and thromboembolism.

References

1. Ziffler AM, Scopp IW, Beck J et al. Profound bleeding after dental extractions during dicumarol therapy. *N Engl J Med.* 1957; 256:351-3.
2. Scopp IW, Fredrics H. Dental extractions in patients undergoing anticoagulant therapy. *Oral Surg Oral Med Oral Pathol.* 1958; 11:470-4.
3. Anon. Discretion in anticoagulant therapy. *N Engl J Med.* 1957; 256:367. Editorial.
4. Tulloch J, Wright IS. Long-term anticoagulant therapy: further experiences. *Circulation.* 1954; 9:823-34.
5. Poller L, Taberner DA. Dosage and control of oral anticoagulants: an international collaborative survey. *Br J Haematol.* 1982; 1:479-85.
6. Loeliger EA. ICSH/ICTH recommendations for reporting prothrombin time in oral anticoagulant control. *Scand J Clin Lab Invest.* 1985; 45:669-70.
7. Hirsh J. Is the dose of warfarin prescribed by American physicians unnecessarily high? *Arch Intern Med.* 1987; 147:769-71.
8. Hirsh J, Levine MN. The optimal intensity of oral anticoagulant therapy. *JAMA.* 1987; 258:2723-6.
9. Hirsh J, Poller L, Deykin D et al. Optimal therapeutic range for oral anticoagulants. *Chest.* 1989; 95:5S-11S.
10. Bussey HI, Force RW, Bianco TM et al. Reliance on prothrombin time ratios causes significant errors in anticoagulation therapy. *Arch Intern Med.* 1992; 152:278-82.
11. Hirsh J. Substandard monitoring of warfarin in North America: time for a change. *Arch Intern Med.* 1992; 152:257-8.
12. Johnson RL. Blood loss in oral surgery. *J Dent Res.* 1956; 35:175-84.
13. Johnson WT, Leary JM. Management of dental patients with bleeding disorders: review and update. *Oral Surg.* 1988; 66:297-303.
14. Sindet-Pedersen S, Ingerslev J, Ramstrom G et al. Management of oral bleeding in haemophilic patients. *Lancet.* 1988; 2:566.
15. Greenberg MS, Miller MF, Lynch MA. Partial thromboplastin time as a predictor of blood loss in oral surgery patients receiving coumarin anticoagulants. *J Am Dent Assoc.* 1972; 84:583-7.
16. Askey JM, Cherry CB. Dental extraction during dicumarol therapy. *Calif Med.* 1956; 84:16-7.
17. Shira RB, Hall RJ, Guernsey LH. Minor oral surgery during prolonged anticoagulant therapy. *J Oral Surg.* 1962; 20:93-9.
18. Behrman SJ, Wright IS. Dental surgery during continuous anticoagulant therapy. *JAMA.* 1961; 175:483-8.
19. Behrman SJ, Wright IS. Dental surgery during continuous anticoagulant therapy. *J Am Dent Assoc.* 1961; 62:172-80.
20. Kwapis BW. Anticoagulant therapy and dental practice. *J Am Dent Assoc.* 1963; 66: 172-5.
21. Frank BW, Dickhaus DW, Claus EC. Dental extractions in the presence of continual anticoagulant therapy. *Ann Intern Med.* 1963; 59:911-3.
22. McIntyre H. Management, during dental surgery, of patients on anticoagulants. *Lancet.* 1966; 2:99-100.
23. Waldrep AC Jr, McKelvey LE. Oral surgery for patients on anticoagulant therapy. *J Oral Surg.* 1968; 26:374-80.
24. Anavi Y, Sharon A, Gutman D et al. Dental extractions during anticoagulant therapy. *Isr J Dent Med.* 1981; 28:9-12.
25. Bailey BM, Fordyce AM. Complications of dental extractions in patients receiving warfarin anticoagulant therapy. *Br Dent J.* 1983; 155:308-10.
26. Rooney TP. General dentistry during continuous anticoagulation therapy. *Oral Surg.* 1983: 56:252-4.
27. Benoliel R, Leviner E, Katz J et al. Dental treatment for the patient on anticoagulant therapy: prothrombin time value—what difference does it make? *Oral Surg.* 1986; 62:149-51.
28. Sindet-Pedersen S, Ramstrom G, Bernvil S et al. Hemostatic effect of tranexamic acid mouthwash in anticoagulant-treated patients undergoing oral surgery. *N Engl J Med.* 1989; 320:840-3.
29. Vinckier F, Vermylen J. Wound healing following dental extractions in rabbits: effects of tranexamic acid, warfarin anticoagulation and socket packing. *J Dent Res.* 1984; 63:646-9.
30. Martinowitz U, Mazar AL, Taicher S et al. Dental extraction for patients on oral anticoagulant therapy. *Oral Surg Oral Med Oral Pathol.* 1990; 70: 274-7.
31. Spouge JD. Hemostasis in dentistry, with special reference to hemocoagulation. *Oral Surg Oral Med Oral Pathol.* 1964; 18:701-11.
32. Mulligan R. Response to anticoagulant drug withdrawal. *J Am Dent Assoc.* 1987; 115:435-8.
33. Mulligan R, Weitzel KG. Pretreatment management of the patient receiving anticoagulant drugs. *J Am Dent Assoc.* 1988; 117:479-83.
34. Yoshimura Y, Oka M, Kishimoto H et al. Hemodynamic changes during dental extraction and post-extraction bleeding in patients with prosthetic heart valves. *Int J Oral Maxillofac Surg.* 1987; 16:425-31.
35. Deron SJ, Kotler MN. Noncardiac surgery in the cardiac patient. *Am Heart J.* 1988; 116:831-8.
36. Cosgriff SW. Prophylaxis of recurrent embolism of intracardiac origin. *JAMA.* 1950; 143:870-2.
37. Sise HS, Moschos CB, Gauthier J et al. The risk of interrupting long-term anticoagulant treatment: a rebound hypercoagulable state following hemorrhage. *Circulation.* 1961; 24:1137-42.
38. Poller L, Thompson J. Evidence for "rebound" hypercoagulability after stopping anticoagulants. *Lancet.* 1964; 2:62-4.
39. Harenberg J, Haas R, Zimmerman R. Plasma hypercoagulability after termination of oral anticoagulants. *Thromb Res.* 1983; 29:627-33.
40. Van Cleve R. The rebound phenomenon—fact or fancy? Experience with discontinuation of long-term anticoagulation therapy after myocardial infarction. *Circulation.* 1965; 32:878-80.

41. Michaels L, Beamish RE. Relapses of thromboembolic disease after discontinued anticoagulant therapy: a comparison of the incidence after abrupt and after gradual termination of treatment. *Am J Cardiol*. 1967; 20:670-3.
42. Kamath VR, Thorne MG. Ischaemic heart-disease and withdrawal of anticoagulant therapy. *Lancet*. 1969; 1:1025-7.
43. Michaels L. Incidence of thromboembolism after stopping anticoagulant therapy: relationship to hemorrhage at the time of termination. *JAMA*. 1971; 215:595-9.
44. Tinker JH, Tarhan S. Discontinuing anticoagulant therapy in surgical patients with cardiac valve prosthesis: experience in 180 operations. *JAMA*. 1978; 239:738-9.
45. Hart RG, Coull BM. Hypercoagulability following coumadin withdrawal. *Am Heart J*. 1983; 111:169-70.
46. Grip L, Blomback, Schulman S. Hypercoagulable state and thromboembolism following warfarin withdrawal in post-myocardial-infarction patients. *Eur Heart J*. 1991; 12:1225-33.
47. DiSesa VJ, Collins JJ Jr., Cohn LH. Hematological complications with the St. Jude valve and reduced-dose Coumadin. *Soc Thorac Surg*. 1989; 48: 280-3.
48. Roser SM, Rosenbloom B. Continued anticoagulation in oral surgery procedures. *Oral Surg*. 1975; 40:448-57.
49. Eckman MH, Beshansky JR, Durand-Zaleski I et al. Anticoagulation for noncardiac procedures in patients with prosthetic heart valves: does low risk mean high cost? *JAMA*. 1990; 263:1513-21.

The postantibiotic effect

J. MICHAEL SPIVEY

Abstract: The factors that affect the presence and duration of the postantibiotic effect (PAE) for different antimicrobial agents are described, and the clinical importance of the PAE is discussed.

Proposed mechanisms by which the PAE occurs include both nonlethal damage induced by the antimicrobial agent and a limited persistence of the antimicrobial agent at the bacterial binding site. The specific microorganism–antimicrobial combination is the most important factor to influence the presence and duration of the PAE. Additional factors are antimicrobial combinations and experimental conditions, including the antimicrobial concentration and the length of the antimicrobial exposure.

Most antimicrobial agents produce a PAE when tested against gram-positive cocci. However, against gram-negative bacilli, β-lactam antibiotics (except for imipenem) have a minimal, or even a negative, PAE. Aminoglycosides, inhibitors of protein and nucleic acid synthesis, and fluoroquinolones have PAEs against gram-negative bacteria that range from one to four hours. In vivo PAEs are generally longer than in vitro PAEs for the same microorganism–antimicrobial combination. In human studies, aminoglycosides, which have an extended PAE against gram-negative bacilli, have been effective when given in once-daily dosing regimens that allow serum drug concentrations to fall below the minimum inhibitory concentration. Extending the dosing interval of an antimicrobial agent that has a PAE has several potential advantages, among them reduced cost, less toxicity, and better compliance among outpatients receiving antimicrobial therapy.

Although data are limited, animal and human studies provide support for the clinical importance of the PAE. Further research into the impact of the PAE on antimicrobial dosing, efficacy, toxicity, and costs is warranted.

Index terms: Anti-infective agents; Antibiotics; Concentration; Dosage schedules; Mechanism of action; Toxicity
Clin Pharm. 1992; 11:865-75

Persistent suppression of bacterial growth after brief exposure to an antimicrobial agent has been noted since the discovery of penicillin. In 1944, Bigger[1] first described a delay in broth turbidity (regrowth) when staphylococci were exposed to benzylpenicillin and later penicillinase to inactivate the penicillin. Later, Parker and Marsh[2] demonstrated that when *Staphylococcus aureus* was exposed to benzylpenicillin for a short period of time there was a lag period before bacterial growth began after penicillin removal. Eagle and colleagues[3,4] further explored the dynamics of bacterial growth after exposure to penicillin. Both in vitro and in vivo experiments with *Streptococcus pneumoniae* provided additional evidence that after exposure to penicillin a bacterial recovery period existed, which was followed by a normal growth phase.[3] Additionally, Eagle et al.[4] demonstrated in a mouse and rabbit infection model that the therapeutic efficacy of penicillin was determined by the aggregate time penicillin remained at bactericidal concentrations plus the recovery period before normal bacterial growth resumed. These researchers were the first to describe the phenomenon known today as the postantibiotic effect (PAE) and to suggest its importance in the design of antimicrobial dosage regimens.

It was not until the mid 1970s that the persistent suppression of bacterial growth after limited exposure to an antimicrobial agent was defined as the PAE.[5] Since that time, research has been directed toward discovering the factors that affect the presence and

J. MICHAEL SPIVEY, PHARM.D. is Assistant Professor, Department of Family Medicine, School of Medicine, East Carolina University, Greenville, NC, and Clinical Assistant Professor of Pharmacy, School of Pharmacy, University of North Carolina, Chapel Hill, NC.

Address reprint requests to Dr. Spivey at the Department of Family Medicine, 4N-80 Brody Building, School of Medicine, East Carolina University, Greenville, NC 27858-4354.

This is **article 680-204-9227** in the **ASHP Continuing Education System**; it qualifies for 1.0 hour of continuing-education credit. See page 893 for learning objectives and test questions.

Reviews in the Clinical Frontiers *section summarize recent research advances, such as those that contribute to an understanding of a disease process or the mechanism of drug action, describe new technologies or medical procedures that are likely to affect drug therapy, or describe likely new modes of drug therapy. Preference is given to articles that assess directions of ongoing research and critically evaluate therapeutic implications in new or rapidly changing areas.*

duration of the PAE for different antimicrobial agents. This review focuses on these factors, as well as on the clinical importance of the PAE.

Mechanism of the PAE

Despite recognition of the PAE for more than 40 years, the mechanism by which it occurs has yet to be fully elucidated. Proposed theories include both nonlethal damage induced by the antimicrobial agent and a limited persistence of the antimicrobial agent at the bacterial binding site, thereby causing a delay in bacterial regrowth after antimicrobial exposure.[6] Understanding the mechanism involved may help explain why fundamental differences in the PAE exist for β-lactam antibiotics and antibiotics that inhibit protein and DNA synthesis when they are tested against gram-positive and gram-negative bacteria. In general, both classes of antibiotics possess a PAE for gram-positive cocci; however, with a few exceptions, only antibiotics that inhibit protein or DNA synthesis possess a PAE for gram-negative bacilli.

Beta-lactam antibiotics covalently bind to penicillin-binding proteins (PBPs), which are enzymes necessary for cell-wall synthesis and growth. Continued binding of the β-lactam–PBP complex, despite removal of unbound antibiotic, may inhibit bacterial regrowth for a short period and be responsible for the PAE seen with gram-positive cocci.[6] However, recent information suggests that the PAE seen with β-lactam antibiotics may coincide with the time it takes to resynthesize new PBPs.[7] Tuomanen[7] demonstrated a rapid synthesis of new PBPs and immediate resumption of cell-wall synthesis by *Escherichia coli* after penicillin exposure and removal, which may explain the absence of a PAE when gram-negative bacilli are exposed to β-lactam antibiotics. It should be noted, however, that Tuomanen[7] showed similar results with streptococci for which an in vitro PAE had been noted with penicillin. Clearly, more research is needed with β-lactam antibiotics to elucidate the relationship between the PAE and resynthesis of PBPs.

In contrast to β-lactam antibiotics, antibiotics that inhibit protein synthesis (chloramphenicol, erythromycin, tetracyclines, clindamycin, and aminoglycosides) bind to ribosomal subunits. Protein synthesis inhibitors possess a PAE for both gram-positive cocci and gram-negative bacilli. For those protein synthesis inhibitors (chloramphenicol, erythromycin, tetracyclines, and clindamycin) that bind reversibly to ribosomal subunits, the PAE is likely due to a delay in the antibiotic dissociating from and diffusing out of the ribosome.[6,8] Conversely, aminoglycoside antibiotics bind irreversibly to ribosomal subunits, and postantibiotic suppression of growth from these agents is probably related to nonlethal damage.[8]

In Vitro Determination of the PAE

Methodology. Several in vitro methods have been developed to determine the PAE. The techniques involve exposing bacteria to an antimicrobial agent for a finite period of time, removing the antimicrobial agent, and quantifying bacterial growth after the antimicrobial exposure until a predetermined increase occurs.

One of the most widely cited in vitro methods, described in detail by Craig and Gudmundsson,[9] exposes an inoculum of bacteria in a logarithmic growth phase to a fixed antimicrobial concentration, usually four times the minimum inhibitory concentration (MIC). After incubation for one to two hours, the antimicrobial agent is removed by repeated washing of the bacteria, broth dilution, or drug inactivation. Penicillinase is the enzyme used to inactivate some β-lactam antibiotics. After antimicrobial removal, the broth culture is again incubated. To characterize the growth kinetics, viable bacterial counts, as measured in colony-forming units (CFU)/milliliter are determined before and after antimicrobial removal and every hour thereafter until turbidity occurs. To ensure that the antimicrobial removal process or subinhibitory antimicrobial concentrations are not contributing to the PAE, an untreated control culture undergoes a similar antimicrobial removal process, subsequent incubation, and viable colony-count determination. This negative-control culture is then used as a reference for comparison of the growth kinetics of it and the treated culture.

Another method of in vitro PAE determination, also described in detail by Craig and Gudmundsson,[9] is the membrane-agar technique. Instead of exposing bacteria to antimicrobial-containing broth, the bacteria are placed on a semipermeable membrane disk on antimicrobial-containing agar. After the antimicrobial exposure time is complete, the antimicrobial agent is removed by placing the disk onto antimicrobial-free agar, which allows diffusion of the drug from the membrane to the agar. Next, the bacteria are suspended in a saline solution at specified times and plated on an agar plate for subsequent viable colony count determination as previously described. With this method, the bacteria are less affected by osmotic pressure than they are with the broth method; however, it is more labor intensive.[9]

Despite the popularity of these in vitro methods, their relevance to an in vivo PAE has been questioned because the bacteria are exposed to a constant antimicrobial concentration, rather than to the fluctuating concentrations seen in vivo.[9] To provide a physiologic reduction of antimicrobial concentrations, broth dilution and dialysis in vitro models that simulate a first-order decline in antimicrobial concentrations have been introduced. With these in vitro models, bacterial growth patterns are determined after a decline in antimicrobial concentrations, as is seen with typical antimicrobial dosing regimens.

Broth dilution models reduce the antimicrobial concentration by adding broth media.[10-12] For example, Gerber et al.[12] demonstrated that exposing *Pseudomonas aeruginosa* to declining gentamicin concentrations produced a PAE of 1.4–1.9 hr after gentamicin concentrations were reduced below the minimal active concentration. One criticism of this model is that it dilutes not only the antimicrobial agent but the microorganism as well; this fact must be taken into account to accurately quantify microbial growth.[9] In vitro dialysis models avoid diluting the bacteria by using a semipermeable membrane to separate the growth media and bacteria while still allowing the bacteria to be exposed to physiologic declining antimicrobial concentrations.[13-15] Both models provide a simulated in vivo environment with respect to antimicrobial concentrations; however, it is difficult to separate the PAE from the effects of subinhibitory antimicrobial concentrations.[9] Additionally, technical differences in each model make quantitative PAE comparisons difficult.

Quantitation of the PAE. Viable colony counts traditionally have been used for determining bacterial growth, independent of the in vitro method used. When viability curves are used, quantitation of the PAE has been standardized as the difference in time required for the test culture (containing antimicrobial) and the control culture (no antimicrobial) to increase one logarithm (CFU/mL) above the number of organisms present at the completion of the drug removal procedure. Figure 1 displays two viability curves for *Staph. aureus* and *Strep. pneumoniae* after exposure to penicillin G and ampicillin, respectively.[6] The PAE is calculated by the equation PAE = $T - C$, where T is the time (hours) for the viable colony count of the test culture to increase by one logarithm above the count observed immediately after completion of the antimicrobial removal procedure, and C is the time for the viable colony count of the control culture to increase by one logarithm above the count observed immediately after completion of the same antimicrobial removal procedure used on the test culture.[6]

Because constructing viable count curves is labor intensive, new methods have been introduced that can considerably reduce the time and effort involved in determining bacterial growth. Spectrophotometric methods have been used to measure PAE, but they have provided inconsistent results.[11,16] Rescott et al.[16] described a good correlation between PAE measured with the Abbott MS-2 research system and viable colony counts for *E. coli* exposed to ampicillin, tobramycin, or ciprofloxacin; whereas Bergan et al.[11] demonstrated a discrepancy between the PAEs measured by optical density and viable colony counts for gram-negative bacteria exposed to aminoglycoside or β-lactam antibiotics. The difference in the spectrophotometric systems used may have accounted for the different results. Also, the PAE has been measured with a bioluminescent assay of bacterial adenosine triphosphate (ATP).[17-19] Because the bioluminescent

Figure 1. In vitro PAEs induced by two-hour exposure of *Staph. aureus* ATCC 6538P (left) and *Strep. pneumoniae* ATCC 27336 (right) to penicillin G 0.4 μg/mL and ampicillin 0.4 μg/mL, respectively. Antimicrobial removal was accomplished by repeated washing, 10^{-3} dilution, or drug inactivation by penicillinase (PENASE). Arrows indicate when the viable colony count had increased 1 logarithm above the count immediately after washing, dilution, or inactivation. The difference in time between the arrows for the control culture versus the test culture represents the PAE. (Reprinted with permission from reference 6.)

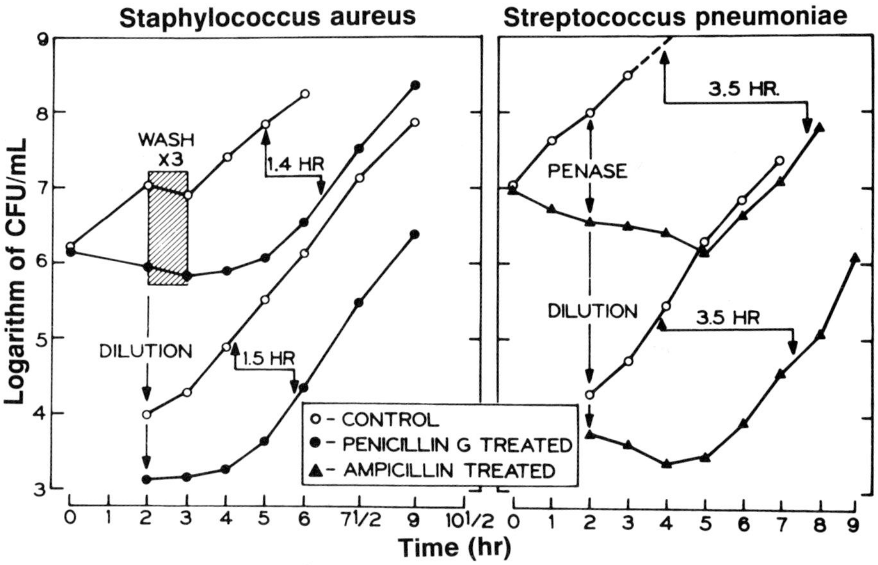

assay detects ATP from surviving and dead bacteria, it may overestimate PAE.[17] Recently, measurement of bacterial carbon dioxide generation by using a blood culture system (BACTEC NR 730, Becton-Dickinson, Sparks, MD) to determine the PAE was compared with viable colony counting. This novel method produced PAEs that correlated well with viable colony counting for a variety of antimicrobials when tested against *Staph. aureus* and *E. coli*.[20] Further research is needed that compares these new, less laborious methods of determining bacterial growth with viable colony counts.

Factors Affecting the PAE

Although various methods have been used to measure the PAE, investigators have consistently demonstrated a PAE for most antimicrobial agents. Nevertheless, several factors that can affect the PAE have been identified. The specific microorganism–antimicrobial combination is the most important factor to influence the presence and duration of the PAE. Additional factors are antimicrobial combinations and experimental conditions, including the antimicrobial concentration and the length of antimicrobial exposure.

Type of Organism and Antimicrobial Agent. Since the early work of Parker and Marsh,[2] which demonstrated a persistent suppression of growth after exposure of staphylococci to benzylpenicillin, many microorganism–antimicrobial combinations have been tested for PAE. Table 1 lists the most common bacteria–antimicrobial combinations tested in vitro.

Most antimicrobials produce a PAE when tested against gram-positive cocci (Table 1). For gram-positive cocci, β-lactam antibiotics (penicillins, cephalosporins, and imipenem) uniformly possess a PAE of one to three hours.[2,3,5,6,9,21-29] Studies with aminoglycosides show a short PAE of two hours or less; however, aminoglycosides' rapid bactericidal action lowers the viable counts too much for accurate detection.[5,6,30] Other inhibitors of protein and nucleic acid synthesis (rifampin, erythromycin, clarithromycin, clindamycin, and tetracyclines) demonstrate a slightly longer PAE (two to four hours) against gram-positive cocci than do β-lactam antibiotics.[5,6,9,31-33] The fluoroquinolones, which inhibit DNA-gyrase, exhibit PAEs of up to 2.5 hours against gram-positive cocci, including methicillin-resistant *Staph. aureus*.[9,24,27,34-36] Also, studies suggest that vancomycin (which inhibits cell-wall synthesis) and trimethoprim (which inhibits folate synthesis) have PAEs of one to three hours for gram-positive cocci.[5,6,9,29,33]

In contrast to data on gram-positive cocci, not all

Table 1.
Maximum in Vitro Postantibiotic Effects for Selected Microorganism–Antimicrobial Combinations[a]

Drug	Microorganism						References
	Staph. aureus	*Strep. pneumoniae*	*Ent. faecalis*	*E. coli*	*K. pneumoniae*	*Ps. aeruginosa*	
Penicillins							
Penicillin G	2, 3	3	3	ND	ND	ND	2, 3, 5, 6, 9, 21, 23, 26
Ampicillin	2	2, 4	1, 2	0	ND	ND	6, 9, 16, 23, 24, 28
Methicillin	2	ND	ND	ND	ND	ND	6, 9
Ticarcillin	ND	ND	ND	ND	ND	0	6, 9
Piperacillin	1	ND	1	0	0	0	9, 24, 25, 28, 38
Cephalosporins							
Cephalothin	2, 3	ND	ND	2	2	ND	6, 9, 22
Cefamandole	1, 2	ND	ND	0	0	ND	6, 9
Ceftriaxone	1	ND	0	0	0	0	9, 25, 28
Cefoperazone	2	ND	ND	0	ND	0	6, 9
Ceftazidime	ND	ND	0	0	0	0	25, 28, 37
Aminoglycosides							
Gentamicin	0, 1	ND	2	3, 4	3, 4	3, 4	5, 6, 9, 12, 17, 26, 28
Tobramycin	ND	ND	ND	3, 4	ND	3, 4	9, 16, 17
Amikacin	2	ND	0	3, 4	3	3, 4	9, 17, 25, 27, 30, 37, 38
Netilmicin	ND	ND	ND	4	ND	3, 4	9, 17
Fluoroquinolones							
Ciprofloxacin	2[b]	ND	1	2	2	2, 3	9, 16, 24, 34-36, 38
Lomefloxacin	2	ND	2	2	2	2	35
Norfloxacin	2	ND	1	2	ND	2	27, 36
Ofloxacin	2	ND	2	2	2	3	35
Miscellaneous							
Erythromycin	3, 4	4	ND	ND	ND	ND	5, 6, 9, 31, 32
Clindamycin	3	3	ND	ND	ND	ND	5, 6, 9, 32
Imipenem	3	ND	1, 2	1, 2	1	2, 3	9, 24, 27, 28, 37
Rifampin	3	ND	ND	4	4	4	6, 9, 33
Trimethoprim	2	ND	ND	1	1	ND	6, 31
Vancomycin	2, 4[b]	ND	0, 3	ND	ND	ND	5, 6, 9, 29

[a]0=PAE of ≤0.5 hr; 1=PAE of 0.6–1.5 hr; 2=PAE of 1.6–2.5 hr; 3=PAE of 2.6–3.5 hr; 4=PAE of >3.5 hr; ND=not determined.
[b]Includes methicillin-resistant *Staph. aureus*.

antimicrobial classes possess a PAE in studies with gram-negative bacilli. Beta-lactam antibiotics have exhibited a minimal PAE, or even a negative PAE, when tested against gram-negative bacilli.[6,9,16,22,23,28,37] A negative PAE results when the growth rate after exposure to antibiotics increases faster for the test culture than for the control culture. This phenomenon is probably related to the formation of gram-negative filamentous forms, induced by β-lactam antibiotics, that divide faster than control organisms on drug removal.[9] An exception to these results is seen with the β-lactam antibiotic imipenem, which exhibits a two- to three-hour PAE against gram-negative bacilli.[9,27,28,37] Binding to PBP 2 and spheroplast induction of gram-negative bacilli by imipenem have been suggested as possible mechanisms for the noted PAE.[19] Unlike β-lactam antibiotics, aminoglycosides demonstrate a two- to four-hour PAE against gram-negative bacilli.[6,9,12,16,17,27,28,30,38,39] Additionally, inhibitors of protein and nucleic acid synthesis (chloramphenicol, rifampin, erythromycin, and the tetracyclines) also show a PAE of one to four hours for gram-negative bacilli.[6,9,33] The fluoroquinolones produce substantial PAEs of three hours or less for gram-negative bacilli, including *Ps. aeruginosa*.[9,16,27,35,38,40]

Limited data exist regarding PAEs for other microorganisms. Against the gram-negative bacillary anaerobe *Bacteroides fragilis*, cefoxitin produced minimal or no PAE, and clindamycin and metronidazole produced a PAE of two to four hours.[41] Amphotericin B and flucytosine suppressed postantimicrobial growth of yeasts, whereas miconazole and ketoconazole exhibited minimal PAEs against *Candida* species.[9]

Antimicrobial Combinations. Recent work suggests that combining antimicrobial agents can have a synergistic, additive, or indifferent effect on the duration of the PAE compared with the PAE of either agent alone.[24-26,29,42] A synergistic PAE has been arbitrarily defined by one author as a PAE for a combination of antimicrobials that is at least one hour greater than the sum of their individual PAEs.[42] For additive or indifferent PAEs, the combination PAEs are approximately equivalent to the mathematical sum of the individual PAEs or no different from the longest of the individual PAEs, respectively.[42]

Because enterococcal infections often require combination antimicrobial treatment, much of the research concerning the effect of combination therapy on the PAE has focused on these pathogens. Fuursted[24] demonstrated a synergistic prolongation of the PAE of one to three hours when isolates of *Enterococcus faecalis* and *Enterococcus faecium* were exposed to streptomycin in combination with either ampicillin or vancomycin; however, an indifferent effect on the PAE was seen when streptomycin was combined with piperacillin, imipenem, or ciprofloxacin. An additive or synergistic increase in the PAE of up to three hours was seen when *Enterococcus faecalis* was tested with either penicillin G plus gentamicin or piperacillin plus amikacin.[25,26,29]

The PAEs of other antimicrobial combinations against gram-positive and gram-negative bacteria have recently been studied.[42] Gudmundsson et al.[42] demonstrated an additive PAE when *Staph. aureus* was tested against a combination of gentamicin plus either dicloxicillin or penicillin G.[42] Additionally, ciprofloxacin or rifampin in combination with dicloxacillin, gentamicin, or each other produced an indifferent or additive prolongation of the PAE against *Staph. aureus*. For the gram-negative bacilli *E. coli* and *Klebsiella pneumoniae*, a β-lactam antibiotic (ampicillin, ceftazidime, or imipenem) combined with an aminoglycoside (gentamicin or tobramycin) resulted in an indifferent PAE. Similar results were seen with the combination of piperacillin and tobramycin against *Ps. aeruginosa*. In contrast to these findings, the combination of imipenem plus tobramycin produced an additive PAE against *Ps. aeruginosa*. A synergistic increase in the PAE of two hours or longer was seen when the combination of rifampin and either imipenem or tobramycin was tested against *Ps. aeruginosa*. An indifferent PAE against *Ps. aeruginosa* was detected when ciprofloxacin was combined with either imipenem or rifampin. These limited data suggest that combining certain antimicrobial agents may result in additive or synergistic prolongations of the PAE. If in vivo studies confirm these results, then the dosing regimens of antimicrobial combinations that produce a synergistic PAE may be designed differently.

Experimental Conditions. Although the specific microorganism–antimicrobial combination is the most important factor influencing the presence and duration of the PAE, the in vitro experimental conditions are also important. The antimicrobial concentration, duration of antimicrobial exposure, and pH of the media are three experimental conditions that substantially affect the PAE. Differing antimicrobial concentrations and durations of exposure can be responsible for differing PAE results among investigators for the same microorganism–antimicrobial combination. It is important to note the antimicrobial concentrations used for in vitro PAE determination, because the concentration may be above the concentrations achievable in vivo and may not be clinically relevant. Additional experimental conditions such as size of the inoculum, type of growth media, and bacterial growth phase have been incompletely studied with respect to their effects on PAE duration.[33]

Antimicrobial Concentrations. Beta-lactam antibiotics display concentration-independent killing, which means that bactericidal activity increases to a maximum response and remains at this plateau despite increasing concentrations.[41,43,44] A similar concentration-independent PAE is seen when gram-positive cocci are exposed to β-lactam antibiotics. The duration of the PAE increases with increasing concentrations to a ceiling level (usually 5–10 times higher than the MIC), and further concentration increases have no effect on the duration of the PAE.[5,6,9,21] Increasing β-lactam antibiotic concentrations against gram-negative bacilli does not induce a PAE.[6,9,44] Vancomycin, another agent that inhibits synthesis of the cell wall, displays concentration-independent bactericidal activity similar to that of β-lactam antibiotics.[45] Likewise, vancomycin produces a concentration-independent PAE against gram-positive bacteria.[45]

In contrast, aminoglycosides and fluoroquinolones display concentration-dependent killing, which means that bactericidal activity increases with increasing concentrations.[26,30,40,41] However, a concentration-independent PAE, similar to that of the β-lactam antibiotics, was demonstrated for these antimicrobials when they were tested against gram-negative bacilli.[6,9,38] This latter outcome may have resulted from the researchers' inability to use viable colony counts to determine the PAEs for these antimicrobials at high concentrations because of the drugs' rapid bactericidal effect. Isaksson et al.[17] was able to demonstrate a concentration-dependent PAE with aminoglycoside concentrations of up to 64 mg/L when the bacterial growth of gram-negative bacilli was assessed by a bioluminescent ATP assay.[17] Other investigators have also demonstrated a concentration-dependent PAE with the aminoglycosides and fluoroquinolones, which is consistent with their concentration-dependent bactericidal activity.[26,30,40]

Antimicrobials that are primarily bacteriostatic, such as erythromycin, tetracycline, and chloramphenicol, appear to produce concentration-independent PAEs against gram-positive and gram-negative bacteria.[5,6,9] Maximum PAEs are seen at concentrations 4–10 times higher than the MIC for most organisms. For rifampin, which inhibits RNA synthesis, maximum prolongation of the PAE has not yet been determined despite increasing the concentration to 200 times higher than the MIC during testing of this agent against *Staph. aureus*.[9]

Duration of Exposure. Several investigators have studied the effect of lengthening the antimicrobial exposure time on the duration of the PAE.[5,6,21,32] Eagle[21] demonstrated that the duration of the postantibiotic recovery period of streptococci exposed to penicillin increased in direct proportion to the duration of the penicillin exposure. Likewise, Bundtzen et al.[6] were able to show prolongation of the PAE, although up to a maximum duration, when the antimicrobial exposure time was increased for several different microorganism–antimicrobial combinations. Additionally, the duration of the PAE for the combinations of penicillin G and *Staph. aureus* and for rifampin and *E. coli* was related linearly to the area under the drug concentration–time curve, up to a maximum PAE duration. Kuenzi et al.[32] demonstrated the same relationship for roxithromycin when tested against *Strep. pneumoniae*. This correlation suggests that the antimicrobial concentration and the duration of antimicrobial exposure are of equal importance in determining the PAE duration.[6]

pH of the Media. The majority of in vitro PAE studies have used culture media with a pH of 7.4, which is the pH of serum. Because alterations in pH may occur at local infection sites, such as an abscess cavity or the urine, the effect of pH on the duration of the PAE has been investigated.[46,47] Neu et al.[46] demonstrated a PAE of four to eight hours for several fluoroquinolones (at concentrations of 100 μg/mL or greater) against gram-positive and gram-negative bacteria, when tested in urine at pH 5.5 or in Mueller-Hinton broth at pH 7.4. Recently, Gudmundsson et al.[47] measured the impact of pH of 5–8 on the PAEs of dicloxacillin, imipenem, gentamicin, tobramycin, and ciprofloxacin against *Staph. aureus*, *E. coli*, and *Ps. aeruginosa*. Shorter PAEs were demonstrated at an acid pH for imipenem, ciprofloxacin, and the aminoglycosides against either *E. coli* or *Ps. aeruginosa*. No consistent effect of pH on the PAE could be determined for dicloxacillin or gentamicin against *Staph. aureus*, whereas ciprofloxacin had a longer PAE against *Staph. aureus* at both ends of the pH spectrum. From these two studies, it appears that high concentrations of fluoroquinolone antimicrobials have a PAE in the urine under acidic conditions; however, an acid pH may shorten the PAE of aminoglycosides, imipenem, or ciprofloxacin against gram-negative bacteria. Further work is needed on the effect of pH on the PAE for different microorganism–antimicrobial combinations.

In Vivo PAE

Although in vitro determination of the PAE has greatly enhanced understanding of this phenomenon, it remains an artificial test. Animal infection models have allowed investigators to test the PAE in vivo. Since the early work of Eagle et al.[4] in the late 1940s, animal models of infection have been used to study bacterial growth kinetics after antimicrobial exposure; however, the majority of data regarding in vivo PAE have been compiled only in the last decade. Two of the more commonly used animal infection models to study the PAE and factors that affect its duration are the murine thigh-infection and rabbit meningitis models.

Eagle et al.[4] first demonstrated in vivo growth suppression of streptococci after various doses of penicillin G in a murine thigh-infection model. A prolonged recovery period was noted before normal growth of streptococci resumed, despite the disappearance of penicillin. The PAEs that Eagle observed for *Strep. pneumoniae* and penicillin G may have been due to a penicillin gamma elimination phase, where inhibitory yet undetectable concentrations of penicillin persisted for extended periods of time.[48] Modifications in the murine infection model have enabled a true in vivo PAE, not affected by residual drug concentrations, to be quantified.[9] In this model, the mouse thigh is injected with a known bacterial inoculum. A single antimicrobial injection is administered, and the thigh muscles are removed frequently from infected mice for determination of both antimicrobial concentration and viable colony count. During the PAE phase, fresh organisms are injected into the opposite thigh of each mouse to ensure that growth is not affected by residual antimicrobial concentrations. Additionally, mice are made granulocytopenic to study only the interactions between the antimicrobial agent and the microorganism without interference from neutrophils.

Gudmundsson et al.[49] demonstrated in vivo PAEs up to 2.1 and 5.6 hours when moxalactam and cefoperazone, respectively, were tested against *Staph. aureus* in neutropenic mice. The PAE for cefoperazone is longer than that reported in vitro (Table 1). Additionally, no in vivo PAE was shown when these β-lactam antibiotics were tested against gram-negative bacilli (*E. coli, K. pneumoniae,* and *Ps. aeruginosa*), which is consistent with in vitro results. Vogelman et al.[50] produced similar results when in vivo PAEs for β-lactam antibiotics were determined against gram-positive cocci and gram-negative bacilli in the murine thigh-infection model. A one- to four-hour in vivo PAE was noted for penicillin G, ampicillin, cefazolin, cefamandole, and cefoperazone when tested against *Staph. aureus*. No PAE was demonstrated for ampicillin, cefamandole, cefazolin, or ticarcillin when tested against *E. coli, K. pneumoniae,* or *Ps. aeruginosa*. In contrast with in vitro results, no PAE was observed for penicillin G or ampicillin against *Strep. pneumoniae* in vivo. When imipenem was tested against *Ps. aeruginosa*, an in vivo PAE of 0.9–4.6 hours was noted, which is also consistent with in vitro results (Table 1).[49] The variation in the PAE duration for imipenem was due to differences in the *Ps. aeruginosa* strains tested. Aminoglycosides have been studied against gram-negative bacilli in the murine thigh-infection model, and a PAE of up to seven hours has been induced.[39,50] Recently, in vivo and in vitro PAEs were determined for aminoglycosides tested against 15 strains of Enterobacteriaceae.[51] In vivo PAEs (1.4–7.3 hours) were consistently greater than in vitro PAEs for all strains studied; however, a twofold to fourfold variation in in vivo PAEs among the same species was noted. Other inhibitors of protein synthesis (erythromycin, clindamycin, tetracycline) also induced in vivo PAEs of up to seven hours when tested against *Staph. aureus* and *Strep. pneumoniae*.[50]

Sande et al.[52] used a rabbit meningitis model to study the in vivo PAE. With this model, the PAE was considerably longer in vivo (6–12 hours) than in vitro (6–7 hours) when ampicillin was tested against *Strep. pneumoniae*. The prolonged in vivo PAEs seen with this model may be due to subinhibitory concentrations present at the site of infection, which have recently been shown to substantially prolong PAEs for β-lactam antibiotics tested against streptococci.[53] Further support for this theory was provided by Tauber et al.,[54] who demonstrated that the PAE of ampicillin against streptococci in the rabbit meningitis model could be reversed when subinhibitory ampicillin concentrations were inactivated by intracisternal administration of β-lactamase. The lack of a true in vivo PAE for ampicillin when tested against streptococci in the rabbit meningitis model is consistent with the in vivo PAE results seen in the murine thigh-infection model. However, Odenholt et al.[55] were able to demonstrate similar in vitro and in vivo PAEs when penicillin was tested against *Strep. pyogenes* in a rabbit tissue cage infection model. Possible explanations for the discrepancy between this in vivo study and others include the use of a different bacterial species and a different animal model, although further research is needed.

Hessen et al.[26] used a rat endocarditis model to study the PAE of penicillin plus gentamicin against *Enterococcus faecalis*. Despite the fact that a synergistic PAE was demonstrated for the antimicrobial combination in vitro, no in vivo PAE could be shown. In a *Ps. aeruginosa* rat endocarditis model, there was a prolonged in vivo PAE for ciprofloxacin; however, no in vivo PAE for ceftazidime was seen.[56] Renneberg and Walder[27] demonstrated a good correlation between in vitro and in vivo PAEs for imipenem, norfloxacin, and amikacin against *Staph. aureus, Strep. faecalis, E. coli,* and *Ps. aeruginosa* when a nonneutropenic murine infection model was used; however, the in vivo PAEs were generally longer than the in vitro PAEs.

Although data are limited, studies show that in vivo PAEs in both nonneutropenic and neutropenic animal models have been longer than in vitro PAEs. The PAE prolongation seen in neutropenic animal models is thought to be the result of a slower growth rate of bacteria in experimental infections than in broth cultures.[8] Additionally, Oshida et al.[57] demonstrated in a neutropenic mouse thigh-infection model that antibiotic concentrations below the MIC may contribute to the prolonged in vivo PAEs. When serum concentrations of aspoxicillin (an acylureidopenicillin) and piperacillin approached the MIC of the *Staph. aureus* isolate tested, penicillinase was injected into the mouse to remove the remaining antibiotic. After penicillinase was injected, the in vivo PAE was reduced from 5.2 to 2.7 hours and 3.3 to 2.0 hours for aspoxicillin and piperacillin, respectively, indicating a sub-MIC effect on the PAE. For the nonneutropenic animal models, the host immune system may partially account for the in vivo PAE prolongation. McDonald et al.[58] demonstrated enhanced bacterial susceptibility to leukocyte phagocytosis and killing in vitro after antimicrobial pretreatment. This phenomenon has been termed postantibiotic leukocyte enhancement. Further support for the hypothesis that the PAE is prolonged by postantibiotic leukocyte enhancement is provided by Fantin et al.,[51] who tested aminoglycosides against gram-negative bacilli and demonstrated an increased in vivo PAE in nonneutropenic mice compared with neutropenic mice.[51]

Antimicrobial concentration, which has been shown to affect the duration of the PAE in vitro, has also been studied in vivo. Aminoglycosides have demonstrated a concentration-dependent PAE when tested against gram-negative bacteria in the murine thigh-infection model.[39,50,51] Although data are limited, the more prolonged in vivo PAEs seen with higher aminoglycoside concentrations are consistent with in vitro PAE results. Because higher serum aminoglycoside concentrations also produce a longer duration of antibiotic exposure in vivo, duration of antimicrobial exposure may be an important factor that has similar effects on in vivo and in vitro PAEs.

In summary, in vivo findings regarding the presence or absence of PAEs for specific microorganism–antimicrobial combinations have been in agreement with in vitro findings. Differences between PAEs in vitro and in vivo have been exhibited for penicillin and ampicillin tested against streptococci. Additionally, in vivo PAEs are generally longer than in vitro PAEs for the same microorganism–antimicrobial combination. Factors such as slower growth in vivo compared with in vitro, sub-MIC effects, and postantibiotic leukocyte enhancement may be responsible for prolonged in vivo PAEs.

Clinical Importance of the PAE

The concordance between in vitro and in vivo PAEs establishes that the PAE is a biological phenomenon and not an experimental apparition. However, is the PAE clinically important? If the PAE is a clinically important event, it is most likely to have an impact on antimicrobial dosing regimens in two ways. For antimicrobial agents with a PAE, dosing intervals could be extended to allow concentrations to fall below the MIC of the organism for the duration of the PAE phase, without loss of efficacy. Conversely, for antimicrobial agents without a PAE, dosing regimens should achieve concentrations above the MIC for the entire dosing interval to ensure efficacy. Both animal and human studies have addressed the clinical importance of the PAE with different antimicrobial dosing regimens.

Animal Data. Animal infection models used to study the in vivo PAE have also been used to determine the impact of dosing regimens on therapeutic efficacy. Gerber et al.[59] used the neutropenic murine thigh-infection model to determine the influence of dosing intervals on the activity of ticarcillin and gentamicin against *Ps. aeruginosa.* For ticarcillin, which does not possess a PAE against *Pseudomonas* species, short dosing intervals are more effective than long dosing intervals that allow ticarcillin concentrations to fall below the MIC. In contrast, gentamicin does have a PAE against *Pseudomonas* species, and it is equally active when given at long and short dosing intervals. Using the murine thigh-infection model, several investigators have demonstrated similar results with gram-negative bacilli: (1) Beta-lactam antibiotics are more effective when given at dosages that maintain concentrations above the MIC, and (2) aminoglycosides are effective when given at dosages that allow concentrations to fall below the MIC for a period of time that does not exceed the PAE.[60-64] In gram-positive infections, antimicrobials that had an in vivo PAE could be administered less frequently than those antimicrobials without an in vivo PAE and still maintain maximum efficacy.[61] Additional animal models of infection (the rat endocarditis, rabbit endocarditis, rat pneumonia, and guinea pig pneumonia models) have yielded results similar to those found with the murine thigh-infection model.[56,65-67] In contrast to antimicrobials without a PAE, the antimicrobials with a PAE could be administered at extended intervals without loss of efficacy. The consistent observations based on different animal infection models support the clinical relevance of the PAE in the treatment of infections.

Human Data. Although animal data support the clinical importance of the PAE in antimicrobial dosing regimens, differences in animal and human pharmacokinetics make extrapolations from the animal model to human infections difficult. Human data addressing the impact of different antimicrobial dosing regimens on therapeutic efficacy are limited, despite the use of antimicrobial agents for more than 40 years. For the most part, antimicrobial agents have been given intermittently to achieve serum concentrations above the MIC for the entire dosing interval.[68] Little consideration has been given to the pharmacodynamics of antimicrobial agents (e.g., PAE), even though Eagle et al.[4] reported the importance of the postantibiotic suppression of growth in the late 1940s.

Anderson et al.[69] demonstrated that for β-lactam antimicrobial agents, which do not have a PAE for gram-negative bacilli, early breakthrough gram-negative bacteremia during antimicrobial therapy is associated with subinhibitory concentrations. The importance of maintaining β-lactam concentrations above the MIC for gram-negative bacilli is further supported by the work of other investigators.[70,71] Bodey et al.[70] demonstrated a higher cure rate (74% versus 59%) in neutropenic cancer patients who received cefamandole continuously versus intermittently. Additionally, Daenen and de Vries-Hospers[71] reported using continuously administered ceftazidime to successfully treat *Ps. aeruginosa* infections in two granulocytopenic patients, when previous intermittent ceftazidime therapy had failed. In one of the cases, subinhibitory serum ceftazidime concentrations were documented during intermittent therapy. These findings are consistent with in vivo animal studies demonstrating the importance of maintaining antimicrobial concentrations above the MIC of the organism when no PAE is present.

Aminoglycoside antibiotics have been the focal point of clinical trials addressing the impact of the PAE on antimicrobial dosing regimens. Because of concentration-dependent bactericidal activity and an extended PAE against gram-negative bacilli, aminoglycosides should be able to be administered in large doses less frequently (once daily versus three times daily) without compromising efficacy. Clinical trials involving a variety of infections have all demonstrated equal, or in one case superior, efficacy when aminoglycoside antibiotics (amikacin, gentamicin, netilmicin, and tobramycin) were administered once daily compared with more than once daily; however, sample sizes have been small (45–144 patients).[72-80] The largest study to date included febrile, granulocytopenic cancer patients randomized to receive a single daily dose of amikacin 20 mg/kg plus ceftriaxone 30 mg/kg or every-eight-hour doses of amikacin 6.5 mg/kg and ceftazidime 33 mg/kg.[81] In 694 evaluable patients, once-daily dosing of amikacin and ceftriaxone was equally efficacious and exhibited similar toxicity compared with multiple daily dosing of amikacin and ceftazidime.

The importance of the PAE in these studies is difficult to interpret because of two factors. First, investigators did not examine the relationship between success or failure and the duration of time that serum concentrations were below the MIC of the infecting organism. Second, several of the studies used broad-spectrum β-lactam antibiotics in combination with aminoglycosides, which may make it difficult to detect differences in dosing regimens.[82] Despite problems with sample size and study design, studies using novel aminoglycoside dosing regimens that allow serum concentrations to fall below the MIC of the organism are promising and support the clinical importance of the PAE. Rigorous examination of the relationship among the PAE duration, the time that serum concentrations remain above the MIC, and clinical cure rates is warranted in human studies investigating once-daily aminoglycoside dosing regimens.

The fluoroquinolones also produce concentration-dependent killing and an extended PAE against gram-negative bacilli. Peloquin et al.[83] documented a higher bacterial eradication rate in patients with gram-negative lower-respiratory-tract infections when plasma ciprofloxacin concentrations were maintained above the MIC of the pathogen for 95% versus 75% of the dosing interval.[83] More recent analysis of these data has suggested that area under the serum concentration–time curve divided by the MIC (AUC/MIC) is a better predictor of efficacy than the time that serum concentrations were maintained above the MIC.[84] This is consistent with other investigators' findings for antimicrobials with concentration-dependent bactericidal activity and a PAE.[39,61] Further evaluation of the importance of the PAE for the fluoroquinolones is warranted.

Despite the need for more research, the implications of the PAE phenomenon may be substantial. For antimicrobial agents that have a PAE, extending the dosing interval has the potential to reduce costs and toxicity. Additionally, compliance in outpatients receiving antimicrobial therapy may be enhanced by reducing the number of daily doses required for treatment.[85] Investigators have also suggested that the PAE is an important pharmacodynamic variable in determining the optimum dosing interval for a given antimicrobial agent.[86,87] Pharmacokinetics and pharmacodynamics have been used together to determine the optimum dosing regimen in individual patients for cefmenoxime, a β-lactam antibiotic without a PAE.[88] Although this method is labor intensive, it substantially shortened the duration of the antimicrobial treatment. Incorporating the PAE into this approach may be useful; however, the PAE cannot be predicted from commonly used in vitro testing, such as the MIC or the minimum bactericidal concentration. Automated methods of in vitro PAE determination will be necessary to provide useful and timely information that can be applied to the clinical setting. Finally, the PAE and other pharmacodynamic variables may be useful in determining the initial dosing regimens of new investigational antimicrobial agents.

Conclusion

Postantimicrobial suppression of bacterial growth has been determined in vitro for virtually all antimicrobial agents tested. A variety of in vitro methods have been used to determine the PAE, and the results can be summarized as follows: (1) Beta-lactam antibiotics possess a PAE for most gram-positive cocci; however, they lack a PAE against gram-negative bacilli, and (2) inhibitors of protein and DNA synthesis have demonstrated a PAE for both gram-positive cocci and gram-negative bacilli. Animal infection models, such as the granulocytopenic murine thigh-infection model, have also been used to quantify the PAE. Concordance between in vitro and in vivo PAEs for different microorganism–antimicrobial combinations provides strong evidence that the PAE is a real biological phenomenon. It should be emphasized that most PAE studies have included only a small number of bacterial strains; therefore, the PAE results for a microorganism–antimicrobial combination reported in the literature may not be applicable to a particular bacterial isolate found in a patient. Although data are limited, animal and human studies provide support for the clinical importance of the PAE. Further research into the impact of the PAE on antimicrobial dosing, efficacy, toxicity, and costs is warranted.

References

1. Bigger JW. The bactericidal actions of penicillin on *Staphylococcus pyogenes*. *Ir J Med Sci*. 1944; 227:553-68.
2. Parker RF, Marsh HC. The action of penicillin on staphylococcus. *J Bacteriol*. 1946; 51:181-6.
3. Eagle H, Fleischman R, Musselman AD. The bactericidal action of penicillin in vivo: the participation of the host, and the slow recovery of the surviving organisms. *Ann Intern Med*. 1950; 33:544-71.
4. Eagle H, Fleischman R, Musselman AD. Effect of schedule of administration on the therapeutic efficacy of penicillin. *Am J Med*. 1950; 9:280-99.
5. McDonald PJ, Craig WA, Kunin CM. Persistent effect of antibiotics on *Staphylococcus aureus* after exposure for limited periods of time. *J Infect Dis*. 1977; 135:217-23.
6. Bundtzen RW, Gerber AU, Cohn DL et al. Postantibiotic suppression of bacterial growth. *Rev Infect Dis*. 1981; 3:28-37.
7. Tuomanen E. Newly made enzymes determine ongoing cell wall synthesis and the antibacterial effects of cell wall synthesis inhibitors. *J Bacteriol*. 1986; 167:535-43.
8. Craig WA, Vogelman B. The postantibiotic effect. *Ann Intern Med*. 1987; 106:900-2.

9. Craig WA, Gudmundsson S. Postantibiotic effect. In: Lorian V, ed. Antibiotics in laboratory medicine. 3rd ed. Baltimore: William & Wilkins; 1991:403-31.
10. Nishida M, Murakawa T, Kamimura T et al. Bactericidal activity of cephalosporins in an in vitro model simulating serum levels. *Antimicrob Agents Chemother*. 1978; 14:6-12.
11. Bergan T, Carlsen IB, Fuglesang JE. An in vitro model for monitoring bacterial responses to antibiotic agents under simulated in vivo conditions. *Infection*. 1980; 8(Suppl 1):96-102.
12. Gerber AU, Wiprachtiger P, Stettler-Spichiger U et al. Constant infusions vs. intermittent doses of gentamicin against *Pseudomonas aeruginosa* in vitro. *J Infect Dis*. 1982; 145:554-60.
13. Zinner SH, Husson M, Klastersky J. An artificial capillary in vitro model of antibiotic bactericidal activity. *J Infect Dis*. 1981; 144:583-7.
14. Blaser J, Stone BB, Zinner SH. Efficacy of intermittent versus continuous administration of netilmicin in a two-compartment in vitro model. *Antimicrob Agents Chemother*. 1985; 27:343-9.
15. Blaser J, Stone BB, Groner MC et al. Comparative study with enoxacin and netilmicin in a pharmacodynamic model to determine importance of ratio of antibiotic peak concentration to MIC for bactericidal activity and emergence of resistance. *Antimicrob Agents Chemother*. 1987; 31:1054-60.
16. Rescott DL, Nix DE, Holden P et al. Comparison of two methods for determining in vitro postantibiotic effects of three antibiotics on *Escherichia coli*. *Antimicrob Agents Chemother*. 1988; 32:450-3.
17. Isaksson B, Nilsson L, Maller R et al. Postantibiotic effect of aminoglycosides on gram-negative bacteria evaluated by a new method. *J Antimicrob Chemother*. 1988; 22:23-33.
18. Hanberger H, Nilsson LE, Maller R et al. Pharmacodynamics of beta-lactam antibiotics on gram-negative bacteria: initial killing, morphology and postantibiotic effect. *Scand J Infect Dis*. 1991; Suppl 74:118-23.
19. Hanberger H, Nilsson LE, Kihlstrom E et al. Postantibiotic effect of β-lactam antibiotics on *Escherichia coli* evaluated by bioluminescence assay of bacterial ATP. *Antimicrob Agents Chemother*. 1990; 34:102-6.
20. Gottfredsson M, Erlendsdottir H, Gudmundsson S. Quantitation of postantibiotic effect by measuring CO_2 generation of bacteria with the BACTEC blood culture system. *Antimicrob Agents Chemother*. 1991; 35:2658-61.
21. Eagle H. The recovery of bacteria from the toxic effects of penicillin. *J Clin Invest*. 1949; 28:832-6.
22. Bodey GP, Pan T. Effect of cephalothin on growth patterns of micro-organisms. *J Antibiot*. 1976; 29:1092-5.
23. Wilson DA, Rolinson GN. The recovery period following exposure of bacteria to penicillins. *Chemotherapy*. 1979; 25:14-22.
24. Fuursted K. Comparative killing activity and postantibiotic effect of streptomycin combined with ampicillin, ciprofloxacin, imipenem, piperacillin, or vancomycin against strains of *Streptococcus faecalis* and *Streptococcus faecium*. *Chemotherapy*. 1988; 34:229-34.
25. Isaksson B, Hanberger H, Maller R et al. Synergistic postantibiotic effect of amikacin and β-lactam antibiotics on *Enterococcus faecalis*. *J Antimicrob Chemother*. 1991; 27(Suppl C):9-14.
26. Hessen MT, Pitsakis PG, Levison ME. Postantibiotic effect of penicillin plus gentamicin versus *Enterococcus faecalis* in vitro and in vivo. *Antimicrob Agents Chemother*. 1989; 33:608-11.
27. Renneberg J, Walder M. Postantibiotic effects of imipenem, norfloxacin, amikacin in vitro and in vivo. *Antimicrob Agents Chemother*. 1989; 33:1714-20.
28. Baquero F, Culebras E, Patron C et al. Postantibiotic effect of imipenem on gram-positive and gram-negative micro-organisms. *J Antimicrob Chemother*. 1986; 18(Suppl E):47-59.
29. Bush LM, Boscia JA, Wendeler M et al. In vitro postantibiotic effect of daptomycin (ly146032) against *Enterococcus faecalis* and methicillin-susceptible and methicillin-resistant *Staphylococcus aureus* strains. *Antimicrob Agents Chemother*. 1989; 33:1198-200.
30. Van der Auwera P, Klastersky J. Serum bactericidal activity and postantibiotic effect in serum of patients with urinary tract infection receiving high-dose amikacin. *Antimicrob Agents Chemother*. 1987; 31:1061-8.
31. Fernandes PB, Swanson RN, Hardy DJ et al. Effect of dosing intervals on efficacy of clarithromycin and erythromycin in mouse infection models. *Drugs Exp Clin Res*. 1988; 14:441-4.
32. Kuenzi B, Segessenmann C, Gerber AU. Postantibiotic effect of roxithromycin, erythromycin, and clindamycin against selected gram-positive bacteria and *Haemophilus influenzae*. *J Antimicrob Chemother*. 1987; 20(Suppl B):39-46.
33. Vogelman BS, Craig WA. Postantibiotic effects. *J Antimicrob Chemother*. 1985; 15(Suppl A):37-46.
34. Smith SM, Eng RH, Berman E. The effect of ciprofloxacin on methicillin-resistant *Staphylococcus aureus*. *J Antimicrob Chemother*. 1986; 17:287-95.
35. Debbia EA, Pesce A, Carlo Schito G. In vitro assessment of the postantibiotic effect of lomefloxacin against gram-positive and gram-negative pathogens. *Am J Med*. 1992; 92(Suppl 4A):45S-47S.
36. Davidson RJ, Zhanel GG, Phillips R et al. Human serum enhances the postantibiotic effect of fluoroquinolones against *Staphylococcus aureus*. *Antimicrob Agents Chemother*. 1991; 35:1261-3.
37. Bustamante CI, Drusano GL, Tatem BA et al. Postantibiotic effect of imipenem on *Pseudomonas aeruginosa*. *Antimicrob Agents Chemother*. 1984; 26:678-82.
38. Fuursted K. Post-antibiotic effect of ciprofloxacin on *Pseudomonas aeruginosa*. *Eur J Clin Microbiol*. 1987; 6:271-4.
39. Craig WA, Redington J, Ebert SC. Pharmacodynamics of amikacin in vitro and in mouse thigh and lung infections. *J Antimicrob Chemother*. 1991; 27(Suppl C):29-40.
40. Pruul H, McDonald PJ. Lomefloxacin-induced modification of the kinetics of growth of gram-negative bacteria and susceptibility to phagocytic killing by human neutrophils. *J Antimicrob Chemother*. 1990; 25:91-101.
41. Craig WA, Ebert SC. Killing and regrowth of bacteria in vitro: a review. *Scand J Infect Dis*. 1991; Suppl 74:63-70.
42. Gudmundsson S, Erlendsdottir H, Gottfredsson M et al. The postantibiotic effect induced by antimicrobial combinations. *Scand J Infect Dis*. 1991; Suppl 74:80-93.
43. Vogelman B, Craig WA. Kinetics of antimicrobial activity. *J Pediatr*. 1986; 108:835-40.
44. Gerber AU, Feller C, Brugger HP. Time course of the pharmacological response to beta-lactam antibiotics in vitro and in vivo. *Eur J Clin Microbiol*. 1984; 3:592-7.
45. Hanberger H, Nilsson LE, Maller R et al. Pharmacodynamics of daptomycin and vancomycin on *Enterococcus faecalis* and *Staphylococcus aureus* demonstrated by studies of initial killing and postantibiotic effect and influence of Ca^{2+} and albumin on these drugs. *Antimicrob Agents Chemother*. 1991; 35:1710-6.
46. Neu HC, Kumada T, Chin NX et al. The post-antimicrobial suppressive effect of quinolone agents. *Drugs Exp Clin Res*. 1987; 13:63-7.
47. Gudmundsson A, Erlendsdottir H, Gottfredsson M et al. Impact of pH and cationic supplementation on in vitro postantibiotic effect. *Antimicrob Agents Chemother*. 1991; 35:2617-24.
48. Ebert SC, Leggett J, Vogelman B et al. Evidence for a slow elimination phase for penicillin G. *J Infect Dis*. 1988; 158:200-2.
49. Gudmundsson S, Vogelman B, Craig WA. The postantibiotic effect of imipenem and other new antimicrobials. *J Antimicrob Chemother*. 1986; 18(Suppl E):67-73.
50. Vogelman B, Gudmundsson S, Turnidge J et al. In vivo postantibiotic effect in a thigh infection in neutropenic mice. *J Infect Dis*. 1988; 157:287-98.
51. Fantin B, Ebert S, Leggett J et al. Factors affecting duration of in-vivo postantibiotic effect for aminoglycosides against gram-negative bacilli. *J Antimicrob Chemother*. 1990; 27:829-36.
52. Sande MA, Korzeniowski OM, Allegro GM et al. Intermittent or continuous therapy of experimental meningitis due to

Streptococcus pneumoniae in rabbits: preliminary observations on the postantibiotic effect in vivo. *Rev Infect Dis*. 1981; 3:98-109.

53. Odenholt-Tornqvist I, Lowdin E, Cars O. Pharmacodynamic effect of subinhibitory concentrations of β-lactam antibiotics in vitro. *Antimicrob Agents Chemother*. 1991; 35:1834-9.
54. Tauber MG, Zak O, Scheld WM et al. The postantibiotic effect in the treatment of experimental meningitis caused by *Streptococcus pneumoniae* in rabbits. *J Infect Dis*. 1984; 149:575-83.
55. Odenholt I, Holm SE, Cars O. An in vivo model for evaluation of the postantibiotic effect. *Scand J Infect Dis*. 1988; 20:97-103.
56. Ingerman MJ, Pitsakis PG, Rosenberg AF et al. The importance of pharmacodynamics in determining the dosing interval in therapy for experimental *Pseudomonas* endocarditis in the rat. *J Infect Dis*. 1986; 153:707-14.
57. Oshida T, Onta T, Nakanishi N et al. Activity of sub-minimal inhibitory concentrations of aspoxicillin in prolonging the postantibiotic effect against *Staphylococcus aureus*. *J Antimicrob Chemother*. 1990; 26:29-38.
58. McDonald PJ, Wetherall BL, Pruul H. Postantibiotic leukocyte enhancement: increased susceptibility of bacteria pretreated with antibiotics to activity of leukocytes. *Rev Infect Dis*. 1981; 3:38-44.
59. Gerber AU, Craig WA, Brugger HP et al. Impact of dosing intervals on activity of gentamicin and ticarcillin against *Pseudomonas aeruginosa* in granulocytopenic mice. *J Infect Dis*. 1983; 147:910-17.
60. Gerber AU, Brugger HP, Feller C et al. Antibiotic therapy of infections due to *Pseudomonas aeruginosa* in normal and granulocytopenic mice: comparison of murine and human pharmacokinetics. *J Infect Dis*. 1986; 153:90-7.
61. Vogelman B, Gudmundsson S, Leggett J et al. Correlation of antimicrobial pharmacokinetic parameters with therapeutic efficacy in an animal model. *J Infect Dis*. 1988; 158:831-47.
62. Leggett JE, Fantin B, Ebert S et al. Comparative antibiotic dose-effect relations at several dosing intervals in murine pneumonitis and thigh-infection models. *J Infect Dis*. 1989; 159:281-92.
63. Fantin B, Leggett J, Ebert S et al. Correlation between in vitro and in vivo activity of antimicrobial agents against gram-negative bacilli in a murine infection model. *Antimicrob Agents Chemother*. 1991; 35:1413-22.
64. Leggett JE, Ebert S, Fantin B et al. Comparative dose-effect relations at several dosing intervals for beta-lactams, aminoglycoside, and quinolone antibiotics against gram-negative bacilli in murine thigh-infection and pneumonitis models. *Scand J Infect Dis*. 1991; Suppl 74:179-84.
65. Gengo FM, Mannion TW, Nightingale CH et al. Integration of pharmacokinetics and pharmacodynamics of methicillin in curative treatment of experimental endocarditis. *J Antimicrob Chemother*. 1984; 14:619-31.
66. Roosendaal R, Bakker-Woudenberg IAJM, van den Berghe-van Raffe M et al. Continuous versus intermittent administration of ceftazidime in experimental *Klebsiella pneumoniae* pneumonia in normal and leukopenic rats. *Antimicrob Agents Chemother*. 1986; 30:403-8.
67. Powell SH, Thompson WL, Luthe MA et al. Once-daily vs continuous aminoglycoside dosing: efficacy and toxicity in animal and clinical studies of gentamicin, netilmicin, and tobramycin. *J Infect Dis*. 1983; 147:918-32.
68. Kunin CM. Dosage schedules of antimicrobial agents: a historical review. *Rev Infect Dis*. 1981; 3:4-11.
69. Anderson ET, Young LS, Hewitt WL. Simultaneous antibiotic levels in "breakthrough" gram-negative rod bacteremia. *Am J Med*. 1976; 61:493-7.
70. Bodey GP, Ketchel SJ, Rodriguez V. A randomized study of carbenicillin plus cefamandole or tobramycin in the treatment of febrile episodes in cancer patients. *Am J Med*. 1979; 67:608-16.
71. Daenen S, de Vries-Hospers H. Cure of *Pseudomonas aeruginosa* infection in neutropenic patients by continuous infusion of ceftazidime. *Lancet*. 1988; 1:937. Letter.
72. Maller R, Isaksson B, Nilsson L et al. A study of amikacin given once daily versus twice daily in serious infections. *J Antimicrob Chemother*. 1988; 22:75-9.
73. Fan ST, Lau WY, Teoh-Chan CH et al. Once daily administration of netilmicin compared with thrice daily, both in combination with metronidazole, in gangrenous and perforated appendicitis. *J Antimicrob Chemother*. 1988; 22:69-74.
74. Hollender LF, Bahnini J, De Manzini N et al. A multicentric study of netilmicin once daily versus thrice daily in patients with appendicitis and other intra-abdominal infections. *J Antimicrob Chemother*. 1989; 23:773-83.
75. Sturm AW. Netilmicin in the treatment of gram-negative bacteremia: single daily versus multiple daily dosage. *J Infect Dis*. 1989; 159:931-7.
76. TerBraak EW, DeVries PJ, Bouter KP et al. Once-daily dosing regimen for aminoglycoside plus β-lactam combination therapy of serious bacterial infections: comparative trial with netilmicin plus ceftriaxone. *Am J Med*. 1990; 89:58-66.
77. Giamarellou H, Yiallouros K, Petrikkos G et al. Comparative kinetics and efficacy of amikacin administered once or twice daily in the treatment of systemic gram-negative infections. *J Antimicrob Chemother*. 1991; 27(Suppl C):73-9.
78. Maller R, Ahrne H, Eilard T et al. Efficacy and safety of amikacin in systemic infections when given as a single daily dose or in two divided doses. *J Antimicrob Chemother*. 1991; 27(Suppl C):121-8.
79. Van der Auwera P, Meunier F, Ibrahim S et al. Pharmacodynamic parameters and toxicity of netilmicin (6 milligrams/kilogram/day) given once daily or in three divided doses to cancer patients with urinary tract infection. *Antimicrob Agents Chemother*. 1991; 35:640-7.
80. Beaucaire G, Leroy O, Beuscart C et al. Clinical and bacteriological efficacy, and practical aspects of amikacin given once daily for severe infections. *J Antimicrob Chemother*. 1991; 27(Suppl C):91-103.
81. The EORTC International Antimicrobial Therapy Cooperative Group. Single vs. multiple daily doses of amikacin combined with ceftriaxone or ceftazidime for empirical therapy of fever in granulocytopenic cancer patients. Program and Abstracts of the 31st Interscience Conference on Antimicrobial Agents and Chemotherapy. Washington, DC: American Society for Microbiology; 1991:292. Abstract 1157.
82. Spivey JM, Schentag JJ. Aminoglycosides revisited. *Curr Opin Infect Dis*. 1990; 3:770-2.
83. Peloquin CA, Cumbo TJ, Nix DE et al. Evaluation of intravenous ciprofloxacin in patients with nosocomial lower respiratory tract infections. *Arch Intern Med*. 1989; 149:2269-73.
84. Forrest A, Ballow CH, Nix DE et al. Population pharmacodynamics of ciprofloxacin. Program and Abstracts of the 31st Interscience Conference on Antimicrobial Agents and Chemotherapy. Washington, DC: American Society for Microbiology; 1991:199. Abstract 602.
85. Gerber AU, Holm SE. Discussion of session II. *Scand J Infect Dis*. 1991; Suppl 74:142-4.
86. McCormack JP, Schentag JJ. Potential impact of quantitative susceptibility tests on the design of aminoglycoside dosing regimens. *Drug Intell Clin Pharm*. 1987; 21:187-92.
87. Turnidge JD. Prediction of antibiotic dosing intervals from in vitro susceptibility, pharmacokinetics and postantibiotic effect: theoretical considerations. *Scand J Infect Dis*. 1991; Suppl 74:137-41.
88. Schentag JJ, Smith IL, Swanson DJ et al. Role for dual individualization with cefmenoxime. *Am J Med*. 1984; 77(Suppl 6A):43-50.

Commentaries

Characterization of the postantibiotic effect

STEVEN C. EBERT

Clin Pharm. 1992; 11:876-7

In his review, Spivey[1] has provided an excellent overview of the literature concerning the theory, methodology, and characterization of the postantibiotic effect (PAE), both in vitro and in vivo. Although the PAE is recognized by most pharmacists as an important factor in the design of antimicrobial dosing regimens, the clinical importance and application of this phenomenon have remained elusive.

PAE in Vitro. As mentioned in the manuscript, antimicrobials that inhibit DNA, RNA, or protein synthesis exhibit a PAE against most bacteria in vitro, whereas agents that inhibit cell wall synthesis demonstrate a PAE against gram-positive bacteria only. The PAE of imipenem against *Pseudomonas* species is an exception. The precise duration of the PAE for any drug–organism pair, however, is quite variable. Enterobacteriaceae usually have shorter PAEs than do *Pseudomonas* species, but strain-to-strain variability exists within the groups. Combining antimicrobials seems to prolong the PAE, but most studies examining this issue have exposed bacteria to both drugs simultaneously rather than in a staggered fashion, which more closely reflects the clinical practice of intermittent dosing.

The duration of the PAE cannot be predicted from the minimum inhibitory concentration (MIC) or the degree of bactericidal activity that occurs during drug exposure.[2] However, supra-MIC concentrations of antimicrobial (usually eight times greater than the MIC) are generally used for PAE studies. Therefore, the MIC would appear to be of some importance. One might argue that in vitro PAE testing would have more clinical relevance if a fixed concentration of drug (e.g., the susceptibility breakpoint concentration) were used for testing rather than a fixed multiple of the MIC.

To use the PAE in dosing antimicrobials in the clinical setting, it may be necessary to develop an automated method for testing. One possibility would be to expose bacterial isolates to drugs possessing PAEs (as is done for microtiter MIC testing) but to remove the drug at some point to allow for regrowth. Clearly, more research into the appropriate concentration, duration of exposure, and method for detecting organism growth is necessary.

PAE in Vivo. For most bacteria, the PAE appears to be longer in vivo than in vitro. As mentioned, this may be due to the presence of host factors such as white blood cells and complement, postantibiotic leukocytic enhancement, and the slower rate of growth of organisms in vivo. It may also be due to the presence of subinhibitory antimicrobial concentrations, which persist for longer periods in in vivo models because of the method of drug removal (i.e., elimination). In fact, the longer the half-life of an antimicrobial, the greater the difference between the in vitro PAE and the in vivo PAE. This may be due to longer periods of exposure to subinhibitory concentrations, inhibitory concentrations, or both.[3]

Streptococcus species may be exceptions to the above difference between in vitro PAE and in vivo PAE. Few data are available to confirm or refute this point.[4,5] Questions have been raised because (1) quinolones such as ciprofloxacin have performed only marginally against streptococci and (2) experimental models of enterococcal endocarditis have shown that aminoglycosides provide greater benefit when administered frequently. Until more data are available, the PAE of antimicrobials against streptococci in vitro should not be extrapolated to the in vivo situation.

For those antimicrobials tested thus far, prolongation of the PAE in vivo is not due to the persistence of inhibitory concentrations of antimicrobial in tissues. However, studies are required with drugs such as the quinolones and macrolides to determine whether this is also the case for these agents.

Clinical Importance of the PAE. The presence of a PAE has not been definitively established in humans. However, as noted by Spivey, results of studies examining the impact of dosing regimens of β lactams[6,7] and quinolones[8] are consistent with concepts shown in animal models.

The most compelling evidence for a PAE in humans

STEVEN C. EBERT, PHARM.D., is Clinical Specialist, Infectious Diseases/Pharmacokinetics, Meriter Hospital, and Clinical Assistant Professor of Pharmacy, University of Wisconsin, Madison, WI.

Address reprint requests to Dr. Ebert at Department of Pharmacy, Meriter Hospital, 202 South Park Street, Madison, WI 53715.

Table 1.
Dosage and Serum Concentration Guidelines for Gentamicin and Tobramycin Based on Elimination Rate Constant

Est. CL_{cr} (mL/min)[a]	k (hr^{-1})[b]	Minimum Dosage (mg/kg/day)	"Equivalent" C_{max}/C_{min} at Indicated Dosing Interval[c]		
			q 8 hr	q 12 hr	q 24 hr
. . .	0.300	4.6	4.7/0.7	6.7/0.3	13.0/0.02
≥100	0.250	4.0	4.3/0.9	5.9/0.4	11.2/0.04
90	0.226	3.6	4.1/0.9	5.5/0.5	10.4/0.06
80	0.202	3.2	3.9/1.0	5.1/0.6	9.5/0.1
70	0.178	2.8	3.7/1.2	4.8/0.7	8.5/0.2
60	0.154	2.4	. . .	4.4/0.9	7.6/0.2
50	0.130	2.1	. . .	4.0/1.0	6.7/0.4
40	0.106	1.7	. . .	3.7/1.2	5.7/0.5
30	0.082	1.3	. . .	. . .	4.8/0.8
20	0.058	1.0	. . .	. . .	4.4/1.1
10	0.034	0.6	. . .	. . .	3.6/1.6

[a] Estimated creatinine clearance.
[b] Estimated or calculated elimination rate constant.
[c] C_{max}=concentration 30 minutes after dose, C_{min}=concentration 30 minutes before dose.

comes from studies demonstrating the efficacy of once-daily administration of aminoglycosides. Pharmacodynamic studies of aminoglycosides suggest that the area under the serum concentration–time curve (AUC) is a more important determinant of efficacy than is the dosing frequency.[9] This has led some clinicians to develop new guidelines for serum concentration monitoring that are designed to achieve a target AUC.[10] One example is shown in Table 1. In the future, pharmacists will be required to vary their target serum drug concentrations on the basis of the drug elimination rate, the dosing interval chosen, the severity of the infection, and the susceptibility of the pathogen.

Finally, the dosing schedules of other agents that exhibit PAEs should be scrutinized. It is likely that agents such as clindamycin and metronidazole, which have reasonably long half-lives and PAEs, could be administered twice daily in most individuals. On the other hand, maintaining serum concentrations of β-lactam antibiotics above the MIC may assist in ensuring efficacy of these agents.

In summary, the PAE is an important pharmacodynamic variable that should remind us that all antimicrobials are not the same. The PAE is one of many pieces of information that may ultimately assist us in individualizing antibiotic dosing regimens at the bedside.

References

1. Spivey JM. The postantibiotic effect. *Clin Pharm.* 1992; 11:865-76.
2. Fantin B, Ebert S, Leggett J et al. Factors affecting duration of in-vivo postantibiotic effect for aminoglycosides against gram-negative bacilli. *J Antimicrob Chemother.* 1990; 27:829-36.
3. Craig WA, Redington J, Ebert SC. Pharmacodynamics of amikacin in vitro and in mouse thigh and lung infections. *J Antimicrob Chemother.* 1991; 27(Suppl C):29-40.
4. Vogelman B, Gudmundsson S, Turnidge J et al. In vivo postantibiotic effect in a thigh infection in neutropenic mice. *J Infect Dis.* 1988; 157:287-98.
5. Odenholt I, Holm SE, Cars O. An in vivo model for evaluation of the postantibiotic effect. *Scand J Infect Dis.* 1988; 20:97-103.
6. Bodey GP, Ketchel SJ, Rodriguez V. A randomized study of carbenicillin plus cefamandole or tobramycin in the treatment of febrile episodes in cancer patients. *Am J Med.* 1979; 67:608-16.
7. Schentag JJ, Smith IL, Swanson DJ et al. Role for dual individualization with cefmenoxime. *Am J Med.* 1984; 77(Suppl 6A):43-50.
8. Forrest A, Ballow CH, Nix DE et al. Population pharmacodynamics of ciprofloxacin. Program and Abstracts of the 31st Interscience Conference on Antimicrobial Agents and Chemotherapy. Washington, DC: American Society for Microbiology; 1991:199. Abstract 602.
9. Vogelman B, Gudmundsson S, Leggett J et al. Correlation of antimicrobial pharmacokinetic parameters with therapeutic efficacy in an animal model. *J Infect Dis.* 1988; 158:831-47.
10. Gilbert DN. Once-daily aminoglycoside therapy. *Antimicrob Agents Chemother.* 1991; 35:399-405.

Regularly scheduled versus as-needed use of inhaled β agonists in the treatment of asthma

MALCOLM R. HILL AND KATHRYN V. BLAKE

Clin Pharm. 1992; 11:877-9

In 1990 Sears et al.[1] suggested that long-term, regularly scheduled administration of an inhaled β agonist is associated with a worsening of asthma compared with as-needed administration. And in 1992, Spitzer et al.[2] reported that excessive use of inhaled β agonists is

MALCOLM R. HILL, PHARM.D., is Clinical Research Pharmacist, Department of Pediatrics, National Jewish Center for Immunology and Respiratory Medicine, Department of Pediatrics and School of Pharmacy, University of Colorado Health Sciences Center, Denver. KATHRYN V. BLAKE, PHARM.D., is Clinical Research Scientist, The Nemours Children's Clinic, Jacksonville FL.

Address reprint requests to Dr. Hill at the Department of Pediatrics, National Jewish Center for Immunology and Respiratory Medicine, 1400 Jackson Street, Denver, CO 80206.

associated with an increased risk of death or near-death from asthma. These findings are provocative and demand that the health-care community re-evaluate the role of β agonists in the pharmacotherapy of asthma.

Constriction of airway smooth muscle leading to airflow obstruction is an important cause of the wheezing and coughing commonly associated with asthma. For many years, a fundamental goal in the treatment of asthma was relief of bronchoconstriction through the application of bronchodilators. Recent evidence from a variety of fields strongly suggests a link between airway inflammation and the pathogenesis of asthma.[3] It is the inflammation within the lung that leads to airway hyperresponsiveness, the characteristic feature of the disease. The airway obstruction observed is a result of this inflammatory process. Pathological characteristics of asthmatic airways include damage to the epithelial lining, the presence of proinflammatory leukocytes, various degrees of mucosal edema, and smooth muscle hypertrophy and constriction. These pathological markers are responsible for the initiation and perpetuation of inflammation[3] and the subsequent development of airway hyperresponsiveness. This underlying hyperresponsiveness predisposes persons with asthma to the bronchoconstriction that is associated with exercise or exposure to cold air, strong odors, or air pollutants such as cigarette smoke.[4] Airway hyperresponsiveness can worsen for days or weeks after viral upper respiratory-tract infection[5] and after allergen exposure in allergic asthmatics.[6] The degree of airway hyperresponsiveness is correlated with the degree of severity of asthma and with medication requirements.[7]

These findings about the pathophysiology of asthma have brought about dramatic changes in the therapeutic strategies employed.[8] The redesigned pharmacotherapeutic approach, together with revised diagnostic guidelines, have been publicized to the medical community by an expert panel of the National Heart, Lung, and Blood Institute as part of the National Asthma Education Program.[9] The goal now is to stem the current increase in morbidity and mortality from asthma.[10] Under the new directives, inhaled β agonists remain first-line agents for the treatment of asthma in its mildest form and are regarded as useful for controlling symptoms as severity increases. Indeed, inhaled β agonists can provide symptomatic relief in patients with the most severe form of chronic asthma. Inhaled glucocorticoids and cromolyn are considered for long-term prophylaxis.

In the Sears et al. study,[1] regular (four times daily) use of the inhaled β agonist fenoterol in addition to an existing antiasthma regimen that included as-needed β agonists was associated with a deterioration of asthma control. The investigators suggested that regular use of inhaled β agonists is a causal factor in the increasing morbidity and mortality from asthma. This idea has been referred to as the chronic effects hypothesis.[11]

There are several possible explanations for these findings. First, increasing airway hyperresponsiveness with continued, regular therapy may account for the observations. In this situation, the use of β agonists to control symptoms is thought to mask the insidious progression of airway inflammation and increases in severity. However, a pattern of increasing airway hyperresponsiveness has not been a consistent finding in clinical studies of inhaled β agonists[12,13] and does not fit the overall clinical impression.

Second, the development of tachyphylaxis or tolerance after prolonged use of β agonists is a well-known phenomenon and is the result of down regulation of β-adrenergic receptors.[14] Clinically, tolerance is manifested by a decrease in response and duration of action, yet it rarely renders inhaled β agonists ineffective. Patients in the Sears et al. study had mild asthma requiring an average of 2.9 puffs per day during the placebo phase of the study and therefore were unlikely to have developed a substantial degree of tolerance before beginning the active-treatment phase. Tolerance could have played a role in the worsening of asthma that was observed during the active-treatment phase.

Finally, the use of fenoterol itself is a potentially important factor. Fenoterol has been associated with death[15] and is thought to be less selective for β_2-receptors than agents such as albuterol[16] and terbutaline. Whether the findings of these investigators can be generalized to include β agonists other than fenoterol is not known.

If regularly scheduled use of inhaled β agonists at traditionally "safe" dosages can increase morbidity, does overuse result in further deleterious consequences? This question was addressed recently in a well-publicized study to determine the association between inhaled β agonists and the risk of death or near-death from asthma.[2] The authors looked for a correlation between the frequency with which prescriptions for various asthma medications were filled and the risk of death or near-death from asthma. There were two startling findings. First, the use of two commonly prescribed inhaled β agonists, albuterol and fenoterol, in excess of one canister per month increased the risk of death or near-death. Second, the risk more than doubled for each additional canister used per month.

The authors were careful to point out that their results do not show whether β agonists cause mortality or are markers of more severe disease. Further evaluation is needed to elucidate the causal factors. It is likely that both increased β-agonist use and increasing disease severity are factors in identifying patients at risk of asthma-related morbidity or mortality. Clearly, the use of inhaled β agonists in the clinical management of asthma patients should be closely monitored. Pharmacists serve a vital role in identifying patients who may be overusing these medications.

Until the optimum dosage schedule for inhaled β agonists is agreed on, some steps can be taken to decrease the reliance on these drugs. Asthma is a chronic disease that is punctuated by acute episodes. An important therapeutic objective is to reduce the frequency of the acute exacerbations as much as possible. Current recommendations for achieving this goal include the institution of anti-inflammatory therapy such as inhaled glucocorticoids or cromolyn.[9] Inhaled glucocorticoids can produce sustained improvement in airway hyperresponsiveness and decrease the requirement for inhaled β agonists.[17] Also, clinicians should evaluate asthmatic patients for overuse of inhaled β agonists. In patients with stable asthma, it may be reasonable to decrease the frequency of administration to the extent that is clinically tolerated. A midday dose could be reduced or eliminated but morning and bedtime doses continued. This strategy will help prevent a decline in pulmonary function during the crucial nighttime hours. Data to guide therapy can be gathered at home by using a hand-held device to monitor the peak expiratory flow rate.[9] Another important step is to recognize and treat exacerbations promptly with short courses of prednisone.[18] This may decrease inhaled β agonist use and the number of hospital admissions.

To settle the issue of regularly scheduled versus as-needed β-agonist therapy for asthma, we will need placebo-controlled clinical trials and careful analysis. Prospective studies to elucidate the mechanism by which any potentially deleterious changes may occur are also required. The health-care community must do whatever is necessary to reduce morbidity and mortality from asthma. The tools required are available; we have only to use them.

References

1. Sears MR, Taylor DR, Print CG et al. Regular inhaled beta agonist treatment in bronchial asthma. *Lancet*. 1990; 336:1391-6.
2. Spitzer WO, Suissa S, Ernst P et al. The use of β-agonists and the risk of death and near death from asthma. *N Engl J Med*. 1992; 326:501-6.
3. Hill MR, Kamada AK. Pathogenesis of asthma: therapeutic implications. *DICP Ann Pharmacother*. 1991; 25:993-1001.
4. Wilson MC, Irvin CG, Larsen GL. Inflammation and asthma. *Semin Respir Med*. 1987; 8:279-86.
5. Empey JW, Laitinen LA, Jacobs L et al. Mechanisms of bronchial hyperreactivity in normal subjects after upper respiratory tract infection. *Am Rev Respir Dis*. 1976; 113:131-9.
6. Cartier A, Thomson NC, Frith PA et al. Allergen-induced increase in bronchial responsiveness to histamine: relationship to the late asthmatic response and change in airway caliber. *J Allergy Clin Immunol*. 1982; 70:170-7.
7. Cockcroft DW. Airway hyperresponsiveness: therapeutic implications. *Ann Allergy*. 1987; 59:405-14.
8. Barnes PJ. A new approach to the treatment of asthma. *N Engl J Med*. 1989; 321:1517-27.
9. National Asthma Education Program Expert Panel. Guidelines for the diagnosis and management of asthma. *J Allergy Clin Immunol*. 1991; 88:425-534.
10. Anon. Asthma—United States, 1980–1987. *MMWR*. 1990; 39:493-7.
11. Pearce N, Crane J, Burgess C et al. Beta-agonists and asthma mortality: deja vu. *Clin Exp Allergy*. 1991; 21:401-10.
12. Salome CM, Schoeffel RE, Yan K et al. Effect of aerosol fenoterol on the severity of bronchial hyperreactivity in patients with asthma. *Thorax*. 1983; 38:854-8.
13. Kerrebijn KF, Van Essen-Sanduliet EEM, Neijens HJ. Effect of long term treatment with inhaled corticosteroids and beta-agonists on the bronchial hyperresponsiveness in children with asthma. *J Allergy Clin Immunol*. 1987; 79:653-9.
14. Fraser CM, Potter PC, Venter JC et al. Adrenergic agents. In: Middleton E, Reed CE, Ellis EF et al., eds. Allergy principles and practice. St. Louis: Mosby; 1988:636-72.
15. Crane J, Pearce N, Flatt A et al. Prescribed fenoterol and death from asthma in New Zealand, 1981–83: case-control study. *Lancet*. 1989; 1:917-22.
16. Crane J, Burgess C, Beasley R. A comparison of the cardiovascular and hypokalemic effects of inhaled salbutamol, fenoterol, and isoprenaline. *Thorax*. 1989; 44:136-2140.
17. Juniper EF, Kline PA, Vanzielghem MA et al. Effect of long-term treatment with an inhaled corticosteroid (budesonide) on airway hyperresponsiveness and clinical asthma in non-steroid dependent asthmatics. *Am Rev Respir Dis*. 1990; 142:832-6.
18. Harris JB, Weinberger MM, Nassif E et al. Early intervention with short courses of prednisone to prevent progression of asthma in ambulatory patients incompletely responsive to bronchodilators. *J Pediatr*. 1987; 110:627-33.

Increasing Prevalence of Asthma

Asthma is among the most common chronic diseases in the United States, afflicting greater than 10 million Americans. The most frequent cause of hospital admissions for children, asthma also leads the list of childhood diseases that cause a significant loss of time from school. The medical and social consequences of asthma are even more severe in the inner city, particularly among black and Hispanic populations. Over 4000 Americans die of asthma each year, and there is mounting evidence that U.S. asthma mortality rates are increasing, following a decade of steady declines during the 1970s. In 1987, asthma mortality rates for children and young adults, ages 5 to 34, exceeded those of 1969. Therefore, research on the mechanisms involved in the pathogenesis, treatment, and prevention of asthma is critical to reducing the morbidity and mortality caused by this disease.

—Prograis LJ Jr, Zunich KM. NIAID programs for asthma research, education, and outreach. *Chest*. 1992; 101(Suppl):357S-358S.

Drug Experience

Straightforward reports of unusual drug experiences are included in this section. These may be confirmations of previously reported drug experiences or brief apparent first reports. While selected references may be cited, the purpose of a Drug Experience *report is not to present an extensive review of the literature.*

A related section, Grand Rounds, *includes papers that are well-documented patient case reports with a thorough review of the important literature to help put the case in perspective.*

Colfosceril in an infant with adult respiratory distress syndrome

C. Y. Jennifer Chan, Terri L. Barton, and Deborah K. Rasch

Clin Pharm. 1992; 11:880-2

Adult respiratory distress syndrome (ARDS) is a form of acute respiratory failure that has been reported in both adults and children and is associated with a high mortality rate.[1] Exogenous surfactant has been shown to be effective in the treatment and prevention of neonatal respiratory distress syndrome (RDS),[2] but limited data are available on its use in ARDS. In this report, we describe an infant with ARDS who showed rapid resolution of symptoms, clinically and roentgenographically, after tracheal administration of colfosceril (exogenous pulmonary surfactant).

Case Report. A three-week-old girl was brought to the clinic because she had had a decreased appetite and loose stools. The infant had been in good health until the morning of admission, when she refused feeding and was inconsolable. She had one episode of emesis that morning before admission. She had been born at full term by spontaneous vaginal delivery without any complications. Her birth weight was 3.0 kg, and her weight on admission was 3.7 kg.

In the clinic, she was cyanotic, cold, and in severe respiratory distress. She also had poor capillary refill and perfusion. Chest examination revealed rales and poor air movement. The vital signs were as follows: rectal temperature, 36.1 °C; heart rate, 172 beats/min; blood pressure, 60/40 mm Hg; and respiratory rate, 68 breaths/min. An endotracheal tube was placed, and a total of 20 mL/kg of 0.9% sodium chloride injection was given i.v. She was then transported to the pediatric intensive-care unit (PICU).

When she arrived at the PICU, the infant was still cyanotic and had poor perfusion and cold extremities. Pulmonary compliance was poor and oxygen saturation, as measured by pulse oximetry, could not be increased above 92% with vigorous hand ventilation. After initial evaluation, she developed paroxysmal supraventricular tachycardia. Her heart rate was 315 beats/min and the blood pressure was not palpable. Sinus rhythm was restored after the third attempt at electrical cardioversion and the administration of a total dose of 15 μg/kg of digoxin i.v. At that time, the patient's heart rate was 165 beats/min and the blood pressure was 79/51 mm Hg. An electrocardiogram revealed sinus rhythm and a right axis deviation of +120° with right ventricular dominance. Despite restoration of sinus rhythm, maintenance of adequate ventilation remained difficult. A ventilator was used at the following settings: rate, 28 breaths/min; inspiration: expiration ratio, 1.25:1; positive end-expiratory pressure (PEEP), 8 cm H_2O, peak inspiratory pressure (PIP), 58–62 cm H_2O; fraction of inspired oxygen (Fio_2), 100%; and tidal volume (TV), 130 mL. The resultant oxygen saturation was 92% to 94%. Chest roentgenograms revealed normal heart size and diffuse alveolar infiltrates throughout the lungs consistent with ARDS.

Colfosceril palmitate intratracheal suspension (Exosurf Neonatal, Burroughs Wellcome Co.) 20 mL (5.4 mL/kg) was administered through an endotracheal tube in four positions to both lungs approximately four hours after admission to the PICU (three hours after the final dose of digoxin). The patient tolerated colfosceril administration well. Four hours after administration, ventilator settings were de-

C.Y. Jennifer Chan, Pharm.D., is Clinical Assistant Professor, College of Pharmacy, The University of Texas at Austin (UT) and Department of Pharmacology, The University of Texas Health Science Center at San Antonio (UTHSC). Terri L. Barton, Pharm.D., is Assistant Professor of Pharmacy Practice, and Director, Drug Information Service, College of Pharmacy, The University of Oklahoma Health Sciences Center, Oklahoma City; at the time this manuscript was prepared, she was Specialty Practice Resident in Drug Information, UTHSC, and Clinical Instructor, College of Pharmacy, UT. Deborah K. Rasch, M.D., is Associate Professor, Department of Anesthesiology and Pediatrics, UTHSC.

Address reprint requests to Dr. Chan at Clinical Pharmacy Programs, The University of Texas Health Science Center at San Antonio, 7703 Floyd Curl Drive, San Antonio, TX 78284-6220.

Presented at the 26th Annual ASHP Midyear Clinical Meeting, New Orleans, LA, December 12, 1991.

creased to the following: rate, 25 breaths/min; PEEP, 6 cm H_2O; PIP, 34 cm H_2O; Fio_2, 40%; and TV, 100 mL. Oxygen saturation was 100%. A chest roentgenogram obtained 10 hours after administration of colfosceril showed clearing of diffuse alveolar infiltrates. The infant's cardiovascular status remained stable. Echocardiography performed four hours after administration of colfosceril showed a normal fractional shortening of the left ventricle (31%) and no structural defects. The patient's respiratory status continued to improve, and the endotracheal tube was removed 40 hours after administration of colfosceril. She was discharged six days after admission in no apparent respiratory distress.

Discussion. ARDS was first described in 1967 in 12 patients with symptoms of tachypnea, hypoxemia, and loss of lung compliance. ARDS occurs in an estimated 150,000 persons each year in the United States, with a mortality rate as high as 50%.[3,4] Because the administration of exogenous surfactant is beneficial in the treatment and prevention of neonatal RDS (a state of quantitative surfactant deficiency), its use has been evaluated in the treatment of ARDS.[2,5,6]

The primary findings in ARDS include arterial hypoxemia that is refractory to oxygen therapy, increased intrapulmonary shunting, decreased lung compliance, and decreased lung volumes, all in the absence of left ventricular failure. Increased alveolar permeability, the primary defect in ARDS, results from injury to the alveolar–capillary membrane and leads to edema in the alveolar space.[4,5] Two of the major precipitants of ARDS, trauma and infection, facilitate activation of the complement and coagulation cascades. The resulting adherence of neutrophils and platelets stimulates the release of a number of toxic substances (e.g., oxygen free radicals, lysosomal enzymes) that promote local inflammatory responses and tissue damage. Also, cellular phospholipases are activated, causing damage to the capillary endothelium and cleaving surfactant phospholipids. This results in a functional surfactant deficiency due to surfactant inactivation.[1,2,4,5,7,8]

Despite the word "adult" in the syndrome's name, the features of ARDS are similar in pediatric and adult patients.[1,4,5,7] The clinical course of ARDS can be divided into four phases. During the first phase the acute injury occurs, with only subtle evidence of the ensuing process. Various conditions have been reported to result in injury to the lung. The insult leading to ARDS in this patient is unclear. However, pneumonia, electrical cardioversion, and shock have been associated with the development of ARDS.[4] In the second phase, the latent period, there is apparent stability lasting 6 to 48 hours. The third phase is the period of acute respiratory failure and progressive pulmonary insufficiency. Signs and symptoms include tachypnea, dyspnea, hypoxemia that is refractory to oxygen therapy, diffuse pulmonary infiltrates, and decreased lung compliance. The final phase results in either resolution of the disease process or hypoxemia and hypercapnia that are unresponsive to treatment and result in death.

Because of the many causes and manifestations of ARDS, treatment is multifaceted. The mainstay of treatment is mechanical ventilatory support with PEEP and appropriate fluid management. If infection develops, antimicrobials are recommended. The benefits of high-dose corticosteroids in the treatment of ARDS have not been proved.[5,7] Preliminary observations suggest that the administration of exogenous surfactant may be beneficial.[6,9]

Pulmonary surfactant serves to lower alveolar surface tension at low lung volumes to prevent alveolar collapse at the end of expiration.[10] It is found along the alveolar epithelium, which is composed of two cell types: type I pneumocytes, which normally cover 95% of the alveolar surface, and type II pneumocytes, which produce pulmonary surfactant. Type II cells also are involved in the repair of the alveolar epithelium after damage to type I cells.[8]

Pulmonary surfactant is primarily composed of phospholipids and apoproteins. Phosphatidylcholine is the most prevalent phospholipid, accounting for 70% to 80% of the total content of endogenous surfactant. Most of the phosphatidylcholine is disaturated with palmitic acid to form dipalmitoylphosphatidylcholine, which appears to be the component responsible for lowering surface tension. Collectively, dipalmitoylphosphatidylcholine and phosphatidylcholine are known as lecithin. Phosphatidylglycerol constitutes 5% to 10% of total surfactant phospholipids. Its role is not clearly defined, but it may promote the association of surfactant apoproteins with phospholipids and the recycling of surfactant by alveolar epithelium. Other phospholipids, including phosphatidylethanolamine, phosphatidylserine, phosphatidylinositol, sphingomyelin, and cholesterol, constitute 10% to 15% of the total lipid content. Their role in surfactant function is unknown.

Several surfactant proteins have been characterized, but most of the available data describe surfactant protein-A (SP-A). SP-A interacts with lipids at body temperature to maintain fluidity. It is involved in regulating the reuptake and secretion of surfactant phospholipids and proteins. SP-A is not incorporated into commercial products since it is not essential for the spreading of surfactants. However, alcohol is added to promote the spreading of phospholipids. Surfactant protein-B (SP-B) and surfactant protein-C (SP-C) have been shown to affect the spreading properties of lipids and accelerate the rate of formation of a surface film at an air–liquid interface.[5,10,11]

Total phospholipid content in patients with ARDS does not differ markedly from that in patients without ARDS. However, several components and ratios of surfactant are altered in ARDS.[12,13] Phophatidylcholine and phosphatidylglycerol are found in decreased amounts, and the lecithin-to-sphingomyelin ratio is decreased. Investigators have attempted to create an ARDS-like injury in animals to study the effects of exogenous surfactant and other agents. While no single animal model exhibits all of the characteristics of clinical ARDS, acute and chronic ARDS-like injuries have been simulated. The administration of exogenous surfactant has led to improved respiratory function in animal models with surfactant depletion and direct lung injury.[14-18]

Currently, there are two surfactant preparations available in the United States. FDA-approved labeling for colfosceril and beractant (Survanta, Ross Laboratories) states that the drugs are indicated for the prevention and treatment of neonatal RDS. Adverse effects reported with exogenous surfactant have been minimal. The frequency of pulmonary hemorrhage and apnea were increased in premature infants who received colfosceril.[19]

Studies of surfactant therapy in humans with ARDS are limited. Using a crossover design, Richman et al.[6] evaluated the effect of 4 g of porcine lung-derived surfactant compared with equal volumes of either 0.9% sodium chloride solution or air in three patients (whose ages were not provided) with ARDS. Maximum increases in arterial Po_2 following transbronchial administration were 31, 37, and 82 mm Hg. In the two patients who exhibited the smallest increases in arterial Po_2, this variable returned to baseline within one hour. However, the increased arterial Po_2 persisted for three days in the third patient. All patients experienced improved pulmonary gas exchange that correlated with increased pulmonary phospholipid concentrations as determined by bronchoalveolar lavage. Neither lung compliance nor functional residual capacity was markedly altered in any of the patients. Surfactant treatment was well tolerated by all of the patients.

Lachmann[9] reported the use of surfactant in a pediatric patient with ARDS. A 4-year-old child with sepsis and severe ARDS was treated with tracheal instillation of natural surfactant (300 mg of phospholipids per kilogram). A dramatic improvement in gas exchange occurred within four hours. Chest roentgenograms obtained 20 minutes before and four hours after surfactant instillation revealed restoration of pulmonary aeration to near normal. The outcome of the patient was not reported.

Currently, only limited data are available concerning the use of surfactant in patients with ARDS. Animal studies and preliminary observations suggest that exogenous surfactant instillation in the management of patients with ARDS deserves further evaluation. Controlled clinical trials to evaluate the efficacy, optimal dosage, and proper administration technique are required before the use of exogenous surfactant in ARDS can be routinely recommended.

Conclusion. Colfosceril therapy appeared to be effective in treating an infant with ARDS.

References

1. Hyers TM, Fowler AA. Adult respiratory distress syndrome: causes, morbidity, and mortality. *Fed Proc.* 1986; 45:25-9.
2. Merritt TA, Hallman M, Spragg R et al. Exogenous surfactant treatments for neonatal respiratory distress syndrome and their potential role in the adult respiratory distress syndrome. *Drugs.* 1989; 38:591-611.
3. Ashbaugh DG, Bigelow DB, Petty TL et al. Acute respiratory distress in adults. *Lancet.* 1967; 2:319-23.
4. Royall JA, Levin DL. Adult respiratory distress syndrome in pediatric patients. I. Clinical aspects, pathophysiology, pathology, and mechanisms of lung injury. *J Pediatr.* 1988; 112:169-80.
5. Holm BA, Matalon S. Role of pulmonary surfactant in the development and treatment of adult respiratory distress syndrome. *Anesth Analg.* 1989; 69:805-18.
6. Richman PS, Spragg RG, Robertson B et al. The adult respiratory distress syndrome: first trials with surfactant replacement. *Eur Respir J.* 1989; 2(Suppl 3):109S-11S.
7. Tse JJ, Brown M, Topf JS. Pathogenesis and treatment of adult respiratory distress syndrome. *J Oral Maxillofac Surg.* 1985; 43:870-5.
8. Cotram RS, Kumar V, Robbins SL, eds. Robbins pathologic basis of disease. 4th ed. Philadelphia: Saunders; 1989.
9. Lachmann B. Animal models and clinical pilot studies of surfactant replacement in adult respiratory distress syndrome. *Eur Respir J.* 1989; 2(Suppl 3):98S-103S.
10. Caminiti SP, Young SL. The pulmonary surfactant system. *Hosp Pract.* 1991; 26:87-100.
11. Jobe A. Metabolism of endogenous surfactant and exogenous surfactants for replacement therapy. *Semin Perinatol.* 1988; 12:231-44.
12. Pison U, Seeger W, Buchhorn R et al. Surfactant abnormalities in patients with respiratory failure after multiple trauma. *Am Rev Respir Dis.* 1989; 140:1033-9.
13. Hallman M, Spragg R, Harrell JH et al. Evidence of lung surfactant abnormality in respiratory failure. *J Clin Invest.* 1982; 70:873-83.
14. Loewen GM, Holm BA, Milanowski L et al. Alveolar hyperoxic injury in rabbits receiving exogenous surfactant. *J Appl Physiol.* 1989; 66:1087-92.
15. Berggren PC, Lachmann B, Curstedt T et al. Gas exchange and lung morphology after surfactant replacement in experimental adult respiratory distress syndrome induced by repeated lung lavage. *Acta Anaesthesiol Scand.* 1986; 30:321-8.
16. Matalon S, Holm BA, Notter RH. Mitigation of pulmonary hyperoxic injury by administration of exogenous surfactant. *J Appl Physiol.* 1987; 62:756-61.
17. Kobayashi T, Kataoka H, Ueda T et al. Effects of surfactant supplement and end-expiratory pressure in lung-lavaged rabbits. *J Appl Physiol.* 1984; 57:995-1001.
18. Harris JD, Jackson F Jr, Moxley MA et al. Effect of exogenous surfactant instillation on experimental acute lung injury. *J Appl Physiol.* 1989; 66:1846-51.
19. Burroughs Wellcome Company. Exosurf Neonatal package insert. Research Triangle Park, NC; 1990 Aug.

Fluconazole failure in a child with burns and candidemia

DEAN C. WILSON

Clin Pharm. 1992; 11:883-4

Every burn wound becomes colonized with microorganisms,[1] and invasion of these microorganisms beyond the eschar is a life-threatening complication. Occasionally fungi are the invading organisms,[1] but obtaining laboratory evidence that this is the case may be delayed because prolonged incubation is required for fungal cultures.[2,3] Burn patients receiving antibacterial agents are ideal hosts for opportunistic fungi.[4] Mortality in burn patients rises with increases in patient age, percentage of total body surface area that is burned, percentage of third-degree burns, and extent of inhalation injury; fungal septicemia contributes further to the likelihood of death.[5] Mortality ranges from 14% to more than 90% in patients with burns and fungal septicemia.[4-6] Thus, it is prudent to institute a comprehensive program of prevention, detection, and treatment of fungal infections to avoid this potentially lethal situation.[7]

Traditional therapy of fungal infections includes the use of amphotericin B, but the drug's potential toxicity sometimes prompts clinicians to seek an alternative antifungal agent. Also, since systemic therapy with amphotericin B can be given only intravenously, an antifungal drug that can be given orally might be of some benefit. This report describes the use of fluconazole in a child with burns and candidemia.

Case Report. An 18-month-old black child was admitted to the burn intensive-care unit with second- and third-degree burns covering 60% of his total body surface area. The boy had jumped into scalding bath water and sustained burns to his head, neck, chest, arms, and legs. The patient's weight was 10 kg, and his body surface area was 0.39 sq m.

During the first two weeks of his hospital stay, the patient underwent three separate operations for escharotomies and skin grafting. Blood cultures yielded *Pseudomonas aeruginosa*, and the child was treated with gentamicin 25 mg (as the sulfate salt) i.v. every eight hours and ceftazidime 200 mg i.v. every eight hours, both for 10 days. Because wound cultures grew *Streptococcus pneumoniae*, therapy with cefazolin 150 mg (as the sodium salt) i.v. every eight hours, which had been started on the first hospital day for prophylaxis, was continued for 14 days. Silver sulfadiazine 1% was applied to the burns, which were also irrigated with 0.5% Dakin's solution. Throughout this time, the white blood cell (WBC) count varied from 2500 to 7500/cu mm, rectal temperature varied from 37.0 to 39.0 °C, the blood urea nitrogen concentration (BUN) remained 4 mg/dL, and the serum creatinine concentration (SCr) was a constant 0.3 mg/dL.

On hospital day 14, a blood culture from a sample collected on hospital day 12 was positive for *Ps. aeruginosa* and *Candida tropicalis*. It was decided that, because of amphotericin B's potential toxicity, oral fluconazole would be used initially. Fluconazole 100 mg was given on hospital day 14, and 50 mg was given on days 15–18; all doses were given through an oral feeding tube. A blood culture collected on hospital day 14 was positive for *C. tropicalis* and negative for bacteria. The WBC count climbed from 16,000 to 23,400/cu mm during hospital days 14–18, and the patient's rectal temperature was 39.0–40.2 °C. The patient's clinical status appeared to be deteriorating.

On hospital day 19, the morning WBC count was 25,300/cu mm and the blood culture from a sample collected on day 17 was positive for *C. tropicalis* (no bacterial elements were found). Fluconazole therapy was discontinued, and amphotericin B 2.5 mg i.v. was given. The blood culture sample obtained on day 19 (before the amphotericin B dose was given) was reported on day 21 to be positive for *C. tropicalis* and negative for bacteria.

The child received amphotericin B 5 mg i.v. on the morning of hospital day 20. A blood culture sample obtained later that day showed no growth on day 22.

On hospital day 21 the WBC count was 13,000/cu mm; SCr, 0.4 mg/dL; and BUN, 6 mg/dL. Amphotericin B 7.5 mg i.v. was administered to the patient on hospital days 21–59, for 41 total days of therapy (total dose, 300 mg).

All blood cultures from samples collected after amphotericin B therapy began were negative for fungal and bacterial growth. The patient improved clinically except for having hesitancy in extending his right hip. On hospital day 32, when the patient was taken to the operating room for more grafting, swelling around the right hip joint was noticed. Aspiration of the joint yielded pus which, when cultured, grew *C. tropicalis* (results of blood cultures at the time were still negative). Roentgenograms showed that the hip was dislocated, and the patient was placed in skeletal traction. All subsequent joint-fluid cultures yielded no growth.

After surgery, all laboratory results were within normal limits, and no adverse effects of amphotericin B were noted. Although the patient experienced a complicated hospital course, no further fungal infection developed. The patient was eventually transferred to another part of the hospital to continue burn rehabilitation.

Discussion. Fluconazole therapy appears to have failed in this patient. After five days of oral therapy, fungal cultures remained positive, WBC counts had

DEAN C. WILSON, PHARM.D., is Intensive Care Specialist and Staff Pharmacist, Department of Pharmacy, Torrance Memorial Medical Center, 3330 Lomita Boulevard, Torrance, CA 90505.

Presented at the 26th Annual ASHP Midyear Clinical Meeting, New Orleans, LA, December 12, 1991.

increased steadily, and the patient's temperature remained elevated. After therapy was switched to amphotericin B, cultures were negative, WBC counts decreased, and the patient's condition improved.

There are some possible explanations for the failure of fluconazole in this patient. Absorption of fluconazole may have been inadequate, but because blood fluconazole concentrations were not measured, this could not be proved. It is unknown whether fluconazole interacts with enteral feedings, which the patient was receiving. The patient did not receive any other drug that is currently considered to interact with fluconazole.[8]

The dosage of fluconazole that we used (10 mg/kg on the first day, followed by 5 mg/kg thereafter) was derived from the dosage (3–6 mg/kg/day) mentioned in the package insert as having been shown to be safe in children.[8] According to the manufacturer, efficacy of the drug in children has not been established, and only limited data are available.[9-12,a] None of the literature on fluconazole discusses its pharmacokinetics in burn patients. It is well documented that the pharmacokinetics of some drugs are altered in burn patients; most notably, the clearance and elimination of the aminoglycosides is increased.[13-15] Some of the physiological alterations that occur in burns are an increase in glomerular filtration rate,[13] an increase in metabolic rate,[13,16] and a decrease in plasma protein concentration.[13,16] Therefore, in this patient the fluconazole dosage may have resulted in subtherapeutic concentrations.

Further evaluation of fluconazole in children and in burn patients is needed to clarify its place in therapy. Fluconazole therapy for systemic candidal infections may be problematical in severely compromised burn patients.

Conclusion. Oral fluconazole failed to control a *C. tropicalis* infection in a child with severe burns.

[a]Jacobson CE, Roerig Division of Pfizer, Inc. Personal communication. 1991 Jan 23.

References

1. Spebar MJ, Lindberg RB. Fungal infection of the burn wound. *Am J Surg*. 1979; 138:879-82.
2. Gauto A, Law EJ, Holder IA et al. Experience with amphotericin B in the treatment of systemic candidiasis in burn patients. *Am J Surg*. 1977; 133:174-8.
3. MacMillan BG, Law EJ, Holder IA. Experience with Candida infections in the burn patient. *Arch Surg*. 1972; 104:509-14.
4. Desai MH, Herndon DN, Abston S. Candida infection in massively burned patients. *J Trauma*. 1987; 27:1186-8.
5. Pensler JM, Herndon DN, Ptak H et al. Fungal sepsis: an increasing problem in major thermal injuries. *J Burn Care Rehabil*. 1986; 7:488-91.
6. Spebar MJ, Pruitt BA. Candidiasis in the burned patient. *J Trauma*. 1981; 21:237-9.
7. Prasad JK, Feller I, Thomson PD. A ten-year review of Candida sepsis and mortality in burn patients. *Surgery*. 1987; 101:213-6.
8. Roerig Division of Pfizer, Inc. Diflucan package insert. New York, NY; 1991 Jan.
9. Arai S, Iguchi K, Kamiya H et al. Experience of fluconazole in pediatric patients. *Jpn J Antibiot*. 1989; 42:170. Abstract.
10. Bunin N, Camitta B. Oral fluconazole for treatment of disseminated fungal infection. *Pediatr Infect Dis J*. 1989; 8:62. Letter.
11. Moncino M, Gutman L. Severe systemic cryptococcal disease in a child: review of prognostic indicators predicting treatment failure and an approach to maintenance therapy with oral fluconazole. *Pediatr Infect Dis J*. 1990; 9:363-8.
12. Viscoli C, Castagnola E, Corsini M et al. Fluconazole therapy in an underweight infant. *Eur J Clin Microbiol Infect Dis*. 1989; 8:925-6.
13. Sawchuk RJ, Rector TS. Drug kinetics in burn patients. *Clin Pharmacokinet*. 1980; 5:548-56.
14. Zaske DE, Sawchuk RJ, Gerding DN et al. Increased dosage requirements of gentamicin in burn patients. *J Trauma*. 1976; 16:824-8.
15. Zaske DE, Sawchuk RJ, Strate RG. The necessity of increased doses of amikacin in burn patients. *Surgery*. 1978; 84: 603-8.
16. Moncrief JA. Burns. *N Engl J Med*. 1973; 288:444-53.

Which Antihypertensive Drugs First

No reasonable observer could argue that diuretics and β-blockers are the last word in antihypertensive treatment. The fact that heart attack, the leading hypertension-related cause of death and disability, responds less well in antihypertensive drug trials than epidemiological experience would have predicted is ample reason to continue the search for more effective therapies. Perhaps the newer drugs can help to close the gap between what treatment might do and what it currently does. But the unpleasant reality is that now, a decade or more after their introduction, we do not know how well calcium channel blockers or converting enzyme inhibitors stack up against their predecessors in ability to extend healthy hypertensive lives! The magnitude of the medical and economic issues merits a clinical trial.

—Alderman MH. Which antihypertensive drugs first—and why! *JAMA*. 1992; 267:2786-7.

DUE Criteria

The DUE Criteria *section of* Clinical Pharmacy *features model drug-use evaluation criteria that may be employed as a component of a comprehensive quality assurance program. The criteria sets are presented in the format used in the ASHP book* Criteria for Drug Use Evaluation. *Some of the criteria sets will have been originally published in that book; others will be presented here for the first time and published in future volumes of the ASHP book. The practitioners who developed a criteria set are acknowledged.*

In selecting drug products for coverage in DUE Criteria, *priority is given to products that have been recently marketed, those that are frequently prescribed, those that have high potential risk associated with their use, and those that are expensive. When feasible, a criteria set will be linked with a Drug Review that appears in the same issue.*

These criteria sets are a starting point for the development of DUE criteria for a specific practice setting. Readers are encouraged to modify the model criteria to fit their own circumstances.

Criteria for use of didanosine in adult and pediatric patients[a]

Element	Standard 100%	Standard 0%	Exception[b] or Critical Preventive/ Responsive Measure[c]		Sources of Information
Justification for Use					
1. Treatment of adult or pediatric patient (over 6 months of age) with advanced human immunodeficiency virus (HIV) infection who is intolerant of zidovudine therapy[1-9]	X		1A. None	1.	History and physical (H&P), laboratory reports, physician orders, progress notes, infectious diseases (ID) consultation report
or					
2. Treatment of adult or pediatric patient (over 6 months of age) with advanced HIV infection who has demonstrated significant clinical or immunologic deterioration during zidovudine therapy[1-9]	X		2A. None	2.	H&P, laboratory reports, physician orders, progress notes, ID consultation report
Critical (Process) Indicators					
3. No history of hypersensitivity to any component of didanosine formulation[1]	X		3A. None	3.	H&P, allergy record
4. Patient not pregnant or breast-feeding [1]	X		4A. Benefits of therapy outweigh risks in woman who was informed and consented (or guardian was informed and consented)	4. 4A.	H&P, laboratory reports, progress notes H&P, laboratory reports, physician orders, progress notes, ID consultation report
5. Baseline laboratory tests obtained before initiation of didanosine therapy[1]: a. Complete blood count (CBC) with differential b. Platelet count c. Liver function tests (aspartate aminotransferase [AST], alanine aminotransferase [ALT],alkaline phosphatase, bilirubin)	X		5A. None	5.	Laboratory reports, physician orders, progress notes

Prepared by Linda M. Cortese, M.S., Clinical Research Pharmacist, Henry M. Jackson Foundation, Rockville, MD, and Darrel C. Bjornson, Ph.D., Associate Professor, Drake University, Des Moines, IA. At the time these criteria were prepared, Dr. Bjornson was assigned to Walter Reed Army Medical Center, Washington, DC, where Ms. Cortese conducts her research.

The assistance of Raymond C.Y. Chung, M.D., is acknowledged.

Element	Standard 100%	Standard 0%	Exception[b] or Critical Preventive/ Responsive Measure[c]	Sources of Information
d. Serum creatinine (SCr) e. Uric acid f. Amylase g. T4 helper/inducer lymphocyte count h. Potassium				
6. Appropriate oral dosage in adult based on patient's weight[1]: a. Given as two-tablet dose (to ensure adequate buffering to prevent degradation of drug in gastric secretions): 300 mg b.i.d. if weight ≥ 75 kg, 200 mg b.i.d. if weight 50–74 kg, and 125 mg b.i.d. if weight 35–49 kg or b. Given as a buffered powder in solution: 375 mg b.i.d. if weight ≥ 75 kg, 250 mg b.i.d. if weight 50–74 kg, and 167 mg b.i.d. if weight 35–49 kg	X		6A. Drug discontinued because of symptoms of neuropathy and resumed at reduced dosage after symptoms resolved 6B. Reduced dosage given to patient with renal impairment 6C. Reduced dosage given to patient with hepatic impairment 6D. Reduced dosage given to patient with phenylketonuria	6. H&P, physician orders, progress notes, medication administration record (MAR) 6A-D. Physician orders, progress notes, ID consultation report, MAR
7. Appropriate oral dosage in pediatric patient based on body surface area[1]: a. Dose given as two chewable (dispersible) buffered tablets (to ensure adequate buffering to prevent degradation of drug in gastric secretions) for child 1 year of age or older; if child is less than 1 year of age, a single tablet is sufficient to provide adequate buffering. Dosage: 100 mg b.i.d. if body surface area (BSA) 1.1–1.4 sq m, 75 mg b.i.d. if BSA 0.8–1.0 sq m, 50 mg b.i.d. if BSA 0.5–0.7 sq m, and 25 mg b.i.d. if BSA ≤ 0.4 sq m. or b. Given as a 10-mg/mL buffered pediatric solution: 125 mg (12.5 mL) b.i.d. if BSA 1.1–1.4 sq m, 94 mg (9.5 mL) b.i.d. if BSA 0.8–1.0 sq m, 62 mg (6 mL) b.i.d. if BSA 0.5–0.7 sq m, and 31 mg (3 mL) b.i.d. if BSA ≤ 0.4 sq m.	X		7A. Drug discontinued because of symptoms of neuropathy and resumed at reduced dosage after symptoms resolved 7B. Reduced dosage given to patient with renal impairment 7C. Reduced dosage given to patient with hepatic impairment 7D. Reduced dosage given to patient with phenylketonuria	7. H&P, physician orders, progress notes, MAR 7A-D. Physician orders, progress notes, ID consultation report, MAR
8. Medication given on empty stomach (one hour before meals or two hours after meals)[1,10]	X		8A. None	8. Physician orders, progress notes
9. Patient or caregiver counseled about a. Major toxicities (i.e., pancreatitis, peripheral neuropathy) and symptoms requiring physician notification (i.e., nausea, vomiting, diarrhea, abdominal pain, tingling in hands or feet) b. Need for decreased alcohol consumption to prevent exacerbation of didanosine toxicity c. Importance of physician follow-up d. Importance of drug compliance and laboratory follow-up	X		9A. None	9. Progress notes, nursing notes
10. Hemoglobin, neutrophil count, platelet count, AST, ALT, serum potassium, alkaline phosphatase, total bilirubin, serum creatinine, uric acid, creatine phosphokinase, and amylase measured and patient assessed for signs of neuropathy 2 weeks after start of therapy and then monthly	X		10A. Monitoring performed more often in patient with family history of pancreatitis, renal or hepatic dysfunction, or unstable laboratory values or in patient receiving other bone-marrow-suppressive drugs	10,10A. H&P, laboratory reports, physician orders, progress notes

Element	Standard 100%	Standard 0%	Exception[b] or Critical Preventive/ Responsive Measure[c]		Sources of Information
11. T4 helper/inducer lymphocyte count measured every 6 months	X		11A. T4 helper/inducer lymphocyte count measured every 3 months when approaching 200/cu mm 11B. If T4 helper/inducer lymphocyte count falls rapidly during didanosine therapy, consider alternative therapy	11,11A,B.	Laboratory reports, physician orders, progress notes
12. Didanosine not given simultaneously with dapsone, ketoconazole, or any form of tetracycline	X		12A. None	12.	H&P, physician orders, progress notes, MAR
Complications					
13. Anaphylaxis (difficulty breathing, hypotension, cardiac arrest)		X	13A. Identify other drug and nondrug causes 13B. Discontinue didanosine 13C. Provide symptomatic and supportive care (re-establish airway, perform cardiopulmonary resuscitation)	13. 13A-C.	Progress notes, nursing notes Physician orders, progress notes, nursing notes, MAR
14. Pancreatitis (moderate to severe pain, oral intake not tolerated, elevated serum amylase levels)[1,3,4,7,8,11,12]		X	14A. Identify other drug and nondrug causes 14B. If serum amylase is 2.1–3.0 times normal and patient is asymptomatic, monitor amylase every 2 weeks 14C. If patient has symptoms and serum amylase is 2.1–3.0 times normal or serum amylase is >5 times upper limit of normal, stop drug until symptoms resolve and/or laboratory values return to baseline; restart didanosine at reduced dosage 14D. If 14A–14C are not successful, discontinue didanosine and consider alternative therapy	14. 14A-D.	Laboratory reports, progress notes, nursing notes Laboratory reports, physician orders, progress notes, ID notes, nursing notes, MAR
15. Peripheral neuropathy[1,3,4,7,8,11,12]		X	15A. Identify other drug and nondrug causes 15B. Reduce dosage of didanosine 15C. If symptoms persist, discontinue didanosine and consider alternative therapy	15. 15A-C.	Progress notes, nursing notes Physician orders, progress notes, nursing notes, MAR
16. Abdominal pain, nausea, vomiting[1,3,4,7,8,11,12]		X	16A. Identify other drug and nondrug causes 16B. Rule out pancreatitis 16C. Treat mild reaction symptomatically; provide supportive care 16D. If reaction severe, reduce didanosine dosage or discontinue didanosine and consider alternative therapy	16. 16A-D.	Progress notes, nursing notes Laboratory reports, physician orders, progress notes, nursing notes, MAR
17. Diarrhea[1]		X	17A. Identify other drug and nondrug causes 17B. Change to chewable tablet formulation	17. 17A-E.	Progress notes, nursing notes Physician orders, progress notes, nursing notes, MAR

Element	Standard 100%	Standard 0%	Exception[b] or Critical Preventive/ Responsive Measure[c]	Sources of Information
			17C. Treat mild reaction symptomatically; provide supportive care	
			17D. Monitor serum potassium and replenish when necessary	
			17E. If reaction severe, discontinue didanosine and consider alternative therapy	
18. Headache, insomnia[1,7,12]			18A. Identify other drug and nondrug causes	18. Progress notes, nursing notes 18A-C. Physician orders, progress notes, nursing notes, MAR
		X	18B. Treat mild reaction symptomatically; provide supportive care	
			18C. If reaction severe, discontinue didanosine and consider alternative therapy	
19. Rash or other dermatologic manifestations[1,4,7,8,12]			19A. Identify other drug and nondrug causes	19. Progress notes, nursing notes 19A-C. Laboratory report, physician orders, progress notes, dermatology consultation report, nursing notes, MAR
		X	19B. Treat reaction symptomatically (antihistamine, anti-inflammatory agent)	
			19C. If reaction severe, discontinue didanosine and consider alternative therapy	
20. Seizures, arrhythmias[1,4,7,12,13]			20A. Identify other drug and nondrug causes	20. Progress notes, nursing notes 20A. Progress notes, nursing notes, MAR
		X	20B. Ensure electrolytes in balance	20B. Laboratory reports, progress notes, nursing notes
			20C. Provide symptomatic and supportive care	20C-D. Physician orders, progress notes, neurology consultation report, cardiology consultation report, nursing notes, MAR
			20D. Discontinue didanosine and consider alternative therapy	
21. Hyperuricemia (serum uric acid ≥ 420 μmol/L in man or ≥ 360 μmol/L in woman or child)[1,4,7,12]		X	21A. Identify other drug and nondrug causes	21. Laboratory reports, progress notes,
			21B. Administer fluids and reduce didanosine dosage	21A-C. Laboratory reports, physician orders, progress notes, nursing notes, MAR
			21C. If hyperuricemia persists or uric acid concentration is >1.25 times upper limit of normal, discontinue didanosine and consider alternative therapy	
22. Constipation[1,4]		X	22A. Identify other drug and nondrug causes	22. Progress notes, nursing notes 22A-C. Physician orders, progress notes, nursing notes, MAR
			22B. Provide symptomatic and supportive care	
			22C. If reaction severe, discontinue didanosine and consider alternative therapy	
23. Hepatotoxicity (elevated liver function test results)[1,4,7,14]		X	23A. Identify other drug and nondrug causes	23. Laboratory reports, progress notes, nursing notes
			23B. Reduce didanosine dosage or interrupt therapy	23A-C. Physician orders, progress notes, nursing notes, MAR
			23C. If hepatotoxicity persists or alkaline phosphatase, ALT, or AST is >5 times upper limit of normal,	

Element	Standard 100%	Standard 0%	Exception[b] or Critical Preventive/ Responsive Measure[c]	Sources of Information	
			discontinue didanosine and consider alternative therapy		
24. Visual effects (retinal depigmentation in child, blurred vision)[1,15]		X	24A. Identify other drug and nondrug causes 24B. Discontinue didanosine and consider alternative therapy	24. 24A,B.	Progress notes, nursing notes Physician orders, progress notes, ophthalmology consultation report, nursing notes, MAR
Outcome Measures					
25. Improvement in Karnofsky performance score and sense of well-being[7,8]	X		25A. Patient died 25B. Patient did not return for follow-up appointment 25C. At baseline patient worked full-time and maintained required life style 25D. Patient's baseline score was 100	25,25A-D.	Progress notes, nursing notes
26. Improvement in patient's and caregiver's subjective assessments of symptoms (e.g., decreased fatigue, increased appetite)[3,4,7,12,16]	X		26A. Patient died 26B. Patient did not return for follow-up appointment 26C. Patient asymptomatic at start of therapy	26,26A-C.	Progress notes, nursing notes
27. Objective improvements (weight gain, changes in CD4 cell count, fewer febrile episodes)[1,4,7,12,16]	X		27A. Patient died 27B. Patient did not return for follow-up appointment 27C. Patient asymptomatic at start of therapy	27,27A-C.	Laboratory reports, progress notes, nursing notes
28. Progression of HIV disease slowed or halted (patient did not develop severe opportunistic infection, neoplasm, or neurological disease)	X		28A. Patient died 28B. Patient did not return for follow-up appointment	28,28A,B.	Laboratory reports, progress notes, nursing notes
29. Patient alive at end of therapy (if didanosine therapy discontinued because of toxicity or treatment failure)	X		29A. Patient did not return for follow-up appointment		Progress notes, nursing notes

[a]Criteria address justification for use (indications), critical (process) indicators, complications of therapy, and patient outcome. Each criterion consists of an element, a standard, exceptions to the standard, and sources of information. The element is the minimum level of evidence needed to show that patient care was optimal. The standard defines the deviation from an element that is acceptable. If no deviation is acceptable, the standard is 100%. Exceptions are circumstances in which deviation is allowable. Sources of information listed are the most reliable sources. Sources pertaining to an element or exception are identified by the number assigned to the element or exception (e.g., 4,4A).
[b]For justification for use, critical (process) indicators, and outcome measures.
[c]For complications.

References

1. Bristol-Myers Squibb. Videx package insert. Princeton, NJ; 1991 Oct.
2. Ahluwalia G, Cooney DA, Mitsuya H et al. Initial studies on the cellular pharmacology of 2',3'-dideoxyadenosine, an inhibitor of HIV infectivity. *Biochem Pharmacol.* 1987; 36:797-800.
3. Butler KM, Husson RN, Balis FM et al. Dideoxyinosine in children with symptomatic human immunodeficiency virus infection. *N Engl J Med.* 1991; 324:137-44.
4. Cooley TP, Kunches LM, Saunders CA et al. Once-daily administration of 2',3'-dideoxyinosine (ddI) in patients with acquired immunodeficiency syndrome or AIDS-related complex: results of phase I trial. *N Engl J Med.* 1990; 322:1340-5.
5. Cooney DA, Ahluwalia G, Mitsuya H et al. Initial studies on the cellular pharmacology of 2',3'-dideoxyadenosine, an inhibitor of HTLV-III infectivity. *Biochem Pharmacol.* 1987; 36:1765-8.
6. Hartman NR, Yarchoan R, Pluda JM et al. Pharmacokinetics of 2',3'-dideoxyadenosine and 2',3'-dideoxyinosine in patients with severe human immunodeficiency virus infection. *Clin Pharmacol Ther.* 1990; 47:647-54.
7. Lambert JS, Siedlin M, Reichman RC et al. 2',3'-dideoxyinosine (ddI) in patients with the acquired immunodeficiency syndrome or AIDS-related complex: a phase I trial. *N Engl J Med.* 1990; 322:1333-40.
8. Merigan TC, Skowron G, Bozzette SA et al. Circulating p24 antigen levels and responses to dideoxycytidine in human immunodeficiency virus (HIV) infections. *Am Coll Physicians.* 1989; 110:189-94.
9. Pizzo PA. Treatment of human immunodeficiency virus-infected infants and young children with dideoxynucleosides. *Am J Med.* 1990; 88(Suppl 58):18S-19S.
10. Shyu Chyi Wen, Knupp C, Pittman K et al. Food induced reduction in bioavailability of didanosine. *Clin Pharmacol Ther.* 1991; 50:503-7.
11. Anon. NIAID updates dideoxyinosine toxicity profile, suggests ways to reduce risk of pancreatitis. *Clin Pharm.* 1990;

9:832,838.
12. Yarchoan R, Pluda JM, Thomas RV et al. Long-term toxicity/ activity profile of 2',3'-dideoxyinosine in AIDS or AIDS-related complex. *Lancet*. 1990; 336:526-9.
13. Katlama C, Tubiana R, Rosenheim M et al. Dideoxyinosine-associated hypokalemia. *Lancet*. 1991; 337:183.
14. Kwan Kew Lai, Gang David L, Zawacki JK et al. Fulminant hepatic failure associated with 2',3'-dideoxyinosine (ddI). *Ann Intern Med*. 1991; 115:283-4.
15. Lafeuillade A, Aubert L, Chaffanjon P et al. Optic neuritis associated with dideoxyinosine. *Lancet*. 1991; 337:615-6. Letter.
16. Bach MC. Clinical response to dideoxyinosine in patients with HIV infection resistant to zidovudine. *N Engl J Med*. 1990; 323:275. Letter.

Current Literature

Drug Reaction Alerts 895

Book Reviews

Applied Therapeutics: The Clinical Use of Drugs, Fifth Edition 897
Edited by Mary Anne Koda-Kimble and Lloyd Yee Young
Reviewed by Vincent F. Mauro and Laurie S. Mauro

Clinical Immunotoxicology 900
Edited by David S. Newcombe, Noel R. Rose, and John C. Bloom
Reviewed by Daniel P. Healy

Handbook of Basic Pharmacokinetics . . . including Clinical Applications, Fourth Edition 901
By W. A. Ritschel
Reviewed by Larry E. Patterson

Neoplastic Diseases: Fundamentals of Clinical Oncology 901
Edited by C. Julian Rosenthal
Reviewed by Bud J. Kane and John G. Kuhn

Books Received 904

Drug Reaction Alerts

Drug Reaction Alerts focuses primarily on serious, unlabeled reactions to new chemical entities. The citations are compiled monthly from International Pharmaceutical Abstracts, which covers over 800 pharmacy and health-related journals worldwide. An address for reprints (when available) follows the name of the corresponding author in each citation.

Pharmacists may use the FDA Adverse Reaction Report form that appears in the January and July issues of Clinical Pharmacy for submitting reports of adverse drug reactions directly to FDA.

Alcohol Deterrents

Fortier-Beaulieu M (Department of Internal Medicine, Hôpital de Boisguillaume, 76233 Boisguillaume, France), Noblet C, Cardot F et al. Possible association of erythema multiforme with **acamprosate**. *Lancet*. 1992; 339:991. Case. (40-year-old woman with alcoholic cirrhosis and ascites; received acamprosate 1.3 g/day for less than two weeks; developed erythema multiforme on trunk and limbs; concomitant spironolactone; laboratory test results confirmed hepatic disease and revealed mild eosinophilia but showed no evidence of viral infection; skin tissue biopsy results characteristic of erythema multiforme; withdrawal of acamprosate and spironolactone led to resolution of symptoms in two weeks)

Angiotensin-Converting-Enzyme Inhibitors

Hedner T (Department of Clinical Pharmacology, Sahlgrenska University Hospital, S-413 45 Göteborg, Sweden), Samuelsson O, Lunde H et al. Angio-oedema in relation to treatment with **angiotensin converting enzyme inhibitors**. *Br Med J*. 1992; 304:941-6. Study. (case series; 38 cases of angioneurotic edema suspected of being caused by angiotensin-converting-enzyme [ACE] inhibitors that were reported to Swedish Adverse Drug Reactions Advisory Committee during 1981–1990; number of reported cases was related to annual use of **captopril, enalapril,** and **lisinopril**; 36 cases were judged to be related to ACE inhibitor use; 28 [77%] of 36 patients developed angioneurotic edema within first three weeks of therapy with ACE inhibitor, with 10 needing hospitalization; 2 of 10 hospitalized patients had life-threatening laryngeal obstruction; withdrawal of ACE inhibitor led to resolution of symptoms in 35 [97%] of 36 patients)

Antibiotics

Fahal IH, Williams PS, Clark RE et al. (Bell GM, Royal Liverpool University Hospital, Liverpool L7 8XP, England). Thrombotic thrombocytopenic purpura due to rifampicin. *Br Med J*. 1992; 304:882. Case. (57-year-old man with renal tuberculosis; received **rifampin** 450 mg daily for three weeks as part of combination therapy; developed severe thrombocytopenic purpura; concomitant isoniazid and ethambutol; platelet count, $13 \times 10^9/L$; withdrawal of rifampin and therapy with fresh frozen plasma, platelets, and whole blood did not stop deterioration in condition; therapy with daily plasma exchange led to platelet count of $188 \times 10^9/L$ and improvement in general condition after nine days)

Anti-inflammatory Agents

Graham LD, Myones BL, Rivas-Chacon RF et al. (Pachman LM, Immunology/Rheumatology No. 50, Children's Memorial Hospital, 2300 Children's Plaza, Chicago, IL 60614). Morbidity associated with long-term **methotrexate** therapy in juvenile rheumatoid arthritis. *J Pediatr*. 1992; 120:468-73. Study. (retrospective; 54 girls and 8 boys, aged 2.3–18.7 years [mean, 9.6 years], with polyarticular juvenile rheumatoid arthritis who received methotrexate 10–20 mg/sq m/wk for 84–296 weeks; monitored for signs of dermatologic, pulmonary, GI, hematologic, and infectious toxicities and for liver function abnormalities; nine children developed transient abnormalities in liver function test results; after receiving 815–2980 mg of methotrexate, 12 children underwent percutaneous liver tissue biopsies; biopsy results showed no signs of fibrosis or cirrhosis; methotrexate therapy discontinued in six children who achieved remission; methotrexate therapy not discontinued permanently in any child because of adverse effects)

Antilipemic Agents

Chrysanthopoulos C, Kounis N (Patras Technical Education Institute, Patras 26221, Greece). Rhabdomyolysis due to combined treatment with **lovastatin** and cholestyramine. *Br Med J*. 1992; 304:1225. Cases. (two men, aged 31 and 42 years, with hyperlipemia and who participated in regular aerobic exercise and received **cholestyramine resin** 12 g daily; received lovastatin 20 mg twice daily as additional antilipemic therapy for two or four weeks; developed rhabdomyolysis; withdrawal of lovastatin and bed rest led to resolution of all symptoms)

Dearing BD, Lavie CJ (Ochsner Clinic, 1514 Jefferson Highway, New Orleans, LA 70121), Lohmann TP et al. **Niacin**-induced clotting factor synthesis deficiency with coagulopathy. *Arch Intern Med*. 1992; 152:861-3. Cases. (three men, aged 44–55 years, with hypercholesterolemia and coronary artery disease; received sustained-action niacin 1 g two or three times daily for two weeks to 10 months; developed clotting factor synthesis deficiency and coagulopathy, with minimal evidence of hepatotoxicity; withdrawal of niacin and therapy with phytonadione or no treatment led to return of prothrombin time to normal range; negative challenge with crystalline niacin in 47-year-old man; positive rechallenge in 55-year-old man)

Antineoplastic Agents

Ching CK, Smith PG, Long RG (City Hospital, Nottingham NG5 1PB, England). **Tamoxifen**-associated hepatocellular damage and agranulocytosis. *Lancet*. 1992; 339:940. Case. (58-year-old woman with advanced invasive adenocarcinoma of breast; received tamoxifen 20 mg twice daily for five months; developed general feeling of unwellness with lethargy, nausea, and retching, and showed signs of jaundice; withdrawal of tamoxifen and conservative therapy did not prevent further deterioration in hepatic function and lowering of white blood cell counts; patient died seven weeks after development of jaundice)

Tolaymat A (Department of Pediatrics, University of Florida Health Science Center, 653 West 8th Street, Building 1, Jacksonville, FL 32209), Leventhal B, Sakarcan A et al. Systemic lupus erythematosus in a child receiving long-term interferon therapy. *J Pediatr*. 1992; 120:429-32. Case. (10.5-year-old boy with juvenile laryngeal papillomatosis; received **interferon alfa-n1** 5 megaunits/sq m daily by i.m. injection for 28 days, then three days per week for 10 months, and followed by 3 megaunits/sq m daily for six years; developed systemic lupus erythematosus [SLE]; withdrawal of interferon alfa and therapy for SLE led to fast recovery)

Antivirals

Torres RA (AIDS Center, Department of Medicine, St. Vincent's Hospital and Medical Center, 153 W. 11th Street, New York, NY 10011), Lin RY, Lee M et al. **Zidovudine**-induced leukocytoclastic vasculitis. *Arch Intern Med*. 1992; 152:850-1. Cases. (two men, aged 33 and 34 years, with human immunodeficiency virus [HIV] infection; received zidovudine for two weeks to one month; developed cutaneous leukocytoclastic vasculitis; concomitant aerosolized pentamidine; withdrawal of zidovudine and therapy with diphenhydramine or with antihistamines plus prednisone led to resolution of symptoms; positive rechallenge)

Whitcup SM, Butler KM, Pizzo PA et al. (Nussenblatt RB, National Institutes of Health, Building 10, Bethesda, MD 20892). Retinal lesions in children treated with dideoxyinosine. *N Engl J Med*. 1992; 326:1226-7. Case. (10-year-old child with human immunodeficiency virus [HIV] infection; received **didanosine** 270 mg/sq m daily; developed atrophic lesions of retinal-pigment epithelium after 78 weeks; didanosine discontinued after cumulative dose of 147 g/sq m because of failure to gain weight, lethargy, mild cerebral atrophy, lower intelligence-quotient score, and retinal lesions)

Drug Interactions

De Klippel N, Sennesael J, Lamote J et al. (De Keyser J, Department of Neurology, Academisch Ziekenhuis, Free University of Brussels, B1090 Brussels, Belgium). Cyclosporin leukoencephalopathy induced by intravenous lipid solution. *Lancet*. 1992; 339:1114. Case. (75-kg, 48-year-old renal transplant recipient who received **cyclosporine** 150 mg, azathioprine, and methylprednisolone for immunosuppression; received propofol dissolved in 10% **fat emulsion** and fentanyl by i.v. infusions after intubation and ventilation for three days that was necessitated by poor initial graft function and development of pulmonary edema; serum triglycerides concentration rose from 3.16 to 6.01 mM; serum cholesterol concentration rose from 3.63 to 5.75 mM; blood cyclosporine concentration, measured by nonspecific fluorescence polarization immunoassay, rose from 250 to 997 ng/mL; graft dysfunction necessitated hemodialysis; after withdrawal of propofol and fentanyl, patient was confused; brain tissue biopsy results suggested cyclosporine nephrotoxicity; withdrawal of cyclosporine led to improvement in strength and mental function and to normalization of renal function after four days)

Longdon P, Henderson A (Intensive Care Unit, Princess Alexandra Hospital, Ipswich Road, Brisbane, Queensland 4102, Australia). Intestinal pseudo-obstruction following the use of enteral charcoal and **sorbitol** and mechanical ventilation with **papaveretum** sedation for theophylline poisoning. *Drug Saf*. 1992; 7:74-7. Cases. (two men, aged 35 and 57 years, who self-poisoned with theophylline; received **activated charcoal** 50 g with 150 mL of 70% sorbitol by enteral administration for four doses and mechanical ventilation assisted by sedation with papaveretum 5 mg/hr; intestinal distention observed after 30 hours in younger man and after 48 hours in older man; concomitant pancuronium 2–4 mg/hr; insertion of flatus tube led to resolution of intestinal pseudo-obstruction in younger man but not in older man; older man developed septicemia and died)

Hypotensive Agents

Bosch X, Sobrino J, Lopez-Soto A et al. (Urbano-Marquez A, Hospital Clínic i Provincial, 08036 Barcelona, Spain). Parotitis due to **nicardipine**. *Br Med J*. 1992; 304:882. Case. (63-year-old man with hypertension and grade I–II hypertensive retinopathy; received nicardipine 30 mg three times daily for two doses; developed transient parotitis after both doses; withdrawal of nicardipine and substitution with captopril did not lead to recurrence of symptoms)

Karim S (Department of Cardiology, Hypertension Research Centre, Mayo Hospital, Lahore, Pakistan), Zubair M. **Urapidil** and enuresis. *Lancet*. 1992; 339:1366. Cases. (one man and one woman, aged <60 years, with hypertension who received urapidil 30 mg twice daily; urapidil dose increased to 60 mg twice daily for treatment of refractory hypertension; complained of enuresis after three days and of persistent and troublesome enuresis one week later; reduction of urapidil dose to 30 mg twice daily and addition of calcium-channel blocker for control of blood pressure led to disappearance of symptoms after three days)

Immunotherapy

Kojima S (Japanese Red Cross Nagoya First Hospital, Nagoya 453, Japan), Tsuchida M, Matsuyama T. Myelodysplasia and leukemia after treatment of aplastic anemia with G-CSF. *N Engl J Med.* 1992; 326:1294-5. Cases. (three children, aged three to five years, with aplastic anemia; received **granulocyte colony-stimulating factor** [G-CSF] for total dose of 33–158 mg; developed myelodysplasia during or after G-CSF therapy; myelodysplasia evolved into acute myelomonocytic leukemia in two children; three children represented about 14% of all children with aplastic anemia who received G-CSF at three institutions and who survived for at least one year without bone marrow transplantation)

Replacement Solutions

Barbier P, Jonville AP, Autret E (Centre Anti-Poisons, Hôpital Bretonneau, 2 bis boulevard Tonnellé, 37044 Tours Cédex, France) et al. Fetal risks with dextrans during delivery. *Drug Saf.* 1992; 7:71-3. Case. (pregnant woman who was undergoing cesarean section because of scarred uterus; received 100 mL of **dextran 40** solution before epidural blockade; experienced fainting and developed urticaria and mild respiratory disturbances without hypotension; sudden lack of fetal cardiac activity led to prompt delivery under general anesthesia of apparently dead baby; immediate and vigorous cardiopulmonary resuscitation revived baby)

Thrombolytic Agents

Barnes D, Hughes RA (Guy's Hospital, London SE1 9RT, England). Guillain-Barré syndrome after treatment with **streptokinase**. *Br Med J.* 1992; 304:1225. Case. (45-year-old man who experienced myocardial infarction; received intravenous streptokinase; developed symptoms of Guillain-Barré syndrome three weeks later; therapy with plasma exchanges led to improvement in neurological condition and to ability to walk independently after three months)

Toxicity

Autti-Ramo I (Peuramaentie 1 H 18, 02700 Kauniainen, Finland), Korkman M, Hilakivi-Clarke L et al. Mental development of 2-year-old children exposed to **alcohol** in utero. *J Pediatr.* 1992; 120:740-6. Study. (case–control; 20 children who were exposed to heavy maternal alcohol intake during first trimester, 20 children who were exposed during first and second trimesters, 20 children who were exposed throughout gestation, and 48 children who were not exposed to alcohol in utero; assessed for mental and language development at mean age of 27 months; children who were exposed to alcohol throughout gestation scored significantly lower on developmental tests than children who were exposed only during first trimester [$p < 0.01$]; number of alcohol-exposed children who showed delayed language development increased with increased duration of intrauterine alcohol exposure [linear trend, $p = 0.0017$]; fetal alcohol syndrome diagnosed in seven children; fetal alcohol effects diagnosed in 13 children)

Wiley JF (Division of Emergency Medicine, St. Christopher's Hospital for Children, Front Street at Erie Avenue, Philadelphia, PA 19134), Gelber ML, Henretig FM et al. Cardiotoxic effects of **astemizole** overdose in children. *J Pediatr.* 1992; 120:799-802. Cases. (five children, 1.5–11 years; ingested overdose of astemizole 1.7–12.2 mg/kg; developed prolonged, corrected Q–T interval, ventricular arrhythmias, and atrioventricular heart block; mean duration of cardiotoxic effects, 2.5 days)

Young JD, Crapo LM (Department of Internal Medicine, Santa Clara Valley Medical Center, 751 S. Bascom Avenue, San Jose, CA 95128). Protracted **phencyclidine** coma from an intestinal deposit. *Arch Intern Med.* 1992; 152:859-60. Case. (29-year-old man; swallowed plastic bag containing phencyclidine; developed coma; received midazolam for 18 days for agitation and diazepam for convulsions; serum phencyclidine concentration decreased on hospital day 20 after plastic bag was rectally excreted; experienced rapid neurologic recovery beginning on day 24)

Book Reviews

Applied Therapeutics: The Clinical Use of Drugs, Fifth Edition

Edited by Mary Anne Koda-Kimble and Lloyd Yee Young.

Published by Applied Therapeutics, Inc., P.O. Box 5077, Vancouver, WA 98668-5077, 1992. xv + 1738 p. Price $85.

In 1975, Young and Kimble edited the first edition of what was then known as *Applied Therapeutics for Clinical Pharmacists*. The mission of that book was to prepare pharmacists to dispense relevant information on pharmacotherapy. Koda-Kimble and Young have now edited the fifth edition of this popular textbook or reference, now known as *Applied Therapeutics: The Clinical Use of Drugs*. One immediately noticeable change is overall size; the fifth edition is more slender than the fourth, which was larger than previous editions. This reduction in size does not affect content—the print is slightly smaller, and the figures and tables are more compact.

With few exceptions, the approximately 100 chapter authors of the fifth edition also contributed to the fourth edition. The chapters have been updated, reflecting knowledge acquired over the past four years; examples of revisions include discussions of the role of *Helicobacter pylori* in peptic ulcer disease, the use of epoetin for anemia of chronic renal failure, and the role of selegiline in Parkinson's disease. Realizing that medical information is constantly changing, the publishers allotted one to three pages in several chapters for the reporting of major developments that occurred between preparation of the chapter and publication of the book.

A chapter on cerebrovascular disease has been added, and a chapter on solid organ transplantation has replaced the one on renal transplantation. Immediately noticeable is the lack of chapters on myocardial infarction and septic shock, common disease states for which there have been recent pharmacotherapeutic advances; these conditions are, however, discussed in other areas of the book. The chapters on infectious disease, which are excellent in their discussion of definitive antimicrobial treatment, do not dwell on empirical treatment.

Each chapter is well referenced and contains a table of contents with subheadings now listed with page numbers. As in previous editions, each chapter presents a case study followed by questions and answers. Although this approach can be criticized as making the practice of pharmacotherapy appear as straightforward as following instructions in a cookbook, a point acknowledged by the editors in the preface, the purpose of this format is to develop problem-solving skills, not to present therapy as

Continued on page 900

Current Literature *Continued from page 897*

consisting of black-and-white decisions.

Compared with other textbooks on pharmacotherapy, *Applied Therapeutics* lacks in-depth discussions of pathophysiology. However, the discussions of pharmacotherapy are extremely well done, with emphasis on practical dosing considerations, monitoring therapy, and determining therapeutic endpoints. Not only is basic information presented in an organized and applicable manner, but the question-and-answer format allows the reader to readily find answers to commonly asked questions. Tables and figures augment the text.

Regardless of the type of pharmacy practice (e.g., community, hospital, nursing home, clinic) or emphasis of practice (e.g., drug distribution, pharmacotherapy), this book should be included in all pharmacy libraries. Its use as a textbook would depend on the focus of the class. If the class combines pathophysiology with pharmacotherapy and only one book is required, *Applied Therapeutics* is not a good choice because of the lack of in-depth discussions of pathophysiology. However, for a pharmacotherapy class in which students already have a good background in pathophysiology, this book would be a good textbook, especially if problem-solving skills will be emphasized.

Reviewed by Vincent F. Mauro, Pharm.D., and Laurie S. Mauro, Pharm.D., College of Pharmacy, The University of Toledo, 2801 West Bancroft Street, Toledo, OH 43606.

Clinical Immunotoxicology

Edited by David S. Newcombe, Noel R. Rose, and John C. Bloom.
Published by Raven Press, 1185 Avenue of the Americas, New York, NY 10036, 1992. xii + 450 p. Price $95.

Twenty-seven nationally and internationally renowned researchers have contributed to this textbook dealing with the toxicology of an increasingly important target organ—the immune system. Most of the authors are academic researchers (10 from The Johns Hopkins University), with the remainder from the Food and Drug Administration, National Institutes of Health, and pharmaceutical industry.

The book focuses on the relatively new discipline of clinical immunotoxicology and explores known and theoretical mechanisms for altered immune function and endogenous and xenobiotic modulators that cause clinical expression of the alterations. The book contains 20 chapters divided into five major parts: "Basic Principles of Immunotoxicology," "Models of Immunotoxic Mechanisms," "Immunotoxic Drugs," "Immunologic Disorders of the Lung," and "Environmental and Occupational Immunotoxins."

The 12 chapters in the first three parts are probably the most useful for expanding the typical pharmacist's knowledge base; examples include a general discussion of the immune system as a specific target for toxicity, toxicity of monoclonal antibodies and conjugates, immunology of cytokines, immunopathogenesis of AIDS, immunosuppressants, drug-induced hematologic disorders, and interactions between antineoplastic agents and the immune system. Most of these chapters are well-written, easy-to-understand overviews that depict the immune system as a target organ for toxic damage. The undergraduate pharmacy student or the general practitioner who already has a general understanding of immune function but does not seek in-depth information will benefit from reading the first 12 chapters; however, the graduate student, academic, or pharmacist who is fairly well-versed in basic and clinical immunology and perhaps practices in a subspecialty area (e.g., hematology–oncology, organ transplantation, infectious diseases) will consider many of these chapters too superficial (e.g., immunotoxicology of cytokines, immunopathogenesis of AIDS). A few chapters stand out as exceptional, though. For example, those that discuss the putative roles of the mast cell in immunotoxicological processes and cyclosporine immunotoxicology are well written and sufficiently detailed to be appealing to the pharmacist specialist. Elaborate discussions on the utility of an in vitro or animal model for evaluation of an in vivo function are not useful to the clinician, but they do provide insight into the methods and formidable problems facing researchers who seek to detect and evaluate toxic responses caused by interactions between chemicals and the human immune system.

The last two parts are well written but poorly edited—they are inappropriately long relative to the other parts, and the chapters are grossly redundant. With the exception of the poison control pharmacist, few pharmacists will consider these sections useful.

The editors state that they designed their book "to enrich the knowledge base of students of medicine, toxicology, immunology and cell and molecular biology." Although pharmacy students and practitioners must be educated in immunotoxicology because many pharmaceuticals produced by recombinant or hybridoma technology exert their pharmacologic and toxicological properties through modulation of the immune system, this book does not optimally meet the needs of most pharmacists.

Most pharmacists will not find the book worth the $95 investment. Graduate students and subspecialists who have a solid grasp of basic and clinical immunology can find primary literature and extensive reviews on specific topics for much less. I look forward to an improved second edition that more adequately meets the specific needs of these groups.

Reviewed by Daniel P. Healy, Pharm.D., College of Pharmacy, University of Cincinnati–Medical Center, Mail Location #4, Cincinnati, OH 45267-0004.

Handbook of Basic Pharmacokinetics . . . including Clinical Applications, Fourth Edition

By W. A. Ritschel.

Published by Drug Intelligence Publications, Inc., 1241 Broadway, Hamilton, IL 62341, 1992. xxi + 588 p. Price $34.

A new edition of *Handbook of Basic Pharmacokinetics* is out. As a clinical pharmacist who uses pharmacokinetics in my daily practice and care of patients, I welcome the inclusion of up-to-date knowledge and nomenclature.

The handbook is a good reference for pharmacy undergraduate and graduate students; it includes basic knowledge and formulas. The tables present information on drug pKa, percentage of drug ionized, calculation of percentage of drug bound to plasma proteins, saliva-to-plasma ratios of drug concentration, and calculations for forensics.

A weakness is the paucity of sample pharmacokinetic calculations, including calculations for drugs that pharmacy practitioners encounter only a couple times a year. Other pharmacokinetics references provide more examples for hands-on experience.

The book is a good reference for background information but needs more examples of calculations typically used in clinical practice.

Reviewed by Larry E. Patterson, Pharm.D., Department of Pharmacy, St. James Community Hospital, P.O. Box 3300, 400 S. Clark Street, Butte, MT 59701.

Neoplastic Diseases: Fundamentals of Clinical Oncology

Edited by C. Julian Rosenthal.

Published by Precept Press, Inc., 160 East Illinois Street, Chicago, IL 60611, 1991. xxvi + 891 p. Price $129.

Believing that existing books on clinical oncology are not easy-to-use reference sources, the editor and authors of *Neoplastic Diseases* set out to present most of the information in a concise format. They intended their brief work to be useful to postgraduate students in oncologic and nononcologic fields as well as to family practitioners caring for patients with cancer.

The topics of the first seven chapters range from epidemiology and carcinogenesis to tumor-growth kinetics and the principles of staging neoplastic diseases. The treatment of these topics is superficial, however, and the authors fail to explain the clinical importance of these topics.

Chapter 8 discusses biologic response modification in cancer, and chapter 9 covers metabolic problems in patients with cancer. Again, the reader is left with little idea of the clinical utility of the information presented.

The next two chapters are the most informative; they deal with diagnostic imaging of tumors and the histopathology of the most common malignant and benign neoplasms. Although these chapters extensively cover their topics, their utility to pharmacists is negligible.

Chapters 12–16 have the most clinical relevance, but they too lack depth. For example, the subject of pain control is covered in a mere two pages, and the entire chapter on supportive care of patients with cancer is only seven pages.

The rest of the book is devoted to specific neoplastic diseases. Each chapter discusses etiology, relevant pathology, diagnosis and staging, prognosis, and therapy of a malignancy. In their attempt to be concise, the authors fail to adequately cover some very complex diagnostic and treatment dilemmas. A notable exception is the chapter on malignant lymphomas; this chapter details well some of the problems with proper diagnosis and treatment.

The textbook includes an appendix that, at first, would seem to be a great asset; it lists currently used combination antineoplastic drug regimens according to disease state. The major drawback is its lack of referencing. It lists regimens that, in the editor's opinion, are among the most effective for a given cancer; the lack of referencing makes it difficult for a clinician to use the information to make decisions regarding the choice of treatment for a patient. However, the appendix might serve as a reference for verifying a question regarding the dose of a given agent in a specific regimen.

Continued on page 904

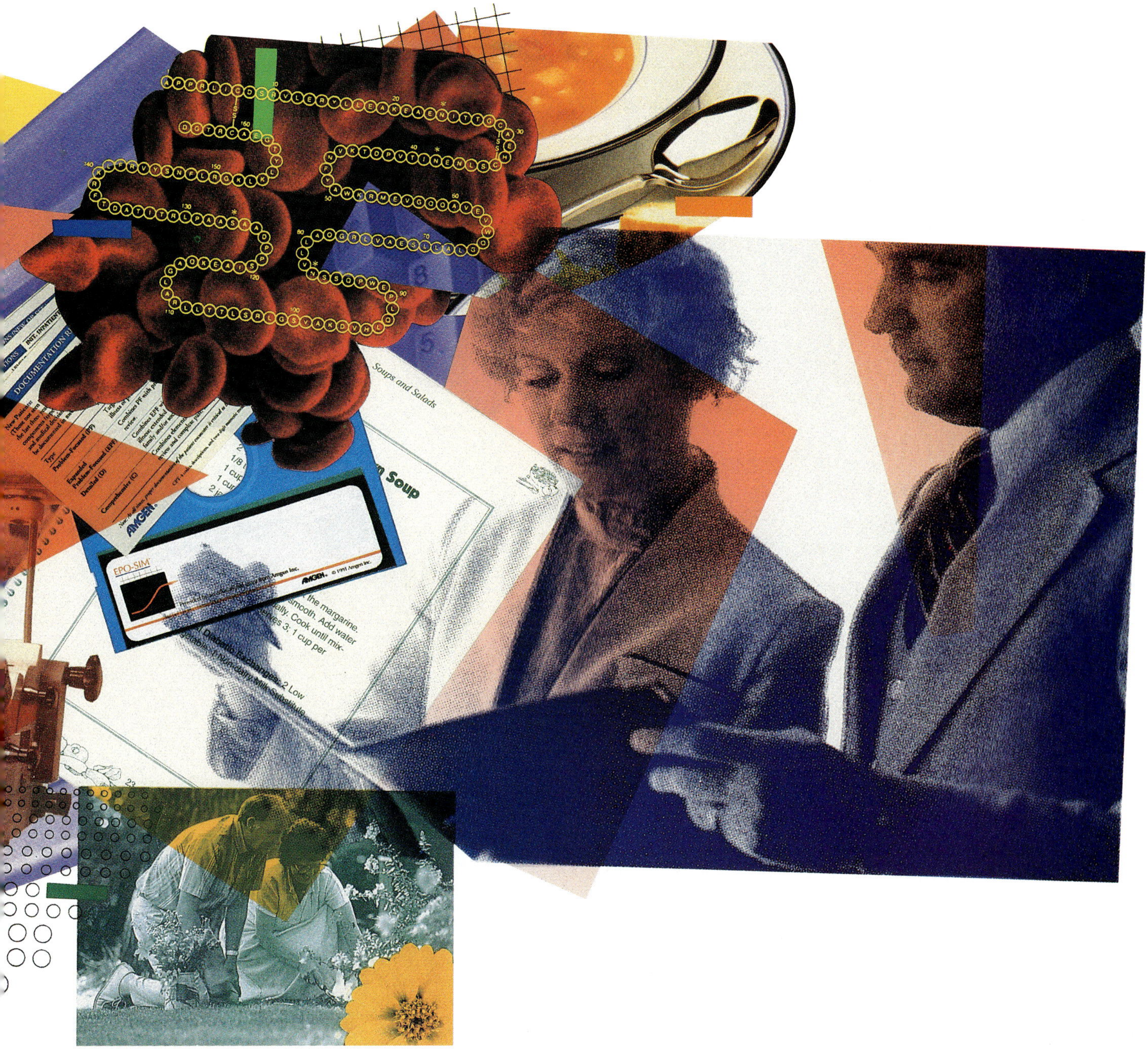
Soups and Salads
EPO-SIM
AMGEN
© 1991 Amgen Inc.
DOCUMENTATION

Continued from page 901

As a result of the editor's desire for conciseness, a large body of background information is left out of the book, detracting from its utility to practitioners who specialize in oncology or who specialize in other fields and need a general reference on oncology. Although no book can be expected to meet the needs of both specialists and generalists, this one is not specific enough for those engaged in the field of clinical oncology yet not informative enough for generalists.

Reviewed by Bud J. Kane, Pharm.D., and John G. Kuhn, Pharm.D., FCCP, Department of Clinical Pharmacy, The University of Texas Health Science Center at San Antonio, 7703 Floyd Curl Drive, San Antonio, TX 78284-6220.

Books Received

Books are listed as soon as received; selected books may be reviewed in Book Reviews in subsequent issues.

Buccal and Nasal Administration as an Alternative to Parenteral Administration, edited by Dominique Duchêne. Published by Editions de Santé, 19 rue Louis-le-Grand, 750002 Paris, France, 1992. 332 p.

Drug Susceptibility in the Chemotherapy of Mycobacterial Infections, by Leonid B. Heifets. Published by CRC Press, Inc., 2000 Corporate Boulevard, N.W., Boca Raton, FL 33431, 1991. 212 p. Price $99.50.

A Handbook on Drug and Alcohol Abuse: The Biomedical Aspects, Third Edition, by Gail Winger, Frederick G. Hofmann, and James H. Woods. Published by Oxford University Press, Inc., 200 Madison Avenue, New York, NY 10016, 1992. xiv + 219 p. Price $49.95 (cloth), $24.95 (paperback).

The Superfamily of *ras*-Related Genes, edited by Demetrios A. Spandidos. Published by Plenum Press, 233 Spring Street, New York, NY 10013, 1991. x + 338 p. Price $89.50.

USAN and the USP Dictionary of Drug Names, 1993 Edition, Carolyn A. Fleeger, editor. Published by the United States Pharmacopeial Convention, Inc., 12601 Twinbrook Parkway, Rockville, MD 20852, 1992. 859 p. Price $100, U.S. and Canada; $140, international.

Advertising Index

American Society of Hospital Pharmacists
ASHP Software, 891
Clinical Pharmacy, 904
Concepts in Immunology and Immunotherapeutics, 864
Understanding Medical Terms, A Guide for Pharmacy Practice, 890
Amgen Inc.
Epogen, 902-903
Monongalia General Hospital
Position Available, 829
Roche Laboratories, Division of Hoffmann-La Roche, Inc.
Rocephin, inside back cover, outside back cover
Roerig, A Division of Pfizer Pharmaceuticals
Cefobid, 831-832
Diflucan, 826-828
Unasyn, 898-900
Scientific Therapeutics Information
Positions Available, 829
Wyeth-Ayerst Laboratories, Inc.
Tubex, inside front cover

News

FDA approves treatment IND protocol for taxol

FDA has approved a treatment IND protocol that will expand patient access to taxol, an antimitotic cytotoxic agent that is derived from the bark of the western yew. The protocol is open to patients with advanced, refractory ovarian cancer who are not candidates for ongoing clinical trials. Eligibility requirements stipulate that the tumor must be resistant to platinum and that the patient must have received and failed to respond to at least two antineoplastic-drug regimens. Queries about the treatment IND protocol or patient eligibility requirements should be directed to the protocol sponsor: Cancer Therapy Evaluation Program, Division of Cancer Treatment, National Cancer Institute, Bethesda, MD 20892.

Three Phase II clinical trials of taxol use in patients with ovarian cancer have been completed. Response rates, recorded over a range of dosages, were 21% to 36%. Clinical trial data suggest that myelosuppression is the dose-limiting toxicity. Peripheral neuropathy, myalgia, mucositis, alopecia, cardiac arrhythmias, and atrioventricular block have been reported. Severe allergic reactions have been attributed to the polyoxyethylated castor oil (Cremophor EL) vehicle.

Patients treated under the protocol will receive taxol at a starting dosage of 135 mg/sq m infused intravenously over 24 hours and repeated every 21 days. The protocol outlines indications, based on hematologic intolerance, for filgrastim administration and for modification of the taxol dosage. Taxol is supplied in 5-mL vials as a concentrated 6-mg/mL solution in Cremophor EL 50% and Dehydrated Alcohol, USP, 50%.

News Briefs

- FDA has approved marketing of **baclofen** (Lioresal Intrathecal, Ciba-Geigy) for intrathecal use in an implantable drug pump for treatment of severe spasticity of spinal cord origin in patients with multiple sclerosis or spinal cord injury. The Medtronic SynchroMed implantable pump was cleared for this use.

- FDA has licensed a new **vaccine against diphtheria, tetanus, and pertussis (DTP) that contains acellular pertussis vaccine adsorbed** (Tripedia, Connaught) for use in children as young as 15 months who have previously received three or four doses of a whole-cell-pertussis DTP vaccine.

- Copies of two statements from NIH consensus development conferences—**Diagnosis and Treatment of Early Melanoma and Diagnosis and Treatment of Depression in Late Life**—are available from the Office of Medical Applications of Research, National Institutes of Health, Federal Building, Room 618, Bethesda, MD 20892.

Upcoming Specialty Meetings

Pain Management in the Pediatric Patient. Indianapolis, IN, December 5; contact Indiana University School of Medicine, Division of Continuing Medical Education, 1226 West Michigan, BR 156, Indianapolis, IN 46202-5178.

1993 Winter Practice and Research Forum. Ft. Lauderdale, FL, February 7–10; contact American College of Clinical Pharmacy, 3101 Broadway, Suite 350, Kansas City, MO 64111; 816-531-2177, (fax) 816-531-4990.

American College of Cardiology. Anaheim, CA, March 14–18; contact ACC, 9111 Old Georgetown Road, Bethesda, MD 20814; 301-897-5400.

Society of Toxicology. New Orleans, LA, March 14–18; contact J. Walsh Cassedy, 1101 14th Street, N.W., Washington, DC 20005; 202-371-1393.

Society for Adolescent Medicine. Chicago, IL, March 18–21; contact E. Moore, 19401 East U.S. Highway 40, Suite 120, Independence, MO 64055; 816-795-8336.

American Society for Clinical Pharmacology and Therapeutics. Honolulu, HI, March 24–27; contact ASCPT, 1718 Gallagher Road, Norristown, PA 19401; 215-825-3838, (fax) 215-834-8652.

Therapy Consultation

The Therapy Consultation *section provides brief advice, in question-and-answer format, on how to handle specific drug-therapy problems. Readers are invited to submit questions, which will be referred to a consultant for an answer. The problems should not be highly specialized or unusual, nor should they be mundane. Questions are answered briefly, based largely on the judgment and personal experience of the consultant, although selected references may be cited to substantiate the consultant's advice.*

Assistance in identifying Therapy Consultation *topics is provided by the drug information centers at Medical College of Virginia Hospitals, Richmond; University of California Medical Center, San Diego; and University of Michigan Medical Center, Ann Arbor.*

Erythromycin, motilin, and gastroparesis

Question: How does erythromycin promote gastrointestinal motility? Is erythromycin effective in the treatment of diabetic gastroparesis or other gastrointestinal disorders?

Answer: Erythromycin can increase gastrointestinal activity in humans[1]; this effect may be related to motilin.[2] While studying the adverse effects of antibiotics on the alimentary tract, Itoh et al.[2] found that intravenous administration of erythromycin induced migrating motor complexes in the stomach and was associated with an increase in the plasma motilin concentration.[2]

Motilin is a linear peptide found primarily in the enterochromaffin cells of the proximal small intestine. The mucosal cells of the duodenum and the antral region of the stomach contain the highest concentration of motilin receptors.[2] Motilin may play an important role in gastric emptying.[3-5] The occurrence of cyclical myoelectric activity in the stomach and duodenum is associated with peaks in plasma motilin.[3] Motilin also induces similar stimulatory activity in both the stomach and duodenum when given exogenously.[4] Administration of antimotilin antibodies, which neutralize circulating endogenous motilin, inhibits this type of activity in the stomach and duodenum.[5]

Motilin infusions accelerate gastric emptying in patients with diabetic gastroparesis.[6,7] However, motilin cannot be used for long-term therapy because it has a short half-life and must be given as a continuous intravenous infusion. Because of its agonistic effect at the motilin receptor, erythromycin may be a useful alternative.

Peeters et al.[8] demonstrated in vitro erythromycin binding to motilin receptors and an ensuing pattern of stimulation in rabbit and human duodenal muscle strips.[8] Erythromycin had no effect on muscle strips of rat or dog duodenum and was totally ineffective on ileal samples. The same anatomical and species specificity is seen with motilin.[8] Other investigators, however, have recently questioned whether motilin agonism can entirely account for erythromycin's prokinetic properties.[9]

Erythromycin has been shown to induce cyclical contractions in the stomachs of healthy volunteers.[10] It appears that this gastrointestinal stimulatory effect is specific for erythromycin and other 14-member-ring macrolides (e.g., oleandomycin). The 16-member and 12-member macrolides exert little or no effect on the gastrointestinal tract.[11] The erythromycin dose needed to induce gastrointestinal activity is much lower than the typical antimicrobial dose. Vantrappen et al.[12] found that an intravenous dose of 40 mg induced contractions that migrated distally in healthy volunteers and diabetic patients.[12] A 350-mg dose, however, produced only a weak contractile effect in healthy volunteers and had no effect in diabetic patients.

Metoclopramide, domperidone, and cisapride have powerful, short-term prokinetic properties in patients with chronic gastroparesis. Although relief of symptoms may persist for some time, the effects of metoclopramide and domperidone on gastric emptying generally wane with continued treatment, particularly when they are administered over several months. Conversely, cisapride has been shown to maintain its effects on gastric emptying, but mixed results have been reported in terms of long-term symptomatic relief.[13,14] Ideally, long-term therapy for gastroparesis should improve gastric emptying and eliminate symptoms of hypomotility.

Gastroparesis often occurs as part of a generalized autonomic neuropathy, as in diabetes, and this may explain why therapies that affect neural control, such as metoclopramide, have had limited long-term efficacy. The direct action of erythromycin at the motilin receptor may, therefore, be of therapeutic advantage. Erythromycin's prokinetic properties, however, may be mediated by way of a cholinergic pathway, as was demonstrated in a canine model following vagotomy and antrectomy.[15]

To date, only preliminary data exist regarding the clinical efficacy of erythromycin. Case reports support the use of erythromycin for gastroparesis associated with chronic intestinal pseudo-obstruction,[16] vagotomy,[17,18] progressive systemic sclerosis,[19] and Ogilvie's syndrome.[20] Erythromycin has been used successfully in facilitating post-pyloric intubation for antroduodenal manometry in children with presumed chronic intestinal pseudo-obstruction.[21] Intraperitoneal administration of erythromycin was also reported to be effective in relieving vomiting associated with gastroparesis in a diabetic patient undergoing continuous ambulatory peritoneal dialysis.[22] Conversely, erythromycin has also been reported to induce ileus in two patients after uncomplicated abdominal surgery.[23]

In the only published placebo-controlled, double-blind study of the use of erythromycin in gastroparesis, Janssens et al.[24] found that a single 200-mg dose of intravenous erythromycin lactobionate administered immediately after meals markedly improved impaired gastric emptying in 10 patients with diabetic gastroparesis.[26] All 10 patients were subsequently treated with 250 mg of oral erythromycin ethylsuccinate, administered three times a day, 30 minutes before meals. After four weeks of oral therapy, gastric emptying improved, but to a lesser degree than with intravenous erythromycin. Four patients had symptoms of gastric obstruction before erythromycin treatment was begun. Of these four patients, one improved and two others, who had tolerated only tube feedings, were able to resume oral feeding. The dosage of insulin required by the patients did not change appreciably over the four-week period, and three patients reported fewer hypoglycemic episodes. The reduced effect of oral erythromycin on gastric emptying may have been related to poor drug absorption, rather than a decline in effect over time. Erythromycin is absorbed in the small intestine, not the stomach, posing an obvious problem in patients with severely impaired gastric emptying.[25]

Although erythromycin is a promising prokinetic agent, its efficacy in the management of gastroparesis must be further investigated. A long-term, controlled trial of oral erythromycin in patients with chronic gastroparesis is warranted. The treatment of gastroparesis may be best accomplished by combining agents that demonstrate additive or synergistic effects. It may be useful to combine an agent that provides adequate symptom control, such as metoclopramide or domperidone, with one that may effectively stimulate gastric emptying for extended periods, such as cisapride. A trial of erythromycin in patients who have not responded to standard therapy may be justified. Erythromycin may be useful in the management of gastroparesis, but its exact role remains to be determined.

1. Lehtola J, Jauhonen P, Kesaniemi A et al. Effect of erythromycin on the oro-caecal transit time in man. *Eur J Clin Pharmacol.* 1990; 39:555-8.
2. Itoh Z, Nakayama M, Suzuki T et al. Erythromycin mimics exogenous motilin in gastrointestinal contractile activity in the dog. *Am J Physiol.* 1984; 247:G688-94.
3. Peeters TL, Vantrappen G, Janssens J. Fasting plasma motilin levels are related to the interdigestive motility complex. *Gastroenterology.* 1980; 79:716.
4. Itoh Z, Honda R, Hiwatashik K et al. Motilin-induced mechanical activity in the canine alimentary tract. *Scand J Gastroenterol.* 1976; 11(Suppl 39):93.
5. Lee KY, Chang TM, Chey WY. Effect of rabbit anti-motilin serum on myoelectric activity and plasma motilin concentration in fasting dogs. *Am J Physiol.* 1983; 245:G547.
6. Schmid R, Schusdziarra V, Allescher HD et al. Effect of motilin on gastric emptying in patients with diabetic gastroparesis. *Diabetes Care.* 1991; 14:65-8.
7. Peeters TL, Muls E, Janssens J et al. Effect of motilin on gastric emptying in patients with diabetic gastroparesis. *Gastroenterology.* 1992; 102:97-101.
8. Peeters T, Matthijs G, Depoortere I et al. Erythromycin is a motilin receptor agonist. *Am J Physiol.* 1989; 257:G470-4.
9. Sarna SK, Soergel KH, Koch TR et al. Gastrointestinal motor effects of erythromycin in humans. *Gastroenterology.* 1991; 101:1488-96.
10. Tomomasa T, Kuroume T, Arai H et al. Erythromycin induces migrating motor complex in human gastrointestinal tract. *Dig Dis Sci.* 1986; 31:157-61.
11. Itoh Z, Suzuki T, Nakaya M et al. Structure-activity relation among macrolide antibiotics in initiation of interdigestive migrating contractions in the canine gastrointestinal tract. *Am J Physiol.* 1985; 248:G320-5.
12. Vantrappen G, Janssens J, Tack J et al. Erythromycin is a potent gastrokinetic in diabetic gastroparesis. *Gastroenterology.* 1989; 96:A525. Abstract.
13. Brown CK, Khanderia U. Use of metoclopramide, domperidone, and cisapride in the management of diabetic gastroparesis. *Clin Pharm.* 1990; 9:357-65.
14. Abell TL, Camilleri M, DiMagno EP et al. Long-term efficacy of oral cisapride in symptomatic upper gut dysmotility. *Dig Dis Sci.* 1991; 36:616-20.
15. Carlson RG, Hocking MP, Sninsky CA et al. Erythromycin acts through a cholinergic pathway to improve canine-delayed gastric emptying following vagotomy and Roux-Y antrectomy. *J Surg Res.* 1991; 50:494-8.
16. Berger SA, Keshavarzian A, DeMeo MT et al. Erythromycin in chronic intestinal pseudo-obstruction. *J Clin Gastroenterol.* 1990; 12:363.
17. Christian RB, Cooke AR. Erythromycin and gastroparesis. *Kans Med.* 1990; 91:259-61.
18. Mozwecz H, Pavel D, Pitrak D et al. Erythromycin stearate as prokinetic agent in postvagotomy gastroparesis. *Dig Dis Sci.* 1990; 35:902-5.
19. Dull JS, Raufman JP, Zakai MD et al. Successful treatment of gastroparesis with erythromycin in a patient with progressive systemic sclerosis. *Am J Med.* 1990; 89:528-30.
20. Armstrong DN, Ballantyne GH, Modlin IM. Erythromycin for reflex ileus in Ogilvie's syndrome. *Lancet.* 1991; 337:378.
21. DiLorenzo C, Lachman R, Hyman PE. Intravenous erythromycin for postpyloric intubation. *J Pediatr Gastroenterol Nutr.* 1990; 11:45-7.
22. Wadhwa NK, Atkins H. Intraperitoneal erythromycin for gastroparesis. *Ann Intern Med.* 1991;114:912.
23. Heyman SN, Stalnikowicz R, Heyman A et al. Erythromycin-induced dynamic ileus? *J Clin Gastroenterol.* 1988; 10:551-4.
24. Janssens J, Peeters TL, Vantrappen G et al. Improvement of gastric emptying in diabetic gastroparesis by erythromycin. *N Engl J Med.* 1990; 322:1028-31.
25. Vantrappen G. Erythromycin—the prokinetic drug of the future. Have we heard this story line before? *Gastroenterology.* 1990; 99:559-60.

Peter J. Yurkowski, Pharm.D.
Pharmacy Practice Resident
University of Cincinnati Hospital
Cincinnati, OH 45267-0791

Karim Anton Calis, Pharm.D.
Coordinator, Drug Information Service
Endocrinology Clinical Pharmacy Specialist
Department of Pharmacy
Warren G. Magnuson Clinical Center
National Institutes of Health
Building 10, Room 1N-257
Bethesda, MD 20892

Drug Reviews

Sumatriptan: A new drug for vascular headache

VAN DOREN HSU

Abstract: The role of serotonin in the pathogenesis of migraine is discussed, and the chemistry, pharmacology, pharmacokinetics, efficacy, adverse effects, and dosage and administration of sumatriptan are reviewed.

Sumatriptan, which is structurally related to the neurotransmitter serotonin, is a serotonin type-1-like-receptor agonist that has a selective but heterogeneous effect on the carotid arterial system. Sumatriptan has a rapid onset of action and a large volume of distribution. Its subcutaneous bioavailability approaches 100%, and its mean terminal half-life is two hours.

Studies have shown that both subcutaneous sumatriptan and oral sumatriptan are superior to placebo in relieving migraine and cluster headaches. Studies comparing oral sumatriptan with either ergotamine tartrate plus caffeine (Cafergot) or aspirin plus metoclopramide indicated that sumatriptan relieved headache more quickly and effectively; however, the dosages of these other agents may have been suboptimal. Sumatriptan is generally well tolerated by patients, and most dose-related effects are mild and transient. The most common adverse effect is pain at the injection site. No drug interactions have been identified so far. Subcutaneous sumatriptan 6 mg and oral sumatriptan 100 mg seem to offer the best benefit-to-risk ratio, although dosage and administration information is limited.

Subcutaneous and oral sumatriptan are effective in aborting moderate to severe migraine and cluster headaches and their associated symptoms. However, more studies are necessary to compare sumatriptan's efficacy with that of other treatments before it can be recommended as first-line therapy for migraine.

Index terms: Dosage; Mechanism of action; Migraine; Pharmacokinetics; Serotonin agonists; Sumatriptan succinate; Toxicity
Clin Pharm. 1992; 11:919-29

Migraine is a common neurological disorder that greatly affects the quality of life and increases work disruption. An average of 9.1% and 16.1% of men and women, respectively, suffer from migraine headache.[1] There are several classes of migraine: common migraine (or migraine without aura), classic migraine (or migraine with aura), ophthalmoplegic migraine, and retinal migraine.[2] Migraine without aura is typically characterized by a unilateral, pulsatile headache of moderate to severe intensity. It can be aggravated by routine physical activity and may be associated with nausea, photophobia, and phonophobia. Migraine with aura, in contrast, is manifested by attacks of neurological symptoms that can be localized to the cerebral cortex or brainstem. Headache, nausea, or photophobia follows the aura immediately or within one hour.[2]

Current abortive treatments for migraine include isometheptene–dichloralphenazone–acetaminophen (Midrin), analgesics with or without antiemetics, and ergot compounds. The response to the various antimigraine therapies is variable. The effectiveness of these drugs largely depends on their use immediately before or early in the course of the headache. Intolerable adverse effects have made some of these drugs unacceptable or unappealing to many patients.

Sumatriptan succinate (Imitrex, Glaxo) is the first of a new class of antimigraine agents known as serotonin type-1-like-receptor agonists. It is currently being evaluated for short-term treatment of migraine with or without aura. New-drug applications for the subcutaneous-injection and oral-tablet formulations were submitted to the FDA in June 1990 and December 1990, respectively. At the time of this writing, approval from the FDA is still pending.

The purpose of this review is to discuss the role of serotonin in the pathogenesis of migraine and the pharmacology, pharmacokinetics, clinical efficacy, pa-

VAN DOREN HSU, PHARM.D., is Clinical Specialist in Neuroscience, Department of Pharmacy Services, University of Maryland Medical System, 22 South Greene Street, Baltimore, MD 21201.

The assistance of Janine Good, M.D., and Paul Weidle, Pharm.D., is acknowledged.

tient tolerance, adverse effects, and dosage and administration of sumatriptan in patients with migraine headaches.

Chemistry

Sumatriptan is structurally related to serotonin; its chemical name is 3-[2-(dimethylamino)ethyl]-*N*-methyl-1*H*-indole-5-methane sulfonamide (Figure 1). The molecular formula of sumatriptan is $C_{14}H_{21}N_3O_2S$, and its molecular weight is 295.40. Although given as the succinate salt, sumatriptan dosage is expressed in terms of the base. Sumatriptan and serotonin share the same basic ring structure; however, they have different side chains. Like serotonin, sumatriptan has low lipophilicity.

Figure 1. Chemical structures of serotonin (top) and sumatriptan (bottom).

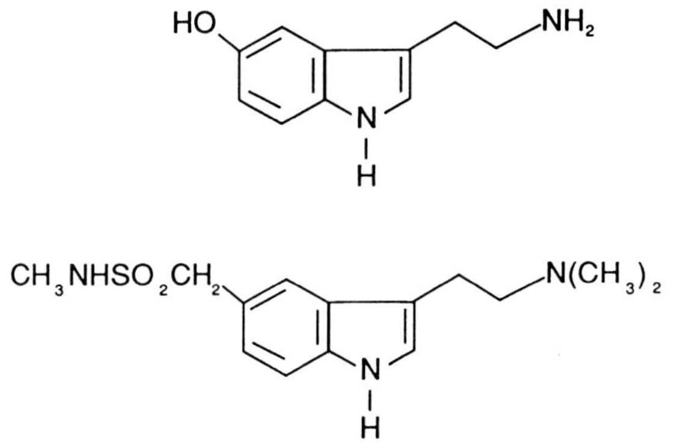

Role of Serotonin in the Pathogenesis of Migraine

Serotonin is a neurotransmitter that is present in most human tissues, with high concentrations in the gastrointestinal tract, brain, and platelets. In brain tissue, serotonin exists in a bound form and is thus protected from destruction by monoamine oxidase. Serotonin is a more potent vasoconstrictor of the external carotid circulation than of the cerebral arteries.[3]

The exact pathogenesis of migraine is still not clearly understood. Researchers have postulated vascular and neurogenic models for migraine.[4-6] It is unlikely that any single theory can explain the disorder.[7]

Certain observations have suggested that serotonin is involved in the pathogenesis of migraine. First, the level of serotonin in platelets has been shown to increase before and decrease during migraine attacks.[8-10] Increased excretion in the urine of 5-hydroxyindoleacetic acid, the main metabolite of serotonin, was noted during an attack. These changes in serotonin levels parallel the symptoms of migraine. Kimball and coworkers[11] reported that intramuscular reserpine, which depletes serotonin, lowered plasma serotonin concentrations and induced a typical headache in migraine patients. In contrast, healthy subjects experienced only a dull, nonspecific headache. These migraine headaches were relieved when intravenous serotonin was infused into the carotid artery.[8,9] Despite serotonin's efficacy in relieving headache, unacceptable adverse effects such as dyspnea, chest tightness, nausea, and dizziness preclude its clinical use. In addition, both methysergide and pizotyline, two medications for migraine prophylaxis, act on serotonin receptors. Likewise, ergotamine exhibits serotonin-like effects on blood vessels. All these observations have led researchers to believe that a structural analogue of serotonin with more specific activity and a more favorable adverse-effect profile would be safe and effective for aborting acute migraine attacks.

Three main classes of serotonin receptors have been identified: type 1 (5-HT_1), type 2 (5-HT_2), and type 3 (5-HT_3). The heterogeneous 5-HT_1 class is further divided into 5-HT_{1A}, 5-HT_{1B}, 5-HT_{1C}, and 5-HT_{1D} receptors, but 5-HT_{1B} receptors have not been identified in humans to date.[12] The 5-HT_{1D} receptor is the most common subtype in the human brain.[13] The 5-HT_1-like receptors are mostly present in the cerebral arteries, whereas 5-HT_2 receptors are more prevalent in temporal arteries. Meningeal arteries, however, have all three classes of serotonin receptors.[14] Recently, there has been a suggestion that a 5-HT_1-like receptor in cranial vasculature may be identical to the 5-HT_{1D} receptor.[15-17]

Pharmacology

Sumatriptan has the highest affinity for 5-HT_{1D} receptors, followed by a fivefold-lower affinity at 5-HT_{1A} receptors, as shown by radioligand-binding studies that used rat, bovine, and porcine brain tissues.[18,19] Sumatriptan is devoid of any activity at other serotonin receptor subtypes, as well as at dopaminergic, β-adrenergic, muscarinic, cholinergic, and benzodiazepine receptors.[18,19]

Sumatriptan, a 5-HT_1-like-receptor agonist, has a selective but heterogeneous vasoconstrictive effect on the carotid arterial circulation. In dogs, Feniuk et al.[15] found that sumatriptan caused a dose-dependent decrease in carotid arterial blood flow, with little or no effect on arterial blood pressure. This reduction in blood flow was associated with an increase in carotid arterial vascular resistance. Little effect was found on total peripheral resistance or resistance in mesenteric, vertebral, and coronary arterial beds. Sumatriptan was also found to be four times less potent than serotonin in contracting isolated saphenous vein from dogs.[17] In anesthetized cats, both sumatriptan and ergotamine caused an increase in carotid vascular resistance, leading to a dose-dependent constriction of arteriovenous anastomoses.[20] In contrast to ergotamine, sumatriptan caused little change in diastolic blood pressure and total peripheral resistance. It also contracts human isolated basilar artery and canine and primate basilar artery by activating the 5-HT_1-like receptors.[16,21] However, no contraction was found in isolated saphenous vein from cats, rabbit aorta, pig coronary artery, greyhound coronary artery, and beagle femoral artery.[17,22] According to the hypothesis proposed by Heyck,[4] an unknown event leads to the opening of carotid arteriovenous anastomoses (and subsequent diversion of blood from capillary beds), ischemia, and hypoxia. Sumatriptan is an effective agent because of its ability to close the shunt and restore blood flow without increasing peripheral resistance.

Another proposed mechanism for migraine is neurogenic inflammation of intracranial blood vessels. Cranial vessels such as the meningeal and large cerebral conducting arteries are innervated by the trigeminal nerve. Stimulation of the trigeminal nerve leads to distention of blood vessels and subsequent protein extravasation and release of vasoactive neuropeptides such as calcitonin gene-related peptide and substance P.[23] Evidence to support this theory includes demonstration of distention of large intracranial vessels during the headache phase and an increase in the plasma concentration of calcitonin gene-related peptide in patients with migraine.[24,25]

Ergotamine has been shown to block the extravasation of plasma protein from dural vessels when the trigeminovascular system is stimulated electrically or by capsaicin.[26] In a later study, sumatriptan produced effects similar to those observed with ergotamine.[27] It selectively blocks the plasma protein extravasation within intracranial tissue but not within extracranial tissue in guinea pigs and rats. Extravasation mediated by substance P or neurokinin A is not blocked by sumatriptan. It is likely that, by activating the 5-HT_1 receptors, sumatriptan constricts the distended cranial vessels and thereby inhibits protein extravasation and pain.

Pharmacokinetics

Absorption. The absorption of sumatriptan is best described by using a two-compartment model. The drug is rapidly absorbed; maximum plasma concentration (C_{max}) is reached approximately 15–20 minutes after subcutaneous injection.[28-31] C_{max} values of 72.4 ng/mL and 53.8 ng/mL are attained after administration of a 6-mg subcutaneous dose and a 100-mg oral dispersible tablet, respectively, in healthy subjects and migraine patients between attacks[32] (see Table 1). Oral absorption of sumatriptan is also rapid; approximately 80% of the C_{max} is achieved within 45 minutes.[32] Compared with the subcutaneous route, the oral route results in a markedly more variable time to reach C_{max} (t_{max}), ranging from 0.5 to 5 hours because of the presence of multiple peaks during the absorption phase. These peaks may be caused by variable rates of gastric emptying and small-bowel transit.[29,34] No difference in the rate and extent of absorption is observed in migraine patients during a migraine attack, compared with a headache-free period.[35]

There is a linear relationship between the dose administered, C_{max}, and area under the plasma concentration–time curve (AUC).[28,33,35,36] Plasma concentrations of sumatriptan associated with a therapeutic response are 8–66 ng/mL, 18–60 ng/mL, and 5–71 ng/mL with subcutaneous, oral, and intravenous administration, respectively.[30,36,37]

Sumatriptan is also quickly absorbed when given intranasally.[38] A C_{max} of 20–25 ng/mL is attained 20 minutes after the first insufflation, but considerable variation is found among patients. This concentration is sustained for up to two hours, which suggests that the nasal solution may have been swallowed and subsequently may have influenced the peak and maintenance levels of sumatriptan. Further studies will be needed to study the pharmacokinetics of intranasal sumatriptan.

Distribution. The mean distribution-phase half-life of sumatriptan given subcutaneously is reported to be 13.1 minutes.[28] The drug is widely distributed throughout the body, as evidenced by its volume of distribution of 170 L.[32] Protein binding is low, ranging from 10% to 21%.[29] Penetration of the blood–brain barrier is poor in mice after intravenous injection.[39]

Metabolism. The bioavailability of subcutaneous sumatriptan approaches 100%.[32] The low oral bioavailability of 14% is presumably due to first-pass hepatic

Table 1.
Mean Pharmacokinetic Values for Sumatriptan[a]

Reference	Dose and Route	Subjects	C_{max} (ng/mL)	t_{max} (hr)	$t_{1/2}$ (hr)	AUC (ng · hr/mL)	V (L)	CL_p (mL/min)	CL_R (mL/min)	F
28	1–16 mg s.c.	Healthy	. . .	0.25[b]	1.8[b]	. . .	201.6[b]	1200.9[b]	. . .	. . .
33	100 mg p.o.	Healthy	42.5	1.2	1.9	159.0	. . .	. . .	. . .	. . .
	200 mg p.o.		80.7	2.5	2.2	335.5	. . .	. . .	. . .	. . .
29	2 mg i.v.	Healthy	37	0.25	1.7	25.5	194	1313	272	. . .
	100 mg p.o.		44	2.3	2.6	180.2	. . .	. . .	242	0.14
32	6 mg s.c.	Migraine and nonmigraine	72.4	0.17[c]	2	. . .	170	1200	260	0.96
	3 mg i.v.		76.8	. . .	. . .	. . .	. . .	. . .	. . .	. . .
	100 mg p.o.		53.8	1.5[c]	2	. . .	. . .	. . .	. . .	0.14

[a]C_{max} = maximum serum drug concentration; t_{max} = time after dose to reach C_{max}; $t_{1/2}$ = half-life; AUC = area under the serum concentration–time curve; V = volume of distribution; CL_p = plasma clearance; CL_R = renal clearance; F = bioavailability.
[b]Overall mean values from sumatriptan 1–16 mg.
[c]Median values.

metabolism.[29] Two metabolites have been identified in humans: the indoleacetic acid analogue and its glucuronide analogue. The indoleacetic acid analogue, which is the main inactive metabolite, has a plasma concentration six to seven times higher than that of the parent compound. Sumatriptan and its indoleacetic acid analogue have similar half-lives, suggesting that the clearance of this metabolite is limited by its rate of formation.[32]

Elimination. After a 2-mg intravenous sumatriptan dose, the mean plasma and renal clearances are 1313 mL/min and 272 mL/min, respectively.[29] This high renal clearance exceeds the normal human glomerular filtration rate of 125 mL/min, which indicates the contribution of active tubular secretion to the elimination process. Comparable results are also seen after a 6-mg subcutaneous dose.[32]

On average, 21% of sumatriptan and 53% of its indoleacetic acid analogue are recovered in the urine. Small amounts of the parent drug and its metabolites are eliminated in the feces.[32]

The mean terminal half-life of sumatriptan is two hours.[28,29,33] An additional terminal phase occurs 12–16 hours after a single oral dose.[32,33] The importance of this terminal phase is still unknown. No pharmacokinetic studies have been conducted in patients with hepatic or renal impairment.

Effect of Food, Age, and Migraine. Food does not affect the oral bioavailability of sumatriptan. No difference has been observed between fed and fasting subjects with respect to pharmacokinetic values.[32]

Twelve healthy elderly subjects (65–86 years of age) were given oral sumatriptan 200 mg and subcutaneous sumatriptan 1–3 mg to investigate the pharmacokinetics in this age group.[32] The C_{max}, t_{max}, and AUC were similar to those in younger subjects.

A study performed in 192 patients with common or classical migraine showed no significant reduction in the rate and extent of oral absorption of sumatriptan 100 mg during a migraine attack, compared with a pain-free state.[35] Similar results were obtained in an early oral dose-ranging study.[37]

Use in Patients with Acute Migraine

Sumatriptan is currently being evaluated as a treatment for acute migraine attacks. So far, no studies have been published on the long-term use of sumatriptan for prophylaxis against migraine. Different routes of administration have been used in trials, but the drug was most often given either subcutaneously or orally because of the ease and feasibility of administration. Intravenous and, more recently, intranasal administration have also been tested.

Sumatriptan was usually compared with placebo, but it was also compared with oral ergotamine plus caffeine (Cafergot, Sandoz)[40] or with aspirin plus metoclopramide.[41] Patients recruited for the studies were generally adults and had migraine with or without aura. Pregnant or nursing women were excluded. Any patient with a history of ischemic heart disease, hypertension (baseline diastolic blood pressure of >95 mm Hg), and other serious systemic diseases such as peripheral vascular disease, renal impairment, or hepatic impairment was excluded. Use of analgesics was not permitted within six hours of the study treatment, and use of ergotamine compounds or narcotics was not permitted within one day of the study treatment. Effectiveness of a drug in relieving migraine headache and associated symptoms was evaluated subjectively, primarily on the basis of information from patients' diary cards. In almost all studies conducted with migraine patients, a standard 4-point grading system was used: 0 = no headache, 1 = mild, 2 = moderate, and 3 = severe. An effective response was defined as a reduction of headache severity from severe or moderate to mild or none after treatment. Other indicators of efficacy included a reduction in functional disability from bed rest or severe impairment to slight or no impairment; absence of pre-existing symptoms including nausea, vomiting, photophobia, and phonophobia; and the need for rescue medications.

Only selective controlled studies are reviewed here. See Tables 2 and 3 for a list of controlled trials. Early open studies[30,31,36,37,50,51] and three placebo-controlled studies[42,48,52] revealed a dose-dependent effect on headache relief in migraine patients. The results from these studies established oral and subcutaneous doses of sumatriptan for further trials.

Intravenous Studies. Several earlier studies had investigated the use of intravenous sumatriptan.[37,53,54] A dose-related effect was found in patients receiving 64 µg/kg or 2 mg either as an intravenous bolus or an infusion.[37,54] Headache and other related symptoms were relieved within 10–30 minutes. This beneficial effect was observed regardless of the interval between the onset of headache and initiation of treatment.[37] However, intravenous sumatriptan was associated with a high frequency of adverse effects, which could have been related to the rapid rise in serum drug concentration.

Subcutaneous Studies. Six hundred thirty-nine patients who had migraine with or without aura were studied in a randomized, double-blind, placebo-controlled, parallel-group trial.[44] Patients with moderate or severe headache were randomized to receive placebo, sumatriptan 6 mg, or sumatriptan 8 mg as a 0.5-mL subcutaneous injection. When headache was still present 60 minutes after the injection, a second double-blind dose of either placebo or sumatriptan 6 mg was given to those who received 6 mg initially. Those who received placebo or sumatriptan 8 mg as the first dose were given placebo as a second injection. Sumatriptan had a rapid onset of action, as evidenced by a response rate of about 50% at 30 minutes compared with about 15% in patients receiving placebo. All sumatriptan regimens were demonstrated to be significantly more effective than placebo in aborting headache at both 60 and 120 minutes ($p < 0.001$ for all comparisons). No differences in effectiveness were observed among the sumatriptan regimens. Secondary measures of efficacy were also favorable: patients receiving sumatriptan required fewer rescue medications, had better functional ability, and had better relief of nausea, vomiting, photophobia, and phonophobia at one and two hours ($p < 0.001$ for all comparisons). Patients responded equally well to sumatriptan regardless of the duration of symptoms before treatment and the type of migraine. Compared with patients receiving placebo, patients receiving sumatriptan had a higher headache recurrence rate within 24 hours (34–38% versus 18%; $p < 0.02$). This higher rate may have been related to the short half-life of sumatriptan. Median time to recurrence was variable, but it appeared to be longer in sumatriptan-treated patients.

Similar response rates were seen in 235 patients who self-injected either subcutaneous sumatriptan 6 mg or placebo at the onset of migraine attacks and a second dose if moderate or severe headache persisted one hour after the initial injection.[45] In contrast to the previously described study,[44] the headache recurrence rate within 48 hours was the same for sumatriptan and placebo (46%). This rate did not take into account whether rescue or other nonstudy medications were given during that period. Thus, the real recurrence rate was still unknown.

Cady and coworkers[43] recruited 1104 migraine patients to participate in a large-scale study with a design similar to that used by the Subcutaneous Sumatriptan International Study Group.[44] Patients were randomized initially to receive either placebo or sumatriptan 6 mg as a 0.5-mL subcutaneous injection.[43] Those patients who had inadequate relief at one hour were randomized to receive a second injection of placebo or sumatriptan 6 mg. Sumatriptan was demonstrated to be superior to placebo in relieving headache at one and two hours ($p < 0.001$). No additional benefit was seen with the administration of a second dose, which confirmed the observation from the Subcutaneous Sumatriptan International Study Group.[44] Likewise, rapid relief was observed as early as 10 minutes after the first injection of sumatriptan. Patients who received active drug had significant improvement in nausea, photophobia, and functional disability ($p < 0.001$ for all comparisons). Patients receiving sumatriptan also required fewer rescue medications than patients receiving placebo. Within 24 hours of headache onset, the percentage of patients who were initially pain free at discharge but experienced some headache recurrence was similar in both groups (sumatriptan, 51%; placebo, 50%).

Oral Studies. Goadsby et al.[46] conducted a study in 61 migraine patients receiving prophylactic antimigraine therapies. Each patient was treated for four attacks: two with oral sumatriptan 100-mg dispersible tablets and two with placebo. The response rate at two

Table 2.
Subcutaneous Sumatriptan in Acute Migraine Treatment[a]

Reference	No. Attacks	Dosing Regimen	First Reported Time of Benefit (min)	Response Rate[b]	Recurrence Rate	Frequency of Adverse Effects
42	277	Pl or Su 1–3 mg; then Su 3 mg at 30 min p.r.n. pain	30	30 min: 48–59% (Su); 26% (Pl)	. . .	. . .
42	242	Pl or Su 1–8 mg	60	60 min: 42–80% (Su); 22% (Pl)	. . .	62% (Su 6 mg); 80% (Su 8 mg); 39% (Pl)
43	1104	Pl or Su 6 mg; repeat at 60 min p.r.n. pain	10	10 min: 14% (Su); 4% (Pl) 1 hr: 70% (Su); 22% (Pl) 2 hr: 81% (Su); 34% (Pl)	Within 24 hr: 51% (Su); 50% (Pl)	85% (Su); 53% (Pl)
44	639	Pl or Su 6 or 8 mg; Pl or Su 6 mg at 60 min p.r.n. pain	30	30 min: 50% (Su 6 mg); 55% (Su 8 mg); 16% (Pl) 1 hr: 73% (Su 6 mg); 80% (Su 8 mg); 26% (Pl) 2 hr: 86% (Su 6 mg); 90% (Su 6 mg + 6 mg); 71% (Su 8 mg); 36% (Pl)	Within 24 hr: 34–38% (Su); 18% (Pl)	50% (Su); 33% (Pl)
45	235	Pl or Su 6 mg; repeat at 60 min p.r.n. pain	60	1 hr: 77% (Su); 26% (Pl) 2 hr: 83% (Su); 30% (Pl)	Within 48 hr[c]: 46% (Su); 46% (Pl)	39% (Su); 19% (Pl)

[a]All cited studies used a double-blind, placebo-controlled, parallel-group design. Su = sumatriptan; Pl = placebo.
[b]Response rate is defined as the percentage of attacks in which there was a reduction of headache severity from severe or moderate to mild or none.
[c]No account of whether rescue or other nonstudy medications had been used within 48 hours.

Table 3.
Oral Sumatriptan in Acute Migraine Treatment[a]

Reference	No. Patients (Attacks)	Dosing Regimen	First Reported Time of Benefit (hr)	Response Rate[b]	Recurrence Rate	Frequency of Adverse Effects
46	61	Pl or Su 100 mg for 4 attacks	2[c]	2 hr: 51% (Su); 10% (Pl)	Within 24 hr[d]: 39% (Su)	. . .
47	94 (194)	Pl or Su 200 mg	2	2 hr[e]: 63% (Su); 33% (Pl)	. . .	27% (Su); 6% (Pl)
48	1130 (3035)	Pl or Su 100–300 mg	2	2 hr[e]: 67% (Su 100 mg); 73% (Su 200 mg); 67% (Su 300 mg); 27% (Pl)	. . .	41% (Su); 15% (Pl)
49	233	Pl or Su 100 mg; repeat at 2 and 24 hr p.r.n.	1	1 hr: 39% (Su); 17% (Pl) 2 hr: 50% (Su); 19% (Pl) 4 hr: 75% (Su); 30% (Pl)	Within 24 hr[f]: 48% (Su); 42% (Pl)	38% (Su); 23% (Pl)
40	577 (1609)	Su 100 mg or 1 capsule of Cafergot	1	1 hr[e]: 33% (Su); 22% (Cafergot) 2 hr[e]: 66% (Su); 48% (Cafergot)	Within 48 hr: 41% (Su); 30% (Cafergot)	By patients: 45% (Su); 39% (Cafergot) By attacks: 31% (Su); 25% (Cafergot)
41	358	Su 100 mg or aspirin 900 mg + metoclopramide 10 mg	2[g]	2 hr: 56% (Su); 45% (A + M)	With 48 hr[d]; 42% (Su); 33% (A + M)	42% (Su); 29% (A + M)

[a]All cited studies used a double-blind parallel-group design, except for the study described in reference 47, which used a double-blind crossover design. Su = sumatriptan; Pl = placebo; A + M = aspirin + metoclopramide.
[b]Response rate is defined as the percentage of attacks in which there was a reduction of headache severity from severe or moderate to mild or none.
[c]Current prophylactic medications were continued.
[d]No account of whether rescue or other nonstudy medications had been used within 48 hours.
[e]Data from first attack.
[f]Recurrence rate was based on the number of pain-free patients at the end of 2 hours.
[g]Not significant (p=0.078).

hours indicated that sumatriptan was superior to placebo. However, 39% (11/28) of sumatriptan-treated patients who were initially pain free at 2 hours eventually experienced recurrence within 24 hours.

Different results were found in a trial specifically for patients suffering from migraine with aura.[47] Significant improvement in headache severity and associated symptoms was seen only two hours after the first attack. No difference between the sumatriptan and placebo groups was detected in subsequent attacks. Because more patients in the sumatriptan group had vomiting before treatment for the second and third attacks, it was postulated that vomiting may have impaired the absorption of oral sumatriptan and hence reduced its efficacy.

In a multicenter trial, 233 migraine patients received a repeated-dose regimen of either sumatriptan 100 mg or placebo.[49] The first dose was taken at the onset of a moderate or severe headache. The dose was repeated two hours later if headache persisted. A third dose was administered to treat those whose headache recurred within 24 hours. Favorable results were seen at two and four hours in those who received sumatriptan regardless of the type of migraine and the time period between onset of headache and initiation of treatment. However, because the second sumatriptan dose was identical to the first dose, it could not be determined whether the second dose offered any additional benefit. Recurrence rates were similar in both groups (sumatriptan, 42%; placebo, 48%). No conclusion could be made about the efficacy of the third dose of sumatriptan because of the small number of subjects.

To date, only two large-scale studies have compared sumatriptan with current migraine-abortive therapy.[40,41] In both trials, a single dose of study drug was administered to abort each attack for up to three attacks. Data from both studies showed that patients who received sumatriptan had their headache relieved more quickly than patients who received other migraine-abortive therapies. Improvement was not as rapid as that seen in the studies that used subcutaneous sumatriptan.[43,44] Patients receiving sumatriptan had consistently better headache relief at two hours than patients receiving ergotamine tartrate 2 mg plus caffeine 200 mg (Cafergot) for all three attacks in that trial. In contrast, the response rates during the first attack did not differ between patients treated with sumatriptan and those treated with aspirin plus metoclopramide, but more sumatriptan-treated patients were completely free of headache (p = 0.016). Sumatriptan was better than either Cafergot or aspirin plus metoclopramide at improving headache during the second and third attacks.[41] The recurrence rate was significantly higher in the sumatriptan group for all attacks in both studies except for the first attack in the study comparing sumatriptan with aspirin plus metoclopramide. The median time to recurrence was 14–24 hours.

These studies raise several important issues. First, the single dose of Cafergot used in the comparative trial was suboptimal. The usual regimen is one capsule at the onset of headache and one capsule every 30–45 minutes if relief is inadequate, up to a maximum of three capsules. Likewise, a single dose of aspirin is suboptimal. Repeated doses may be necessary, especially in patients with moderate or severe migraine attacks. Second, the dispersible sumatriptan tablets used in the studies were associated with a high frequency of vomiting. These tablets have been replaced by film-coated, tasteless tablets that will reduce vomiting and consequently enhance the absorption of oral sumatriptan. These film-coated tablets should be used in future trials. Information on headache recurrence was based on the patients' diary cards. No information regarding how many rescue medications were used or whether patients used other nonstudy medications during the study period was recorded. Hence, the reported recurrence rates may not be accurate.

Intranasal Studies. In patients who suffer from gastric stasis, nausea, or vomiting, intranasal administration of sumatriptan provides a noninvasive alternate route of administration. The Finnish Sumatriptan Group and the Cardiovascular Clinical Research Group[38] reported a randomized, double-blind, placebo-controlled trial involving 74 migraine patients who received intranasal sumatriptan or placebo. Patients received a 0.1-mL insufflation of either sumatriptan 20 mg or placebo in one nostril. A second dose was given 15 minutes after the first one. Significantly more patients in the sumatriptan group than in the placebo group had improvement in headache at one and two hours after administration ($p = 0.004$ at one hour; $p < 0.001$ at two hours). Headache relief was also achieved earlier in sumatriptan-treated patients. Moreover, the change in the mean headache severity score after treatment was also significantly greater in patients who received sumatriptan than in patients who received placebo. In addition, the functional disability score and percentage of patients requiring rescue medication were also lower at all assessments in patients receiving active drug. No difference was observed in the number of migraine recurrences after 24 hours. Despite the favorable result from this preliminary study, further studies will be needed to determine the pharmacokinetics and optimal dose of intranasal sumatriptan.

Use in Patients with Cluster Headache

Cluster headache is characterized by recurrent, unilateral headache attacks of great intensity but brief duration. It is commonly accompanied by symptoms of autonomic dysfunction. The attacks tend to occur in cluster periods, which can last from weeks to months.[2] Treatment of cluster headache is difficult and should be initiated at the start of the attack.

Although the exact cause of cluster headache remains unknown, the disorder shares certain similarities with migraine. Because subcutaneous sumatriptan has a rapid onset of action and has successfully reduced the symptoms of migraine, a pilot study was carried out to evaluate its effectiveness in patients with cluster headache.[55] Relief of headache and disappearance of autonomic symptoms were experienced by four of six patients within 8–17 minutes after receiving subcutaneous sumatriptan 3 or 6 mg.[55]

A randomized, double-blind, placebo-controlled, crossover study was then conducted in 39 evaluable patients who had a documented history of cluster headache.[56] All patients received their first subcutaneous injection of either sumatriptan 6 mg or placebo within 10 minutes of the onset of an attack. Alternate treatment was given at the next attack, at least 24 hours afterwards. Sumatriptan was shown to be significantly more effective than placebo (74% versus 26%; $p < 0.001$) in reducing headache severity within 15 minutes of administration. At 10 and 15 minutes, more patients receiving sumatriptan than patients receiving placebo were pain free ($p < 0.001$). Other evidence of efficacy included shortening of the duration of the attack, fewer patients requiring rescue medication, reduction in ipsilateral conjunctival injection, and reduction of functional disability.

Patient Acceptance and Adverse Effects

Sumatriptan was rated significantly better than both placebo and the usual treatment of migraine (aspirin or acetaminophen) in terms of efficacy, speed of relief, and quantity of doses required for relief in a survey performed by Osterhaus.[57] All of the survey respondents were patients who had received a single dose of subcutaneous sumatriptan in previous trials. However, patients indicated that sumatriptan caused more tingling and numbness than placebo. In comparative tolerability studies, more volunteers preferred the use of an autoinjector to an injection given by physicians because of a lower frequency of local irritation.[32]

A recent study published by the Sumatriptan Auto-Injector Study Group[45] evaluated the efficacy and tolerability of subcutaneous sumatriptan when self-administered with an autoinjector. Sumatriptan 12 mg/mL or placebo was given in a 0.5-mL prefilled syringe using an autoinjector. Patients were instructed to inject the drug into the thigh when they experienced a moderate or severe migraine attack. An optional injection could be given if headache was still present after one hour of the initial injection. Seventy-nine percent of the sumatriptan-treated patients graded their therapy as good or excellent, compared with only 22% of the placebo group. Six percent of all patients could not treat their attacks completely because of broken syringes, and one patient had trouble reading the instructions during an attack. Overall, self-injection of sumatriptan was well tolerated, as reflected by only two withdrawals from the trial. The frequency of injection site reactions was 10% for one dose of sumatriptan, 8% for two doses of sumatriptan, and 3% for two doses of placebo. This study provided evidence that use of an autoinjector for self-administration of subcutaneous sumatriptan is safe and efficacious.

In the United Kingdom and several other countries, packs of prefilled syringes with an autoinjector are now available by prescription for subcutaneous administration by patients at the onset of migraine attacks.[58] No published literature is available at this time to determine drug acceptance or safety in these patients.

In a report that pooled data from almost 5000 participants in previous sumatriptan studies, adverse effects occurred in 50% and 69% of the patients receiving oral and subcutaneous sumatriptan, respectively.[59] The frequency was higher than that in the placebo groups. Severe adverse events occurred twice as often with sumatriptan as with placebo. Nevertheless, sumatriptan is generally well tolerated by patients. These dose-related effects are generally mild and transient. Brief pain at the injection site is the most commonly reported adverse effect in patients receiving intravenous or subcutaneous injections (40% versus 17% in controls). Taste disturbance (11%) and nausea and vomiting (14%) have commonly been experienced in patients who took oral dispersible tablets. These symptoms would be minimized with the use of film-coated tablets instead of the dispersible tablets, which are known to cause such problems.[59] Other untoward effects include tingling in the head, flushing, warm or hot sensation, and chest tightness and pressure. These effects occur more often in patients taking subcutaneous sumatriptan, possibly because of the rapid absorption and higher blood levels. Malaise, fatigue, dizziness, drowsiness, and weakness are also reported, but they are typical after migraine attack. These symptoms usually resolve within 2–5 minutes of the start of an intravenous infusion, 10–30 minutes after a subcutaneous injection, or up to one hour after oral administration. The frequency of adverse effects increases with the number of doses.[35,37,45,51]

Visual disturbances were reported in 1.1% and 1.6% of patients who received one 6-mg subcutaneous injection and two 6-mg subcutaneous injections, respectively, in a large, controlled trial.[43] It was postulated that relative ischemia due to posterior ciliary artery or central retinal artery vasoconstriction contributed to this bothersome effect.[60]

Compared with Cafergot and with aspirin plus metoclopramide, sumatriptan was associated with a significantly higher frequency of adverse effects (Cafergot, $p = 0.008$; aspirin plus metoclopramide, $p = 0.009$).[40,41] There was no difference in the frequency when 53 reports that listed bad taste caused by the dispersible tablets as the only adverse effect were excluded. More patients in the Cafergot group than in the sumatriptan group experienced nausea, vomiting, dizziness, vertigo, and abdominal discomfort. Aspirin plus metoclopramide, on the other hand, caused more diarrhea and disorder of nasal cavity or sinus.

No significant changes in blood pressure, heart rate, electrocardiogram (ECG), or routine blood variables were observed in the majority of the study trials. Several patients had nonspecific asymptomatic changes on the ECG after treatment.[40,44] One patient was reported to experience severe chest pain and ST-segment elevation on the ECG within minutes after receiving subcutaneous sumatriptan on two occasions.[61] Therefore, sumatriptan should be used cautiously in patients with ischemic heart disease. In two subjects, liver enzymes were transiently elevated but returned to normal after the completion of the study.[33] Increases in systolic and diastolic blood pressure have been noted after sumatriptan administration in hypertensive and elderly subjects.[32,59] Therefore, cautious use in these patients is warranted. In addition, because stimulation of 5-HT_1-like receptors may cause peripheral vasoconstriction, caution must be exercised in patients with symptomatic ischemic heart disease.[59] Medical supervision may be required for initial treatments if sumatriptan is used at all in these patients.

No information is available on the teratogenicity of sumatriptan in humans. In animal studies, no teratogenic, genotoxic, or oncogenic effect has been identified.

Drug Interactions

No drug interactions involving sumatriptan have been identified so far.[62] Fowler et al.[63] performed three studies in patients taking propranolol hydrochloride 80 mg three times a day, pizotyline (a 5-HT_2 antagonist) 0.5 mg three times a day, or flunarizine (a calcium-channel blocker) 10 mg daily for prophylaxis of migraine. No change was observed in the pharmacokinetic values of sumatriptan, blood pressure, or pulse with the coadministration of these prophylactic medications.

The effect on blood pressure of subcutaneous sumatriptan 2 or 4 mg was examined in 38 patients with migraine who were pretreated with intravenous dihydroergotamine 1 mg.[32] The maximal increase in blood pressure was no higher in the group receiving both medications than it was in the group receiving dihydroergotamine alone.

A crossover study in 16 volunteers who received oral sumatriptan 200 mg after being pretreated with alcohol 0.8 mg/kg or placebo did not demonstrate any changes in the pharmacokinetic data.[32] However, more studies may be necessary to determine any changes after long-term alcohol intake.

Dosage and Administration

No information is available on the dosage form that will be marketed if sumatriptan is approved by the FDA. Judging from the doses used in clinical trials, subcutaneous sumatriptan 6 mg and oral sumatriptan

100 mg offer the best benefit-to-risk ratio. The dispersible tablets used in the original trials caused taste disturbances and have been replaced by film-coated tablets. Repeated dosing may be necessary if headache is only partially relieved by the initial dose.

Recently, sumatriptan was approved in Canada for treatment of acute migraine. The dosage forms available there include a prefilled syringe of 0.5 mL of injectable sumatriptan at a concentration of 12 mg/mL and 100-mg film-coated tablets. Along with the prefilled syringes, an autoinjector is available for subcutaneous administration by patients. Patients can repeat treatment up to a maximum of two subcutaneous injections or three oral doses per day with a minimum of one hour between subcutaneous doses and two hours between oral doses.[a] If no relief is experienced after the initial dose, a second dose should not be given.

Cost of Drug

In Canada the cost for each 100-mg tablet is approximately $14 Canadian (approximately $12 U.S.). Each 0.5-mL prefilled syringe costs $34 Canadian ($29 U.S.), with an additional $7.50 Canadian ($6 U.S.) for each autoinjector. The autoinjector is made to last approximately two years.[a]

Role of Sumatriptan in Headache Therapy

An ideal agent for migraine attacks should be quick and easy to use, be well tolerated with few adverse effects, and have a rapid onset of action regardless of the duration of symptoms before starting treatment. Subcutaneous sumatriptan has a rapid onset of action (as early as 10 minutes after administration). Studies have demonstrated the superiority of sumatriptan over placebo and Cafergot in relieving headache and its associated symptoms. An effective response is found in 48–80% of patients at one hour and 81–91% at two hours after subcutaneous injection. The corresponding rates for oral sumatriptan are 33–39% and 50–73% at one and two hours, respectively. The ergot compounds and analgesics with or without antiemetics that are currently used to treat migraine are most effective when treatment is initiated soon after the onset of attack. In contrast, sumatriptan has been shown to be equally effective when administered before an attack or four hours after the onset of an attack. Even though a substantial portion of patients experience adverse effects, patient tolerance and preference are not compromised. Sumatriptan's adverse-effect profile is much more favorable and acceptable to patients than that of the ergot compounds.[40] Its selective vasoconstriction in the cranial arteries allows its use in patients in whom ergot compounds are contraindicated, including patients with peripheral vascular disease and ischemic heart disease.

Currently, there are several effective treatments for acute cluster headache attacks. Oxygen therapy has the advantages of having no serious adverse effects and few contraindications to use. However, it is inconvenient and may not be accessible when needed. Adverse effects from ergot compounds are not uncommon. Intravenous dihydroergotamine requires a visit to a clinic or emergency room. Sumatriptan presents an alternative for cluster headache because of its proven clinical efficacy over placebo and its ease of administration. However, more comparative studies with current migraine abortive therapies, including dihydroergotamine and ergot compounds, will be necessary to further determine its exact place in antimigraine therapy.

If the autoinjector with prefilled syringes is approved, patients currently going to a clinic or hospital for drug injections may be able to self-administer subcutaneous sumatriptan at home. Both the duration of attacks and the number of emergency room and clinic visits may be reduced.

Intranasal sumatriptan will also be a breakthrough for migraine patients if this dosage form is marketed in the future. It will be particularly beneficial for those who experience gastrointestinal disturbances with migraine and for those who cannot manage to use the autoinjector for self-administration.

Instructions to the Patient

Demonstration of competent subcutaneous injection technique by patients or caregivers is necessary before sumatriptan treatment is initiated. Patients should be instructed to either take one sumatriptan 100-mg oral tablet or inject 0.5 mL of sumatriptan (at a concentration of 12 mg/mL) subcutaneously into the deltoid muscle at the earliest sign of headache or aura. Subsequent doses should be taken a minimum of one hour after the initial subcutaneous dose and a minimum of two hours after the initial oral dose, up to a daily maximum of two subcutaneous injections or three oral tablets. If no relief is obtained one or two hours after the subcutaneous or oral administration of sumatriptan, the dose should not be repeated.[a] Other rescue medications or medical advice should be sought at that time.

Formulary Considerations

High-volume use of sumatriptan will be expected in emergency rooms and clinics because of the acute nature of migraine. Even though sumatriptan will probably be more expensive than current drug therapies, its high cost can be offset by the savings from fewer emergency room and clinic visits and less disruption of work time. The quality of life and daily function will also be enhanced for those who suffer from migraine.

Use of sumatriptan should be limited to patients who experience infrequent moderate to severe migraine and cluster headache attacks but do not get adequate relief from current abortive therapies. Sumatriptan may also be useful in patients in whom ergot compounds or other antimigraine drugs are contraindicated. Use of sumatriptan as a long-term prophylactic medication for migraine is not recommended at this time. The safety and efficacy of sumatriptan have not been established in patients with impaired renal or hepatic function.

Conclusion

Subcutaneous and oral sumatriptan are effective in relieving moderate to severe migraine and cluster headache and associated symptoms such as nausea, vomiting, photophobia, and phonophobia. Sumatriptan is a good alternative for patients who do not respond well to current headache-abortive drugs or those for whom such drugs are contraindicated. More studies are necessary to compare sumatriptan's efficacy with that of other treatments before it can be recommended as the first-line therapy for migraine attack.

[a] Quinn B, Glaxo Canada Ltd. Personal communication. 1992 Jun 30.

References

1. Goldstein ME, Chen TC. The epidemiology of disabling headaches. *Adv Neurol*. 1982; 33:377-90.
2. Headache Classification Committee of the International Headache Society. Classification and diagnostic criteria for headache disorders, cranial neuralgias and facial pain. *Cephalalgia*. 1988; 8(Suppl 7):1-96.
3. Lance JW, Anthony M, Gonski AG. Serotonin, the carotid body and cranial vessels in migraine. *Arch Neurol*. 1967; 16:533-8.
4. Heyck H. Pathogenesis of migraine. *Res Clin Stud Headache*. 1969; 2:1-28.
5. Graham JR, Wolff HG. Mechanism of migraine headache and action of ergotamine tartrate. *Arch Neurol Psychiatry*. 1938; 39:737-63.
6. Moskowitz MA. Basic mechanisms in vascular headache. *Neurol Clin*. 1990; 8:801-15.
7. Lance JW, Lambert GA, Goadsby PJ et al. 5-Hydroxytryptamine and its putative aetiological involvement in migraine. *Cephalalgia*. 1989; 9(Suppl 9):7-13.
8. Anthony M, Hinterberger H, Lance JW. Plasma serotonin in migraine and stress. *Arch Neurol*. 1967; 16:544-52.
9. Sicuteri F, Testi A, Anselmi B. Biochemical investigations in headaches: increase in 5-hydroxyindoacetic acid excretion during migraine attacks. *Int Arch Allergy Appl Immunol*. 1961; 19:55-8.
10. Curran DA, Hinterberger H, Lance JW. Total plasma serotonin, 5-hydroxyindoacetic acid and p-hydroxy-m-methoxymandelic acid secretion in normal and migrainous subjects. *Brain*. 1965; 88:997-1010.
11. Kimball RW, Friedman AP, Valeejo E. Effect of serotonin in migraine patients. *Neurology*. 1960; 10:107-11.
12. Pazos A, Probst A, Palacio JM. Serotonin receptors in the human brain: III. Autoradiographic mapping of serotonin-1 receptors. *Neuroscience*. 1987; 21:97-122.
13. Peroutka SJ, Switzer JA, Hamik A. Identification of 5-hydroxytryptamine 1D binding sites in human brain membrane. *Synapse*. 1989; 3:61-6.
14. Edvinsson L, Jansen I. Characterization of 5-HT receptors mediating contraction of human cerebral, meningeal and temporal arteries: target for GR43175 in acute treatment of migraine? *Cephalalgia*. 1989; 9(Suppl 10):39-40. Abstract.
15. Feniuk W, Humphrey PPA, Perren MJ. The selective carotid vasoconstrictor action of GR43175 in anaesthetized dogs. *Br J Pharmacol*. 1989; 96:83-90.
16. Connor HE, Feniuk W, Humphrey PPA. Characterization of 5-HT receptors mediating contraction of canine and primate basilar artery by use of GR43175, a selective 5-HT_1-like receptor agonist. *Br J Pharmacol*. 1989; 96:379-87.
17. Humphrey PPA, Feniuk W, Perren MJ et al. GR43175, a selective agonist for the 5-HT_1-like receptor in dog isolated saphenous vein. *Br J Pharmacol*. 1988; 94:123-32.
18. McCarthy BG, Peroutka SJ. Comparative neuropharmacology of dihydroergotamine and sumatriptan (GR43175). *Headache*. 1989; 29:420-2.
19. Peroutka SJ, McCarthy BG. Sumatriptan (GR43175) interacts selectively with 5-HT1B and 5-HT1D binding sites. *Eur J Pharmacol*. 1989; 163:133-6.
20. Feniuk W, Humphrey PPA, Perren MJ. Selective vasoconstrictor action of GR43175 on arteriovenous anastomoses (AVAS) in the anaesthetised cats. *Br J Pharmacol*. 1987; 92:756P. Abstract.
21. Parsons AA, Whalley ET, Feniuk W et al. 5-HT_1-like receptors mediate 5-hydroxytryptamine-induced contraction of human isolated basilar artery. *Br J Pharmacol*. 1989; 96:434-49.
22. Feniuk W, Humphrey PPA, Perren MJ et al. A comparison of 5-hydroxytryptamine receptors mediating contraction on rabbit aorta and dog saphenous vein: evidence for different receptor types obtained by use of selective agonist and antagonist. *Br J Pharmacol*. 1985; 86:697-704.
23. Moskowitz MA, Buzzi MG. Neuroeffector functions of sensory fibres: implications for headache mechanisms and drug actions. *J Neurol*. 1991; 238:S18-S22.
24. Friberg L, Olesen J, Iversen HK et al. Migraine pain associated with middle cerebral artery dilatation: reversal by sumatriptan. *Lancet*. 1991; 338:13-7.
25. Goadsby PJ, Edvinsson L, Ekman R. Vasoactive peptide release in the extracerebral circulation of humans during migraine headaches. *Ann Neurol*. 1990; 28:183-7.
26. Saito K, Markowitz S, Moskowitz MA. Ergot alkaloids block neurogenic extravasation in dura mater: proposed action in vascular headaches. *Ann Neurol*. 1988; 24:732-7.
27. Buzzi MG, Moskowitz MA. The anti-migraine drug, sumatriptan (GR43175), selectively blocks neurogenic plasma extravasation from blood vessels in dura mater. *Br J Pharmacol*. 1990; 99:202-6.
28. Gutterman DL, Plachetka JR, Donn K et al. Evaluation of the safety and pharmacokinetic properties of single subcutaneous doses of GR43175 in healthy adult, male volunteers. *Cephalalgia*. 1989; 9(Suppl 10):412-3. Abstract.
29. Fowler PA, Thomas M. Lacey LF et al. Early studies with the novel 5-HT_1-like agonist GR 43175 in healthy volunteers. *Cephalalgia*. 1989; 9(Suppl 9):57-62.
30. Tfelt-Hansen P, Brand J, Dano P et al. Early clinical experience with subcutaneous GR43175 in acute migraine: an overview. *Cephalalgia*. 1989; 9(Suppl 9):73-7.
31. Baar HA, Doenicke A, Melchart D et al. Treatment of acute migraine with subcutaneous GR43175 in West Germany. *Cephalalgia*. 1989; 9(Suppl 9):83-7.
32. Fowler PA, Lacey LF, Thomas M et al. The clinical pharmacology, pharmacokinetics and metabolism of sumatriptan. *Eur Neurol*. 1991; 31:291-4.
33. Busch MA, Plachetka JR, Donn KH et al. Evaluation of the pharmacokinetics and safety of ascending single oral doses of GR43175 administered to healthy male volunteers. *Cephalalgia*. 1989; 9(Suppl 10):414-5. Abstract.
34. Feniuk W, Humphrey PPA, Perren MJ et al. Rationale for the use of 5-HT_1-like agonists in the treatment of migraine. *J Neurol*. 1991; 238(Suppl 1):S57-S61.
35. Cutler NR, Hussey EK, Sramek JJ et al. Oral sumatriptan in pharmacokinetics in the migrainous state. *Cephalalgia*. 1991; 11(Suppl 11):222-3. Abstract.
36. Doenicke A, Melchart D, Bayliss EM. Effective improvement of symptoms in patients with acute migraine by GR43175 administered in dispersible tablets. *Cephalalgia*. 1989; 9(Suppl 9):89-92.
37. Perrin VL, Farkkila M, Goasguen J et al. Overview of initial clinical studies with intravenous and oral GR43175 in acute migraine. *Cephalalgia*. 1989; 9(Suppl 9):63-72.

38. The Finnish Sumatriptan Group and the Cardiovascular Clinical Research Group. A placebo-controlled study of intranasal sumatriptan for the acute treatment of migraine. *Eur Neurol.* 1991; 31:332-8.
39. Humphrey PPA, Feniuk W, Perren MJ et al. Serotonin and migraine. *Ann NY Acad Sci.* 1990; 600:587-600.
40. The Multinational Oral Sumatriptan and Cafergot Comparative Study Group. A randomized, double-blind comparison of sumatriptan and Cafergot in the acute treatment of migraine. *Eur Neurol.* 1991; 31:314-22.
41. The Oral Sumatriptan and Aspirin plus Metoclopramide Comparative Study Group. A study to compare oral sumatriptan with oral aspirin plus oral metoclopramide in the acute treatment of migraine. *Eur Neurol.* 1992; 32:177-84.
42. Ensink FBM. Subcutaneous sumatriptan in the acute treatment of migraine. *J Neurol.* 1991; 238(Suppl 1):S66-S69.
43. Cady RK, Wendt JK, Kirchner JR et al. Treatment of acute migraine with subcutaneous sumatriptan. *JAMA.* 1991; 265:2831-5.
44. The Subcutaneous Sumatriptan International Study Group. Treatment of migraine attacks with sumatriptan. *N Engl J Med.* 1991; 325:316-21.
45. The Sumatriptan Auto-Injector Study Group. Self-treatment of acute migraine with subcutaneous sumatriptan using an auto-injector device. *Eur Neurol.* 1991; 31:323-31.
46. Goadsby PJ, Zagami AS, Donnan GA et al. Oral sumatriptan in acute sumatriptan. *Lancet.* 1991; 338:782-3.
47. Banerjee M, Findley LJ. Sumatriptan in the treatment of acute migraine with aura. *Cephalalgia.* 1992; 12:39-44.
48. The Oral Sumatriptan Dose-Defining Study Group. Sumatriptan—an oral dose-defining study. *Eur Neurol.* 1991; 31:300-5.
49. The Oral Sumatriptan International Multiple-Dose Study Group. Evaluation of a multiple-dose regimen of oral sumatriptan for the acute treatment of migraine. *Eur Neurol.* 1991; 31:306-13.
50. Brion N, Bons JP, Bayliss EM et al. Initial clinical experience with the use of subcutaneous GR43175 in treating acute migraine. *Cephalalgia.* 1989; 9(Suppl 9):79-82.
51. Byer J, Gutterman DL, Plachetka et al. Dose response study for subcutaneous GR43175 in the treatment of acute migraine. *Cephalalgia.* 1989; 9(Suppl 10):349-50. Abstract.
52. Patten JP, for the Oral Sumatriptan Dose-Defining Study Group. Clinical experience with oral sumatriptan: a placebo-controlled, dose-ranging study. *J Neurol.* 1991; 238(Suppl 1):S62-S65.
53. Doneicke A, Brand J, Perrin VL. Possible benefit of GR43175, a novel 5-HT_1-like receptor agonist, for the acute treatment of severe migraine. *Lancet.* 1988; 1(8598):1309-11.
54. Friberg L, Olesen J, Iversen HK et al. Migraine pain associated with middle cerebral artery dilatation: reversal by sumatriptan. *Lancet.* 1991; 338:13-7.
55. Krabbe A. Early clinical experience with subcutaneous GR43175 in acute cluster headache attacks. *Cephalalgia.* 1989; 9(Suppl 10):406. Abstract.
56. The Sumatriptan Cluster Headache Study Group. Treatment of acute cluster headache with sumatriptan. *N Engl J Med.* 1991; 325:322-6.
57. Osterhaus JT. The performance of sumatriptan and other acute migraine treatments from the patient's perspective. *Cephalalgia.* 1991; 11(Suppl 11):220-1. Abstract.
58. Anon. Sumatriptan, serotonin, migraine, and money. *Lancet.* 1992; 339:151-2. Editorial.
59. Brown EG, Endersby CA, Smith RN et al. The safety and tolerability of sumatriptan: an overview. *Eur Neurol.* 1991; 31:339-44.
60. Korenfeld MS. Subcutaneous sumatriptan in acute migraine. *JAMA.* 1991; 266:2703. Letter.
61. Willett F, Curzen N, Adams J et al. Coronary vasospasm induced by subcutaneous sumatriptan. *Br Med J.* 1992; 304:1415.
62. Humphrey PPA, Feniuk W, Marriott AS et al. Preclinical studies on the anti-migraine drug, sumatriptan. *Eur Neurol.* 1989; 31:282-90.
63. Fowler PA, Lacey LF, Keene ON et al. Effect of prophylactic migraine medications on the pharmacokinetic and pharmacodynamic profiles of sumatriptan. *Cephalalgia.* 1991; 11 (Suppl 11):228-9. Abstract.

Serotonin Receptors and Headache

. . . Today, there is renewed interest in 5-hydroxytryptamine, due almost entirely to the introduction of a new drug, sumatriptan, that has proved effective for the treatment of both migraine and cluster headache. . . . of perhaps greater interest is that sumatriptan is a designer drug, synthesized to activate selectively a particular subpopulation of 5-hydroxytryptamine receptors. But where are these receptors? Are they vascular or neural?

. . . The development of sumatriptan, no doubt to be followed by other drugs that activate particular types and subtypes of serotoninergic receptors, should lead to further understanding of the mechanisms of headache, in addition to providing new therapeutic agents for its treatment.

—Raskin NH. Serotonin receptors and headache. *N Engl J Med.* 1991; 325:353-4. Editorial.

Paroxetine, sertraline, and fluvoxamine: New selective serotonin reuptake inhibitors

SARA R. GRIMSLEY AND MICHAEL W. JANN

Abstract: The pharmacology and pharmacokinetics, adverse effects, drug interactions, efficacy, and dosage and administration of the new selective serotonin reuptake inhibitors paroxetine, sertraline, and fluvoxamine are reviewed.

Paroxetine, sertraline, and fluvoxamine all have large volumes of distribution and are highly bound to plasma proteins. In contrast to fluoxetine, these three drugs possess shorter elimination half-lives of approximately one day and are metabolized to clinically inactive compounds. Nausea was the most commonly reported adverse effect for all three agents. Other reported adverse effects are headache, sedation, dry mouth, insomnia, sexual dysfunction, and constipation. Because of their favorable pharmacokinetic profiles, paroxetine, sertraline, and fluvoxaetine are less likely than fluoxamine to interact with other drugs.

Paroxetine has been found to be superior to placebo and equivalent to amitriptyline, imipramine, clomipramine, and doxepin in treatment of depression. Sertraline has been found to be superior to placebo and equivalent to amitriptyline in treatment of depression. Fluvoxamine has been found to be superior to placebo and equivalent to imipramine, clomipramine, desipramine, mianserin, and maprotiline in the treatment of depression. Fluvoxamine and sertraline have been shown to be superior to placebo in the treatment of obsessive-compulsive disorder.

Clinical experience has demonstrated all three drugs to be effective in treatment of depression. They may be especially useful in elderly patients, in those who cannot tolerate alternative treatments, and in those who do not respond to adequate trials of other antidepressant therapies.

Index terms: Antidepressants; Depression; Dosage; Drug administration; Drug interactions; Fluvoxamine; Paroxetine; Pharmacokinetics; Sertraline hydrochloride; Toxicity
Clin Pharm. 1992; 11:930-57

The role of serotonin in the biology and treatment of various neurological and psychiatric illnesses has been the subject of intensive research. Serotonergic dysfunction has been implicated in disorders such as depression, anxiety, obsessive-compulsive disorder, sleep and eating disorders, schizophrenia, Alzheimer's dementia, personality disorders, alcoholism, autism, pain, and aggression and impulse disorders. Agents that modulate serotonergic activity may be useful in the treatment of these illnesses. In the past few years, a new class of drugs that selectively block the reuptake of serotonin into presynaptic neurons has demonstrated antidepressant action. Members of this class of selective serotonin reuptake inhibitors (SSRIs) include fluoxetine, sertraline, paroxetine, fluvoxamine, zimeldine, citalopram, ifoxetine, and indalpine. Of these, fluoxetine and sertraline are the only agents currently marketed in the United States. Fluoxetine (Prozac, Dista) has been available since January 1988, and sertraline (as the hydrochloride salt, Zoloft, Pfizer) appeared on the U.S. market recently after receiving FDA approval for the treatment of depression in December 1991. The new drug applications for paroxetine (SmithKline Beecham) and fluvoxamine (Solvay Pharmaceuticals) have been submitted and are currently under FDA review. Zimeldine, although shown to be an effective antidepressant, was withdrawn from clinical use in 1983 because of its association with Guillain-Barré syndrome, and the other mentioned agents are in various stages of development.

This review will examine the roles of three SSRIs—paroxetine, sertraline, and fluvoxamine—in the treatment of depression, as well as explore other therapeutic areas where these drugs may have potential benefit. Basic background information necessary for understanding the many implications of these agents will be provided.

Neuropharmacology of Serotonin

Serotonin, or 5-hydroxytryptamine (5-HT), is a regulatory neurotransmitter with generally inhibitory effects. The cell bodies of the serotonergic system are primarily concentrated in the raphe or midline section of the brainstem, but the neuronal axons are quite expansive in their projections, making this network the largest chemical system contained in the mammalian brain.[1] Because serotonergic innervation extends to

SARA R. GRIMSLEY, PHARM.D., is Assistant Professor, Department of Pharmacy Practice, and MICHAEL W. JANN, PHARM.D., is Director, Center for Clinical Research, and Associate Professor, Departments of Pharmacy Practice and Pharmaceutical Sciences, Mercer University Southern School of Pharmacy, Atlanta, GA.
Address reprint requests to Dr. Grimsley at Mercer University Southern School of Pharmacy, 3001 Mercer University Drive, Atlanta, GA 30341.

This is **article 680-204-9228** in the **ASHP Continuing Education System**; it qualifies for 1.0 hour of continuing-education credit. See page 976 for learning objectives and test questions.

such a great number of central structures, this system is believed to play an important role in the modulation of a variety of psychobiological functions, such as mood, sleep, consumption behavior, sexual activity, motor activity, neuroendocrine function, and cognitive processes.[2] Various neurotransmitter systems, including that of serotonin, are involved in certain regulatory or signaling processes during fetal development that are completely different from those in the mature brain.[3] During early fetal development, serotonin is believed to be fundamental in regulating certain neuronal maturation processes in the brain, and disturbances in these regulatory processes during the prenatal and neonatal periods could be a key factor in various types of psychopathology that appear later in life.[1] Pharmacological manipulation of the serotonergic system in the mature adult brain may "reactivate" some of these developmental mechanisms, which in turn can result in clinical improvements in various types of neuropsychiatric illnesses.[1]

Radioligand-binding studies have allowed for the identification and characterization of specific serotonin receptor subtypes. Three categories of serotonin receptors have been identified: types 5-HT_1, 5-HT_2, and 5-HT_3.[4,5] The 5-HT_1 group has been further delineated into subtypes A, B, C, D, and E.[4] A subclassification has also been proposed for the 5-HT_2 group: subtypes A and B.[6] Therapeutic agents that have mechanisms involving the different serotonin receptor subtypes and their potential clinical indications are shown in Table 1.

The highest concentrations of 5-HT_{1A} sites in the CNS are located in the raphe nuclei, hippocampus, and dentate gyrus. Electrophysiological studies suggest that dorsal raphe 5-HT_{1A} receptors are located presynaptically and function as autoreceptors.[6,7] Cloning of the 5-HT_{1A} receptor has allowed for the development of potential therapeutic agents that act as pure agonists, partial agonists, or pure antagonists. The 5-HT_{1B} and 5-HT_{1D} receptors have not been cloned, but these subtypes are pharmacologically distinct and are suggested to function also as autoreceptors.[6,8] Although the clinical utility of agents that interact with 5-HT_{1B} receptors is currently unknown, potential selective agonists of 5-HT_{1D} receptors, such as sumatriptan, produce vasoconstriction of cerebral arteries, and clinical trials examining their usefulness for migraine headaches are under way.[6,9] Possible effectiveness of these agents in the treatment of depression and anxiety remains to be determined.

Extracellular signals detected by 5-HT_1 and 5-HT_2 receptors are transported across the cellular membrane by interactions with guanosine triphosphate-binding proteins (G proteins) that are coupled to the receptors. In contrast to ion channel-mediated neurotransmission (e.g., γ-aminobutyric acid, glutamate, acetylcholine receptors), which generates synaptic potentials within milliseconds, neurotransmission by G protein activation results in complex chains of events involving various secondary messengers as well as ion channels.[10] These secondary messengers, or cellular effectors, include enzymes such as adenylate cyclase, phospholipase A, and phospholipase C. The 5-HT_{1A}, 5-HT_{1B}, and 5-HT_{1D} receptors are pharmacologically similar in that they are believed to elicit cellular responses through inhibition of adenylate cyclase, which is coupled with the pertussis-sensitive Gi protein.[6] The 5-HT_{1C} receptor is different in this respect and is classified with the 5-HT_2 receptor because of their pharmacological similarities. These receptor types generate cellular effects through the secondary messenger system involving the phosphoinoside pathway.

The greatest density of 5-HT_{1C} receptors is in the choroid plexus; other notable areas include the spinal cord, basal ganglia, hippocampus, and hypothalamus.[6] At present, there are no postulated roles for 5-HT_{1C} receptor-specific agents in neuropsychiatric disorders. The differentiation between 5-HT_{2A} and 5-HT_{2B} receptors is based on their binding affinity for the ligand ^{3}H-

Table 1.
Characteristics of Serotonin Receptor Subtypes[a]

Characteristic	5-HT_{1A}	5-HT_{1B}	5-HT_{1C}	5-HT_{1D}	5-HT_{2A}	5-HT_{2B}	5-HT_3
Molecular biology	Cloned	. . .	Cloned	. . .	. . .	Cloned	. . .
Pharmacological ligands	5-HT RU 24969 *d*-LSD	5-HT RU 24969	Mianserin	5-CT	Ketanserin Spiperone LSD	Ketanserin Spiperone LSD	. . .
Therapeutic agents	Buspirone Ipsapirone Gepirone Tandospirone	. . .	. . .	Sumatriptan	. . .	. . .	Zacopride Ondansetron Granisetron
Potential clinical indications	Anxiety Depression Obsessive-compulsive disorder Panic disorder Alcoholism Appetite regulation Hypertension	. . .	. . .	Migraine (acute treatment) Anxiety Depression	Schizophrenia Depression Anxiety Migraine (prophylaxis) Hypertension Rhinitis	Schizophrenia Depression Anxiety Migraine (prophylaxis) Hypertension Rhinitis	Migraine Nausea and vomiting Anxiety Schizophrenia Dementia

[a]5-HT = serotonin; 5-CT = 5-carboxyamidotryptamine; LSD = lysergic acid diethylamide.

labeled ketanserin. The high-affinity state is designated as the 5-HT_{2A} site, and the low-affinity state is designated as the 5-HT_{2B} site.[6] Functional differences between these two 5-HT_2 receptor subtypes have not been clearly distinguished; however, it appears that the 5-HT_{2B} receptor subtype corresponds to the classic 5-HT_2 receptor based on binding affinity likenesses.[11] The 5-HT_{2B} receptor has also been cloned, and 51% of its cDNA is homologous to that of the 5-HT_{1C} receptor.[6] Agents that act at these receptor subtypes may have utility for the treatment of a variety of mental and physical disorders, as shown in Table 1.

The 5-HT_3 receptors are located in both the periphery and the CNS. Antagonists of peripheral 5-HT_3 receptors such as ondansetron, granisetron, and zacopride are used in the treatment of nausea and vomiting.[9,12] Activation of the 5-HT_3 receptor in the CNS is believed to produce the release of dopamine from rat striatal slices and inhibit acetylcholine release from rat cortex.[6,13] Based on various pharmacological effects, at least three subtypes of 5-HT_3 receptors have been suggested, but differentiation of these subtypes has not been accomplished because of a lack of specific ligands.[6] Clinical trials examining the efficacy of 5-HT_3 compounds in the treatment of anxiety, schizophrenia, dementia, and migraine are currently under way.

A fourth subtype of serotonin receptor, 5-HT_4, has been suggested. Although its pharmacology and distinction from the other serotonin receptor subtypes remain to be determined, this subtype is thought to stimulate adenylate cyclase through G protein mechanisms.[6,14]

Basic Pharmacology of Selective Serotonin Reuptake Inhibitors

The SSRIs are pharmacologically distinct in that they do not bind to any specific neuroreceptor system but produce antidepressant effects through selective blockade of serotonin reuptake.[15] Reuptake is a major inactivating mechanism for serotonin after its release into the synaptic cleft. Inhibition of the serotonin uptake carrier produces an increased concentration of serotonin in the synapse.[16] This carrier, which is responsible for serotonin reuptake through cellular membranes, was recently determined, and its cDNA was cloned.[17] As a result of the increased serotonin available to act on both presynaptic autoreceptors and postsynaptic receptors, serotonergic turnover is reduced, which can be measured by a decrease in 5-hydroxyindoleacetic acid concentrations. Two notable effects result from the increase in synaptic serotonin concentrations, both of which involve desensitization of presynaptic serotonin autoreceptors and ultimate enhancement of serotonergic neurotransmission. Desensitization of presynaptic serotonin terminal autoreceptors causes a greater amount of serotonin to be released into the synaptic cleft per impulse, and desensitization of somatodendritic serotonin autoreceptors, which are located on the cell body, allows for regularity of the firing rate of serotonergic neurons in spite of sustained blockade of serotonin reuptake.[18] Animal studies have shown that during the first several days of administration of SSRIs the serotonergic neuronal firing rate decreases markedly.[16] But as a result of somatodendritic autoreceptor desensitization, firing rates partially recovered within 7 days and returned to normal baseline firing rates by day 14.[19] The net result of these adaptations is increased serotonin release and neurotransmission, but this outcome does not occur until the neurons resume their normal firing rates. This observation is pertinent because of a potential correlation with the delayed onset of antidepressant efficacy.

In addition to the SSRIs' activity at the dorsal raphe, long-term administration of these agents (as well as all other major classes of antidepressant agents) has been reported to decrease the activity of tyrosine hydroxylase (the rate-limiting enzyme in the synthesis of norepinephrine) at the locus ceruleus.[20] Further actions of the SSRIs at the locus ceruleus remain to be investigated.

Toward a Common Linkage for Depression and Other Neuropsychiatric Disorders

Theories about the biological basis for depression have continually evolved over the past 20 years. Mass[21] proposed in 1975 that, based on biochemical and pharmacological evidence, two types of depression existed: types A and B. Type A was caused by a disturbance of norepinephrine metabolism, and type B was caused by a disturbance in serotonin metabolism. Dopamine metabolism remained unaltered in both types. This basic hypothesis was expanded by Akiskal and McKinney,[22,23] who proposed that depressive symptoms represented a final common pathway that developed from physiological stressors, genetic predisposition, psychosocial stressors, and developmental predisposition. These stressors and predispositions resulted in alterations in neurotransmitter function or metabolism, which caused the depressive symptomatology.

Neuroreceptor Alterations after Antidepressant Treatment. The first-generation tricyclic antidepressants such as amitriptyline and imipramine are relatively nonspecific agents that affect both norepinephrine and serotonin. Other effective treatments for depression include the monoamine oxidase inhibitors and electroconvulsive therapy. It is well accepted that successful antidepressant treatment does not take place until three to four weeks after initiation of therapy. This observation, coupled with evidence that various types of antidepressant treatments seemingly resulted in certain consistent changes in measures of neuroreceptor function, provided a basis for the proposal of a common neuropharmacological mechanism for antidepressant activity.[24] The primary consistent change that occurred after long-term administration of tricyclic antidepressants or monoamine oxidase inhibitors was a reduction in the density of β-adrenergic receptors in the brain and a resulting decrease in receptor-mediated adenosine 3',5'-cyclic phosphate (cAMP) response; thus, the hypothesis was formed that antidepressant activity resulted from down-regulation of β-adrenergic receptors.[25] Since that time, however, it has been discovered that the SSRI antidepressants do not share this property. Most animal studies have found that fluoxetine,[26] fluvoxamine,[18] and paroxetine[27] do not down-regulate β-adrenergic receptors after repeated treatment. Certainly, these findings weaken the hypothesis that β-adrenergic receptor down-regulation is a common mechanism for antidepressant action.

Other types of neuroreceptor alterations that have been observed after long-term antidepressant treatment include desensitization of presynaptic α_2-adrenergic autoreceptors, sensitization of postsynaptic α_1-adrenergic receptors, and changes in postsynaptic α_2-adrenergic receptor binding.[25] However, none of these changes are constantly observed across all classes of antidepressant agents; therefore, they cannot be postulated as essential components for antidepressant efficacy. Net enhancement of serotonergic neurotransmission results from long-term administration of most effective antidepressant agents, although the means to this end are varied.[25] As described, the SSRIs mainly affect presynaptic autoreceptors; the tricyclic antidepressants promote serotonin transmission by reducing 5-HT_2 receptor density and by inducing supersensitivity of postsynaptic serotonin receptors. This ultimate magnification of serotonergic neurotransmission may be critically related to therapeutic antidepressant activity.[25]

Serotonergic and noradrenergic neurons overlap in the brain, and there is evidence that these two systems interact in a complicated manner. One supporting finding is that antidepressant treatment has not been observed to reduce the number of β-adrenergic receptors in the absence of serotonergic input.[28] This observation may imply that without intact serotonergic neuronal function, β-adrenergic receptors become less functional or perhaps are resistant to antidepressant therapy.

Dysregulation Hypothesis. Because of the neuropharmacological evidence for altered receptor (noradrenergic or serotonergic) function in depression and the indications for a serotonergic-noradrenergic linkage, it has been hypothesized that a dysregulated neurotransmitter system underlies depression.[29] Six criteria for dysregulation were established: (1) the system is impaired in one or more regulatory or homeostatic mechanisms; (2) basal output of the system is erratic; (3) normal periods of functioning are disrupted; (4) the system is less responsive to environmental stimuli; (5) a slow return to basal activity occurs after a disturbance; and (6) effective agents restore or reregulate the system.

Much research into the dysregulation hypothesis has focused on the abnormal activities of the postsynaptic receptors. To provide an example of this hypothesis, abnormal functioning of α_2 receptors, which are located both presynaptically and postsynaptically, has been suggested.[29] Abnormal or subsensitive postsynaptic α_2 receptors have been reported to reflect a dysregulated noradrenergic pathway.[30] As early as 1978, animal models showed that the presynaptic α_2 autoreceptors also underwent a reduction in sensitivity after long-term antidepressant treatment.[31] It was suggested that down-regulation of presynaptic neurons resulted in a resetting of the "braking" mechanism that could lead to proper neuronal functioning. Postsynaptic receptor effects would then play a compensatory role to allow for increased noradrenergic release.

Although the dysregulation hypothesis was initially implicated in depression, this theory can also be applied to other neuropsychiatric disorders such as panic and phobic disorders and schizophrenia.[32,33] Research based on advanced mathematical modeling techniques, such as the chaotic attractor theory using electrophysiological data, is under way in an attempt to predict drug response.[34]

Figure 1 illustrates the sites of the various presynaptic and postsynaptic receptor types for the different neurotransmitter systems. Serotonergic receptor subtypes could also be located with α and β receptors; however, for clarity, the serotonergic tract is separated. Antidepressants could act through the various neuroreceptors at several different areas to restore the neuronal firing rate of a dysregulated system. As previously described, this restoration could be accomplished by a variety of different adaptational changes, depending on the pharmacological effects of the specific antidepressant agents. Finally, although different neuroreceptors are involved, the common pharmacological mechanisms that result intraneuronally must occur through the interplay of various secondary messenger systems.[35-37]

Clinical Pharmacology and Pharmacokinetics

Unlike tricyclic antidepressants, the SSRIs are structurally diverse. There are minimal structural similarities among fluvoxamine, sertraline, paroxetine, and

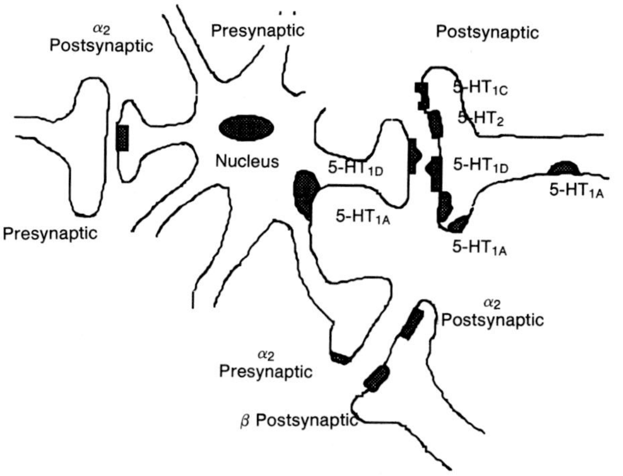

Figure 1. Schematic representation of sites of neuroreceptors in the CNS.

fluoxetine (Figure 2).[38] Results from numerous animal studies reveal that these agents are potent and selective inhibitors of serotonin reuptake. Inhibition of norepinephrine and dopamine reuptake occurs only with high drug concentrations, and in normally used doses these effects are virtually absent. Among compared agents, paroxetine demonstrates the most potent and selective inhibition of serotonin reuptake in vitro. Inhibition of radioligand binding to histamine type 1, α_1, α_2, β, muscarinic, 5-HT_1, 5-HT_2, and dopamine type 2 receptors is extremely weak for these compounds, which accounts largely for their different and favorable adverse-effect profiles compared with those of other classes of antidepressants.

As a group, these three agents undergo extensive metabolism to clinically inactive compounds, possess relatively large volumes of distribution, and are highly bound to plasma proteins. A summary of select pharmacokinetic properties of these agents in healthy and diseased populations is shown in Table 2.

Paroxetine. The pharmacokinetic behavior of oral and intravenous paroxetine has been studied in animals and humans. When a single 30-mg dose of paroxetine labeled with carbon 14 was given to healthy volunteers, the compound was reported to be efficiently absorbed from the gastrointestinal tract.[39] Paroxetine is highly lipophilic, as evidenced by the fact that only 1% of the drug resides in the systemic circulation, and its plasma protein binding is approximately 95%. The reported distribution volume in animals ranges from 3.1 to 28.0 L/kg.[40] Oxidation of paroxetine at the methylenedioxy carbon atom forms an unstable catechol intermediate.[39] The intermediate is converted to various polar sulphate and glucuronide metabolites. These polar metabolites possess significantly weaker binding affinities for serotonin reuptake and are considered to be clinically inactive.[41] The mean terminal elimination half-life of paroxetine is approximately 24

Figure 2. Chemical structures of selective serotonin reuptake inhibitors.

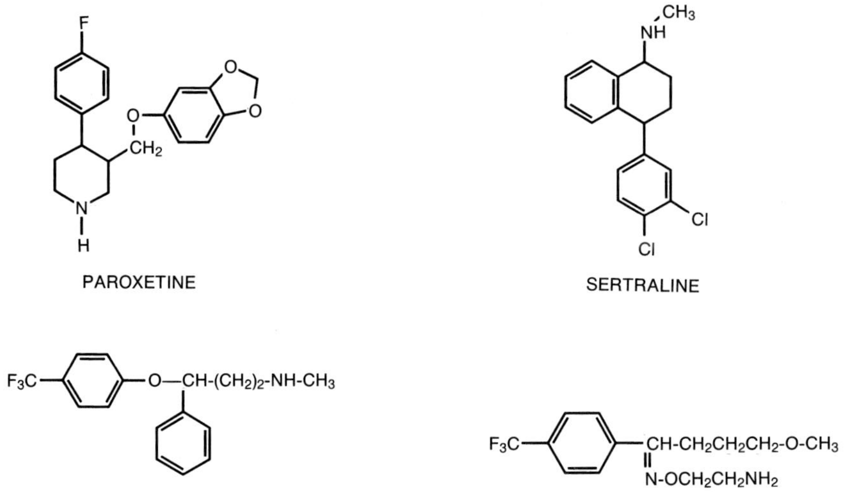

Table 2.
Summary of Pharmacokinetic Variables of Paroxetine, Sertraline, and Fluvoxamine[a]

Drug and Patient Population	C_{max} (ng/mL)	C_{min} (ng/mL)	t_{max} (hr)	$t_{1/2}$ (hr)	AUC (ng · hr/mL)	Time to Steady State (days)	Protein Binding (%)
Paroxetine 20 mg p.o.							
Young, healthy (*n* = 29)	10.7 ± 10.4	5.1 ± 7.2	5.8 ± 1.7	21.1 ± 17.8	454 ± 792	7–14	95
Elderly (*n* = 16)	16.7 ± 13.5	6.9 ± 6.0	5.3 ± 0.9	21.2 ± 17.7	546 ± 771	...	...
Hepatic disease (*n* = 12)	4.3	...	2.8	18.8	146.2	...	...
Severe renal impairment (*n* = 6)	46.2 ± 8.6	...	6.5 ± 2.5	29.7 ± 18.9	2046 ± 1348	...	...
Sertraline (as the hydrochloride salt) 100 mg p.o.							
Healthy (*n* = NR)	20	...	6–8	26	...	7–14	98.6
Fluvoxamine maleate 100 mg p.o.							
Healthy (*n* = 8)	31–87	...	2–8	14.6	...	10	77

[a]Adapted from references 39, 45, 46, 47, 49, and 54. Reported as mean, mean ± S.D., or range.

hours, and studies with administration of paroxetine 20–30 mg/day reported that steady-state plasma concentrations are achieved within 7–14 days.[27,39] Wide interpatient variability in maximum plasma concentrations was observed in both single-dose and multiple-dose studies. These findings indicate the possibility of nonlinear pharmacokinetics in some patients treated with paroxetine.[39] This effect, which can result in disproportionately high plasma drug concentrations after an increase in dosage, has been found to occur primarily in those with relatively low initial plasma paroxetine concentrations. Conversely, linear pharmacokinetics were observed in those who had relatively high initial plasma drug concentrations.[40]

Steady-state plasma paroxetine concentrations measured in 94 depressed patients ranged between 1 and 150 ng/mL. No correlations were found between clinical response or adverse effects and plasma drug concentrations.[42] In addition, no significant differences in pharmacokinetic values were observed when paroxetine was administered under fasting and nonfasting conditions, with a low-fat versus a high-fat diet, or with milk, water, or antacids.[43]

The effects of age and disease states on paroxetine pharmacokinetics are shown in Table 2. Generally, the values for younger and elderly volunteers did not differ significantly. However, because of the wide interpatient variability in both age groups, it is suggested that the maximum daily dosage of paroxetine in the elderly be 40 mg.[44] In a single-dose (20-mg) study of paroxetine in patients with hepatic cirrhosis, the elimination half-life was considerably longer than that in the control group (89.2 versus 36.0 hr); however, the difference was not significant.[45] As indicated in Table 2, paroxetine disposition is altered in patients with severe renal impairment (creatinine clearance of <30 mL/min). But studies involving mild (60–80 mL/min) and moderate (30–60 mL/min) renal impairment found pharmacokinetic values to be similar to those in healthy controls.[46] Paroxetine may be a safe choice for antidepressant therapy in patients with renal dysfunction; however, decreased dosages are still recommended because of safety considerations.

Sertraline. Sertraline is slowly absorbed after oral administration. Peak plasma concentrations occur six to eight hours after a single 100-mg dose, and the elimination half-life is approximately 26 hours, allowing for once-daily dosing.[47,48] Accordingly, achievement of steady-state plasma concentrations could be anticipated to occur within one to two weeks. Sertraline is 98.6% bound to plasma proteins, including albumin and α_1-acid glycoprotein, and its volume of distribution in animals exceeds 20 L/kg.[47,49] Biotransformation of sertraline occurs via *N*-demethylation to produce the primary metabolite, desmethylsertraline, which possesses an elimination half-life of approximately 66 hours. Although this desmethyl metabolite is a selective inhibitor of serotonin reuptake, it is considered to be relatively inactive clinically because its potency is 5 to 10 times less than that of the parent compound.[49,50] Sertraline and desmethylsertraline are subsequently metabolized to the ketone form and then hydroxylated to the primary metabolites, which are eliminated in both urine and feces.[49] Less than 0.2% of a sertraline dose is excreted unchanged in the urine.[48] Although considerable variability in plasma concentrations has been observed after a single oral dose, these concentrations have been positively correlated with the dose administered, indicating the probable linearity of sertraline pharmacokinetics.[48] The maximum plasma concentration of sertraline is 32% greater when sertraline is administered with food than when sertraline is administered without food, but the clinical importance of this difference is not known.[51]

Fluvoxamine. The absorption of fluvoxamine after oral administration is almost complete and reportedly unaffected by the presence of food.[52,53] After a single 100-mg oral dose of fluvoxamine maleate, peak plasma concentrations of 31–87 μg/L were observed between two and eight hours after the dose in eight healthy volunteers.[54] There has been wide interpatient variability in plasma fluvoxamine concentrations. Most clinical trials have reported a lack of any correlation between plasma concentration and antidepressant efficacy. One study, however, suggested that clinical response may be associated with steady-state plasma fluvoxamine concentrations of 160–220 ng/mL.[55] The elimination half-life has been reported to be 14.6 hours after a single oral dose, 16.9 hours during multiple dosing in healthy volunteers,[54,56] and 23.2 hours during multiple dosing in depressed individuals.[56] Steady-state plasma fluvoxamine concentrations are achieved after about 10 days of therapy, and the drug can be administered as a once-daily dose.[52] A double-blind investigation into the efficacy and tolerability of 100 mg taken once daily during the day, 100 mg taken once daily at bedtime, and 50 mg taken twice daily found no difference in efficacy among the three dosing regimens. However, those receiving the single nighttime dose experienced fewer adverse effects and had a lower dropout rate from the study.[56] Plasma protein binding in humans is approximately 77%, and the volume of distribution is thought to be greater than 5 L/kg.[52] Single-dose and multiple-dose pharmacokinetic studies in healthy elderly subjects indicate that variables such as peak plasma concentration, time to peak concentration, and elimination half-life are unchanged in aged populations compared with younger controls. Thus, no adjustments in fluvoxamine dosage are usually required in older depressed patients.[52]

Studies in both humans and animals using fluvoxamine labeled with carbon 14 have isolated 11 metabolites, of which 9 were identified and none were pharmacologically active.[57,58] The primary routes of degradation involve oxidative elimination of the methoxyl and amino groups of the parent compound. A single-dose study using radiolabeled drug indicated that excretion of fluvoxamine is mainly (94%) by renal mechanisms.[52] Excretion of fluvoxamine in breast milk has been reported to be negligible.[59]

Adverse Effects

The SSRIs differ substantially from the tricyclic antidepressants with respect to anticholinergic, sedative, cardiovascular, and weight-gain adverse effects. As previously described, these differences can be attributed to the SSRIs' relative lack of interaction with muscarinic, adrenergic, and histaminic receptors.

A summary of the adverse-effect profiles of paroxetine, sertraline, and fluvoxamine is provided in Table 3. Also included is information for fluoxetine, with which these newer agents can be compared.[60] The most commonly reported acute adverse effect of this class of drugs appears to involve gastrointestinal disturbances. Anxiety, agitation, and anorexia, which are frequently reported with fluoxetine, appear to occur less commonly with the agents discussed here. On the other hand, these newer SSRIs may be associated with a higher frequency of headache, sedation, dry mouth, and constipation than fluoxetine.

Paroxetine. Adverse-effect information from worldwide paroxetine clinical trials is shown in Table 3.[61] Nausea (27%), headache (19%), and dry mouth (18%) were among the most common occurrences. Both sedation (21%) and insomnia (14%) were freqently reported during paroxetine treatment, and although paroxetine is usually administered during the day, bedtime administration may be preferable if sedation is a problem. Other notable effects with paroxetine include general weakness, constipation, sweating, and dizziness. Sexual dysfunction was reported as a combination of decreased libido (3%) and abnormal ejaculation (3%). With long-term use for more than six weeks, the adverse-effect profile of paroxetine differs (n = 934).[62] Headache (15%) was the most commonly reported problem, followed by sweating (12%), weight gain (9%), weakness (8%), constipation (8%), insomnia (8%), and somnolence (6%). The following adverse effects were reported in 3% of the patients: pruritus, diarrhea, dry mouth, agitation, dizziness, and sexual dysfunction. Perhaps most important is the virtual absence of nausea in this report, suggesting that this most common adverse effect during initial paroxetine therapy subsides with continued treatment.

Elevated hepatic enzymes were reported in less than 2% of a group of 714 paroxetine-treated patients.[62] Significant (but not clinically important) reductions in hemoglobin, hematocrit, and white blood cell count have been observed in paroxetine-treated patients in both long-term and short-term studies.[63] Both animal and human studies indicate that paroxetine is less likely to cause seizures than other standard antidepressant treatments, and the drug has been safely administered to epileptic patients whose epilepsy was controlled by anticonvulsant medications without change in seizure frequency.[64] During worldwide clinical trials only 2 of 2963 patients (0.07%) treated with paroxetine experienced seizures.[65]

In comparative clinical trials the overall incidence of anticholinergic and cardiovascular adverse effects has consistently been lower with paroxetine than with tricyclic antidepressants.[63] In 14 healthy male volunteers, paroxetine 30 mg was administered for 14 days without any significant changes in cardiovascular function as measured by ECG recordings.[66] In addition, paroxetine 30–40 mg/day produced no significant changes in heart rate or blood pressure.[67] In a single-dose study with paroxetine 30 mg in 10 healthy female volunteers, no significant effects were observed on various psychomotor function tests.[68] On coadministration of paroxetine 30 mg with alcohol 0.5 g/kg, there were significant increases in reaction-time test results obtained at 1.5 and 4.0 hours postadministration.[68]

Quantitative pharmacoelectroencephalogram (QPEEG) analyses provide information for classification of psychotropic drugs according to their effects on

Table 3.
Summary of Adverse-Effect Profiles of Paroxetine, Sertraline, Fluvoxamine, and Fluoxetine[a]

Adverse Effect	Paroxetine[61] (n = 2,683)	Sertraline[71] (n = 861)	Fluvoxamine[83] (n = 24,624)	Fluoxetine[60] (n = 1,034)
Nausea	27.0	26.1	15.7	24.3
Headache	19.0	20.3	4.7	10.4
Sedation	21.0	13.4	6.9	10.1
Insomnia	14.0	16.4	4.5	15.0
Dry mouth	18.0	16.3	4.6	11.2
Constipation	13.0	8.4	2.9	5.4
Diarrhea	11.0	17.7	2.2	12.6
Tremor	10.0	10.7	3.3	10.1
Dizziness	12.0	11.7	3.8	10.0
Weakness or fatigue	15.0	10.6	6.2	10.1
Increased sweating	12.0	8.4	1.7	8.4
Anxiety or agitation	8.0	5.6	1.4	15.3
Vision disturbances	5.0	4.2	...	4.7
Sexual dysfunction	3.0	17.2	<0.1	...
Vomiting	2.0	3.8	3.2	...
Anorexia	4.0	2.8	2.1	11.7
Taste perversion	2.0	1.2	...	4.9
Urinary disturbances	2.0	1.4	...	0.6

[a] Percentage of patients reporting adverse effect.

various measures of brain function. Antidepressant agents typically produce one of two primary types of QPEEG profiles: the "thymeretic" profile is characteristic of desipramine-type agents and indicates CNS-activating effects; the "thymoleptic" profile implies sedating properties and is observed with imipramine and amitriptyline-like antidepressants.[69] The effects of paroxetine on QPEEG analysis were examined in eight healthy volunteers (four female, four male) who each received a single dose of placebo, amitriptyline hydrochloride 75 mg, or paroxetine 30 mg in a single-blind method.[70] In contrast to placebo, both amitriptyline and paroxetine produced effects consistent with those of sedative-type antidepressants, suggesting that paroxetine does possess sedative properties.

Data are available on 15 patients who ingested overdoses of paroxetine alone or in combination with other agents. The largest amount consumed was reported to be 850 mg, and symptoms consisted of gastrointestinal and CNS disturbances.[62] Specific details about symptoms were not provided. No cardiovascular problems or seizures were reported, and all patients recovered with supportive care.[63]

Sertraline. During placebo-controlled clinical trials with sertraline, the most common adverse effects were nausea (26.1%), headache (20.3%), diarrhea and loose stools (17.7%), insomnia (16.4%), dry mouth (16.3%), sedation (13.4%), and sexual dysfunction (17.2%), the latter of which was substantially more common in males (15.5%) than in females (1.7%)[71] These effects were significantly more frequent with sertraline than with placebo. Other adverse effects related to sertraline treatment can be found in Table 3.

In general, sertraline is considered to be devoid of effects on heart rate or blood pressure; however, one group of investigators reported a significant increase in supine systolic blood pressure after a single 100-mg dose in healthy volunteers over 50 years of age.[72] Sertraline produces no apparent effects on intraventricular conduction or ECG time intervals.[73,74] Sertraline was reported to induce hypomania (after nine days of treatment) in two previously depressed patients (unipolar depression) who were receiving dosages of 200 mg/day.[75] In premarketing clinical trials, sertraline treatment was associated with activation of mania or hypomania in approximately 0.4% of patients.[71] Mild elevations of hepatic aminotransferases are infrequently reported.[76,77] Information regarding sertraline's epileptogenic potential in humans is lacking.

QPEEG studies indicate that the CNS effects of sertraline are dose-related.[78-80] A single 100-mg dose was associated with slight alerting or "vigilance-enhancing" effects, but at higher doses (200 and 400 mg) EEG changes were consistent with sedative effects.[79] Low therapeutic doses (≤100 mg) of sertraline improve or have no effect on psychomotor function, whereas doses of 200 to 400 mg may cause some impairment.[72,79,81,82] Concomitant administration of alcohol (0.5 g/kg of body weight) with sertraline 200 mg/day in elderly volunteers produced no changes in performance ability (compared with sertraline alone) on a number of psychometric evaluations, indicating an absence of enhanced depressant effects when sertraline is combined with moderate doses of alcohol.[81] Results from another study, which examined the effects of concomitant administration of alcohol (0.8 g/kg) with sertraline (150 mg/day) in healthy volunteers, also support this conclusion.[49] Three patients who ingested overdoses of 750–2100 mg of sertraline recovered completely.[71]

Fluvoxamine. A recent review examined the safety and tolerability of fluvoxamine in 24,624 patients who had been treated in uncontrolled clinical trials worldwide.[83] The data represent 54 studies, the majority of which were open trials that were conducted in Europe and enrolled patients with depression. The most common adverse effect with fluvoxamine was nausea (15.7%), followed by sedation (6.9%), weakness (6.2%), headache (4.7%), dry mouth (4.6%), and insomnia (4.5%). The frequencies of other effects appear in Table 3. Overall, fluvoxamine was well tolerated by these patients; however, it should be kept in mind that 23,500 of these patients were participating in open, uncontrolled studies.

When pooled data from several controlled studies involving 222 patients were used, the frequencies of the adverse effects reported with fluvoxamine treatment were much higher: nausea and vomiting (37%), sedation (26%), dry mouth (26%), headache (22%), constipation (18%), agitation (16%), insomnia (15%), dizziness (14%), tremor (11%), and sweating (11%).[52] The discrepancies between the two data sets are likely caused in part by differences in numbers of patients and designs of the studies. Although it is difficult to draw conclusions about adverse-effect frequencies with fluvoxamine, examination of results from individual studies reveals that nausea, sedation, headache, dry mouth, and constipation are invariably the most commonly reported occurrences during fluvoxamine treatment. Although adverse-effect frequencies vary widely among studies, they generally fall between the extremes of these two reports.[52,83]

The cardiovascular effects of fluvoxamine have been compared with those of various tricyclic agents in studies involving both animals and humans.[84-88] Fluvoxamine has consistently failed to show clinically important effects on heart rate, blood pressure, or ECG readings, although there are some reports of benign decreases in heart rate. Fluvoxamine may be relatively safe to use in depressed individuals with cardiovascular disease; however, more clinical data regarding its use in this population are needed. The autonomic effects of fluvoxamine have been compared with those of amitriptyline, doxepin, and placebo in a controlled study in healthy volunteers.[88] Amitriptyline and doxepin produced significant decreases in salivation and pupil diameter, whereas the effects associated with fluvoxamine were not significantly different from those associated with placebo.

Fluvoxamine has been reported to have a lower epileptogenic potential than tricyclic and other antidepressants. Animal studies have suggested either an absence of proconvulsant activity at normal therapeutic dosages[89] or only slight potentially convulsive activity.[90] Information on fluvoxamine's proconvulsive potential in humans is limited. In the previously described review of more than 24,000 patients, seizures were reported during fluvoxamine therapy in only 11 patients (0.0004%).[83] One investigator reported on the use of fluvoxamine in 35 depressed epileptic patients who were maintained on anticonvulsant medications.[91] Twenty-eight patients completed the open study and received fluvoxamine maleate 50–200 mg/day for a mean treatment period of 87 days. Compared with pretreatment levels, there was no change in seizure frequency or in EEG readings during fluvoxamine treatment. Although seizures have been reported during fluvoxamine treatment,[92] current evidence suggests that fluvoxamine is relatively safe in this respect.

There are several reports of elevated liver enzymes (e.g., γ-glutaryl transferase, alkaline phosphatase, and bilirubin) in patients taking fluvoxamine, which returned to normal when drug therapy was discontinued.[93,94] Administration of fluvoxamine to patients with compromised renal function has not been found to produce any further dysfunction after six weeks of treatment.[95] Other adverse effects that have been reported with fluvoxamine treatment include mania,[96-98] apathy and indifference,[99] and akathisia.[100] Weight loss has been reported and is suggested to occur as a result of an increase in resting metabolic rate.[101,102]

Some QPEEG studies have found that a single 75-mg dose of fluvoxamine maleate produces a typical thymoleptic profile; however, its sedative effects were less than those of the reference agent, imipramine.[69,103] In contrast, in an earlier investigation that used QPEEG techniques Itil et al.[104] observed that fluvoxamine's EEG profile more closely resembled that of desipramine and predicted that fluvoxamine possessed predominantly stimulant-type properties. These investigators also observed large biological variability in the EEG profiles among individual patients, which could partially explain the differences. In several studies, a 75-mg dose of fluvoxamine maleate had little effect on, or slightly improved, attention, concentration, and psychomotor activity.[69,103,105] During eight days of fluvoxamine maleate administration (50 mg twice a day), no effects on memory or learning performance were observed,[106] and there were very few effects on measures of psychomotor performance.[107]

The neuroendocrine effects of fluvoxamine have been studied in both animals and humans. In rats, fluvoxamine did not significantly affect plasma prolactin concentrations in one study[52] and produced significant elevations in another.[108] The latter study also found that fluvoxamine did not alter plasma luteinizing-hormone concentrations in female rats. In 10 healthy men, short-term fluvoxamine administration produced no changes in basal luteinizing hormone, follicle-stimulating hormone, prolactin, growth hormone, thyrotropin, or cortisol, as well as no alterations in hormonal responses to hypoglycemia or thyrotropin-releasing hormone.[109] In healthy volunteers, administration of fluvoxamine maleate 150 mg at night led to significant increases in plasma melatonin concentrations measured the following morning, both after a single dose and during subchronic (three weeks) administration.[110,111] In contrast, no changes in plasma melatonin levels were observed during administration of tranylcypromine, pirlindole (a reversible, type A monoamine oxidase inhibitor), maprotiline, or mianserin.[111]

Fluvoxamine appears to be relatively safe in overdose situations. According to the product monograph, there have been at least 58 reported cases of fluvoxamine maleate overdose, with 8.6 g being the maximum amount ingested.[112] There have been nine deaths, all associated with ingestion of multiple medications. The most commonly reported symptom has been drowsiness. One elderly patient who ingested fluvoxamine maleate 3 g and temazepam 250 mg was unconscious for five days but recovered fully.[113]

Summary. Overall, the adverse-effect profiles of the different SSRIs are comparable. Paroxetine and sertraline appear to be associated with greater incidences of adverse effects than fluvoxamine; however, as previously mentioned, the incidences reported for fluvoxamine may be underestimated because of the open-label design of the studies included in the analysis. Sertraline may be more likely to be associated with insomnia than sedation, whereas the reverse is true for paroxetine and fluvoxamine. Also, the incidence of sexual dysfunction, especially in males, seems to be substantially greater with sertraline than with the other two agents. It is not clear whether this adverse effect has been properly examined in fluvoxamine-treated patients, however, because no information on sexual dysfunction was included in the report cited.[83] Many patients would be hesitant to reveal this type of adverse effect unless specifically questioned. A review of double-blind, controlled antidepressant trials involving 185 patients found the incidence of fluoxetine-associated sexual dysfunction to be 5%.[114] Clinicians at one center have reported treatment-emergent sexual dysfunction in 5 of 60 fluoxetine-treated patients (8.3%).[115] Individuals who experience drug-related sexual problems can become distressed, and some may be inclined to discontinue their medication. Early recognition of such problems and proper patient education are essential. Fluoxetine-associated adverse effects such as ejaculatory disturbances, impotence, decreased libido, and anorgasmia have been successfully treated with agents such as yohimbine, cyproheptadine, and amantadine.[115-117] These treatments could potentially prove useful for sexual adverse effects of other SSRIs as well.

Drug Interactions

A potentially serious interaction between fluoxetine and monoamine oxidase inhibitors has been documented.[118] This serotonergic syndrome, characterized by excitement, diaphoresis, rigidity, hyperthermia, and autonomic hyperactivity, has led to coma and death. Although this interaction has not been reported with the agents discussed here, it may be assumed that a similar potential exists. Therefore, it is recommended that a period of at least two weeks separate the use of any SSRI and a monoamine oxidase inhibitor. A more extended washout period is necessary for cases in which the parent compound or active metabolite possesses an especially long elimination half-life; for example, a washout period of five weeks is recommended after fluoxetine therapy.

Paroxetine. The effects of various drugs on the pharmacokinetics of paroxetine have been examined.[39,119] Phenytoin, which induces hepatic enzymes, was reported to decrease the paroxetine area under the concentration–time curve (AUC) by 28%.[39] No significant changes occurred when paroxetine was given with diazepam, phenobarbital, or digoxin.[39,119] Cimetidine was reported to increase the paroxetine AUC by 50%, but the importance of this effect is unclear. Although no significant pharmacokinetic changes were observed with warfarin, an increased bleeding time was noted when both drugs were coadministered.[119] Careful monitoring of prothrombin time is recommended when warfarin and paroxetine are used concurrently. No clinically important interactions were observed during coadministration of paroxetine with haloperidol, amobarbital, oxazepam, or alcohol, indicating that paroxetine does not potentiate the CNS depressant effects of such agents.[120] Plasma lithium concentrations were unaffected by concurrent paroxetine therapy in a five-week open study, and the drug combination was well tolerated.[121]

Sertraline. In a placebo-controlled study in 16 healthy volunteers, sertraline produced a slight decrease (1.4%) in steady-state lithium levels and an increase (6.9%) in the renal clearance of lithium; however, neither change was statistically or clinically significant.[122] Administration of sertraline also had no clinically important effects on the pharmacokinetics and protein binding of diazepam or on the plasma concentration and renal clearance of digoxin in healthy volunteers.[123,124] In a placebo-controlled trial involving healthy subjects, prothrombin time and warfarin plasma protein binding were determined after a single oral dose of warfarin.[125] After 22 days of sertraline treatment a second dose of warfarin was administered, and a significant increase in the prothrombin time AUC and a decrease in warfarin plasma protein binding were observed. Although these changes were deemed to be clinically unimportant in this study, coadministration of sertraline with anticoagulants should be accompanied by careful monitoring of prothrombin time. Coadministration of sertraline has been found to have only minimal, clinically unimportant effects on steady-state desipramine levels in healthy volunteers.[126]

Fluvoxamine. Coadministration of fluvoxamine with atenolol had no effects on plasma atenolol concentrations, but concomitant use of fluvoxamine with propranolol caused a five-fold increase in propranolol concentrations.[52] This interaction produced only a small potentiation of propranolol-induced reductions in heart rate and decreases in diastolic blood pressure during excercise. Coadministration of fluvoxamine with warfarin has been accompanied by a 65% increase in plasma warfarin concentrations, with resultant increases in prothrombin time.[52] In a double-blind, placebo-controlled study in healthy volunteers, fluvoxamine had no significant influence on digoxin pharmacokinetics.[127] Addition of fluvoxamine maleate (100–300 mg/day) to an existing tricyclic antidepressant regimen has been reported to produce marked elevations in plasma concentrations of tricyclic antidepressants.[128,129] Such cases have been described with desipramine, imipramine, clomipramine, and amitriptyline, and they were accompanied by pronounced symptoms of tricyclic antidepressant toxicity in three patients who were taking desipramine or imipramine.[128] This type of interaction is well documented between fluoxetine and tricyclic antidepressants; however, the effect would be expected to be substantially more prolonged with fluoxetine compared with fluvoxamine because of the extended half-lives of fluoxetine and its metabolite.[118] Elevated serum theophylline concentrations, from 14.2 mg/L to 27.4 mg/L, accompanied by symptoms of toxicity were reported after one week of fluvoxamine coadministration in an 11-year-old asthmatic boy being treated for depression.[130] Fluvoxamine maleate (100–300 mg/day) has been used in combination with lithium (600–3000 mg/day) without any documented interactions.[131]

Clinical Studies in Depression

Double-blind, placebo-controlled, parallel-group studies with other antidepressants have examined the efficacy of the SSRIs in the treatment of depression (Tables 4–6). These clinical trials have typically been six weeks long, but some studies extended more than one year. Although several clinical rating scales can be used to evaluate and assess antidepressant drug efficacy, the 21-item Hamilton Rating Scale for Depression (HAMD) is considered the professional standard. A clinical response is usually designated as a 25–50% reduction in the total HAMD score at the end of the treatment period. Other commonly used assessment scales include the Clinical Global Impression (CGI) scales for improvement and severity of illness, the Montgomery-Asberg Depression Rating Scale (MADRS), the Raskin Depression Scale (RDS), and the 56-item Hopkins Symptom Checklist (HSCL).

Paroxetine. *Placebo-Controlled Studies.* In the double-blind, placebo-controlled trials summarized in Table 4, paroxetine was found to be superior to placebo in three studies[132-134] and slightly more effective than placebo in two studies.[135,136] Four of these comparisons with placebo were identical in study design; the paroxetine dosage was flexible (10–50 mg/day), and the study duration was six weeks.[132-134,136] Three studies found paroxetine to be significantly more effective than placebo in reducing depressive symptomatology by the end of six weeks as determined by the standard clinical rating scales used.[132-134] In two studies, this effect was evident by week 2 of treatment, and improvements continued until week 6.[132,133] Paroxetine was also shown to be significantly more effective than placebo in reducing symptoms of anxiety in three of these investigations.[132-134]

The fourth study found a nonsignificant trend to-

Table 4.
Summary of Controlled, Parallel-Group Clinical Trials of Paroxetine in the Treatment of Depression

Reference	Study Type and Patient Population[a]	Comparative Agents, Daily Dosage Range (Mean),[b] and No. Patients	Duration (wk)	Clinical Rating Scales[c]	Overall Results
132	R, DB, PC Depressed outpatients	PRX 10–50 mg/day (31.5); $n = 36$ PL; $n = 40$	6	HAMD, MADRS, CGI, RDS, HSCL	PRX > PL
133	R, DB, PC Depressed outpatients	PRX 10–50 mg/day (30.7); $n = 34$ PL; $n = 32$	6	HAMD, MADRS, CGI, RDS, CAS, HSCL	PRX > PL
134	R, DB, PC Depressed outpatients	PRX 10–50 mg/day (28.3); $n = 32$ PL; $n = 26$	6	HAMD, MADRS, CGI, RDS, CAS, HSCL	PRX > PL
136	R, DB, PC Depressed outpatients	PRX 10–50 mg/day (33.8); $n = 33$ PL; $n = 33$	6	HAMD, MADRS, CGI, HSCL	PRX = PL
135	R, DB, PC Depressed outpatients	PRX 30 mg/day; $n = 22$ PL; $n = 25$	4	HAMD, CGI	PRX = PL
140	R, DB, PC Depressed outpatients	PRX 10–50 mg/day (28.7); $n = 38$ IMI 65–275 mg/day (135.2); $n = 37$ PL; $n = 36$	6	HAMD, MADRS, CGI, RDS, HSCL	PRX > PL, IMI > PL, PRX = IMI
141	R, DB, PC Depressed outpatients	PRX 10–50 mg/day (45.5[d]); $n = 33$ IMI 65–275 mg/day (204.1[d]); $n = 38$ PL; $n = 36$	6	HAMD, MADRS, CGI, RDS, HSCL	PRX > PL PRX > IMI, IMI = PL
142	R, DB, PC Depressed outpatients	PRX 10–50 mg/day (25.6); $n = 39$ IMI 65–275 mg/day (111.3); $n = 40$ PL; $n = 37$	6	HAMD, MADRS, CGI, RDS, CAS, HSCL	PRX > PL, PRX > IMI, IMI > PL
143	R, DB, PC Depressed outpatients	PRX 10–50 mg/day (30.9); $n = 35$ IMI 65–275 mg/day (144.9); $n = 31$ PL; $n = 36$	6	HAMD, MADRS, CGI, RDS, HSCL	PRX > PL, IMI > PL, PRX = IMI
144	R, DB, PC Depressed outpatients	PRX 20–50 mg/day (38); $n = 40$ IMI 65–275 mg/day (210); $n = 40$ PL; $n = 42$	6	HAMD, MADRS, CGI, RDS	PRX > PL, IMI > PL, IMI > PRX
145	R, DB Depressed inpatients	PRX 30 mg/day; $n = 56$ CMI 150 mg/day; $n = 46$	6	HAMD, MES	CMI > PRX, both agents effective
181	R, DB Elderly depressed outpatients	PRX 10–40 mg/day (23.4); $n = 136$ DOX ≤200 mg/day (105.2); $n = 135$	6	HAMD, MADRS, CGI, HSCL	PRX = DOX, both agents effective
180	R, DB Elderly depressed outpatients	PRX 30 mg/day; $n = 40$ CMI 75 mg/day; $n = 39$	6	HAMD, CGI	PRX = CMI, both agents effective

[a]R = randomized; DB = double blind; PC = placebo controlled.
[b]CMI = clomipramine hydrochloride; DOX = doxepin (as the hydrochloride salt); IMI = imipramine hydrochloride; PL = placebo; PRX = paroxetine. Mean dosage is the mean daily dosage used throughout the study unless otherwise indicated.
[c]CAS = Covi Anxiety Scale; CGI = Clinical Global Impression; HAMD = Hamilton Rating Scale for Depression; HSCL = Hopkins Symptom Checklist; MADRS = Montgomery-Asberg Depression Rating Scale; MES = Bech-Rafaelson Melancholia Scale; RDS = Raskin Depression Scale.
[d]Mean daily dosage at endpoint.

Table 5.
Summary of Controlled, Parallel-Group Clinical Trials of Sertraline in the Treatment of Depression

Reference	Study Type and Patient Population[a]	Comparative Agents, Daily Dosage Range (Mean),[b] and No. Patients	Duration (wk)	Clinical Rating Scales[c]	Overall Results
149	R, DB, PC Depressed outpatients	SER fixed, 50, 100, or 150 mg/day; $n = 213$ PL; $n = 76$	6	HAMD, CGI	SER > PL
150	Phase I: OL sertraline Depressed outpatients	SER 50–200 mg/day; $n = 467$	8	HAMD, CGI	
	Phase II: R, DB, PC Phase I responders	SER 50–200 mg/day (100); $n = 185$ PL; $n = 110$	44	HAMD, CGI	SER > PL
76	R, DB, PC Depressed outpatients	SER 50–200 mg/day (159); $n = 149$ AMI 50–150 mg/day (111); $n = 149$ PL; $n = 150$	8	HAMD, CGI, RDS, CAS, HSCL	SER > PL, AMI > PL, SER = AMI
77	R, DB Elderly depressed outpatients	SER 50–200 mg/day (116.2); $n = 161$ AMI 50–150 mg/day (88.3); $n = 80$	8	HAMD, CGI, RDS, CAS, HSCL	SER = AMI, both agents effective

[a]R = randomized; DB = double blind; PC = placebo controlled; OL = open label.
[b]AMI = amitriptyline hydrochloride; PL = placebo; SER = sertraline (as the hydrochloride salt). Mean dosage is the mean daily dosage used throughout the study.
[c]CAS = Covi Anxiety Scale; CGI = Clinical Global Impression; HAMD = Hamilton Rating Scale for Depression; HSCL = Hopkins Symptom Checklist; RDS = Raskin Depression Scale.

ward superiority of paroxetine over placebo on all clinical rating scales.[136] However, a considerable portion of patients did show substantial improvement with paroxetine; at the end of six weeks 45% of paroxetine-treated patients had HAMD score reductions of 50% or greater, compared with 24% of those who received placebo. Paroxetine was significantly more effective than placebo in the subgroup of 33 patients who had been ill for longer than one year than in those who had shorter durations of depressive illness. Compared with placebo, paroxetine significantly reduced suicidal thoughts.

In another placebo-controlled trial the paroxetine dosage was fixed at 30 mg/day, and the study duration was only four weeks.[135] Both placebo and paroxetine resulted in similar clinical improvements based on HAMD assessments. When baseline CGI scores were compared with week 4 CGI scores, paroxetine-treated patients showed significant improvement. The reasons for the nonsuperiority over placebo in this study may be related to either the fixed dosage (because some patients may have responded to a higher dosage) or the four-week duration of the trial. This time period is generally considered to be too short for full evaluation of potential efficacy in clinical antidepressant drug trials.

Comparisons with Other Antidepressants. Paroxetine has been compared with several tricyclic agents, including amitriptyline, imipramine, clomipramine, and doxepin. In these studies, a placebo washout period of 4–14 days usually preceded the random assignment to treatment with paroxetine or the other antidepressant drug. Clinical assessments were conducted on a weekly basis using standardized rating scales, as shown in Table 4.

In a fixed-dose study comparing amitriptyline hydrochloride 75 mg/day with paroxetine 30 mg/day, paroxetine was equivalent to amitriptyline in clinical efficacy.[137] At six weeks, both agents were associated with a 19-point decrease in HAMD scores. It appeared that amitriptyline hydrochloride 75 mg/day was the minimum dosage necessary to achieve a therapeutic response. This study was conducted in the Philippines and most likely used an Asian population. Tricyclic antidepressant metabolism and clearance have been reported to be decreased by approximately 50% in Asian groups.[138] Therefore, the amitriptyline dosage could be in a moderate therapeutic range for this population. Differences in paroxetine disposition among various ethnic groups have not been reported.

Another fixed-dosage comparative study that used amitriptyline hydrochloride 150 mg/day and paroxetine 30 mg/day was conducted in Germany.[139] As in the previous study, both agents showed equal clinical efficacy with an 18-point reduction in HAMD scores. Adverse effects associated with amitriptyline included dry mouth and constipation. Nausea and vomiting were the most noted adverse effects with paroxetine.[137,139]

Five trials compared the antidepressant effectiveness of paroxetine with that of imipramine and placebo in depressed outpatients.[140-144] These studies were similar in design and lasted six weeks. Maximum daily dosages were paroxetine 50 mg/day and imipramine hydrochloride 275 mg/day, and response to treatment was defined as a reduction of 50% or more in HAMD scores. Paroxetine was significantly more effective than placebo in reducing depressive symptomatology in all five of these studies, whereas imipramine demonstrated this effect in all except one

Table 6.
Summary of Controlled, Parallel-Group Clinical Trials of Fluvoxamine in the Treatment of Depression

Reference	Study Type and Patient Population[a]	Comparative Agents, Daily Dosage Range (Mean),[b] and No. Patients	Duration (wk)	Clinical Rating Scales[c]	Overall Results
171	R, DB, PC Depressed inpatients	FVX 150–300 mg/day (273); $n = 23$ PL; $n = 22$	4	HAMD, CGI, BPRS	FVX > PL
172	R, DB Depressed inpatients	FVX 100–300 mg/day (221); $n = 74$ IMI 50–200 mg/day (112); $n = 77$	4	HAMD, CGI	FVX = IMI, both agents effective
173	R, DB, PC Depressed outpatients and inpatients	FVX 100–300 mg/day (155); $n = 161$ IMI 100–300 mg/day (156); $n = 153$ PL; $n = 150$	4, 6[d]	HAMD, CGI	FVX > PL, IMI > PL, FVX = IMI
174	R, DB, PC Depressed inpatients	FVX 150–300 mg/day (180); $n = 22$ IMI 150–300 mg/day (176); $n = 21$ PL; $n = 20$	6	HAMD, CGI, BPRS, HSCL	FVX > PL, IMI > PL, FVX = IMI
175	R, DB, PC Depressed outpatients	FVX 100–300 mg/day; $n = 18$ IMI 100–300 mg/day; $n = 18$ PL; $n = 18$	6	HAMD, MADRS, CGI, HSCL	FVX > PL, IMI > PL, FVX = IMI
176	R, DB, PC Depressed inpatients	FVX 150–300 mg/day (145); $n = 31$ IMI 150–300 mg/day (159); $n = 36$ PL; $n = 19$	6	HAMD, CGI, BPRS	FVX > PL, FVX > IMI, IMI = PL
177	R, DB, PC Depressed outpatients	FVX 100–300 mg/day (240); $n = 17$ IMI 100–300 mg/day (180); $n = 18$ PL; $n = 17$	6	HAMD, MADRS, CGI	IMI > PL, FVX = PL, FVX = IMI
178	R, DB, q.d. dosing schedule Depressed outpatients	FVX 150–300 mg/day (281); $n = 21$ CMI 150–300 mg/day (137); $n = 23$	4	HAMD, CGI	FVX = CMI, both agents effective
178	R, DB, t.i.d. dosing schedule Depressed outpatients	FVX 150–300 mg/day (214); $n = 15$ CMI 150–300 mg/day (191); $n = 15$	6	HAMD, CGI	FVX = CMI, both agents effective
179	R, DB, PC	FVX 100–300 mg/day (218); $n = 30$ DMI 100–300 mg/day (224); $n = 30$ PL; $n = 30$	6	HAMD, CGI, MADRS	FVX = PL, DMI = PL
95	R, DB, PC Elderly depressed outpatients	FVX 150–300 mg/day (161); $n = 33$ IMI 150–300 mg/day (160); $n = 29$ PL; $n = 14$	4	HAMD, CGI	FVX > PL, IMI > PL, FVX = IMI

[a]R = randomized; DB = double blind; PC = placebo controlled.
[b]DMI = desipramine hydrochloride; FVX = fluvoxamine maleate; IMI = imipramine hydrochloride; PL = placebo. Mean dosage is the mean daily dosage used throughout the study.
[c]BPRS = Brief Psychiatric Rating Scale; CGI = Clinical Global Impression; HAMD = Hamilton Rating Scale for Depression; HSCL = Hopkins Symptom Checklist; MADRS = Montgomery-Asberg Depression Rating Scale.
[d]Trial duration extended to six weeks in U.S. sites.

of the studies.[141] In two of the trials paroxetine and imipramine were determined to be equally superior to placebo, with no significant differences in antidepressant efficacy between the two treatments.[140,143] Another study found paroxetine, but not imipramine, to be superior to placebo on most clinical rating scales used.[141] Compared with the imipramine group, the paroxetine group also had significantly larger reductions in HAMD scores. The lack of positive findings with imipramine was possibly because of the large number of imipramine-treated patients who withdrew from the study ($n = 17$) because of adverse effects, but whose scores were still included in the efficacy analysis. The last two placebo-controlled comparative trials of paroxetine and imipramine found superior antidepressant effectiveness compared with placebo for both active treatments.[142,144] In one of these studies, imipramine was associated with significantly greater improvement than paroxetine on most measures,[144] whereas the opposite was true for the other study, in which paroxetine-treated patients had larger reductions in HAMD scores than those who received imipramine.[142] In this last study, significant improvements were evident by week 1 with paroxetine but not until week 6 with imipramine.[142]

Paroxetine was generally better tolerated than imipramine in the above-described trials, and this difference in adverse effects was significant in three of the five studies.[140,141,143] As expected, the primary adverse effects with imipramine were anticholinergic. The only adverse experiences that were significantly more frequent with paroxetine than with placebo were ejaculation difficulties in one study[144] and nausea in another.[140]

One of the above studies included a brief analysis of data pooled from six sites in the multicenter trial of which it was a part.[144] It is unclear whether the other previously described studies were also part of the multicenter trial. In this multisite analysis comparing paroxetine (n = 234), imipramine (n = 233), and placebo (n = 235), both drugs were superior to placebo in the treatment of depression. No significant differences were found at the endpoint analysis between paroxetine and imipramine. The most frequently reported adverse effects from paroxetine were sedation, nausea, and reduced appetite, and imipramine produced the typical anticholinergic adverse effects.

Paroxetine also has been compared with the serotonergic antidepressant clomipramine in the treatment of depression.[145] After a seven-day placebo treatment period, patients were randomized to receive a fixed dosage of paroxetine 30 mg/day or clomipramine hydrochloride 150 mg/day. Patients were evaluated weekly with the HAMD scale and other depression rating scales commonly used in Europe. Plasma levels of both drugs were also measured weekly. At six weeks, the response rate was higher with clomipramine (87%) than with paroxetine (52%). Both drugs produced significant HAMD score reductions at week 6 compared with baseline. Correlations between clinical response and plasma drug levels were not found for either agent. Adverse effects reported by clomipramine-treated patients included tremor, dry mouth, orthostatic dizziness, and increased sweating. Few adverse effects were reported by paroxetine-treated patients. In a preliminary data analysis from 100 patients, paroxetine 20–40 mg/day was compared with fluoxetine (as the hydrochloride salt) 40–60 mg/day in a six-week, double-blind, parallel-group study.[146] Both drugs were reported to be therapeutically equivalent, and paroxetine-treated patients experienced fewer adverse effects.

In a continuation of a previous study,[144] 44 nonresponding patients were given the option to cross over to the other treatment. Ten patients who did not respond to imipramine were crossed over to paroxetine, 15 patients who did not respond to paroxetine were crossed over to imipramine, and 19 patients who did not respond to placebo were treated with paroxetine.[147] The response rates for the three groups were 50%, 73%, and 32%, respectively. The 65 responding patients from all of the treatment groups, including the previous study and the crossover phase, were allowed to continue therapy for up to one year.[144,147] A relapse rate of approximately 50% was noted during the year for both the imipramine-treated and paroxetine-treated groups. In another long-term study, preliminary data analysis showed that paroxetine-treated patients continued to maintain a therapeutic response after one year of treatment.[148]

Sertraline. Results from four double-blind, multicenter trials indicate the effectiveness of sertraline in the treatment of depression. One of these trials was conducted in a population of elderly patients and will be discussed in a later section.[77] The first study, for which only preliminary results are available, compared the effectiveness of various fixed dosages of sertraline (50, 100, or 200 mg/day) with placebo in 369 depressed outpatients.[149] After a seven-day washout period, patients were randomized to receive one of the established sertraline dosages or placebo for six weeks. All three sertraline-treated groups had significant improvements in depressive symptoms, which were superior to those in the placebo-treated group. Sertraline treatment was generally well tolerated and was associated with a small (0.6 kg) but significant decrease in body weight, compared with placebo treatment.

A second double-blind, multicenter study compared the effectiveness of sertraline with that of amitriptyline and placebo in 448 outpatients with major depression.[76] The trial length was eight weeks, and during the first three weeks dosages of active medication were adjusted to an optimum dosage (50, 100, or 200 mg for sertraline and 50, 100, or 150 mg for amitriptyline hydrochloride), which was maintained for the remainder of the study. In addition to standard weekly evaluations for antidepressant efficacy, a "side effect burden" score was established for each treatment group to evaluate overall frequencies and severities of adverse effects. Although comparison of some clinical rating scale scores indicated that amitriptyline had superior antidepressant efficacy at weeks 1 and 2, by week 3 significant differences between the two treatment groups were not detected. During weeks 3–8, both sertraline and amitriptyline were significantly more effective than placebo, according to all clinical rating scales used. The amitriptyline-treated group had a significantly higher side effect burden throughout the study than those treated with sertraline or placebo.

Preliminary data are also available from a trial that investigated sertraline in the prevention of depressive relapse.[150] During the first eight weeks of the study 467 patients with major depression were treated in an open-label manner with sertraline. After this initial treatment period, those patients who had a satisfactory response to sertraline were randomly assigned to double-blind treatment with either sertraline (n = 185) or placebo (n = 110) for 44 weeks. The relapse rate of depressive episodes during the 44-week period, as measured by HAMD and CGI assessments, was considered to be the primary efficacy variable. The placebo-treated group had a significantly higher relapse rate than the sertraline group (39.0% vs. 6.5%); thus, sertraline appears to possess long-term efficacy in the prevention of depressive relapse.

Fluvoxamine. Fluvoxamine, which is currently available in 27 countries under the trade names Luvox, Faverin, and Floxyfral, has been involved in an extensive number of worldwide clinical trials including more than 25,000 patients.[151] Results of at least 14 open trials and 31 controlled trials examining the efficacy of fluvoxamine in the treatment of depression have been published. It is beyond the scope of this article to review each of these investigations in detail. Early open noncomparative trials found fluvoxamine to be moderately to markedly effective in treating patients with major depressive disorder.[152-154] Fluvoxamine has also been compared with placebo,[155] imipramine,[156] oxaprotiline,[157] and flupentixol[158] in open or single-blind trials; the results showed that fluvoxamine was superior to placebo,[155] was comparable in efficacy to imipramine and oxaprotiline,[156,157] and was less effective than flupentixol.[158] These trials generally involved a treatment period of four to six weeks, but two studies lasted up to a year or longer.[152,154]

The largest of the open studies was conducted in Europe and involved treatment of 6258 depressed patients with fluvoxamine maleate 50–300 mg/day for six weeks.[159] Results from 5625 patients (90%) were analyzable; of these, 73% satisfactorily completed the study. Based on MADRS, CGI, and Psychosomatic Symptom Scale scores, there was an overall improvement of approximately 65% at week 6. Suicidal ideation showed the most marked improvement (81%) at the end of the treatment period. This study included a subgroup of 1096 patients over the age of 60 years who improved slightly less than the younger patients according to MADRS scores (61% versus 68%). In general, fluvoxamine was well tolerated by both age groups, with comparable incidences of adverse effects; however, there was a higher dropout rate because of adverse effects in the elderly subgroup. A comparison of the overall incidences of adverse effects at week 1 and week 6 suggested that drug-related adverse occurrences diminish substantially with continued fluvoxamine treatment.

Double-blind Studies. The larger and more rigidly controlled double-blind comparative studies of fluvoxamine have been selected for discussion, the details of which are included in Table 6. Additional double-blind trials have found fluvoxamine to be as effective as imipramine[160-162] or superior to imipramine[163] and as effective as desipramine,[55] mianserin,[164] maprotiline,[165,166] and clomipramine[167-169] in the treatment of depressive disorder. Fluvoxamine was also demonstrated to have efficacy similar to that of lorazepam in relieving both anxious and depressive symptoms in the treatment of mixed anxiety-depression.[170]

One double-blind trial compared fluvoxamine with placebo in the treatment of 45 depressed inpatients.[171] Subjects, all female, were randomized to receive fluvoxamine or placebo for four weeks, and efficacy was measured weekly by CGI, HAMD, and the Brief Psychiatric Rating Scale (BPRS). Global improvement according to CGI scores was significantly better in the fluvoxamine-treated group (72.2%) than in the placebo-treated group (52.6%), which itself showed considerable improvement. HAMD and BPRS scores were substantially reduced in both treatment groups, with the fluvoxamine group showing a significantly greater improvement than the placebo group only on the HAMD factors related to cognitive and sleep disturbances. Those BPRS items related to depressive symptomatology were reported to be especially influenced by fluvoxamine treatment, but only the item pertaining to guilt improved more significantly in the fluvoxamine group than in the placebo group. Details about baseline scores of or improvements in those BPRS items related to thought disorder and suspiciousness and hostility were not provided. Interestingly, 14 patients in the fluvoxamine group (61%) and 13 patients in the placebo group (59%) dropped out before completion of the four-week treatment period; the primary reason cited was treatment ineffectiveness. Only one patient in the fluvoxamine group terminated treatment prematurely because of adverse effects.

Fluvoxamine was compared with imipramine in a double-blind, multicenter study involving 151 hospitalized patients with primary unipolar or bipolar depression.[172] Patients were randomly assigned to treatment with fluvoxamine maleate 100–300 mg/day or imipramine hydrochloride 50–200 mg/day for four weeks, during which time weekly assessments were done using HAMD and CGI rating scales. Both treatment groups exhibited substantial improvement, and there was no significant difference between the two groups. HAMD scores decreased 67.2% in those treated with fluvoxamine and 62.1% in those treated with imipramine by the end of week 4. The maximum daily dosage of imipramine hydrochloride allowed in this study was only 200 mg, although the maximum recommended dosage in clinical practice and that generally used in clinical trials is 300 mg/day. This study also permitted rather liberal use of concomitant psychotropic medications. During week 4, 94% of imipramine-treated patients and 85% of fluvoxamine-treated patients received concomitant medications for complaints such as insomnia, anxiety, and agitation.

There have been five double-blind, placebo-controlled trials comparing fluvoxamine with imipramine in the treatment of depression,[173-177] three of which involved severely ill inpatients.[173,174,176] As indicated in Table 6, each of these studies involved a six-week active treatment period and used comparable dosage ranges for both medications, with maximum allowable dosages of 300 mg/day for each drug. Three of the trials demonstrated that both active treatments were superior to placebo in relieving depression, with no significant difference between active treatments.[173-175] The other studies showed that imipramine, but not fluvoxamine, was superior to placebo[177] and that fluvoxamine was superior to both imipramine and placebo.[176] In general, these comparative studies with fluvoxamine and imipramine reported more anticholinergic effects and adverse cardiovascular effects with imipramine, higher incidences of nausea and vomiting with fluvoxamine, and notable degrees of sedation, tremor, and dry mouth with both drug treatments.

Preliminary data have been reported from the largest of these studies, which was a multicenter, international trial and involved treatment of 464 depressed inpatients and outpatients.[173] HAMD and CGI scores at week 4 revealed significant improvement over baseline for both fluvoxamine-treated and imipramine-treated groups. At week 6 HAMD scores were reduced by 59% in those receiving fluvoxamine, by 52% in those receiving imipramine, and by 32% in the placebo-treated group. These results appear positive; however, details regarding the significance of the differences between treatment groups were not included in the preliminary report.

Two double-blind studies have demonstrated that both imipramine and fluvoxamine are superior to placebo and do not differ significantly in efficacy.[174,175] Both groups of researchers observed a nonsignificant trend toward superiority of fluvoxamine over imipramine. The first study, conducted in 63 depressed inpatients, found that after six weeks of treatment HAMD scores had decreased by 75% in the fluvoxamine group, by 55% in the imipramine group, and by only 6% in the placebo group.[174] CGI and BPRS scores also improved significantly more in the fluvoxamine group but not in the imipramine group, compared with those in the placebo group. Only 32 of 63 patients completed the study and were included in the six-week analysis. The most common reason cited for premature withdrawal was ineffectiveness of treatment. The fluvoxamine group had the fewest dropouts ($n = 7$) compared with 12 and 13 dropouts in the imipramine-treated and placebo-treated groups, respectively. The second study involved treatment of 54 outpatients with major depression.[175] At the end of the six-week treatment period MADRS scores in both the imipramine-treated and fluvoxamine-treated groups were significantly improved compared with scores in the placebo-treated group. The difference in HAMD score improvements between those receiving fluvoxamine and those receiving placebo was also significant in favor of fluvoxamine.

One study comparing fluvoxamine with placebo and imipramine, which involved 81 severely depressed hospitalized patients, found that fluvoxamine provided superior antidepressant efficacy compared with imipramine.[176] Sixty patients completed at least two weeks of the trial and were included in the analysis: 12 receiving placebo, 21 receiving fluvoxamine, and 27 receiving imipramine. Compared with both the placebo-treated and imipramine-treated groups, those receiving fluvoxamine had significantly greater improvements in depressive symptomatology as measured by CGI, BPRS, and HAMD scores. Imipramine was not shown to be statistically superior to placebo on any of the three clinical rating scales. Also, the number of patients who did not tolerate imipramine was significantly higher than the number who did not tolerate placebo, whereas this difference was not exhibited in the fluvoxamine group.

In contrast to the findings of that inpatient study, another study involving 54 depressed outpatients described superior antidepressant efficacy of imipramine, but not of fluvoxamine, over placebo according to overall response rates in each treatment group.[177] Responders were designated as those showing a ≤50% reduction in HAMD scores in addition to a much improved or better rating on the CGI at the end of the six-week treatment period. Of the 52 patients included in the efficacy analysis, the percentages of responders according to the above criteria were 67% for imipramine, 53% for fluvoxamine, and 30% for placebo. Based on this definition of response, imipramine but not fluvoxamine was determined to be significantly superior to placebo. Consideration of each clinical rating scale independently yielded no significant differences in HAMD, CGI, or MADRS score improvements among the three treatment groups. Factors that may have contributed to these findings include the 30% placebo response rate and the relatively small sample size.

Two double-blind trials compared the antidepressant efficacy of fluvoxamine with that of clomipramine, both of which were described in the same report.[178] Although clomipramine's only labeled indication in the United States is for the treatment of obsessive-compulsive disorder, it has been widely used in other countries for the treatment of depression for a number of years. These two studies were similar except for the dosing regimens used. In the first investigation, 30 depressed outpatients were randomly assigned to receive clomipramine hydrochloride or fluvoxamine maleate 150–300 mg/day in three divided doses for four weeks. In the second study, 43 depressed outpatients received once-daily (evening) dosages of fluvoxamine maleate or clomipramine hydrochloride 150–300 mg/day in a six-week trial. According to HAMD scores, both drugs caused a significant and comparable improvement in depressive symptomatology in both studies. However, there was a slight trend toward superiority of clomipramine over fluvoxamine in the three-times-daily dosing study, whereas the opposite was true for the once-daily dosing study. There was no significant difference in efficacy between the two dosing schedules of fluvoxamine; however, it appeared that those who received three daily doses tolerated the drug better.

There were no dropouts in either study.

The antidepressant efficacy of fluvoxamine has also been compared with that of desipramine and placebo in a double-blind, multicenter trial that lasted six weeks.[179] Ninety depressed outpatients were randomly assigned to one of the three treatment groups, and 81 of these patients completed three weeks of the study and were included in efficacy analyses. Patients in all three treatment groups improved substantially over the course of the study; however, there was no significant difference in efficacy between either active treatment and placebo as measured by HAMD, MADRS, or CGI scores. However, at six weeks the percentage of patients who were markedly ill was noticeably greater in the placebo group (62%) than in the fluvoxamine (37%) or desipramine (33%) groups. The authors concluded by suggesting that perhaps six weeks is too short a time period to evaluate comparative antidepressant drug efficacies and that even higher (300–400 mg/day) dosages of fluvoxamine maleate may be necessary to realize this drug's full antidepressant potential.

Depression in the Elderly

Clinical depression occurs frequently among aged individuals, but oftentimes these patients cannot tolerate the adverse effects of available antidepressant agents or may have medical conditions that discourage the use of these medications. The SSRIs appear to offer an advantage over the tricyclic antidepressants with respect to those adverse effects that are often especially bothersome in the elderly. Therefore, the SSRIs may be particularly useful in the treatment of this group of depressed persons. Paroxetine, sertraline, and fluvoxamine have all been shown to be effective in the treatment of depression in the elderly. Details of these clinical trials are also included in Tables 4–6.

Paroxetine. The antidepressant effectiveness of paroxetine in patients over the age of 60 years has been compared with that of clomipramine and doxepin in two double-blind, randomized, six-week studies.[180,181] In the trial that compared paroxetine with clomipramine, the paroxetine dosage was fixed at 20 mg/day for the first week and 30 mg/day during the remaining weeks.[180] The clomipramine hydrochloride dosage was increased from 25 mg/day to 50 mg/day during the first week and then fixed at 75 mg/day during weeks 2–6. Both agents were equally effective in decreasing HAMD scores from baseline: 19.5 points for the paroxetine group and 19.3 points for the clomipramine group at week 6. The most frequently reported adverse effects with paroxetine were tremors and somnolence, whereas anticholinergic adverse effects accounted for most of the problems with clomipramine. Paroxetine was compared with doxepin in a multicenter trial in which combined data were reported involving 271 geriatric patients (mean age = 68 years).[181] Dosing schedules were flexible and allowed increases to a maximum of 40 mg/day for paroxetine and 200 mg/day for doxepin (as the hydrochloride salt). Both treatments produced significant reductions in total HAMD scores at week 6 compared with baseline. Overall, there was no significant difference between the two drugs; however, superiority of paroxetine over doxepin was indicated by two efficacy measures: the CGI severity of illness scale and the HAMD depressed mood item. Paroxetine treatment was associated with significantly more nausea and headache than doxepin treatment; however, doxepin therapy was associated with more anticholinergic effects and sedation.

Sertraline. Sertraline was compared with amitriptyline in the treatment of 241 depressed outpatients over the age of 65 years in a multicenter, double-blind, eight-week trial.[77] Evaluations of safety and efficacy were performed biweekly, and sertraline was found to be similar to amitriptyline in clinical efficacy. An antidepressant response was experienced by 69.4% of sertraline-treated and 62.5% of amitriptyline-treated patients based on HAMD scores and by 79.5% of sertraline-treated and 73.4% of amitriptyline-treated patients based on CGI scores. Twenty-eight percent of sertraline-treated patients and 35% of amitriptyline-treated patients discontinued participation because of adverse effects, primarily dizziness and nausea with sertraline and dry mouth, dizziness, sedation, and constipation with amitriptyline. Sertraline-related adverse effects experienced by this elderly group were comparable to those described in younger populations.

Fluvoxamine. As described in the preceding section, a large, open-label study conducted in Europe reported that fluvoxamine was effective and well tolerated in the subgroup of 1096 depressed patients who were over the age of 60 years.[159] In addition, there have been several controlled trials of fluvoxamine in this age group.

The antidepressant effectiveness of fluvoxamine was studied in 76 severely depressed patients between the ages of 60 and 71 years in a double-blind comparative trial involving imipramine and placebo.[95] After four weeks, both active treatments resulted in improvements on HAMD and CGI scores that were superior to those seen with placebo. A clinically important response to fluvoxamine was observed at week 2, whereas this effect was seen at week 3 in the imipramine-treated group. Cardiovascular effects of fluvoxamine were comparable to those of placebo, but imipramine produced orthostatic hypotension in this elderly group. The adverse effect most frequently associated with fluvoxamine was nausea. Effective dosages of fluvoxamine in these elderly patients were similar to those used in younger groups, although the mean dosage was slightly lower.

In a double-blind comparison of fluvoxamine maleate (100–200 mg/day) with mianserin hydrochloride (40–80 mg/day) in the treatment of 57 depressed individuals over the age of 65 years, both treatments produced significant improvements in MADRS and CGI scores after six weeks.[182] The overall response rates were "not outstanding." Although this study used a lower-than-usual dosage range for fluvoxamine maleate, the mean daily dosage, 170 mg, was comparable to that used in other studies. Fluvoxamine treatment was not associated with nausea in this study. In another preliminary report of data pooled from two double-blind, placebo-controlled studies involving fluvoxamine treatment of 51 elderly depressed individuals, fluvoxamine was effective and well tolerated.[183]

Treatment-Resistant Depression

Treatment-resistant depression or treatment-refractory depression are ambiguous phrases often used to denote a depression that has not responded to previous trials of antidepressant medications. A problem with the use of these terms is that there are no well-established guidelines for determining how many previous treatment trials, and at what dosages and durations, should fail before a depressed individual is labeled as being resistant to treatment. It is likely that a large portion of those who are considered refractory have not actually received adequate initial antidepressant trials with regard to dosages or durations of treatment and are not really resistant to treatment. In spite of these confounding issues, antidepressants are sometimes investigated for their efficacy in treatment-resistant depression. Several of these trials have been conducted with fluvoxamine and have yielded both positive and negative results.

In an open comparative trial of fluvoxamine and oxaprotiline (a serotonergic versus a noradrenergic agent), patients who were nonresponders to either initial treatment after three weeks were crossed over to the alternative agent for a subsequent treatment period of three weeks.[157] Initial responders continued to receive the initial treatment for a period of seven weeks. Overall, there was no significant difference in efficacy between the two treatments. Only 20% of those who were initial nonresponders to their first treatment responded to therapy with the alternative compound. Ninety percent of those who initially responded to treatment maintained that response at seven weeks. Although the sample size was small ($n = 24$) and the treatment periods short, these results suggest that individuals who do not respond to one type of selective antidepressant (e.g., serotonergic) are unlikely to respond to an agent with a different selectivity (e.g., noradrenergic).

Another similarly designed study of fluvoxamine and oxaprotiline reached a similar conclusion.[184] Seventy patients with resistant depression were assigned to receive fluvoxamine or oxaprotiline on a double-blind basis for the first treatment period of four weeks. Overall, the response rate during this period (13%) was unusually low; none of the 35 patients treated with fluvoxamine responded, and 27% of the 35 patients treated with oxaprotiline responded, based on significant improvements in HAMD scores. Poor treatment results were also obtained during the crossover phase; 2 of the 21 patients (10%) who completed at least two weeks of fluvoxamine treatment responded, and 12 of the 31 patients (38%) crossed over to oxaprotiline responded. Mean daily dosages of fluvoxamine maleate and oxaprotiline hydrochloride appeared to be adequate, 288 mg and 260 mg, respectively. It was suggested that the negative results may have been because of the treatment-resistant nature of the patients included.

There are other reports of successful fluvoxamine treatment of depressed patients who had not responded to trials of various tricyclic antidepressants.[185-187] In a double-blind continuation phase of a comparative study of fluvoxamine, desipramine, and placebo, fluvoxamine showed significant antidepressant efficacy after eight weeks of treatment in 9 of 11 patients who had previously failed to respond to a six-week trial of desipramine.[186] In another open study of four weeks' duration involving 11 severely depressed patients who had not responded to a variety of antidepressant treatments, fluvoxamine was markedly effective in six, minimally effective in four, and produced no change in one individual, as measured by HAMD and CGI scores.[185] Fluvoxamine was also reported to be effective, either alone or in combination with perphenazine, lithium, or both in 18 (64%) of 28 patients with severe refractory depression.[187] Treatment with fluvoxamine alone was accompanied by significant improvements in HAMD scores in eight individuals. Another 10 individuals required augmentation with lithium ($n = 8$) or lithium plus perphenazine ($n = 2$) before a significant antidepressant response was achieved. Although reports of fluvoxamine's efficacy in treatment-resistant depression are conflicting, current evidence suggests that a fluvoxamine trial may be warranted in depressed patients who show an unsatisfactory response to tricyclic antidepressant agents.

Obsessive-Compulsive Disorder

The effectiveness of the tricyclic antidepressant clomipramine in the treatment of obsessive-compulsive disorder (OCD) provided preliminary evidence that this disorder may be largely related to some type of dysregulation in serotonergic function. Subsequent clinical trials have found that all pharmacological agents that are consistently effective in relieving OCD symptomatology are potent inhibitors of serotonin reuptake. Although these agents fall within the therapeutic class of antidepressants, their antiobsessional activity is considered to be independent of their antidepressant effects. This knowledge allows for rational pharmacological choices in the treatment of OCD; however, the precise etiological abnormalities that are present in OCD remain to be determined.[188,189]

Although early clinical studies commonly lasted only four to six weeks, it has since been recognized that in evaluating treatments for OCD, much longer trials may be necessary to allow for identification of late responders. It is generally recommended that clinical trials extend for a minimum of 8 weeks, and preferably 10 weeks. It is also important that these trials allow for use of the maximum recommended dosages for each agent. The most widely used rating scale for measuring drug efficacy in clinical OCD trials is the Yale-Brown Obsessive-Compulsive Scale (Y-BOCS). Other commonly used rating scales include the National Institute of Mental Health's General Obsessive-Compulsive Scale (NIMH-GOC), the self-rated Maudsley Obsessive-Compulsive Inventory (MOC), and the CGI severity of illness and improvement scales. Clinical response in OCD trials is often defined as a reduction in symptoms by 50% or more, an outcome generally characterized by varying degrees of residual symptomatology. In addition to monitoring for improvement in obsessive-compulsive symptoms, these trials also commonly monitor for changes in depressive symptomatology by use of the standard rating scales previously described.

Clomipramine is the only agent currently approved by FDA for the treatment of OCD in the United States. However, fluoxetine has also been shown to be effective for this indication in some, but not all, clinical trials.[190-195] Not surprisingly, fluvoxamine and sertraline have also been examined for their antiobsessional efficacy, as shown in Table 7. Results of clinical trials with paroxetine have not yet been published.

Sertraline. One double-blind, controlled multicenter trial compared the efficacy of sertraline with that of placebo in the treatment of OCD.[196] Eighty-seven OCD patients were randomized to treatment with sertraline or placebo for a period of 10 weeks. During the first two weeks, the sertraline dosage was increased to an optimum dosage (maximum of 200 mg/day), which was maintained through week 8. During the last two weeks the medications were decreased and discontinued; thus, the actual duration of the comparative phase of the study was eight weeks. According to most rating scales used, sertraline was significantly superior to placebo. Results of the MOC scale indicated a trend in favor of sertraline that did not reach significance.

The results from one site in the multicenter trial described above, which involved only 19 patients, failed to indicate significant superiority of sertraline over placebo.[197] Subsequent to this report, several errors resulting from incorrect computer data entry were discovered, and the appropriate corrections appeared in a later publication.[198] The overall conclusions of the original report were unchanged, however, and the authors suggested that the lack of positive findings was possibly because of the small sample size.

Fluvoxamine. There are several accounts of successful fluvoxamine treatment of OCD. A single-blind trial involving 10 patients[199] and a case report[200] have reported that fluvoxamine is effective in treating OCD patients who had been refractory to conventional pharmacological and psychotherapeutic treatments. There are also reports of the clinical effectiveness of fluvoxamine in treating concurrent OCD and Tourette's syndrome[201] and coexisting OCD and autistic disorder.[202] Other reports indicate that fluvoxamine was successfully augmented with fenfluramine[203] and neuroleptic agents[204] in the treatment of OCD patients who had not responded to fluvoxamine therapy alone. One controlled trial found that lithium augmentation of fluvoxamine in 30 treatment-refractory OCD patients was ineffective.[205] In addition to these reports, several double-blind, controlled studies have investigated the usefulness of fluvoxamine in treating OCD (Table 7).

Three double-blind studies have found fluvoxamine to be superior to placebo in treating OCD. The first involved 38 patients, and at the end of the 10-week treatment period the fluvoxamine-treated group had

Table 7.
Summary of Controlled Clinical Trials of Selective Serotonin Reuptake Inhibitors in the Treatment of Obsessive-Compulsive Disorder

Reference	Study Type[a]	Comparative Agents, Daily Dosage Range (Mean),[b] and No. Patients	Duration (wks)	Clinical Rating Scales[c]	Overall Results
196	R, DB, PC, parallel	SER 50–200 mg/day (180); *n* = 43 PL; *n* = 44	10	Y-BOCS, CGI, MOC, NIMHOCS	SER > PL
206	R, DB, PC, parallel	FVX 200–300 mg/day (294[d]); *n* = 18 PL; *n* = 20	10	Y-BOCS, CGI, NIMHOCS	FVX > PL
97	R, DB, PC, crossover	FVX 50–300 mg/day; *n* = 16 PL; *n* = 16	20	SCL-OCS, GRS-OC, MOC, OCC, HAMD, HAMA	FVX > PL
207	R, DB, PC, parallel	FVX 100–300 mg/day (255[d]); *n* = 21 PL; *n* = 21	6–8	Y-BOCS, CGI, MOC, HAMD, HAMA	FVX > PL
209	R, DB, parallel	FVX 100–300 mg/day; *n* = 21 DMI 100–300 mg/day; *n* = 19	8	Y-BOCS, CGI, HAMD	FVX > DMI

[a]R = randomized; DB = double blind; PC = placebo controlled.
[b]DMI = desipramine hydrochloride; FVX = fluvoxamine maleate; PL = placebo; SER = sertraline (as the hydrochloride salt). Mean dosage is the mean daily dosage throughout study unless otherwise indicated.
[c]CGI = Clinical Global Impression; GRS-OC = General Rating Scale for Obsessions and Compulsions; HAMA = Hamilton Rating Scale for Anxiety; HAMD = Hamilton Rating Scale for Depression; MOC = Maudsley Obsessive-Compulsive Inventory; NIMHOCS = National Institute of Mental Health Obsessive-Compulsive Scale; OCC = Obsessive-Compulsive Checklist; SCL-OCS = Symptom Checklist 90-Obsessive-Compulsive Scale; Y-BOCS = Yale-Brown Obsessive-Compulsive Scale.
[d]Mean daily dosage at endpoint.

significantly greater improvements in OCD symptomatology, as measured by the Y-BOCS and NIMH-GOC scales, than those who were treated with placebo.[206] In the second study, which used a crossover design and lasted 20 weeks, 16 OCD patients were treated with both placebo and fluvoxamine.[97] The study design involved a two-week, single-blind placebo period, followed by random assignment to treatment with either fluvoxamine or placebo for eight weeks, and then a two-week washout period before crossover to the opposite treatment for eight weeks. Thirteen patients (81%) improved significantly while receiving fluvoxamine maleate at dosages of up to 300 mg/day, and three (19%) showed some response to placebo. For the group as a whole, fluvoxamine treatment was accompanied by significant improvements over baseline on various measures of OCD, depression, and anxiety symptoms, but placebo treatment produced no significant changes on any of the 10 measures.

In a third study, 42 patients were randomly assigned to treatment with fluvoxamine or placebo for six to eight weeks.[207] Approximately one-half of these patients had concurrent depressive disorder. In the fluvoxamine-treated group, 9 of 21 patients exhibited significant clinical antiobsessional response, whereas none of those who received placebo were responders. A significant reduction in Y-BOCS scores was evident at week 2 in the fluvoxamine group, and improvement continued until the end of treatment. In support of fluvoxamine's differential antidepressant and antiobsessional effects, response was not correlated with the baseline severity of depression. The fluvoxamine responders included three depressed and six nondepressed patients. However, in those depressed patients who did respond to fluvoxamine, there was a significant correlation between reductions in Y-BOCS and HAMD scores. This association was also noted in the previously described crossover study.[97] In some patients, depression may exist secondary to OCD, so that successful treatment of obsessive-compulsive symptoms is accompanied by an antidepressant effect.[208]

Fluvoxamine has also been compared with desipramine in the treatment of 40 outpatients with OCD.[209] In this double-blind, eight-week study, fluvoxamine was significantly more effective than desipramine in decreasing the severity of obsessive-compulsive symptoms as measured by Y-BOCS and CGI ratings. Eleven of the 21 patients treated with fluvoxamine and 2 of the 19 who received desipramine were considered to be responders. Consistent with the findings of other studies, there was no correlation between the initial severity of the depression and the decrease in severity of obsessive-compulsive symptoms. Interestingly, fluvoxamine was effective in relieving depressive symptoms in these patients with primary OCD, whereas desipramine was not. Only those who had significant improvements in OCD symptoms showed a significant antidepressant response.

Fluvoxamine has also been compared with a form of behavioral therapy in the treatment of OCD.[210] In this long-term study, 60 patients were randomly assigned to one of three treatment groups for a treatment period of 24 weeks: fluvoxamine plus antiexposure therapy, fluvoxamine plus exposure therapy, or placebo plus exposure therapy. Exposure therapy involved guided exposure to the feared object or situation followed by response prevention. Antiexposure involved avoidance of feared situations and use of relaxation techniques, coupled with minimal resistance to obsessive thoughts and compulsive behaviors. Measures of efficacy, which included both self-ratings and assessor ratings of severity and duration of rituals each day as well as measures of depression (HAMD, MADRS, BDI), were assessed at weeks 8 and 24, and again at week 48 for follow-up. At week 8, both groups who had received fluvoxamine showed significant reductions in rituals compared with baseline and also had significantly greater reduction in the daily duration of rituals compared with those who were treated with placebo plus exposure. At week 24, the fluvoxamine-treated groups had significantly greater reductions in depressive symptoms compared with the placebo-treated group, which was not observed at week 8. A comparison of the two fluvoxamine groups at week 24 showed no difference in effects on rituals between exposure and antiexposure therapy; however, poor compliance with antiexposure instructions was noted among this treatment group. There was a slight but nonsignificant trend toward superiority of the combined fluvoxamine–exposure treatment at week 24. At week 48, there were no differences among the three groups with respect to depression or rituals, and improvements that had been achieved at week 24 were maintained six months after cessation of treatment in all three groups.

Other Potential Indications

Favorable outcomes also resulted when fluvoxamine was investigated for a wide variety of other uses, including panic disorder with and without agoraphobia,[211-214] cataplexy,[215] bipolar depression,[131,178] psychocutaneous disorders,[216] and depersonalization disorder.[217] Fluvoxamine administration has been found to reduce voluntary ethanol consumption in both animals and humans,[218,219,220] and there are reports of its effectiveness in improving memory in patients with alcoholic organic brain syndrome.[220-223] There is also preliminary evidence for its possible utility in treating obesity.[224,225] Sertraline has also been demonstrated to reduce voluntary food and ethanol consumption in animals.[226-230] Case reports have described successful fluvoxamine treatment of the hypokinetic rigid syndrome associated with Parkinson's disease[231] and marked hyperphagia in an elderly patient with dementia.[232] Fluvoxamine has been reported to have beneficial effects on symptoms of late luteal phase dysphoric disorder (premenstrual syndrome), but these effects were not significantly different from those associated with placebo treatment.[233] The results of some of these controlled studies appear in Table 8.

Dosage and Administration

The usual dosage range for paroxetine in the treatment of depression is 20–50 mg/day. The recommended starting dosage is 20 mg/day, which can be increased in 10-mg increments no more often than weekly if the response is unsatisfactory after the first several weeks of therapy. Worldwide clinical trials have established 20 mg/day as the minimum effective dosage.[234] Study results indicate that paroxetine is best tolerated when administered as a single morning dose. However, alternative dosing times may be appropriate in some patients, depending on the adverse effects experienced. Patients who experience gastrointestinal disturbances should benefit from administration of paroxetine with food. In elderly patients, the maximum recommended daily dosage is 40 mg.

Clinical studies of sertraline have initiated treatment at 50 mg/day followed by increases, if needed, up to a maximum of 200 mg/day. Sertraline may be taken once daily, with or without food. The time of administration is flexible and may depend on the occurrence of adverse effects (e.g., sedation) in a particular patient.

The usual effective dosage range of fluvoxamine maleate is 100–200 mg/day. Therapy should begin with 50 mg/day at bedtime and be gradually increased by 50-mg increments according to patient response, up to a maximum of 300 mg/day. Fluvoxamine may be administered as a single daily dose or a divided dose; however, the manufacturer recommends that no more than 150 mg be given as a single dose.[112] Bedtime dosing appears to cause fewer adverse effects, and the tablets should be taken with meals to minimize stomach upset, which is especially frequent during the initial weeks of therapy.

Table 8.
Summary of Controlled Clinical Trials of Fluvoxamine in the Treatment of Various Neuropsychiatric Disorders

Reference	Study Type and Patient Population[a]	Comparative Agents, Daily Dosage or Dosage Range,[b] and No. Patients	Duration (wk)	Overall Results and Comments
214	DB, PC, parallel Panic disorder	FVX 150 mg/day; $n = 20$ RIT 20 mg/day; $n = 20$ PL; $n = 19$	8	FVX > RIT and FVX > PL Significant reduction in frequency of panic attacks in 15 of 20 FVX-treated, 2 of 20 RIT-treated, and 1 of 19 PL-treated patients
213	DB, parallel Panic disorder with agoraphobia, generalized anxiety disorder, and obsessive-compulsive disorder	FVX 100 mg/day; $n = 24$ CMI 150 mg/day; $n = 26$	6	FVX = CMI Both agents significantly decreased symptoms of anxiety and panic attacks; 14 of 24 in FVX group and 15 of 26 in CMI group were symptom-free after treatment
212	DB, parallel Panic disorder with and without agoraphobia	FVX 150 mg/day; $n = 20$ MAP 150 mg/day; $n = 24$	6	FVX > MAP FVX, but not MAP, significantly decreased frequency of panic attacks and symptoms of anxiety and depression
216	DB, PC, parallel Anxiety and depression associated with psychocutaneous disorders (psychogenic pruritus, urticaria, dermatitis artefacta, alopecia areata, glossodynia)	FVX 100–300 mg/day; $n = 37$ PL; $n = 33$	4	FVX = PL Both treatments significantly reduced symptoms of anxiety and depression
224	DB, PC, parallel Refractory obesity	FVX 100–200 mg/day; $n = 16$ PL; $n = 13$	12	FVX = PL 14 of 16 FVX-treated patients lost a mean of 3.5 kg and 11 of 13 PL-treated patients lost a mean of 2.8 kg
223	DB, crossover Alcoholic chronic organic brain disease (Korsakoff's psychosis, $n = 6$; alcoholism-associated dementia, $n = 3$; alcoholic liver disease, $n = 1$)	FVX 100–200 mg/day; $n = 10$ PL; $n = 10$	4 each treatment	FVX > PL FVX treatment produced significant improvement in episodic memory in patients with Korsakoff's psychosis, but not in those with alcoholism-associated dementia

[a]DB = double blind; PC = placebo controlled.
[b]CMI = clomipramine hydrochloride; FVX = fluvoxamine maleate; MAP = maprotiline hydrochloride; PL = placebo; RIT = ritanserin.

Formulary Considerations

At the present time only sertraline has been FDA approved and is available for the treatment of depression. It is speculated that fluvoxamine and paroxetine will be approved in 1992 or 1993. Although there have been no comparative studies with these three agents, it appears that they possess similar efficacies in the treatment of depression, as well as similar onsets of action.

Based on the available information, these three agents also have comparable adverse-effect profiles. As stated previously, it remains to be determined whether fluvoxamine is truly associated with the overall more favorable adverse-effect profile presented in Table 3 or whether the incidences reported there are underestimated. Also, it appears that sertraline may be less likely to cause sedation than the other two agents but may be more likely to produce sexual dysfunction. This observation, too, needs to be confirmed.

The SSRIs offer distinct advantages over tricyclic and other available antidepressant agents in terms of anticholinergic, sedative, and cardiovascular adverse effects. These differences may be especially important in the elderly population, in whom each of these agents has been reported to be an effective antidepressant. Another primary advantage of the SSRIs is their apparent safety in overdose situations, whereas the potential lethality of tricyclic antidepressants in such cases is well recognized. As a group, paroxetine, sertraline, and fluvoxamine also possess slightly different profiles than that of fluoxetine. One main distinction is that these agents appear to cause substantially less anxiety and anorexia, which are often associated with fluoxetine therapy. Also, these compounds, especially paroxetine and fluvoxamine, can produce notable sedative effects in some patients. Other adverse effects such as headache, dry mouth, and constipation may occur more frequently with the agents discussed here than with fluoxetine. These newer SSRIs may represent useful therapeutic alternatives in patients who cannot tolerate fluoxetine or in the growing population of patients for whom negative media publicity about fluoxetine presents a problem.

Paroxetine, sertraline, and fluvoxamine all possess pharmacokinetic advantages over fluoxetine that translate to an expected lower potential for drug interactions. In contrast to fluoxetine, these three drugs possess shorter elimination half-lives of approximately one day and are metabolized to clinically inactive compounds. Although there have been minimal reports of clinically important drug interactions with the newer SSRIs, it is unknown whether such interactions actually exist. Such information is often evident only after a period of clinical experience. For example, with fluoxetine's widespread use, it is now known that this compound can interact in a clinically important way with tricyclic antidepressants,[118] antipsychotic agents,[235] and anticonvulsants.[236,237] The mechanism of these interactions could be related to the potent inhibiting actions of fluoxetine and norfluoxetine on the cytochrome P 450-2D6 isoenzyme, which is one of the primary isoenzyme systems involved in the metabolism of many psychoactive drugs.[238,239] Paroxetine, sertraline, and fluvoxamine have also been reported to be inhibitors of this isoenzyme system and so may possess similar drug interactions.[240] As previously described, fluvoxamine has been reported to increase plasma tricyclic antidepressant concentrations substantially on coadministration,[128,129] whereas sertraline had minimal effects.[126] Certainly, as information becomes available about the potential of each of these drugs to interact with other medications, it will aid the process of selection among this class of agents.

Another primary factor in formulary consideration will be the costs of these drugs. Currently, the average wholesale prices of both 50-mg and 100-mg sertraline are similar to that of fluoxetine. A survey of several local independent and chain retail pharmacies showed that the average retail costs to the patient for one month's treatment of sertraline 50 mg/day, sertraline 100 mg/day, or fluoxetine 20 mg/day were comparable: $64.91, $66.40, or $67.78, respectively. At present, sertraline should be considered a worthwhile formulary addition, based on its described differences from other available antidepressant agents. When paroxetine and fluvoxamine are marketed, the costs of these agents will be a consideration in recommendations for their use.

Conclusion

The SSRIs are an unconventional and exciting class of antidepressant medications. The development and characterization of these compounds have considerably expanded our knowledge concerning the underlying biological processes in depression, as well as other neuropsychiatric disorders. There is substantial evidence that the SSRIs may possess therapeutic utility in a variety of illnesses. Clinical experience has demonstrated these drugs to be effective in the treatment of depression. They may be particularly useful in elderly depressed patients, in those who cannot tolerate alternate treatments, and in those who do not respond to adequate trials of other antidepressant therapies.

References

1. Azmitia EC, Whitaker-Azmitia PM. Awakening the sleeping giant: anatomy and plasticity of the brain serotonergic system. *J Clin Psychiatry.* 1991; 52(Suppl 12):4-16.
2. Siever LJ, Kahn RS, Lawlor BA et al. Critical issues in defining the role of serotonin in psychiatric disorders. *Pharmacol Rev.* 1991; 43:509-25.
3. Whitaker-Azmitia PM. Role of serotonin and other neurotransmitter receptors in brain development: basis for developmental pharmacology. *Pharmacol Rev.* 1991; 43:553-61.
4. Glennon RL. Serotonin receptors: clinical implications. *Neurosci Biobehav Rev.* 1990; 14:35-47.
5. Bradley PB, Engel G, Feniuk W et al. Proposals for the classification and nomenclature of functional receptors for 5-hydroxytryptamine. *Neuropharmacology.* 1986; 25:563-76.
6. Gonzalez-Heydrich J, Peroutka SJ. Serotonin receptor and reuptake sites: pharmacologic significance. *J Clin Psychiatry.* 1990; 51(Suppl 4):5-12.

7. Jann MW. Buspirone: an update on a unique anxiolytic agent. *Pharmacotherapy*. 1988; 8:100-16.
8. Yocca FD. Neurochemistry and neurophysiology of buspirone and gepirone: interactions at presynaptic and postsynaptic 5-HT-1A receptors. *J Clin Psychopharmacol.* 1990; 10:6S-12S.
9. Peroutka SJ. Serotonin receptor subtypes and neuropsychiatric diseases: focus on 5-HT_{1D} and 5-HT_3 receptor agents. *Pharmacol Rev.* 1991; 43:579-86.
10. Manji HK. G proteins: implications for psychiatry. *Am J Psychiatry*. 1992; 149:746-60.
11. McKenna DJ, Peroutka SJ. Differentiation of 5-HT receptor subtypes using 125-I R-(-)2,5-demethoxy-4-iodophenylisopropylamine (DOI) and ^{3}-H ketanserin. *J Clin Neurosci.* 1989; 9:3482-90.
12. Kohler DR, Goldspiel BR. Ondansetron: a serotonin receptor 5-HT-3 antagonist for antineoplastic chemotherapy-induced nausea and vomiting. *DICP Ann Pharmacother.* 1991; 25:367-80.
13. Barnes JM, Barnes NM, Costall B et al. 5-HT-3 receptors mediate the release of acetylcholine release in cortical tissues. *Nature*. 1989; 338:762-3.
14. Clake DE, Craig DA, Fozard JR. The 5-HT-4 receptor, naughty, but nice. *Trends Pharmacol Sci.* 1989; 10:385-6.
15. Wong DT, Bymaster FP, Reid LR et al. Fluoxetine and two other serotonin uptake inhibitors without affinity for neuronal receptors. *Biochem Pharmacol.* 1983; 32:1287-93.
16. Fuller RW, Wong DT. Serotonin reuptake blockers in vitro and in vivo. *J Clin Psychopharmacol.* 1987; 7:14-20.
17. Hoffman BJ, Mezey E, Brownstein MJ. Cloning of a serotonin transporter affected by antidepressants. *Science*. 1991; 254:579-80.
18. Hrdina PD. Pharmacology of serotonin uptake inhibitors: focus on fluvoxamine. *J Psychiatr Neurosci.* 1991; 16(Suppl 1):10-8.
19. Blier P, de Montigny C, Chaput Y. A role for the serotonin system in the mechanism of action of antidepressant treatments: preclinical evidence. *J Clin Psychiatry*. 1990; 51(Suppl 4):14-20.
20. Nestler EJ, McMahon A, Sabban EL et al. Chronic antidepressant administration decreases the expression of tyrosine hydroxylase in the rat locus ceruleus. *Proc Natl Acad Sci.* 1990; 87:7522-6.
21. Maas JW. Biogenic amines and depression. *Arch Gen Psychiatry*. 1975; 32:1357-61.
22. Akiskal HS, McKinney WT. Depressive disorders: towards a unified hypothesis. *Science*. 1973; 182:20-9.
23. Akiskal HS, McKinney WT. Overview of recent research in depression: integration of ten conceptual models into a comprehensive clinical frame. *Arch Gen Psychiatry*. 1975; 32:285-305.
24. Charney DS, Menkes DB, Henninger GR. Receptor sensitivity and the mechanism of action of antidepressant treatment. *Arch Gen Psychiatry*. 1982; 38:1160-80.
25. Charney DS, Southwick SM, Delgado PL et al. Current status of the receptor sensitivity hypothesis of antidepressant action: implications for the treatment of severe depression. In: Amsterdam JD, ed. Pharmacotherapy of depression: applications for the outpatient. New York: Dekker; 1990:13-35.
26. Beasley CM, Masica DN, Potvin JH. Fluoxetine: a review of receptor and functional effects and their clinical implications. *Psychopharmacology*. 1992; 107:1-10.
27. Tulloch IF, Johnson AM. The pharmacologic profile of paroxetine, a new selective serotonin reuptake inhibitor. *J Clin Psychiatry*. 1992; 53(Suppl 2):7-12.
28. Susler F. Deamplication of noradrenergic signal transfer by antidepressants: a unified catecholamine-serotonin hypothesis of affective disorders. *Psychopharmacol Bull.* 1983; 19:300-4.
29. Siever LJ, Davis KL. Overview: toward a dysregulation hypothesis of depression. *Am J Psychiatry*. 1985; 142:1017-31.
30. Price LH, Charney DS, Rubin L et al. Alpha-two adrenergic receptor function in depression. *Arch Gen Psychiatry*. 1986; 43:849-58.
31. Finberg JPM. Antidepressant drugs and down-regulation of presynaptic receptors. *Biochem Pharmacol.* 1987; 36:3557-62.
32. Jann MW, Kurtz NM. Treatment of panic and phobic disorders. *Clin Pharm.* 1987; 6:947-64.
33. Ereshefsky L, Tran-Johnson TK, Watanabe MD. Pathophysiologic basis for schizophrenia and the efficacy of antipsychotics. *Clin Pharm.* 1990; 9:682-707.
34. Goldberger AL, Rigney DR, West BJ. Chaos and fractals in human physiology. *Sci Am.* 1990; 262:43-9.
35. Koe BK. Preclinical pharmacology of sertraline: a potent and specific inhibitor of serotonin reuptake. *J Clin Psychiatry*. 1990; 51(Suppl 12):13-7.
36. Berridge M. The molecular basis of communication within the cell. *Sci Am.* 1985; 253:142-52.
37. Sanders-Bush E, Conn PJ. Neurochemistry of serotonin neuronal systems: consequences of serotonin receptor activation. In: Meltzer HY, ed. Psychopharmacology: third generation of progress. New York: Saunders; 1987:95-103.
38. Rickels K, Schweizer E. Clinical overview of serotonin reuptake inhibitors. *J Clin Psychiatry*. 1990; 51(Suppl 12):9-12.
39. Kaye CM, Haddock RE, Langley PF et al. A review of the metabolism and pharmacokinetics of paroxetine in man. *Acta Psychiatr Scand.* 1989; 80(Suppl 350):60-75.
40. DeVane CL. Pharmacokinetics of the selective serotonin reuptake inhibitors. *J Clin Psychiatry*. 1992; 53(Suppl 2):13-20.
41. Haddock RE, Johnson AM, Langley PF et al. Metabolic pathway of paroxetine in animals and the comparative pharmacological properties of its metabolites. *Acta Psychiatr Scand.* 1989; 80(Suppl 350):24-6.
42. Tasker TCG, Kaye CM, Zussman BD et al. Paroxetine plasma levels: lack of correlation with efficacy or adverse effects. *Acta Psychiatr Scand.* 1989; 80(Suppl 350):152-5.
43. Greb WH, Brett MA, Buscher G et al. Absorption of paroxetine under various dietary conditions and following antacid intake. *Acta Psychiatr Scand.* 1989; 80(Suppl 350):99-101.
44. Bayer AJ, Roberts NA, Allen EA et al. The pharmacokinetics of paroxetine in the elderly. *Acta Psychiatr Scand.* 1989; (Suppl 350):85-6.
45. Dalhoff K, Almdal TP, Bjerrum K et al. Pharmacokinetics of paroxetine in patients with cirrhosis. *Eur J Clin Pharmacol.* 1991; 41:351-4.
46. Doyle GD, Laher M, Kelly JG et al. The pharmacokinetics of paroxetine in renal impairment. *Acta Psychiatr Scand.* 1989; 80(Suppl 350):89-90.
47. Ronfeld RA, Shaw GL, Tremaine LM. Distribution and pharmacokinetics of the selective 5-HT uptake blocker sertraline in man, rat and dog. *Psychopharmacology*. 1988; 96:269. Abstract.
48. Pages LJ, Garg DC, Martinez JJ et al. Safety and pharmacokinetics of sertraline in healthy young males. *J Clin Pharmacol.* 1988; 28:920. Abstract.
49. Doogan DP, Caillard V. Sertraline: a new antidepressant. *J Clin Psychiatry*. 1988; 49:(Suppl 8)46-51.
50. Heym J, Koe BK. Pharmacology of sertraline: a review. *J Clin Psychiatry*. 1988; 495:40-5.
51. Anon. Pfizer's sertraline clears FDA advisory committee on Nov 19: NDA review awaits finish of dissolution, food effects and dosing work; Phase IV on tap. *FDC Reports ("The Pink Sheet")*. 1990; 52(Nov 26):3-5.
52. Benfield P, Ward A. Fluvoxamine: a review of its pharmacodynamic and pharmacokinetic properties, and therapeutic efficacy in depressive illness. *Drugs*. 1986; 32:313-34.
53. Wheeler SC, Vlasses PH, Dobinska MR et al. Plasma fluvoxamine levels in fasted and fed subjects. *J Clin Pharmacol.* 1985; 25:463.
54. DeBree H, Van der Schoot JB, Post LC. Fluvoxamine maleate; disposition in man. *Eur J Drug Metab Pharmacokinet.* 1983; 8:175-9.

55. Nathan RS, Perel JM, Pollock BG et al. The role of neuropharmacologic selectivity in antidepressant action: fluvoxamine versus desipramine. *J Clin Psychiatry*. 1990; 51:367-72.
56. Siddiqui UA, Chakravarti SK, Jesinger DK. The tolerance and antidepressive activity of fluvoxamine as a single dose compared to a twice daily dose. *Curr Med Res Opin*. 1985; 9:681-91.
57. Overmars H, Scherpenisse PM, Post LC. Fluvoxamine maleate: metabolism in man. *Eur J Drug Metab Pharmacokinet*. 1983; 8:269-80.
58. Ruijten HM, DeBree HD, Borst JM et al. Fluvoxamine: metabolic fate in animals. *Drug Metab Dispos*. 1984; 12:82-92.
59. Wright S, Dawling S, Ashford JJ. Excretion of fluvoxamine in breast milk. *Br J Clin Pharmacol*. 1991; 209:31.
60. Sommi RW, Crismon ML, Bowden C. Fluoxetine: a serotonin-specific second generation antidepressant. *Pharmacotherapy*. 1987; 7:1-15.
61. Dunbar GC: An interim overview of the safety and tolerability of paroxetine. *Acta Psychiatr Scand*. 1989; 80(Suppl 350):135-7.
62. Dechant KL, Clissold SP. Paroxetine. *Drugs*. 1991; 41:225-53.
63. Boyer WF, Blumhardt CL. The safety profile of paroxetine. *J Clin Psychiatry*. 1992; 53(Suppl 2):61-6.
64. Rasmussen JGC, Johnson AM. Reduced seizure potential in animals and reduced incidence of seizures in depressed patients during treatment with the selective serotonin reuptake inhibitor paroxetine. *Biol Psychiatry*. 1991; 29:634S. Abstract.
65. Waalinder J, Feighner JP. Novel selective serotonin reuptake inhibitors: Part 1. *J Clin Psychiatry*. 1992; 53:107-12.
66. Warrington SJ, Dana-Haeri J, Sinclair AJ. Cardiovascular and psychomotor effects of repeated doses of paroxetine: comparison of amitriptyline and placebo in healthy men. *Acta Psychiatr Scand*. 1989; 80(Suppl):42-4.
67. McClelland GR, Raptopoulos P. Cardiovascular effects of paroxetine and amitriptyline and repeated administration to normal volunteers. *Br J Clin Pharmacol*. 1985; 19:282. Abstract.
68. Hindmarch I, Harrison C. The effects of paroxetine and other antidepressants in combination with alcohol on psychomotor activity related to car driving. *Hum Psychopharmacol. 1988; 3:13-20.*
69. Saletu B, Grunberger J, Rajna P. Pharmaco-EEG profiles of antidepressants. Pharmacodynamic studies with fluvoxamine. *Br J Clin Pharmacol*. 1983; 15:369S-384S.
70. McClelland GR, Raptopoulos P, Jackson D. The effect of paroxetine on the quantitative EEG. *Acta Psychiatr Scand*. 1989; 80(Suppl):50-2.
71. Pfizer Pharmaceuticals. Zoloft package insert. New York, NY; 1992 Jan.
72. Mattila MJ, Saarialho-Kere U, Mattila M. Acute effects of sertraline, amitriptyline, and placebo on the psychomotor performance of healthy subjects over 50 years of age. *J Clin Psychiatry*. 1988; 49:52-8.
73. Guy S, Silke B. The electrocardiogram as a tool for therapeutic monitoring: a critical analysis. *J Clin Psychiatry*. 1990; 51:37-9.
74. Fisch C. Effects of sertraline on the ECG in non-elderly and elderly patients with major depression. *Biol Psychiatry*. 1991; 29:353S. Abstract.
75. Laporta M, Chouinard G, Goldbloom D et al. Hypomania induced by sertraline, a new serotonin reuptake inhibitor. *Am J Psychiatry*. 1987; 144:1513-4. Letter.
76. Reimherr FW, Chouinard G, Cohn CK et al. Antidepressant efficacy of sertraline: a double-blind, placebo-and amitriptyline-controlled, multicenter comparison study in outpatients with major depression. *J Clin Psychiatry*. 1990; 51(Suppl B):18-27.
77. Cohn CK, Shrivastava R, Mendels J et al. Double-blind, multicenter comparison of sertraline and amitriptyline in elderly depressed patients. *J Clin Psychiatry*. 1990; 51(Suppl B):28-33.
78. Saletu B, Grunberger J, Linzmayer L. On central effects of serotonin reuptake inhibitors: quantitative EEG and psychometric studies with sertraline and zimelidine. *J Neural Transm*. 1986; 67:241-66.
79. Saletu B, Grunberger J. Drug profiling by computed electroencephalography and brain maps, with special consideration of sertraline and its psychometric effects. *J Clin Psychiatry*. 1988; 49:59-71.
80. Itil TM, Mukherjee S, Dayican Gulay et al. Mode of action and dose finding of sertraline, a new antidepressant based on CEEG-brain mapping technology. *Psychopharmacology*. 1988; 96:281. Abstract.
81. Hindmarch I, Shillingford J, Shillingford C. The effects of sertraline on psychomotor performance in elderly volunteers. *J Clin Psychiatry*. 1990; 51:34-6.
82. Hindmarch I, Bhatti JZ. Psychopharmacological effects of sertraline in normal, healthy volunteers. *Eur J Clin Pharmacol*. 1988; 35:221-3.
83. Wagner W, Plekkenpol B, Gray TE et al. Review of fluvoxamine safety database. *Drugs*. 1992; 43(Suppl 2):48-54.
84. Saletu B, Schjerve M, Grunberger J et al. Fluvoxamine—a new serotonin reuptake inhibitor: first clinical and psychometric experiences in depressed patients. *J Neural Transm*. 1977; 41:17-36.
85. Claassen V. Review of the animal pharmacology and pharmacokinetics of fluvoxamine. *Br J Clin Pharmacol*. 1983; 15:349S-355S.
86. Roos JC. Cardiac effects of antidepressant drugs. A comparison of the tricyclic antidepressants and fluvoxamine. *Br J Clin Pharmacol*. 1983; 15:440S-449S.
87. Robinson JF, Doogan DP. A placebo controlled study of the cardiovascular effects of fluvoxamine and clovoxamine in human volunteers. *Br J Clin Pharmacol*. 1982; 14:805-8.
88. Wilson WH, Higano H, Papadatos Y et al. A double-blind placebo-controlled study to compare the autonomic effects of fluvoxamine with those of amitriptyline and doxepin in healthy volunteers. *Br J Clin Pharmacol*. 1983; 15:385S-392S.
89. Krijzer F, Snelder M, Bradford D. Comparison of the (pro) convulsive properties of fluvoxamine and clovoxamine with eight other antidepressants in an animal model. *Neuropsychobiology*. 1984; 12:249-54.
90. Warter JM, Tranchant C, Marescaux C et al. Immediate effects of 14 non MAOI antidepressants in rats with spontaneous petit mal-like seizures. *Prog Neuropsychopharmacol Biol Psychiatry*. 1990; 14:261-70.
91. Harmant J, van Rijckevorsel-Harmant K, de Barsy TH. Fluvoxamine: an antidepressant with low (or no) epileptogenic effect. *Lancet*. 1990; 336:386. Letter.
92. Naldi L, Zucchi A, Brevi A et al. Fluvoxamine and epilepsy. *Lancet*. 1990; 336:947. Letter.
93. Bamrah J, Benbow S, McKenna J. Fluvoxamine and liver enzymes. *Br J Psychiatry*. 1990; 156:287. Letter.
94. Green BH. Fluvoxamine and hepatic function. *Br J Psychiatry*. 1988; 153:130-1. Letter.
95. Wakelin JS. Fluvoxamine in the treatment of the older depressed patient; double-blind, placebo-controlled data. *Int Clin Psychopharmacol*. 1986; 1:221-30.
96. Jefferson JW, Greist JH, Perse TL et al. Fluvoxamine-associated mania/hypomania in patients with obsessive compulsive disorder. *J Clin Psychopharmacol*. 1991; 11:391-2. Letter.
97. Perse TL, Greist JH, Jefferson JW et al. Fluvoxamine treatment of obsessive-compulsive disorder. *Am J Psychiatry*. 1987; 144:1543-8.
98. Burrai C, Bocchetta A, Zompo MD. Mania and fluvoxamine. *Am J Psychiatry*. 1991; 148:1263-4.
99. Hoehn-Saric R, Lipsey J, McLeod D. Apathy and indifference in patients on fluvoxamine and fluoxetine. *J Clin Psychopharmacol*. 1990; 10:343-5.
100. Baldwin D, Fineberg N, Montgomery S. Fluoxetine, fluvoxamine and extrapyramidal tract disorders. *Int Clin Psychopharmacol*. 1991; 6:51-8.
101. Fernstrom MH, Massoudi M, Kupfer DJ. Fluvoxamine and

weight loss. *Biol Psychiatry.* 1988; 24:948-9. Letter.

102. Fernstrom MH. Depression, antidepressants and body weight change. *Ann NY Acad Sci.* 1989; 575:31-9.
103. Saletu B, Grunberger J, Rajna P et al. Clovoxamine and fluvoxamine-2 biogenic amine re-uptake inhibiting antidepressants: quantitative EEG, psychometric and pharmacokinetic studies in man. *J Neural Transm.* 1980; 49:63-86.
104. Itil TM, Bhattachyaryya A, Polvan N et al. Fluvoxamine (DU-23,000), a new antidepressant. Quantitative pharmaco-electroencephalography and pilot clinical trials. *Prog Neuropsychopharmacol.* 1977; 1:309-22.
105. Curran HV, Lader M. The psychopharmacological effects of repeated doses of fluvoxamine, mianserin and placebo in healthy human subjects. *Eur J Clin Pharmacol.* 1986; 29:601-7.
106. Curran HV, Shine P, Lader M. Effects of repeated doses of fluvoxamine, mianserin and placebo on memory and measures of sedation. *Psychopharmacology.* 1986; 89:360-3.
107. Lader MH, Curran HV. Psychotropic effects of repeated doses of fluvoxamine in normal subjects. *Clin Neuropharmacol.* 1984; 7:S316. Abstract.
108. Cella S, Penalva A, Locatelli V et al. Neuroendocrine studies with fluvoxamine: animal data. *Br J Clin Pharmacol.* 1983; 15:357S-363S.
109. Kletzky OA, St. Michel P, Mashchak CA. Lack of effect of fluvoxamine, a new serotonin reuptake inhibitor, on hypothalamic-pituitary function. *Curr Ther Res.* 1983; 33:394-400.
110. Demisch K, Demisch L, Bochnik HJ et al. Melatonin and cortisol increase after fluvoxamine. *Br J Clin Pharmacol.* 1986; 22:621-2. Letter.
111. Demisch K, Demisch L, Nickelsen T et al. The influence of acute and subchronic administration of various antidepressants on early morning melatonin plasma levels in healthy subjects: increases following fluvoxamine. *J Neural Transm.* 1987; 68:257-70.
112. Solvay Kingswood, Inc. Luvox (fluvoxamine maleate) product monograph. Scarborough, Ontario, Canada.
113. Banerjee AK. Recovery from prolonged cerebral depression after fluvoxamine overdose. *Br Med J.* 1988; 296:1774.
114. Stark P, Hardison CD. A review of multicenter controlled studies of fluoxetine vs. imipramine and placebo in outpatients with major depressive disorder. *J Clin Psychiatry.* 1985; 46:53-8.
115. Herman JB, Brotman AW, Pollack MH et al. Fluoxetine-induced sexual dysfunction. *J Clin Psychiatry.* 1990; 51:25-7.
116. Hollander E. McCarley A. Yohimbine treatment of sexual side effects induced by serotonin reuptake blockers. *J Clin Psychiatry.* 1992; 53:207-9.
117. Balogh S, Hendricks SE, Kang J. Treatment of fluoxetine-induced anorgasmia with amantadine. *J Clin Psychiatry.* 1992; 53:212-3.
118. Ciraulo DA, Shader RI. Fluoxetine drug-drug interactions: I. Antidepressants and antipsychotics. *J Clin Psychopharmacol.* 1990; 10:48-50.
119. Bannister SJ, Houser VP, Hulse JD et al. Evaluation of the potential interactions of paroxetine with diazepam, cimetidine, warfarin, and digoxin. *Acta Psychiatr Scand.* 1989; 90(Suppl 350):102-6.
120. Boyer WF, Feighner JP. An overview of paroxetine. *J Clin Psychiatry.* 1992; 53(Suppl 2):3-6.
121. Stellamans G. A study to investigate the efficacy, adverse events, safety, and pharmacokinetic effects of co-administration of paroxetine and lithium. *Biol Psychiatry.* 1991; 29:628S. Abstract.
122. Wilner KD, Lazar JD, Deutsch DA et al. The effects of sertraline on steady-state lithium levels and renal clearance of lithium. *Biol Psychiatry.* 1991; 29:354S. Abstract.
123. Gardner MH, Ronfeld RA, Wilner KD et al. The effects of sertraline on the pharmacokinetics of diazepam in healthy volunteers. *Biol Psychiatry.* 1991; 29:354S. Abstract.
124. Forster PL, Dewland PM, Muirhead D et al. The effects of sertraline on plasma concentration and renal clearance of digoxin. *Biol Psychiatry.* 1991; 29:355S. Abstract.
125. Wilner KD, Lazar JD, Apseloff G et al. The effects of sertraline on the pharmacodynamics of warfarin in healthy volunteers. *Biol Psychiatry.* 1991; 29:354S. Abstract.
126. Preskorn SH, Alderman J, Harris S et al. Desipramine levels after sertraline or fluoxetine. Paper presented at 32nd Annual NCDEU Meeting. Boca Raton, FL; 1992 May 26–29.
127. Ochs HR, Greenblatt DJ, Verburg-Ochs B et al. Chronic treatment with fluvoxamine, clovoxamine, and placebo: interaction with digoxin and effects on sleep and alertness. *J Clin Pharmacol.* 1989; 29:91-5.
128. Spina E, Campo GM, Avenoso A et al. Interaction between fluvoxamine and imipramine/desipramine in four patients. *Ther Drug Monit.* 1992; 14:194-6.
129. Bertschy G, Vandel S, Vandel B et al. Fluvoxamine-tricyclic antidepressant interaction. *Eur J Clin Pharmacol.* 1991; 40:119-20.
130. Sperber AD. Toxic interaction between fluvoxamine and sustained release theophylline in an 11-year-old boy. *Drug Safety.* 1991; 6:460-2.
131. Hendrickx B, Floris M. A controlled pilot study of the combination of fluvoxamine and lithium. *Curr Ther Res.* 1991; 49:106-10.
132. Rickels K, Amsterdam J, Clary C et al. A placebo-controlled double-blind clinical trial of paroxetine in depressed outpatients. *Acta Psychiatr Scand.* 1989; 80(Suppl 350):117-23.
133. Kiev A. A double-blind, placebo-controlled study of paroxetine in depressed outpatients. *J Clin Psychiatry.* 1992; 53(Suppl 2):27-9.
134. Claghorn JL. The safety and efficacy of paroxetine compared with placebo in a double-blind trial of depressed outpatients. *J Clin Psychiatry.* 1992; 53(Suppl 2):33-5.
135. Miller SM, Naylor GJ, Murtagh M et al. A double-blind comparison of paroxetine and placebo in the treatment of depressed patients in a psychiatric outpatient clinic. *Acta Psychiatr Scand.* 1989; 80(Suppl 350):143-4.
136. Smith WT, Glaudin V. A placebo-controlled trial of paroxetine in the treatment of major depression. *J Clin Psychiatry.* 53(Suppl 2):36-9.
137. Bascara L. A double-blind study to compare the effectiveness and tolerability of paroxetine and amitriptyline in depressed patients. *Acta Psychiatr Scand.* 1989; 80(Suppl 350):141-2.
138. Wood AJJ, Zhou HH. Ethnic differences in drug disposition and responsiveness. *Clin Pharmacokinet.* 1991; 20:350-73.
139. Kuhs H, Rudolf GAE. A double-blind study of the comparative antidepressant effect of paroxetine and amitriptyline. *Acta Psychiatr Scand.* 1989; 80(Suppl 350):145-6.
140. Fabre LF. A 6-week, double-blind trial of paroxetine, imipramine, and placebo in depressed outpatients. *J Clin Psychiatry.* 1992; 53(Suppl 2):40-3.
141. Shrivastava RK, Shrivastava SHP, Overweg N et al. A double-blind comparison of paroxetine, imipramine, and placebo in major depression. *J Clin Psychiatry.* 1992; 53(Suppl 2):48-51.
142. Feighner JP, Boyer WF. Paroxetine in the treatment of depression: a comparison with imipramine and placebo. *Acta Psychiatr Scand.* 1989; 80(Suppl 350):125-9.
143. Cohn JB, Crowder JE, Wilcox CS et al. A placebo and imipramine controlled study of paroxetine. *Psychopharmacol Bull.* 1990; 26:185-8.
144. Peselow ED, Filippi AM, Goodnick P et al. The short and long-term efficacy of paroxetine from a six week double-blind parallel design trial vs imipramine and placebo. *Psychopharmacol Bull.* 1989; 25:267-71.
145. Danish University Antidepressant Group. Paroxetine: a selective serotonin reuptake inhibitor showing better tolerance, but weaker antidepressant effect than clomipramine in a controlled multicenter study. *J Affective Disord.* 1990; 18:289-99.
146. DeWilde J, Mertens C, Bartholome F. A double-blind multicenter study comparing paroxetine 20–40 mg with fluoxetine 20–60 mg in depressed patients. *Biol Psychiatry.* 1991;

29:255S. Abstract.
147. Peselow ED, Fillippi AM, Goodnick P et al. The short and long-term efficacy of paroxetine HCL: B. Data from a double-blind crossover study from a year long trial vs imipramine and placebo. *Psychopharmacol Bull.* 1989; 25:272-6.
148. Claghorn J. Paroxetine: long-term efficacy and tolerability. *Biol Psychiatry.* 1991; 29:255S. Abstract.
149. Fabre LF. A double-blind multicenter study comparing the safety and efficacy of sertraline with placebo in major depression. *Biol Psychiatry.* 1991; 29:353S. Abstract.
150. Doogan DP, Caillard V. Sertraline in the prevention of relapse in major depression. *Psychopharmacology.* 1988; 96(Suppl):271. Abstract.
151. Freeman CP. Fluvoxamine: clinical trials and clinical use. *J Psychiatr Neurosci.* 1991; 16(Suppl 1):19-25.
152. Feldmann HS, Denber HCB. Long-term study of fluvoxamine: a new rapid-acting antidepressant. *Int Pharmacopsychiatry.* 1982; 17:114-22.
153. Brasseur R, Van Moffaert M, Mesotten F et al. A Belgian multicentre study of fluvoxamine in depressive outpatients. *Acta Psychiatr Belg.* 1985; 85:636-43.
154. Martin AJ, Wakelin J. Fluvoxamine—a baseline study of clinical response, long term tolerance and safety in a general practice population. *Br J Clin Pract.* 1986; 40:95-9.
155. Porro V, Fiorenzoni S, Menga C et al. Single-blind comparison of the efficacy of fluvoxamine versus placebo in patients with depressive syndrome. *Curr Ther Res.* 1988; 43:621-9.
156. Bramanti P, Ricci RM, Roncari R et al. An Italian multicenter experience with fluvoxamine, a new antidepressant drug, versus imipramine. *Curr Ther Res.* 1988; 43:718-24.
157. Emrich HM, Berger M, Riemann D et al. Serotonin reuptake inhibition vs. norepinephrine reuptake inhibition: a double-blind differential-therapeutic study with fluvoxamine and oxaprotiline in endogenous and neurotic depressives. *Pharmacopsychiatry.* 1987; 20:60-3.
158. Hamilton BA, Jones PG, Hoda AN et al. Flupenthixol and fluvoxamine in mild to moderate depression: a comparison in general practice. *Pharmatherapeutica.* 1989; 5:292-7.
159. Martin AJ, Tebbs VM, Ashford JJ. Affective disorders in general practice. Treatment of 6000 patients with fluvoxamine. *Pharmatherapeutica.* 1987; 5:40-9.
160. Gonella G, Baignoli G, Ecari U. Fluvoxamine and imipramine in the treatment of depressive patients: a double-blind controlled study. *Curr Med Res Opin.* 1990; 12:177-84.
161. Guy W, Wilson W, Ban T et al. A double-blind clinical trial of fluvoxamine and imipramine in patients with primary depression. *Psychopharmacol Bull.* 1984; 20:73-8.
162. Amore M, Bellini M, Berardi D et al. Double-blind comparison of fluvoxamine and imipramine in depressed patients. *Curr Ther Res.* 1989; 46:815-20.
163. Guelfi JD, Dreyfus JF, Pichot P et al. Fluvoxamine and imipramine: results of a long-term controlled trial. *Int Clin Psychopharmacol.* 1987; 2:103-9.
164. Perez A, Ashford JJ. A double-blind, randomized comparison of fluvoxamine with mianserin in depressive illness. *Curr Med Res Opin.* 1990; 12:234-41.
165. De Jonghe F, Swinkels J, Tuynman-Qua H. Randomized double-blind study of fluvoxamine and maprotiline in treatment of depression. *Pharmacopsychiatry.* 1991; 24:21-7.
166. Kasper S, Voll G, Vieira A et al. Response to total sleep deprivation before and during treatment with fluvoxamine or maprotiline in patients with major depression—results of a double-blind study. *Pharmacopsychiatry.* 1990; 23:135-42.
167. De Wilde JEM, Doogan DP. Fluvoxamine and chlorimipramine in endogenous depression. *J Affective Disord.* 1982; 4:249-59.
168. Klok CJ, Brouwer GH, van Pragg HM et al. Fluvoxamine and clomipramine in depressed patients. *Acta Psychiatr Scand.* 1981; 64:1-11.
169. Dick P, Ferrero E. A double-blind comparative study of the clinical efficacy of fluvoxamine and chlorimipramine. *Br J Clin Pharmacol.* 1983; 15:419S-425S.
170. Laws D, Ashford JJ, Anstee JA. A multicentre double-blind comparative trial of fluvoxamine versus lorazepam in mixed anxiety and depression treated in general practice. *Acta Psychiatr Scand.* 1990; 81:185-9.
171. Conti L, Dell'osso L, Re F et al. Fluvoxamine maleate: double-blind clinical trial vs placebo in hospitalized depressed patients. *Curr Ther Res.* 1988; 43:468-80.
172. Guelfi JD, Dreyfus JF, Pichot P et al. A double-blind controlled clinical trial comparing fluvoxamine with imipramine. *Br J Clin Pharmacol.* 1983; 15:411S-417S.
173. Amin MM, Ananth JV, Coleman BS et al. Fluvoxamine: antidepressant effects confirmed in a placebo-controlled international study. *Clin Neuropharmacol.* 1984; 7:580. Abstract.
174. Lapierre YD, Browne M, Horn E et al. Treatment of major affective disorder with fluvoxamine. *J Clin Psychiatry.* 1987; 48:65-8.
175. March JS, Kobak KA, Jefferson JW et al. A double-blind, placebo-controlled trial of fluvoxamine versus imipramine in outpatients with major depression. *J Clin Psychiatry.* 1990; 51:200-2.
176. Feigner JP, Boyer WF, Meredith CH et al. A placebo-controlled inpatient comparison of fluvoxamine maleate and imipramine in major depression. *Int Clin Psychopharmacol.* 1989; 4:239-44.
177. Lydiard RB, Laird LK, Morton WA et al. Fluvoxamine, imipramine and placebo in the treatment of depressed outpatients: effects on depression. *Psychopharmacol Bull.* 1989; 25:68-70.
178. Wilde JE, Mertens C, Wakelin JS. Clinical trials of fluvoxamine vs chlorimipramine with single and three times daily dosing. *Br J Clin Pharmacol.* 1983; 15:427S-431S.
179. Roth D, Mattes J, Sheehan KH et al. A double-blind comparison of fluvoxamine, desipramine and placebo in outpatients with depression. *Prog Neuropsychopharmacol Biol Psychiatry.* 1990; 14:929-39.
180. Guillibert E, Pelicier Y, Archambault JC et al. A double-blind multicenter study of paroxetine versus clomipramine in depressed elderly patients. *Acta Psychiatr Scand.* 1989; 80(Suppl):132-4.
181. Dunner DL, Cohn JB, Walshe T et al. Two combined, multicenter double-blind studies of paroxetine and doxepin in geriatric patients with major depression. *J Clin Psychiatry.* 1992; 53(Suppl 2):57-60.
182. Phanjoo AL, Wonnacott S, Hodgson A. Double-blind comparative multicentre study of fluvoxamine and mianserin in the treatment of major depressive episode in elderly people. *Acta Psychiatr Scand.* 1991; 83:476-9.
183. Ashford JJ. Fluvoxamine in elderly depressed patients. *Biol Psychiatry.* 1991; 29:632S. Abstract.
184. Nolen WA, van de Putte JJ, Dijken WA et al. Treatment strategy in depression. I. Non-tricyclic and selective reuptake inhibitors in resistant depression: a double-blind partial crossover study on the effects of oxaprotiline and fluvoxamine. *Acta Psychiatr Scand.* 1988; 78:668-75.
185. Lapierre YD, Oyewumi LK, Coleman B. The efficacy of fluvoxamine as an antidepressant. *Clin Trials.* 1981; 18:313-20.
186. White K, Wykoff W, Tynes LL et al. Fluvoxamine in the treatment of tricyclic-resistant depression. *Psychiatr J Univ Ottawa.* 1990; 15:156-8.
187. Delgado PL, Price LH, Charney DS et al. Efficacy of fluvoxamine in treatment-refractory depression. *J Affective Disord.* 1988; 15:55-60.
188. Murphy DL, Zohar J, Benkelfat C et al. Obsessive-compulsive disorder as a 5-HT subsystem-related behavioural disorder. *Br J Psychiatry.* 1989; 155:15-24.
189. Winslow JT, Insel TR. Neurobiology of obsessive compulsive disorder: a possible role of serotonin. *J Clin Psychiatry.* 1990; 51:27-31.
190. Levine R, Hoffman JS, Knepple ED et al. Long-term fluoxetine treatment of a large number of obsessive-compulsive patients. *J Clin Psychopharmacol.* 1989; 9:281-3.
191. Pigott TA, Pato MT, Bernstein SE et al. Controlled compari-

sons of clomipramine and fluoxetine in the treatment of obsessive-compulsive disorder. *Arch Gen Psychiatry.* 1990; 47:926-32.
192. Modell JG, Himle J, Nesse RM et al. Sequential trials of fluoxetine, phenelzine, and tranylcypromine in the treatment of obsessive-compulsive disorder. *J Anxiety Disord.* 1989; 3:287-93.
193. Turner SM, Jacob RG, Beidel DC et al. Fluoxetine treatment of obsessive-compulsive disorder. *J Clin Psychopharmacol.* 1985; 5:201-12.
194. Fontaine R, Chouinard G. Fluoxetine in the treatment of obsessive-compulsive disorder. *Prog Neuropsychopharmacol Biol Psychiatry.* 1985; 9:605-8.
195. Jenike MA, Buttol PHL, Baer L et al. Fluoxetine in obsessive-compulsive disorder: a positive open trial. *Am J Psychiatry.* 1989; 146:909-11.
196. Chouinard G, Goodman W, Greist J et al. Results of a double-blind placebo controlled trial of a new serotonin uptake inhibitor, sertraline, in the treatment of obsessive-compulsive disorder. *Psychopharmacol Bull.* 1990; 26:279-84.
197. Jenike MA, Baer L, Summergrad P et al. Sertraline in obsessive-compulsive disorder: a double-blind comparison with placebo. *Am J Psychiatry.* 1990; 147:923-8.
198. Jenike MA, Baer L. Correction. *Am J Psychiatry.* 1990; 147:1393. Letter.
199. Price LH, Goodman WK, Charney DS et al. Treatment of severe obsessive-compulsive disorder with fluvoxamine. *Am J Psychiatry.* 1987; 144:1059-61.
200. Solyom L, Solyom CA. Successful fluvoxamine treatment of a case of refractory obsessive-compulsive disorder. *Can J Psychiatry.* 1990; 35:696-7.
201. Delgado PL, Goodman WK, Price LH et al. Fluvoxamine/pimozide treatment of concurrent Tourette's and obsessive-compulsive disorder. *Br J Psychiatry.* 1990; 157:762-5.
202. McDougle CJ, Price LH, Goodman WK. Fluvoxamine treatment of coincident autistic disorder and obsessive-compulsive disorder: a case report. *J Autism Dev Disord.* 1990; 20:537-43.
203. Hollander E, DeCaria CM, Schneier FR et al. Fenfluramine augmentation of serotonin reuptake blockade antiobsessional treatment. *J Clin Psychiatry.* 1990; 51:119-23.
204. McDougle CJ, Goodman WK, Price LH et al. Neuroleptic addition in fluvoxamine-refractory obsessive-compulsive disorder. *Am J Psychiatry.* 1990; 147:652-4.
205. McDougle CJ, Price LH, Goodman WK et al. A controlled trial of lithium augmentation in fluvoxamine-refractory obsessive-compulsive disorder: lack of efficacy. *J Clin Psychopharmacol.* 1991; 11:175-84.
206. Jenike MA, Hyman S, Baer L et al. A controlled trial of fluvoxamine in obsessive-compulsive disorder: implications for a serotonergic theory. *Am J Psychiatry.* 1990; 147:1209-15.
207. Goodman WK, Price LH, Rasmussen SA et al. Efficacy of fluvoxamine in obsessive-compulsive disorder. *Arch Gen Psychiatry.* 1989; 46:36-44.
208. Goodman WK, Price LH, Rasmussen SA et al. Serotonergic agents in obsessive-compulsive disorder. *Psychopharmacol Bull.* 1989; 25:31-5.
209. Goodman WK, Price LH, Delgado PL et al. Specificity of serotonin reuptake inhibitors in the treatment of obsessive-compulsive disorder. *Arch Gen Psychiatry.* 1990; 47:577-85.
210. Cottraux J, Mollard E, Bouvard M et al. A controlled study of fluvoxamine and exposure in obsessive-compulsive disorder. *Int Clin Psychopharmacol.* 1990; 5:17-30.
211. Servant D, Bailly D, Parquet PJ. Fluvoxamine in the treatment of panic disorder with obsessive-compulsive symptoms. *Am J Psychiatry.* 1988; 145:174-5. Letter.
212. Den Boer J, Westenberg HG. Effect of a serotonin and noradrenaline uptake inhibitor in panic disorder: a double-blind comparative study with fluvoxamine and maprotiline. *Int Clin Psychopharmacol.* 1988; 3:59-74.
213. Den Boer J, Westenberg H, Kamerbeek W et al. Effect of serotonin uptake inhibitors in anxiety disorders; a double-blind comparison of clomipramine and fluvoxamine. *Int Clin Psychopharmacol.* 1987; 2:21-32.
214. Den Boer JA, Westenberg HGM. Serotonin function in panic disorder: a double blind placebo controlled study with fluvoxamine and ritanserin. *Psychopharmacology.* 1990; 102:85-94.
215. Schachter M, Parkes JD. Fluvoxamine and clomipramine in the treatment of cataplexy. *J Neurol Neurosurg Psychiatry.* 1980; 43:171-4.
216. Hendrickx B, Van Moffaert M, Spiers R et al. The treatment of psychocutaneous disorders: a new approach. *Curr Ther Res.* 1991; 49:111-9.
217. Hollander E, Liebowitz MR, DeCaria C et al. Treatment of depersonalization with serotonin reuptake blockers. *J Clin Psychopharmacol.* 1990; 10:200-3.
218. Alvarado R, Contreras S, Segovia-Riquelme N et al. Effects of serotonin uptake blockers and of 5-hydroxytryptophan on the voluntary consumption of ethanol, water and solid food by UChA and UChB rats. *Alcohol.* 1989; 7:315-9.
219. Murphy JM, Waller MB, Gatto GJ et al. Monoamine uptake inhibitors attenuate ethanol intake in alcohol-preferring (P) rats. *Alcohol.* 1985; 2:349-52.
220. Tollefson GD. Serotonin and alcohol: interrelationships. *Psychopathology.* 1989; 22:37-48.
221. McEntee WJ, Mair RG. Memory improvement in Korsakoff's disease with fluvoxamine. *Arch Gen Psychiatry.* 1990; 47:978-9. Letter.
222. Martin PR, Adinoff B, Bone GAH et al. Fluvoxamine (F) treatment of alcoholic chronic organic brain syndromes (COBS). *Clin Pharmacol Ther.* 1987; 41:211. Abstract.
223. Martin PR, Adinoff B, Eckardt M et al. Effective pharmacotherapy of alcoholic amnestic disorder with fluvoxamine. *Arch Gen Psychiatry.* 1989; 46:617-21.
224. Abell CA, Farquhar DL, Galloway SM et al. Placebo controlled double-blind trial of fluvoxamine maleate in the obese. *J Psychosom Res.* 1986; 30:143-6.
225. Bagiella E, Cairella M, Del Ben M et al. Changes in attitude toward food by obese patients treated with placebo and serotonergic agents. *Curr Ther Res.* 1991; 50:205-10.
226. Nielsen JA, Krupp MN, Heym J et al. Sertraline inhibits feeding and body weight gain in rodents. *Psychopharmacology.* 1988; 96:271. Abstract.
227. Simansky KJ, Vaidya AH. Behavioral mechanisms for the anorectic action of the serotonin (5-HT) uptake inhibitor sertraline in rats: comparison with directly acting 5-HT agonist. *Brain Res Bull.* 1990; 25:953-60.
228. Lucki I, Kreider MS, Simansky KJ. Reduction of feeding behavior by the serotonin uptake inhibitor sertraline. *Psychopharmacology.* 1988; 96:289-95.
229. Gill K, Filion Y, Amit Z. A further examination of the effects of sertraline on voluntary ethanol consumption. *Alcohol.* 1988; 5:355-8.
230. Gill K, Amit Z, Koe BK. Treatment with sertraline, a new serotonin uptake inhibitor, reduces voluntary ethanol consumption in rats. *Alcohol.* 1988; 5:349-54.
231. Meerwaldt JD. Treatment of hypokinetic rigid syndrome with fluvoxamine maleate. *Lancet.* 1986; 1:977-8. Letter.
232. Hope RA, Allman P. Hyperphagia in dementia: fluvoxamine takes the biscuit. *J Neurol Neurosurg Psychiatry.* 1991; 54:88. Letter.
233. Veeninga AT, Westenberg H, Weusten JT. Fluvoxamine in the treatment of menstrually related mood disorders. *Psychopharmacology.* 1990; 102:414-6.
234. Dunner DL, Dunbar GC. Optimal dose regimen for paroxetine. *J Clin Psychiatry.* 1992; 53(Suppl 2):21-6.
235. Goff DC, Midha KK, Brotman AW et al. Elevation of plasma concentrations of haloperidol after addition of fluoxetine. *Am J Psychiatry.* 1991; 148:190-2.
236. Grimsley SR, Jann MW, Carter JG et al. Increased carbamazepine plasma concentrations after fluoxetine coadministration. *Clin Pharmacol Ther.* 1991; 50:10-5.
237. Sovner R, Davis JM. A potential drug interaction between

fluoxetine and valproic acid. *J Clin Psychopharmacol.* 1991; 11:389. Letter.

238. Brosen K. Recent developments in hepatic drug oxidation. Implications for clinical pharmacokinetics. *Clin Pharmacokinet.* 1990; 18:220-39.
239. Brosen K, Skjelbo E. Fluoxetine and norfluoxetine are potent inhibitors of P450IID6—the source of the sparteine/debrisoquine oxidation polymorphism. *Br J Clin Pharmacol.* 1991; 32:136-7. Letter.
240. Crewe HK, Lennard MS, Tucker GT et al. The effect of paroxetine and other specific 5-HT reuptake inhibitors on cytochrome P450IID6 activity in human liver microsomes. In: Proceedings of the British Pharmacology Society. *Br J Clin Pharmacol.* 1991:658P-9P. Abstract.

Research Notes

Intrathecal administration of morphine followed by patient-controlled intravenous administration for postoperative analgesia

ROBERT W. WETMORE, MARK A. KALT, JOHN W. SYBERT, AND EARL T. HECKER

Clin Pharm. 1992; 11:958-61

Efficacious, safe, and cost-effective postoperative analgesia can be provided when narcotics are given perioperatively by intrathecal injection or postoperatively by i.v. patient-controlled analgesia (PCA).[1-4] Intrathecal narcotic injection is simple and reliable, requires small doses, and can be performed conveniently at the time of spinal anesthesia.[5] We, like others,[6-9] have found that a single intrathecal dose of morphine provides reliable and prolonged analgesia after most thoracoabdominal and orthopedic procedures.

A single intrathecal dose of morphine provides analgesia for approximately 12–36 hours, but repeated intrathecal injection of narcotics is impractical and increases the risk of cephalalgia, paralysis, paresthesia, infection, and epidural hemorrhage.[3] Thus, another narcotic-administration method may be necessary in patients whose pain outlasts the single intrathecal dose. Intravenous PCA with narcotics offers advantages over i.m. injection and could provide pain control as the effects of intrathecal morphine diminish.[5]

We evaluated the safety and analgesic efficacy of morphine in the treatment of postoperative pain when the drug was given by two regimens: (1) a single intrathecal dose injected immediately before surgery, followed by postoperative i.v. PCA and (2) postoperative i.v. PCA only.

Methods. *Patients Receiving Sequential Intrathecal and I.V. PCA Morphine.* We retrospectively examined the medical records of patients who had received intrathecal morphine and subsequent i.v. morphine by PCA for the treatment of postoperative pain; we called these patients the sequential group and included patients who had been treated from January through April 1991. The attending anesthesiologist selected the patients to receive this regimen of analgesia. A single intrathecal dose of preservative-free morphine (Astramorph/PF, Astra) was given immediately before initiation of anesthesia; the morphine was diluted with the patient's cerebrospinal fluid or combined with tetracaine or bupivacaine. The dose of morphine was determined by the anesthesiologist.

Patients could be given supplemental postoperative doses of i.v. morphine before PCA was started; the need for and dose of supplemental morphine was determined by an anesthesiology resident. Morphine administration by i.v. PCA was started when the intrathecal morphine was judged to have stopped providing adequate analgesia and when the high-risk period for delayed respiratory depression associated with intrathecal morphine (12–18 hours) had passed. A PCA device (Lifecare 4100 PCA Plus, Abbott) was used to deliver as-needed i.v. bolus doses of morphine sulfate 0.5 mg with a 10-minute lock-out interval and a four-hour limit of 12 mg; there was no basal morphine infusion.

Nurses and other health professionals asked patients to rate their comfort every two hours for the first eight hours after surgery and at least as often as every four hours thereafter. Patients rated their comfort during the past interval with the following scale: 1 = comfortable, 2 = in mild discomfort, 3 = in pain, 4 = in bad pain, and 5 = in very bad pain. The PCA regimen was adjusted to maintain a score of ≤2 or to lessen adverse effects. Clinicians based the decision to discontinue PCA on numerous patient-specific factors, including the ability to tolerate oral analgesics, tolerance of advances in diet, bowel function, severity of pain, need for i.v. access, and degree of activity.

Data collected for these patients for the period preceding PCA included (1) the length of time between the patients' return to the general nursing unit after

ROBERT W. WETMORE, PHARM.D., is Assistant Director of Clinical Pharmacy; MARK A. KALT, D.O., is Anesthesia Resident; JOHN W. SYBERT, D.O., is Staff Anesthesiologist; and EARL T. HECKER, D.O., F.A.C.O.S., is Chief of Surgery, Botsford General Hospital, Farmington Hills, MI.

Address reprint requests to Dr. Wetmore at Botsford General Hospital, 28050 Grand River Avenue, Farmington Hills, MI 48336.

The clerical assistance of Ms. Debra Renauer and Mrs. Kerri Sochocki is acknowledged.

Presented at the 26th Annual ASHP Midyear Clinical Meeting, New Orleans, LA, December 9, 1991.

surgery and the first supplemental dose (if any) of i.v. morphine, (2) times and doses of supplemental i.v. morphine, and (3) length of time between the intrathecal morphine dose and the start of PCA. Data collected for the period after PCA initiation included (1) the total amount of morphine given, (2) the duration of PCA, and (3) pain scores. Adverse effects and associated treatments that occurred during the entire length of morphine therapy were recorded.

Patients Receiving I.V. PCA Morphine Only. We selected patients whose postoperative analgesia was provided only by i.v. morphine via PCA and who closely matched the sequential group with respect to surgical procedure, age, sex, and weight; these patients had also been treated from January through April 1991. We called these patients the PCA-only group. The initial regimen for the PCA-only patients consisted of a basal morphine sulfate infusion of 0.5–1.0 mg/hr and as-needed bolus doses of 1.0–1.6 mg with a 10-minute lock-out interval. This dosage is similar to those described by other authors.[10,11] PCA was started within one hour of the patients' arrival at the recovery room, and dosage was adjusted as it was for the sequential group. Decisions to discontinue PCA were made as for those in the sequential group. The data collected for these patients were the same as those collected for the sequential group after PCA initiation.

Results. The sequential group comprised 27 consecutive patients, and the PCA-only group comprised 13 matched patients (Table 1).

More than half of the patients who received intrathecal morphine required supplemental morphine sulfate within 24 hours after surgery (Table 2). The average amount of supplemental morphine sulfate was 3 mg per patient (range, 2–9 mg). PCA was started 25.4 ± 3.0 hours (mean ± S.D.) after the intrathecal dose of morphine. The mean total PCA morphine sulfate dose was 31 mg (range, 7–127 mg), and the mean ± S.D. total duration of sequential therapy (intrathecal plus PCA) was 70.4 ± 14.6 hours (range, 45–106 hours). The initial PCA regimen was adequate in 23 (85%) of the 27 patients in the sequential group. The other four patients required adjustment of the morphine sulfate boluses to 0.8 mg/dose (with no change in the lock-out interval or the four-hour limit).

Table 3 shows the morphine requirements of patients in both groups who underwent the same type of surgery. The requirements in the PCA-only group after the first 24 postoperative hours were about twice the total PCA requirements for those in the sequential group (whose PCA was started about 25 hours postoperatively). Because of the small sample we did not determine whether the differences in morphine requirements were statistically significant. Table 3 also shows that the duration and efficacy of morphine therapy were similar between groups.

Table 4 shows that adverse effects were more common in the sequential group. Nausea, the most common adverse effect, was usually well controlled with droperidol. Again, whether differences were statistically significant was not determined.

Discussion. We did not intend our study to be particularly rigorous in the evaluation of pain-control methods; our sample was small and data were collected retrospectively. In addition, patient selection was

Table 1.
Comparison of Treatment Groups[a]

Characteristic	Sequential Group	PCA-Only Group
n	27	13
Mean ± S.D. age (yr)	63 ± 14	61 ± 15
Mean ± S.D. weight (kg)	81 ± 18	81 ± 10
No. (%) women	18 (67)	9 (69)
Type of surgery (no. [%])		
Knee	13 (48)	7 (54)
Hip	7 (26)	1 (8)
Colon	4 (15)	5 (38)
TAH-BSO[b]	1 (4)	0
Exploratory laparotomy	1 (4)	0
Pyeloplasty	1 (4)	0

[a] Patients in the sequential group received one preoperative dose of intrathecal morphine and postoperative i.v. morphine by patient-controlled analgesia (PCA). Patients in the PCA-only group received only postoperative i.v. morphine by PCA.
[b] Total abdominal hysterectomy with bilateral salpingo-oophorectomy.

Table 2.
Postoperative Pain Control Associated with Intrathecal Morphine ($n = 27$)

Type of Surgery	Intrathecal Morphine Sulfate Dose (mg)[a]	Pain-free Interval (hr)[a,b]	No. (%) Pts. Given Supplemental Morphine[c]	Time to Start of PCA (hr)[a,d]
Knee ($n = 13$)	0.28 ± 0.06	16.7 ± 8.0	8 (62)	24.6 ± 2.4
Hip ($n = 7$)	0.29 ± 0.09	22.7 ± 7.0	2 (29)	26.4 ± 2.9
Colon ($n = 4$)	0.35 ± 0.06	22.7 ± 12.1	2 (50)	27.0 ± 5.4
TAH-BSO[e] ($n = 1$)	0.4	24.0	1 (100)	24.0
Exploratory laparotomy ($n = 1$)	0.3	7.0	1 (100)	24.0
Pyeloplasty ($n = 1$)	0.4	24.0	0	24.0

[a] Data reported as mean ± S.D. when $n > 1$.
[b] Interval between time patient arrived at general nursing unit postoperatively and time of first supplemental dose of i.v. morphine (before start of PCA).
[c] Supplemental i.v. morphine given before start of PCA.
[d] Time from dose of intrathecal morphine to start of PCA.
[e] Total abdominal hysterectomy with bilateral salpingo-oophorectomy.

Table. 3
Pain Control in Patients Receiving Sequential and PCA-Only Morphine Therapy[a]

Type of Surgery and Pain-Control Method	PCA Morphine Sulfate Dose (mg)[b]	Duration of Morphine Therapy (hr)[c]	Mean Pain Score[d]
Knee, sequential ($n = 13$)	34.6 ± 32.1	69.3 ± 13.1	1.7 ± 0.4
Knee, PCA-only ($n = 7$)	73.5 ± 40.9	66.1 ± 11.3	1.4 ± 0.4
Hip, sequential ($n = 7$)	19.2 ± 12.3	68.6 ± 16.2	1.6 ± 0.4
Hip, PCA-only ($n = 1$)	61.0	73.0	1.1
Colon, sequential ($n = 4$)	39.7 ± 24.0	80.3 ± 17.3	1.5 ± 0.3
Colon, PCA-only ($n = 5$)	90.2 ± 35.5	74.8 ± 10.0	1.3 ± 0.1

[a] Sequential therapy consisted of one preoperative dose of intrathecal morphine and postoperative i.v. morphine by patient-controlled analgesia (PCA). PCA-only therapy consisted of postoperative PCA initiated within one hour of arrival at the recovery room. Data presented as mean ± S.D. when $n > 1$.

[b] For the PCA-only group, data for the first 24 postoperative hours are excluded. This allows comparison with PCA requirements of the sequential group, in which PCA was started at an average of 25.4 hours after the intrathecal morphine dose.

[c] For sequential group, time from intrathecal morphine dose to discontinuation of PCA. For PCA-only group, duration of PCA.

[d] Mean ± S.D. (when $n > 1$ patient) of mean pain scores for each patient during PCA. Mean scores for each patient were derived from ≥14 pain ratings, where 1 = comfortable, 2 = in mild discomfort, 3 = in pain, 4 = in bad pain, and 5 = in very bad pain.

not random. Intrathecal narcotic administration is the preferred method of postoperative analgesia at our institution and is generally offered to the patient unless the risk of respiratory depression or intrathecal injection is thought to be unreasonable. The decision to offer intrathecal morphine is left to the individual anesthesiologist and may be influenced by the availability of health professionals to provide adequate monitoring after surgery.

Regardless of these limitations, our findings suggest that the sequential use of morphine via intrathecal injection and i.v. PCA is effective and fairly safe. Mean pain scores (Table 3) indicate that analgesia was adequate in both the sequential and PCA-only groups. To our knowledge, other authors have not described the sequential use of intrathecal and i.v. PCA morphine for postoperative analgesia.

The average patient who received intrathecal morphine required supplemental i.v. morphine about 19 hours after arriving at the general nursing unit. This suggests that PCA therapy could be started earlier than 25.4 hours after the intrathecal morphine dose (the average time in this study). Because intrathecal morphine can cause delayed respiratory depression, however, a protocol that called for relatively early PCA initiation would have to specify that low PCA doses be used at first. Delayed respiratory depression is a consequence of slow rostral spread of an intrathecally injected narcotic and occurs when the drug concentration reaches a critical level in the respiratory center of the central nervous system.[12] Several factors, one of which is the supplemental use of systemic narcotics, can substantially increase the risk of respiratory depression associated with intrathecal morphine.

PCA morphine requirements varied with the type of surgery (Table 3). Explanation of this finding is beyond the scope of this study, but clinicians should be aware that postoperative analgesic requirements may not be independent of the surgical procedure.

Patients who had received intrathecal morphine required about half as much PCA morphine as did matched patients (after the first 24 postoperative hours) who had not received intrathecal morphine. Although the pain control offered by intrathecal morphine might be expected to be limited after 24 hours, we believe that the dose did somehow decrease analgesic requirements well after 24 hours. We cannot explain the apparent prolonged influence of intrathecal morphine, but the phenomenon has clinical importance. If PCA is used after intrathecal morphine administration, the initial PCA dosage should be low. Our PCA regimen for patients who had received intrathecal morphine called for morphine bolus doses that were about half those that were used in the PCA-only group. We recommend that clinicians consider reducing initial standard PCA bolus doses and that they use slow, methodical dosage escalation.

Table 4.
Adverse Reactions in Patients Receiving Sequential and PCA-Only Morphine Therapy[a]

Reaction	No. (%) Patients
Sequential Group ($n = 27$)	
Nausea, emesis	12 (44)[b]
Pruritus	8 (30)[b]
Hypotension	3 (11)[b, c]
Somnolence, confusion	2 (7)[c]
Apnea	1 (4)[c]
PCA-Only Group ($n = 13$)	
Nausea, emesis	5 (39)
Pruritus	2 (15)

[a] Sequential therapy consisted of one preoperative dose of intrathecal morphine and postoperative i.v. morphine by patient-controlled analgesia (PCA). PCA-only therapy consisted of postoperative PCA initiated within one hour of arrival at the recovery room.

[b] Reaction occurred after start of PCA in two patients.

[c] Reaction occurred before start of PCA in one patient.

The most common adverse effects—nausea, vomiting, and pruritus—occurred with a frequency consistent with that reported by other authors.[13,14] Hypotension occurred in 3 of the 27 patients in the sequential group; in 1 of these patients, hypotension occurred before PCA was started. Most authors have not mentioned this reaction as an adverse effect of intrathecal morphine, so we are unsure about a cause-and-effect relationship in our patients. One patient who had received intrathecal morphine developed apnea in the recovery room, but the relatively early onset of apnea makes it unclear whether intrathecal morphine was responsible. One patient from the sequential group became somnolent before PCA was begun, but this condition was mild and disappeared within several hours. Another patient from the same group became confused after PCA initiation. The PCA regimen was adjusted, and the confusion disappeared.

Conclusion. Adequate postoperative pain control can be provided by a single preoperative dose of intrathecal morphine followed by postoperative morphine given by i.v. PCA. Preoperative intrathecal morphine appears to decrease the amount of i.v. morphine that is required after the first 24 postoperative hours.

References

1. Ma CSJ, Lin D. Patient controlled analgesia: drug options, infusion schedules, and other considerations. *Hosp Formul.* 1991; 26:198-206.
2. Rapp RP, Bivins BA, Littrell RA et al. Patient controlled analgesia: a review of effectiveness of therapy and an evaluation of currently available devices. *DICP Ann Pharmacother.* 1989; 23:899-904.
3. Cousins MJ, Mather LE. Intrathecal and epidural administration of opioids. *Anesthesiology.* 1984; 61:276-310.
4. Morgan M. The rational use of intrathecal and extradural opioids. *Br J Anaesth.* 1989; 63:165-88.
5. Stoelting RK. Intrathecal morphine—an underused combination for postoperative pain management. *Anesth Analg.* 1989; 68:707-9.
6. Jacobson L, Chabal C, Brody MC. A dose-response study of intrathecal morphine: efficacy, duration, optimal dose, and side effects. *Anesth Analg.* 1988; 67:1082-8.
7. Yamaguchi H, Wantanabe S, Motokawa K et al. Intrathecal morphine dose-response data for pain relief after cholecystectomy. *Anesth Analg.* 1990; 70:168-71.
8. Yamaguchi H, Wantanabe S, Fukada T et al. Minimal effective dose of intrathecal morphine for pain relief following transabdominal hysterectomy. *Anesth Analg.* 1989; 68:537-40.
9. Gray Jr, Fromme GA, Nauss LA et al. Intrathecal morphine for post-thoracotomy pain. *Anesth Analg.* 1986; 65:873-6.
10. Wong EY, Thompson MV, Dudgeon MA et al. Hospital pharmacy-based service for patient-controlled analgesia. *Am J Hosp Pharm.* 1990; 47:364-9.
11. McCall LJ, Dierks DR. Pharmacy-managed patient-controlled analgesia service. *Am J Hosp Pharm.* 1990; 47:2706-10.
12. Bragg CL. Practical aspects of epidural and intrathecal narcotic analgesia in the intensive care setting. *Heart Lung.* 1989; 18:599-608.
13. Gustafsson LL, Schildt B, Jacobsen K. Adverse effects of extradural and intrathecal opiates: report of a nationwide survey in Sweden. *Br J Anaesth.* 1982; 54:479-86.
14. Abbound TK, Shnider SM, Dailey PA et al. Intrathecal administration of hyperbaric morphine for the relief of pain in labour. *Br J Anaesth.* 1984; 56:1351-60.

Pharmacokinetics and safety of intramuscular injection of concentrated ceftriaxone in children

JOHN S. BRADLEY, LISA S. COMPOGIANNIS, WILLIAM E. MURRAY, MARK A. ACOSTA, AND GLORIA L. TSU

Clin Pharm. 1992; 11:961-4

Ceftriaxone has been used extensively to treat infections in children.[1,2] Its extended elimination half-life allows for once-daily dosing for the treatment of invasive bacterial infections, including meningitis.[3,4] Outpatient therapy with once-daily dosing (using either intravenous or intramuscular injection) has been described.[5-7] The i.m. route has important uses in both ambulatory-care pediatric medicine and outpatient therapy in children who were initially hospitalized. Using 1% lidocaine hydrochloride, instead of water, to reconstitute ceftriaxone sodium to a ceftriaxone concentration of 250 mg/mL significantly reduced the pain associated with i.m. injection without significantly altering the pharmacokinetic values.[8] The volume of solution injected is an important determinant of the discomfort associated with i.m. injection.[9] Following the manufacturer's directions for reconstitution gives a final ceftriaxone concentration of approximately 250 mg/mL, which often necessitates giving a child two or three injections per dose to avoid injecting too much fluid into any single site.[10] Injection of the smaller volume associated with a more concentrated solution may therefore be less painful than multiple injections of a dilute solution, even though the more concentrated solution has a higher tonicity.[11]

We have previously described the use of i.m. ceftriaxone reconstituted with 1% lidocaine hydrochloride to a volume that is half the volume recommended by the manufacturer.[12] We now describe the pharmacoki-

JOHN S. BRADLEY, M.D., is Associate Clinical Professor of Pediatrics, Department of Pediatrics, Division of Infectious Diseases, University of California at San Diego; LISA S. COMPOGIANNIS, B.S.N., is Infectious Diseases Research Nurse, Division of Infectious Diseases, Children's Hospital–San Diego; WILLIAM E. MURRAY, PHARM.D., is Clinical Pharmacokineticist, Pharmacy Department, Children's Hospital–San Diego; MARK A. ACOSTA, PHARM.D., is Pediatric Hematology Clinical Pharmacist, Pharmacy Department, Children's Hospital–San Diego; and GLORIA L. TSU, PHARM.D., is Pediatric Clinical Pharmacist, Pharmacy Department, Children's Hospital–San Diego.

Address reprint requests to Dr. Bradley at Department of Pediatrics, Division of Infectious Diseases, Children's Hospital–San Diego, 8001 Frost Street, San Diego, CA 92123.

Sue Kohlhepp, Ph.D., is acknowledged for performing the HPLC analyses and assisting in manuscript preparation.

Dr. Bradley is a participant in the speakers' bureau of Roche Laboratories.

netics and safety of concentrated ceftriaxone following i.m. injection in children.

Methods. Children between two months and 18 years of age who were being treated at Children's Hospital–San Diego (CHSD) with injectable antimicrobials for infections due to organisms deemed susceptible to ceftriaxone were considered for this study. The children were required to have indwelling i.v. catheters large enough for blood sampling to avoid multiple venipunctures. Written informed consent was obtained from a parent or guardian. Assent was obtained from the child, when applicable (i.e., children over seven years old). Patients with known renal or hepatic dysfunction were excluded, as were patients with markedly elevated serum concentrations of creatinine (normal, 0.5–1.5 mg/dL), alanine aminotransferase (normal, 5–40 U/L), or aspartate aminotransferase (normal, 4–40 U/L). No children received concomitant β-lactam therapy during the study period.

Vials of ceftriaxone sodium[a] were diluted with a volume of 1% lidocaine hydrochloride[b] that was half that recommended by the manufacturer; 0.45, 0.9, 1.8, and 3.6 mL of diluent were used for 250-mg, 500-mg, 1-g, and 2-g vials, respectively.

One i.m. dose of ceftriaxone (50 mg/kg as the sodium salt; maximum, 2 g) was substituted during the 24-hour study interval for all i.v. antimicrobial therapy already being administered. We based the volume of injection on an assumed ceftriaxone concentration of 450 mg/mL. Blood samples were collected from most children at the following times after injection: 1, 2, 3, 6, 12, and 24 hours. For children already receiving ceftriaxone, a preinjection blood sample was obtained to measure the serum ceftriaxone concentration before i.m. antimicrobial administration.

Serum samples were stored at –20 °C before assay and were assayed within four days of collection. Serum ceftriaxone concentrations were measured by high-performance liquid chromatography (HPLC) by an outside laboratory.[c] The method of Patel et al.,[13] a reversed-phase ion-pairing technique, was adapted for quantitation of ceftriaxone in sera. An isocratic HPLC[d] was equipped with a reversed-phase C_{18} column[e] (5-μm particles, 2.5 cm × 4.6 mm internal diameter) and a variable wavelength detector set at 280 nm.[f] Mobile phase consisted of 500 mL of acetonitrile, 10 mL of 1 M phosphate buffer (pH 7), 3 g of hexadecyltrimethylammonium bromide,[g] and water to 1 L. Retention time of ceftriaxone was six to seven minutes with a flow rate of 1 mL/min. Serum samples were either diluted 1:10 with cold methanol or filtered through a PLGC ultrafiltration membrane[h] to remove serum proteins. Sensitivity was 5 μg/mL for the diluted sample and 0.5 μg/mL for the filtered sample. Mean ± S.D. sample recovery, determined with spiked normal sera, was 97 ± 7% for both sample preparation methods.

Pharmacokinetic values were calculated by using a microcomputer program developed by Chan and Wnuck.[14] Bioavailability was assumed to be 1.0.[15] In the children from whom we had obtained a sufficient number of evaluable serum ceftriaxone concentrations, individual pharmacokinetic variables including volume of distribution (V), terminal half-life ($t_{1/2}$), clearance (CL), and area under the serum concentration–time curve (AUC) were estimated. The trapezoidal rule was used for calculating AUC. Estimation of $t_{1/2}$ was performed by using samples obtained after six hours, assuming absorption to have been complete by that time.[8] In patients already receiving ceftriaxone, the AUC values were corrected by subtracting the contribution of previous doses. The elimination rate constant (k) was calculated from the terminal slope of the concentration–time curve (from 6 to 24 hours). Peak serum concentration (C_{max}) and time to peak concentration (t_{max}) were also determined.

To assess muscle toxicity[16,17] serum creatine kinase (CK) concentrations were measured 24 hours after i.m. injection. Normal CK values at CHSD are less than 188 U/L for children over one year of age and 376 U/L for children one year of age and younger. Adverse events were evaluated by study personnel 24 hours after injection.

We had previously determined the concentration of ceftriaxone when reconstituted with one half the recommended volume of diluent. To verify the lower-than-expected concentrations in that study, we reconstituted single vials (500 mg, 1 g, 2 g) with 1% lidocaine according to the manufacturer's instructions. Multiple aliquots of each reconstituted ceftriaxone vial were assayed by HPLC.

Results. Reconstitution of ceftriaxone sodium with 1% lidocaine hydrochloride according to the manufacturer's directions yielded the concentrations of ceftriaxone given in Table 1; results from our previous study[12] are also given.

Eleven children were enrolled in the study. The average age of the children was seven years, five months, and the range was five months to 17 years. Six of the children were female. Data from two children were subsequently excluded from the complete pharmacokinetic analysis. A six-year-old girl who had a normal serum creatinine at the time of study entry was later

Table 1.
Effect of Diluent Volume on Ceftriaxone Concentration

Vial Size	*n*	Volume of Diluent (mL)[a]	Mean Ceftriaxone Concentration (mg/mL)
Standard Solution[b]			
500 mg	3	1.8	233
1 g	3	3.6	244
2 g	3	7.2	216
Concentrated Solution[c]			
250 mg	3	0.45	444
500 mg	3	0.9	476
1 g	4	1.8	416
2 g	5	3.6	467

[a]Diluent was 1% lidocaine.
[b]Reconstituted according to manufacturer's directions.
[c]Reconstituted with half the diluent recommended by the manufacturer. Data previously reported, reference 12.

found to have markedly abnormal renal function, confirmed by abnormal vancomycin pharmacokinetics. A nine-month-old boy was inadvertently given one half the prescribed dose of ceftriaxone and is therefore included only in the time-to-peak-concentration data analysis.

Of the remaining nine patients, six had a sufficient number of ceftriaxone determinations to allow calculation of pharmacokinetic values. In the three excluded patients, one or more samples critical to determining the pharmacokinetic values were not available because of missed samples, mislabeled samples, and a broken serum container. Of the six children available for pharmacokinetic analysis, three were receiving i.v. ceftriaxone at the time of i.m. injection. Preinjection ceftriaxone concentrations in these children were 45, 50.5, and 85 µg/mL. Pharmacokinetic values are given in Table 2. Peak serum ceftriaxone concentration and time to peak concentration were available from some children who had insufficient data for complete pharmacokinetic analysis. These data are also given in Table 2.

Seven children enrolled in this study had CK concentrations obtained 24 hours after injection. The mean ± S.D. serum CK concentration was 155 ± 120 U/L (Table 3).

Eight children required only one injection (73%). Three children who weighed more than 40 kg received two injections (27%). No child required three injections. The only adverse event occurred in a 12-year-old girl with Wiskott-Aldrich syndrome who described local tenderness at one of two injection sites for two hours after the injection. No objective method was used to assess pain associated with i.m. injection.

Table 2.
Ceftriaxone Pharmacokinetic Values after I.M. Administration of Concentrated Injection[a]

Variable	n	Mean ± S.D.	Range
AUC (mg · hr/L)	6	2021 ± 870	1092–3208
CL (L/kg/hr)	6	0.029 ± 0.012	0.016–0.046
V (L/kg)	6	0.341 ± 0.081	0.260–0.477
$t_{1/2}$ (hr)	6	9.0 ± 2.8	5.1–12.7
C_{max} (mg/L)			
in children with no prior ceftriaxone	5	175.4 ± 33.9	123–200.5
t_{max} (hr)	9	2.1 ± 0.8	1–3

[a]AUC = area under the serum concentration–time curve, CL = clearance, V = volume of distribution, $t_{1/2}$ = terminal half-life, C_{max} = peak concentration, t_{max} = time to reach C_{max}.

Discussion. The recommended ceftriaxone concentration for i.m. injection (250 mg/mL) and the dose of 50 mg/kg necessitate a large injection volume. The volume required to deliver a daily 80-mg/kg dose to treat meningitis has been considered impractical.[18]

When the drug is reconstituted with half the volume of diluent suggested by the manufacturer, a solution with an average ceftriaxone concentration of approximately 450 mg/mL is achieved. This concentrated ceftriaxone solution is somewhat more difficult to prepare than the standard concentration. At room temperature, it may take as long as five minutes for the powder to dissolve into a viscous solution. Also, if refrigerated after reconstitution, it may require warming back to room temperature to resolubilize.

Using half the recommended volume of diluent would presumably result in a ceftriaxone concentration of 500 mg/mL. We showed previously that the resultant concentration is 450 mg/mL.[12] Possible explanations for this discrepancy are that (1) the solubility of ceftriaxone is less than 500 mg/mL, (2) the HPLC assay system detects less ceftriaxone than other assays, and (3) the amount of ceftriaxone present in each vial varies. In the present study, we reconstituted vials according to the manufacturer's directions and produced solutions with a mean concentration of 231 mg/mL (8% less than the expected 250 mg/mL). Because we have found that the concentration of ceftriaxone solutions is consistently lower than that suggested by the package insert, regardless of the vial size, and because the ceftriaxone concentration in a saturated solution is 477 mg/mL,[i] we assumed that the ceftriaxone concentration was 450 mg/mL for this study. We also assume that this is the drug concentration in our everyday use of concentrated ceftriaxone. We believe that variations in solution concentration above and below this average value are not clinically significant.

Table 3.
Creatine Kinase (CK) Concentrations after I.M. Injection of Concentrated Ceftriaxone

Patient	No. Injections	Total Volume of Injection (mL)	Ceftriaxone Dose	Patient Weight (kg)	CK Concentration 24 Hours after Injection (U/L)[a]	Adverse Events
1	2	2.2	2 g	45.3	90	None
2	1	2.5	1.125 g	25	24	None
3	1	0.88	400 mg	8	82	None
4	1	1.22	550 mg	11.49	248[b]	None
5	2	2.2	2 g	42.5	315	Muscle soreness for 2 hr
6	2	2.2	2 g	66.5	276	None
7	1	0.77	350 mg	7	50	None

[a]No patient had i.m. injections in the previous three days. Normal, <188 U/L for children older than one year and <376 U/L for children up to one year old.

[b]CK concentration one day before study was 265 U/L and four days after study was 72 U/L. A subcutaneously tunneled central catheter was surgically placed four days before this study.

Potential problems with the increased tonicity of concentrated ceftriaxone are (1) decreased absorption of ceftriaxone, potentially affecting blood and tissue concentrations of antimicrobial, and (2) increased muscle toxicity (as defined by serum CK concentrations) due to the higher osmotic load delivered i.m. Serum ceftriaxone concentrations determined in our patients demonstrated pharmacokinetic characteristics similar to those previously published for the 250-mg/mL reconstitution concentration.[15,19,20] The range of CK concentrations was consistent with those for other intramuscularly injected drugs.[9,16,17] One of the study subjects reported prolonged pain at one injection site. No reports of significant pain or other adverse reactions have been noted by the CHSD passive-reporting system for adverse drug reactions after more than 1000 injections with high-concentration ceftriaxone, which has been used routinely since December 1988. Our subjective overall assessment is that ceftriaxone appears to be as well tolerated at high reconstitution concentration as other injectable antimicrobials.

Given the advantages of a smaller volume of injected antibiotic and our data suggesting similar serum concentrations, we advocate the use of the concentrated preparation for i.m. injection in children, with the dose calculated on the basis of the average ceftriaxone reconstitution concentration of 450 mg/mL.

Conclusion. A concentrated ceftriaxone sodium injection prepared with 1% lidocaine hydrochloride appears to be safe for i.m. injection and to have i.m. pharmacokinetic values similar to those of nonconcentrated injection.

---

[a]Rocephin, Roche Laboratories, Hoffmann-La Roche, Inc., Nutley, NJ.

[b]Xylocaine, Astra Pharmaceutical Products Inc., Westboro, MA.

[c]Infectious Diseases Reference Laboratory, Portland, OR.

[d]Beckman Instruments, Inc., Fullerton, CA.

[e]Serva Feinbiochemica, Heidelberg, Germany.

[f]Model 100-10, Hitachi, Tokyo, Japan.

[g]Sigma Chemical Company, St. Louis, MO.

[h]Millipore Corporation, Bedford, MA.

[i]Billstein S, Roche Laboratories. Personal communication, 1988.

References

1. Chadwick EG, Connor EM, Shulman ST et al. Efficacy of ceftriaxone in treatment of serious childhood infections. *J Pediatr.* 1983; 103:141-5.
2. Harrison CJ, Welch W, Marks MI. Ceftriaxone therapy in pediatric patients. *Am J Dis Child.* 1983; 137:1048-51.
3. Yogev R, Shulman ST, Chadwick EG et al. Once daily ceftriaxone for central nervous system infections and other serious pediatric infections. *Pediatr Infect Dis.* 1986; 5:298-303.
4. Frenkel LD. Once-daily administration of ceftriaxone for the treatment of selected serious bacterial infections in children. *Pediatrics.* 1988; 82:486-92.
5. Powell KR, Mawhorter SD. Outpatient treatment of serious infections in infants and children with ceftriaxone. *J Pediatr.* 1987; 110:898-901.
6. Dagan R, Phillip M, Watemberg NM. Outpatient treatment of serious community acquired pediatric infections using once daily intramuscular ceftriaxone. *Pediatr Infect Dis J.* 1987; 6:1080-4.
7. Bradley JS, Ching DK, Phillips SE. Outpatient therapy of serious pediatric infections with ceftriaxone. *Pediatr Infect Dis J.* 1988; 7:160-4.
8. Patel IH, Weinfeld RE, Konikoff J et al. Pharmacokinetics and tolerance of ceftriaxone in humans after single-dose intramuscular administration in water and lidocaine diluents. *Antimicrob Agents Chemother.* 1982; 21:957-62.
9. Greenblatt DJ, Koch-Weser J. Intramuscular injection of drugs. *N Engl J Med.* 1976; 295:542-6.
10. Howry LB, Bindler RM, Tso Y. Pediatric medications. Philadelphia: Lippincott; 1981:62.
11. Rockwell K, Burch K. Intramuscular antibiotic preparation and administration using a 1% lidocaine diluent: policies for the pediatric patient. *Hosp Pharm.* 1991; 26:634-5.
12. Bradley JS, Ching DLK, Wilson TA et al. Once-daily ceftriaxone to complete therapy of uncomplicated group B streptococcal infection in neonates: a preliminary report. *Clin Pediatr.* 1992; 31:274-8.
13. Patel IH, Chen S, Parsonnet M et al. Pharmacokinetics of ceftriaxone in humans. *Antimicrob Agents Chemother.* 1981; 20:634-41.
14. Chan KKH, Wnuck K. Microcomputer based pharmacokinetics for calculating absorption rate. *Comput Programs Biomed.* 1983; 16:27-34.
15. Delsignore R, Baroni CM, Crotti G et al. Absolute bioavailability of ceftriaxone after intramuscular administration to healthy volunteers. *Chemotherapy.* 1983; 29:157-62.
16. Sidell FR, Culver DL, Kaminskis A. Serum creatine phosphokinase activity after intramuscular injection. *JAMA.* 1974; 229:1894-7.
17. Meltzer HY, Mrozak S, Boyer M. Effect of intramuscular injections on serum creatine phosphokinase activity. *Am J Med Sci.* 1970; 259:42-8.
18. Plotkin SA, Daum RS, Giebink GS. Treatment of bacterial meningitis. *Pediatrics.* 1988; 81:904-7.
19. Pickup ME, Bird HA, Lowe JR et al. A pharmacokinetic and tolerance study of Ro13-9904, a new cephalosporin antibiotic. *Br J Clin Pharmacol.* 1981; 12:111-5.
20. Scully BE, Ru KP, Neu HC. Pharmacokinetics of ceftriaxone after intravenous infusion and intramuscular injection. *Am J Med.* 1984; 77(suppl 4C):112-6.

Nausea and vomiting after abdominal surgery

John M. Benson, Joseph T. DiPiro, Cathy L. Coleman, Jan D. Hirsch, L. Deane Donnigan, Johnny A. Stanfield, and Talmadge A. Bowden, Jr.

Clin Pharm. 1992; 11:965-7

In patients who have undergone general anesthesia, postoperative nausea and vomiting pose potential problems. No common denominator or specific indicator has been identified that will consistently predict which patients will be affected postoperatively. Often nausea and vomiting have been attributed to nasogastric tubes, general anesthetics, analgesics, and demographic characteristics.[1,2] Nausea and vomiting not only cause discomfort to the patient but also can adversely affect perception of the hospital experience and may lead to serious complications. First, vomiting may result in aspiration, leading to pneumonitis or pneumonia. This problem occurs more frequently in elderly, mentally debilitated, or recumbent patients. Second, the patient experiencing nausea is less likely to ambulate; thus recovery is delayed. The vomiting patient may become dehydrated, and persistent vomiting can interfere with oral drug therapy. Last, factors associated with nausea and vomiting have the potential to increase the hospital stay.

There is little objective information describing the incidence and etiology of postoperative nausea and vomiting after abdominal surgery or the effect of nausea and vomiting on hospital stay. If such information were available, it would help the clinician to choose potential interventions for this problem. The objectives of this study were (1) to determine the incidence of postoperative nausea and vomiting, (2) to identify the relationship between intraoperative and postoperative factors and the occurrence and duration of postoperative nausea or vomiting, and (3) to determine the relationship between nausea or vomiting and length of hospital stay in our institution for patients undergoing abdominal surgery.

Methods. We prospectively evaluated 101 patients who were admitted to the Medical College of Georgia Hospital for abdominal surgery and required general anesthesia. All patients were at least 18 years of age. Those who experienced nausea and vomiting within 48 hours before surgery were excluded. The study was approved by the human assurance committee of the Medical College of Georgia. Preoperative data collection included patient demographic characteristics (age, weight, sex, and race), type of operation, and a medical history from the hospital record. After the patient returned from surgery, the duration of operation, preoperative medications, anesthetic and induction agents used, placement of nasogastric tube, and analgesics used in the recovery room were recorded. Thereafter, the administration of analgesic and antiemetic agents was recorded. At the same time each day, one of the investigators interviewed patients about the occurrence of nausea or vomiting during the preceding 24 hours. Nausea and vomiting were not defined for the patients; they were simply asked if they had experienced nausea or vomiting, and any occurrence was considered a positive response for that day. Time until resumption of a regular diet was also noted. Patients were followed for seven days postoperatively or until hospital discharge, whichever came first.

The a priori level of significance was set at 0.05. Differences in incidence of nausea or vomiting among patient groups were investigated using chi-square analysis. Duration of nausea or vomiting was defined as the number of days in which nausea or vomiting occurred, as opposed to the duration of individual episodes. Mean ± S.D. duration (days) of nausea or vomiting was compared among groups by using an analysis of variance (ANOVA) procedure for multiple-group comparisons and Student's *t* test or Mann-Whitney *U* test, as appropriate, for two-group comparisons. Since many variables affect a surgery patient's length of hospitalization, a multiple-regression procedure was used to explore the relative contribution of the duration of nausea or vomiting to the length of hospital stay.

Results. The intent of the analyses was to explore the clinical importance of postoperative nausea and vomiting. Therefore, trends in the data are noted and discussed even though statistical significance was not attained, possibly because of the small sample sizes of some groups. The demographic characteristics of the 101 patients in this study are presented in Table 1. The mean ± S.D. age of the study patients was 43.2 ± 15.7

John M. Benson, Pharm.D., is Clinical Coordinator, Perinatology Team, Department of Pharmacy Services, University Hospital, and Clinical Assistant Professor of Pharmacy, University of Utah, Salt Lake City; at the time of this study, he was Assistant Professor of Pharmacy, University of Georgia, Athens. Joseph T. DiPiro, Pharm.D., is Professor of Pharmacy, University of Georgia, and Clinical Professor and Director of Clinical Research, Department of Surgery, Medical College of Georgia, Augusta. Cathy L. Coleman, Pharm.D., is Staff Development Specialist, Department of Pharmaceutical Services, Emory University Hospital, Atlanta. Jan D. Hirsch, Ph.D., is Assistant Director, Pharmacoeconomic Research, Glaxo Inc., Research Triangle Park, NC. L. Deane Donnigan, Pharm.D., is Drug Information Specialist, Emory University Hospital. Johnny A. Stanfield is Research Nurse, Department of Surgery, Medical College of Georgia. Talmadge A. Bowden, Jr., M.D., is Professor of Surgery, Medical College of Georgia. At the time of this study, Dr. Coleman was Clinical Pharmacy Resident and Dr. Donnigan was Staff Pharmacist, Medical College of Georgia Hospital.

Address reprint requests to Dr. Benson at Department of Pharmacy Services (A-050), University Hospital, 50 North Medical Drive, Salt Lake City, UT 84132.

Supported by a grant from Glaxo Inc.

Presented in part at the ASHP Midyear Clinical Meeting, Las Vegas, NV, December 5, 1990.

Table 1.
Demographic and Clinical Data (n = 101)

Variable	No. (%) Patients
Age (yr)[a]	43.2 ± 15.7
Weight (kg)[a]	77.4 ± 23.1
Duration of operation (hr)[a]	3.69 ± 1.78
Duration of hospitalization (days after surgery)[a]	3.31 ± 1.86
Race	
White	58 (57.4)
Black	43 (42.6)
Gender	
Female	73 (72.3)
Male	28 (27.7)
Nausea or vomiting	42 (41.6)
Promethazine administered[b]	30 (71.4)
Anesthetic or induction agents used	
Isoflurane or enflurane	98 (97.0)
Narcotic (e.g., sufentanil)	92 (91.1)
Thiopental sodium	84 (83.2)
Nitrous oxide	64 (63.4)
Surgical procedure	
Cholecystectomy	56 (55.4)
Colostomy closure	13 (12.9)
Gastrectomy	7 (6.9)
Splenectomy	4 (4.0)
Colostomy	4 (4.0)
Other	17 (16.8)
Nasogastric tube placed postoperatively	64 (63.4)
Histamine H_2-receptor blocking agent given preoperatively	55 (54.5)

[a]Expressed as mean ± S.D.
[b]Of 42 patients with nausea or vomiting.

years; 73 were women and 28 were men. The most common procedure was cholecystectomy, which accounted for 55.4% of all surgeries.

The overall incidence of nausea or vomiting was 41.6%, with a duration ranging from one to at least seven days (in two patients) after surgery. The incidence of nausea alone was 23.8% and that of nausea with vomiting was 16.8%. Because only one patient had vomiting alone, data on nausea or vomiting were combined in all analyses. Of the 42 patients who had nausea or vomiting, the onset in 34 (81%) was on the first postoperative day. The onset of nausea or vomiting in the other eight patients was on the second day for four, the third day for three, and the seventh day for one. An antiemetic agent (promethazine) was used postoperatively in 30 patients who had nausea or vomiting. Interestingly, promethazine was also administered to six patients with neither symptom.

The incidence of nausea or vomiting did not appear to differ according to such descriptive variables as age, race, weight, type of surgery, or anesthetic or induction agents. There was an apparent trend in the incidence of nausea or vomiting between males and females (28.6% versus 46.6%, respectively), but it was not significant ($p = 0.10$).

Duration of nausea or vomiting was found to differ with patient weights. A significantly longer mean ± S.D. duration of nausea or vomiting was observed among patients weighing less than 100 kg (0.93 ± 1.46 days, $n = 84$) as opposed to patients weighing 100 kg or more (0.18 ± 0.39 days, $n = 17$; $p = 0.036$). Trends that were not significant included a longer duration of nausea or vomiting in patients who received postoperative meperidine as compared with morphine or buprenorphine ($p = 0.24$) and a tendency for patients 40–60 years of age to have a longer duration of nausea or vomiting than those aged 18–39 or 60–81 ($p = 0.12$). The duration of nausea or vomiting did not appear to differ according to other patient variables.

No significant difference was detected in the mean ± S.D. duration of hospitalization between those patients who had nausea or vomiting and those who did not (3.28 ± 1.76 versus 3.33 ± 1.94 days, respectively; $p = 0.92$). However, when only those patients who experienced postoperative nausea or vomiting were considered, there was a significant correlation between the duration of hospitalization and the duration of nausea or vomiting ($r = 0.56$, $p = 0.0009$).

A multiple-regression analysis was conducted using duration of hospitalization as the dependent variable. Age, weight, surgical procedure, duration of surgery, presence of nasogastric tube, duration of nausea or vomiting, postoperative analgesic agent used, use of a histamine H_2-receptor blocking agent preoperatively, and number of days until patients resumed a regular diet were entered as independent variables. ANOVA revealed significantly shorter periods until regular diet was resumed for cholecystectomy procedures compared with all other surgeries ($p < 0.05$). Mean ± S.D. number of days to regular diet was 2.2 ± 1.1 for cholecystectomy patients and 5.8 ± 1.6, 5.0 ± 0.8, 6.6 ± 1.1, 5.0 ± 1.0, and 5.4 ± 1.9 for patients with colostomy closure, splenectomy, gastrectomy, colostomy, and other surgical procedures, respectively. The mean ± S.D. duration of hospitalization was also significantly different ($p < 0.05$, ANOVA) for cholecystectomy patients (2.5 ± 1.4 days) as compared with other surgeries (4.9 ± 2.0, 5.0 ± 1.0, 5.5 ± 0.7, 5.7 ± 0.6, and 4.9 ± 1.9 days, respectively). Therefore, surgical procedure was treated as a two-level variable (cholecystectomy or noncholecystectomy) in the regression model. The resultant model was significant (adjusted $R^2 = 0.65$, $p = 0.0001$). Number of days until a regular diet was tolerated was the only variable with a beta coefficient significantly different from zero ($p = 0.0001$), indicating a significant correlation between days until a regular diet was resumed and duration of hospital stay. The standardized beta coefficient for this variable indicated that 72% of the variance in duration of hospital stay was explained by the delay until a regular diet was resumed. Duration of nausea or vomiting was the next most prominent variable (14%) but was not significant ($p = 0.07$). When noncholecystectomy procedures were analyzed separately, the contribution of delay until regular diet to the model was not significant.

Discussion. The incidence of nausea or vomiting after abdominal surgery has been sparsely reported; the incidence in this study (41.6%) was slightly higher than in previous reports (25–35%).[3] This difference may be partly due to our data collection criteria. We considered the presence of either nausea or vomiting to be a positive result, whereas previous investigators have reported incidences as both nausea and vomiting.

Perioperative administration of meperidine has been reported by other investigators to cause more postoperative nausea and vomiting than administration of other injectable analgesic agents.[1] We noted a trend toward greater duration of nausea or vomiting among patients treated with meperidine compared with morphine or buprenorphine.

The finding of a significant difference in duration of nausea or vomiting among patients of differing weights confirmed our clinical observations. However, this conflicts with previous reports in the literature.[1,3] A possible explanation is the difference in anesthetic agents used among studies.[1] A correlation between weight and duration of nausea or vomiting implies that certain subpopulations of patients may be at increased risk of postoperative gastrointestinal symptoms.

Higher incidences of postoperative nausea and vomiting have previously been reported in females and in middle-aged patients.[1,3] In fact, the higher incidence in middle-aged patients has been attributed to selection of surgical procedures that primarily affect women in this age group.[3] We noted trends (higher incidences of nausea or vomiting in women and in patients between 40 and 60 years) in our data that support these previous reports, but the differences were not significant. If such differences exist, this may alert the clinician to alter the selection of anesthetic or analgesic agents or to be more aggressive with antiemetic drugs in middle-aged female patients. Use of nasogastric tubes, duration of surgery, and number or type of anesthetic agents used during surgery, which are frequently cited as causes of postoperative nausea and vomiting, were not found to have a significant correlation with either incidence or duration of nausea or vomiting in our study, suggesting that these perioperative factors may not be reliable predictors of postoperative nausea and vomiting for many patients.

An important finding was the relationship between time until resumption of a regular diet and duration of hospitalization after cholecystectomy. Future research needs to be directed at managing factors that delay resumption of a regular diet; such research could result in cost savings by shortening hospital stay. Other gastrointestinal surgical procedures will require further study to determine whether such a relationship exists.

A related finding was the correlation between duration of nausea or vomiting and duration of hospitalization in patients who had at least one episode of nausea or vomiting. Given the obvious relationship between nausea or vomiting and ability to resume a regular diet, controlling nausea or vomiting appears to have the potential for decreasing hospital stay in some patients. Unfortunately, it is still unknown what characteristics will identify patients most likely to have a shortened hospital stay as a result of antiemetic therapy. The lack of a difference in duration of hospitalization between patients with and without nausea or vomiting was surprising but may be due to the effects of other variables on hospital stay for patients without nausea or vomiting.

A limitation of this study was the way in which the data on nausea and vomiting were collected. Since patients were interviewed once each day regarding their nausea or vomiting, only a positive or negative result was recorded each day, and the severity of symptoms (e.g., number of vomiting episodes, duration of each episode) was not recorded. This precluded the use of an interval-level variable for nausea or vomiting in the analyses and examination of the intensity of nausea or vomiting by procedure.

Conclusion. In this study, the incidence of nausea or vomiting after abdominal surgery was 41.6%. Patient weight and type of surgery correlated with the incidence or duration of nausea or vomiting. There was a direct correlation between nausea or vomiting and length of hospital stay in those patients who had at least one episode of nausea or vomiting. Time until resumption of a regular diet was the strongest determinant of length of hospital stay.

References

1. Bellville JW, Bross ID, Howland WS. Postoperative nausea and vomiting. IV: factors related to postoperative nausea and vomiting. *Anesthesiology.* 1960; 21:186-93.
2. Hovorka J, Korttila K, Erkola O. The experience of the person ventilating the lungs does influence postoperative nausea and vomiting. *Acta Anaesthesiol Scand.* 1990; 34:203-5.
3. Purkis IE. Factors that influence postoperative vomiting. *Can Anaesth Soc J.* 1964; 11:335-53.

Commentary

Lowering the plasma fibrinogen concentration with drugs

Edzard Ernst

Clin Pharm. 1992; 11:968-71

There is little doubt that a high plasma fibrinogen concentration is a major, independent cardiovascular risk factor[1-4]; many clinical studies strongly support this view.[5-12] In most of these studies fibrinogen had as much influence as cholesterol and other accepted cardiovascular risk factors. Several preconditions of a cause-and-effect relationship between fibrinogen and atherosclerosis are fulfilled. The degree of hyperfibrinogenemia is correlated with the degree of cardiovascular risk,[5-11] and there are plausible pathophysiological mechanisms through which fibrinogen could harm the cardiovascular system. High fibrinogen levels are associated with a state of hypercoagulability that predisposes individuals to thrombotic events. Fibrinogen is a cofactor for platelet aggregation, and it is an important determinant of the properties of blood flow through its effects on plasma viscosity and red blood cell aggregation. Finally, fibrinogen directly affects the vessel wall by enhancing the proliferation of smooth muscle cells.[1-4]

It seems possible or even likely that a high fibrinogen concentration is causally related to cardiovascular events. Using drugs to lower fibrinogen levels deliberately might therefore become a practice in the future.[13] This paper summarizes the published data on oral fibrinogen-lowering drugs. The aim is to describe these agents and to discuss problems that must first be resolved before the drugs are used to lower fibrinogen therapeutically.

Fibrates. Clofibrate reduced the plasma fibrinogen concentration from 4.3 g/L to 3.3 g/L on average when given at a dosage of 2 g/day to patients with peripheral arterial occlusive disease.[14] The basic findings of this controlled study have been confirmed repeatedly. For example, a World Health Organization trial also showed a significant decline in fibrinogen levels with clofibrate.[15] This effect may have been related to an observed decline in mortality from cardiovascular disease; the reduction was greatest in individuals with high fibrinogen levels at the beginning of the study.

Bezafibrate,[16] fenofibrate,[17] and ciprofibrate[18] also lower fibrinogen concentrations. Of these, bezafibrate has been the most thoroughly investigated. Winocour et al.[19] conducted a placebo-controlled, double-blind trial in hyperlipoproteinemic patients with type I diabetes. The researchers reported an average reduction in the plasma fibrinogen concentration from 4.1 g/L to 2.9 g/L after administering bezafibrate 400 mg/day for three months. Most other studies of bezafibrate have shown similar reductions in fibrinogen. When patients with an excessively high plasma fibrinogen concentration are treated, the decline may be more marked,[20] but this might be due to the phenomenon of regression toward the mean.

Etofibrate did not have a significant influence on plasma fibrinogen levels in a placebo-controlled trial.[21] One open study showed that fibrinogen levels fell significantly when gemfibrozil was given for 90 days to patients with type IV hyperlipoproteinemia.[22]

We do not know how fibrates lower fibrinogen, but two possibilities have been discussed: an interaction with apolipoprotein A and an inhibition of the hepatic synthesis of this protein.[19] Fibrates frequently have adverse effects. Their fibrinogen-lowering potential is therefore best reserved for hypercholesterolemic patients with high fibrinogen levels.

Other Lipid-Lowering Agents. Simvastatin does not have a notable effect on fibrinogen levels in hypercholesterolemic patients,[23] and lovastatin was reported to increase fibrinogen in an open study involving familial hypercholesterolemia.[24] The latter finding was not confirmed in a similar trial.[25] The discrepancy cannot be explained on the basis of the published data.

Beta-Adrenergic-Receptor Blockers. Propranolol[26] and celiprolol[27] have been shown to lower plasma fibrinogen concentrations in angina pectoris patients in open studies. Metoprolol tartrate 100 mg, given to healthy volunteers twice daily for two weeks, did not significantly lower plasma fibrinogen.[28] An analysis of survivors of myocardial infarction showed that patients treated with various β blockers had a lower plasma fibrinogen concentration three to six months after infarction than those who did not take such medications.[29] Even though the designs of these studies can be

Edzard Ernst, Ph.D., M.D., is Professor and Head, Department of Physical Medicine and Rehabilitation, University of Vienna, Währinger Gürtel 18-20, A-1097 Vienna, Austria.

criticized, the fibrinogen-lowering potential of β blockers is worth investigating in detail.

Antiplatelet Drugs. Ticlopidine has repeatedly been shown to reduce plasma fibrinogen. It was given for 12 months to patients with intermittent claudication and led to an 11% reduction in the plasma fibrinogen concentration.[30] It induced a 20% decrease when administered for 12 months to patients with cerebrovascular disorders.[31] When ticlopidine hydrochloride 500 mg/day or placebo was given for three weeks to stroke patients, fibrinogen levels fell (by 17%) only in the treated group.[32]

Dipyridamole[33] and aspirin[34] have both been found to lower fibrinogen, but these studies require confirmation with a more rigorous design. The use of antiplatelet drugs for the mere purpose of lowering fibrinogen levels would be highly questionable—first, because the effect is only marginal; second, because of the well-known adverse effects of these substances; and third, because it has not yet been shown that reducing the fibrinogen concentration changes the risk of adverse cardiovascular events.

Pentoxifylline. The literature on the relation between pentoxifylline and fibrinogen is extensive but contradictory.[35] For instance, when pentoxifylline was given to patients with cerebral ischemia at a dosage of 1200 mg/day for 25 days, fibrinogen levels fell significantly.[36] Other investigators have used the same dosage for four or five weeks in patients with intermittent claudication without finding significant alterations in fibrinogen levels.[37,38] Then again, others have found significant changes when giving patients with intermittent claudication the same dosage for 90 days.[39] These discrepancies cannot be explained, and an answer to whether pentoxifylline truly has an effect on plasma fibrinogen must await a well-designed trial.

The clinical effectiveness of pentoxifylline in peripheral arterial occlusive disease is mediated by its rheologic actions on red and white blood cells rather than by the changes it may induce in plasma fibrinogen.[40]

Other Vasodilators. Other vasoactive medications that (under a variety of clinical conditions) have been found to reduce fibrinogen are nafronyl oxalate,[41] suloctidil,[42] troxerutin,[43] xanthinol niacinate,[44] prazosin,[45] isoxsuprine,[46] and niceritrol.[47] These findings need to be confirmed in controlled trials by independent groups. Vinburnine significantly lowered fibrinogen levels in a placebo-controlled, double-blind trial conducted in patients with diabetic microangiopathy.[48]

Calcium Dobesilate. Calcium dobesilate lowered fibrinogen concentrations when given to patients with diabetic retinopathy at a dosage of 1.5 g/day for three months.[49] This finding was confirmed in a randomized, placebo-controlled trial with similar patients.[50] The fibrinogen concentration fell from 3.3 g/L to 2.7 g/L during three months of treatment. Thus, the fibrinogen-lowering effect of calcium dobesilate is relatively well established, although the mechanism is not known. Since the drug has only a few adverse effects, its potential as a fibrinogen-lowering agent should be investigated further.

Anabolic Steroids. Stanozolol lowered fibrinogen levels in healthy volunteers[51] and in patients with Raynaud's phenomenon.[52] The drug was recently found to be effective in the treatment of skin ulcers caused by cryofibrinogenemia; it is believed to break down cryofibrinogens.[53] Other anabolic compounds have exhibited similar effects on fibrinogen.[34,54] The use of anabolic steroids to reduce fibrinogen would, however, be limited to rare clinical situations.

Other Medications. Other agents that have been shown to reduce fibrinogen in various clinical situations are *Allium sativum* (garlic),[55] sulodexide,[56] sulfinpyrazone,[57] and β-benzalbutyrate.[34] When given to hyperthyroid patients, methimazole lowered the plasma fibrinogen concentration from 4.6 g/L to 3.3 g/L.[58] When given to women after breast cancer operations, tamoxifen reduced fibrinogen from 3.2 g/L to 2.7 g/L.[59] It is questionable whether the drug treatment per se or the successful treatment of the illness resulted in the reduction in fibrinogen levels.

The calcium-channel blocking agent nisoldipine was reported to reduce fibrinogen in a double-blind, crossover trial when given to patients with coronary heart disease at a dosage of 10 mg twice daily for four weeks.[60] One can only estimate mean values from the data; they were around 6 g/L at baseline, did not change during the placebo phase, and dropped to around 5 g/L by the end of treatment. Thus, the baseline values were excessively high and were not brought into the normal range by the treatment. This trial (even though double-blind) needs to be confirmed. Other calcium antagonists do not seem to influence fibrinogen levels.[a]

In an open placebo-controlled study, defibrotide, an oral "profibrinolytic and antithrombotic" drug, lowered the fibrinogen concentration from 3.9 g/L to 3.0 g/L during six months of therapy.[61] The drug was given at 400 mg twice daily to patients with intermittent claudication.

Finally, a study in rabbits showed that fibrinogen can be lowered by powder of the seaweed *Laminaria digitata* (1 g daily for two weeks).[62]

Discussion. The substances that have been reported to lower the plasma fibrinogen concentration are many and heterogeneous. Interpretation of the data is difficult because, with only a few exceptions, the drugs were given to patients with the intention of treating a defined disease or symptom. Therefore, the lowering of fibrinogen could have been a mere by-product of the intended clinical effect of the therapy. For example, if the fibrinogen level is elevated because of bacterial infection, the elimination of the bacteria by, for instance, penicillin would indirectly cause a reduction in fibrinogen. Yet nobody would suggest that penicillin has fibrinogen-lowering properties. Thus, it is difficult to decide to what extent the fibrinogen level was lowered by the drug and to what extent it decreased because some underlying disease process was successfully inhibited.

A simple way out of this dilemma is to conduct trials in healthy volunteers with normal baseline fibrinogen levels. Another approach would be valuable when using cholesterol-lowering medications: A controlled trial could be performed in which subjects received either one such agent with no effect on fibrinogen or another one with fibrinogen-lowering properties; both agents would have similar effects on blood lipids. Comparing the rates of cardiovascular events for the two groups might indicate the clinical value of fibrinogen-lowering strategies.

Further research is needed to (1) test whether lowering fibrinogen independently reduces the occurrence of cardiovascular events, (2) define how fibrinogen levels are controlled physiologically and the mechanism by which drugs might lower them, and (3) identify agents that specifically reduce fibrinogen. At present, it seems premature to use any medication solely or even preferentially because of its fibrinogen-lowering effect.

Conclusion. Hyperfibrinogenemia is a major cardiovascular risk factor, and many drugs are associated with lowering of the plasma fibrinogen concentration. Further research is needed, however, to determine whether medications should be used for their fibrinogen-lowering effect.

[a]Ernst E, unpublished data.

References

1. Ernst E. Plasma fibrinogen—an independent cardiovascular risk factor. *J Intern Med*. 1990; 227:365-72.
2. Cook NS, Ubben D. Fibrinogen as a major risk factor in cardiovascular disease. *Trends Pharmacol Sci*. 1990; 11:444-51.
3. DiMinno G, Mancini M. Measuring plasma fibrinogen to predict stroke and myocardial infarction. *Arteriosclerosis*. 1990; 10:1-7.
4. Ernst E. Fibrinogen as a major risk factor. *Br Med J*. 1991; 303:596-7.
5. Meade TW, Mellows W, Brozovic M et al. Haemostatic function and ischemic heart disease: principal results of the Northwick Park Heart Study. *Lancet*. 1986; 2:533-7.
6. Wilhelmsen L, Svärdsudd K, Korsan-Bengtsen K et al. Fibrinogen as a risk factor for stroke and myocardial infarction. *N Engl J Med*. 1984; 311:501-5.
7. Stone MC, Thorp JM. Plasma fibrinogen—a major coronary risk factor. *J R Coll Gen Pract*. 1985; 35:565-9.
8. Breddin HK, Krzywanek HJ, Althoff P. Spontaneous platelet aggregation and coagulation parameters as risk factors for arterial occlusions in diabetics. Results of the PARD study. *Int Angiol*. 1986; 5:181-95.
9. Kannel WB, Wolf PA, Castelli WP et al. Fibrinogen and risk of cardiovascular disease. *JAMA*. 1987; 258:1183-6.
10. Balleisen L, Schulte H, Assmann G et al. Coagulation factors and the progress of coronary heart disease. *Lancet*. 1987; 2:461. Letter.
11. Yarnell JWG, Baker JA, Sweetnam PM et al. Fibrinogen, viscosity, and white blood cell count are major risk factors for ischemic heart disease. *Circulation*. 1991; 83:836-44.
12. Kannel WB, D'Agostino RB, Wilson PWF et al. Diabetes, fibrinogen, and risk of cardiovascular disease: the Framingham experience. *Am Heart J*. 1990; 120:672-6.
13. Ernst E. Orale, fibrinogensenkende Medikation. *Munch Med Wochenschr*. 1983; 125:94-6.
14. Dormandy JA, Gutteridge JMC, Hoare E et al. Effect of clofibrate on blood viscosity in intermittent claudication. *Br Med J*. 1974; 4:259-61.
15. Green KG, Heady A, Oliver MF. Blood pressure, cigarette smoking and heart attack in the WHO cooperative trial of clofibrate. *Int J Epidemiol*. 1989; 18:355-60.
16. Zimmermann R, Ehlers W, Walter E. The effect of bezafibrate on the fibrinolytic system. *Atherosclerosis*. 1978; 29:477-85.
17. Leschke M, Hoffken H, Schmidtsdorff A. Einfluss von Fenofibrat auf Fibrinogenkonzentration und Blutfluidität. *Dtsch Med Wochenschr*. 1989; 114:939-44.
18. Simpson JA, Lorimer AR, Walker JD et al. Effect of ciprofibrate on platelet aggregation and fibrinolysis in patients with hypercholesterolaemia. *Thromb Haemost*. 1985; 54:442-4.
19. Winocour PH, Durrington PN, Bhatnagar D et al. Double blind placebo-controlled study of the effects of bezafibrate on blood lipids, lipoproteins, and fibrinogen in hyperlipidaemic type 1 diabetes mellitus. *Diabetic Med*. 1990; 7:736-43.
20. Niort G, Bulgarelli A, Cassader M et al. Effect of short term treatment with bezafibrate on plasma fibrinogen, fibrinopeptide A, platelet activation and blood filterability in atherosclerotic hyperfibrinogenemic patients. *Atherosclerosis*. 1988; 71:113-9.
21. Ernst E, Matrai A. Die Effekte von Etofibrat auf die Fliesseigenschaften des Blutes. *Therapiewoche*. 1988; 38:45-7.
22. Avellone G, DiGarbo V, Panno AV et al. Changes induced by gemfibrozil on lipidic, coagulative and fibrinolytic pattern in patients with type IV hyperlipoproteinemia. *Int Angiol*. 1988; 7:270-7.
23. Bo M, Bonino F, Neirotti et al. Hemorheologic and coagulative pattern in hypercholesterolemic subjects treated with lipid lowering drugs. *Angiology*. 1991; 42:106-13.
24. Beigel Y, Fuchs J, Snir M et al. Lovastatin therapy in heterozygous familial hypercholesterolaemic patients: effect on blood rheology and fibrinogen levels. *J Intern Med*. 1991; 230:23-7.
25. Koppensteiner R, Hinar E, Ehringer H. Effect of lovastatin on hemorheology in type II hyperlipoproteinemia. *Atherosclerosis*. 1990; 83:53-8.
26. Mehrotra TN, Mital HS, Singh VS et al. Platelet adhesiveness, plasma fibrinogen and fibrinolytic activity in angina pectoris before and after propranolol treatment. *J Assoc Physicians India*. 1983; 31:641-3.
27. Herrmann JM, Mayer EO. A long term study of the effects of celiprolol on blood pressure and lipid-associated risk factors. *Am Heart J*. 1988; 116:1416-21.
28. Ernst E, Roloff C, Marshall M. Betablocker erhöht Blutfluidität. *Herz Gefässe*. 1984; 4:447-8.
29. Berglund U, Wallentin L, von Schenk H. Platelet function and plasma fibrinogen and their relations to gender, smoking habits, obesity and beta-blocker treatment in young survivors of myocardial infarction. *Thromb Haemost*. 1988; 60:21-4.
30. Aukland A, Hurlow RA, George AJ et al. Platelet inhibition with ticlopidine in atherosclerotic intermittent claudication. *J Clin Pathol*. 1982; 35:740-3.
31. Cornad J, Lecrubier C, Scarabin P et al. Effects of long term administration of ticlopidine on platelet function and hemostatic variables. *Thromb Res*. 1980; 20:143-8.
32. Ciuffetti G, Aisa G, Mercuri M et al. Effects of ticlopidine on the neurologic outcome and the hemorheologic pattern in the postacute phase of ischemic stroke: a pilot study. *Angiology*. 1990; 41:505-11.
33. Passero S, Giannini F, Nardini M et al. Effetti della reductione della viscosita ematica adematocrito constante sul flusso ematico cerebrale. *Ric Clin Lab*. 1985; 15(Suppl 1):301-5.
34. Pickart LR, Thaler MM. Fatty acids, fibrinogen and blood flow: a general mechanism for hyperfibrinogenemia and its pathologic consequences. *Med Hypotheses*. 1980; 6:545-57.
35. Ward A, Clissold SP. Pentoxifylline. *Drugs*. 1987; 34:50-97.
36. Ott E, Lechner H. Hemorheologic conditions in patients with pentoxifylline. *Ric Clin Lab*. 1981; 11(Suppl 1):253-6.
37. Ernst E, Matrai A, Weihmayr T et al. Behandlung der arteriellen verschlusskrankheit. *Munch Med Wochenschr*. 1985; 127:917-9.
38. Triebe G, Münnich U, Liebold F. Haemodilution or pentoxifylline in the treatment of peripheral vascular disease. *Dtsch Med Wochenschr*. 1992; 117:523-30.

39. Bachet P, Lancrenon S, Chassoux G. Fibrinogen and pentoxifylline. *Thromb Res.* 1989; 55:161-3.
40. Ernst E. Hemorheological therapy. In: Chien S, Dormandy J, Ernst E, eds. Clinical hemorheology. Dordrecht, Netherlands: Nijhoff; 1987.
41. Kiesewetter H, Jung F, Schwab J et al. Periphere arterielle Verschlusskrankheit. *Munch Med Wochenschr.* 1987; 129:21-4.
42. Roba J, Roncucci R, Lambelin G. Pharmacological properties of suloctidil. *Acta Clin Belg.* 1977; 32:3-7.
43. LeDevehat C, Lemoine A. Hemorheological changes induced by troxerutin in patients affected by venous insufficiency of lower legs. *Clin Hemorheol.* 1985; 5:740. Abstract.
44. Davis E, Rozov H. The effect of xantinol nicotinate on small blood vessels. *Bibl Anat.* 1973; 11:334-9.
45. Letcher RL, Chien S, Laragh JH. Changes in blood viscosity accompanying the response to prazosin in patients with essential hypertension. *J Cardiovasc Pharmacol.* 1979; 1(Suppl 6):S8-S20.
46. DiPerri T, Forconi S, Agnusdei D et al. The effects of intravenous isoxsuprine on blood viscosity in patients with occlusive peripheral arterial disease. *Br J Clin Pharmacol.* 1978; 5:225-60.
47. Hamazaki T, Hasunuma K, Kobayashi S et al. The effects on lipids, blood viscosity and platelet aggregation of combined use of niceritrol and a low dose of acetylsalicylic acid. *Atherosclerosis.* 1985; 55:107-13.
48. LeDevehat, Vimeux M. Pharmacological study of the action of vinburnine versus placebo. *Int Angiol.* 1989; 8:57-61.
49. Barras JP, Graf C. Behandlung der Hyperviskosität bei diabetischer Retinopathie mit Doxium. *Vasa.* 1980; 9:161-4.
50. Benarroch JS, Brodsky M, Rubinstein A et al. Treatment of blood hyperviscosity with calcium dobesilate in patients with diabetic retinopathy. *Ophthalmic Res.* 1985; 17:131-8.
51. Preston FE, Burakowski BK, Portes NR et al. The fibrinolytic response to stanozolol in normal subjects. *Thromb Res.* 1981; 22:543-51.
52. Jarret PEM, Morland, Browse NL. Treatment of Raynaud's phenomenon by fibrinolytic enhancement. *Br Med J.* 1978; 2:523-5.
53. Falanga V, Kirsner RS, Eaglstein WH et al. Stanozolol in treatment of leg ulcers due to cryofibrinogenaemia. *Lancet.* 1991; 338:347-8.
54. Charkabarti R, Faernley GR. Phenphormin plus ethylestrenol in survivors of myocardial infarction. *Lancet.* 1976; 2:556-8.
55. Harenberg J, Giese C, Zimmermann R. Effect of dried garlic on blood coagulation, fibrinolysis, platelet aggregation and serum cholesterol levels in patients with hyperlipoproteinaemia. *Atherosclerosis.* 1988; 74:247-9.
56. Castelluccio A, Bologna E. Effect of solodexide on blood viscosity in patients with peripheral vascular disease. *Curr Med Res Opin.* 1991; 12:325-31.
57. Johnston RV, Lowe GDO, Drummond MM et al. A study of the effect of sulphinpyrazone ("Anturan") on blood viscosity. *Curr Med Res Opin.* 1979; 6:271-3.
58. Conti ML, Mameli G, Sorano GG et al. Fibrinogen, FPA in hyperthyroidism before and after treatment. *Thromb Res Suppl.* 1991; 64(Suppl 13):22. Abstract.
59. Love RR, Surawicz TS, Williams EC. Antithrombin III level, fibrinogen level, and platelet count changes with adjuvant tamoxifen therapy. *Arch Intern Med.* 1992; 152:317-20.
60. Salmasi AM, Salmasi S, MacDonald G et al. Improvement of silent myocardial ischaemia and reduction of plasma fibrinogen during nisoldipine therapy in occult coronary arterial disease. *Int J Cardiol.* 1991; 31:71-80.
61. Marelli C, Belcaro G, Girardello R. Defibroside in patients with intermittent claudication. *Curr Ther Res.* 1990; 47:459-65.
62. Tang ZL, Shen SF. A study of *Laminaria digitata* powder on experimental hyperlipoproteinemia and its hemorheology. *Chung Hsi I Chieh Ho Tsa Chih.* 1989; 9:223-5.

“

Failure of Controlled Clinical Trial Data To Reach the Literature

Not too long ago clinicians could read the peer-reviewed literature and decide whether there was scientific justification for using a drug. The pharmaceutical firms were as interested in publishing the results of their clinical trials as the physicians who performed those trials. Although in general this may remain so, there appears to be an increasing number of exceptions. . . .

When the practicing physician no longer has access to the scientific data, he or she becomes dependent on an FDA evaluation. . . .

The FDA should be a strong link in the chain of protections to the patient. However, it should not be the only link. The FDA should insist that the data from controlled clinical trials be sent to peer-reviewed journals as well. The clinicians who perform therapeutic studies should have the right, as part of their contractual agreements with the pharmaceutical firms, to have their findings submitted for publication. Until then, clinicians deciding whether or not to use a new drug may remain uncomfortably reliant on the simple fact that the FDA approved it.

—Mindel JS. Failure of controlled clinical trial data to reach the literature. *Clin Pharmacol Ther.* 1992; 52:4-5.

”

DUE Criteria

The DUE Criteria *section of* Clinical Pharmacy *features model drug-use evaluation criteria that may be employed as a component of a comprehensive quality assurance program. The criteria sets are presented in the format used in the ASHP book* Criteria for Drug Use Evaluation. *Some of the criteria sets will have been originally published in that book; others will be presented here for the first time and published in future volumes of the ASHP book. The practitioners who developed a criteria set are acknowledged.*

In selecting drug products for coverage in DUE Criteria, *priority is given to products that have been recently marketed, those that are frequently prescribed, those that have high potential risk associated with their use, and those that are expensive. When feasible, a criteria set will be linked with a Drug Review that appears in the same issue.*

These criteria sets are a starting point for the development of DUE criteria for a specific practice setting. Readers are encouraged to modify the model criteria to fit their own circumstances.

Criteria for use of sumatriptan in adult inpatients and outpatients[a]

Element	Standard 100%	Standard 0%	Exception[b] or Critical Preventive/ Responsive Measure[c]		Sources of Information
Justification for Use					
1. Abortive treatment of migraine attacks in patients with infrequent moderate to severe headache[1-5] a. Who do not respond to their current abortive regimen or b. In whom other treatments for migraine abortion (e.g., ergot-containing compounds, nonsteroidal anti-inflammatory drugs) are contraindicated or	X		1A. None	1.	History and physical (H&P), physician orders, progress notes, emergency room record (ER)
2. Abortive treatment of cluster headache attacks in patients who do not respond to current therapies[6]	X		2A. None	2.	H&P, physician orders, progress notes, ER
Critical (Process) Indicators					
3. No history of hypersensitivity to sumatriptan	X		3A. None	3.	H&P, ER, allergy record
4. Sumatriptan not used in pregnant or lactating women	X		4A. Benefit outweighs risk to fetus or baby	4,4A.	H&P, progress notes, laboratory reports (human chorionic gonadotropin)
5. Sumatriptan not used for long-term migraine prophylaxis	X		5A. None	5.	H&P, physician orders, progress notes, ER
6. Blood urea nitrogen, serum creatinine, alanine aminotransferase, aspartate aminotransferase, alkaline phosphatase, lactate dehydrogenase obtained before initiation of therapy and if there is any suspected renal or hepatic impairment	X		6A. None	6.	Physician orders, progress notes, laboratory reports
7. Sumatriptan not used in patients with[7] a. Uncontrolled hypertension b. Ischemic heart disease c. Previous myocardial infarction or Prinzmetal's angina	X		7A. None	7.	Physician orders, progress notes, electrocardiogram (ECG), medication administration record (MAR)

Prepared by Van Doren Hsu, Pharm.D., Clinical Specialist, Neuroscience, University of Maryland Medical System, 22 South Greene Street, Baltimore, MD 21201.

Element	Standard 100%	Standard 0%	Exception[b] or Critical Preventive/ Responsive Measure[c]	Sources of Information	
d. Concurrent therapy with monoamine oxidase inhibitors, selective serotonin-reuptake inhibitors, or lithium					
e. Acute-phase (21 days) subarachnoid hemorrhage due to aneurysm rupture					
8. Demonstration of competent subcutaneous injection technique by patient before self-injection of sumatriptan[8]	X		8A. Proper injection technique demonstrated by a caregiver	8,8A.	Progress notes, nursing notes
9. Appropriate subcutaneous dosage in adult using the autoinjector: 6 mg per injection at the onset of headache, with maximum of two injections daily with a minimum of one hour between injections[1,2,6,d]	X		9A. Headache relief obtained after one injection	9,9A.	Physician orders, progress notes, MAR
10. Appropriate oral dosage in adult: one 100 mg tablet at onset of headache, up to three tablets daily, with a minimum of two hours between tablets[3-5,d]	X		10A. Headache relief obtained after one or two tablets	10,10A.	Physician orders, progress notes, MAR
11. Subsequent doses of sumatriptan not administered if there is no response to the initial dose[d]	X		11A. None	11.	Physician orders, progress notes, MAR
Complications					
12. Injection-site reaction: pain, erythema, irritation[1,2,6,9]		X	12A. Identify other drug or nondrug causes	12,12B.	Progress notes, nursing notes
			12B. Rotate injection sites	12A.	Physician orders, progress notes, MAR
13. Gastrointestinal: taste disturbances, nausea, vomiting, transient elevation of liver function test results[3-5,10]		X	13A. Identify other drug or nondrug causes	13,13A.	Progress notes, laboratory reports, MAR, nursing notes
			13B. Change to subcutaneous injection if nausea or vomiting precludes adequate absorption of oral sumatriptan (provided that proper injection technique is used)	13B.	Physician orders, progress notes, MAR
14. Neurologic: tingling in the head, flushing, dizziness, drowsiness, vertigo, weakness[1-6,9]		X	14A. Identify other drug or nondrug causes	14,14A,B.	Progress notes, MAR, nursing notes
			14B. Discontinue if severe		
15. Cardiovascular: change in blood pressure and heart rate, ECG changes, chest tightness and pressure[1,4,7,9,11,12]		X	15A. Identify other drug or nondrug causes	15,15A-D.	Progress notes, ECG, MAR, nursing notes
			15B. Discontinue sumatriptan if chest pain occurs		
			15C. Obtain ECG if chest pain occurs		
			15D. Administer sublingual nitroglycerin if chest pain occurs		
16. Miscellaneous: malaise, fatigue, flushing, burning, warm or hot sensation, visual disturbances[1-6,9]		X	16A. Identify other drug or nondrug cause	16,16A.	Progress notes, MAR, nursing notes
Outcome Measures					
17. Subjective rating of headache severity reduced from severe or moderate to mild or none	X		17A. None	17.	Physician orders, progress notes
18. Absence of associated symptoms (nausea, vomiting, photophobia, or phonophobia) if present before treatment	X		18A. None	18.	Physician orders, progress notes
19. Improvement in functional disability to none or slight impairment of working ability	X		19A. None	19.	Physician orders, progress notes

Element	Standard 100%	Standard 0%	Exception[b] or Critical Preventive/ Responsive Measure[c]	Sources of Information
20. No recurrence of headache within 24 hours	X		20A. Patient has atypical nonmigrainous or noncluster headaches	20,20A. Physician orders, progress notes

[a]Criteria address justification for use (indications), critical (process) indicators, complications of therapy, and patient outcome. Each criterion consists of an element, a standard, exceptions to the standard, and sources of information. The element is the minimum level of evidence needed to show that patient care was optimal. The standard defines the deviation from an element that is acceptable. If no deviation is acceptable, the standard is 100%. Exceptions are circumstances in which deviation is allowable. Sources of information listed are the most reliable sources. Sources pertaining to an element or exception are identified by the number assigned to the element or exception (e.g., 4,4A).

[b]For justification of use, critical (process) indicators, and outcome measures.

[c]For complications.

[d]Quinn B, Glaxo Canada Ltd. Personal communication. 1992. Jun 30.

References

1. The Subcutaneous Sumatriptan Study Group. Treatment of migraine attacks with sumatriptan. *N Engl J Med.* 1991; 325:316-21.
2. Cady RK, Wendt JK, Kirchner JR et al. Treatment of acute migraine with subcutaneous sumatriptan. *JAMA.* 1991; 265:2831-5.
3. The Oral Sumatriptan International Multiple-Dose Study Group. Evaluation of a multiple-dose regimen of oral sumatriptan for the acute treatment of migraine. *Eur Neurol.* 1991; 31:306-13.
4. The Oral Sumatriptan and Cafergot Comparative Study Group. A randomized, double-blind comparison of sumatriptan and Cafergot in the acute treatment of migraine. *Eur Neurol.* 1991; 31:314-22.
5. The Oral Sumatriptan and Aspirin plus Metoclopramide Comparative Study Group. A study to compare oral sumatriptan with oral aspirin plus oral metoclopramide in the acute treatment of migraine. *Eur Neurol.* 1992; 32:177-84.
6. The Sumatriptan Cluster Headache Study Group. Treatment of acute cluster headache with sumatriptan. *N Engl J Med.* 1991; 325:322-6.
7. Glaxo UK. Imigran prescribing information. Uxbridge, Middlesex, England. 1992.
8. The Sumatriptan Auto-Injector Study Group. Self-treatment of acute migraine with subcutaneous sumatriptan using an auto-injector device. *Eur Neurol.* 1991; 31:323-31.
9. Brown EG, Endersby CA, Smith RN et al. The safety and tolerability of sumatriptan: an overview. *Eur Neurol.* 1991; 31:339-44.
10. Busch MA, Plachetka JR, Donn KH et al. Evaluation of the pharmacokinetics and safety of ascending single doses of GR43175 administered to healthy male volunteers. *Cephalalgia.* 1989; 9(Suppl 10):414-5. Abstract.
11. Fowler PA, Lacey LF, Thomas M et al. The clinical pharmacology, pharmacokinetics and metabolism of sumatriptan. *Eur Neurol.* 1991; 31:291-4.
12. Willett F, Curzen N, Adams J et al. Coronary vasospasm induced by subcutaneous sumatriptan. *Br Med J.* 1992; 304:1415.

in the elderly because of

a. Fewer anticholinergic adverse effects.
b. Fewer cardiovascular adverse effects.
c. Fewer gastrointestinal adverse effects.
d. Alternatives a and b are both correct.

9. What length of time should be allowed between discontinuation of sertraline therapy and initiation of monoamine oxidase inhibitor therapy?

a. One week.
b. Two weeks.
c. Three weeks.
d. Five weeks.

10. In addition to depression, the SSRIs have been effectively used for the treatment of all of the following neuropsychiatric disorders except

a Obsessive-compulsive disorder.
b Panic disorder.
c. Simple phobias.
d Alcoholism.

Answer Sheet

November 1992 ***Clinical Pharmacy***

Note: An enrollment form for the ASHP Continuing Education System appears in the June and December issues. Please accumulate all the answer sheets you wish to use in one enrollment and submit them at one time with a completed enrollment form.

The American Society of Hospital Pharmacists is approved by the American Council on Pharmaceutical Education as a provider of continuing pharmaceutical education. ACPE®

Place an X in the box(es) at the top of the column(s) corresponding to the test(s) you are taking. Darken the boxes corresponding to the correct answers.

☐ ACPE 680-204-9228

	a	b	c	d
1.	☐	☐	☐	☐
2.	☐	☐	☐	☐
3.	☐	☐	☐	☐
4.	☐	☐	☐	☐
5.	☐	☐	☐	☐
6.	☐	☐	☐	☐
7.	☐	☐	☐	☐
8.	☐	☐	☐	☐
9.	☐	☐	☐	☐
10.	☐	☐	☐	☐

ASHP Use Only
(1.0)9228_____(3)

Current Literature

Drug Reaction Alerts

Drug Reaction Alerts focuses primarily on serious, unlabeled reactions to new chemical entities. The citations are compiled monthly from International Pharmaceutical Abstracts, *which covers over 800 pharmacy and health-related journals worldwide. An address for reprints (when available) follows the name of the corresponding author in each citation.*

Pharmacists may use the FDA Adverse Reaction Report form that appears in the January and July issues of Clinical Pharmacy *for submitting reports of adverse drug reactions directly to FDA.*

Angiotensin-Converting-Enzyme Inhibitors

Mets T, De Bock V, Praet JP (Division of Geriatrics, Academic Hospital, Free University of Brussels [V.U.B.], 1090 Brussels, Belgium). First-dose hypotension, ACE inhibitors, and heart failure in the elderly. *Lancet.* 1992; 339:1487. Study. (case series; 97 elderly inpatients, mean age 83.7 years, with chronic heart failure who received **captopril** 6.25 mg; after one dose of captopril, 52 patients experienced a decrease in systolic blood pressure of ≥15%, and 5 of these patients experienced a decrease of >30%; mean decrease in blood pressure was small; maximum decrease in blood pressure occurred after 60 minutes; 3 patients experienced mild, transient symptoms from decrease in blood pressure)

Antifungals

Juhlin L (Department of Dermatology, University Hospital, S 751 85 Uppsala, Sweden). Loss of taste and **terbinafine**. *Lancet.* 1992; 339:1483. Case. (46-year-old woman with toenail infection; received terbinafine 250 mg daily for six weeks; experienced loss of taste for salty and bitter substances followed by loss of taste for sour and sweet substances one week later; withdrawal of terbinafine led to return of taste sensations in same order as they disappeared, but full ability to taste sweet substances did not return for five weeks; toenail was normal four months after start of terbinafine therapy)

Anti-infective Agents

Forster DJ, Causey DM, Rao NA (Doheny Eye Institute, University of Southern California, Los Angeles, CA 90033). Bull's eye retinopathy and **clofazimine**. *Ann Intern Med.* 1992; 116:876-7. Case. (42-year-old man with AIDS and *Mycobacterium avium–Mycobacterium intracellulare* infection; received clofazimine for 10 months; developed epithelial degeneration of retinal pigment; concomitant foscarnet, pentamidine, ethionamide, ciprofloxacin, and epoetin; withdrawal of clofazimine did not lead to subjective improvement in vision, but areas of depigmentation in fundus began to increase slightly in degree of pigmentation; died six months later from progressive cytomegalovirus and human immunodeficiency virus encephalopathy)

Zec N, Donovan JW, Aufiero TX et al. (Demers LM, Milton S. Hershey Medical Center, Hershey, PA 17033). Seizures in a patient treated with continuous **povidone–iodine** mediastinal irrigation. *N Engl J Med.* 1992; 326:1784. Case. (62-year-old man with sternal-wound infection after quadruple coronary bypass surgery; received continuous mediastinal irrigation with 1:10 solution of povidone–iodine for five days; experienced generalized seizure that lasted two minutes, then developed renal failure; serum iodide concentration, 1200 μg/dL [normal range, 5.7–7.6]; EEG showed no evidence of epileptic activity or other abnormality; replacement of povidone–iodine irrigation with neomycin–polymyxin B irrigation led to improvement in renal function)

Anti-inflammatory Agents

Vallerand H, Cossart C, Milosevic D et al. (Leone J, Departments of Respiratory Disease and Medicine, CHRU de Reims, 51092 Reims, France). Fatal pneumocystis pneumonia in asthmatic patient treated with **methotrexate**. *Lancet.* 1992; 339:1551. Case. (61-year-old patient with asthma; received weekly dose of methotrexate 15 mg by i.m. injection for total dose of 90 mg; developed opportunistic *Pneumocystis carinii* pneumonia; extensive therapy with anti-infectives and mechanical ventilation did not lead to improvement in asthma or pneumonia; died 72 hours later because of hypoxia)

Antilipemic Agents

Bannwarth B, Miremont G, Papapietro PM. Lupuslike syndrome associated with **simvastatin**. *Arch Intern Med.* 1992; 152:1093. Case. (70-year-old woman with primary hypercholesterolemia; received simvastatin 10 mg/day; developed syndrome of fever and symmetrical polyarthritis of upper limbs resembling systemic lupus erythematosus; withdrawal of simvastatin and therapy with prednisone led to relief of joint pain within three days and complete resolution of syndrome within two weeks; therapy with prednisone was tapered and discontinued two weeks later)

Antituberculars

Tajima A, Mine T, Ogata E (Tokyo University School of Medicine, Tokyo 112, Japan). **Rifampin-**associated ulcerative colitis. *Ann Intern Med.* 1992; 116:778-9. Case. (40-year-old man with pulmonary tuberculosis; received rifampin for three months; exacerbated ulcerative colitis; therapy with sulfasalazine for 10 days led to aggravation of symptoms; withdrawal of rifampin led to resolution of symptoms; positive rechallenge twice; attempt at desensitization was unsuccessful)

Benzodiazepine Antagonists

Katz Y, Boulos M, Singer P et al. (Rosenberg B, Rambam Medical Center, P.O. Box 9602, 31096 Haifa, Israel). Cardiac arrest associated with **flumazenil**. *Br Med J.* 1992; 304:1415. Case. (60-year-old man who had received diazepam for sedation during intubation; received flumazenil 0.4 mg by i.v. injection for reversal of diazepam-caused sedation; experienced cardiac arrest; died 20 minutes later despite resuscitation attempts)

Corticosteroids

Wong J, Black P (Auckland Hospital, Auckland 1, New Zealand). Acute adrenal insufficiency associated with high dose

Continued on page 980

Current Literature *Continued from page 978*

inhaled steroids. *Br Med J.* 1992; 304:1415. Case. (38-year-old man with bronchopulmonary aspergillosis; received **budesonide** 1.6 mg/day initially, then 4.8 mg/day for two weeks and increased to 6.4 mg/day for two weeks, then 3.2 mg/day for six weeks and decreased to 2.4 mg/day; complained of lethargy, malaise, nausea, vomiting, and dizziness; cosyntropin test results and blood endogenous steroid concentrations determined three weeks after dose reduction showed decreased adrenal activity; studies repeated one month later were within normal ranges)

Drug Interactions

Azana JR (Servicio de Farmacología Clínica, Clínica Universitaria de Navarra, Avda. Pio XII s/n, 31080 Pamplona, Spain), Catalán M, Alvarez MP et al. Possible interaction between **cyclosporine** and **josamycin:** description of three cases. *Clin Pharmacol Ther.* 1992; 51:572-5. Cases. (three men, aged 23, 42, and 55 years, who received cyclosporine as immunosuppressive therapy after heart transplantation; received josamycin 1 g three times daily for treatment of atypical pneumonia or *Toxoplasma* infection; developed greatly increased blood cyclosporine concentrations; withdrawal of josamycin or reduction of josamycin dosage led to progressive decrease in blood cyclosporine concentration)

Barbui T, Rambaldi A, Parenzan L et al. (Remuzzi G, Mario Negri Institute for Pharmacological Research, 24100 Bergamo, Italy). Neurological symptoms and coma associated with **doxorubicin** administration during chronic cyclosporin therapy. *Lancet.* 1992; 339:1421. Case. (49-year-old man who received **cyclosporine** 2 mg/kg/day as immunosuppressive therapy after heart transplantation and developed lymphoproliferative disease that was noticed 22 months after transplantation; received doxorubicin 60 mg as part of antineoplastic regimen; developed major neurological signs followed by coma on two occasions soon after doxorubicin dose; spontaneously recovered from first episode of coma 12 hours after onset; concomitant vincristine, cyclophosphamide, and prednisone; cyclosporine was discontinued when doxorubicin was given; computed tomographic scan of brain was normal; sepsis documented a few days after second development of coma; died eight days later; examination at autopsy showed no evidence of ischemic or hemorrhagic damage of CNS)

Redington K, Wells C, Petito F (The New York Hospital, New York, NY 10021). **Erythromycin** and valproate interaction. *Ann Intern Med.* 1992; 116:877-8. Case. (38-year-old woman who received **valproic acid** 3.5 g/day for seizure disorder; received erythromycin 250 mg four times daily for one week as treatment for upper-respiratory-tract infection; developed anxiety and confusion; concomitant clorazepate dipotassium and lithium carbonate; serum valproic acid concentration, 260.4 mg/L [therapeutic range, 50–100]; withdrawal of valproic acid and erythromycin led to gradual decrease in serum valproic acid concentration; reinstitution of valproic acid 3.5 g/day led to no further incident and improvement in symptoms over next 24 hours)

Hypotensive Agents

Milavetz JJ (Department of Internal Medicine, University of Arizona Medical Center, 1501 N. Campbell Avenue, Tucson, AZ 85724), Popovtzer MM. Angiotensin-converting enzyme inhibitors and glycosuria. *Arch Intern Med.* 1992; 152:1081-3. Case. (29-year-old man with renal transplant and increasing hypertension; received **lisinopril** 20 mg/day for three days; developed oliguria and fluid volume overload; concomitant terazosin hydrochloride, cyclosporine, prednisone, and azathioprine; withdrawal of lisinopril and therapy with temporary hemodialysis led to eventual improvement; developed

Continued on page 987

Current Literature *Continued from page 980*

glycosuria three weeks after hospitalization for oliguria; no rechallenge)

Immunosuppressive Agents

Zijlmans JM (University Medical Center of Leiden, 2300 RC Leiden, Netherlands), van Rijthoven AW, Kluin PM et al. Epstein-Barr virus-associated lymphoma in a patient with rheumatoid arthritis treated with **cyclosporine.** *N Engl J Med.* 1992; 326:1363. Case. (58-year-old man with long-standing, seropositive, erosive rheumatoid arthritis; received cyclosporine 5 mg/kg/day for four months, then 2.5 mg/kg/day for 3.7 years; developed GI symptoms that necessitated discontinuation of cyclosporine; histologic examination of ulcerations and tumors in small bowel showed Burkitt's-type lymphoma and DNA sequences from Epstein-Barr virus; therapy with antineoplastic agents led to remission of tumor; recurrence of therapy-resistant tumor led to death 16 months after tumors were initially found)

Pediatrics

Anderson KJ, Rivers RP (Department of Pediatrics, St. Mary's Hospital Medical School, London W2 1PG, England). Desferrioxamine in acute iron poisoning: 2. *Lancet.* 1992; 339:1602. Case. (22-month-old boy who ingested unknown quantity of ferrous sulfate tablets; received one 2-g dose of oral **deferoxamine** then i.m. injections every six to eight hours with one six-hour trial of s.c. infusion during second 24-hour period for total of 64 hours [total dose, 553 mg/kg; mean dose, 184 mg/kg/24 hours]; developed cough and lethargy; chest roentgenogram showed diffuse shadowing in right upper lobe of lungs; therapy with antibiotic led to progressive recovery)

Chan KW, Bond M, Fernandez W (Department of Pediatrics, Division of Hematology/Oncology, Children's Hospital, Vancouver, British Columbia V6H 3V4, Canada). Desferrioxamine in acute iron poisoning: 1. *Lancet.* 1992; 339:1601-2. Study. (case series; 13 children, mean age of nine years, with thalassemia major; received **deferoxamine** 15 mg/kg/hr by infusion for up to 48 hours; total of 193 courses of deferoxamine therapy; no child developed respiratory symptoms or significant obstructive or restrictive disease; no significant toxicity observed)

Progestins

Panwalker AP (Veterans Affairs Medical Center, Wilmington, DE 19805). Hyperglycemia induced by **megestrol acetate.** *Ann Intern Med.* 1992; 116:878. Case. (25-year-old man with AIDS and 13-kg weight loss; received oral megestrol acetate 80 mg twice daily and increased to 160 mg twice daily when weight loss resumed; continued to lose weight and developed signs of diabetes mellitus; withdrawal of megestrol acetate led to blood glucose concentrations in normal range; therapy with pentamidine isethionate and corticosteroids for treatment of respiratory infection led to recurrence of hyperglycemia)

Serotonin Agonists

Willett F, Curzen N, Adams J et al. (Armitage M, Royal Bournemouth Hospital, Bournemouth, England). Coronary vasospasm induced by subcutaneous **sumatriptan.** *Br Med J.* 1992; 304:1415. Case. (47-year-old man with migraine headache; received two doses of sumatriptan by s.c. injection; developed chest pain within minutes; therapy with sublingual nitroglycerin did not relieve chest pain; positive rechallenge under controlled conditions showed ECG changes consistent with coronary vasospasm; symptoms resolved and ECG tracings returned to normal 22 minutes after sumatriptan injection)

Continued on page 988

Current Literature *Continued from page 987*

Teratogenicity

Ghidini A, Sicherer S, Willner J (Division of Medical and Molecular Genetics, Mount Sinai School of Medicine, New York, NY 10029). Congenital abnormalities (VATER) in baby born to mother using **lovastatin**. *Lancet*. 1992; 339:1416-7. Case. (3.55-kg baby girl born at 39 weeks' gestation with vertebral anomalies, anal atresia, tracheoesophageal fistula with esophageal atresia, and renal and radial dysplasias; 32-year-old mother, whose last normal menstrual period was six weeks previous, received lovastatin 10 mg/day and dextroamphetamine 10 mg/day for treatment of hypercholesterolemia, progressive weight gain, and increased abdominal girth for five weeks when pregnancy was not known; lovastatin and dextroamphetamine were discontinued when urine pregnancy test results confirmed suspicion of pregnancy; ultrasound scan of fetus at 21 weeks' gestation showed no fetal abnormalities; pregnancy was unremarkable)

Tranquilizers

Safferman AZ, Lieberman JA, Alvir JM et al. (Howard A, Hillside Hospital, Long Island Jewish Medical Center, Albert Einstein College of Medicine, Glen Oaks, NY 11004). Rechallenge in **clozapine**-induced agranulocytosis. *Lancet*. 1992; 339:1296-7. Study. (case series; nine patients, mean age of 39.2 years, who had recovered from clozapine-induced agranulocytosis; received retreatment with clozapine; maximum daily clozapine dose was 336 mg at first onset of agranulocytosis and 375 mg at second onset; mean time to onset of agranulocytosis was 24.4 weeks for first episode and 14.6 weeks for second episode; interval between first and second exposure to clozapine ranged from two months to two years)

Advertising Index

American Society of Hospital Pharmacists
AHFS Drug Information 93, 988
Basic Skills in Interpreting Laboratory Data, 975
Concepts in Immunology and Immunotherapeutics, 911
Handbook of Institutional Pharmacy Practice, 979
Handbook on Injectable Drugs, 7th Edition, 986
Understanding Medical Terms, A Guide for Pharmacy Practice, 957
Amgen, Inc.
Epogen, 984-985
Neupogen, 907-910
ASHP Research and Education Foundation
Institutional, 983
Burroughs Wellcome Company
Exosurf Neonatal, 913-916
Eisenhower Medical Center
Position Available, 980
National Osteoporosis Foundation
Institutional, 977
Ohio State University–Columbus
Positions Available, 987
Roche Laboratories, Division of Hoffmann-La Roche, Inc.
Rocephin, 981-982
Saint Barnabas Medical Center
Position Available, 987
Scientific Therapeutics Information
Positions Available, 977
SmithKline Beecham
Timentin, inside back cover, outside back cover
Wyeth-Ayerst Laboratories, Inc.
Tubex, inside front cover

News

CDC advises on management of persons exposed to multiple-drug-resistant tuberculosis 991

Three studies examine angiotensin-converting-enzyme-inhibitor prevention of heart failure 999

Cefpodoxime marketing approved by FDA 999

Free drug programs for indigent patients should be more accessible, says Senate committee on aging 1000

News Briefs 1000

Upcoming Specialty Meetings 1000

CDC advises on management of persons exposed to multiple-drug-resistant tuberculosis

The Centers for Disease Control (CDC) recently released a report advising clinicians on the management of persons exposed to multiple-drug-resistant tuberculosis (MDR-TB), which is defined as tuberculosis caused by a strain of *Mycobacterium tuberculosis* that is resistant to both isoniazid and rifampin.[1] The CDC's advice for preventing active disease is summarized here.

Active tuberculosis caused by resistant bacterial strains carries a high mortality rate. In recent outbreaks of MDR-TB in Florida and New York, most of the exposed persons who developed active disease also had human immunodeficiency virus (HIV) infection, and 72–89% of persons who developed active disease died.[2,3]

Evaluation of Persons Exposed to Tuberculosis. The evaluation of persons exposed to tuberculosis should include consideration of the likelihood that (1) the exposed person is newly infected with *M. tuberculosis*, (2) the infecting strain is resistant to multiple drugs, and (3) the exposed person will develop active tuberculosis.

Likelihood of New Infection. Contacts who have had a positive tuberculin skin-test result documented in the past and who are not likely to be immunosuppressed are probably not newly infected. They should be evaluated for preventive therapy on the basis of the earlier tuberculin test result; they do not need to be evaluated further for tuberculosis exposure unless they have symptoms of active disease.

If the contact is likely to be immunosuppressed and he or she has no history of a positive tuberculin skin-test result, a tuberculin skin test should be administered, along with a chest roentgenogram and sputum examination, if indicated. If the induration at the skin-test site is ≥5 mm, the person should be considered newly infected. Active disease should be excluded, and the contact should then be evaluated for preventive therapy. A high-risk contact (defined as the immediate family, close social contacts, others who spent substantial time in an indoor area with the infectious patient) who has a negative tuberculin skin-test reaction and is not anergic should receive a follow-up skin test 12 weeks after the end of the exposure period. The high-risk contact should have a chest roentgenogram, and preventive therapy should be considered during the follow-up period if the contact is a child or if others who had similar exposure to the infectious patient exhibit skin-test reactivity or active tuberculosis. If the follow-up skin-test result is negative, preventive therapy can be discontinued.

Contacts who are infected with HIV, are likely to be infected with HIV, have another cause of marked immu-

Continued on page 994

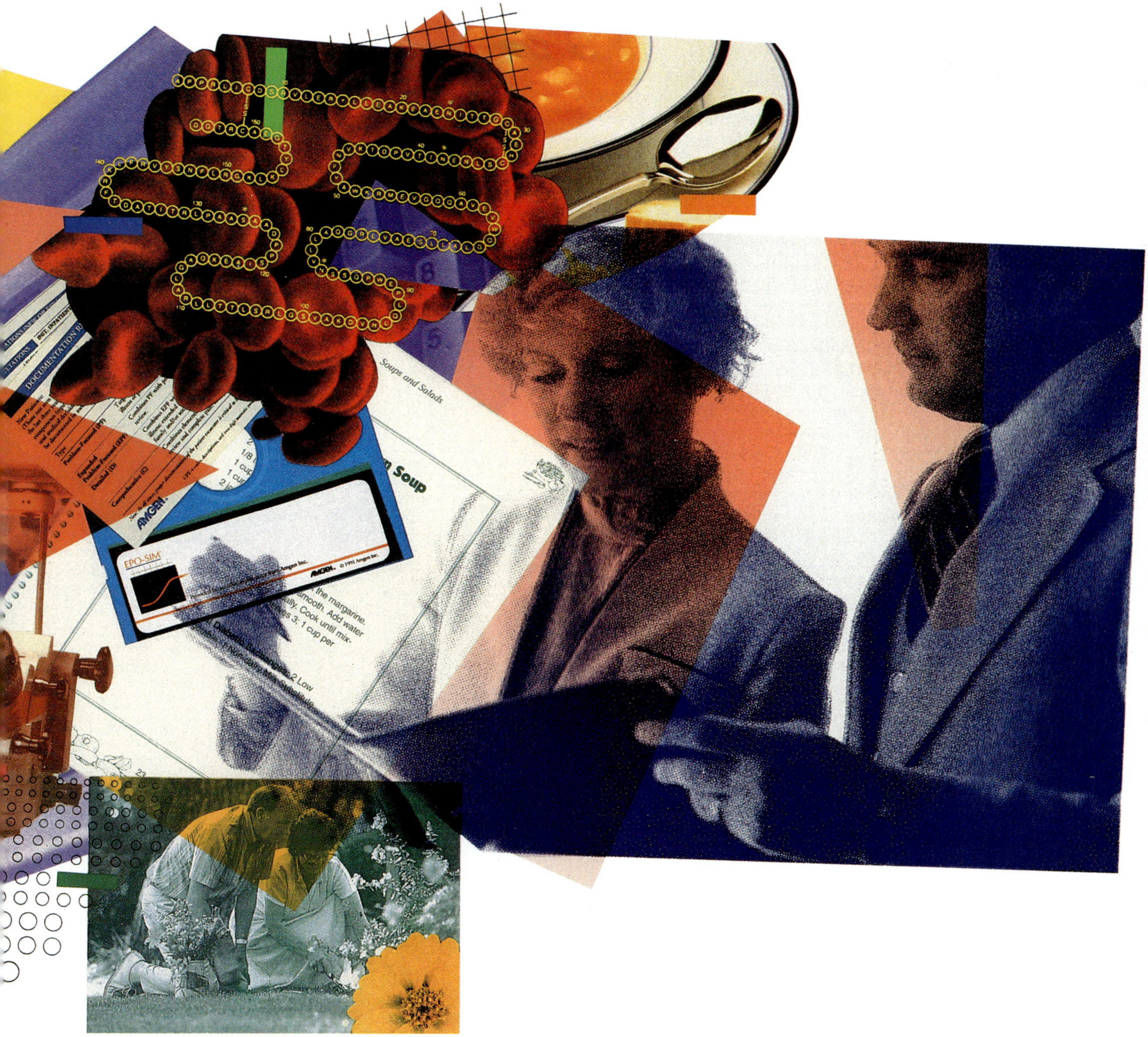
Soups and Salads
EPO-SIM
AMGEN

Continued from page 991

nosuppression, or are immunosuppressed and have a previous positive tuberculin skin-test result should receive a tuberculin skin test and be tested for anergy. Individuals who are not anergic can be evaluated in the same manner as those who are not likely to be immunosuppressed. Persons who are anergic should be considered "probably newly infected" if they are high-risk contacts or if others with comparable exposure show evidence of contagion. Active disease should be excluded, and they should be evaluated for preventive therapy.

Likelihood of Resistant Strain. If new infection is considered likely and the person has been exposed to a patient with infectious MDR-TB, the likelihood that the person is infected with a multiple-drug-resistant strain should be assessed according to the guidelines shown in the table.

Likelihood of Active Disease. Immunodeficiency is the most important determinant of whether a person infected with *M. tuberculosis* will develop active tuberculosis. Therefore, counseling and voluntary HIV antibody testing should be offered routinely to all patients known or likely to be infected with *M. tuberculosis*. Other conditions that cause immunosuppression also increase the risk of active disease, but to a lesser extent than HIV infection. Other factors associated with a greater risk of active disease are infection within the past two years (this time limit may not hold for HIV-infected persons) and age less than 5 years or greater than 60 years.

Preventive Therapy. All preventive regimens for MDR-TB should be administered under the direct observation of a health-care provider. To the extent possible, regimens should be tried in a systematic manner. Clinicians who are not familiar with the management of MDR-TB should consult with experts.

In selecting a drug regimen, clinicians should consider the results of susceptibility tests of the isolate taken from the presumed source case. General guidelines for selecting a preventive regimen, excerpted from the CDC statement, are as follows:

- Newly infected contacts who are thought to have a low to low-intermediate likelihood of infection with multiple-drug-resistant *M. tuberculosis* (see table) should be managed according to standard recommendations for infected contacts of non-MDR-TB patients. Infected contacts who are thought to have an intermediate to high likelihood of being infected with a multiple-drug-resistant strain of *M. tuberculosis* need to be further categorized according to their risk of developing active tuberculosis. Those at high risk for disease include persons who are HIV infected, persons with risk factors for HIV infection who have unknown HIV status, and persons with other conditions known to cause severe immunosuppression. Preventive therapy regimens with at least two antituberculosis drugs should be strongly considered for persons likely to be infected with multiple-drug-resistant *M. tuberculosis* who have a high risk of developing active disease. This suggestion is based on considerations of the extraordinarily high likelihood of progression to clinically active tuberculosis, especially in persons with advanced HIV disease; the severe consequences of clinically active MDR-TB in persons with HIV infection; and the possibility that MDR-TB may be more amenable to cure if treated when the bacterial burden is low rather than when the disease becomes clinically apparent and the bacterial burden is substantially higher. No clinical data exist on the risks and benefits of regimens that do not include isoniazid or rifampin; however, preventive therapy with more than one drug is recommended, since efficacy of preventive monotherapy with alternative drugs has not been demonstrated.
- For contacts who are not HIV infected, who do not have risk factors for HIV infection with unknown HIV status, who do not have another condition that substantially increases the likelihood of progression to active tuberculosis, and who are believed to be infected with a strain of *M. tuberculosis* that is 100% resistant (by the proportion method of susceptibility testing) to isoniazid and rifampin, other considerations apply. For these persons, two options are available to the clinician: (1) administer no preventive therapy and provide careful clinical follow-up for the appearance of signs and symptoms of tuberculosis, or (2) consider multiple-drug preventive therapy with drugs other than isoniazid or rifampin. If the infecting strain of *M. tuberculosis* from the source patient is less than 100% resistant to isoniazid, isoniazid should be used for preventive therapy for contacts; alternatively, if the infecting strain is less than 100% resistant to rifampin, rifampin should be used.
- Because the efficacy of preventive therapy with drugs other than isoniazid and rifampin is unknown, persons placed on alternative multiple-drug preventive therapy regimens should receive periodic medical and radiographic evaluation for the first two years after tuberculous infection (e.g., every three months for persons who are HIV positive or who for some other reason have a substantially

Continued on page 999

Likelihood of Infection with Multiple-Drug-Resistant *Mycobacterium tuberculosis* among Contacts Thought To Be Newly Infected[a,b]

Infectiousness of the Source MDR-TB Case[c]	Closeness and Intensity of MDR-TB Exposure	Contact's Risk of Exposure to Drug-Susceptible TB	Estimated Likelihood of Infection with Multiple-Drug-Resistant *M. tuberculosis*[d]
+	+	−	High
+	−	−	High-intermediate
−	+	−	High-intermediate
−	−	−	Intermediate
+	+	+	Intermediate
+	−	+	Low-intermediate
−	+	+	Low-intermediate
−	−	+	Low

[a]+ = high, − = low, MDR-TB = multiple-drug-resistant tuberculosis (adapted from reference 1).
[b]Anergic contacts should be considered likely to be newly infected if there is evidence of contagion among contacts with comparable exposure.
[c]Indicators of increased infectivity include exposure to patients who cough and have sputum smears positive for acid-fast bacilli and evidence of tuberculin skin-test conversions among other contacts.
[d]Multiple-drug preventive therapy should be considered for persons in the high, high-intermediate, and intermediate categories.

Continued from page 994

higher risk of developing active disease; every six months for persons who are HIV negative or are not at increased risk). Sputum examination should be done if tuberculosis symptoms are present.

Persons with HIV infection or other immunosuppressive conditions that greatly increase their risk of active disease should receive 12 months of continuous preventive therapy. Others should be treated continuously for six months.

One possible preventive regimen for MDR-TB is pyrazinamide 25–30 mg/kg/day plus ethambutol 15–25 mg/kg/day. Another is pyrazinamide plus a fluoroquinolone with in vitro activity against *M. tuberculosis*. Inclusion of an aminoglycoside or capreomycin could be considered. Use of aminosalicylic acid, ethionamide, or cycloserine is not recommended because adverse effects are common and efficacy against *M. tuberculosis* is low. Clinicians who are interested in enrolling patients in a pilot study of fluoroquinolone preventive therapy should call the Clinical Research Branch, Division of Tuberculosis Elimination, CDC, 404-639-2530.

1. Centers for Disease Control. Management of persons exposed to multidrug-resistant tuberculosis. *MMWR*. 1992; 41(RR-11):59-71.
2. Centers for Disease Control. Nosocomial transmission of multidrug-resistant tuberculosis to health-care workers and HIV infected patients in an urban hospital—Florida. *MMWR*. 1990; 39:718-22.
3. Centers for Disease Control. Nosocomial transmission of multidrug-resistant tuberculosis among HIV-infected persons—Florida and New York, 1988–1991. *MMWR*. 1991; 40:585-91.

Three studies examine angiotensin-converting-enzyme-inhibitor prevention of heart failure

Three recent studies provide insights into possible approaches to the prevention of heart failure through the use of angiotensin-converting-enzyme (ACE) inhibitors.[1-3]

The Studies of Left Ventricular Dysfunction (SOLVD) prevention trial compared the effects of enalapril and placebo in preventing progression to overt heart failure in 4228 patients with left ventricular dysfunction (ejection fraction, ≤0.35) but no symptoms of heart failure. Enalapril did not significantly affect survival over the three-year trial but did reduce the incidence of heart failure and related hospitalizations. These findings suggest that ACE inhibitor therapy can alter the course of left ventricular dysfunction, presumably by alleviating symptoms that would otherwise be present or by slowing progression of the disease.[4]

In the Survival and Ventricular Enlargement (SAVE) trial, treatment with captopril or placebo was begun 3 to 16 days after myocardial infarction in 2231 patients with ejection fractions of ≤0.40 but without symptoms of myocardial ischemia or overt heart failure.[2] After an average follow-up of 42 months, captopril was associated with improved survival (19% reduction in the risk of death) and with reduced morbidity and mortality from cardiovascular causes.

The patient populations studied in both the SOLVD and SAVE trials are likely to develop congestive heart failure eventually. In the third study, prevention was tested at a more fundamental step.[3] This trial attempted to stop the myocardial remodeling process before left ventricular dilation occurred. In this six-month placebo-controlled study, enalaprilat was begun within 24 hours of the onset of chest pain, followed by oral administration of enalapril. No survival benefit from therapy was evident. The trial was stopped prematurely because of safety concerns involving elderly patients who experienced early hypotensive reactions. It is possible that early treatment with an ACE inhibitor may be beneficial only if the subgroup of patients who are likely to develop left ventricular dilation can be identified.[4]

According to Cohn in an accompanying editorial,[4] the SOLVD results justify, but do not require, the use of ACE inhibitors in patients with asymptomatic left ventricular dysfunction. Physicians should be "strongly encouraged" to prescribe an ACE inhibitor for patients with left ventricular systolic dysfunction who are recovering from a myocardial infarction. However, he notes that the dosages used in these and other clinical trials are higher than those frequently prescribed for patients with heart failure.

1. The SOLVD investigators. Effect of enalapril on mortality and the development of heart failure in asymptomatic patients with reduced left ventricular ejection fractions. *N Engl J Med*. 1992; 327:685-91.
2. Pfeffer MA, Braunwald E, Moyé LA et al. Effect of captopril on mortality and morbidity in patients with left ventricular dysfunction after myocardial infarction: results of the Survival and Ventricular Enlargement Trial. *N Engl J Med*. 1992; 327:669-77.
3. Swedberg K, Held P, Kjekshus J et al. Effects of the early administration of enalapril on mortality in patients with acute myocardial infarction: results of the Cooperative New Scandinavian Enalapril Survival Study II (CONSENSUS II). *N Engl J Med*. 1992; 327:678-84.
4. Cohn JN. The prevention of heart failure—a new agenda. *N Engl J Med*. 1992; 327:725-7. Editorial.

Cefpodoxime marketing approved by FDA

The Upjohn Company has introduced a new oral cephalosporin, cefpodoxime proxetil (Vantin), for treatment of the following mild to moderate infections caused by susceptible bacterial strains: acute community-acquired pneumonia caused by *Streptococcus pneumoniae* and non-β-lactamase-producing strains of *Haemophilus influenzae*; acute, uncomplicated urethral and cervical gonorrhea caused by *Neisseria gonorrhoeae* (including penicillinase-producing strains); acute, uncomplicated anorectal gonorrhea in women caused by *N. gonorrhoeae* (including penicillinase-producing strains); uncomplicated skin and skin-structure infections caused by *Staphylococcus aureus* (including penicillinase-producing strains) or *Streptococcus pyogenes*; acute otitis media caused by *Strep. pneumoniae, H. influenzae* (including β-lactamase-producing strains), or *Moraxella (Branhamella) catarrhalis*; pharyngitis or tonsillitis caused by *Strep. pyogenes*; uncomplicated urinary-tract infections caused by *Escherichia coli, Klebsiella pneumoniae, Proteus mirabilis*, or *Staphylococcus saprophyticus*.

Cefpodoxime proxetil, a prodrug, is de-esterified to cefpodoxime. About 50% of an orally administered dose is absorbed and 29–33% of a dose is excreted unchanged in the urine in 12 hours. The elimination half-life is two to three hours. Cefpodoxime undergoes minimal metabolism. Cefpodoxime is 21–29% bound to plasma proteins.

The most common adverse effects reported with the film-coated tablets are diarrhea (7.1%) and nausea (3.8%); diarrhea (7.0%) and diaper rash (3.5%) are associated with use of the suspension.

A single dose of cefpodoxime is adequate treatment for gonorrhea. For other indications, cefpodoxime is given every 12 hours for 7 to 14 days. The dosing interval should be extended to 24 hours in patients with a creatinine clearance of 30 mL/min or less. The dose depends on the indication and ranges from 100 to 400 mg.

Vantin is supplied as 100- and 200-mg tablets (of cedpodoxime equivalent) in bottles of 20 and 100 and unit dose packages of 100. When mixed as directed, each bottle of oral suspension provides 100 mL of cefpodoxime 50 mg/5 mL or 100 mg/5 mL.

Free drug programs for indigent patients should be more accessible, says Senate committee on aging

Pharmaceutical company programs providing free drugs to indigent patients need to be made more accessible, says a U.S. Senate Special Committee on Aging report on the accessibility and affordability of prescription drugs for older Americans. Pharmacists, says the report, could help to (1) identify patients who would benefit from these programs and (2) distribute the free drug products in a timely manner.

The report includes an alphabetical list of drugs covered under programs sponsored by the 36 pharmaceutical manufacturers surveyed and a directory of the programs that lists the products covered, quantities supplied, patient eligibility criteria, restrictions, and other information. The report can be obtained by calling 202-512-2470 or writing to the U.S. Government Printing Office, Washington, DC 20402-9315 and asking for stock number 552-070-13026-8; single copies are $3.50 each.

The Pharmaceutical Manufacturers Association responded to the committee report by compiling a directory of 59 available programs from 44 companies and establishing a toll-free telephone number for up-to-date information on specific products: 800-PMA-INFO (800-762-4636). To receive PMA's *1992 Directory of Pharmaceutical Indigent Programs,* written requests must be sent to PMA, 1100 15th Street, N.W., Washington, DC 20005.

News Briefs

• The $10,000 **Astra Clinical Pharmacy Research Award** for 1992 has been awarded to Michael R. Ujhelyi, Pharm.D., College of Pharmacy, University of Cincinnati, for a proposal entitled "The Influence of Age on Stereoselective Renal Excretion and Organic Cation/Proton Antiport Activity." His coinvestigators are Michael B. Bottorff, Pharm.D., William Cacini, Ph.D., and Michael L. Markel, M.D. Applications for the 1993 award will be accepted until April 1, 1993. For more information, contact an Astra medical representative or Joseph M. Scavone, M.S., Pharm.D., Massachusetts College of Pharmacy and Allied Health Sciences, 179 Longwood Avenue, Boston, MA 02115.

• An updated version of **Cancer Chemotherapy Guidelines: Recommendations for the Management of Vesicant Extravasation, Hypersensitivity, and Anaphylaxis** is available from the Oncology Nursing Society for $6 to members and $7 to nonmembers; to obtain a copy, write to the Oncology Nursing Society, Attn: Publications, 501 Holiday Drive, Pittsburgh, PA 15220, or call 412-921-7373.

• Indications for **didanosine** (Videx, Bristol-Myers Squibb) now include treatment of adult patients with advanced human immunodeficiency virus (HIV) infection who have received prior, prolonged therapy with zidovudine. The new indication reflects findings of a study published in the August 27, 1992, issue of the *New England Journal of Medicine*. New, lower dosages for adults were approved: patients weighing ≥60 kg should receive 200 mg (tablet) or 250 mg (powder) twice daily; patients weighing <60 kg should receive 125 mg (tablet) or 167 mg (powder) twice daily.

• **Clemastine fumarate 1.34 mg** (Tavist-1, Sandoz) and **clemastine fumarate 1.34 mg with phenylpropanolamine hydrochloride 75 mg** (Tavist-D) have been switched from prescription to nonprescription status. Tavist syrup and Tavist-2 (2.68-mg tablets) will remain available by prescription only.

• A 7.5% **metronidazole vaginal gel** (MetroGel-Vaginal, Curatek) has been approved by FDA for the treatment of bacterial vaginosis. The recommended dosage is one applicator full of gel (approximately 37.5 mg of metronidazole) administered twice daily for five days.

• Mononine (Armour), a **factor IX concentrate purified using monoclonal antibody technology,** has been approved for marketing.

• Labeled indications for **estradiol** (Estrace, Mead Johnson) have been expanded to include prevention of postmenopausal osteoporosis.

• **Fialuridine** (Oclassen Pharmaceuticals), an antiviral compound in clinical trials for the treatment of chronic active hepatitis B, has been designated an orphan drug.

Upcoming Specialty Meetings

American College of Physicians. Washington, DC, April 1–4; contact ACP, Sixth and Race Streets, Philadelphia, PA 19106-1572; 215-351-2400.

American College of Preventive Medicine. St. Louis, MO, April 17–20; contact ACPM, 1015 15th Street, N.W., Suite 304, Washington, DC 20005; 202-789-0003.

Second Annual Spring Clinical Nephrology Meetings. Chicago, IL, April 22–25; contact National Kidney Foundation, 30 East 33rd Street, New York, NY 10016; 800-622-9010, (fax) 212-689-9261.

American Academy of Neurology. New York, NY, April 25–May 1; contact J. W. Kolehmainen, 2221 University Avenue S.E., Suite 335, Minneapolis, MN 55414; 612-623-8115.

American Society of Addiction Medicine. Los Angeles, CA, April 29–May 2; contact ASAM, 5225 Wisconsin Avenue, N.W., Suite 409, Washington, DC 20015; 202-244-8948.

American Society for Clinical Investigation. Washington, DC, April 30–May 3; contact C. Malin, 6900 Grove Road, Thorofare, NJ 08086; 609-848-1000.

Therapy Review

Antipyretic therapy in the febrile child

LAUREEN A. DRWAL-KLEIN AND STEPHANIE J. PHELPS

Abstract: General principles of thermoregulation, the pathophysiology of fever, controversies concerning the use of antipyretic therapy, and nonpharmacologic and pharmacologic treatments commonly used for antipyresis in the pediatric population are reviewed.

Several arguments can be made for not ameliorating the febrile response. Fever is an important diagnostic and prognostic clinical sign that may have beneficial effects for the host. In addition, body temperatures of ≤41 °C (105.8 °F) are relatively harmless. Reasons for treating fever include patient discomfort, the potential for adverse sequelae, the possibility of seizures, and the possibility that fever could affect the pharmacokinetic profiles of drugs. Nonpharmacologic treatment for fever includes environmental measures to enhance dissipation of body heat and sponging.

Aspirin and acetaminophen are the agents used most frequently for antipyresis in pediatric patients. However, aspirin use in children with a viral illness has been associated with development of Reye's syndrome. As a result, its use in children has declined in the United States. Acetaminophen is relatively free of adverse effects and is considered first-line pharmacologic antipyresis therapy. Ibuprofen suspension should be considered as second-line antipyretic therapy. Combination therapy with acetaminophen and aspirin may be considered if the patient fails to respond to other nonpharmacologic and pharmacologic therapies; however, combination therapy may result in increased risk of drug toxicity, increased probability of adverse reactions, and increased risk of intoxication.

Aspirin, acetaminophen, and ibuprofen are equally effective for antipyresis in pediatric patients. However, because acetaminophen is the safest medication, it is currently the therapy of choice.

Index terms: Acetaminophen; Analgesics and antipyretics; Aspirin; Combined therapy; Dosage; Fever; Ibuprofen; Pediatrics; Pharmacokinetics; Reye's syndrome; Toxicity
Clin Pharm. 1992; 11:1005-21

The presence of fever in children provokes a great deal of anxiety in parents. In fact, fever is one of the most common reasons that parents seek medical attention for their children. In a 1980 survey Schmitt[1] found that 63% of parents suffer from fever phobia, whereas 52% of parents believe that serious adverse effects, including brain damage, could occur with fevers of 40 °C (104 °F). Schmitt also reported that fever phobia frequently leads parents to aggressively seek treatments that decrease temperature in their febrile children. He found that 56% of parents give antipyretics for temperatures of 37.0 to 37.8 °C (98.6 to 100 °F), a range that includes normal body temperature, and 85% give antipyretics before body temperature reaches 38.9 °C (102 °F). Schmitt's findings were subsequently confirmed by Kramer et al.,[2] who demonstrated that fever phobia exists among parents of all socioeconomic classes.

Although parents frequently treat their febrile child, there is considerable debate in the medical community on the appropriate management of the febrile child.[3-7] In this review we will discuss general principles of thermoregulation, pathophysiology of fever, controversies in fever management, and nonpharmacologic

LAUREEN A. DRWAL-KLEIN, PHARM.D., is Assistant Professor, Department of Pharmacy Practice, Massachusetts College of Pharmacy and Allied Health Sciences, and Clinical Pharmacist, Children's Hospital, Boston, MA; at the time of this writing, she was Assistant Professor, Department of Pharmacy Practice and Administration, College of Pharmacy, Rutgers University, Piscataway, NJ, and Clinical Pharmacist, Department of Pharmacy, Robert Wood Johnson University Hospital, New Brunswick, NJ. STEPHANIE J. PHELPS, PHARM.D., is Associate Professor of Clinical Pharmacy and Pediatrics, Colleges of Pharmacy and Medicine, The University of Tennessee, Memphis, and Director of Therapeutic Drug Monitoring, Le Bonheur Childrens Medical Center, Memphis.

Address reprint requests to Dr. Drwal-Klein at the Massachusetts College of Pharmacy and Allied Health Sciences, 179 Longwood Avenue, Boston, MA 02115.

Supported in part by a Center of Excellence grant from the state of Tennessee.

and pharmacologic treatments used to decrease body temperature.

Thermoregulation

Despite a continuously changing environment, humans usually maintain a fairly constant body temperature. The preoptic anterior region of the hypothalamus is the center of the body's thermoregulatory system and is responsible for maintaining the body at a specific set-point temperature. The preoptic anterior region contains thermosensitive neurons whose rate of discharge is affected by the temperature of blood flowing through the hypothalamus and by feedback from the cold and warmth receptors that are located in the skin and muscle. If the hypothalamus senses the need to preserve the set-point temperature, it stimulates the autonomic nervous system, via norepinephrine and serotonin, to initiate physiologic processes that alter heat production or dissipation. Heat production occurs as a result of metabolic processes and thermogenic processes, particularly peripheral vasoconstriction and shivering. Heat loss occurs via radiation, conduction, convection, and evaporation. Physiologically, heat loss is accomplished mainly by sweating and peripheral vasodilation.[5,8-10]

Fever is defined as an increase in body temperature due to an elevated thermoregulatory set-point temperature.[10,11] Body temperature may also be elevated due to excessive heat production or defective heat loss.[3,4,9,11] It is important to differentiate between these causes of increased body temperature because the appropriate treatment varies with the cause of temperature elevation. This review will address only those increases in body temperature caused by an elevated thermoregulatory set point.

Pathophysiology

Endogenous pyrogens are thought to mediate the febrile response. Although interleukin-1, tumor necrosis factor, platelet-activating factor, interleukin-6, and interferon are all endogenous pyrogens, interleukin-1 is generally considered the prototypic endogenous pyrogen.[5,8-11] Many substances—including bacteria, viruses, fungi, toxins, antigen–antibody complexes, complement components, lymphocyte products, androgenic steroid metabolites, and inflammatory bile acids—can stimulate the production of endogenous pyrogens.[8,10,12] Macrophages, leukocytes, Kupffer cells, astrocytes, and microglia are among the many types of cells that may secrete pyrogens when stimulated.[9,12] Although it is generally agreed that endogenous pyrogens mediate the febrile response, the mechanism by which they increase the thermoregulatory set point is unclear. Endogenous pyrogens may elevate the thermoregulatory set point directly; however, it appears more likely that they elevate the thermoregulatory set point indirectly via increased production of prostaglandin E_2.[8-12] Prostaglandin E_2 may increase body temperature by increasing the production of adenosine 3′, 5′-cyclic phosphate.[13] Once the set-point temperature in the hypothalamus is raised, the body responds by increasing heat production and decreasing heat dissipation.[13,14] Maintaining an increased body temperature is a costly process because every 1 °C increase in body temperature results in about a 10% increase in metabolic rate.[13]

Clinically, the average normal body temperature corresponds to an oral temperature reading of 37 °C (range of 36–38 °C).[5,9] Rectal temperatures are approximately 0.5 °C higher and axillary temperatures are approximately 0.5 °C lower than oral temperatures.[5] As a result of diurnal variation normal body temperature may fluctuate daily by approximately 0.5 °C, with peak temperatures occurring in the early evening and nadir temperatures occurring in the early morning. This fluctuation is usually greater in children than in adults.[8,9] Fever is usually defined clinically as any temperature above the normal range.[15]

When possible, it is important to determine the source of fever because it is preferable to treat the cause of the fever rather than the fever itself. The most common cause of fever in a child is an acute viral infection. Less common causes of fever include bacterial infections, dehydration, malignancy, allergies, central nervous system lesions, radiation, immunizations, and various medications.[4,5] Infants younger than four months are at increased risk for serious diseases secondary to immature immune systems. Because it is often difficult to assess the subtle signs of a serious disease in these patients, they should be examined by a physician when febrile.[15]

Controversies in Treatment

Arguments against Treating Fever. Although fever has been managed with nonpharmacologic and pharmacologic therapies for years, the use of measures to lower body temperature remains controversial. Several reasons have been cited for not treating most febrile patients. Fever is an important diagnostic and prognostic clinical sign. Masking fever with antipyretics may delay initiation of necessary antibiotic therapy and may limit the use of a temperature curve to determine therapeutic response. Many also argue that the risks associated with antipyretics do not outweigh the benefits gained in treating fever.[3-7,15] Contrary to the belief of many parents, body temperatures of ≤41 °C (105.8 °F) are relatively harmless, and body temperatures rarely exceed 41 °C unless thermoregulatory mechanisms are compromised.[1,3,15-18]

Furthermore, several recent reviews[13,19] cite multiple studies that support the beneficial effects of fever on the host. In addition to animal studies, several studies in humans have shown that the presence of fever may be associated with decreased morbidity and mortality from bacterial infections.[20-25] Studies in febrile animals have demonstrated increased mortality when the animals were given antipyretic therapy.[26-28]

Several excellent reviews have been published on the immunological consequences of fever.[13,29-32] Increases in body temperature have been shown to result in increased white blood cell activity and mobility, activation of T-lymphocytes, activation of B-cells, and stimulation of interferon production and function.[33-46] Additionally, it has been shown that fever and hypoferremia act synergistically to inhibit bacterial growth.[47-49] It should be noted that many of the beneficial effects of fever on the host defense system diminish at 42 °C. Thus, extreme pyrexia is not beneficial to the host.

A few studies have specifically examined the clinical aspects of the effect of antipyretic treatment on the immune system. In a study of children with chicken pox it was found that children who received acetaminophen had a longer time to total crusting of lesions than placebo-treated patients.[50] Stanley et al.[51] found that adults infected with rhinovirus exhibited more nasal viral shedding when they received aspirin compared with placebo. Similarly, Graham and colleagues[52] reported that there was a trend toward a longer duration of rhinovirus shedding in patients who received aspirin or acetaminophen compared with controls. In addition, the use of aspirin or acetaminophen was associated with suppression of the serum neutralizing antibody response and increased nasal symptoms and signs. Conversely, Munzenberger and colleagues[53] found no difference in the length of hospital stay between children who received more than two doses of antipyretics during their stay and children who received no doses or one dose. This study can be criticized, however, because hospital stay is a weak discriminator. A recent study that compared acetaminophen with placebo in febrile children who had a presumed viral infection found no difference in mean duration of fever or symptoms between the two treatment groups. In addition, no difference in comfort level of the patients was noted between groups.[54]

Arguments for Fever Reduction. Despite arguments against treating most febrile patients, in practice many patients receive therapies to decrease body temperature. Schmitt[1] found that most textbooks recommend antipyretic treatment in children with temperatures of ≥39–39.5 °C (102.2–103.1 °F). Those clinicians supporting fever management cite patient discomfort, the potential for adverse sequelae, and the possibility of seizures as reasons for treatment.[3-5,15]

Although interpatient variability exists, fever alone usually does not produce discomfort until the body temperature exceeds 39.5 °C.[1] Temperatures of this magnitude may occur after strenuous exercise.[16] Steele et al.[55] noted that even with fevers of ≥ 39.4 °C, 74% of pediatric patients receiving only placebo for fever reduction were comfortable. Although parental fever phobia stems from concerns about the adverse sequelae associated with fever,[1,2] most fevers are harmless.[16] Fever may cause confusion, delirium, irritability, disorientation, or hallucinations.[1] In addition, the 10% increase in metabolic rate seen with each 1 °C increase in temperature results in increases in oxygen consumption, carbon dioxide production, requirements for fluids and calories, and cardiac output.[13] Although most patients can tolerate these adverse effects, patients who are malnourished or dehydrated, patients with cardiac or respiratory compromise, and patients with neurologic disease may not. In the rare case where body temperature exceeds 41 °C, heat stroke and brain damage may occur.[1,15] In summary, although fever may be associated with adverse sequelae, fevers of ≤41 °C are well tolerated and relatively harmless in most patients.[1,3,15,16]

Febrile Seizures. An important concern in any febrile child less than 6 years of age is the possibility of febrile seizures. Approximately 4% of children between the ages of three months and five years will experience a febrile seizure.[56,57] Most febrile seizures occur in patients who have a temperature of at least 39 °C; however, it has been postulated that the rate of temperature escalation may be more important than the absolute temperature in the development of febrile seizures.[58] This hypothesis may explain why in many children a seizure is the first sign of a febrile episode. Most febrile seizures are simple seizures characterized by generalized tonic–clonic convulsions that last for less than 15 minutes. Although most children will have normal health after a febrile seizure, these seizures are associated with some risks, including recurrence of febrile seizures, injury during the seizure, and development of epilepsy.[57] Because of these risks, the prevention of febrile seizures is often cited as justification for management of fever.

Although many clinicians advocate the use of antipyretics to prevent febrile seizures in children, there are no studies to support this bias. In a study that compared counseling on the appropriate use of aspirin therapy plus continuous maintenance therapy with phenobarbital versus aspirin therapy counseling and placebo, 5% of the patients receiving phenobarbital plus aspirin therapy counseling experienced a febrile seizure, whereas 25% of the patients who received aspirin therapy counseling without anticonvulsants experienced a seizure during a 12-month period.[59] Because a 25% recurrence rate is similar to the natural course for untreated children, this study suggests that antipyretic treatment is not helpful in preventing febrile seizures. This is the only study that has evaluated antipyretics in prevention of febrile seizures; additional studies may help clarify the role of antipyretics in febrile-seizure prophylaxis.

Despite the absence of studies in this area, many clinicians believe that any child with a history of febrile seizures or epilepsy should receive aggressive antipyretic therapy while febrile.[5,15,56] Those recommending the use of antipyretics for febrile-seizure prophylaxis suggest that children receive an antipyretic at the first sign of fever and continue to receive treatment for at least 48 hours. Unfortunately, in many cases this plan is difficult to execute because parents may not realize their child is febrile until after a seizure has occurred. Once a febrile seizure has begun, sponging with tepid water may be instituted to decrease the temperature below the seizure threshold.

Anticonvulsant therapy may be considered in addition to antipyretic therapy in patients at increased risk for recurrent febrile seizures or epilepsy (i.e., patients who have abnormal neurologic development, patients who have had a febrile seizure that lasted more than 15 minutes, patients who have had a focal seizure, patients whose seizure was followed by transient or persistent neurologic abnormalities, patients who were less than one year of age at the time of their first febrile seizure, patients with a family history of nonfebrile seizures, and patients who have had repeated seizures within a 24-hour period).[57,60,61] Although daily administration of phenobarbital has been the traditional treatment of choice for the prevention of febrile seizures, a recent report of decreased cognitive performance in patients who received phenobarbital therapy for febrile-seizure prophylaxis has prompted a reevaluation of this treatment.[62] Daily administration of valproic acid and intermittent administration of diazepam have also been used for the prevention of febrile seizures; however, their role in this therapy is controversial.[58,63] Currently there is controversy about the role of both antipyretics and anticonvulsants in the prevention of febrile seizures.

Pharmacokinetic Effects of Fever. Finally, some would argue theoretically that a sustained fever should be treated in some patients to prevent or minimize the effects of fever on the pharmacokinetic profiles of drugs. Ballard[64] and more recently Mackowiak[65] have reviewed the effects of fever on pharmacokinetics. Fever may affect the gastrointestinal absorption of drugs. Chang[66] demonstrated that gastric acid output is inversely correlated with body temperature. Beresford et al.[67] made the clinical observation that febrile illnesses result in a reduced transit time through the gastrointestinal tract. In addition, increases in cardiac output that are associated with fever may lead to an increase in perfusion of the gastrointestinal tract.[65] Theoretically, all of these changes could affect the gastrointestinal absorption of drugs. The intramuscular absorption of drugs may also be affected by the presence of fever because increases in cardiac output also increase perfusion of the musculoskeletal system.[65]

Fever may also affect drug distribution. For a number of drugs, increases in temperature result in an increase in the unbound fraction of drug and a decrease in the protein-binding constant.[64] Such changes in protein binding may result in decreased total serum concentrations of highly protein bound drugs (e.g., many of the anticonvulsants).[68] In addition, it has been suggested that fever may enhance diffusion of some drugs into the peripheral compartment. For example, Pennington et al.[69] demonstrated that fever was associated with an increase in the volume of distribution of gentamicin, a poorly protein bound drug.

The effect of fever on drug clearance appears to be variable. Studies have demonstrated that fever may accelerate some pathways of drug elimination and retard others.[70,71] Because of the narrow therapeutic range of theophylline, the reports of decreased clearance of theophylline in the presence of fever are important.[72-76] Although there are many unanswered questions concerning the relationship between body temperature and the pharmacokinetic profiles of many drugs, it would appear that the effect of fever on the pharmacokinetic profiles of drugs deserves consideration in the febrile child.

Nonpharmacologic Treatment

Several simple measures may be used in all febrile patients to enhance dissipation of body heat. These measures include removing excessive clothing and blankets, maintaining a cool environmental temperature, avoiding excessive activity, and providing adequate hydration. Removing excessive clothing and blankets will enable more efficient dissipation of body heat through the skin. Maintaining an environmental temperature of 21–22 °C (69.8–71.6 °F) will enhance conduction. Vigorous activities should be discouraged because additional body heat may be generated; however, total bed rest is not required. The increased insensible water losses that occur with elevated body temperature increase maintenance fluid requirements in the febrile patient. For each degree of temperature above 37.2 °C (99 °F) there is an increase in insensible water loss of 7 mL per kilogram of body weight per 24 hours; thus, maintenance fluids must be increased accordingly.[77] Providing adequate fluids to the febrile patient is essential because proper hydration is required to maintain the blood flow necessary for heat dissipation.[5,15] One should ensure that these general measures have been taken before antipyretic medications are begun.

External cooling via topical sponging may be used to decrease body temperature. Sponging increases evaporation and therefore promotes heat loss. Sponging does not affect the thermoregulatory set point; hence, when sponging is used without an antipyretic, patients may experience discomfort as the hypothalamus attempts to offset the decreased body temperature produced by sponging. In addition, body temperature will rise when sponging is discontinued.[15] The efficacy of sponging for decreasing body temperature is controversial. Several researchers[55,78,79] demonstrated that continuous sponging with tepid water was effective in decreasing body temperature. In contrast, Newman[80] did not note a significant degree of temperature reduction when patients were sponged with tepid water. In the studies by Friedman et al.[79] and Newman[80] patients were sponged for 20 minutes, whereas Steele and colleagues[55] and Hunter[78] may have sponged for as long as two and four hours, respectively. Although sponging was more effective than placebo for temperature reduction in Hunter's and Friedman et al.'s studies, in both studies acetaminophen therapy was more effective for temperature reduction than sponging.

To enhance evaporation when sponging, the child should be placed in a bathtub containing approximately two inches of tepid water. All skin surfaces should be intermittently wet with a thin layer of water. Some suggest gently rubbing the child with a wash cloth while applying water, because the rubbing action may produce cutaneous vasodilation that further enhances heat dissipation.[5,15] Tepid water should be used for sponging. Cold water causes greater discomfort for the patient because it results in more peripheral vasoconstriction and shivering as the body attempts to maintain a higher temperature. In addition, cold water may increase the core body temperature.[55] Although sponging with tepid water is generally a safe procedure, it should be used cautiously in severely dehydrated patients because it may enhance vasoconstriction and thereby promote heat retention.[81] In the past, isopropyl alcohol was used for sponging; however, its use is discouraged because inhalation of its vapors may result in toxicity (e.g., headache, seizures, dizziness, and coma) and because it may cause a rapid cooling that produces vasoconstriction and an increase in body temperature.[82-86]

Pharmacologic Treatment

Aspirin, acetaminophen, ibuprofen, phenacetin, choline salicylate, naproxen, indomethacin, diclofenac, and fenoprofen are among the agents that can decrease the set-point temperature, thereby decreasing body temperature in the febrile child.[3-4,87] In the pediatric population the majority of these agents are rarely used for antipyresis because they are not available in a convenient dosage form, have not been extensively studied in pediatric patients, or possess toxicity profiles that cause their risk to outweigh their benefit. Traditionally, aspirin and acetaminophen have been the medications most frequently used for antipyresis in the pediatric population. Recently, ibuprofen suspension was approved by the FDA for use as an antipyretic in the pediatric population.

Aspirin

Although aspirin was synthesized in 1853, its antipyretic efficacy was not demonstrated in children until around 1900 and it did not become available in the United States until 1915.[88] For more than 70 years aspirin was used extensively for antipyresis in the pediatric population; however, in recent years its use has declined because of reports of an association between aspirin therapy and Reye's syndrome.[89,90]

Aspirin inhibits cyclooxygenase, an enzyme that catalyzes the conversion of arachidonic acid to prostaglandin E_2. The resulting decrease in brain concentrations of prostaglandin E_2 is thought to lower the hypothalamic set-point temperature. In addition to its antipyretic effects, aspirin also possesses anti-inflammatory activity that may be fortuitous in patients with an inflammatory process and fever.[87,91,92]

Pharmacokinetics. The pharmacokinetic profile of aspirin has been reviewed recently.[93,94] When aspirin is given in tablet form, the rate-limiting step in its absorption is dissolution; therefore, the absorption rate depends on the tablet formulation.[95-98] Because increases in gastric pH may increase the dissolution rate of aspirin tablets, concomitant administration of antacid and aspirin may increase the rate of dissolution.[97-100] Gastric emptying time also influences the absorption of aspirin; thus, in overdose situations where gastric emptying is decreased, the rate of absorption of aspirin may also be decreased.[95,101-103] When using a children's 80-mg aspirin tablet, Wilson et al.[88] noted aspirin absorption as early as 0.25 hour and a peak concentration at 2.3 hours after dosing. Compared with orally administered products, rectally administered aspirin has a decreased rate of absorption.[104-106] One study demonstrated that rectal retention of at least 10 hours was required for complete (82–98%) absorption of a cocoa butter-based aspirin suppository.[104]

Once absorbed, aspirin is rapidly hydrolyzed by esterases to salicylate.[107] The biological half-life of aspirin in adults is 14–20.5 minutes.[107] Windorfer et al.[108] demonstrated that infants and children have esterase activity similar to that of adults. Thus, one would expect the biological half-life of aspirin in infants and children to be similar to that seen in an adult. Neonates, however, convert aspirin to salicylate more slowly than adults because of comparatively lower esterase activity.[108] Once aspirin is hydrolyzed, the pharmacokinetics depend on the salicylate moiety. At therapeutic serum concentrations salicylate is highly protein bound (90%).[109-112] The volume of distribution of salicylate is approximately 0.08–0.3 L/kg in neonates, 0.12 L/kg in children, and 0.157–0.167 L/kg in adults.[88,113-116] The fraction of salicylate bound to protein decreases and the volume of distribution increases with increasing plasma salicylate concentrations.[108,109,111,117-119] Decreases in serum concentrations of albumin (e.g., in neonates and patients with chronic inflammatory joint disease, hepatic disease, or renal disease) may also result in an increase in the unbound fraction of salicylate and an increase in the volume of distribution.[108-111,115,120-123] In addition, salicylate protein binding may be decreased in neonates and patients with renal dysfunction because of endogenous substances that may affect the affinity or the number of protein-binding sites.[108,109,120,124,125]

Salicylate is eliminated from the body by direct renal excretion of unchanged drug or is biotransformed to salicyluric acid, salicyl phenolic glucuronide, salicyl acyl glucuronide, and gentisic acid. Gentisic acid and salicyluric acid may be further metabolized to gentisuric acid, which is renally eliminated. The metabolic pathways involving the formation of salicyluric acid and salicyl phenolic glucuronide, the pathways primarily responsible for salicylate elimination at low doses, are saturable and therefore can be characterized by Michaelis-Menten elimination processes. It is because these pathways are saturable that total serum salicylate concentrations increase disproportionately compared with the dose.[126-128] Levy and Garrettson[113] demonstrated that like adults, neonates eliminate aspirin primarily by formation of salicyluric acid and glucuronide conjugates. Neonates, however, have a much lower capacity than adults to metabolize salicylate. A study of a single newborn exposed to large doses of aspirin in utero indicated that prolonged fetal exposure to salicylate may increase the rate of maturation of the pathway involving the formation of salicyluric acid.[114]

Renal elimination of salicylates becomes important when higher doses of salicylate are used because the salicyluric acid and salicyl phenolic glucuronide pathways are saturable.[128] Urinary excretion is pH dependent, with more excretion occurring when the urine is alkaline.[129,130] Medications that increase the urine pH (e.g., magnesium and aluminum antacids) may enhance the renal elimination of salicylate.[131,132] Because of immaturity of the renal system, neonates eliminate salicylate slower than adults do and excrete less unmetabolized salicylic acid than adults who receive a comparable dose of aspirin.[113,114]

Efficacy. Multiple studies have demonstrated the antipyretic efficacy of aspirin in the pediatric population.[78,88,133-138] Salicylic acid concentrations of 5–10 mg/dL have been associated with antipyretic efficacy.[88] Aspirin begins to decrease body temperature within one hour after oral administration. The maximum degree of temperature reduction (i.e., 0.8–1.4 °C) generally occurs three hours after administration. Body temperature begins to re-elevate about three to four hours after the administration of aspirin; thus, doses should be given every four hours.[4,78,88,133-138]

Dosage Recommendations. A variety of pediatric dosage schedules that use age, body surface area, and weight have been published. Before 1979, aspirin dosing was based on age, and doses were given every three hours. Recognizing the discrepancy between product labeling and physician prescribing of aspirin, Done et al.[139,140] conducted a study to determine the optimal dosing regimen for aspirin. Using pharmacokinetic data and computer modeling, the investigators developed the regimen shown in Table 1. Although the study suggested that body weight provides an effective and consistent means of dosing aspirin, the recommendations are based on age rather than weight for ease of parental administration. The current age-related dosing recommendations correspond to a dose of approximately 10–15 mg/kg. In 1979, the FDA adopted Done et al.'s regimen for labeling of all aspirin products.

Using computer modeling, Wilson et al.[88] confirmed that when Done et al.'s dosing regimen (Table 1) is used, the first dose of aspirin will produce therapeutic salicylate concentrations. However, Wilson et al. also demonstrated that salicylic acid may accumulate to concentrations in excess of those needed for antipyresis when Done et al.'s dosing guidelines are used for repeated dosing. Consequently, Wilson proposed several new dosing regimens for aspirin that need to be validated in clinical studies before they can be recommended. In addition, a recent study that examined the relationship between aspirin dose and antipyretic response in infants and children demonstrated that 10 mg/kg is the optimal single dose for antipyresis.[141] Repeated dosing of aspirin in neonates is not suggested until serum concentration monitoring is performed because aspirin elimination in neonates is decreased.[113,114] Thus, the pediatric dosing of aspirin may require further refinement to provide optimal efficacy and minimal toxicity.

Table 1.
Dosing of Aspirin[139,140]

Age (yr)	No. 81-mg Tablets	Dose (mg)[a]
<2	As directed by physician	As directed by physician
2–3	2	162
4–5	3	243
6–8	4	324
9–10	5	405
11	6	486
≥12	8	648

[a] Doses may be repeated every 4 hours, not to exceed five doses in 24 hours.

Dosing of aspirin in young children is also limited by the absence of a convenient liquid dosage form; therefore, dosing recommendations are generally not provided for children less than two years of age.

Adverse Effects. A disadvantage of aspirin is its toxicity profile. Aspirin use can be associated with disturbances in platelet function, gastrointestinal disorders, hypersensitivity reactions, hepatotoxicity, and salicylism.[91] Salicylate intoxication can result in tinnitus, hyperpyrexia, hyperventilation, respiratory failure, alteration in acid–base balance, fever, nausea, dehydration, coma, seizures, cardiovascular collapse, hemorrhagic phenomena, hepatotoxicity, renal failure, hyperglycemia, and hypoglycemia.[91] Toxic salicylate concentrations may occur as a result of overdose, drug interactions, dehydration, or an impaired ability to eliminate the drug.

Aspirin use has decreased substantially since its association with Reye's syndrome, a disorder characterized by encephalopathy and fatty infiltration of the viscera.[89,90,142] Between 1980 and 1982 four studies in the United States demonstrated an association between the use of aspirin in children during a viral illness, particularly influenza or chicken pox, and the development of Reye's syndrome.[143-145] Based on the results of these studies, in 1982 the FDA, the Surgeon General, and the American Academy of Pediatrics issued warnings concerning a possible association between the development of Reye's syndrome and salicylate use in children suffering from influenza or chicken pox.[146-148] Many argued, however, that because of methodologic problems these studies did not conclusively demonstrate an association between the ingestion of aspirin and the development of Reye's syndrome. Major criticisms of these studies, as described in Table 2, include such biases as selection, recall, data collection, and temporal precedence.[149-152]

Because of the intense criticisms of these studies, the Public Health Service undertook its own study to investigate the potential hazard of salicylate ingestion in pediatric patients suffering from influenza or chicken pox. This study was carefully designed to address many of the problems cited in the previous studies. In 1985 the results of the pilot phase of the Public Health Service study were published. Again, an association was established between the use of aspirin during an antecedent illness and the subsequent development of Reye's syndrome.[153] Despite continued controversy, in 1986 the FDA mandated that warning labels be placed on all packages of products containing salicylates. Subsequent to the mandatory labeling requirements, the U.S. Public Health Service published its main study, the results of which were in agreement with the pilot study.[154] Further evidence for the association between aspirin use and Reye's syndrome was provided by a carefully designed study published by Forsyth and colleagues in 1988.[155]

Although the controversy continues, there clearly has been a decrease in reported cases of Reye's syndrome in the United States since 1980.[156] This decrease in the number of cases of Reye's syndrome has paralleled the decrease in the use of aspirin in children.[90,157,158] However, at the present time there still is not enough evidence to definitively say that aspirin use is associated with the development of Reye's syndrome. Trends in Reye's syndrome cases will need to be followed for an extended period of time to rule out causes other than aspirin use. In addition, biological evidence demonstrating the mode of action by which aspirin precipitates Reye's syndrome is needed. Currently it is prudent to avoid salicylate use in the pediatric population.

Table 2.
Criticisms of Initial Studies on the Association of Aspirin Use with the Development of Reye's Syndrome

Selection Bias
- Absence of standardized entry criteria for cases and controls
- Inadequate matching of cases and controls for the severity of the prodromal illness

Recall Bias
- Lack of amnestic equivalence between groups
- Control interviews took place a longer time after the onset of illness than did case interviews

Data Collection Bias
- Interviewers were not blinded to the classification of subjects
- Unstructured style of interview
- Parents of controls were interviewed at home, whereas parents of cases were interviewed at the hospital, thereby altering the ability of the interviewer to ascertain the accuracy of the reported medication use

Temporal Precedence Bias
- Exposure to aspirin may have followed rather than preceded the onset of Reye's syndrome

Acetaminophen

Although the antipyretic activity of acetaminophen was first described in humans in the 1890s, it was not until 1956 that its antipyretic efficacy was demonstrated in children.[159,160] Since 1982, the use of acetaminophen in the United States has increased as the use of aspirin in children has declined.[89,90]

As with aspirin, the antipyretic effects of acetaminophen are believed to result from its ability to decrease prostaglandin synthesis in the brain. Unlike aspirin, acetaminophen is not an effective inhibitor of the peripheral formation of prostaglandins and therefore does not possess the anti-inflammatory effects of aspirin.[87,91,161]

Pharmacokinetics. There have been several recent reviews of the pharmacokinetic profile of acetaminophen in pediatric patients.[162-164] Peak acetaminophen concentrations occur about 30 minutes to one hour after healthy febrile children or adults ingest acetaminophen syrup.[88,165-167] When adults ingest acetaminophen tablets, peak serum concentrations occur approximately 30 minutes to two hours after ingestion.[167-172] Published data are not available on the absorption of acetaminophen tablets in children. Because acetaminophen absorption depends on the rate of gastric emptying, concomitant administration of propantheline with acetaminophen may decrease the rate of acetaminophen absorption, and administration of acetaminophen with metoclopramide may increase the rate of acetaminophen absorption.[169,170,173] Similarly, the administration of opiates may delay the absorption of acetaminophen.[174] Prolonged gastric emptying may also explain the slow rate of absorption of acetaminophen noted in neonates.[175] Acetaminophen absorption may also be affected by the dose; the rate of absorption appears to decrease and the bioavailability increases with increasing doses.[88,168] Acetaminophen administered orally is subject to first-pass metabolism.[168] Absorption of acetaminophen from rectal suppositories depends on the base used. In general, compared with orally administered products, rectally administered acetaminophen has a decreased rate of absorption; hence, lower blood concentrations are achieved.[167,174,176-179]

Wilson et al.[88] reported an apparent volume of distribution for acetaminophen of 0.8–1 L/kg in febrile children. Similarly, the mean volume of distribution in adults has been reported as 0.9–1.1 L/kg.[180,181] At therapeutic plasma concentrations, acetaminophen protein binding is negligible. However, protein binding of up to 43% has been reported in patients who have taken toxic overdoses.[181]

The reported elimination half-life of acetaminophen in children has ranged from 1.8 to 4 hours,[88,166,174,182-184] whereas a mean half-life of 2.8 to 4.7 hours has been reported in neonates.[174,175,182] The mean half-life of acetaminophen in adults is 1.6–3.8 hours.[168,171,180,182,185-189] Severe intoxication with acetaminophen may be associated with a prolonged half-life.[188,190] Less than 2% to 4% of acetaminophen is excreted unchanged in the urine in both pediatric and adult patients given therapeutic doses.[175,182,185,186,189,191] The major route of elimination is hepatic metabolism. In contrast to adults, in whom the major metabolite of acetaminophen is the glucuronide conjugate, the major metabolite in infants and children is the sulfate conjugate.[175,182,186,189,192] In addition to the glucuronide and sulfate conjugates of acetaminophen, a reactive intermediate metabolite formed by oxidation through the P-450 mixed-function oxidase system, *N*-acetyl-benzoquinoneimine, has also been identified. This reactive intermediate is usually detoxified by conjugation with hepatic glutathione and then excreted as cysteine and mercaptopurate conjugates.[191,193] Studies in adults have demonstrated that with overdoses the proportion of an acetaminophen dose eliminated by the P-450 mixed-function oxidase system increases as the sulfation and glucuronidation pathways become saturated.[194-196] When a large proportion of acetaminophen is eliminated via the P-450 system, hepatic glutathione may become depleted. If hepatic glutathione is unavailable for binding to the reactive intermediate metabolite of acetaminophen, the metabolite may covalently bind to the liver, resulting in hepatic necrosis.[191,193,197-199]

Compared with adult patients, pediatric patients seem to have a lower incidence of hepatotoxicity from acetaminophen overdose.[190,200-202] Preliminary data suggest that the lower incidence of hepatotoxicity in pediatric patients may be related to differences in elimination of acetaminophen in this population. It has been demonstrated in rats that the rate of synthesis of glutathione declines with age.[203] Thus, children may have more glutathione available for protection against acetaminophen-induced hepatoxicity. In mice, hepatic glutathione stores increase more rapidly than P-450 levels with increasing age. Therefore, the hepatoprotective effect of glutathione may develop more rapidly than the enzyme producing the toxic metabolite.[204] A recent study of acetaminophen elimination in a neonate after maternal overdose demonstrated that human neonates do appear to have a lower capacity than adults to form the reactive intermediate metabolite.[205] Finally, a study of the elimination of acetaminophen in a pediatric patient who ingested a massive overdose of acetaminophen demonstrated that children may have a larger capacity for sulfation than adults.[190] As a result of the larger capacity for sulfation, the proportion of acetaminophen metabolized by the P-450 system in the intoxicated pediatric patient may be less than that in an adult patient.

Efficacy. Most studies comparing acetaminophen with aspirin have not demonstrated any significant differences between the two drugs in temperature reduction.[78,88,134-138] In several studies there seemed to be a trend toward a quicker onset of action and a shorter duration of action with acetaminophen than with aspirin, but this trend may have been influenced by the difference in dosage forms used in these studies (acetaminophen elixir was compared with aspirin tablets).[78,133,138] Walker et al.[137] compared acetaminophen tablets with aspirin tablets and reported no difference in time to onset of action between the two products. However, they did note that for patients with an initial rectal temperature of 40.0–40.5 °C the duration of the effect of acetaminophen seemed to be shorter than that of aspirin. No differences were noted between the two products in patients who had an initial temperature of 38.8–39.9 °C. Plasma acetaminophen concentrations of 0.4–1.8 mg/dL have been associated with antipyretic efficacy.[88]

Dosage Recommendations. Acetaminophen (Table 3) and aspirin dosing (Table 1) are similar (10–15 mg/kg every four hours) because of the similar pharmacokinetic and pharmacodynamic profiles of the drugs and because 80-mg dosing units are marketed for both products.[139,140,206] Theoretically, the conformity in dosing schedules for these two antipyretics should prevent confusion regarding antipyretic dosing in children, thereby preventing or decreasing the likelihood of underdosing or overdosing. In a single-dose study comparing the efficacy of 5, 10, and 20 mg/kg of acetaminophen in febrile children, Windorfer and Vogel[165] noted dose-dependent efficacy and concluded that the ideal dose of acetaminophen for antipyresis is between 10 and 20 mg/kg. In summarizing studies that have used doses of 5–20 mg/kg of acetaminophen, Temple[207] noted that as the dose of acetaminophen is increased, the maximum degree of temperature reduction and the duration of the antipyretic effect are also increased. Therefore, when a dose of 10 mg/kg is used, an interval of four hours is necessary; however, when a dose of 20 mg/kg is used, acetaminophen should be administered every six hours.

Adverse Effects. Acetaminophen, unlike aspirin, is relatively free of adverse reactions. Rarely, hypersensitivity reactions and hematological abnormalities have been associated with acetaminophen use.[91,151] When taken in excessive amounts, acetaminophen can produce serious hepatotoxicity.[91,208] The incidence of seri-

Table 3.
Dosing of Acetaminophen[206]

Age	Weight in lb (kg)	No. Dropperfuls[a,b]	No. Teaspoonfuls of Elixir[a,c]	No. Chewable Tablets[a,d]
0–3 mo	6–11 (2.5–5.4)	½	. . .	. . .
4–11 mo	12–17 (5.5–7.9)	1	½	1
12–23 mo	18–23 (8.0–10.9)	1½	¾	1½
2–3 yr	24–35 (11.0–15.9)	2	1	2
4–5 yr	36–47 (16.0–21.9)	. . .	1½	3
6–8 yr	48–59 (22.0–26.9)	. . .	2	4
9–10 yr	60–71 (27.0–31.9)	. . .	2½	5
11 yr	72–95 (32.0–43.9)	. . .	3	6
≥12 yr	≥96 (≥44.0)	. . .	. . .	8

[a] Doses may be repeated every 4 hours, not to exceed five doses in 24 hours.
[b] 80 mg/0.8-mL dropperful.
[c] 160 mg/5 mL.
[d] 80 mg/tablet.

ous hepatotoxicity from acetaminophen overdose in children, however, is very low compared with that seen in adults, even when acetaminophen is taken in equivalent overdoses.[200-208]

Ibuprofen

Ibuprofen tablets have been commercially available for prescription use in the United States since 1974. In 1984, the FDA approved ibuprofen 200-mg tablets for nonprescription use. Recently, ibuprofen has become available by prescription only as a 20-mg/mL oral suspension. Although ibuprofen's antipyretic efficacy in children was reported in 1976, ibuprofen suspension was not approved by the FDA as an antipyretic for use in children until 1989. Like aspirin, ibuprofen inhibits central and peripheral prostaglandin synthesis; hence, it possesses both antipyretic and anti-inflammatory activity.[87,91]

Pharmacokinetics. Walson and Mortensen[163] recently reviewed the pharmacokinetics of ibuprofen in children. Peak plasma ibuprofen concentrations occur one to two hours after oral administration of ibuprofen powder, tablets, or suspension in children.[166,209-212] Similarly, peak plasma concentrations of ibuprofen have been reported about one to two hours after adults ingested ibuprofen tablets.[213-217] Studies in adults have demonstrated that ibuprofen is highly protein bound, approximately 99%.[215,218] The protein binding of ibuprofen is nonlinear at high concentrations.[216,219] Ibuprofen has a volume of distribution of approximately 0.2 L/kg in children and 0.16–0.21 L/kg in adults.[212,215,217,220] Brown et al.[220] reported that the volume of distribution of ibuprofen is age dependent in febrile children: Children who were less than 2.5 years old had a larger volume of distribution than children who were 2.5 years or older. In the same population it was noted that the volume of distribution of ibuprofen was also dose dependent, with a larger volume of distribution seen with a 10-mg/kg dose than with a 5-mg/kg dose.

In children ibuprofen has a mean half-life of 0.9–2.3 hours, which is similar to the half-life of 1.3–2.7 hours reported in adults.[163,209-212,216,217,220] Ibuprofen is eliminated mainly by hepatic metabolism via oxidation. The two main metabolites are (+)-2[4'-(2-hydroxy-2-methylpropyl)phenyl]propionic acid and (+)-2-[4'-(2-carboxypropyl)phenyl]propionic acid.[218] Mills et al.[218] reported that with repeated dosing ibuprofen did not appear to affect its own metabolism. Renal elimination of unchanged ibuprofen is minimal.[218] Wilson et al.[220] reported a more rapid clearance of ibuprofen in children who were less than 2.5 years old compared with children who were 2.5 years or older. In evaluating the pharmacokinetic profile of ibuprofen, it is important to remember that ibuprofen suspension is marketed as a racemic mixture. The pharmacokinetic profiles of the enantiomers have not been studied in febrile children, and the antipyretic activity of the individual enantiomers is not known.

Efficacy. Many studies have been published comparing the antipyretic effects of ibuprofen with those of acetaminophen or aspirin in the pediatric population. Most of these studies have shown no difference between ibuprofen and acetaminophen or aspirin in terms of rate, degree, or duration of temperature reduction. Serum ibuprofen concentrations of >1 mg/dL have been correlated with effective antipyresis.[163] In the majority of these studies, a single dose of 5–10 mg/kg was administered in an unblinded manner.[221-229] These unblinded comparative studies are described in Table 4.

To date, three randomized, double-blind studies comparing the antipyretic efficacy of ibuprofen with that of acetaminophen have been published.[166,230,231] Walson et al.[166] compared the safety and efficacy of placebo, ibuprofen 5 mg/kg, ibuprofen 10 mg/kg, and acetaminophen 10 mg/kg in 118 febrile children ages 2–11 years. All treatments decreased temperature significantly compared with placebo. Ibuprofen 10 mg/kg lowered temperature significantly more than acetaminophen 10 mg/kg for the entire population as well as a subset of patients with an initial temperature of 39.2 °C. Ibuprofen 10 mg/kg also produced a significantly greater reduction in temperature than ibuprofen 5 mg/kg in the subgroup with higher temperatures. The investigators reported that the duration of action of ibuprofen 10 mg/kg was greater than that of ibuprofen 5 mg/kg. The durations of action of both doses of ibuprofen were greater than that of acetaminophen. No significant differences in adverse effects were reported among the groups.

More recently, Wilson et al.[230] compared the antipyretic efficacy of placebo, ibuprofen 5 mg/kg, ibuprofen 10 mg/kg, and acetaminophen 10 mg/kg in a modified double-blind study. This study enrolled 178 patients between the ages of 3 months and 11 years. Patients were randomly assigned to a treatment group based on age and initial rectal temperature. All treatments, including placebo, decreased temperature significantly. However, the temperatures of those receiving either dose of ibuprofen or acetaminophen were lower than the temperatures of those receiving placebo at all time periods studied, excluding baseline measurements. The higher dose of ibuprofen was the most effective treatment for normalizing body temperature. In addition, ibuprofen 10 mg/kg had significantly greater antipyretic effectiveness than ibuprofen 5 mg/kg in children with the highest initial temperatures (39.5–40.5 °C). The time to onset of effectiveness was significantly longer for the placebo group (1.38 hours) compared with any of the treatment groups (0.72-0.76 hour). The maximum temperature reduction was 1.79 °C with ibuprofen 10 mg/kg, 1.68 °C with ibuprofen 5 mg/kg, and 1.58 °C with acetaminophen. Maximum antipyresis occurred at about four hours for all treatment groups. Ibuprofen 10 mg/kg had the longest duration of action compared with the other treatments. Two episodes of hypothermia were reported. One child who received ibuprofen 10 mg/kg had transient hypothermia during profuse night sweats

Table 4.
Unblinded Comparative Studies of the Antipyretic Efficacy of Ibuprofen[a]

Reference	Study Design	Age (yr)	*n*	Drug and Dose (mg/kg)	Temperature Reduction		
					Rate	Magnitude	Duration
221	SD	0.25–11	175	IB 7 A 8	...[b]	IB = A	...
222	MD[c]	0.17–12	96	IB 6 AS 10	IB = A	IB = A	IB = A
223	MD	2–12	45	IB 7 A dosed by age[d]	IB = A	IB = A	IB = A
224	SD	2–12	39	IB 7 A 8	IB = A	IB = A	IB = A
225	SD	Mean age = 4.3	28	IB 7 AS 15	IB = AS[e] IB = AS[f]	IB > AS[e] IB = AS[f]	IB = A[e] IB = AS[f]
226	MD	0.17–10	30	IB dosed by age[g] A dosed by age[h]	...	IB = A	IB > A
227	MD	0.17–12	46	IB 6 A 12 mg/kg	...	IB = A	...
228	SD	2–8	22	IB dosed by Young's rule[i] A dosed by Young's rule[j]	IB = A	IB = A	IB > A
229	SD	0.25–13	79	IB 6 IB 0.5 A 12.5 IN 0.5 AS 10 AM 5	...	IB 0.5 < IB 6 = A = IN = AS = AM	...

[a] MD = multiple dose; SD = single dose; IB = ibuprofen; A = acetaminophen; AS = aspirin; IN = indomethacin; AM = aminophenazone.
[b] Results were not analyzed statistically.
[c] Single blind.
[d] Acetaminophen: 2–3 years, 62.5 mg; 3–6 years, 125 mg; 6–12 years, 250 mg.
[e] Patients with pyrexia due to upper-respiratory-tract infection.
[f] Patients with pyrexia due to other causes.
[g] Ibuprofen: <12 months, 50 mg every eight hours; 12–59 months, 100 mg every eight hours; 60–120 months, 200 mg every eight hours.
[h] Acetaminophen: <12 months, 125 mg every eight hours; 12–59 months, 250 mg every eight hours; 60–120 months, 500 mg every eight hours.
[i] Based on adult dose of 400 mg.
[j] Based on adult dose of 300 mg.

that resulted from pulmonary tuberculosis. Another child had a transient drop in temperature to 36.1 °C 12 hours after administration of ibuprofen 5 mg/kg, which was judged to be unrelated to the ibuprofen dosing.

Finally Sidler et al.[231] examined the effectiveness of ibuprofen and acetaminophen in 89 children, 5 months to 13 years old, with a rectal temperature of ≥38.5 °C. All patients received a single dose of ibuprofen 7 mg/kg, ibuprofen 10 mg/kg, or acetaminophen 10 mg/kg. Two additional doses were permitted at eight-hour intervals if fever persisted. Body temperature was recorded for 24 hours. All three treatments significantly decreased body temperature at three hours. At three hours patients in the ibuprofen 10-mg/kg group had a significantly lower temperature than those in the acetaminophen group. The difference, however, was less than 1 °C. The authors reported that 59% of the children in the acetaminophen group received a second dose, whereas 38% and 44% of children in the ibuprofen 7-mg/kg and ibuprofen 10-mg/kg groups, respectively, received a second dose. When the mean body temperatures of the groups over the 24-hour study period were compared, the overall mean body temperature was significantly lower for both of the ibuprofen groups compared with the acetaminophen group. However, the magnitude of the differences among groups varied significantly over time. Four patients who received ibuprofen complained of adverse effects, whereas two patients who received acetaminophen complained of adverse effects.

These controlled studies clearly demonstrate that ibuprofen is at least as effective an antipyretic as acetaminophen. Although the controlled studies that were cited demonstrate some advantages in using ibuprofen, further comparative studies are needed to fully assess the relative antipyretic efficacy of the two agents. Because the antipyretic efficacy of acetaminophen is dose dependent,[165,207] future studies should compare ibuprofen with higher doses of acetaminophen.

Dosage Recommendations. When ibuprofen is used for antipyresis, the current recommendations for pediatric dosing are 5 mg/kg every six to eight hours for fever of ≤ 39.1 °C (102.5 °F) and 10 mg/kg every six to eight hours for fever of >39.1 °C.[232,233] Although the current dosing recommendations for ibuprofen are based on weight, corresponding age-related dosing can be calculated, as demonstrated in Table 5. As is the case for aspirin and acetaminophen, ibuprofen antipyretic dosing recommendations will likely be revised as more experience with the drug is obtained.

Adverse Effects. All studies of ibuprofen for fever

Table 5.
Dosing of Ibuprofen Suspension (100 mg/5 mL)[232,233]

Age	Weight in lb (kg)	Dose (teaspoonfuls)[a] ≤102.5 °F (39.1 °C)[b]	Dose (teaspoonfuls)[a] >102.5 °F (39.1 °C)[c]
6–11 mo	13–17 (6.0–7.9)	¼	½
12–23 mo	18–23 (8.0–10.9)	½	1
2–3 yr	24–35 (11.0–15.9)	¾	1½
4–5 yr	36–47 (16.0–21.9)	1	2
6–8 yr	48–59 (22.0–26.9)	1¼	2½
9–10 yr	60–71 (27.0–31.9)	1½	3
≥11 yr	≥72 (≥32.0)	2	4

[a] Doses may be repeated every 6–8 hours, not to exceed 40 mg/kg in 24 hours.
[b] Approximately 5 mg/kg.
[c] Approximately 10 mg/kg.

control have reported infrequent adverse effects.[166,221-231,234,235] Adverse effects that have been reported in these studies include diarrhea, vomiting, rash, agitation, abdominal pain, nervousness, hypothermia, and irritability. However, it is known that ibuprofen may cause other adverse effects, including hypersensitivity reactions, renal dysfunction, aseptic meningitis, platelet dysfunction, hepatotoxicity, and gastrointestinal ulceration.[238] As more experience is acquired in using ibuprofen for antipyresis, these other more serious adverse reactions may also be seen.

Several reviews that summarize the experience with ibuprofen overdoses in children have documented the occurrence of gastrointestinal disturbances, bleeding disorders, central nervous system depression, metabolic acidosis, hypotension, bradycardia, seizures, apnea, drowsiness, diaphoresis, liver dysfunction, renal dysfunction, and death.[237-239] Hall et al.[238] found that children less than five years old are particularly susceptible to developing apnea, coma, and seizures after toxic ingestions of ibuprofen. Hall and associates also reported that children who ingest more than 400 mg of ibuprofen per kilogram have the greatest risk of developing serious toxicity. The only pediatric death reported occurred after an ingestion of 469 mg/kg.

Combination Regimens

Some clinicians have suggested administering a combination of antipyretic treatments to enhance temperature reduction. Two studies have demonstrated that concurrent sponging and acetaminophen are more effective in reducing body temperature than either treatment alone.[55,79] The clinical importance of the observed less than 1 °F difference between acetaminophen alone and acetaminophen and sponging, however, is debatable. In addition, in a study by Hunter[78] no additional antipyresis was noted when acetaminophen and tepid sponging were combined. If these two treatments are used in combination, acetaminophen should be given at least 30 minutes before the initiation of sponging to allow a decrease of the hypothalamic set-point temperature.[15]

Several antipyretic regimens have combined acetaminophen and aspirin. Two studies have compared aspirin, acetaminophen, and a combination of aspirin and acetaminophen.[133,134] Steele and colleagues[133] reported no differences among the three groups with respect to the rate and degree of temperature reduction. The combination therapy, however, produced a more sustained temperature reduction than either agent alone. This study may be criticized because of the low age-related doses of acetaminophen and aspirin used when either agent was given alone.[15,240] Although the three treatment groups were not statistically compared in the second study, a trend toward a greater degree of temperature reduction with combination therapy was evident.[134] However, this study too can be faulted for the dosing used; the combination of aspirin 11 mg/kg and acetaminophen 14 mg/kg was compared with aspirin 12.5 mg/kg and acetaminophen 10 mg/kg.

Although no clinical studies support their use, regimens employing alternate dosing of acetaminophen and aspirin every two to four hours have been used for antipyresis in pediatric patients.[241] Using computer simulations, Wilson et al.[88] demonstrated the difficulty in maintaining therapeutic serum concentrations of acetaminophen and aspirin with an every-four-hour alternating schedule of the two drugs. This group further demonstrated that if the two drugs are alternated every two hours, salicylic acid may accumulate to toxic concentrations. The computer simulation work by Wilson et al. illustrates the need for clinical studies with this alternating regimen before its use can be advocated.

Several other concerns have been expressed about the use of either of these combined regimens.[3,15] The concomitant use of salicylates with acetaminophen theoretically may increase the risk of drug toxicity. The combination of acetaminophen and aspirin results in plasma concentrations that are higher than those produced by equivalent doses of aspirin or acetaminophen administered alone.[242] In addition, in mice the administration of aspirin before acetaminophen has been shown to alter the percentage of a dose of acetaminophen excreted as sulfate, glucuronide, mercaptopurate, and cysteine conjugates.[243] Such changes in acetaminophen metabolism may increase a patient's risk for acetaminophen hepatotoxicity. Furthermore, the depletion of hepatic glutathione that may occur with salicylate administration may also increase the risk of acetaminophen hepatotoxicity.[244] Another concern is the increased probability of an adverse drug reaction whenever polytherapy is used. In addition, if a parent runs out of aspirin or acetaminophen he or she may inadvertently increase the dose of the other medication, thereby increasing the risk of intoxication.[3,4,15]

Conclusion

Before any discussion of antipyretic treatment, one should consider the questionable benefit of decreasing body temperature. It is also important to remember that in many cases antipyretics will decrease, but will not "normalize," body temperature. Before instituting any antipyretic therapy, one should ensure that the general environment promotes heat loss.

If the decision is made to pursue pharmacologic therapy, one must consider the benefits and risks associated with the three medications that have been discussed. Currently, acetaminophen, aspirin, and ibuprofen should be regarded as equally effective. However, the efficacy of aspirin and acetaminophen is supported by more than 50 years of experience, whereas ibuprofen has been approved for use as an antipyretic in children for less than 5 years.

Because these treatments appear equally effective, one must carefully consider their adverse-effect profiles when selecting an antipyretic. Acetaminophen is the safest medication and should be regarded as first-line pharmacologic antipyretic therapy. Although the current literature suggests that few adverse effects are associated with ibuprofen when it is used for antipyresis, multiple serious adverse effects have been reported when ibuprofen was used for other indications. Because of limited experience with ibuprofen for antipyresis in the pediatric population and the documented risk of serious toxicity, ibuprofen should not be used as first-line antipyretic therapy. Because aspirin has been associated with Reye's syndrome and numerous other adverse effects, ibuprofen appears safer and therefore should be considered as second-line antipyretic therapy at this time. When suggesting ibuprofen for use as an antipyretic, one should be aware that ibuprofen suspension is available only by prescription and that it is substantially more costly than acetaminophen or aspirin. If a patient fails to respond to nonpharmacologic therapies and the appropriate doses of acetaminophen, ibuprofen, and aspirin, then combination antipyretic therapy may be considered. In using combination therapy one must remember that there are no definitive clinical studies to support the efficacy of combination regimens and that concurrent use of two medications increases the risk for adverse effects.

References

1. Schmitt BD. Fever phobia. *Am J Dis Child.* 1980; 134:176-81.
2. Kramer MS, Naimark L, Leduc DG. Parental fever phobia and its correlates. *Pediatrics.* 1985; 75:1110-3.
3. Done AK. Treatment of fever in 1982: a review. *Am J Med.* 1983; 74(Suppl 6A):27-35.
4. Lovejoy FH. Aspirin and acetaminophen: a comparative view of their antipyretic and analgesic activity. *Pediatrics.* 1978; 62(Suppl):904-9.
5. Kaufmann RD. Fever. In: Shirkey HC, ed. Pediatric therapy. 6th ed. St. Louis: Mosby; 1980:287-91.
6. Linakis JG, Lovejoy SH Jr. Antipyretics. In: Yaffe SJ, Aranda JV, eds. Pediatric pharmacology. Philadelphia: Saunders; 1992:335-44.
7. Gupta AK, Mohan M. Antipyretics in pediatric practice. *Indian Pediatr.* 1990; 27:216-22.
8. Dinarello CA, Wolff SM. Pathogenesis of fever in man. *N Engl J Med.* 1978; 298:607-12.
9. Boulant JA. Thermoregulation. In: Mackowiak PA, ed. Fever: basic mechanisms and management. New York: Raven; 1991:1-22.
10. Dinarello CA, Cannon JG, Wolff SM. New concepts on the pathogenesis of fever. *Rev Infect Dis.* 1988; 10:168-89.
11. Stitt JT. Prostaglandin E as the neural mediator of the febrile response. *Yale J Biol Med.* 1986; 59:137-49.
12. Bernheim HA. Is Prostaglandin E_2 involved in the pathogenesis of fever? Effects of interleukin-l on the release of prostaglandins. *Yale J Biol Med.* 1986; 59:151-8.
13. Kluger MJ. Is fever beneficial? *Yale J Biol Med.* 1986; 59:89-95.
14. Dinarello CA. Endogenous pyrogens: the role of cytokines in the pathogenesis of fever. In: Mackowiak PA, ed. Fever: basic mechanisms and management. New York: Raven; 1991:23-47.
15. Schmitt BD. Fever in childhood. *Pediatrics.* 1984; 74(Suppl):929-36.
16. DuBois EF. Why are fever temperatures over 106 °F rare? *Am J Med Sci.* 1949; 217:361-8.
17. McCarthy PL, Dolan TF. Hyperpyrexia in children: eight-year emergency room experience. *Am J Dis Child.* 1976; 130:849-51.
18. Tomlinson WA. High fever experience in private practice. *Am J Dis Child.* 1975; 129:693-6.
19. Kluger MJ. The adaptive value of fever. In: Mackowiak PA, ed. Fever: basic mechanisms and management. New York: Raven; 1991:105-24.
20. Hoefs J, Sapico FL, Canawati HN et al. The relationship of white blood cell and pyrogenic response to survival in spontaneous bacterial peritonitis. *Gastroenterology.* 1980; 78:1308. Abstract.
21. Weinstein MP, Iannini PB, Stratton CW et al. Spontaneous bacterial peritonitis. A review of 28 cases with emphasis on improved survival and factors influencing prognosis. *Am J Med.* 1978; 64:592-8.
22. Mackowiak PA, Browne RH, Souther PM et al. Polymicrobial sepsis: an analysis of 184 cases using log linear models. *Am J Med Sci.* 1980; 280:73-80.
23. Bryant RE, Hood AF, Hood CE et al. Factors affecting mortality of gram-negative rod bacteremia. *Arch Intern Med.* 1971; 127:120-8.
24. Kreger BE, Craven DE, McCabe WR. Gram-negative bacteremia: IV. Re-evaluation of clinical features and treatment in 612 patients. *Am J Med.* 1980; 68:344-55.
25. Richter RW, Brust JCM. Pneumococcal meningitis at Harlem hospital. *NY State J Med.* 1971; 71:2747-54.
26. Vaughn LK, Veale WL, Cooper KE. Antipyresis: its effects on mortality rate of bacterially infected rabbits. *Brain Res Bull.* 1980; 5:69-73.
27. Bernheim HA, Kluger MJ. Fever: effect of drug-induced antipyresis on survival. *Science.* 1976; 193:237-9.
28. Kurosawa S, Kobune F, Okuyama K et al. Effects of antipyretics in rinderpest virus infection in rabbits. *J Infect Dis.* 1987; 155:991-7.
29. Duff GW. Is fever beneficial to the host: a clinical perspective. *Yale J Biol Med.* 1986; 59:125-30.
30. Roberts NJ. Temperature and host defenses. *Microbiol Rev.* 1979; 43:241-59.
31. Roberts NJ. Immunological consequences of fever. In: Mackowiak PA, ed. Fever: basic mechanisms and management. New York: Raven; 1991:125-42.
32. Roberts NJ. Impact of temperature elevation on immunologic defenses. *Rev Infect Dis.* 1991; 13:462-72.
33. Bernheim HA, Bodel PT, Askenase PW et al. Effects of fever on host defense mechanisms after infection in the lizard

Dipsosaurus dorsalis. *Br J Exp Pathol*. 1978; 59:76-84.

34. Nahas GG, Tannieres ML, Lennon JF. Direct measurement of leukocyte motility: effect of pH and temperature. *Proc Soc Exp Biol Med*. 1971; 138:350-2.
35. Bryant RE, DesPrez RM, VanWay MH et al. Studies on human leukocyte mobility: I. Effects of alteration of pH, electrolyte concentrations, and phagocytosis on leukocyte migration, adhesiveness, and aggregation. *J Exp Med*. 1966; 124:483-99.
36. Phelps A, Stanislaw D. Polymorphonuclear leukocyte mobility in vitro: I. Effect of pH, temperature, ethyl alcohol, and caffeine, using a modified Boyden chamber technique. *Arthritis Rheum*. 1969; 12:181-8.
37. Sebag J, Reed WP, Williams RC. Effect of temperature on bacterial killing by serum and by polymorphonuclear leukocytes. *Infect Immun*. 1977; 16:947-54.
38. Ashman RB, Nahmias AJ. Enhancement of human lymphocyte responses to phytomitogens in vitro by incubation at elevated temperatures. *Clin Exp Immunol*. 1977; 29:464-7.
39. Smith JB, Knowlton RP, Agarwal SS. Human lymphocyte responses are enhanced by culture at 40 °C. *J Immunol*. 1978; 1121:691-4.
40. Roberts NJ, Steigbigel RT. Hyperthermia and human leukocyte functions: effects on response of lymphocytes to mitogen and antigen and bactericidal capacity of monocytes and neutrophils. *Infect Immun*. 1977; 18:673-9.
41. Gupta S, Agarwal SS. Effect of hyperthermia on in vitro proliferative response of lymphocyte subpopulations. *Fed Proc*. 1980; 39:916. Abstract.
42. Duff GW, Durum SK. Fever and immunoregulation: hyperthermia, interleukins 1 and 2, and T-cell proliferation. *Yale J Biol Med*. 1982; 55:437-42.
43. Hanson DF, Murphy PA, Silican R et al. The effect of temperature on the activation of thymocytes by interleukins I and II. *J Immunol*. 1983; 130:216-21.
44. Jampel HD, Duff GW, Gershon RK et al. Fever immunoregulation: III. Hyperthermia augments the primary in vitro humoral immune response. *J Exp Med*. 1983; 157:1229-38.
45. Heron I, Berg K. The actions of interferon are potentiated at elevated temperatures. *Nature*. 1978; 274:508-10.
46. Yerushalmi A, Tovery MG, Gresser I. Antitumor effect of combined interferon and hyperthermia in mice. *Proc Soc Exp Biol Med*. 1982; 169:413-5.
47. Garibaldi JA. Influence of temperature on the biosynthesis of iron transport compounds by *Salmonella typhimurium*. *J Bacteriol*. 1972; 110:262-5.
48. Grieger TA, Kluger MJ. Fever and survival: the role of serum iron. *J Physiol*. 1978; 279:187-96.
49. Kluger MJ, Rothenburg BA. Fever and reduced iron: their interaction as a host defense response to bacterial infection. *Science*. 1979; 203:374-6.
50. Doran TF, DeAngelis C, Baumgardner RA et al. Acetaminophen: more harm than good for chicken pox? *J Pediatr*. 1989; 114:1045-8.
51. Stanley ED, Jackson GG, Panusarn C et al. Increased viral shedding with aspirin treatment of rhinovirus infection. *JAMA*. 1975; 231:1248-51.
52. Graham MH, Burrell CJ, Douglas RM et al. Adverse effects of aspirin, acetaminophen, and ibuprofen on immune function, viral shedding, and clinical status in rhinovirus-infected volunteers. *J Infect Dis*. 1990; 162:1277-82.
53. Munzenberger PJ, Robayo JR, del Valle J. Effect of antipyretics on the length of hospital stay of pediatric patients with bacterial infection. *Am J Hosp Pharm*. 1981; 38:861-3.
54. Kramer MS, Naimark LE, Roberts-Brauer R et al. Risks and benefits of paracetamol antipyresis in young children with fever of presumed viral origin. *Lancet*. 1991; 337:591-4.
55. Steele RW, Tanaka PT, Lara RP et al. Evaluation of sponging and of oral antipyretic therapy to reduce fever. *J Pediatr*. 1970; 77:824-9.
56. Hirtz DG. Generalized tonic-clonic and febrile seizures. *Pediatr Clin North Am*. 1989; 36:365-82.
57. Consensus Development Panel. Febrile seizures: long-term management of children with fever-associated seizures. *Pediatrics*. 1980; 66:1009-12.
58. Applegate MS, Lo W. Febrile seizures: current concepts concerning prognosis and clinical management. *J Fam Pract*. 1989; 29:422-8.
59. Camfield PR, Camfield CS, Shapiro SH et al. The first febrile seizure—antipyretic instruction plus either phenobarbital or placebo to prevent recurrence. *J Pediatr*. 1980; 97:16-21.
60. Annegers JF, Hauser WA, Shirts SB et al. Factors prognostic of unprovoked seizures after febrile convulsions. *N Engl J Med*. 1987; 316:493-8.
61. Berg AT, Shinnar S, Hauser AW et al. Predictors of recurrent febrile seizures: a metaanalytic review. *J Pediatr*. 1990; 116:329-37.
62. Farwell JR, Lee YJ, Hirtz DG et al. Phenobarbital for febrile seizures—effects on intelligence and on seizure recurrence. *N Engl J Med*. 1990; 322:364-9.
63. Knudsen FU. Intermittent diazepam prophylaxis in febrile convulsions: pros and cons. *Acta Neurol Scand*. 1991; 83(Suppl 135):1-24.
64. Ballard BE. Pharmacokinetics and temperature. *J Pharm Sci*. 1974; 63:1345-58.
65. Mackowiak PA. Influence of fever on pharmacokinetics and pharmacodynamics. In: Mackowiak PA, ed. Fever: basic mechanisms and management. New York: Raven; 1991:341-51.
66. Chang HC. Gastric secretion in fever and infectious diseases. *J Clin Invest*. 1933; 12:155-69.
67. Beresford CH, Neale RJ, Brooks OG. Iron absorption and pyrexia. *Lancet*. 1971; 1:568-72.
68. Goulden KJ. Effect of febrile illness and its treatment on anticonvulsant levels in children. *Can Med Assoc J*. 1986; 134:1337-9. Editorial.
69. Pennington JE, Dale DC, Reynolds HY et al. Gentamicin sulfate pharmacokinetics: lower levels of gentamicin in blood during fever. *J Infect Dis*. 1975; 132:270-5.
70. Song CS, Gelb NA, Wolff SM. The influence of pyrogen-induced fever on salicylamide metabolism in man. *J Clin Invest*. 1972; 51:2959-66.
71. Elin RJ, Vesell ES, Wolff SM. Effects of etiocholanolone-induced fever on plasma antipyrine half-lives and metabolic clearance. *Clin Pharmacol Ther*. 1975; 17:447-57.
72. Matthay RA, Matthay MA, Weinberger MW. Grand mal seizure induced by oral theophylline. *Thorax*. 1976; 31:470-1.
73. Chang KC, Lauuer BA, Bell TD et al. Altered theophylline pharmacokinetics during acute respiratory viral illness. *Lancet*. 1978; 1:1132-3.
74. Fleetham JA, Nakatsu K, Munt PW. Theophylline pharmacokinetics and respiratory infections. *Lancet*. 1978; 2:898. Letter.
75. Clark CJ, Boyd G. Theophylline pharmacokinetics during respiratory viral infection. *Lancet*. 1979; 1:492. Letter.
76. Kraemer MJ, Furukawa CT, Koup JR et al. Altered theophylline clearance during an influenza B outbreak. *Pediatrics*. 1982; 69:476-80.
77. Boineau FG, Lewy JE. Estimation of parenteral fluid requirements. *Pediatr Clin North Am*. 1990; 37:257-64.
78. Hunter J. Study of antipyretic therapy in current use. *Arch Dis Child*. 1973; 48:313-5.
79. Friedman AD, Barton LL, Sponging Study Group. Efficacy of sponging vs acetaminophen for reduction of fever. *Pediatr Emerg Care*. 1990; 6:6-7.
80. Newman J. Evaluation of sponging to reduce body temperature in febrile children. *Can Med Assoc J*. 1985; 132:641-2.
81. Aynsley-Green A, Pickering D. Tepid sponging in pyrexia. *Br Med J*. 1975; 2:393. Letter.
82. McFadden SW, Haddow JE. Coma produced by topical application of isopropanol. *Pediatrics*. 1969; 43:622-3.

83. Senz EH, Goldfarb DK. Coma in a child following use of isopropyl alcohol in sponging. *J Pediatr.* 1958; 53:322-3.
84. Garrison RF. Acute poisoning from use of isopropyl alcohol in tepid sponging. *JAMA.* 1958; 152:317-8.
85. Moss MH. Alcohol-induced hypoglycemia and coma caused by alcohol sponging. *Pediatrics.* 1970; 46:445-7.
86. Arditi M, Killner MS. Coma following use of rubbing alcohol for fever control. *Am J Dis Child.* 1987; 141:237-8. Letter.
87. Clark WG. Antipyretics. In: Mackowiak PA, ed. Fever: basic mechanisms and management. New York: Raven; 1991:297-40.
88. Wilson JT, Brown RD, Bocchini JA et al. Efficacy, disposition and pharmacodynamics of aspirin, acetaminophen and choline salicylate in young febrile children. *Ther Drug Monit.* 1982; 4:147-180.
89. Rahwan GL, Rahwan RG. Aspirin and Reye's syndrome: the change in prescribing habits of health professionals. *Drug Intell Clin Pharm.* 1986; 20:143-5.
90. Arrowsmith JB, Kennedy DL, Kuritsky JN et al. National patterns of aspirin use and Reye syndrome reporting, United States, 1980 to 1985. *Pediatrics.* 1987; 79:858-63.
91. Insel P. Analgesic-antipyretics and anti-inflammatory agents; drugs employed in the treatment of rheumatoid arthritis and gout. In: Goodman and Gilman's the pharmacological basis of therapeutics. 8th ed. Gilman AG, Rall TW, Nies AS et al., eds. New York: Pergamon; 1990:638-81.
92. Clissold SP. Aspirin and related derivates of salicylic acid. *Drugs.* 1986; 32(Suppl 4):8-26.
93. Levy G. Clinical pharmacokinetics of aspirin. *Pediatrics.* 1978; 62(Suppl):867-72.
94. Needs CJ, Brooks PM. Clinical pharmacokinetics of the salicylates. *Clin Pharmacokinet.* 1985; 10:164-77.
95. Levy G, Gumtow RH, Rutowski JM. The effect of dosage form upon the gastrointestinal absorption of salicylates. *Can Med Assoc J.* 1961; 85:414-19.
96. Levy G. Comparison of dissolution and absorption rates of different commercial aspirin tablets. *J Pharm Sci.* 1961; 50:388-92.
97. Leonards JR. The influence of solubility on the rate of gastrointestinal absorption of aspirin. *Clin Pharmacol Ther.* 1963; 4:476-9.
98. Levy G, Leonards JR, Procknal JA. Development of in vitro dissolution tests which correlate quantitatively with dissolution rate-limited drug absorption in man. *J Pharm Sci.* 1965; 54:1719-22.
99. Levy G, Hayes BA. Physiochemical basis of the buffered acetylsalicylic acid controversy. *N Engl J Med.* 1960; 262:1053-8.
100. Lieberman SV, Wood JH. Aspirin formulation and absorption rate: II. Influence on serum levels of tablets, antacids, and solutions. *J Pharm Sci.* 1964; 53:1492-6.
101. Levy G, Hollister LE. Dissolution rate limited absorption in man. *J Pharm Sci.* 1965; 54:1121-5.
102. Matthew H, Mackintosh TF, Tompsett SL et al. Gastric aspiration and lavage in acute poisoning. *Br Med J.* 1966; 1:1333-7.
103. Ferguson RK, Boutros AR. Death following self-poisoning with aspirin. *JAMA.* 1970; 213:1186-8.
104. Nowak MM, Brundhofer B, Gibaldi M. Rectal absorption from aspirin suppositories in children and adults. *Pediatrics.* 1974; 54:23-6.
105. Connolly K, Lam L, Ward OC. Rectal aspirin—absorption and antipyretic effect. *Arch Dis Child.* 1979; 54:713-5.
106. Gibaldi M, Grundhofer B. Bioavailability of aspirin from commercial suppositories. *J Pharm Sci.* 1975; 64:1064-6.
107. Rowland M, Riegelman S, Harris PA et al. Absorption kinetics of aspirin in man following oral administration of an aqueous solution. *J Pharm Sci.* 1972; 61: 379-85.
108. Windorfer A, Kuenzer W, Urbanek R. The influence of age on the activity of acetylsalicylic acid-esterase and protein-salicylate binding. *Eur J Clin Pharmacol.* 1974; 7:227-31.
109. Borga O, Odar-Cederlöf I, Ringberger VA et al. Protein binding of salicylate in uremic and normal plasma. *Clin Pharmacol Ther.* 1976; 20:464-75.
110. Yacobi A, Levy G. Intraindividual relationships between serum protein binding of drugs in normal human subjects, patients with impaired renal function, and rats. *J Pharm Sci.* 1977; 66:1285-8.
111. Wosilait WD. Theoretical analysis of the binding of salicylate by human serum albumin: the relationship between free and bound drug and therapeutic levels. *Eur J Clin Pharmacol.* 1976; 9:285-90.
112. McArthur JN, Smith MJH. The determination of the binding of salicylate to serum proteins. *J Pharm Pharmacol.* 1969; 21:589-94.
113. Levy G, Garrettson LK. Kinetics of salicylate elimination by newborn infants of mothers who ingested aspirin before delivery. *Pediatrics.* 1974; 53:201-10.
114. Garrettson LK, Procknal JA, Levy G. Fetal acquisition and neonatal elimination of a large amount of salicylate. *Clin Pharmacol Ther.* 1975; 17:98-103.
115. Hollister L, Levy G. Some aspects of salicylate distribution and metabolism in man. *J Pharm Sci.* 1965; 54:1126-9.
116. Graham GG. Champion GD, Day RO et al. Patterns of plasma concentrations and urinary excretion of salicylate in rheumatoid arthritis. *Clin Pharmacol Ther.* 1977; 22:410-20.
117. Ekstrand R, Alvan G, Borga O. Concentration dependent plasma protein binding of salicylate in rheumatoid patients. *Clin Pharmacokinet.* 1979; 4:137-43.
118. Levy G, Tsuchiya T. Salicylate accumulation kinetics in man. *N Engl J Med.* 1972; 287:430-2.
119. Levy G, Yaffe SJ. Relationship between dose and apparent volume of distribution of salicylate in children. *Pediatrics.* 1974; 54:713-7.
120. Perez-Mateo M, Erill S. Protein binding of salicylates and quinidine in plasma from patients with renal failure, chronic liver disease and chronic respiratory insufficiency. *Eur J Clin Pharmacol.* 1977; 11:225-31.
121. Wallace S, Brodie MJ. Decreased drug binding in serum from patients with chronic hepatic disease. *Eur J Clin Pharmacol.* 1976; 9:429-32.
122. Costello PB, Green FA, Jung CY. Free versus bound salicylate concentration in adults and children with chronic inflammatory joint disease. *Arthritis Rheum.* 1982; 25:32-7.
123. Levy G, Baliah T, Procknal JA. Effect of renal transplantation on protein binding of drugs in serum of donor and recipient. *Clin Pharmacol Ther.* 1976; 20:512-6.
124. Windorfer A, Karitzky K, Gasteiger U et al. Investigations on salicylate protein binding in newborns and infants. *Eur J Pediatr.* 1978; 127:163-72.
125. Lowenthal DT, Briggs WA, Levy G. Kinetics of salicylate elimination by anephric patients. *J Clin Invest.* 1974; 54:1221-6.
126. Levy G. Pharmacokinetics of salicylate elimination in man. *J Pharm Sci.* 1965; 54:959-67.
127. Levy G, Tsuchiya T, Amsel LP. Limited capacity for salicyl phenolic glucuronide formation and its effect on the kinetics of salicylate elimination in man. *Clin Pharmacol Ther.* 1972; 13:258-68.
128. Tsuchiya T, Levy G. Biotransformation of salicylic acid to its acyl and phenolic glucuronides in man. *J Pharm Sci.* 1972; 61:800-1.
129. MacPherson CR, Milne MD, Evans BM. The excretion of salicylate. *Br J Pharmacol.* 1955; 10:484-9.
130. Levy G, Leonard JR. Urine pH and salicylate therapy. *JAMA.* 1971; 217:81. Letter.
131. Levy G, Lampman T, Kamath BL et al. Decreased serum salicylate concentrations in children with rheumatic fever treated with antacid. *N Engl J Med.* 1975; 293:323-5.
132. Hansten PD, Hayton WL. Effect of antacid and ascorbic acid on serum salicylate concentration. *J Clin Pharmacol.* 1980; 20:326-31.
133. Steele RW, Young FS, Bass JW et al. Oral antipyretic therapy evaluation of aspirin-acetaminophen combination. *Am J Dis Child.* 1972; 123:204-6.

134. Similä S, Keinanen S, Kouvalainen K. Oral antipyretic therapy: evaluation of benorylate, an ester of acetylsalicylic acid and paracetamol. *Eur J Pediatr.* 1975; 121:15-20.
135. Eden AN, Kaufman A. Clinical comparison of three antipyretic agents. *Am J Dis Child.* 1967; 114:284-7.
136. Tarlin L, Landrigan P, Babineau R et al. A comparison of the antipyretic effect of acetaminophen and aspirin. *Am J Dis Child.* 1972; 124:880-2.
137. Walker PC, Helms RA, Wall HP et al. Comparative efficacy study of chewable aspirin and acetaminophen in the antipyresis of children. *J Clin Pharmacol.* 1986; 26:106-11.
138. Colgan MT, Mintz AA. The comparative antipyretic effect of *N*-acetyl-*p*-aminophenol and acetylsalicylic acid. *J Pediatr.* 1957; 50:552-5.
139. Done AK, Yaffe SJ, Clayton JM. Aspirin dosage for infants and children. *J Pediatr.* 1979; 95:617-25.
140. Done AK, Yaffe JS, Clayton JM. New dosage for aspirin—long overdue but wrong. *Pediatr Alert.* 1979; 4:93-4.
141. Vigano A, Dalla Villa A, Cecchini I et al. Correlation between dosage and antipyretic effect of aspirin in children. *Eur J Clin Pharmacol.* 1986; 31:359-61.
142. Reye RDK, Morgan G, Baral J. Encephalopathy and fatty degeneration of the viscera. A disease entity in childhood. *Lancet.* 1963; 2:749-52.
143. Starko KM, Ray CG, Dominguez LB et al. Reye's syndrome and salicylate use. *Pediatrics.* 1980; 66:859-64.
144. Halpin TJ, Holtzhauer FJ, Campbell RJ et al. Reye's syndrome and medication use. *JAMA.* 1982; 248:687-91.
145. Waldman RJ, Hall WN, McGee H et al. Aspirin as a risk factor in Reye's syndrome. *JAMA.* 1982; 247:3089-4.
146. Anon. Salicylate labeling may change. *FDA Drug Bull.* 1982; 12:9-10.
147. Centers for Disease Control. Surgeon General's advisory on the use of salicylates and Reye syndrome. *MMWR.* 1982; 31:289-90.
148. Committee on Infectious Diseases. Aspirin and Reye syndrome. *Pediatrics.* 1982; 69:810-2.
149. Daniels SR, Greenberg RS, Ibrahim MA. Scientific uncertainties in the studies of salicylate use and Reye's syndrome. *JAMA.* 1983; 249:1311-6.
150. Reye Syndrome Working Group. Reye syndrome and salicylates: a spurious association. *Pediatrics.* 1982; 70:158-60. Editorial.
151. Wilson JT, Brown RD. Reye syndrome and aspirin use: the role of the prodromal illness severity in the assessment of relative risk. *Pediatrics.* 1982; 69:822-5.
152. Hoekelman RA. Take two aspirin and call me in the morning: salicylate use and Reye's syndrome. *Am J Dis Child.* 1982; 136:973-4.
153. Hurwitz ES, Barrett MJ, Bregman D et al. Public Health Service study on Reye's syndrome and medications: report of the pilot phase. *N Engl J Med.* 1985; 313:849-57.
154. Hurwitz ES, Barrett MJ, Bregman D et al. Public Health Service study of Reye's syndrome and medications: report of the main study. *JAMA.* 1987; 257:1905-11.
155. Forsyth BW, Horwitz RI, Acampora D et al. New epidemiologic evidence confirming that bias does not explain the aspirin/Reye's syndrome association. *JAMA.* 1989; 261:2517-24.
156. Centers for Disease Control. Reye syndrome surveillance—United States, 1989. *MMWR.* 1991; 40:88-90.
157. Remington PL, Rowley D, McGee H et al. Decreasing trends in Reye syndrome and aspirin use in Michigan, 1979 to 1984. *Pediatrics.* 1986; 77:93-8.
158. Barrett MJ, Hurwitz ES, Schonberger LB et al. Changing epidemiology of Reye syndrome in the United States. *Pediatrics.* 1986; 77:598-602.
159. Spooner JB, Harvey JG. The history and usage of paracetamol. *J Int Med Res.* 1976; 4(Suppl 4):1-6.
160. Cornely DA, Ritter JA. *N*-acetyl-*p*-aminophenol (Tylenol elixir) as pediatric antipyretic-analgesic. *JAMA.* 1956; 160:1219-22.
161. Koch-Weser J. Acetaminophen. *N Engl J Med.* 1976; 295:1297-300.
162. Peterson RG, Rumack BH. Pharmacokinetics of acetaminophen in children. *Pediatrics.* 1978; 62(Suppl):877-9.
163. Walson PD, Mortensen ME. Pharmacokinetics of common analgesics, anti-inflammatories and antipyretics in children. *Clin Pharmacokinet.* 1989; 17(Suppl 1):116-37.
164. Forrest JAH, Clements JA, Prescott LF. Clinical pharmacokinetics of paracetamol. *Clin Pharmacokinet.* 1982; 7:93-107.
165. Windorfer A, Vogel C. Untersuchungen über Serumkonzentrationen und Temperaturverlauf nach einer neuen oral applizierbaren flussigen Paracetamolzuberertung. *Klin Padiatr.* 1976; 188:430-4.
166. Walson PD, Galletta G, Braden NJ et al. Ibuprofen, acetaminophen, and placebo treatment of febrile children. *Clin Pharmacol Ther.* 1989; 46:9-17.
167. Eandi M, Viano I, Ricci Gamalero S. Absolute bioavailability of paracetamol after oral or rectal administration in healthy volunteers. *Arzneim Forsch.* 1984; 34:903-7.
168. Rawlins MD, Henderson DB, Hibjab AR. Pharmacokinetics of paracetamol (acetaminophen) after intravenous and oral administration. *Eur J Clin Pharmacol.* 1977; 11:283-6.
169. Nimmo J, Heading RC, Tothill P et al. Pharmacological modification of gastric emptying: effects of propantheline and metoclopramide on paracetamol absorption. *Br Med J.* 1973; 1:587-9.
170. Heading RC, Nimmo J, Prescott LF et al. The dependence of paracetamol absorption on the rate of gastric emptying. *Br J Pharmacol.* 1973; 47:415-21.
171. McGilveray IJ, Mattock GL. Some factors affecting the absorption of paracetamol. *J Pharm Pharmacol.* 1972; 24:615-9.
172. Dordoni B, Wilson RA, Thompson RPH et al. Reduction of absorption of paracetamol by activated charcoal and cholestyramine: a possible therapeutic measure. *Br Med J.* 1973; 3:86-7.
173. Clements JA, Heading RC, Nimmo WS et al. Kinetics of acetaminophen absorption and gastric emptying in man. *Clin Pharmacol Ther.* 1978; 24:420-31.
174. Hopkins CS, Underhill S, Booker PD. Pharmacokinetics of paracetamol after cardiac surgery. *Arch Dis Child.* 1990; 65:971-6.
175. Levy G, Khanna NN, Soda DM et al. Pharmacokinetics of acetaminophen in the human neonate: formation of acetaminophen glucuronide and sulfate in relation to plasma bilirubin concentration and D-glucaric acid excretion. *Pediatrics.* 1975; 55:818-25.
176. Moolenaar F, Schoonen AJM, Everts A et al. Biopharmaceutics of rectal administration of drugs in man. Absorption rate and bioavailability of paracetamol from fatty suppositories. *Pharm Weekbl.* 1979; 114:689-94.
177. Keinänen S, Hietula M, Similä S et al. Antipyretic therapy comparison of rectal and oral paracetamol. *Eur J Clin Pharm.* 1977; 12:77-80.
178. Seideman P, Alvan G, Andrews RS et al. Relative bioavailability of a paracetamol suppository. *Eur J Clin Pharmacol.* 1980; 17:465-8.
179. Cullen S, Kenny D, Ward OC et al. Paracetamol suppositories: a comparative study. *Arch Dis Child.* 1989; 64:1504-5.
180. Perucca E, Richens A. Paracetamol disposition in normal subjects and in patients treated with antiepileptic drugs. *Br J Clin Pharmacol.* 1979; 7:201-6.
181. Gazzard BG, Fort-Hutchinson AW, Smith MJH et al. The binding of paracetamol to plasma proteins of man and pig. *J Pharm Pharmacol.* 1973; 25:964-7.
182. Miller RP, Robert RJ, Fischer LJ. Acetaminophen elimination kinetics in neonates, children, and adults. *Clin Pharmacol Ther.* 1976; 19:284-94.
183. Keinänen-Kiukaanniemi S, Similä S, Luoma P et al. Antipyretic effect and plasma concentrations of rectal acetaminophen and diazepam in children. *Epilepsia.* 1979; 20:607-12.
184. Nahata MC, Powell DA, Durrell DE et al. Acetaminophen accumulation in pediatric patients after repeated therapeutic doses. *Eur J Clin Pharmacol.* 1984; 27:57-9.

185. Nelson E, Morioka T. Kinetics of the metabolism of acetaminophen by humans. *J Pharm Sci.* 1963; 52:864-8.
186. Cummings AJ, King ML, Martin BK. A kinetic study of drug elimination: the excretion of paracetamol and its metabolites in man. *Br J Pharmacol Chemother.* 1967; 29:150-7.
187. Prescott LF, Sansur M, Levin W et al. The comparative metabolism of phenacetin and *N*-acetyl-*p*-aminophenol in man, with particular reference to effects on the kidney. *Clin Pharmacol Ther.* 1968; 9:605-14.
188. Prescott LF, Wright N, Roscoe P et al. Plasma-paracetamol half-life and hepatic necrosis in patients with paracetamol overdosage. *Lancet.* 1971; 1:519-22.
189. Levy G, Regardh C. Drug biotransformation interaction in man. V: acetaminophen and salicylic acid. *J Pharm Sci.* 1971; 60:608-11.
190. Leih-Lai MW, Sarnaik AP, Newton JF et al. Metabolism and pharmacokinetics of acetaminophen in a severely poisoned young child. *J Pediatr.* 1984; 105:125-8.
191. Mitchell JR, Thorgeirsson SS, Potter WZ et al. Acetaminophen-induced hepatic injury: protective role of glutathione in man and rationale for therapy. *Clin Pharmacol Ther.* 1974; 16:676-84.
192. Alam SN, Robert RJ, Fischer LJ. Age-related differences in salicylamide and acetaminophen conjugation in man. *J Pediatr.* 1977; 90:130-5.
193. Mitchell JR, Jollow DJ, Potter WZ et al. Acetaminophen-induced hepatic necrosis. IV. Protective role of glutathione. *J Pharmacol Exp Ther.* 1973; 187:211-7.
194. Slattery JT, Levy G. Acetaminophen kinetics in acutely poisoned patients. *Clin Pharmacol Ther.* 1979; 25:184-95.
195. Davis M, Simmons CJ, Harrison NG et al. Paracetamol overdose in man: relationship between pattern of urinary metabolites and severity of liver damage. *Q J Med.* 1976; 178:181-91.
196. Davis M, Lavadarios D, Williams RS. Metabolism of paracetamol after therapeutic and hepatotoxic doses in man. *J Int Med Res.* 1976; 4(Suppl 4):40-5.
197. Mitchell JR, Jollow DJ, Potter WZ et al. Acetaminophen-induced hepatic necrosis. I. Role of drug metabolism. *J Pharmacol Exp Ther.* 1973; 187:285-94.
198. Jollow DJ, Mitchell JR, Potter WZ et al. Acetaminophen-induced hepatic necrosis. II. Role of covalent binding in vivo. *J Pharmacol Exp Ther.* 1973; 187:195-202.
199. Jollow DJ, Thorgeirsson SS, Potter WZ et al. Acetaminophen-induced hepatic necrosis: VI. Metabolic disposition of toxic and nontoxic doses of acetaminophen. *Pharmacology.* 1974; 12:251-71.
200. Peterson RG, Rumack BH. Age as a variable in acetaminophen overdose. *Arch Intern Med.* 1981; 141:390-3.
201. Rumack BH, Peterson RG. Acetaminophen overdose: incidence, diagnosis, and management in 416 patients. *Pediatrics.* 1978; 62(Suppl):898-903.
202. Meredith TJ, Newman B, Goulding R. Paracetamol poisoning in children. *Br Med J.* 1978; 2:478-9.
203. Lauterburg BH, Vaishnav Y, Stillwell WG et al. The effects of age and glutathione depletion on hepatic glutathione turnover in vivo determined by acetaminophen probe analysis. *J Pharmacol Exp Ther.* 1980; 213:54-8.
204. Hart JG, Timbrell JA. The effect of age on paracetamol hepatotoxicity in mice. *Biochem Pharmacol.* 1979; 28:3015-7.
205. Roberts I, Robinson MJ, Mughal MZ et al. Paracetamol metabolites in the neonate following maternal overdose. *Br J Clin Pharmacol.* 1984; 18:201-6.
206. McNeil Consumer Products Company. Tylenol product information. Fort Washington, PA; 1988.
207. Temple AR. Review of comparative antipyretic activity in children. *Am J Med.* 1983; 75(Suppl 5A):38-46.
208. Rumack BH. Acetaminophen overdose. *Am J Med.* 1983; 75(Suppl 5A):104-12.
209. Mäkela AL, Lempiäinen M, Ylijoki H. Ibuprofen levels in serum and synovial fluid. *Scand J Rheumatol.* 1981; Suppl 39:15-7.
210. Mäkela AL, Lempiäinen M, Yrjana T. Ibuprofen in the treatment of juvenile rheumatoid arthritis: metabolism and concentrations in synovial fluid. *Br J Clin Pract.* 1980; 6(Suppl):23-7.
211. Nahata MC, Durrell DE, Powell DA et al. Pharmacokinetics of ibuprofen in febrile children. *Eur J Clin Pharmacol.* 1991; 40:427-8.
212. Konstan MW, Hoppel CL, Chai BL et al. Ibuprofen in children with cystic fibrosis: pharmacokinetics and adverse effects. *J Pediatr.* 1991; 118:956-64.
213. Adams SS. Some biological properties of 2(4-isobutylphenyl)propionic acid. *J Pharm Sci.* 1967; 56:1686.
214. Kaiser DG. GLC determination of ibuprofen in plasma. *J Pharm Sci.* 1976; 63:219.
215. Abernathy DR, Greenblatt DJ. Ibuprofen disposition in obese individuals. *Arthritis Rheum.* 1985; 28:1117-21.
216. Lockwood GF, Albert KS, Gillespie WR et al. Pharmacokinetics of ibuprofen in man: I. Free and total area/dose relationships. *Clin Pharmacol Ther.* 1983; 34:97-103.
217. Benvenuti C, Cancellieri V, Gambaro V et al. Pharmacokinetics of two new oral formulations of ibuprofen. *Int J Clin Pharmacol Ther Toxicol.* 1986; 24:308-12.
218. Mills RFN, Adams SS, Cliffe EE et al. The metabolism of ibuprofen. *Xenobiotica.* 1973; 3:589-98.
219. Lockwood GF, Albert KS, Szpunar GJ et al. Pharmacokinetics of ibuprofen in man: III. Plasma protein binding. *J Pharmacokinet Biopharm.* 1983; 11:469-82.
220. Brown RD, Wilson JT, Kearns GL et al. Single-dose pharmacokinetics of ibuprofen and acetaminophen in febrile children. *J Clin Pharmacol.* 1992; 32:231-41.
221. Joshi YM, Sovani VB, Joshi VV et al. Comparative evaluation of the antipyretic efficacy of ibuprofen and paracetamol. *Indian Pediatr.* 1990; 27:803-6.
222. Heremans G, Dehaen F, Rom N et al. A single-blind parallel group study investigating the antipyretic properties of ibuprofen syrup versus acetylsalicylic acid syrup in febrile children. *Br J Clin Pract.* 1988; 42:245-7.
223. Phadke MA, Paranjape PV, Joshi AS. Ibuprofen in children with infective disorders—antipyretic efficacy. *Br J Clin Pract.* 1985; 39:437-40.
224. Amdekar YK, Desai RZ. Antipyretic activity of ibuprofen and paracetamol in children with pyrexia. *Br J Clin Pract.* 1985; 39:140-3.
225. Kandoth PW, Joshi MK, Joshi VR et al. Comparative evaluation of antipyretic activity of ibuprofen and aspirin in children with pyrexia of varied aetiology. *J Int Med Res.* 1984; 12:292-7.
226. Wilson G, Guerra AJ, Santos NT. Comparative study of the antipyretic effect of ibuprofen (oral suspension) and paracetamol (suppositories) in paediatrics. *J Int Med Res.* 1984; 12:250-4.
227. Brown DA, Pruitt AW. A comparison of aluminum ibuprofen suspension and acetaminophen elixir in the treatment of fever in children. *Clin Res.* 1984; 32:881A. Abstract.
228. Sheth UK, Gupta K, Paul T et al. Measurement of antipyretic activity of ibuprofen and paracetamol in children. *J Clin Pharmacol.* 1980; 20:672-5.
229. Similä S, Kouvalainen K, Keinanen S. Oral antipyretic therapy: evaluation of ibuprofen. *Scand J Rheumatol.* 1976; 5:81-3.
230. Wilson JT, Brown RD, Kearns GL et al. Single-dose, placebo-controlled comparative study of ibuprofen and acetaminophen antipyresis in children. *J Pediatr.* 1991; 119:803-11.
231. Sidler J, Frey B, Baerlocher K. A double-blind comparison of ibuprofen and paracetamol in juvenile pyrexia. *Br J Clin Pract.* 1990; 44(Suppl 70):22-5.
232. McNeil Consumer Products Company. Pedia Profen package insert. Fort Washington, PA; 1989 Jul.
233. Whitehall Laboratories, Inc. Children's Advil Suspension package insert. New York, NY; 1989 Sep.
234. Kotob A. A comparative study of two dosage levels of ibuprofen syrup in children with pyrexia. *J Int Med Res.*

1985; 13:122-6.

235. Marriott SC, Stephenson TJ. A double-blind dose-ranging trial with paediatric ibuprofen. *Br J Clin Pract.* 1990; 44(Suppl 70):15-8.
236. Royer GL, Seckman CE, Welshman IR. Safety profile: fifteen years of clinical experience with ibuprofen. *Am J Med.* 1984; 77:25-34.
237. Barry WS, Meinzinger MM, Howse CR. Ibuprofen overdose and exposure in utero: results from a postmarketing voluntary reporting system. *Am J Med.* 1984; 77:35-9.
238. Hall AH, Smolinske SC, Conrad FL et al. Ibuprofen overdose: 126 cases. *Ann Emerg Med.* 1986; 15:1308-13.
239. Hall AH, Smolinske SC, Kulig KW et al. Ibuprofen overdose—a prospective study. *West J Med.* 1988; 148:653-6.
240. Wolman IJ. Oral antipyretic therapy. *Am J Dis Child.* 1973; 126:564. Letter.
241. Yaffe SJ. Alternate doses of aspirin and acetaminophen. *Pediatr Alert.* 1978; 3:19-20.
242. Gennaro AR, Packman EW, DeLong AF. Plasma levels of aspirin and acetaminophen produced by a single combined dose of aspirin and acetaminophen in man. *Am J Pharm.* 1981; 153:12-8.
243. Whitehouse LW, Paul CJ, Wong TJ et al. Effect of aspirin on a subtoxic dose of ^{14}C-acetaminophen in mice. *J Pharm Sci.* 1977; 66:1399-403.
244. Kaplowitz N, Kuhlenkamp J, Goldstein L et al. Effect of salicylates and phenobarbital on hepatic glutathione in the rat. *J Pharmacol Exp Ther.* 1980; 212:240-5.

Statement of Ownership, Management and Circulation (Required by 39 U.S.C. 3685) 1. Title of publication, Clinical Pharmacy. 1A. Publication No. 02782677. 2. Date of filing, October 1, 1992. 3. Frequency of issue, Monthly. 3A. No. issues published annually, 12. 3B. Annual subscription price, $49.00. 4. Location of known office of publication, 7272 Wisconsin Avenue, Bethesda, Montgomery County, MD 20814. 5. Location of the headquarters or general business offices of publishers, 7272 Wisconsin Avenue, Bethesda, MD 20814. 6. Publisher, American Society of Hospital Pharmacists, Inc., 7272 Wisconsin Avenue, Bethesda, MD 20814. Editor, C. Richard Talley, 7272 Wisconsin Avenue, Bethesda, MD 20814. 7. Owner, American Society of Hospital Pharmacists, Inc., 7272 Wisconsin Avenue, Bethesda, MD 20814. 8. Known bondholders, mortgagees, and other security holders owning 1% or more of total amount of bonds, mortgages, and other securities, None. 9. For completion by nonprofit organizations authorized to mail at special rates (Section 132.122, PSM). The purpose, function, and nonprofit status of this organization and the exempt status for federal income tax purposes have not changed during preceding 12 months. 10. Extent and nature of circulation, A. Total no. copies printed, 9,816/10,200*; B. Paid circulation, 1. Sales through dealers and carriers, street vendors and counter sales, 300/0. 2. Mail subscriptions, 8,009/8,507; C. Total paid circulation, 8,309/8,507; D. Free distribution by mail, carrier or other means, samples, complimentary and other free copies, 519/495; E. Total distribution, 8,828/9,002; F. Copies not distributed, 1. Office use, left over, unaccounted, spoiled after printing, 988/1,198. Returns from news agents, 0, 0; G. Total, 9,816/10,200. I certify that the statements made by me are correct and complete, signed C. Richard Talley.

*First figure, average no. of copies each issue during preceding 12 months; second figure, actual no. of copies single issue published nearest to filing date.

Research Notes

Toxicity of rapidly infused concentrated intravenous immune globulin

CINDY IPPOLITI, LORETTA ANN WILLIAMS, AND STEVEN HUBER

Clin Pharm. 1992; 11:1022-6

Bone marrow transplantation (BMT) after myeloablative therapy offers curative potential to patients with otherwise fatal hematologic and nonhematologic malignancies.[1] Bacterial, fungal, and viral infections account for substantial morbidity and mortality in the posttransplant period and limit the success of allogeneic and autologous marrow transplantation.[2-5] Administration of intravenous immune globulin (IVIG) to BMT patients has been shown to reduce the incidence of bacterial infections, decrease the incidence and severity of cytomegalovirus pneumonitis, and, when combined with ganciclovir, effectively treat cytomegalovirus pneumonia.[6-11] Additionally, compared with placebo, IVIG has been reported to decrease the incidence of acute graft-versus-host disease in allogeneic BMT patients.[12,13]

In the M. D. Anderson Cancer Center Bone Marrow Transplant Unit, IVIG is administered prophylactically to all allogeneic BMT patients, to selected autologous BMT patients deemed at high risk for infection, and to patients with documented autoimmune thrombocytopenia after transplantation. The administration of IVIG is complex and time-consuming for both the patient and nursing personnel. Based on current manufacturer recommendations, the rate of IVIG infusions must be started slowly and increased every 15–30 minutes based on patient tolerance. Administration may take up to eight hours in some patients. In addition, the volume of fluid delivered with IVIG is intolerable in a subset of fluid-restricted patients with transplant-related complications such as capillary leak syndrome, congestive heart failure, veno-occlusive disease, or renal failure.

To simplify the administration process for nursing staff while limiting the volume of fluid infused, we assigned patients to receive a concentrated formulation of IVIG infused at a constant rate (without rate titration) over five, four, three, or two hours.

The aims of the study reported here were to (1) determine the maximum tolerated rate of infusion of concentrated IVIG, (2) determine the incidence and severity of adverse reactions in patients who received concentrated IVIG without initial rate titration, and (3) determine whether premedication lessened the severity of adverse reactions during subsequent infusions.

Methods. Commercially available IVIG (Venoglobulin-I, Alpha Therapeutic Corporation, Los Angeles, CA) was used to prepare the concentrated IVIG. A 5-g vial of Venoglobulin-I was reconstituted with Sterile Water for Injection, USP, to 10% solution. The resulting solution was a slightly viscous, yellowish, clear solution with an osmolarity of approximately 510 mOsm.

To assess the stability of the concentrated solution, two lots of a 10% solution of Venoglobulin-I were tested after 0, 8, and 24 hours at room temperature after reconstitution. Anticomplementary activity, measured by hemolysin-sensitized sheep-erythrocyte assay, was used to assess polymer formation and Fc functional activity; kallikrein activity was determined by a chromogenic enzymatic assay and compared with a standard preparation; prekallikrein activator was determined by chromogenic assay and compared with the Center for Biologics Evaluation and Research standard; measles antibody activity was assessed by using microtitration hemagglutination inhibition techniques; high-performance liquid chromatography was used to measure immunoglobulin fragments and polymers; and pH was monitored. The results of these studies indicated that the concentrated Venoglobulin-I prepa-

---

CINDY IPPOLITI, PHARM.D., is Clinical Research Specialist, Bone Marrow Transplantation, University of Texas M. D. Anderson Cancer Center, Houston, and Assistant Clinical Professor, School of Pharmacy, University of Houston. LORETTA ANN WILLIAMS, M.S.N., is Clinical Nurse Specialist in Bone Marrow Transplantation, Department of Hematology, and STEVEN HUBER, M.S., is Deputy Division Head for Pharmacy Patient Care Services, Division of Pharmacy, University of Texas M. D. Anderson Cancer Center.

Address reprint requests to Dr. Ippoliti at the Division of Pharmacy, Box 90, M. D. Anderson Cancer Center, University of Texas, 1515 Holcombe Boulevard, Houston, TX 77030.

The assistance of Christine Chow, Pharm.D., at Alpha Therapeutic Corporation in evaluating the concentrated intravenous immune globulin preparation used in these studies is acknowledged.

Support for these studies was provided by an educational grant from Alpha Therapeutic Corporation.

ration was chemically and functionally stable at room temperature for at least 24 hours after reconstitution (Table 1). However, it is not recommended that reconstituted product remain at room temperature for extended periods of time because of the possibility of microbial contamination.

Treatment Protocol. Adult patients (>15 years of age) who received autologous or allogeneic bone marrow transplants between February 1989 and November 1990 were eligible for the study if they had not previously received IVIG. Recipients of allogeneic transplants received concentrated IVIG prophylaxis for infection at a dose of 0.5 g/kg of body weight intravenously every 7 days starting 2 days before transplantation and continuing until 100 days post-transplantation. This dose was then administered monthly for nine months. Selected autologous marrow transplant patients treated before January 1990 received concentrated IVIG at a dosage of 0.5 g/kg of body weight every 14 days for the duration of their hospitalization. Bone marrow recipients who had thrombocytopenia that was refractory to platelet transfusions were given a trial of concentrated IVIG 0.5 g/kg/day for five consecutive days.

This study was designed as a phase I rate-escalation study. Forty patients were enrolled in the study. Patients were entered into one of four treatment groups. Patients 1–10 were assigned to group 1, patients 11–20 to group 2, patients 21–30 to group 3, and patients 31–40 to group 4. An IMED pump (IMED Corporation, San Diego, CA) was used to administer concentrated IVIG. For the first concentrated IVIG infusion, the pump was adjusted to deliver the total dose over a period of six hours; rate titration was not used for any of the infusions. Administration times for the second and all subsequent infusions were five, four, three, and two hours for groups 1, 2, 3, and 4, respectively.

All procedures followed were in accordance with the ethical standards of the M. D. Anderson Cancer Center's committee on human experimentation.

Assessment and Treatment of Adverse Reactions. Patients were monitored by staff nurses continuously throughout each concentrated IVIG infusion and every one to two hours by a BMT clinical nurse specialist. Objective assessment included temperature, vital signs, and auscultation of heart and lungs. Patients were asked for a subjective assessment of symptoms such as headache, nausea, chills, and flushing. The severity of adverse reactions was graded on a toxicity scale that was modified for the present study from the approved standard at M. D. Anderson Cancer Center (Table 2).

According to predetermined criteria, the infusion rate was not altered and no medications were administered when a grade 1 adverse reaction occurred. For adverse reactions of grade 2 or above, the concentrated IVIG infusion was stopped, and appropriate medications were administered (Table 3). When the reaction resolved, the infusion was resumed at one half the rate at which the reaction occurred. If no further reactions occurred after 30 minutes, the infusion rate was increased to the rate of the patient's group assignment.

Patients with grade 3 fever, chills, or flushing received acetaminophen 650 mg by mouth and diphenhydramine hydrochloride 25 mg i.v. over 15 minutes before all subsequent infusions of concentrated IVIG. Patients were removed from the study if a grade 4 reaction occurred.

Results. Between February 1989 and November 1990, 40 patients who required IVIG for prophylaxis of infection or for thrombocytopenia that was refractory to platelet transfusions were enrolled in the study (Table 4). Six of 40 patients (15%) had grade 2 or greater reactions during the first six-hour infusion (Table 5). Adverse reactions consisted of fever, chills, and flushing. All adverse reactions occurred within one to three hours after the start of the infusion.

The incidence of grade 2 or greater reactions during the second infusion was 10% in group 2 (four-hour infusion period) and 60% in group 4 (two-hour infu-

Table 1.
Stability of Reconstituted Venoglobulin-I[a,b]

Storage Time (hr)	ACA ($C'H_{50}$ units/mg)	Kallikrein (%)	PKA (%)	Measles Antibody (CBER units/mL)	pH	HPLC: Fragments (%)	HPLC: Polymers (%)	HPLC: Monomers Plus Dimers (%)
Lot GV9042A								
0	0.42	7.19	<2.5	0.67	6.65	0.1	0.6	99.3
8	0.35	6.01	None	ND	6.73	0.2	0.7	99.1
24	0.34	5.43	<2.5	0.67	6.71	0.0	0.7	99.3
Lot GV0001A								
0	0.18	4.03	<2.5	0.67	6.71	0.0	0.7	99.3
8	0.14	3.78	None	ND	6.68	0.0	0.7	99.3
24	0.13	3.01	<2.5	0.67	6.74	0.0	0.8	99.2

[a] ACA = anticomplementary activity, measured by reduction in hemolytic complement ($C'H_{50}$) units per milligram of intravenous immune globulin; PKA = prekallikrein activator; CBER = Center for Biologics Evaluation and Research, FDA; HPLC = high-performance liquid chromotography; ND = not determined.
[b] Values are based on single determination.

Table 2.
Adverse Reaction Grading Scale

Signs or Symptoms	Patient Manifestations			
	Grade 1	Grade 2	Grade 3	Grade 4
Chills	Feels cold	Shaking	Severe shaking	Uncontrolled shaking
Headache	Slight to moderate	Severe, relieved by nonnarcotic analgesic	Severe, relieved by narcotic	Not relieved by narcotic
Flushing	Face feels warm, no observable redness	Face pink in some areas	Diffuse facial redness	Diffuse facial redness
Shortness of breath, RR[a] increased, dyspnea	Shortness of breath with exertion, no dyspnea, RR stable	RR increased by >6 breaths/min with exertion, return to baseline with 5 min of rest	Shortness of breath at rest, RR increased by >6 breaths/min	Obvious dyspnea with nasal flare, need for oxygen
Fever	38.3 °C	39 °C	39.5 °C	40° C
Pulmonary congestion	Faint unilateral or bilateral crackles	Marked unilateral or bilateral crackles	Diffuse unilateral crackles	Diffuse bilateral crackles
Cardiac	Tachycardia of <30 beats/min above baseline	Development of S_3 gallop, resting tachycardia of ≥30 beats/min above baseline	Same as grade 2	Same as grade 2 with pulmonary findings

[a]RR = respiratory rate.

Table 3.
Treatments for Grades 2–4 Adverse Reactions

Reaction	Stop Infusion	Medication
Chills	Yes	Meperidine hydrochloride 25 mg IVPB[a]
Headache	No	Analgesic
Flushing	Yes	Diphenhydramine hydrochloride 25 mg IVPB
Fever	Yes	Acetaminophen 650 mg orally
Shortness of breath and dyspnea	Yes	Oxygen
Pulmonary congestion	Yes	Diuretics with or without oxygen
Cardiac	Yes	Diuretics as indicated

[a] IVPB = intravenous piggyback.

Table 4.
Patient Characteristics

Characteristic	No. Patients			
	Group 1 (*n* = 10)	Group 2 (*n* = 10)	Group 3 (*n* = 10)	Group 4 (*n* = 10)
Diagnosis				
Lymphoma	2	5	3	0
Acute leukemia	3	0	2	3
Chronic leukemia	2	3	5	5
Multiple myeloma	1	2	0	0
Metastatic breast cancer	1	0	0	1
Aplastic anemia	1	0	0	1
Transplant type				
Allogeneic	4	2	5	9
Autologous	6	8	5	1
Mean age in yr (range)	40.5 (30–55)	33.5 (17–59)	34 (32–44)	33 (16–49)

Table 5.
Reactions of Grade 2 or Greater after First Six-Hour Infusion of Intravenous Immune Globulin

Group	Age (yr)	Transplant Type	Disease	Reaction (Grade)
1	36	Autologous	Hodgkin's disease	Chills (3)[a]
1	40	Autologous	Multiple myeloma	Chills (2), headache (2)
1	46	Autologous	Chronic myelogenous leukemia	Chills (2)
2	59	Autologous	Multiple myeloma	Chills (2)[a]
2	43	Autologous	Non-Hodgkin's lymphoma	Chills (2)
2	17	Autologous	Hodgkin's disease	Chills (4),[a] fever (3)

[a] Received premedication for all subsequent doses.

sion period). The type and severity of the reactions experienced by these seven patients are shown in Table 6. No adverse reactions occurred in groups 1 (five-hour infusion) and 3 (three-hour infusion) during the second infusion.

Of the 40 patients, 38 went on to receive the third dose of concentrated IVIG at the assigned infusion rate. None of these patients experienced any adverse reactions. The patient in group 2 who developed severe shaking, chills, and fever of 40 °C during the first six-hour infusion was premedicated with acetaminophen and meperidine for the second infusion. After only one hour of the second concentrated IVIG infusion, originally scheduled to last four hours, he again developed shaking, chills, and fever. The infusion was terminated, and he was removed from the study. The patient in group 4 who developed shortness of breath with the two-hour infusion had clinical and radio-

Table 6.
Adverse Reactions to Second Concentrated Intravenous Immune Globulin (IVIG) Infusion

Group	Age (yr)	Transplant Type	Disease	Reaction (Grade)
2[a]	17	Autologous	Hodgkin's disease	Chills (4), fever (3)
4[b,c]	46	Allogeneic	Multiple myeloma	Shortness of breath (3), flushing (3)
4[b]	49	Allogeneic	Chronic myelogenous leukemia	Chills (3)
4	32	Allogeneic	Chronic myelogenous leukemia	Chills (2)
4	33	Allogeneic	Chronic myelogenous leukemia	Chills (2)
4	34	Allogeneic	Acute leukemia	Chills (2), fever (2)
4	28	Allogeneic	Chronic myelogenous leukemia	Chills (2)

[a] Removed from study.
[b] Premedicated for subsequent infusions.
[c] Subsequent doses of concentrated IVIG infused over four hours.

graphic evidence of congestive heart failure. She was treated with oxygen, fluid restriction, diuretics, and digoxin. To avoid rapid fluid challenges, she received all subsequent doses of concentrated IVIG over a four-hour period.

Discussion. Overall, concentrated IVIG administered over a period of three hours or longer was well tolerated; the incidence of toxicity was 3.3%. However, the high rate (60%) of adverse reactions seen in group 4 (two-hour infusion) may be misleading. Because patients were consecutively entered, the groups were not matched for underlying disease, transplant type, or frequency of IVIG administration. Nine of the 10 patients in group 4 received an allogeneic BMT, compared with 5 or fewer patients in the other groups. No data exist to suggest that patients receiving an allogeneic BMT may have a higher incidence of adverse reactions to IVIG, so allogeneic BMT cannot be ruled out as an explanation for the discrepancies seen in our current study.

The incidence of adverse reactions to the first concentrated IVIG infusion (six hours for all study participants) was 15%. The reported incidence of adverse reactions for standard IVIG concentrations is 5–10% based on information included in the package inserts. Several features of the patient population and of the concentrated IVIG treatment may have contributed to the higher incidence observed in this study: (1) It was a condition of study entry that patients had no prior IVIG therapy, and such patients may have a higher incidence of adverse reactions than patients who have had prior therapy. (2) The total IVIG dosages used in this study were higher than those used for immune globulin replacement therapy. (3) The IVIG concentration was 10%. (4) The dose was administered at a constant infusion rate, without rate titration. (5) Patients received no premedication for the first infusion. It is not possible to determine from this study whether the incidence of adverse effects was significantly increased by any of the variables indicated. Although the figure was higher than that reported elsewhere, the incidence of serious adverse experiences was judged to be acceptable, and substantial benefits can accrue with the infusion conditions used in this study.

In 1986, Ochs and colleagues[12] reported a successful program that enabled patients with primary immunodeficiency diseases to self-administer IVIG at home. Although details of the infusion process were not given, the authors concluded that "home administration of IVIG is both feasible and safe." Furthermore, the authors pointed out that home administration saved approximately $2400 to $3600 per patient per year.

Also in 1986, Ashida and Saxon[13] reported the long-term self-administration of IVIG by patients with hypogammaglobulinemia. After an initial period of rate titration during which a portable infusion pump was used, the maximum tolerated infusion rate was similar to that reported in the current study. With the portable pump, the maximum rate was 2.4 mL/hr; thus, the total infusion time for a patient receiving a dose of 400 mg/kg was approximately three hours. In the current study, an infusion period of two hours provoked an unacceptable incidence of adverse reactions in patients who were receiving 500 mg/kg, whereas infusion over a three-hour period was acceptable.

The concentrated fluid volume allows a substantial decrease in fluid load (approximately 350 mL/dose for a 70-kg patient rather than 700 mL/dose). The shortened administration period allows more efficient use of resources such as nursing time and clinic facilities. For patients who are receiving IVIG on an outpatient basis, rapid administration of concentrated IVIG will shorten the time of administration, reduce hospital costs, and enhance compliance.

Conclusion. The administration of concentrated solutions of Venoglobulin-I over a period of three hours was safe and well tolerated in BMT patients. Patients should continue, however, to receive the first infusion over a six-hour period with close monitoring.

References

1. Champlin RE. Bone marrow transplantation: introduction and overview. In: Champlin R, ed. Bone marrow transplantation. Norwell, MA: Kluwer Academic Publishers; 1990:1-7.
2. Deeg HJ. Delayed complications and long-term effects after bone marrow transplantation. *Hematol Oncol Clin North Am.* 1990; 4:641-57.
3. Karp JE, Merz WG, Dick JD et al. Strategies to prevent or control infections after bone marrow transplants. *Bone Marrow Transplant.* 1991; 8:1-6.
4. Lum LG. Recapitulation of immune ontogeny: a vital component for the success of bone marrow transplantation. In: Champlin R, ed. Bone marrow transplantation. Norwell, MA: Kluwer Academic Publishers; 1990:27-54.
5. Reusser P, Riddell SR, Meyers JD et al. Cytotoxic T-lymphocyte response to cytomegalovirus after human allogeneic

bone marrow transplantation: pattern of recovery and correlation with cytomegalovirus infection and disease. *Blood.* 1991; 78:1373-80.

6. Winston DJ, Ho WG, Champlin RE. Ganciclovir and intravenous immunoglobulin in bone marrow transplants. In: Champlin RE, Gale RP, eds. New strategies in bone marrow transplantation. New York: Wiley-Liss; 1991:337-48.
7. Sullivan KM, Kopecky K, Jocom J et al. Antimicrobial and immunomodulatory effects of intravenous immunoglobulin in bone marrow transplantation. In: Program and abstracts of the Twenty-eighth Conference on Antimicrobial Agents and Chemotherapy. Washington, DC: American Society for Microbiology; 1988:216. Abstract.
8. Petersen FB, Bowden RA, Thornquist M et al. The effect of prophylactic intravenous immune globulin on the incidence of septicemia in marrow transplant recipients. *Bone Marrow Transplant.* 1987; 2:141-8.
9. Graham-Pole J, Camitta B, Casper J et al. Intravenous immunoglobulin may lessen all forms of infection in patients receiving allogeneic bone marrow transplantation for acute lymphoblastic leukemia: a pediatric oncology group study. *Bone Marrow Transplant.* 1988; 3:559-66.
10. Sullivan KM, Kopecky KJ, Jocom J et al. Immunomodulatory and antimicrobial efficacy of intravenous immunoglobulin in bone marrow transplantation. *N Engl J Med.* 1990; 323:705-12.
11. Winston DJ, Ho WG, Lin C-H et al. Intravenous immune globulin for prevention of cytomegalovirus infection and interstitial pneumonia after bone marrow transplantation. *Ann Intern Med.* 1987; 106:12-18.
12. Ochs HD, Fischer SH, Lee ML et al. Intravenous immunoglobulin home treatment for patients with primary immunodeficiency diseases. *Lancet.* 1986; 1:610-11.
13. Ashida ER, Saxon A. Home intravenous immunoglobulin therapy by self-administration. *J Clin Immunol.* 1986; 6:306-9.

Pharmacokinetics of ondansetron in patients receiving cisplatin therapy

MICHAEL D. PARR, WILLIAM J. MCINTYRE, LISA M. HENDERSON, JOHN S. MACDONALD, AND MARY H. H. CHANDLER

Clin Pharm. 1992; 11:1026-9

Treatment of chemotherapy-induced nausea and vomiting is one of the more difficult challenges in hematology and oncology practice. Patients who develop chemotherapy-induced nausea and vomiting may have a decrease in their quality of life, and some patients may refuse further therapy because of this adverse effect.[1]

Ondansetron (Zofran; Glaxo Inc., Research Triangle Park, NC) has demonstrated antiemetic properties in animal and human studies.[2-6] In a trial comparing ondansetron with placebo, ondansetron decreased the number of episodes of emesis (median of 1.5 with ondansetron and 5.5 with placebo) and delayed the first episode of emesis by a median of 11.6 hours.[7] In a double-blind crossover study comparing ondansetron with metoclopramide, 75% of the patients had two or fewer episodes of nausea during ondansetron therapy compared with 42% of patients during metoclopramide therapy.[8] Ondansetron (as the hydrochloride salt) was administered as an 8-mg i.v. loading dose, followed by continuous infusion of 1 mg/hr for 24 hours. Metoclopramide (as the hydrochloride salt) was given as a 5-mg/kg i.v. loading dose followed by continuous infusion of metoclopramide 0.5 mg/hr for 8 hours and then placebo for 16 hours. In addition to its antiemetic effects, ondansetron may have anxiolytic and antipsychotic properties.[2]

In healthy volunteers the terminal half-life of ondansetron is reported to be three hours. Ondansetron is almost totally eliminated by metabolism, with less than 3% of an i.v. dose excreted unchanged in the urine.[9]

This report describes a pilot study of the pharmacokinetics of ondansetron in patients receiving high-dose cisplatin therapy.

Methods. *Patient Enrollment and Study Procedures.* Six patients were enrolled in the prospective, open-label, nonrandomized study. All were at least 18 years of age, were receiving a cisplatin-containing regimen for the first time, and were receiving high doses of cisplatin (^{3}60 mg/sq m). None of the patients gave a history of anticipatory nausea or vomiting. Patients were excluded if daily activity was limited (Karnofsky performance status less than 50%[10]), if renal or hepatic function was impaired (serum creatinine >2 mg/dL or serum bilirubin >1.5 mg/mL), or if the patient vomited within 24 hours before the start of the study. A complete blood count with differential, liver function tests, and serum electrolyte, creatinine, cholesterol, and triglyceride determinations were performed at baseline and were repeated at 24 hours to monitor for toxicity. Signed informed consent was obtained from all patients.

All patients had two peripheral intravenous catheters placed (one in each arm). One catheter was used for administration of ondansetron, antineoplastic agents, and any fluid flushes required. The other catheter was used exclusively to draw blood samples for

MICHAEL D. PARR, PHARM.D., is Assistant Director, Department of Pharmacy, University Hospital of Arkansas, Little Rock. WILLIAM J. MCINTYRE, PHARM.D., is Fellow, Cancer Immunology, College of Pharmacy, University of Texas Health Science Center, San Antonio. LISA M. HENDERSON, PHARM.D., is Glaxo Pharmacy Fellow in Gastroenterology and Clinical Assistant Professor, College of Pharmacy, University of Michigan, Ann Arbor. JOHN S. MACDONALD, M.D., is Professor of Medicine and Chief, Division of Medicine, Temple University Comprehensive Cancer Center, Philadelphia, PA. MARY H. H. CHANDLER, PHARM.D., is Associate Professor, College of Pharmacy, University of Kentucky Medical Center, Lexington.

Address reprint requests to Dr. Parr at Department of Pharmacy, University Hospital of Arkansas, 4301 West Markham, Slot 571, Little Rock, AR 72205.

Supported by a grant from Glaxo Inc.

Presented at the 23rd Annual ASHP Midyear Clinical Meeting, Dallas, TX, December 5, 1988.

the study.

Each patient received three 4-mg doses of ondansetron. Each dose was diluted in 50 mL of 0.9% sodium chloride injection and was administered over 15 minutes using an infusion pump (Abbott, Chicago, IL). Ondansetron was administered 30 minutes before and at 3.5 and 7.5 hours after the start of the cisplatin infusion. Vital signs were monitored at baseline and at 30, 60 and 120 minutes after each dose of ondansetron was given.

Blood samples were obtained before and at 5, 15, 30, 60, 120, and 180 minutes after the first ondansetron infusion. Additional blood samples were obtained 5 minutes before and 5 minutes after the second and third ondansetron infusions and at 10, 12, and 24 hours after the start of the cisplatin infusion. All samples were collected in heparin-containing evacuated containers (Becton-Dickinson, Rutherford, NJ) and centrifuged at 4000 rpm. The plasma was then harvested and frozen at –70 °C until analysis.

During the 24-hour study period, any episodes of nausea or vomiting were recorded and the amount of vomitus was estimated. The patients were also monitored and interviewed for any adverse reactions.

Pharmacokinetic Analysis. Pharmacokinetic analysis was performed using compartmental and noncompartmental methods. Compartmental analysis was performed with the PCNONLIN computer program (Statistical Consultants Inc., Lexington, KY). Pharmacokinetic variables were estimated using a two-compartment model with constant i.v. input and first-order output and with a one-compartment model with constant i.v. input and first-order output.[11] Both models have the capability for multiple-dose analysis. These models estimated the best Akaike information criterion values.[12] The area under the curve estimated by the multiple-dose analysis may be biased.[11] Therefore, the area under the concentration–time curve (AUC) was determined by using the trapezoidal rule. The AUC after the first dose was extrapolated from time 0 to infinity by dividing the last measured plasma concentration (at 3.67 hours) by 2. Clearance (CL) was calculated by dose/AUC and was standardized to body weight.

Analytical Method. A high-performance liquid chromatography procedure employing solid-phase extraction was used to quantitate plasma ondansetron concentrations. The method used a cyanoanalytical column with ultraviolet detection at 305 nm.[7] The recovery from solid-phase extraction was greater than 95%. The assay is quantitatively accurate to 1 ng/mL and is sensitive to 0.5 ng/mL. The procedure is linear in the range of 1–250 ng/mL. Subject sample concentrations greater than 250 ng/mL were diluted to fit within the standard curve range and normalized by multiplying by an appropriate dilution factor. The intraday coefficients of variation at concentrations of 1, 5, 10, 25, 50, 100, and 250 ng/mL were 0.06, 0.1, 0.076, 0.039, 0.092, 0.071, and 0.057, respectively. The interday coefficients of variation at concentrations of 2, 80, and 200 ng/mL were 0.35, 0.07, and 0.05, respectively. Plasma samples were frozen for 6 to 12 months. The patient samples were analyzed on consecutive days.

Results. All six subjects completed the study, although two subjects required droperidol for management of severe nausea and vomiting during the 24-hour study period. Demographic data are summarized in Table 1.

The plasma ondansetron concentration–time profiles for each patient are represented in Figures 1 and 2, and the pharmacokinetic values are listed in Table 2.

The concentration data best fit a two-compartment model for four of the six patients. Data from subjects 5 and 6 were best described by a one-compartment model. The models of best fit were obtained when data points were weighted to the reciprocal of the plasma concentrations. The mean ± S.D. terminal elimination rate constant λ_2 was 0.318 ± 0.189 hr^{-1}. All data points were used to calculate λ_2. The harmonic mean for half-life was 2.18 hours.

One patient experienced more than two episodes of vomiting during the 24-hour period. None of the patients experienced retching, extrapyramidal symptoms, or a major adverse event. Vital signs remained stable, and laboratory values did not change appreciably. The most frequent adverse reaction was mild sedation. One patient complained of dry mouth, and another experienced heartburn.

Discussion. Our pharmacokinetic data are limited by the small sample size. Ondansetron appears to best

Table 1.
Demographic Characteristics of Study Patients

Patient	Age (yr)[a]	Sex	Wt (kg)	Cisplatin Dose (mg/sq m)[b]	Concurrent Antineoplastic Therapy
1	69	M	66	60	Cyclophosphamide, doxorubicin
2	54	M	66	100	None
3	58	M	56	60	Cyclophosphamide, doxorubicin
4	56	M	80	60	Cyclophosphamide, doxorubicin
5	61	M	53	60	Etoposide
6	64	M	86	80	Doxorubicin

[a]Mean ± S.D. age was 60.5 ± 5.9 years.
[b]Mean ± S.D. dose was 67.8 ± 13.0 mg/sq m.

Figure 1. Plasma ondansetron concentration-versus-time profiles for patients 1, 2, and 3.

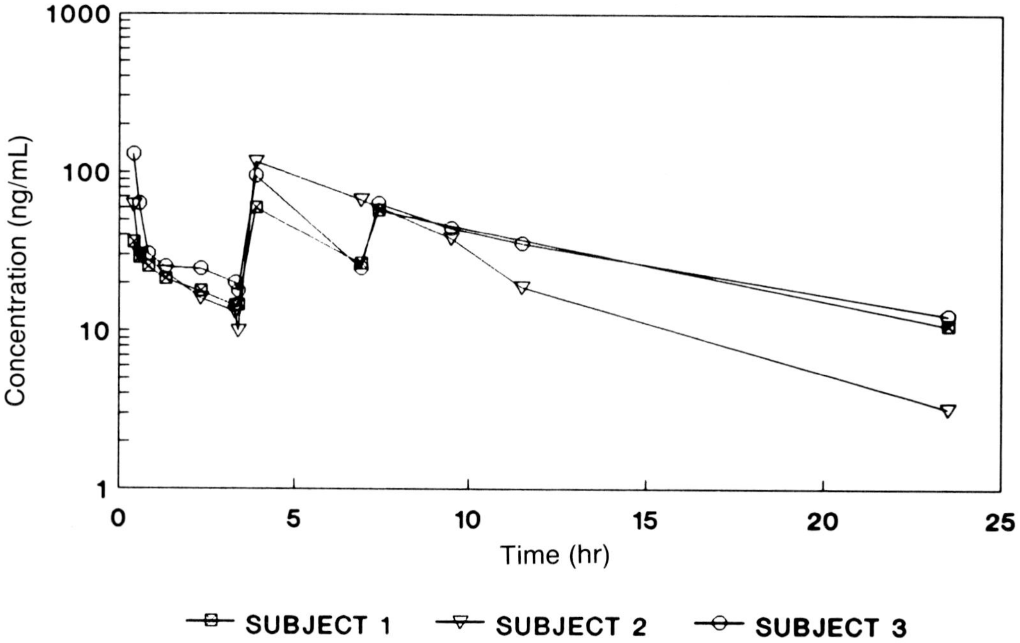

Figure 2. Plasma ondansetron concentration-versus-time profiles for patients 4, 5, and 6.

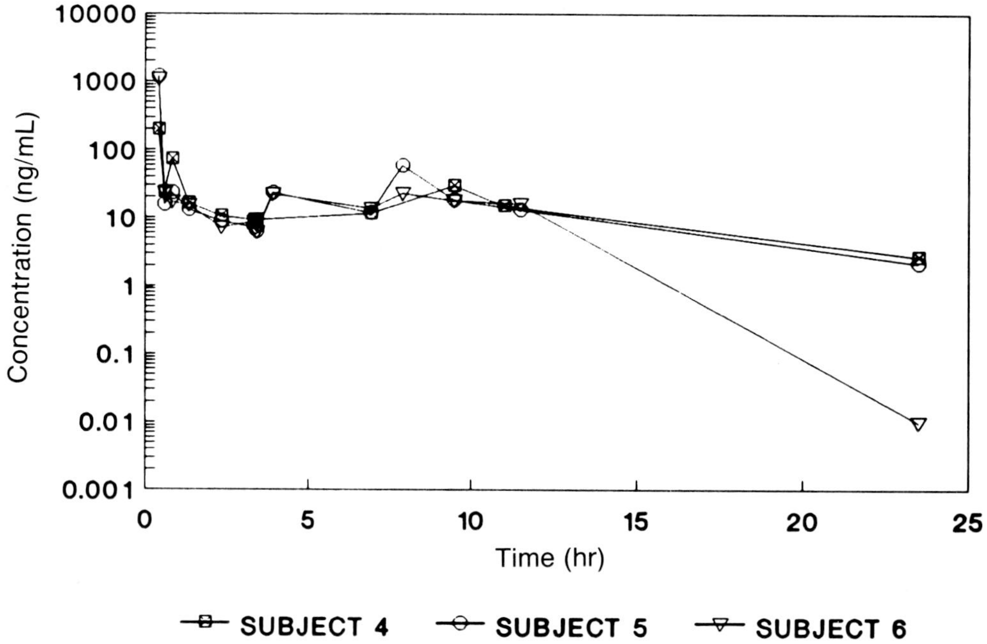

fit a two-compartment model in patients receiving high-dose cisplatin therapy. If we consider subject 3 (in whom $\lambda_2 = 0.722\ hr^{-1}$) an outlier, the mean λ_2 would be $0.237\ hr^{-1}$ instead of $0.318\ hr^{-1}$, which is more consistent with values reported by other investigators.[2,6,9] However, several studies have demonstrated a decrease in ondansetron clearance with an increase in patient age.[13,14] The average age of the subjects in our study was 60.5 years, but no age-related decrease in clearance was evident. The average λ_2 in our study is closer to the λ_2 reported in young, healthy subjects.[14] The pharmacokinetic estimates were based on plasma samples obtained after multiple doses and it was not possible to obtain samples far into the terminal elimination phase. Therefore, the elimination rate constant determined in this study may overestimate the true elimination rate constant. This is reflected by the fact that the mean λ_2 based on plasma samples obtained

Table 2.
Pharmacokinetic Values for Ondansetron[a]

Subject	λ_2 (hr^{-1})	AUC ($\mu g \cdot hr/L$)	CL (L/hr/kg)
1	0.253	128.2	0.473
2	0.221	111.2	0.544
3	0.722	231.6	0.306
4	0.257	99.5	0.502
5	0.241	198.3	0.381
6	0.215	202.6	0.229
Mean ± S.D.	0.318 ± 0.189	161.9 ± 55.6	0.403 ± 0.124

[a] λ_2 = terminal elimination rate constant, AUC = area under the plasma concentration–time curve, CL = clearance.

after the third dose (at 10, 12 and 24 hours after the start of the cisplatin infusion) was 0.148 hr^{-1}. However, definitive conclusions cannot be made because of the limited number of data points in the terminal distribution phase. In future studies, more samples should be obtained after the first dose and at steady state to better characterize ondansetron's pharmacokinetic profile.

Ondansetron appeared to provide protection against nausea and vomiting at the dosage used. The number of episodes of emesis were similar to those reported in the literature for metoclopramide.[15] However, our study was not designed to evaluate the efficacy of ondansetron.

Further studies are needed to determine appropriate dosage regimens in patient subpopulations.

Conclusion. The pharmacokinetics of ondansetron were best described by a two-compartment model.

References

1. Wilcox PM, Fetting JH, Nettesheim KM et al. Anticipatory vomiting in women receiving cyclophosphamide, methotrexate and 5-FU (CMF) adjuvant chemotherapy for breast carcinoma. *Cancer Treat Rep.* 1982; 66:1601-4.
2. Costall B, Domeney AM, Gunning SJ et al. GR-38032F: a potent and novel inhibitor of cisplatin induced emesis in the ferret. *Br J Pharmacol.* 1987; 90:90P. Abstract.
3. Kris MG, Gralla RJ, Clark RA et al. Dose-ranging evaluation of the serotonin antagonist GR-C507/75 (GR 38032F) when used as an antiemetic in patients receiving anticancer chemotherapy. *J Clin Oncol.* 1988; 6:659-62.
4. Kris MG, Gralla RJ, Clark RA et al. Phase II trials of the serotonin antagonist GR 38032F for the control of vomiting caused by cisplatin. *J Natl Cancer Inst.* 1989; 81:42-6.
5. Hesketh PJ, Murphy WK, Lester EP et al. GR 38032F (GR-C507/75): a novel compound in the prevention of acute cisplatin-induced emesis. *J Clin Oncol.* 1989; 7:700-5.
6. Grunberg SM, Stevenson LL, Russell CA et al. Dose ranging phase I study of the serotonin antagonist GR 38032F for prevention of cisplatin-induced nausea and vomiting. *J Clin Oncol.* 1989; 7:1137-41.
7. Cubeddu LX, Hoffmann IS, Fuenmayor NT et al. Efficacy of ondansetron (GR 38032F) and the role of serotonin in cisplatin induced nausea and vomiting. *N Engl J Med.* 1990; 322:810-6.
8. Marty M, Pouillart P, Scholl S et al. Comparison of the 5-hydroxytryptamine$_3$ (serotonin) antagonist ondansetron (GR 38032F) with high-dose metoclopramide in the control of cisplatin-induced emesis. *N Engl J Med.* 1990; 322:816-21.
9. Colthup PV, Palmer JL. The determination in plasma and pharmacokinetics of ondansetron. *Eur J Cancer Clin Oncol.* 1989; 25(Suppl 1):S71-4.
10. Karnofsky DA. Triethyliene melamine in treatment of neoplastic disease. *Arch Intern Med.* 1951; 87:477-516.
11. Metzler CM, Weiner DL. PCNONLIN. 3rd ed. Lexington, KY: Statistical Consultants; 1989.
12. Akaike H. An information criteria (AIC). *Math Sci.* 1976; 14:5-9.
13. Colthup PV, Felgate CC, Palmer JL et al. Determination of ondansetron in plasma and its pharmacokinetics in the young and elderly. *J Pharm Sci.* 1991; 80:868-71.
14. Pritchard JF, Bryson JC, Kernodle AE et al. Age and gender effects on ondansetron pharmacokinetics: evaluation of healthy aged volunteers. *Clin Pharmacol Ther.* 1992; 51:51-5.
15. Grunberg SM, Akerley WL, Krailo MD et al. Comparison of metoclopramide and metoclopramide plus dexamethasone for complete protection from cisplatinum induced emesis. *Cancer Invest.* 1986; 4:379-85.

Drug Experience

Straightforward reports of unusual drug experiences are included in this section. These may be confirmations of previously reported drug experiences or brief apparent first reports. While selected references may be cited, the purpose of a Drug Experience *report is not to present an extensive review of the literature.*

A related section, Grand Rounds, *includes papers that are well-documented patient case reports with a thorough review of the important literature to help put the case in perspective.*

Removal of ethosuximide and phenobarbital by peritoneal dialysis in a child

ERIC D. MARQUARDT, DENIS Y. ISHISAKA, KUMAR K. BATRA, AND BARBARA CHIN

Clin Pharm. 1992; 11:1030-1

Ethosuximide and phenobarbital are frequently used as anticonvulsants in children. In adults, ethosuximide is removed by hemodialysis, and phenobarbital is removed by peritoneal dialysis and hemodialysis.[1,2] There is one case report of the removal of phenobarbital by peritoneal dialysis in a neonate.[3] We are unaware of any other literature on the removal of these medications by peritoneal dialysis in children.

A child at our hospital underwent peritoneal dialysis while receiving ethosuximide and phenobarbital. This report describes the concentration of these medications in peritoneal dialysis effluent.

Case Report. A 10-year-old, 23.8-kg Asian girl was admitted to the hospital complaining of abdominal pain. She had a history of polycystic kidney disease and had received a renal transplant 18 months before admission. The transplanted kidney was removed two months later, after being rejected. She had been treated with ambulatory peritoneal dialysis for renal failure since then and was currently receiving eight hours of peritoneal dialysis by cycler daily. The patient had a similar episode of pain six months before admission and was treated for *Proteus mirabilis* peritonitis. The patient also had a history of hemosiderosis, elevated liver enzymes, and growth retardation.

She was receiving ethosuximide syrup 400 mg three times daily and phenobarbital elixir 72 mg every 12 hours. She had been treated with these drugs for 22 months. Although she had a seven-year history of absence seizures, she had not had a seizure in more than one year. Serum phenobarbital and ethosuximide concentrations one month before admission were 24 mg/L and 136 mg/L, respectively.

On the day of admission, the peritoneal fluid was yellow and cloudy. The patient was afebrile and in moderate distress. A sample of the peritoneal fluid was cultured and subsequently grew *Pseudomonas aeruginosa*. The patient was given one intravenous dose of gentamicin 80 mg (as the sulfate salt), and then gentamicin 6 mg (as the sulfate salt) and cefazolin 250 mg (as the sodium salt) were added to each liter of peritoneal dialysis fluid (Dianeal PD-2 with 2.5% dextrose, Baxter Healthcare Corp., Deerfield, IL). The patient received a 1-L exchange of dialysis fluid approximately every four hours. The patient continued to receive her anticonvulsant medications at preadmission dosages.

On hospital day 2 the patient had a seizure, which was witnessed by members of the nursing and medical staffs. The patient cried out, she had bilateral eyelid twitching, and both eyes deviated to the left. The patient was unresponsive to shaking by the physician. The seizure stopped spontaneously after approximately three minutes. The serum phenobarbital concentration on that day was 16 mg/L. She was given phenobarbital sodium 75 mg intravenously, and the route of maintenance phenobarbital therapy was changed from oral to intravenous. On hospital day 3 the serum ethosuximide concentration was 38 mg/L. On hospital day 5 the route of phenobarbital therapy was changed back to oral, and the dosage was increased to 90 mg every 12 hours because the serum concentration on day 4 was 12 mg/L. On hospital day 6 the phenobarbital dosage was increased to 105 mg

---

ERIC D. MARQUARDT, PHARM.D., and DENIS Y. ISHISAKA, PHARM.D., are Clinical Pharmacists, Department of Pharmacy, University of California Davis Medical Center (UCDMC), Sacramento, and Assistant Clinical Professors, School of Pharmacy, University of California, San Francisco. KUMAR K. BATRA, PH.D., is Director of Toxicology Laboratory, Department of Pathology, and BARBARA CHIN, M.D., is Resident in Pediatrics, Department of Pediatrics, UCDMC.

Address reprint requests to Dr. Marquardt at the Department of Pharmacy, University of California Davis Medical Center, 2315 Stockton Boulevard, Sacramento, CA 95817.

The assistance of Ron Wade, M.S., is acknowledged.

Supported in part by a research grant from the Pharmacy Sciences Liaison unit of the Upjohn Company, Kalamazoo, MI.

Presented at the 49th ASHP Annual Meeting, Washington, DC, June 3, 1992.

every 12 hours because the serum concentration on the previous day was 15 mg/L. The serum phenobarbital concentration on day 6 was 21 mg/L.

Measurement of Anticonvulsant Concentrations in Dialysis Effluent. We suspected that the patient's anticonvulsant medications were being removed during peritoneal dialysis, so we measured their concentrations in the dialysis effluent. Samples of peritoneal dialysis effluent from five exchanges were frozen immediately after collection and then thawed just before analysis.

Phenobarbital concentrations were measured by high-performance liquid chromatography (HPLC). We added 200 μL of acetonitrile, which contained cyclopentobarbital 12.5 μg/mL as an internal standard, to 100 μL of dialysis effluent. The mixture was centrifuged, and 10 μL of the supernate was injected onto a 5-μm particle size, Spherisorb ODS-2 HPLC column (15 cm × 4.6 mm, Alltech Associates, Deerfield, IL) at 50 °C. The phenobarbital and internal standard were eluted by a mobile phase consisting of 33% (v/v) methanol and 14% (v/v) acetonitrile in 0.01 M potassium phosphate buffer at a flow rate of 1.5 mL/min, by using a Perkin-Elmer series 10 pump (Mountain View, CA). Phenobarbital and the internal standard were detected by using a Perkin-Elmer LC-95 ultraviolet–visible-light detector set at 210 nm. All determinations were run in duplicate.

Ethosuximide concentrations were determined by the enzyme-multiplied immunoassay method (EMIT, Syva Corp., Palo Alto, CA) on the Roche COBAS FARA analyzer (Roche Diagnostic Systems, Belleville, NJ). All determinations were run in duplicate.

Phenobarbital concentrations in dialysis effluent ranged from 10 to 13 mg/L, and ethosuximide concentrations ranged from 59 to 111 mg/L (Table 1). About 14 mg of phenobarbital and 106 mg of ethosuximide, on average, were removed from the body per four-hour dwell. Therefore, if the five exchanges were typical, approximately 82 mg of phenobarbital and 630 mg of ethosuximide were removed in a 24-hour period. These amounts correspond to about 40% of the phenobarbital dose (on day 6) and about 50% of the ethosuximide dose removed daily.

Discussion. Before admission this patient was receiving only eight hours of dialysis daily. She had serum anticonvulsant concentrations that were in the usual therapeutic range and had not had a recent seizure. After admission, her dialysis time increased to 24 hours per day and her serum anticonvulsant concentrations dropped. The removal of these medications by peritoneal dialysis, along with not giving the patient any supplemental doses, might have contributed to the development of seizure activity. Unfortunately, we did not measure steady-state serum drug concentrations, which might have helped define the extent of drug clearance by peritoneal dialysis. Furthermore, the dosage of phenobarbital was changing while we were collecting samples, and the dialysis times for which we obtained samples did not have a consistent temporal relationship to the anticonvulsants' administration times. Also, it is possible that inflammation of our patient's peritoneum contributed to drug removal during dialysis.

Further studies and steady-state serum concentrations are required to accurately determine the amounts of these drugs removed by peritoneal dialysis. Our data suggest that substantial amounts of phenobarbital and ethosuximide are removed by peritoneal dialysis. It may be necessary to increase the dosage of both drugs for children undergoing peritoneal dialysis. Also, peritoneal dialysis may prove to be an alternate method for treating acute overdoses of these medications.

Conclusion. Increasing the daily duration of peritoneal dialysis apparently caused decreases in serum phenobarbital and ethosuximide concentrations and may have contributed to seizure activity.

References

1. Marbury TC, Lee CC, Perchalski RJ et al. Hemodialysis clearance of ethosuximide in patients with chronic renal disease. *Am J Hosp Pharm.* 1981; 38:1757-60.
2. Anderson RJ, Gambertoglio JG, Schrier RW. Clinical use of drugs in renal failure. Springfield, IL: Charles C Thomas; 1976.
3. Chow-Tung E, Lau AH, Vidyasagar D et al. Clearance of phenobarbital by peritoneal dialysis in a neonate. *Clin Pharm.* 1982; 1:268-71.

Table 1.
Removal of Anticonvulsant Drugs by Peritoneal Dialysis[a]

Hospital Day	Dialysis Time	Volume of Dialysis Effluent (L)	Drug Concentration in Dialysis Effluent (mg/L)[b]	
			Phenobarbital	Ethosuximide
5	0800–1200	1.14	10	59
6	0800–1230	1.01	13	90
	1245–1615	1.23	12	111
	1635–2015	1.07	12	104
7	0415–0800	1.33	12	92

[a]Ethosuximide syrup 400 mg was given daily at 0800, 1200, and 2000; this regimen was started 22 months before admission and continued throughout hospitalization. Phenobarbital elixir 72 mg had been given daily at 0800 and 2000 from 22 months before admission until hospital day 2. On hospital day 2, one 75-mg dose of phenobarbital sodium was given i.v., and the maintenance dosage was changed to phenobarbital sodium 72 mg i.v. daily at 0800 and 2000. On hospital day 5, the dosage was changed to phenobarbital 90 mg orally daily at 0800 and 2000. On hospital day 6, the dosage was changed to phenobarbital 105 mg orally daily at 0800 and 2000.
[b]Means of duplicate determinations.

ASHP Report

Acknowledgment to reviewers—October 1, 1991, to September 30, 1992

This year, approximately 158 manuscripts were submitted for publication consideration to *Clinical Pharmacy*, including papers solicited by the editors. Approximately 44% of the papers received were ultimately accepted. During this same period, we received critiques from 195 reviewers who evaluated the merit of *Clinical Pharmacy* submissions. Readers are indebted to these reviewers, who contributed their time in this advisory capacity. Their efforts have helped maintain the high standards of *CP*. Several referees reviewed more than one paper during the year, and their extra contributions are especially appreciated.

Lori J. Acuncius
Brian K. Alldredge
Nancy M. Allen
Guy W. Amsden
Robert K. Ausman
Brian A. Baker
Charles H. Ballow
Carol E. Balmer
Randal L. Batenhorst
Jerry L. Bauman
Angela Benson
John M. Benson
Rosemary R. Berardi
Richard C. Berchou
Roger G. Berlin
Varsha Bhatt-Mehta
Mary C. Birmingham
Robert A. Blum
John A. Bosso
Michael B. Bottorff
Bradley A. Boucher
Eric G. Boyce
Barbara W. Brandom
Cynthia Brennan
Dennis G. Brierton
Candace S. Brown
Rex O. Brown
Reginald Bruskewitz
Robert G. Buice
Kelly Joan Burch
Michael E. Burton
Henry I. Bussey
R. Keith Campbell
Suzanne Campbell
Patrice Carmichael
Barry L. Carter
Ladia Cheng
Thomas J. Comstock
Richard E. Crass
William R. Crom
Kent B. Crossley
Larry H. Danziger
Robin Davis
Francine G. Dela Cruz
Richard Dettloff
Roland N. Dickerson
Joseph T. DiPiro
Robert E. Dupuis
Steven C. Ebert
Mark J. Ellison
Susan C. Fagan
Martha P. Fankhauser
Kelly Faulkner
Richard C. Fiscella
John F. Flaherty
Richard J. Fleck
Courtney V. Fletcher
Peter Gal
Amy Galip
William R. Garnett
Susan Gorman
Kathryn L. Grant
Sara R. Grimsley
David R. Guay
Sally K. Guthrie
Robert A. Hamilton
Edward M. Hampton
Christine Hansen
Thomas C. Hardin
Evelyn Hermes
Malcolm R. Hill
Beverly J. Holcombe
John R. Horn
Denise L. Howrie
Robert J. Ignoffo
Timothy J. Ives
Marie W. Jackson
Martin L. Job
Cary E. Johnson
Curtis A. Johnson
June Felice Johnson
Joan E. Kapusnik-Uner
James A. Karboski
Steven R. Kayser
William A. Kehoe
Deborah Kiely
Terrance A. Killilea
Bruce J. Kimelblatt
Julie Kirk
David F. Kisor
Rachel L. Kleiman-Wexler
Margaret Knapp
Philip R. Kohls
Wayne A. Kradjan
Daniel W. Krichbaum
Peggy G. Kuehl
John G. Kuhn
Kenneth C. Lamp
Alan H. Lau
R. David Lauper
Mary W. L. Lee
Richard D. Leff
Marc Levine
Robert A. Littrell
James Mack
Allan Mailloux
Robert A. Mangione
C. Randall Marchbanks
Kathryn M. Martin
Dayna L. McCauley
Barbara A. McGee
Betty J. McGrath
James M. McKenney
David McKindley
Fred L. Meister
Donald R. Miller
Lucinda G. Miller
Jorge R. Miranda-Massari
Jay M. Mirtallo
Michael A. Montwill
James B. Mowry
Bruce A. Mueller
John E. Murphy
Jean M. Nappi
David E. Nix
Paul E. Nolan
Julie Oki
Frank P. Paloucek
Roy C. Parish
Robert B. Parker
Rakesh Patel
Larry E. Patterson
Mark D. Peters
Karen I. Plaisance
Roy A. Pleasants
Ron E. Polk
William R. Porter
Rebecca Rogers Prevost
Arden Prince
Randall A. Prince
Mark C. Pugh
Michael D. Reed
Danny Rodman
Keith A. Rodvold
Ronald J. Ruggiero
David R. Rutledge
Patrick B. Ryan
Michael J. Rybak
Kevin Rynn
Rosalie Sagraves
Jan V. Sahai
Judith J. Saklad
Paula L. Sanders
William T. Sawyer
Gary Schmidt
Robert E. Schumacher
Arthur A. Schuna
Charles F. Seifert
Amy L. Shafer
Pamela A. Simon
Gary E. Sloskey
Ralph E. Small
Laurie Jo Smith
Steven P. Smith
William J. Spruill
Gary E. Stein
Robert C. Stevens
Clinton F. Stewart
Arthur B. Straughn
Lisa Sunyecz
Robert L. Talbert
Joseph A. Tami
Jerry W. Taylor
Philip D. Thomson
James E. Tisdale
Timothy J. Van Mouwerik
Eva M. Vasquez
Donna F. Veal
Thomas G. Vondracek
Michael E. Ward
David W. Waterhouse
D. Raymond Weber
Paul J. Weidle
Sophy P. Weinroth
Lynda S. Welage
Timothy E. Welty
Andrea Wendrow
Dennis M. Williams
James E. Wilson
Allison Winecoff
David R. Witmer
Gary C. Yee
Peter J. Yurkowski
Alan J. Zametkin
Barbara J. Zarowitz

DUE Criteria

The DUE Criteria *section of* Clinical Pharmacy *features model drug-use evaluation criteria that may be employed as a component of a comprehensive quality assurance program. The criteria sets are presented in the format used in the ASHP book* Criteria for Drug Use Evaluation. *Some of the criteria sets will have been originally published in that book; others will be presented here for the first time and published in future volumes of the ASHP book. The practitioners who developed a criteria set are acknowledged.*

In selecting drug products for coverage in DUE Criteria, *priority is given to products that have been recently marketed, those that are frequently prescribed, those that have high potential risk associated with their use, and those that are expensive. When feasible, a criteria set will be linked with a Drug Review that appears in the same issue.*

These criteria sets are a starting point for the development of DUE criteria for a specific practice setting. Readers are encouraged to modify the model criteria to fit their own circumstances.

Criteria for use of theophylline (aminophylline) in inpatients and outpatients with pulmonary disease[a]

Element	Standard 100%	Standard 0%	Exception[b] or Critical Preventive/ Responsive Measure[c]	Sources of Information
Justification for Use[1-10,d]				
1. Prophylaxis of chronic asthma in outpatient (especially with nocturnal symptoms) already receiving optimum doses of ß-adrenergic agonists or	X		1A. Beta agonists contraindicated	1, 1A. History and physical (H&P), progress notes, outpatient profile
2. Treatment of acute exacerbation of asthma, requiring an emergency department visit, in patient receiving maintenance therapy with oral theophylline or	X		2A. Initial serum theophylline concentration, ≥15 µg/mL	2. H&P, progress notes 2A. Laboratory reports
3. Treatment of patient hospitalized because of asthma or	X		3A. None	3. H&P, progress notes
4. Continuation of outpatient maintenance therapy for chronic asthma in patient hospitalized for an unrelated condition or	X		4A. None	4, H&P, progress notes
5. Adjunctive treatment of partially reversible chronic obstructive pulmonary disease in patient already receiving a ß agonist or an anticholinergic drug	X		5A. Beta agonists and anticholinergics contraindicated	5. H&P, progress notes, medication administration record (MAR) 5A. Progress notes
Critical (Process) Indicators[1,3,8,9]				
6. Pretreatment assessment consists of medical history and physical examination with assessment of lung function, including spirometry (forced expiratory volume in one second, forced vital capacity, maximum	X		6A. None	6. H&P, progress notes, respiratory therapy reports

Prepared by Marjorie Shaw Phillips, M.S., QI/DUE Pharmacist, Department of Pharmacy, Medical College of Georgia Hospital and Clinics, 1120 Fifteenth Street, Augusta, GA 30912.

Element	Standard 100%	Standard 0%	Exception[b] or Critical Preventive/ Responsive Measure[c]	Sources of Information
midexpiratory flow rate, or peak expiratory flow rate)[1]				
7. No history of anaphylaxis or hypersensitivity reaction to theophylline, caffeine, theobromine, ethylenediamine, or sulfites	X		7A. Only theophylline may be used in patient with ethylenediamine allergy 7B. Sulfite-free product used for patient with sulfite allergy	7. H&P, allergy reports 7A, B. Physician orders, MAR
8. Appropriate initial dosage for oral therapy in ambulatory adult or child over one year of age: the lesser of 400 mg/day or 16 mg/kg/day, given in divided doses[3]	X		8A. If patient obese, dosage based on ideal body weight	8. Physician orders, progress notes, MAR, outpatient profile 8A. Progress notes, nursing notes
9. Appropriate initial dosage (mg/kg/day) for oral therapy in child less than one year of age: 5 + (0.2 × age in weeks), given in divided doses[9,11]	X		9A. Initial mg/kg/day dosage less than 8 + (0.3 × age in weeks)[11]	9, 9A. H&P, physician orders, progress notes, MAR, outpatient profile
10. Route of administration and dosage formulation selected on the basis of patient condition: a. Intravenous theophylline or aminophylline used in patient who cannot take medication orally or when rapid achievement of therapeutic concentrations is vital b. Immediate-release oral formulation used for initial doses and for patients who cannot swallow extended-release preparation c. Extended-release preparation used to improve efficacy, safety, and compliance during maintenance therapy	X		10A. Extended-release formulation used for initial doses in patient for whom the theophylline dosage is being slowly adjusted	10, 10A. Physician orders, progress notes, MAR, outpatient profile
11. Extended-release formulations are swallowed whole (not crushed or chewed)	X		11A. Tablets split on score marking, or bead-filled capsules opened and sprinkled on food	11, 11A. Progress notes, nursing notes, MAR
12. Immediate-release oral theophylline product given q 6–8 hr	X		12A. Shorter dosage interval because of high elimination rate (determined from serum theophylline levels)	12, 12A. Physician orders, progress notes, laboratory reports
13. Extended-release oral theophylline product given q 12 hr	X		13A. Longer dosage interval because of slow drug metabolism (half life, >10 hr) (e.g., heart failure, liver disease) or products with indication for once-daily administration (e.g., Theo-24, Uniphyl) 13B. Shorter dosage interval because of increased drug metabolism (e.g., smoker, child, or subtherapeutic serum theophylline trough level) 13C. Once daily at bedtime for nocturnal asthma	13. Physician orders, MAR, outpatient profile 13A. Progress notes, MAR, outpatient profile, laboratory reports 13B. Progress notes, laboratory reports 13C. Physician orders, progress notes, MAR, outpatient profile
14. Appropriate loading dose for inpatient i.v. therapy administered at a rate not to exceed 20 mg/min (usually over 20–30 min)[1]: a. If no previous theophylline, theophylline 4.7 mg/kg (aminophylline 6 mg/kg) b. If serum theophylline level known, theophylline 0.5 mg/kg for every 1-	X		14A. In a patient being switched to i.v. therapy, loading dose not required if current serum concentration on oral theophylline is effective	14, 14A Physician orders, progress notes, MAR, i.v. flow sheet, laboratory reports

Element	Standard 100%	0%	Exception[b] or Critical Preventive/ Responsive Measure[c]	Sources of Information
μg/mL increase in serum theophylline needed to reach target of 15 μg/mL c. If serum theophylline level unknown, theophylline 2.5 mg/kg (aminophylline 3 mg/kg)				
15. Appropriate initial maintenance dosage for inpatient i.v. therapy by continuous infusion[1]: a. For adult patient, theophylline 0.4 mg/kg/hr (aminophylline 0.6 mg/kg/hr) b. For infant 1–6 mo old, theophylline 0.4 mg/kg/hr (aminophylline 0.5 mg/kg/hr) c. For infant 6–12 mo old, theophylline 0.8 mg/kg/hr (aminophylline 1 mg/kg/hr) d. For child 1–9 yr old, theophylline 1.2 mg/kg/hr (aminophylline 1.5 mg/kg/hr) e. For child 10–16 yr old, theophylline 0.96 mg/kg/hr (aminophylline 1.2 mg/kg/hr)	X		15A. If patient is obese, dosage based on ideal body weight 15B. If patient smokes, theophylline 0.6 mg/kg/hr (aminophylline 0.75 mg/kg/hr) 15C. If patient has severe liver, cardiac, or pulmonary dysfunction, theophylline 0.2 mg/kg/hr (aminophylline 0.25 mg/kg/hr) 15D. If therapeutic level with oral theophylline, dosage (mg/hr) of i.v. theophylline equals total daily oral dosage divided by 24 (multiply by 1.25 for mg/hr of aminophylline) 15E. Alternative maintenance dosage indicated on basis of previous i.v. therapy	15. Physician orders, MAR, i.v. flow sheet 15A–E. Progress notes
16. Serum theophylline levels monitored[1,3,4]: a. One hour after i.v. loading dose b. Approximately 6 to 12 hr after i.v. infusion initiated c. Twenty-four hours after initiating or modifying i.v. therapy to assess steady-state levels d. Within three days after each oral dosage adjustment e. At 6–12-mo intervals during maintenance therapy f. If smoker (tobacco, marijuana) discontinues habit	X		16A. Symptoms controlled without adverse effects by initial maintenance dosage (or maximum of 600 mg/day for adults and children weighing >45 kg)[3] (maximum of 16 mg/kg or 400 mg/day for children weighing ≤45 kg)	16. Physician orders, progress notes, MAR, laboratory reports 16A. Progress notes, nursing notes
17. Serum theophylline determinations made at correct time relative to drug administration[4]: a. Two hours after solution or uncoated (immediate-release) tablet given b. Four hours after extended-release tablet given	X		17A. Serum determinations made 3–7 hr after dose of Theo-Dur given	17. Laboratory reports, nursing notes, MAR
18. Theophylline (aminophylline) dosage adjusted to achieve steady-state serum theophylline concentrations of 5–15 μg/mL[1]	X		18A. Patient requires higher serum drug concentrations (15–20 μg/mL) for relief of symptoms	18. Physician orders, laboratory reports 18A. Progress notes
19. If adverse reaction to theophylline at usual dosage, serum levels checked	X		19A. None	19. Physician orders, progress notes, nursing notes
20. If expected bronchodilator effect not achieved, serum levels checked	X		20A. None	20. Physician orders, progress notes, nursing notes
21. Patient receiving concomitant fluroquinolone antimicrobial, cimetidine, high-dose allopurinol (e.g., 600 mg/day), or erythromycin monitored for[4,12]: a. Clinical signs of supratherapeutic theophylline levels (e.g., increased heart rate and blood	X		21A. Serum drug concentration monitoring not required for erythromycin therapy duration of 5 days or less[12]	21, 21A. Physician orders, progress notes, nursing notes, laboratory reports, MAR, outpatient profile

Element	Standard 100%	Standard 0%	Exception[b] or Critical Preventive/ Responsive Measure[c]	Sources of Information
pressure, increased anxiety and insomnia) b. Serum theophylline levels at least once during concomitant therapy				
22. Patient receiving concomitant rifampin, phenobarbital, or phenytoin monitored for[4,12]: a. Clinical signs of subtherapeutic theophylline levels (lack of control of symptoms) b. Serum theophylline levels at least once during concomitant therapy	X		22A. None	22. Physician orders, progress notes, nursing notes, laboratory reports, MAR, outpatient profile
23. Patient receiving concomitant lithium has serum lithium levels and drug effectiveness monitored closely[4,12]	X		23A. None	23. Physician orders, progress notes, MAR, outpatient profile
24. Patient educated about role of theophylline in prevention and control of symptoms[1]	X		24A. If patient incompetent or incapable, caregiver educated	24. Physician orders, progress notes, nursing notes, patient education notes, respiratory function notes, pharmacy consultation notes
Complications[4,8,e]				
25. Gastrointestinal effects: nausea, vomiting, epigastric pain, abdominal cramps, anorexia, diarrhea		X	25A. Identify other drug and nondrug causes 25B. Evaluate serum theophylline level and decrease theophylline dosage if indicated 25C. If symptoms severe and not controlled by adjusting dosage, discontinue theophylline	25. Progress notes, nursing notes 25A. Physician orders, progress notes, nursing notes, MAR 25B. Physician orders, MAR, laboratory reports 25C. Physician orders, progress notes, nursing notes, MAR
26. CNS effects: headache, irritability, restlessness, nervousness, insomnia, dizziness, reflex hyperexcitability, seizures		X	26A. Unless symptoms minor, discontinue theophylline 26B. Identify other drug and nondrug causes 26C. Evaluate serum theophylline level and decrease theophylline dosage if indicated 26D. Treat seizures symptomatically 26E. If theophylline overdosage (>40 μg/mL or seizures),[3,4] repeatedly administer activated charcoal (50–100 g initially with 75–100 mL of sorbitol; may repeat doses of at least 20 g of activated charcoal every 2 hr)[13]	26. Progress notes, nursing notes 26A. Physician orders, progress notes, nursing notes, MAR 26B. Physician orders, progress notes, nursing notes, MAR 26C. Physician orders, MAR, laboratory reports 26D. Physician orders, progress notes, nursing notes, MAR 26E. Physician orders, progress notes, MAR, laboratory reports
27. Cardiopulmonary toxicity: tachycardia, arrhythmias, tachypnea		X	27A. Unless symptoms minor, discontinue theophylline 27B. Identify other drug and nondrug causes 27C. Evaluate serum theophylline level and decrease theophylline dosage if indicated 27D. Treat symptomatically with or without supportive care, which may include supplemental oxygen and cardiopulmonary resuscitation	27. Progress notes, nursing notes 27A. Physician orders, progress notes, nursing notes 27B. Physician orders, progress notes, nursing notes, MAR 27C. Physician orders, MAR, laboratory reports 27D. Physician orders, progress notes, nursing notes, MAR
28. Metabolic effects: hyperglycemia, hypokalemia		X	28A. Identify other drug and nondrug causes 28B. Evaluate serum	28. Progress notes, nursing notes, laboratory reports 28A. Physician orders, progress

Element	Standard 100%	Standard 0%	Exception[b] or Critical Preventive/ Responsive Measure[c]	Sources of Information
			theophylline level and decrease theophylline dosage if indicated	notes, nursing notes, MAR 28B. Physician orders, MAR, laboratory reports
			28C. If symptoms severe and not controlled by adjusting dosage, discontinue theophylline	28C. Physician orders, progress notes, nursing notes, MAR, laboratory reports
			28D. Treat electrolyte disturbances symptomatically	28D. Physician orders, MAR, laboratory reports
29. Hypersensitivity reactions: urticaria, pruritus, angioedema		X	29A. Identify other drug and nondrug causes	29. Progress notes, nursing notes
			29B. Identify ethylenediamine sensitivity and discontinue aminophylline	29A–D. Physician orders, progress notes, nursing notes, MAR
			29C. Treat symptomatically with antihistamine or epinephrine with or without supportive care, which may include fluids, cardiopulmonary resuscitation, and assisted ventilation	
			29D. If severe reaction, discontinue theophylline	
Outcome Measures				
30. Improvement in or control of asthma symptoms	X		30A. Nonasthmatic indication for use	30. Progress notes, nursing notes
31. Reduced variability in peak expiratory flow rate	X		31A. None	31. Respiratory function reports
32. Improvement in tests of pulmonary function	X		32A. None	32. Respiratory function reports
33. Prevention of acute exacerbations of asthma	X		33A. Nonasthmatic indication for use	33, 33A. Progress notes, emergency department records
34. Maintenance of normal activity levels	X		34A. Concomitant condition(s) limit activity levels	34, 34A. Progress notes
35. Fewer or no emergency department visits required for exacerbation of asthma	X		35A. Nonasthmatic indication for use	35, 35A. Emergency department records
36. Decreased nocturnal asthma symptoms (patient is rarely awakened at night)	X		36A. Nonasthmatic indication for use	36, 36A. Progress notes, nursing notes
37. Decreased corticosteroid requirements in corticosteroid-dependent patient (lower oral corticosteroid requirements or ability to control symptoms with high inhaled doses rather than oral doses)	X		37A. None	37. Physician orders, progress notes, MAR, outpatient

[a]Criteria address justification for use (indications), critical (process) indicators, complications of therapy, and patient outcome. Each criterion consists of an element, a standard, exceptions to the standard, and sources of information. The element is the minimum level of evidence needed to show that patient care was optimal. The standard defines the deviation from an element that is acceptable. If no deviation is acceptable, the standard is 100%. Exceptions are circumstances in which deviation is allowable. Sources of information listed are the most reliable sources. Sources pertaining to an element or exception are identified by the number assigned to the element or exception (e.g., 3, 3A).

[b]For justification for use, critical (process) indicators, and outcome measures.

[c]For complications.

[d]Many clinicians, particularly outside the United States, believe that methylxanthines should be used "selectively, cautiously, and with close patient supervision and serum theophylline monitoring" only after a trial of optimum doses of aerosol bronchodilators and prophylactic anti-inflammatory aerosols in those patients who show objective evidence of additional benefit from methylxanthines.[5]

[e]Unless there is a strong suspicion of an alternative cause, theophylline therapy should be suspended while adverse reactions are evaluated. Some patients may experience signs and symptoms of theophylline toxicity at therapeutic serum drug concentrations (<20 μg/mL).

References

1. National asthma education program coordinating committee guidelines for the diagnosis and management of asthma. *J Allergy Clin Immunol.* 1991; 88(3, part 2):425-534.
2. Addis GJ. Theophylline in the management of airflow obstruction: 1. Much evidence to suggest theophylline is valuable. *Br Med J.* 1990; 300:928-9.
3. Weinberger M. The pharmacology and therapeutic use of theophylline. *J Allergy Clin Immunol.* 1984; 73(5, part 1):525-40.
4. Hendeles L, Massanari M, Weinberger M. Theophylline. In: Evans WE, Schentag JJ, Jusko WJ, eds. Applied pharma-

cokinetics: principles of therapeutic drug monitoring. 2nd ed. Spokane, WA: Applied Therapeutics; 1986:1105-88.

5. Lam A, Newhouse MT. Management of asthma and chronic airflow limitation. Are methylxanthines obsolete? *Chest.* 1990; 98:44-52.
6. Tandon MK, Kailis SG. Bronchodilator treatment for partially reversible chronic obstructive airways disease. *Thorax.* 1991; 46:248-51.
7. Jenne JW. Theophylline is no more obsolete than 'two puffs q.i.d' of current $beta_2$ agonists. *Chest.* 1990; 98:2-3.
8. Grant JA, Ellis EF, eds. Update on theophylline: symposium proceedings. *J Allergy Clin Immunol.* 1986; 78:669-824.
9. Hendeles L, Weinberger M, Szefler S et al. Safety and efficacy of theophylline in children with asthma. *J Pediatr.* 1992; 120(2, part 1):177-83.
10. Rogers R, Owens G, Pennock B. The pendulum swings again towards rational use of theophylline. *Chest.* 1985; 87:280-2.
11. Nassif EG, Weinberger MM, Shannon D et al. Theophylline disposition in infancy. *J Pediatr.* 1981; 98:158-61.
12. Jonkman JHG. Therapeutic consequences of drug interactions with theophylline pharmacokinetics. *J Allergy Clin Immunol.* 1986; 78:736-42.
13. Goldberg MJ, Park GD, Berlinger WG. Treatment of theophylline intoxication. *J Allergy Clin Immunol.* 1986; 78:811-7.

CP Continuing Education

ASHP journal continuing-education instructions and enrollment form

Instructions

1. The system is flexible. You may select any combination of tests from *AJHP* and *Clinical Pharmacy* to give you the number of credits you need.
2. An answer sheet is published at the end of each installment of the Continuing Education column. This enrollment form is published in the June and December issues of *AJHP* and *CP*.
3. Complete only one enrollment form, but note on the form all the tests you are taking. Staple together all answer sheets for one enrollment.
4. Tests included must have been published within the past 18 months. Once a particular test is included in an enrollment, it may not be included in a subsequent enrollment.
5. The passing score on each test is 70%. Within four weeks of receiving your enrollment, ASHP will mail you a CE certification or notify you that certain tests were failed. Failed tests may be retaken only one time, without additional cost. There are no refunds for failed tests.
6. ASHP is approved by the American Council on Pharmaceutical Education as a provider of continuing pharmaceutical education (Provider Number 680-204.) Most states that recognize ACPE-approved providers will accept credit earned through journal CE programs; however, since some states have restrictions on the number of credit hours or CE units they will accept toward the total requirement, it is advised that readers check with their respective state board of pharmacy if they are uncertain about the board's regulations.
7. Send your enrollment form, answer sheet(s), and check (made payable to ASHP) to:

ASHP CE
Customer Service Department
American Society of Hospital Pharmacists
7272 Wisconsin Avenue
Bethesda, MD 20814

Enrollment Form

Name ______________________________

Address ______________________________

City ____________ State ____________ Zip ________

Fee Schedule

$5/hour

$20 minimum/enrollment

Tests included in this enrollment must have been published within the past 18 months.

Test Number	*Hours of Credit**
________	________
________	________
________	________
________	________
________	________
________	________
________	________
________	________
________	________
Total hours	________
Total fee ($) enclosed	________

(Write additional numbers and hours on a separate sheet and attach it to this form.)

*10 hours = 1.0 C.E.U.

ACPE® *The American Society of Hospital Pharmacists is approved by the American Council on Pharmaceutical Education as a provider of continuing pharmaceutical education*

Current Literature

Drug Reaction Alerts

Drug Reaction Alerts focuses primarily on serious, unlabeled reactions to new chemical entities. The citations are compiled monthly from International Pharmaceutical Abstracts, *which covers over 800 pharmacy and health-related journals worldwide. An address for reprints (when available) follows the name of the corresponding author in each citation.*

Pharmacists may use the FDA Adverse Reaction Report form that appears in the January and July issues of Clinical Pharmacy *for submitting reports of adverse drug reactions directly to FDA.*

Analgesics and Antipyretics

Rotenberg FA, Giannini VS (Pharmacy Services, Rhode Island Hospital, 593 Eddy Street, Providence, RI 02903). Hyperkalemia associated with **ketorolac**. *Ann Pharmacother*. 1992; 26:778-9. Case. (59-year-old man with pain following excision of upper lobe of right lung; received single dose of ketorolac 30 mg as i.m. injection; developed hyperkalemia [5.7 mM] and slight respiratory acidosis about 3.5 hours after injection; concomitant postoperative infusion of dextrose, sodium chloride, and potassium chloride [<6 meq] for hydration; discontinuation of postoperative infusion and therapy with insulin, glucose, sodium bicarbonate, and furosemide led to stabilization of patient)

Antiandrogens

Markus H, Polkey M, Harrison M (Department of Neurology, Middlesex Hospital, London W1N 8AA, England). Visual loss and optic atrophy associated with **cyproterone acetate**. *Br Med J*. 1992; 305:159. Case. (80-year-old man with prostatic neoplasm; received cyproterone acetate 100 mg three times daily for nine months, then a lower dosage because of malaise and nausea, for a total of more than 2.5 years of therapy; developed bilateral visual loss; withdrawal of cyproterone acetate and substitution with goserelin led to improved vision over three months, with return of visual evoked potentials to left eye)

Antibiotics

Frye RF, Job ML (DeKalb Medical Center, Department of Pharmaceutical Services, 2701 N. Decatur Road, Decatur, GA 30033), Dretler RH et al. **Teicoplanin** nephrotoxicity: first case report. *Pharmacotherapy*. 1992; 12:240-2. Case. (71-year-old man with type 1 diabetes mellitus and osteomyelitis of left great toe caused by methicillin-resistant *Staphylococcus aureus*; received teicoplanin 1200 mg every 12 hours by i.v. injection for three doses followed by 1200 mg every 24 hours over 40 days in accordance with investigational protocol; developed acute interstitial nephritis; concomitant insulin; blood urea nitrogen and serum creatinine concentrations were markedly elevated; therapy with furosemide and hemodialysis did not lead to improvement in renal function; referred for long-term dialysis)

Antifungals

Lavrijsen AP (Department of Dermatology, University Hospital, Leiden, Netherlands), Balmus KJ, Nugteren-Huying WM et al. Hepatic injury associated with **itraconazole**. *Lancet*. 1992; 340:251-2. Cases. (three patients, aged 57–75 years, with fungal infections; received itraconazole 100–200 mg twice daily; incurred hepatic injury; withdrawal of itraconazole led to recovery)

Anti-inflammatory Agents

Dent MT, Ganapathy S, Holdsworth CD et al. (Channer KC, Royal Hallamshire Hospital, Sheffield, England). **Mesalazine** induced lupus-like syndrome. *Br Med J*. 1992; 305:159. Case. (38-year-old woman with proctitis who had developed adverse effects from receiving sulfasalazine 1.5 g/day; received mesalamine 1.2 g/day for seven months; developed clinical symptoms and immunoserological findings consistent with diagnosis of lupus-like syndrome; withdrawal of mesalamine led to decrease in body temperature within 24 hours, slow resolution of other symptoms, and return of immune profile to normal but did not lead to disappearance of antinuclear factor after two months)

Gentric A, Pennec YL (Harvier Medical Clinic, Central University Hospital, 29609 Brest Cedex, France). **Diclofenac**-induced pseudomembranous colitis. *Lancet*. 1992; 340:126-7. Case. (80-year-old woman with acute lumbago; received diclofenac 75 mg twice daily by i.m. injection; developed pseudomembranous colitis; withdrawal of diclofenac did not lead to stoppage of diarrhea; histological examination confirmed diagnosis of pseudomembranous colitis; therapy with vancomycin led to rapid improvement)

Parodi A, Rivara G, Guarrera M (University of Genoa, Genoa, Italy). Possible **naproxen**-induced relapse of subacute cutaneous lupus erythematosus. *JAMA*. 1992; 268:51-2. Case. (59-year-old woman with history of subacute cutaneous lupus erythematosus [SCLE]; received naproxen sodium 250–500 mg/day for one month; developed relapse of SCLE; therapy with azathioprine and hydroxychloroquine did not lead to resolution of SCLE; withdrawal of naproxen led to clearing of skin lesions)

Antimanic Agents

Collings S (Bethlem and Maudsley Joint Hospital, London, England). Thrombocytopenia associated with **lithium carbon-**

ate. *Br Med J*. 1992; 305:159. Case. (24-year-old patient with bipolar disorder; received lithium carbonate 750 mg/day for 17 days; developed thrombocytopenia; withdrawal of lithium carbonate led to recovery of platelet count; positive rechallenge with lithium carbonate 500 mg/day)

Antineoplastic Agents

Kamthan AG (Department of Neoplastic Diseases, Mount Sinai Hospital, 1 Gustave L. Levy Place, New York, NY 10029-6574), Bruckner HW, Hirschman SZ et al. *Clostridium difficile* diarrhea induced by cancer chemotherapy. *Arch Intern Med*. 1992; 152:1715-7. Cases. (four women, aged 41–53 years, with carcinoma of colon, rectum, or adrenal cortex; received various combination therapies with **fluorouracil, levamisole hydrochloride, leucovorin calcium, methotrexate, cisplatin,** and **doxorubicin hydrochloride;** developed diarrhea associated with *Clostridium difficile;* no concomitant antibiotic; therapy with vancomycin hydrochloride and metronidazole, alone or in combination with i.v. replacement fluids, led to recovery)

Cardiac Drugs

Dutertre JP, Machet L, Codjovi P et al. (Autret E, Department of Clinical Pharmacology, Centre Hospitaliere Regional et Universitaire de Tours, Hôpital Bretonneau, 2, Bis Boulevard Tonnellé, 37044 Tours Cedex, France). Severe chronic diarrhea secondary to **celiprolol**. *Ann Pharmacother*. 1992; 26:842-3. Case. (61-year-old man with angina pectoris; received celiprolol hydrochloride 200 mg/day for two weeks; developed severe diarrhea; withdrawal of celiprolol hydrochloride and substitution with bisoprolol led to stoppage of diarrhea within seven days)

Contamination

Riddick FA Jr (Ochsner Clinic, New Orleans, LA 70121), Jordan JD. Cruise ship anisocoria. *Ann Intern Med*. 1992; 117:95. Case. (woman with soft contact lenses who was on a trip aboard a cruise ship; applied transdermal **scopolamine** patch behind her ear and wore it for four days; developed photophobia and eye pain; removal of scopolamine patch and contact lenses led to resolution of symptoms)

Drug Interactions

Walker R, Milford D, Derbyshire P (Department of Hematology, Children's Hospital, Ladywood Middleway, Birmingham, B16 8ET, England). Bradycardia after amphotericin, irradiation, and **anthracycline**. *Lancet*. 1992; 340:380. Case. (5.5-year-old boy with acute lymphoblastic leukemia previously treated with an anthracycline [total dose, 350 mg/sq m] who received autologous bone-marrow transplant after conditioning with cyclophosphamide and body irradiation; received **amphotericin B** at increasing dosage of 0.25–1.0 mg/kg/day by i.v. infusion for treatment of persistent pyrexia; developed profound bradycardia; withdrawal of amphotericin B led to recovery of heart rate; positive rechallenge with amphotericin B at half-strength dose by slow infusion)

Immunotherapy

Park JW (Hematology/Oncology Clinic, Ambulatory Care Center, A-502, 400 Parnassus Avenue, University of California, San Francisco, CA 94143-0324), Mehrotra B, Barnett BO et al. The Sweet syndrome during therapy with granulocyte colony-stimulating factor. *Ann Intern Med*. 1992; 116:996-8. Case. (41-year-old woman with leukopenia induced by antineoplastic agents; received **filgrastim** 300 mg/day for three days by s.c. injection, followed by no filgrastim for 48 hours around time of antineoplastic drug administration, and then two more doses of filgrastim; developed acute febrile neutrophilic dermatosis; no therapy led to resolution of lesions; additional antineoplastic therapy but without filgrastim did not lead to problems)

Quinolones

Aoun M (Infectious Diseases Clinic and Microbiology Laboratory, Institute Jules Bordet, 1000 Brussels, Belgium), Jacquy C, Debusscher L et al. Peripheral neuropathy associated with fluoroquinolones. *Lancet*. 1992; 340:127. Case. (37-year-old man with chronic vertebral osteomyelitis; received oral **pefloxacin** 400 mg twice daily for five months; developed paresthesia of lower legs followed by progressive weakness of right foot and difficulty in walking; withdrawal of pefloxacin led to dramatic improvement of peripheral neuropathy within 10 days; developed recurrence of osteomyelitis six months later; therapy with **ofloxacin** 200 mg twice daily led to relapse of peripheral neuropathy within 15 days; withdrawal of ofloxacin led to decrease in severity of peripheral neuropathy within seven days; therapy with oral **ciprofloxacin** 250 mg twice daily for two months led to minimal limb paresthesia; development of unbearable symptoms led to withdrawal of ciprofloxacin)

Tocolytics

Minakami H (Department of Obstetrics and Gynecology, Jichi Medical School, Minamikawachi-machi, Tochigi 329-04, Japan), Takahashi T, Izumi A et al. Enlargement of the salivary gland after **ritodrine** treatment in pregnant women. *Br Med J*. 1992; 304:1668. Cases. (six pregnant women with premature labor; received ritodrine hydrochloride by i.v. injection for a total of 184–2900 mg over 0.5–29 days; developed parotitis; resolution of swelling occurred within five days; results of serological tests performed on five women ruled out possibility of mumps; all infants were born healthy)

Topical Preparations

Payne CM, Bladin C, Colchester AC et al. (Lane D, William Harvey Hospital, Ashford, Kent TN24 0LZ, England). Argyria from excessive use of topical **silver sulfadiazine**. *Lancet*. 1992; 340:126. Case. (59-year-old man with recurrent extensive venous leg ulcers; applied 1% silver sulfadiazine cream to ulcers for five months in such quantities that a 50-g tube was used every two days; developed argyria with ulcer surfaces appearing tarnished and thighs becoming light blue and experienced loss of sensation over forearms and legs, although ulcers did not improve)

Tranquilizers

Frankenburg FR, Kando J (McLean Hospital, Belmont, MA 02178-9106). Eosinophilia, **clozapine**, and pancreatitis. *Lancet*. 1992; 340:251. Case. (17-year-old woman with psychotic symptoms; received clozapine 100 mg/day; developed eosinophilia and pancreatitis; withdrawal of clozapine led to resolution of somatic symptoms within a few days but deterioration of psychiatric status; positive rechallenge)

Vasoconstricting Agents

Redfield MM (Mayo Clinic, 200 First Street, S.W., Rochester, MN 55905), Nicholson WJ, Edwards WD et al. Valve disease associated with ergot alkaloid use: echocardiographic and pathologic correlations. *Ann Intern Med*. 1992; 117:50-2. Study. (case series; five patients, aged 34–62 years, who had used caffeine plus **ergotamine tartrate** combination or **methysergide maleate** for treatment of headaches for 6–20 years and developed heart-valve disorders; no history suggestive of rheumatic fever, collagen vascular disease, or infective endocarditis, and no extracardiac signs or symptoms of carcinoid syndrome; one patient had peripheral vascular disease consistent with diagnosis of ergotism; all patients developed valvular disease that was sufficiently symptomatic to necessitate heart-valve replacement; one woman continued to use ergotamine tartrate after initial surgery for heart-valve replacement and developed severe tricuspid regurgitation)

Continued on page 1042

Current Literature *Continued from page 1041*

Books Received

Books are listed as soon as received; selected books may be reviewed in Book Reviews in subsequent issues.

Applied Pharmacokinetics: Principles of Therapeutic Drug Monitoring, Third Edition, edited by William E. Evans, Jerome J. Schentag, William J. Jusko et al. Published by Applied Therapeutics, Inc., P.O. Box 5077, Vancouver, WA 98668-5077, 1992. Price $82.50 (U.S.), $90 (elsewhere).

Drug Regimen Review: A Process Guide for Pharmacists. Published by the American Society of Consultant Pharmacists and Sandoz Pharmaceuticals Corporation, 1992. Available from ASCP, 1321 Duke Street, Alexandria, VA 22314. viii + 372 p. Price $95 (ASCP members), $135 (nonmembers).

Patient Recruitment in Clinical Trials, by Bert Spilker and Joyce A. Cramer. Published by Raven Press, 1185 Avenue of the Americas, New York, NY 10036, 1992. xix + 346 p. Price $80.

Psychotropic Drug Handbook, 6th Edition, by Paul J. Perry, Bruce Alexander, and Barry I. Liskow. Published by Harvey Whitney Books Company, 4906 Cooper Road, P.O. Box 42696, Cincinnati, OH 45242 1991. vi + 358 p. Price $38.75.

Advertising Index

American Society of Hospital Pharmacists
Criteria for Drug Use Evaluation, Volumes 1, 2, and 3, 1042
The Elements of Quality in Pharmaceutical Care, 995
Amgen Inc.
Epogen, 992-993
Neupogen, 1001-1004
HealthInfusion
Position Available, 995
Immunex Corporation
Position Available, 1038
Jackson Memorial Hospital
Position Available, 995
Roche Laboratories, Division of Hoffmann-La Roche, Inc.
Rocephin, inside back cover, outside back cover
Roerig, A Division of Pfizer Pharmaceuticals
Diflucan, 996-998
Wyeth-Ayerst Laboratories, Inc.
Tubex, inside front cover

Index to Volume 11

The index to Volume 11 is composed of three parts: a subject index, an author index, and an advertising index.

The subject index is made up mainly of terms constructed by *International Pharmaceutical Abstracts*. The *IPA* index is an alphabetical, open-ended, controlled-vocabulary index that makes use of standardized headings. (The primary index terms for each article are listed routinely in *Clinical Pharmacy* as "index terms" after abstracts.) *IPA* covers all authored papers and editorials in *Clinical Pharmacy,* as well as selected letters and news reports. The subject index also notes all regular columns and, under the respective column headings, the titles of items in the "News," "Therapy Consultation," "Letters," "Editorials," and "Book Reviews" sections. The subject index also contains, under the heading "Correction Notices," the title and issue of publication of items for which corrections were printed, as well as the page numbers on which the corrections appear.

Issue	*Pages*	*Issue*	*Pages*
January	1–92	July	571–656
February	93–204	August	657–742
March	205–280	September	743–822
April	281–374	October	823–904
May	375–454	November	905–988
June	455–570	December	989–1052

Subject Index

A

Absorption
anti-infective agents; intraperitoneal, CAPD, 246
metoclopramide hydrochloride; peritoneal dialysis, 174
Acetaminophen; fever; therapy, pediatrics, review, 1005
Acquired immunodeficiency syndrome
didanosine; therapy, FDA approvals, 4
566C80; *P. carinii* pneumonia, treatment IND, FDA approvals, 99
foscarnet sodium; cytomegalic inclusion disease therapy, FDA approvals, 4
ganciclovir; cytomegalic inclusion disease therapy, liver toxicity, 432
zidovudine; therapy, DUE criteria, 63
Adenosine; use; evaluation, criteria, 727
Administration; Food and Drug Administration; procedures, changes, new-drug approvals, 574
Adolescents
antihistamines; DUE criteria, therapy, extrapyramidal side effects, 553
antiparkinson agents; DUE criteria, therapy, extrapyramidal side effects, 553
benzodiazepines; DUE criteria, therapy, extrapyramidal side effects, 553
parasympatholytic agents; DUE criteria, therapy, extrapyramidal side effects, 553
Adrenergic agents, see **Sympathomimetic agents**
Adverse drug reactions report form, 85, 649
Advertising Index, 92, 204, 280, 374, 454, 570, 656, 742, 822, 904, 988, 1042
Aerosols; β agonists; regular vs. as-needed, asthma therapy, 877
Age; patients; home parenteral nutrition therapy, toxicity, 543
Agency for Health Care Policy and Research; protocols; pain therapy, 309, 391
AIDS, see **Acquired immunodeficiency syndrome**
Alcohols, cetyl; combination, colfosceril palmitate, tyloxapol; adult respiratory distress syndrome therapy, neonate, 880; use evaluation criteria, 355
Aldesleukin; marketing; FDA approvals, 669
Allergies; fentanyl; diffuse rash, transdermal patches, 222
Aluminum; blood levels; sucralfate toxicity, deferoxamine therapy, 636
Amantadine; hyperprolactinemia; therapy, psychotropic toxicity, 851
American Society of Hospital Pharmacists; protocols; antimicrobial prophylaxis, surgery, 483; globulin immune, i.v. therapy, 117
Amino acids
choline; cognition disorders therapy, FDA disapprovals, 467
marketing; cognition disorders therapy, FDA disapprovals, 467
Aminoglycosides; intraperitoneal; absorption, CAPD, 246
Aminophylline
availability; liquid, enteral administration, 428
use; evaluation, criteria, 1033
Amphotericin B
candidiasis; therapy, burns, infant, 883
use; evaluation, bladder irrigation, criteria, 809
Anabolic agents; steroids; hyperfibrinogenemia therapy, 968
Analgesics and antipyretics
acetaminophen; fever therapy, pediatrics, review, 1005
aspirin; fever therapy, pediatrics, review, 1005
fentanyl; adverse reactions, transdermal patches, 222; transdermal patches, 22
ibuprofen; fever therapy, pediatrics, review, 1005
morphine sulfate; Baxter Infusor, PCA, postoperative pain therapy, 342; intrathecal and i.v. PCA vs. PCA alone, postoperative pain, 958; toxicity, muscle spasticity, midazolam therapy, 57
pain; protocols, therapy, 309, 391
Anemia; dapsone; hemolytic, toxicity, therapy, 800
Anesthetics; toxicity; nausea and vomiting, abdominal surgery, 965
Anesthetics, local
lidocaine, combination, prilocaine; pain therapy, s.c. injection sites, 347
pain; protocols, therapy, 391
Angiotensin-converting enzyme inhibitors; labeling; warnings, risks, pregnancy, 467
Antiarrhythmic drugs, see **Cardiac drugs**
Anti-infective agents
dosage schedules; therapy, postantibiotic effect, 876
566C80; *P. carinii* pneumonia, treatment IND, FDA approvals, 99
surgery; prophylaxis, ASHP protocols, 483
toxicity; endocrine disorders, HIV infections, therapy, 705; postantibiotic effect, factors, 865
Antibiotics
dosage schedules; therapy, postantibiotic effect, 876
mechanism of action; postantibiotic effect, 865
toxicity; endocrine disorders, HIV infections, therapy, 705
vancomycin; intraperitoneal, absorption, CAPD, 246
Antibodies; monoclonal; antiendotoxin, DUE criteria, 257; sepsis therapy, 223; sepsis therapy, criteria, 255
Anticoagulants
heparin; vs. sodium chloride, i.v. lock flushing, 797
ticlopidine hydrochloride; FDA approvals, 99
toxicity; hemorrhage, dental surgery, 857
warfarin sodium; interactions, tetracycline, potentiation, prothrombin time, 806; toxicity, intramural hematoma of the small intestine, 632
Anticonvulsants
eclampsia; and preeclampsia therapy, 236
ethosuximide and phenobarbital; clearance, peritoneal dialysis, 1030
phenobarbital and ethosuximide; clearance, peritoneal dialysis, 1030
Antidepressants
depression; therapy, geriatrics, 96
fluvoxamine; therapy, review, 930
paroxetine; therapy, review, 930
sertraline hydrochloride; FDA approvals, 381; therapy, review, 930
Antidotes
charcoal activated and methylene blue; therapy, dapsone toxicity, 800
methylene blue and charcoal activated; therapy, dapsone toxicity, 800
Antiemetics
metoclopramide hydrochloride; pharmacokinetics, CAPD, 174
ondansetron hydrochloride; pharmacokinetics, therapy, cisplatin toxicity, 1026
scopolamine; transdermal patches, hyperemesis gravidarum therapy, 830
Antifungals
amphotericin B; bladder irrigation, DUE criteria, 809; candidiasis therapy, burns, infant, 883
fluconazole; candidiasis therapy, lack, burns, infant, 883
toxicity; endocrine disorders, HIV infections, therapy, 705
Antihistamines
astemizole; toxicity, cardiovascular, labeling, warnings, 825
diphenhydramine hydrochloride; therapy, fentanyl adverse reactions, 222
drug use; evaluations, criteria, therapy, extrapyramidal side effects, 553
terfenadine; toxicity, cardiovascular, labeling, warnings, 825
Anti-inflammatory agents
nabumetone; FDA approvals, 381
nonsteroidal; toxicity, ulcers, therapy, review, 690
oxaprozin; nonsteroidal, therapy, 591
Antilipemic agents
hyperfibrinogenemia; therapy, 968
pravastatin sodium; FDA approvals, 99; hypercholesterolemia therapy, review, 677
simvastatin; FDA approvals, 290
Antineoplastic agents
aldesleukin; FDA approvals, 669
cisplatin; toxicity, ondansetron therapy, pharmacokinetics, 1026
finasteride; FDA approvals, 825
idarubicin; acute nonlymphocytic leukemia therapy, 152
leukemia; acute, adult, therapy, review, 767
taxol; treatment IND, FDA approvals, 912
Antiparkinson agents; drug use; evaluation, criteria, therapy, extrapyramidal side effects, 553

Antivirals
didanosine; AIDS therapy, FDA approvals, 4; DUE criteria, 885
foscarnet sodium; cytomegalic inclusion disease therapy, AIDS, FDA approvals, 4
ganciclovir; liver toxicity, cytomegalic inclusion disease therapy, AIDS, 432
toxicity; endocrine disorders, HIV infections, therapy, 705
zalcitabine; AIDS buyers groups, FDA actions, 385; marketing, FDA approvals, accelerated drug review policy, 747
zidovudine; DUE criteria, 63
zidovudine and zalcitabine; combined therapy, HIV infections, 747
Anxiolytics, sedatives and hypnotics; triazolam; labeling changes, package inserts, FDA approvals, 467; product withdrawal, United Kingdom, 9
Arrhythmia; therapy; toxicity, review, 714
Arthritis
nabumetone; rheumatoid, therapy, FDA approvals, 381
oxaprozin; rheumatoid, therapy, 591
ASHP Commission on Therapeutics; protocols; antimicrobial prophylaxis, surgery, 483; i.v. globulin immune, 117
Asians; Koreans; phenylpropanolamine, toxicity, hypertension, lack, 168
Aspirin
eclampsia; and preeclampsia therapy, 236
fever; therapy, pediatrics, review, 1005
Astemizole; toxicity; cardiovascular, labeling, warnings, 825
Asthma
β agonists; therapy, aerosols, dosage schedules, 877
sympathomimetic agents; β agonists, therapy, controversies, 13
Atracurium besylate; use; evaluation, criteria, 435
Availability, drugs, see **Drugs, availability**
Azithromycin
marketing; delay, Pfizer, 218; FDA approvals, 98
pharmacology, 137

B

Bacterial infections
antibodies; antiendotoxin monoclonal, therapy, 223; antiendotoxin monoclonal, therapy, criteria, 255; antiendotoxin monoclonal, therapy, DUE criteria, 257
anti-infective agents; prophylaxis, surgery, ASHP protocols, 483
cefpodoxime proxetil; bacterial, therapy, FDA approvals, 999
cefprozil; therapy, FDA approvals, 295
lomefloxacin hydrochloride; therapy, FDA approvals, 458
temafloxacin hydrochloride; therapy, FDA approvals, 381
Barbiturates; pain; protocols, therapy, 391
Basal ganglia diseases; psychotherapeutic agents; toxicity, therapy, DUE criteria, 553
Benzodiazepine antagonists; flumazenil; FDA approvals, 287
Benzodiazepines
drug use; evaluation, criteria, therapy, extrapyramidal side effects, 553
overdose; toxicity, flumazenil therapy, 287
pain; protocols, therapy, 391
Beractant; use; evaluation, criteria, 357
Bioavailability, see **Drugs, availability**
Biologicals; approvals; FDA, 1991, 208
Blood levels
aluminum; sucralfate toxicity, deferoxamine therapy, 636
ceftriaxone; i.m., concentrated, pediatrics, 961
cholesterol; and HDL monitoring, coronary disease, 378
ciprofloxacin; and milk levels, 352
ethosuximide and phenobarbital; decreased, peritoneal dialysis, 1030
fentanyl; transdermal patches, pain therapy, 22
ondansetron hydrochloride; pharmacokinetics, therapy, cisplatin toxicity, 1026
phenobarbital and ethosuximide; decreased, peritoneal dialysis, 1030
theophylline; aminophylline availability, enteral administration, 428
Book Reviews, 92, 277, 373, 565, 655, 742, 897,
Advances in Pain Research and Therapy, Volume 18: The Design of Analgesic Clinical Trials, 92
Applied Therapeutics: The Clinical Use of Drugs, Fifth Edition, 897
The Biochemical Basis of Neuropharmacology, Sixth Edition, 655
Clinical Immunotoxicology, 900
Combined Modality Cancer Therapy: Radiation and Infusional Chemotherapy, 565
Data Collection Forms in Clinical Trials, 373
Drugs in Gastroenterology, 565
Guide to Clinical Trials, 277
Handbook of Basic Pharmacokinetics . . .including Clinical Applications, Fourth Edition, 901
Manual of Antibiotics and Infectious Diseases, Seventh Edition, 742
Neoplastic Diseases: Fundamentals of Clinical Oncology, 901
Pharmacokinetics and Pharmacodynamics, Volume 3: Peptides, Peptoids, and Proteins, 277
Books Received, 198, 374, 454, 570, 655, 742, 904, 1042
Bromocriptine; hyperprolactinemia; therapy, psychotropic toxicity, 851
Burns
amphotericin B; candidiasis therapy, infant, 883
fluconazole; candidiasis therapy, lack, infant, 883

C

Calcium antagonists
hyperfibrinogenemia; therapy, 968
new drugs; advantages, 549
nimodipine; cerebrovascular ischemia therapy, 350
verapamil hydrochloride; pharmacokinetics, intact capsules vs. sprinkled on food, 539
Calcium regulators; pamidronate disodium; hypercalcemia therapy, FDA approvals, 220
Cancer, see **Antineoplastic agents**
Cancer drugs, see **Antineoplastic agents**
Candidiasis
amphotericin B; therapy, burns, infant, 883
fluconazole; therapy, lack, burns, infant, 883
Capsules; verapamil hydrochloride; intact vs. sprinkled on food, equivalency, pharmacokinetics, 539
Carbamazepine; concomitant therapy, 632
Carcinoma; aldesleukin; renal cell, therapy, FDA approvals, 669
Cardiac drugs
adenosine; DUE criteria, 727
antiarrhythmic agents; therapy, toxicity, review, 714
dobutamine; congestive heart failure, long-term therapy, 618
flecainide; interactions, implanted cardiac devices, 48
moricizine; interactions, implanted cardiac devices, 48
Cefazolin sodium; toxicity; seizures, intraventricular injections, 104
Cefpodoxime proxetil; marketing; FDA approvals, 999
Cefprozil; marketing; FDA approvals, 295
Ceftriaxone; reconstitution; i.m., pharmacokinetics and toxicity, pediatrics, 961
Cellulose; hemorrhage; prophylaxis, dental surgery, anticoagulant toxicity, 857
Central nervous system drugs; cognition activators; FDA disapprovals, 467
Cephalosporins
cefazolin sodium; toxicity, seizures, intraventricular injections, 104
cefpodoxime proxetil; FDA approvals, 999
cefprozil; FDA approvals, 295
ceftriaxone; concentrated, pharmacokinetics, toxicity, pediatrics, 961
intraperitoneal; absorption, CAPD, 246
Cerebral ischemia; nimodipine; therapy, 350
Cerebrovascular disorders
nimodipine; ischemic stroke therapy, 350
ticlopidine hydrochloride; prophylaxis, FDA approvals, 99; therapy, review, 603
Charcoal activated; and methylene blue; therapy, dapsone toxicity, 800
Cholelitholytic agents; ursodiol; pruritus therapy, biliary cirrhosis, 672
Cholesterol; tests, laboratory; and HDL monitoring, coronary disease, 378
Choline; marketing; cognition disorders therapy, FDA disapprovals, 467
Ciprofloxacin hydrochloride; body distribution; blood and milk levels, 352
Cisplatin; toxicity; ondansetron therapy, pharmacokinetics, 1026
Clarithromycin
marketing; FDA approvals, 98
pharmacology, 137
Clearance, see **Excretion**
Clinical Pharmacy
acknowledgment to reviewers—October 1, 1991, to September 30, 1992, 1032
instructions for submitting computer disks with revised manuscripts, 62
procedure for submission of manuscripts to journals published by the American Society of Hospital Pharmacists, 60
Clinical studies
dobutamine; congestive heart failure, long-term therapy, 618
pravastatin sodium; hypercholesterolemia therapy, review, 677
Cognition disorders; therapy; amino acids, vitamins, marketing, FDA disapprovals, 467
Colfosceril palmitate; combination, alcohols, cetyl, tyloxapol; adult respiratory distress syndrome therapy, neonate, 880; use evaluation criteria, 355
Collagen; hemorrhage; microcrystalline, prophylaxis, dental surgery, anticoagulant toxicity, 857
Combined therapy
acetaminophen and aspirin; fever, pediatrics, review, 1005
aspirin and acetaminophen; fever, pediatrics, review, 1005
zalcitabine and zidovudine; HIV infections, FDA approvals, 747
zidovudine and zalcitabine; HIV infections, FDA approvals, 747
Commentaries, 350, 549, 714, 797, 876, 968
Complexes
Haemophilus b oligosaccharide conjugate vaccines; equivalency, immunogenicity, pediatrics, 332
Haemophilus b polysaccharide conjugate vaccines; equivalency, immunogenicity, pediatrics, 332
Compliance; patients; calcium antagonists therapy, 549
Concentration
antibiotics; postantibiotic effect, 865
ceftriaxone; i.m., pharmacokinetics, toxicity, pediatrics, 961
globulin immune; injections, administration rate, toxicity, 1022; reconstitution, dextrose vs. water for injection, 628
Control, quality; zalcitabine; problems, AIDS buyers groups, 385
Coronary disease; tests, laboratory; cholesterol and HDL monitoring, 378
Correction Notices, 14, 308, 585, 750, 829
Advances in the treatment of unstable angina pectoris (Nov 1991, Therapy Review), 14
American Academy of Pediatrics issues recommendations on treatment of Lyme disease (Oct 1991, News), 14
Clarithromycin and azithromycin: New macrolide antibiotics (Feb 1992, Drug Review), 308
Parenteral nutrition in pediatric patients (May 1988, Therapy Review), 750
Retreatment with digoxin immune Fab (Nov 1991, Letters), 14
Review of 1991 shows 30 new drugs, several important biologics cleared for marketing (Mar 1992, News), 585
Table of contents (Aug 1992), 829
Cost
Haemophilus b oligosaccharide conjugate vaccines; immunization, pediatrics, 332
Haemophilus b polysaccharide conjugate vaccines; immunization, pediatrics, 332
zalcitabine; therapy, 747
***CP* Continuing Education,** 77, 189, 261, 442, 559, 640, 731, 811, 892, 976, 1039
Creams; lidocaine, combination, prilocaine; anesthesia, pain, s.c. injection sites, 347
Current Literature, 87, 197, 273, 368, 448, 562, 652, 735, 819, 895, 978, 1040
Cytomegalic inclusion disease
foscarnet sodium; therapy, AIDS, FDA approvals, 4
ganciclovir; therapy, liver toxicity, AIDS, 432
Cytotoxic agents, see **Antineoplastic agents**

D

Dapsone; toxicity; hemolytic anemia, methemoglobinemia, therapy, 800
ddI, see **Didanosine**
Deferoxamine mesylate; therapy; aluminum overload, sucralfate toxicity, CAPD, 636
Depression
serotonin reuptake inhibitors; therapy, review, 930
sertraline hydrochloride; therapy, FDA approvals, 381
therapy; geriatrics, 96

Devices
Baxter Infusor; morphine PCA, postoperative pain therapy, 342
implants; cardiac, interactions, antiarrhythmic agents, 48
metrology; cups, spoons, droppers, drug overdose, 220
Dextrose; comparison, water for injection; globulin immune reconstitution, toxicity, 628
Diabetes mellitus
electrolytes, combination, polyethylene glycol; gastric lavage, protocols, 751
metoclopramide hydrochloride; pharmacokinetics, CAPD, 174
Dialysis; peritoneal; clearance, ethosuximide and phenobarbital, 1030; continuous ambulatory, anti-infective agents absorption, 246; metoclopramide pharmacokinetics, 174; sucralfate, toxicity, aluminum overload, 636
Diazepam; eclampsia; and preeclampsia therapy, 236
Didanosine
marketing; FDA approvals, 4
use; evaluation, criteria, 885
Diluents; lidocaine; ceftriaxone, i.m., reconstitution, pediatrics, 961
Diphenhydramine hydrochloride; allergies; therapy, fentanyl adverse reactions, 222
Diphtheria and tetanus toxoids and pertussis vaccines; marketing; FDA approvals, 290
Diuretics; hydrochlorothiazide; hypertension therapy, phenylpropanolamine effects, lack, 168
Dobutamine; heart failure; congestive, long-term therapy, 618
Dosage
adenosine; DUE criteria, 727
alcohols, cetyl, combination, colfosceril palmitate, tyloxapol; DUE criteria, 355
aldesleukin, 669
aminophylline; DUE criteria, 1033
amphotericin B; DUE criteria, 809
analgesics and antipyretics; fever therapy, pediatrics, review, 1005
antibodies; monoclonal antiendotoxin, DUE criteria, 257
antihistamines; DUE criteria, therapy, extrapyramidal side effects, 553
anti-infective agents; intraperitoneal, absorption, CAPD, 246
antiparkinson agents; DUE criteria, therapy, extrapyramidal side effects, 553
azithromycin, 98, 137
benzodiazepines; DUE criteria, therapy, extrapyramidal side effects, 553
beractant; DUE criteria, 357
cefpodoxime proxetil, 999
cefprozil, 295
cisplatin; high, toxicity, ondansetron therapy, 1026
clarithromycin, 98, 137
didanosine, 4; DUE criteria, 885
diphtheria and tetanus toxoids and pertussis vaccines; immunization, pediatrics, 290
dobutamine; congestive heart failure, long-term therapy, 618
doxazosin mesylate, 415
ethosuximide and phenobarbital; clearance, peritoneal dialysis, 1030
felodipine, 9
fentanyl; adverse reactions, transdermal patches, 222
finasteride, 825
flumazenil, 287
foscarnet sodium, 4
Haemophilus b oligosaccharide conjugate vaccines; immunization, pediatrics, 332
Haemophilus b polysaccharide conjugate vaccines; immunization, pediatrics, 332
idarubicin, 152
γ-interferon; review, 834
interferon gamma-1b; review, 834
lactase; lactose intolerance, reduced symptoms, 533
lomefloxacin hydrochloride, 458; review, 753
morphine sulfate; Baxter Infusor, PCA, postoperative pain therapy, 342
nabumetone, 381
omeprazole; ulcers, peptic esophagitis, DUE criteria, 177
overdose; benzodiazepines, flumazenil therapy, 287; dapsone, toxicity, hemolytic anemia, methemoglobinemia, 800; measuring cups, spoons, droppers, toxicity, 220
oxaprozin, 591
pamidronate disodium, 220
parasympatholytic agents; DUE criteria, therapy, extrapyramidal side effects, 553
phenobarbital and ethosuximide; clearance, peritoneal dialysis, 1030
pravastatin sodium, 99; hypercholesterolemia therapy, review, 677
quinapril hydrochloride, 220
serotonin reuptake inhibitors; depression therapy, review, 930
sertraline hydrochloride, 381
simvastatin, 290
skeletal muscle relaxants; DUE criteria, 435
sumatriptan; DUE criteria, 972
sumatriptan succinate; therapy, review, 919
temafloxacin hydrochloride, 381; review, 753
theophylline; DUE criteria, 1033
ticlopidine hydrochloride, 99; review, 603
ursodiol; pruritus therapy, biliary cirrhosis, 672
zalcitabine, 747
zidovudine; DUE criteria, 63
Dosage forms
drug administration systems; measuring cups, spoons, droppers, overdose, 220
fentanyl; transdermal patches, adverse reactions, 222; transdermal patches, pain therapy, 22
Dosage schedules
β agonists; aerosols, regular vs. as-needed, asthma therapy, 877
antibiotics; postantibiotic effect, 865; therapy, postantibiotic effect, 876
anti-infective agents; prophylaxis, surgery, ASHP protocols, 483; therapy, postantibiotic effect, 876
calcium antagonists; therapy, 549
dobutamine; congestive heart failure, long-term therapy, 618
nutrition; parenteral, chronic home therapy, toxicity, 543
oxaprozin, 591
triazolam; labeling changes, FDA approvals, 467
Doxacurium chloride; use; evaluation, criteria, 435
Doxazosin mesylate; pharmacology; review, 415
Drug administration
alcohols, cetyl, combination, colfosceril palmitate, tyloxapol; intratracheal, adult respiratory distress syndrome, neonate, 880
γ-interferon; chronic granulomatous disease therapy, 834
interferon gamma-1b; chronic granulomatous disease therapy, 834
serotonin reuptake inhibitors; depression therapy, review, 930
verapamil hydrochloride; equivalency, intact capsules vs. sprinkled on food, 539
Drug administration rate; globulin immune; i.v. infusion, concentrated, toxicity, 1022
Drug administration routes
β agonists; regular vs. as-needed, asthma, 877
aminophylline; enteral administration, availability, 428
anti-infective agents; prophylaxis, surgery, ASHP protocols, 483
cefazolin sodium; intraventricular, toxicity, seizures, 104
deferoxamine mesylate; intraperitoneal, i.v., aluminum overload therapy, 636
fentanyl; transdermal patches, pain therapy, 22
intraperitoneal; anti-infective agents, absorption, CAPD, 246
mesalamine; rectal, inflammatory bowel disease therapy, 514
methotrexate; intramuscular, ectopic pregnancy therapy, 529
metoclopramide hydrochloride; i.p. vs. i.v. oral, pharmacokinetics, CAPD, 174
morphine sulfate; intrathecal and i.v. PCA vs. PCA alone, postoperative pain therapy, 958
olsalazine sodium; oral, inflammatory bowel disease therapy, 514
roentgenographic agents; ionic, epidural, toxicity, inadvertent intrathecal injection, 105
scopolamine; transdermal patches, hyperemesis gravidarum therapy, 830
Drug administration sites
fentanyl; transdermal patches, adverse reactions, 222
lidocaine, combination, prilocaine; anesthesia, pain, s.c. injections, 347
Drug administration systems
Baxter Infusor; morphine PCA, postoperative pain therapy, 342
devices; measuring cups, spoons, droppers, overdose, 220
Drug interactions
antiarrhythmic agents and devices; cardiac implants, impaired functioning, 48
azithromycin, 137
cisplatin and ondansetron hydrochloride; pharmacokinetics, 1026
clarithromycin, 137
devices and antiarrhythmic agents; cardiac implants, impaired functioning, 48
food and verapamil hydrochloride; equivalency, intact capsules vs. sprinkled, 539
lomefloxacin hydrochloride; review, 753
ondansetron hydrochloride and cisplatin; pharmacokinetics, 1026
serotonin reuptake inhibitors; depression therapy, review, 930
sucralfate and tests, laboratory; occult blood, interference, 625
temafloxacin hydrochloride; review, 753
tests, laboratory and sucralfate; occult blood, interference, 625
tetracycline hydrochloride and warfarin sodium; potentiation, prothrombin time, 806
verapamil hydrochloride and food; equivalency, intact capsules vs. sprinkled, 539
warfarin sodium and tetracycline hydrochloride; potentiation, prothrombin time, 806
Drug Reaction Alerts, 87, 197, 273, 368, 448, 562, 652, 735, 819, 895, 978, 1040
Drugs
new; marketing, FDA approvals, 1991, 208
reconstitution; ceftriaxone, i.m., pharmacokinetics, toxicity, pediatrics, 961; globulin immune, dextrose vs. water for injection, 628
selection; antimicrobial prophylaxis, surgery, ASHP protocols, 483
Drugs, adverse reactions, see **Toxicity**
Drugs, availability; aminophylline; liquid, enteral administration, 428
Drugs, body distribution
ciprofloxacin hydrochloride; blood and milk levels, 352
metoclopramide hydrochloride; peritoneal dialysis, 174
Drugs, investigational
investigational new drugs; 566C80, *P. carinii* pneumonia, protocols, 99; taxol, ovarian neoplasms therapy, protocols, 912; zalcitabine, FDA actions, premarketing access, 385
new-drug applications; approvals, changes, FDA processing, 574
Drug use
evaluation; adenosine, criteria, 727; aminophylline, theophylline, criteria, 1033; amphotericin B, bladder irrigation, criteria, 809; antiendotoxin monoclonal antibodies, criteria, 257; beractant, criteria, 357; didanosine, criteria, 885; Exosurf Neonatal, criteria, 355; omeprazole, criteria, 177; skeletal muscle relaxants, criteria, 435; sumatriptan criteria, 972; therapy, extrapyramidal side effects, 553; zidovudine, criteria, 63
fentanyl; diffuse rash, transdermal patches, 222
DUE Criteria, 63, 177, 257, 355, 435, 553, 727, 809, 885, 972, 1033
adenosine, 727
agents for extrapyramidal adverse effects, 553
amphotericin B bladder irrigation, 809
antiendotoxin monoclonal antibodies (HA-1A and E5), 257
beractant (Survanta), 357
colfosceril (Exosurf Neonatal), 355
didanosine, 885
omeprazole, 177
pancuronium bromide, vecuronium bromide, atracurium besylate, tubocurarine chloride, metocurine iodide, pipecuronium bromide, and doxacurium chloride, 435
sumatriptan, 972
theophylline (aminophylline), 1033
zidovudine, 63

E

Eclampsia; therapy, 236
Editorial; Who should receive antiendotoxin monoclonal antibody therapy? 255
Electrolytes; combination, polyethylene glycol; gastric lavage, diabetes mellitus, protocols, 751
Endocrine diseases; therapy; HIV infections related, 705
Enzymes; lactase; lactose intolerance, reduced symptoms, 533
Epidemiology; leukemia; adult acute, therapy, review, 767
Epilepsy
ethosuximide and phenobarbital ; absence, clearance, peritoneal dialysis, 1030
phenobarbital and ethosuximide; absence, clearance,

peritoneal dialysis, 1030
Equivalency
Haemophilus b oligosaccharide conjugate vaccines; immunogenicity, pediatrics, 332
Haemophilus b polysaccharide conjugate vaccines; immunogenicity, pediatrics, 332
verapamil hydrochloride; pharmacokinetics, intact capsules vs. sprinkled on food, 539
Equivalency, generic; globulin immune; formulary selection, ASHP protocols, 117
Errors, medication; dosage; measuring devices, 220
Erythromycin; gastroparesis; therapy, effects, motilin, 917
Esophageal and gastric varices; β blockers; gastrointestinal hemorrhage prophylaxis, 337
Esophagitis; omeprazole; peptic, therapy, DUE criteria, 177
Ethosuximide; and phenobarbital; clearance, peritoneal dialysis, 1030
Excretion
ethosuximide and phenobarbital; clearance, peritoneal dialysis, 1030
metoclopramide hydrochloride; clearance, CAPD, 174
phenobarbital and ethosuximide; clearance, peritoneal dialysis, 1030

F

Felodipine; marketing; FDA approvals, 9
Fentanyl
adverse reactions; diffuse rash, transdermal patches, 222
patches transdermal; pain therapy, 22
Fever; analgesics and antipyretics; therapy, pediatrics, review, 1005
Finasteride; marketing; FDA approvals, 825
566C80; pneumonia; *P. carinii*, treatment IND, FDA approvals, 99
Flecainide; interactions; implanted cardiac devices, 48
Fluconazole; candidiasis; therapy, lack, burns, infant, 883
Flumazenil; marketing; FDA approvals, 287
Fluvoxamine; depression; therapy, review, 930
Food; interactions; verapamil, open vs. intact capsules, pharmacokinetics, 539
Food and Drug Administration (U.S.)
approvals; aldesleukin marketing, 669; azithromycin, clarithromycin, marketing, 98; cefpodoxime marketing, 999; cefprozil marketing, 295; didanosine, foscarnet, marketing, 4; DTP vaccines marketing, 290; felodipine marketing, 9; finasteride marketing, 825; flumazenil marketing, 287; lomefloxacin marketing, 458; nabumetone marketing, 381; new-drug applications, changes, processing, 574; new drugs and biologicals, 1991, 208; pamidronate, marketing, 220; pravastatin, marketing, 99; quinapril, marketing, 220; sertraline marketing, 381; simvastatin marketing, 290; temafloxacin marketing, 381; ticlopidine, marketing, 99; triazolam labeling changes, package inserts, 467; zalcitabine, marketing, accelerated drug review policy, 747
azithromycin; actions, toxicity reports, marketing delay, 218
cognition activators; disapprovals, marketing, 467
566C80; *P. carinii* pneumonia, treatment IND approvals, 99
labeling; drug measuring devices, overdose, 220
regulations; astemizole, terfenadine, warning labels, cardiovascular toxicity, 825; temafloxacin, toxicity, product withdrawal, 747
taxol; treatment IND approvals, 912
triazolam; actions, toxicity reports, 9
zalcitabine; actions, AIDS buyers groups, quality problems, 385
Formularies; globulin immune; product selection, ASHP protocols, 117
Foscarnet sodium; marketing; FDA approvals, 4

G

Ganciclovir; toxicity; liver, cytomegalic inclusion disease therapy, AIDS, 432
Gastric lavage; electrolytes, combination, polyethylene glycol; diabetes mellitus, protocols, 751
Gastrointestinal drugs
histamine H_2 antagonists; ulcer therapy, NSAID toxicity, review, 690
mesalamine; inflammatory bowel disease therapy, 514
misoprostol; ulcer therapy, NSAID toxicity, review, 690
olsalazine sodium; inflammatory bowel disease therapy, 514
omeprazole; DUE criteria, 177; ulcer therapy, NSAID toxicity, review, 690
sucralfate; interference, occult blood tests, 625; toxicity, aluminum overload, deferoxamine therapy, CAPD, 636
Gastrointestinal hemorrhage; β blockers; prophylaxis, cirrhosis, esophageal varices, 337
Gastroparesis; erythromycin; therapy, 917
Gelatin; sponges; hemorrhage prophylaxis, dental surgery, anticoagulant toxicity, 857
Geriatrics
depression; therapy, 96
pain; therapy, protocols, 391
Globulin immune
reconstitution; dextrose vs. water for injection, toxicity, 628
therapy; i.v., ASHP protocols, 117
toxicity; side effects, concentrated injections, 1022
Granulomatous disease
γ-interferon; chronic, therapy, 834
interferon gamma-1b; chronic, therapy, 834
Guidelines, treatment, see **Protocols**

H

HA-1A
see also **Nebacumab**
sepsis; antiendotoxin monoclonal antibodies, therapy, 223
***Haemophilus* b oligosaccharide conjugate vaccines;** immunization; equivalency, immunogenicity, pediatrics, 332
***Haemophilus influenzae*;** immunization; conjugate vaccines, immunogenicity, pediatrics, 332
Headache; sumatriptan; therapy, DUE criteria, 972
Health care; home; parenteral nutrition, toxicity, 543
Heart failure; dobutamine; congestive, long-term therapy, 618
Heavy metal antagonists; deferoxamine mesylate; therapy, aluminum overload, sucralfate toxicity, CAPD, 636
Hematoma; warfarin sodium; toxicity, intramural, small intestine, 632
Hemorrhage; anticoagulants; toxicity, dental surgery, 857
Hemostatics; therapy; anticoagulant toxicity, dental surgery, 857
Heparin; flushes; toxicity, thrombocytopenia, thromboembolism, 797
HIV infections
didanosine; therapy, DUE criteria, 885
therapy; associated endocrine disorders, 705
zalcitabine; therapy, Roche premarketing access programs, 385
zalcitabine and zidovudine; combined therapy, FDA approvals, 747
zidovudine and zalcitabine; combined therapy, FDA approvals, 747
Hoffmann-La Roche Pharmaceuticals; zalcitabine; investigational new drugs, premarketing access programs, 385
Hospitals; length of stay; nausea and vomiting, anesthetics toxicity, surgery, 965
Hydrochlorothiazide; hypertension; phenylpropanolamine effects, lack, 168
Hyperalimentation, see **Nutrition; parenteral**
Hypercalcemia; pamidronate disodium; therapy, neoplasms, FDA approvals, 220
Hypercholesterolemia
pravastatin sodium; therapy, FDA approvals, 99; therapy, review, 677
simvastatin; therapy, FDA approvals, 290
Hyperemesis gravidarum; scopolamine; transdermal patches, 830
Hyperfibrinogenemia; therapy, 968
Hyperprolactinemia; psychotherapeutic agents; toxicity, therapy, 851
Hypertension
doxazosin mesylate; therapy, review, 415
felodipine; therapy, FDA approvals, 9
phenylpropanolamine hydrochloride; toxicity, lack, 168
quinapril hydrochloride; therapy, FDA approvals, 220
Hypotensive agents
doxazosin mesylate; review, 415
eclampsia; and preeclampsia therapy, 236
felodipine; FDA approvals, 9
quinapril hydrochloride; marketing, FDA approvals, 220

I

Ibuprofen; fever; therapy, pediatrics, review, 1005
Idarubicin; leukemia; nonlymphocytic, acute, therapy, 152
Immunization
diphtheria and tetanus toxoids and pertussis; vaccines, FDA approvals, 290
Haemophilus influenzae; conjugate vaccines, immunogenicity, pediatrics, 332
rabies; vaccines, human rabies immune globulin, 37
Immunogenicity
Haemophilus b oligosaccharide conjugate vaccines; equivalency, pediatrics, 332
Haemophilus b polysaccharide conjugate vaccines; equivalency, pediatrics, 332
Immunosuppressive agents; methotrexate; ectopic pregnancy therapy, 529
Immunotherapy
globulin immune; i.v. therapy, ASHP protocols, 117; reconstitution, dextrose vs. water for injection, 628; toxicity, concentrated injections, bone marrow transplantation, 1022
γ-interferon; chronic granulomatous disease, 834
interferon gamma-1b; chronic granulomatous disease, 834
nebacumab; sepsis, criteria, 255; sepsis, DUE criteria, 257
sepsis; antiendotoxin monoclonal antibodies, 223
Xomen-E5; sepsis, criteria, 255; sepsis, DUE criteria, 257
Implants; heart; interactions, antiarrhythmic agents, 48
Inflammatory bowel disease
mesalamine; therapy, 514
olsalazine sodium; therapy, 514
Injections
cefazolin sodium; intraventricular, toxicity, seizures, 104
ceftriaxone; i.m., concentrated, pharmacokinetics and toxicity, pediatrics, 961
dobutamine; intravenous, congestive heart failure, long-term therapy, 618
globulin immune; concentrated, i.v. infusion rate, toxicity, 1022; reconstitution, dextrose vs. water for injection, 628; i.v. therapy, ASHP protocols, 117
heparin, comparison, sodium chloride; lock flushing, 797
morphine sulfate; intrathecal and i.v. PCA vs. PCA alone, postoperative pain, 958
pamidronate disodium; marketing, FDA approvals, 220
patient-controlled analgesia; morphine, Baxter Infusor, postoperative pain therapy, 342
roentgenographic agents; ionic, epidural, toxicity, inadvertent intrathecal administration, 105
sodium chloride, comparison, heparin; lock flushing, 797
subcutaneous; pain, lidocaine–prilocaine therapy, 347
Insomnia; triazolam; therapy, labeling, changes, package inserts, FDA approvals, 467
γ-Interferon; granulomatous disease; chronic, therapy, review, 834
Interferon gamma-1b; granulomatous disease; chronic, therapy, review, 834
Irrigating solutions; amphotericin B; bladder, urinary anti-infectives, DUE criteria, 809

K

Kidney failure
metoclopramide hydrochloride; pharmacokinetics, CAPD, 174
sucralfate; toxicity, aluminum overload, deferoxamine therapy, CAPD, 636

L

Labeling
angiotensin-converting enzyme inhibitors; warnings, risks, pregnancy, 467
astemizole; warnings, cardiovascular toxicity, 825
devices; dosage measuring, overdose, 220
terfenadine; warnings, cardiovascular toxicity, 825
triazolam; changes, FDA approvals, 467

Lactase; lactose intolerance; effects, reduced symptoms, 533
Lactation; ciprofloxacin hydrochloride; milk and blood levels, 352
Lactose intolerance; lactase; effects, reduced symptoms, 533
Letters, 13, 104, 222, 308, 386, 583, 674, 767
Asthma in children, 386
Beta-adrenergic agonists in asthma, 13
Danger of epidural use of ionic contrast media, 105
Diffuse rash associated with transdermal fentanyl, 222
Potential interaction between terfenadine and macrolide antibiotics, 675
Seizures after intraventricular cefazolin adminstration, 104
Topical capsaicin for osteoarthritis, 308
Use of cytomegalovirus immune globulin, 674
Use of succimer, 387
Use of surfactant products, 583
Value of transdermal fentanyl, 584
Leukemia; therapy; acute, adult, review, 767
Lidocaine
combination, prilocaine; anesthesia, pain, s.c. injection sites, 347
diluents; ceftriaxone, reconstitution, concentrated, pediatrics, 961
Liver cirrhosis
β blockers; gastrointestinal hemorrhage prophylaxis, 337
ursodiol; biliary, pruritus therapy, 672
Liver diseases; effects; astemizole, terfenadine toxicity, 825
Lomefloxacin hydrochloride
marketing; FDA approvals, 458
pharmacology; review, 753
Lung diseases
aminophylline; therapy, DUE criteria, 1033
theophylline; therapy, DUE criteria, 1033

M

Macrolides
azithromycin; FDA approvals, 98; marketing delay, Pfizer, 218; pharmacology, 137
clarithromycin; FDA approvals, 98; pharmacology, 137
erythromycin; gastroparesis therapy, effects, motilin, 917
Magnesium sulfate; eclampsia; and preeclampsia therapy, 236
Marketing
aldesleukin; FDA approvals, 669
azithromycin; delay, Pfizer, 218; FDA approvals, 98
cefpodoxime proxetil; FDA approvals, 999
cefprozil; FDA approvals, 295
clarithromycin; FDA approvals, 98
cognition activators; FDA disapprovals, 467
diphtheria and tetanus toxoids and pertussis vaccines; FDA approvals, 290
felodipine; FDA approvals, 9
finasteride; FDA approvals, 825
flumazenil; FDA approvals, 287
lomefloxacin hydrochloride; FDA approvals, 458
nabumetone; FDA approvals, 381
new drugs; and biologicals, FDA approvals, 1991, 208
pamidronate disodium; FDA approvals, 220
pravastatin sodium; FDA approvals, 99
quinapril hydrochloride; FDA approvals, 220
sertraline hydrochloride; FDA approvals, 381
simvastatin; FDA approvals, 290
temafloxacin hydrochloride; FDA approvals, 381
ticlopidine hydrochloride; FDA approvals, 99
zalcitabine; FDA approvals, accelerated drug review policy, 747
Mechanism of action
antibiotics; postantibiotic effect, 865
azithromycin, 137
clarithromycin, 137
idarubicin, 152
lomefloxacin hydrochloride; review, 753
sertraline hydrochloride, 381
sumatriptan succinate; migraine therapy, review, 919
temafloxacin hydrochloride; review, 753
ticlopidine hydrochloride; cerebrovascular disorders therapy, review, 603
Mesalamine; inflammatory bowel disease; therapy, 514
Methemoglobinemia; dapsone; toxicity, therapy, 800
Methotrexate; pregnancy; ectopic, therapy, 529
Methylene blue; and charcoal activated; therapy, dapsone toxicity, 800
Metoclopramide hydrochloride; pharmacokinetics; peritoneal dialysis, 174
Metocurine iodide; use; evaluation, criteria, 435
Metrology; devices; dosage measuring, overdose potential, 220
Midazolam hydrochloride; muscle spasticity; therapy, morphine toxicity, 57
Migraine
sumatriptan; therapy, DUE criteria, 972
sumatriptan succinate; therapy, review, 919
Misoprostol; ulcers; therapy, NSAID toxicity, review, 690
Monoamine oxidase inhibitors; depression; therapy, geriatrics, 96
Moricizine; interactions; implanted cardiac devices, 48
Morphine sulfate
pain; postoperative, intrathecal and i.v. PCA vs. PCA, 958
patient-controlled analgesia; Baxter Infusor, postoperative pain therapy, 342
toxicity; muscle spasticity, midazolam therapy, 57
Mortality
β agonists; regular vs. as-needed, asthma therapy, 877
antiarrhythmic agents; toxicity, 714
Mouthwashes; tranexamic acid; hemorrhage prophylaxis, anticoagulant toxicity, dental surgery, 857
Muscle spasticity; morphine sulfate; toxicity, midazolam therapy, 57

N

Nabumetone; marketing; FDA approvals, 381
Nadolol; gastrointestinal hemorrhage; prophylaxis, cirrhosis, esophageal varices, 337
Nausea
anesthetics; and vomiting, toxicity, surgery, 965
ondansetron hydrochloride; and vomiting, therapy, cisplatin toxicity, 1026
Nebacumab
sepsis; antiendotoxin monoclonal antibodies, therapy, criteria, 255
use; evaluation, criteria, 257
Neoplasms; pamidronate disodium; hypercalcemia therapy, FDA approvals, 220
News, 4, 96, 208, 287, 378, 458, 574, 669, 747, 825, 912, 991
Acellular pertussis vaccine approved by FDA, 290
Adverse effects prompt withdrawal of temafloxacin, 747
Benzodiazepine antagonist approved by FDA, 287
Call for applications to conduct research on patient outcomes associated with pharmaceutical therapy in ambulatory-care setting, 467
CDC advises on management of persons exposed to multiple-drug-resistant tuberculosis, 991
Cefpodoxime marketing approved by FDA, 999
Cefprozil enters oral antibiotic market, 295
Cognitive enhancers illegal, says FDA, 467
Depression in elderly is common but undertreated, says expert panel, 96
Didanosine and foscarnet marketed for use by patients with AIDS, 4
EPA seeks information on efficacy of sterilants and disinfectants, 295
Expert panel issues guidelines on asthma management, 295
False-positive viral antibody test results reported in influenza vaccine recipients, 220
FDA announces four initiatives for drug approval system, 574
FDA approves release of recombinant interleukin-2 product, 669
FDA approves treatment IND protocol for taxol, 912
FDA seeks changes in benzodiazepine packaging and labeling, 295
FDA seizes cold sterilizing solution, 220
FDA warns of overdose risk from dosage cups, 220
FDA warns quality of underground zalcitabine is poor; Roche expands premarketing access programs, 385
Federal task force revises recommendations for PCP prophylaxis, 670
Felodipine marketed as antihypertensive agent, 9
Finasteride approved for treatment of benign prostatic hyperplasia, 825
Free drug programs for indigent patients should be more accessible, says Senate committee on aging, 1000
Guidelines address systemic glucocorticosteroid use for infection management, 295
HDL testing should be routine part of assessments of coronary heart disease risk, says consensus panel, 378
Heavy use of inhaled β agonists associated with increased risk of fatal or near-fatal asthma, study shows, 458
Lomefloxacin reaches U.S. market, 458
Nabumetone marketed for osteoarthritis, rheumatoid arthritis, 381
New labeling and patient insert for triazolam approved by FDA, 467
News Briefs, 9, 103, 221, 296, 385, 467, 576, 670, 750, 829, 912, 1000
Oral temafloxacin approved for U.S. market, 381
Pamidronate released for management of hypercalcemia of malignancy, 220
Pediatrics academy issues new guidelines for acellular pertussis vaccine use, 576
Pfizer delays marketing azithromycin, 218
Pravastatin reaches U.S. market, 99
Quinapril marketed as antihypertensive agent, 220
Results of ISIS-3 published, 576
Review of 1991 shows 30 new drugs, several important biologics cleared for marketing, 208
Sertraline cleared for marketing as antidepressant, 381
Tacrine made available under treatment IND protocol, 385
Talley to succeed Zellmer as editor of *AJHP* and *Clinical Pharmacy*, 750
Terfenadine and astemizole pose cardiovascular risks to certain patients, health professionals warned, 825
Third HMG-CoA reductase inhibitor marketed for cholesterol reduction, 290
Three studies examine angiotensin-converting-enzyme-inhibitor prevention of heart failure, 999
Ticlopidine approved for stroke prevention, 99
Treatment IND protocol announced for *Pneumocystis carinii* pneumonia, 99
Two macrolide antimicrobials approved for marketing, 98
United Kingdom suspends sales of triazolam; FDA to review safety data, 9
Upcoming Specialty Meetings, 9, 103, 221, 296, 385, 470, 576, 670, 750, 912, 1000
Warnings about use of angiotensin-converting-enzyme inhibitors in advanced pregnancy strengthened, 467
Working group issues report on aluminum contamination of parenteral nutrient solutions, 6
Zalcitabine approved under accelerated drug review policy, 747
Nimodipine; cerebrovascular disorders; ischemic stroke therapy, 350
Nutrition
diet; lactose intolerance, lactase effects, reduced symptoms, 533
parenteral; home therapy, side effects, 543

O

Occult blood; tests, laboratory; Gastroccult vs. Hemoccult, interference, sucralfate, 625
Olsalazine sodium; inflammatory bowel disease; therapy, 514
Omeprazole
ulcers; therapy, NSAID toxicity, review, 690
use; evaluation, criteria, 177
Ondansetron hydrochloride; pharmacokinetics; therapy, cisplatin toxicity, 1026
Opiates; pain; protocols, therapy, 391
Osteoarthritis
nabumetone; therapy, FDA approvals, 381
oxaprozin; therapy, 591
Ovarian neoplasms; taxol; treatment IND, FDA approvals, 912
Oxaprozin; arthritis; rheumatoid, and osteoarthritis, therapy, 591

P

Package inserts; patients; triazolam, changes, FDA approvals, 467
Paclitaxel, see **Taxol**
Pain
analgesics; protocols, therapy, 309
lidocaine, combination, prilocaine; anesthesia, s.c. injection sites, 347
morphine sulfate; postoperative, Baxter Infusor PCA, 342; postoperative, intrathecal and i.v. PCA vs. PCA alone, 958
therapy; protocols, 391
Pamidronate disodium; marketing; FDA approvals, 220

Pancuronium bromide; use; evaluation, criteria, 435
Parasympatholytic agents; drug use; evaluation, criteria, therapy, extrapyramidal side effects, 553
Parenterals, see **Injections**
Paroxetine; depression; therapy, review, 930
Patches transdermal
fentanyl; adverse reactions, diffuse rash, 222; pain therapy, 22
scopolamine; hyperemesis gravidarum therapy, 830
Patient-controlled analgesia; morphine sulfate; and intrathecal vs. PCA alone, postoperative pain therapy, 958; Baxter Infusor, postoperative pain therapy, 342
Patients
inpatients; amphotericin B, DUE criteria, 809; antiendotoxin monoclonal antibodies, DUE criteria, 257; DUE criteria, therapy, extrapyramidal side effects, 553; omeprazole, DUE criteria, 177; zidovudine, DUE criteria, 63
outpatients; aminophylline, theophylline, DUE criteria, 1033; DUE criteria, therapy, extrapyramidal side effects, 553; omeprazole, DUE criteria, 177; sumatriptan, DUE criteria, 972; zidovudine, DUE criteria, 63
Pediatrics
amphotericin B; candidiasis therapy, burns, infant, 883
analgesics and antipyretics; fever therapy, review, 1005
antibodies; monoclonal antiendotoxin, DUE criteria, 257
antihistamines; DUE criteria, therapy, extrapyramidal side effects, 553
antiparkinson agents; DUE criteria, therapy, extrapyramidal side effects, 553
benzodiazepines; DUE criteria, therapy, extrapyramidal side effects, 553
ceftriaxone; i.m., concentrated, pharmacokinetics, toxicity, 961
didanosine; DUE criteria, 885
diphtheria and tetanus toxoids and pertussis vaccines; marketing, FDA approvals, 290
ethosuximide and phenobarbital; clearance, peritoneal dialysis, 1030
fluconazole; candidiasis therapy, lack, burns, infant, 883
Haemophilus b oligosaccharide conjugate vaccines; equivalency, immunogenicity, 332
Haemophilus b polysaccharide conjugate vaccines; equivalency, immunogenicity, 332
neonates; beractant, DUE criteria, 357; ciprofloxacin blood levels, maternal administration, 352; Exosurf Neonatal, DUE criteria, 355; pulmonary surfactant, adult respiratory distress syndrome therapy, 880
pain; therapy, protocols, infants and neonates, 391
parasympatholytic agents; DUE criteria, therapy, extrapyramidal side effects, 553
phenobarbital and ethosuximide; clearance, peritoneal dialysis, 1030
zidovudine; DUE criteria, 63
Pfizer Pharmaceuticals; azithromycin; marketing delay, 218
Pharmacokinetics
acetaminophen; fever therapy, pediatrics, review, 1005
aldesleukin, 669
anti-infective agents; absorption, intraperitoneal, CAPD, 246
aspirin; fever therapy, pediatrics, review, 1005
azithromycin, 98, 137
cefpodoxime proxetil, 999
cefprozil, 295
ceftriaxone; i.m., concentrated, pediatrics, 961
clarithromycin, 98, 137
didanosine, 4
diphtheria and tetanus toxoids and pertussis vaccines; pediatrics, 290
doxazosin mesylate; review, 415
felodipine, 9
fentanyl; transdermal patches, pain therapy, 22
finasteride, 825
flumazenil, 287
foscarnet sodium, 4
ibuprofen; fever therapy, pediatrics, review, 1005
idarubicin, 152
γ-interferon; review, 834
interferon gamma-1b; review, 834
lomefloxacin hydrochloride, 458; review, 753
mesalamine, 514
metoclopramide hydrochloride; peritoneal dialysis, 174
nabumetone, 381
olsalazine sodium, 514
ondansetron hydrochloride; therapy, cisplatin toxicity, 1026
oxaprozin, 591
pamidronate disodium, 220
pravastatin sodium, 99; hypercholesterolemia therapy, review, 677
quinapril hydrochloride, 220
serotonin reuptake inhibitors; depression, therapy, review, 930
sertraline hydrochloride, 381
simvastatin, 290
sumatriptan succinate; migraine therapy, review, 919
temafloxacin hydrochloride, 381; review, 753
ticlopidine hydrochloride, 99; review, 603
verapamil hydrochloride; equivalency, intact capsules vs. sprinkled on food, 539
Pharmacy, institutional, hospital
quality assurance; programs, adenosine, DUE criteria, 727; programs, aminophylline, theophylline, DUE criteria, 1033; programs, amphotericin B, DUE criteria, 809; programs, antiendotoxin monoclonal antibodies, DUE criteria, 257; programs, beractant, DUE criteria, 357; programs, didanosine, DUE criteria, 885; programs, DUE criteria, therapy, extrapyramidal side effects, 553; programs, Exosurf Neonatal, DUE criteria, 355; programs, omeprazole, DUE criteria, 177; programs, skeletal muscle relaxants, DUE criteria, 435; programs, sumatriptan DUE criteria, 972; programs, zidovudine, DUE criteria, 63
Phenobarbital; and ethosuximide; clearance, peritoneal dialysis, 1030
Phenylpropanolamine hydrochloride; toxicity; hypertension, lack, 168
Phenytoin; eclampsia; and preeclampsia therapy, 236
Pipecuronium bromide; use; evaluation, criteria, 435
Placental transfer; scopolamine; transdermal patches, hyperemesis gravidarum therapy, 830
Plants; herbs; cognition disorders therapy, FDA disapprovals, 467
Platelet aggregation inhibitors
hyperfibrinogenemia; therapy, 968
ticlopidine hydrochloride; cerebrovascular disorders therapy, review, 603
Pneumonia; 566C80; *P. carinii*, treatment IND, FDA approvals, 99
Poisoning; dapsone; therapy, 800
Polyethylene glycol; combination, electrolytes; gastric lavage, diabetes mellitus, protocols, 751
Pravastatin sodium
hypercholesterolemia; therapy, review, 677
marketing; FDA approvals, 99
Preeclampsia; therapy, 236
Pregnancy
angiotensin-converting enzyme inhibitors; risks, labeling, warnings, 467
methotrexate; ectopic, therapy, 529
scopolamine; hyperemesis gravidarum therapy, transdermal patches, 830
Prilocaine; combination, lidocaine; anesthesia, pain, s.c. injection sites, 347
Product withdrawal
azithromycin; Pfizer, marketing delay, 218
temafloxacin hydrochloride; toxicity, FDA regulations, 747
triazolam; United Kingdom, 9
Prolactin inhibitors
amantadine; hyperprolactinemia therapy, psychotropic toxicity, 851
bromocriptine; hyperprolactinemia therapy, psychotropic toxicity, 851
Propranolol; gastrointestinal hemorrhage; prophylaxis, cirrhosis, esophageal varices, 337
Prostatic hypertrophy; finasteride; therapy, FDA approvals, 825
Prothrombin time
tetracycline hydrochloride; interactions, warfarin, potentiation, 806
warfarin sodium; interactions, tetracycline, potentiation, 806
Protocols
adenosine; DUE criteria, 727
alcohols, cetyl, combination, colfosceril palmitate, tyloxapol; DUE criteria, 355
American Society of Hospital Pharmacists; antimicrobial prophylaxis, surgery, 483; globulin immune, i.v. therapy, 117
aminophylline; DUE criteria, 1033
amphotericin B; bladder irrigation, DUE criteria, 809
antibodies; monoclonal antiendotoxin, DUE criteria, 257
antihistamines; DUE criteria, therapy, extrapyramidal side effects, 553
antiparkinson agents; DUE criteria, therapy, extrapyramidal side effects, 553
benzodiazepines; DUE criteria, therapy, extrapyramidal side effects, 553
beractant; DUE criteria, 357
didanosine; DUE criteria, 885
electrolytes, combination, polyethylene glycol; gastric lavage, diabetes mellitus, 751
566C80; *P. carinii* pneumonia, treatment IND, FDA approvals, 99
omeprazole; ulcers, peptic esophagitis, therapy, DUE criteria, 177
pain; therapy, 309, 391
parasympatholytic agents; DUE criteria, therapy, extrapyramidal side effects, 553
skeletal muscle relaxants; DUE criteria, 435
sumatriptan; DUE criteria, 972
taxol; treatment IND, FDA approvals, 912
theophylline; DUE criteria, 1033
zidovudine; DUE criteria, 63
Pruritus; ursodiol; therapy, biliary cirrhosis, 672
Psychotherapeutic agents
toxicity; extrapyramidal side effects, therapy, DUE criteria, 553
toxicity; hyperprolactinemia, therapy, 851
Pulmonary surfactants
alcohols, cetyl, combination, colfosceril palmitate, tyloxapol; adult respiratory distress syndrome therapy, neonate, 880; DUE criteria, 355
beractant; DUE criteria, 357
Purchasing; zalcitabine; quality problems, AIDS buyers groups, 385

Q

Quality assurance; hospital pharmacy; programs, adenosine, DUE criteria, 727; programs, aminophylline, theophylline, DUE criteria, 1033; programs, amphotericin B, DUE criteria, 809; programs, antiendotoxin monoclonal antibodies, DUE criteria, 257; programs, beractant, DUE criteria, 357; programs, didanosine, DUE criteria, 885; programs, DUE criteria, therapy, extrapyramidal side effects, 553; programs, Exosurf Neonatal, DUE criteria, 355; programs, omeprazole, DUE criteria, 177; programs, skeletal muscle relaxants, DUE criteria, 435; programs, sumatriptan DUE criteria, 972; programs, zidovudine, DUE criteria, 63
Quinapril hydrochloride; marketing; FDA approvals, 220
Quinolones
ciprofloxacin hydrochloride; blood and milk levels, 352
lomefloxacin hydrochloride; FDA approvals, 458; pharmacology, review, 753
temafloxacin hydrochloride; FDA approvals, 381; pharmacology, review, 753; product withdrawal, toxicity, FDA regulations, 747

R

Rabies; immunization; vaccines, human rabies immune globulin, 37
Rabies immune globulin; immunization, 37
Rabies vaccines; human diploid cell; immunization, 37
Rational therapy; antiarrhythmic agents, 714
Regulations
Food and Drug Administration; astemizole, terfenadine, warning labels, cardiovascular toxicity, 825; cognition activator marketing, 467; zalcitabine, quality problems, premarketing access, 385
labeling; ACE inhibitors, warnings, risks, pregnancy, 467
new-drug applications; approvals, changes, FDA processing, 574
temafloxacin hydrochloride; product withdrawal, FDA, 747
Respiratory distress syndrome
alcohols, cetyl, combination, colfosceril palmitate, tyloxapol; adult, therapy, neonate, 880; therapy, DUE criteria, 355
beractant; therapy, DUE criteria, 357
Respiratory smooth-muscle relaxants
aminophylline; availability, enteral administration, 428; DUE criteria, 1033
theophylline; DUE criteria, 1033
Respiratory tract infections
azithromycin; therapy, FDA approvals, 98; therapy, marketing delay, Pfizer, 218
clarithromycin; therapy, FDA approvals, 98
Reye's syndrome; aspirin; toxicity, fever therapy, pediatrics, 1005
Roentgenographic agents; ionic; epidural, toxicity, inadvertent intrathecal injection, 105

S

Sales; triazolam; product withdrawal, United Kingdom, 9
Saline, see **Sodium chloride**
Scopolamine; hyperemesis gravidarum; transdermal patches, 830
Seizures; cefazolin sodium; toxicity, intraventricular injections, 104
Self-study Materials; *Concepts in Oncology Therapeutics, A Self-Instructional Course,* 568
Sepsis; antibodies; antiendotoxin monoclonal, therapy, 223; antiendotoxin monoclonal, therapy, criteria, 255; antiendotoxin monoclonal, therapy, DUE criteria, 257
Serotonin agonists
sumatriptan; DUE criteria, 972
sumatriptan succinate; migraine therapy, review, 919
Sertraline hydrochloride
depression; therapy, review, 930
marketing; FDA approvals, 381
Shock; antibodies; septic, antiendotoxin monoclonal, therapy, 223
Simvastatin; marketing; FDA approvals, 290
Skeletal muscle relaxants
atracurium besylate; DUE criteria, 435
doxacurium chloride; DUE criteria, 435
metocurine iodide; DUE criteria, 435
midazolam hydrochloride; muscle spasticity therapy, morphine toxicity, 57
pancuronium bromide; DUE criteria, 435
pipecuronium bromide; DUE criteria, 435
tubocurarine chloride; DUE criteria, 435
vecuronium bromide; DUE criteria, 435
Skin diseases
azithromycin; therapy, FDA approvals, 98
clarithromycin; FDA approvals, 98
Sodium chloride; comparison, heparin; i.v. lock flushing, 797
Sucralfate
interference; occult blood tests, Gastroccult vs. Hemoccult, 625
toxicity; aluminum overload, deferoxamine therapy, CAPD, 636
Sumatriptan; use; evaluation, criteria, 972
Sumatriptan succinate; migraine; therapy, review, 919
Surgery
anesthetics; abdominal, toxicity, nausea and vomiting, 965
anti-infective agents; prophylaxis, ASHP protocols, 483
dental; hemorrhage prophylaxis, anticoagulant toxicity, 857
protocols; pain therapy, 309, 391
Sustained-action medications
calcium antagonists; therapy, improved patient compliance, 549
verapamil hydrochloride; intact capsules vs. sprinkled on food, pharmacokinetics, 539
Sympatholytic agents
β blockers; hyperfibrinogenemia therapy, 968
nadolol; gastrointestinal hemorrhage, prophylaxis, cirrhosis, esophageal varices, 337
propranolol; gastrointestinal hemorrhage, prophylaxis, cirrhosis, esophageal varices, 337
Sympathomimetic agents
β agonists; aerosols, dosage schedules, asthma therapy, 877; asthma therapy, controversies, 13
phenylpropanolamine hydrochloride; toxicity, hypertension, lack, 168

T

Tachycardia; adenosine; paroxysmal supraventricular, therapy, DUE criteria, 727
Taxol; ovarian neoplasms; treatment IND, FDA approvals, 912
Temafloxacin hydrochloride
marketing; FDA approvals, 381
pharmacology; review, 753
product withdrawal; toxicity, FDA regulations, 747
Teratogenicity
angiotensin-converting enzyme inhibitors; pregnancy, labeling, warnings, 467
scopolamine; placental transfer, hyperemesis gravidarum transdermal therapy, 830
Terfenadine; toxicity; cardiovascular, labeling, warnings, 825
Tests, laboratory
cholesterol; and HDL monitoring, coronary disease, 378
occult blood; Gastroccult vs. Hemoccult, interference, sucralfate, 625
Tetracycline hydrochloride; interactions; warfarin, potentiation, prothrombin time, 806
Tetracyclines; tetracycline hydrochloride; interactions, warfarin, potentiation, prothrombin time, 806
Theophylline
blood levels; aminophylline availability, enteral administration, 428
use; evaluation, criteria, 1033
Therapy Consultation, 672, 751, 830, 917
Diabetes control during bowel cleansing with PEG–electrolyte solution, 751
Erythromycin, motilin, and gastroparesis, 917
Transdermal scopolamine for hyperemesis gravidarum, 830
Use of ursodiol in a patient with biliary cirrhosis, 672
Thrombocytopenia; heparin; toxicity, i.v. lock flushing, 797
Thromboembolism; heparin; toxicity, i.v. lock flushing, 797
Ticlopidine hydrochloride
cerebrovascular disorders; therapy, review, 603
marketing; FDA approvals, 99
Topical preparations
fentanyl; transdermal patches, pain therapy, 22
lidocaine, combination, prilocaine; creams, anesthesia, pain, s.c. injection sites, 347
Toxicity
acetaminophen; fever therapy, pediatrics, review, 1005
adenosine; DUE criteria, 727
β agonists; regular vs. as-needed, asthma, 877
alcohols, cetyl, combination, colfosceril palmitate, tyloxapol; DUE criteria, 355
aldesleukin, 669
aminophylline; DUE criteria, 1033
amphotericin B; DUE criteria, 809
anesthetics; nausea and vomiting, abdominal surgery, 965
angiotensin-converting enzyme inhibitors; pregnancy, labeling, warnings, 467
antiarrhythmic agents, 714; interactions, implanted cardiac devices, 48
antibodies; monoclonal antiendotoxin, DUE criteria, 257
anticoagulants; hemorrhage, dental surgery, 857
antihistamines; DUE criteria, therapy, extrapyramidal side effects, 553
anti-infective agents; postantibiotic effect, factors, 865
anti-inflammatory agents; nonsteroidal, ulcers, therapy, review, 690
antiparkinson agents; DUE criteria, therapy, extrapyramidal side effects, 553
aspirin; Reye's syndrome, fever therapy, pediatrics, 1005
astemizole; cardiovascular, labeling, warnings, 825
azithromycin; side effects, 98, 137; side effects, marketing delay, Pfizer, 218
benzodiazepines; DUE criteria, therapy, extrapyramidal side effects, 553; overdose, flumazenil therapy, 287
beractant; DUE criteria, 357
β blockers; side effects, gastrointestinal hemorrhage prophylaxis, 337
calcium antagonists; side effects, 549
cefazolin sodium; seizures, intraventricular injections, 104
cefpodoxime proxetil, 999
cefprozil, 295
ceftriaxone; side effects, lack, i.m., concentrated, pediatrics, 961
cisplatin; ondansetron therapy, pharmacokinetics, 1026
clarithromycin; side effects, 98, 137
dapsone; hemolytic anemia, methemoglobinemia, therapy, 800
didanosine, 4; DUE criteria, 885
diphtheria and tetanus toxoids and pertussis vaccines; side effects, pediatrics, 290
doxazosin mesylate; side effects, 415
drugs; endocrine disorders, HIV infections, therapy, 705; measuring cups, spoons, droppers, dosing problems, 220
felodipine, 9
fentanyl; transdermal, side effects, 22
finasteride, 825
flumazenil, 287
foscarnet sodium, 4
ganciclovir; liver, cytomegalic inclusion disease therapy, AIDS, 432
globulin immune; reconstitution, dextrose vs. water for injection, lack, 628; side effects, concentrated injections, 1022
Haemophilus b oligosaccharide conjugate vaccines; side effects, pediatrics, 332
Haemophilus b polysaccharide conjugate vaccines; side effects, pediatrics, 332
heparin; flushes, thrombocytopenia, thromboembolism, 797
ibuprofen; fever therapy, pediatrics, review, 1005
idarubicin; side effects, 152
injections; pain, lidocaine–prilocaine topical anesthesia, 347
γ-interferon; side effects, review, 834
interferon gamma-1b; side effects, review, 834
lomefloxacin hydrochloride; side effects, 458, 753
mesalamine; side effects, 514
methotrexate; side effects, ectopic pregnancy therapy, 529
morphine sulfate; Baxter Infusor, PCA, postoperative pain therapy, 342; muscle spasticity, midazolam therapy, 57; side effects, intrathecal and i.v. PCA vs. PCA alone, 958
nabumetone, 381
nutrition; parenteral, home therapy, 543
olsalazine sodium; side effects, 514
omeprazole; side effects, DUE criteria, 177
oxaprozin; side effects, 591
pamidronate disodium, 220
parasympatholytic agents; DUE criteria, therapy, extrapyramidal side effects, 553
phenylpropanolamine hydrochloride; hypertension, lack, 168
pravastatin sodium; side effects, 99; side effects, hypercholesterolemia therapy, review, 677
psychotherapeutic agents; extrapyramidal side effects, therapy, DUE criteria, 553; hyperprolactinemia, therapy, 851
quinapril hydrochloride, 220
roentgenographic agents; ionic, inadvertent intrathecal injection, 105
scopolamine; placental transfer, hyperemesis gravidarum transdermal therapy, 830
serotonin reuptake inhibitors; side effects, depression therapy, review, 930
sertraline hydrochloride, 381
simvastatin, 290
skeletal muscle relaxants; DUE criteria, 435
sucralfate; aluminum overload, deferoxamine therapy, CAPD, 636
sumatriptan; DUE criteria, 972
sumatriptan succinate; side effects, migraine therapy, review, 919
temafloxacin hydrochloride, 381; side effects, 753
terfenadine; cardiovascular, labeling, warnings, 825
tetracycline hydrochloride; interactions, warfarin, potentiation, prothrombin time, 806
theophylline; DUE criteria, 1033
ticlopidine hydrochloride; side effects, 99; side effects, review, 603
triazolam; side effects, product withdrawal, United Kingdom, 9
verapamil hydrochloride; side effects, lack, intact capsules vs. sprinkled on food, 539
warfarin sodium; interactions, tetracycline, potentiation, prothrombin time, 806; intramural hematoma of the small intestine, 632
zalcitabine, 747
zidovudine; DUE criteria, 63
Tranexamic acid; hemorrhage; prophylaxis, dental surgery, anticoagulant toxicity, 857
Transplantation; bone marrow; adult acute leukemia, therapy, review, 767; globulin immune, concentrated injections, toxicity, 1022
Triazolam
labeling; changes, FDA approvals, 467
product withdrawal; United Kingdom, 9
Tubocurarine chloride; use; evaluation, criteria, 435
Tyloxapol; combination, alcohols, cetyl, colfosceril palmitate; adult respiratory distress syndrome therapy, neonate, 880; use evaluation criteria, 355

U

Ulcers
anti-inflammatory agents; nonsteroidal, toxicity, review, 690
omeprazole; duodenal, gastric, therapy, DUE criteria, 177
United Kingdom; triazolam; product withdrawal, 9
Urinary tract infections; amphotericin B; therapy, DUE criteria, 809
Ursodiol; pruritus; therapy, biliary cirrhosis, 672

V

Vaccines
diphtheria and tetanus toxoids and pertussis; marketing, FDA approvals, 290
Haemophilus b oligosaccharide conjugate; equivalency, immunogenicity, pediatrics, 332
Haemophilus b polysaccharide conjugate; equivalency, immunogenicity, pediatrics, 332
rabies; human diploid cell, immunization, 37
Vancomycin; intraperitoneal; absorption, CAPD, 246
Vasodilating agents; hyperfibrinogenemia; therapy, 968
Vecuronium bromide; use; evaluation, criteria, 435
Vehicles
dextrose, comparison, water for injection; globulin immune reconstitution, toxicity, 628
water for injection, comparison, dextrose; globulin immune reconstitution, toxicity, 628
Verapamil hydrochloride; pharmacokinetics; equivalency, intact capsules vs. sprinkled on food, 539
Vitamins; marketing; cognition disorders therapy, FDA disapprovals, 467
Volume of distribution, see **Drugs, body distribution**
Vomiting
anesthetics; and nausea, toxicity, surgery, 965
ondansetron hydrochloride; and nausea, therapy, cisplatin toxicity, 1026

W

Warfarin sodium
interactions; tetracycline, potentiation, prothrombin time, 806
toxicity; intramural hematoma of the small intestine, 632
Water for injection; comparison, dextrose; globulin immune reconstitution, toxicity, 628
Weight; patients; nausea and vomiting, anesthetics toxicity, surgery, 965
Wounds and injuries; protocols; pain therapy, 309, 391

X

Xomen-E5
sepsis; antiendotoxin monoclonal antibodies, therapy, 223; antiendotoxin monoclonal antibodies, therapy, criteria, 255
use; evaluation, criteria, 257

Z

Zalcitabine
marketing; FDA approvals, accelerated drug review policy, 747
purchasing; AIDS buyers groups, quality problems, 385
Zidovudine
and zalcitabine; HIV infections, combined therapy, 747
use; evaluation, criteria, 63

Author Index

A

Acosta, Mark A. see Bradley, John S., 961
Adams, Margaret A. see Kozloski, Gary D., 539
Agency for Health Care Policy and Research Acute pain management: operative or medical procedures and trauma, part 1, 309; part 2, 391
Anderson, Douglas C. Jr. see Sagraves, Rosalie, 830
ASHP Commission on Therapeutics ASHP therapeutic guidelines for intravenous immune globulin, 117
ASHP Commission on Therapeutics ASHP therapeutic guidelines on antimicrobial prophylaxis in surgery, 483
Avent, Minyon L. Warfarin-induced intramural hematoma of the small intestine, 632

B

Babamoto, Kenneth S. Doxazosin: a new α_1-adrenergic antagonist, 415
Bagwell, J. Todd see Martin, Emory S. III, 104
Bailie, George R. see Figge, Helen L., 432
Banner, William Jr. Use of succimer (letter), 388
Barone, Joseph A. see Frenia, Maureen L., 37
Barriere, Steven L. Gram-negative sepsis, the sepsis syndrome, and the role of antiendotoxin monoclonal antibodies, 223
Barton, Terri L. see Chan, C. Y. Jennifer, 880
Batra, Kumar K. see Marquardt, Eric D., 1030
Bauman, Jerry L. see Tworek, Deborah A., 48
Bay, William see Gora, Mary Lea, 174
Benson, John M. Nausea and vomiting after abdominal surgery, 965
Bernstein, Linda R. see Herfindal, Eric T., 543
Bezarro, Edward R. see Wermeling, Daniel P., 342
Bhatt-Mehta, Varsha Criteria for use of colfosceril (Exosurf Neonatal) in neonates, 355
Birmingham, William E. see Littrell, Robert A., 57
Bjornson, Darrel C. see Cortese, Linda M., 675, 885
Blake, Kathryn V. see Hill, Malcolm R., 877
Bolinger, Ann M. Recombinant interferon gamma for treatment of chronic granulomatous disease and other disorders, 834
Boucher, Bradley A. see Wermeling, Daniel P., 342
Bowden, Talmadge A. Jr. see Benson, John M., 965
Bradley, John S. Pharmacokinetics and safety of intramuscular injection of concentrated ceftriaxone in children, 961
Briceland, Laurie L. see Figge, Helen L., 432
Briggs, Gerald G. see Wermeling, Daniel P., 342
Brocavich, Joseph M. see Etzel, Joseph V., 705
Bush-Veith, Stacie see Martin, Emory S. III, 104

C

Calis, Karim Anton Transdermally administered fentanyl for pain management, 22
Calis, Karim A. see also Kohler, David R., 584
Calis, Karim Anton see also Yurkowski, Peter J., 917
Canaday, Bruce R. see Avent, Minyon L., 632
Cantral, Kimberly A. see Jungnickel, Paul W., 677
Capparelli, Edmund V. New calcium-channel blockers: improved therapy? 549
Cersosimo, Robert J. Idarubicin: an anthracycline antineoplastic agent, 152
Chan, C. Y. Jennifer Colfosceril in an infant with adult respiratory distress syndrome, 880
Chandler, Mary H. H. see Parr, Michael D., 1026
Chin, Barbara see Marquardt, Eric D., 1030
Coleman, Cathy L. see Benson, John M., 965
Compogiannis, Lisa S. see Bradley, John S., 961
Coonce, Shannon L. Beta-adrenergic agonists in asthma (letter), 14
Coonce, Shannon L. see also Simon, Pamela A., 387
Corso, Diane M. see Calis, Karim Anton, 22
Corso, Diane M. see also Kohler, David R., 584
Cortese, Linda M. Criteria for use of didanosine in adult and pediatric patients, 885
Cortese, Linda M. Potential interaction between terfenadine and macrolide antibiotics (letter), 675

D

Danos, Erica A. Apparent potentiation of warfarin activity by tetracycline, 806
Danziger, Larry H. see Piscitelli, Stephen C., 137
Darbinian, Jeanne A. see Herfindal, Eric T., 543
D'Elia, John A. see Min, David I., 636
De Vito, Joseph M. see Kozloski, Gary D., 539
DeVane, C. Lindsay Book review, 277
DiPiro, Joseph T. see Benson, John M., 965
DiPiro, Joseph T. see also Hardin, Thomas C., 255
Donnelly, Andrew J. Criteria for use of pancuronium bromide, vecuronium bromide, atracurium besylate, tubocurarine chloride, metocurine iodide, pipecuronium bromide, and doxacurium chloride in adults, 435
Donnigan, L. Deane see Benson, John M., 965
Drwal-Klein, Laureen A. Antipyretic therapy in the febrile child, 1005

E

Ebert, Steven C. Characterization of the postantibiotic effect, 876
Elder, Cheryl A. β-Adrenergic antagonists for primary prevention of gastrointestinal hemorrhage in patients with cirrhosis and esophageal varices, 337
Ernst, Edzard Lowering the plasma fibrinogen concentration with drugs, 968
Ernst, Edzard Treating ischemic stroke: is nimodipine the answer? 350
Erstad, Brian L. Dapsone-induced methemoglobinemia and hemolytic anemia, 800
Etzel, Joseph V. Endocrine complications associated with human immunodeficiency virus infection, 705
Ezell, Jeanne R. see Marken, Patricia A., 553
Ezri, Marilyn see Tworek, Deborah A., 48

F

Fankhauser, Martha P. Book review, 655
Figge, Helen L. Possible ganciclovir-induced hepatotoxicity in patients with AIDS, 432
Fisher, Joseph N. see Marken, Patricia A., 851
Flynn, Patrice L. Topical capsaicin for osteoarthritis (letter), 308
Foster, Thomas S. see Wermeling, Daniel P., 342
Frenia, Maureen L. Features and treatment of rabies, 37

G

Gabbe, Steven G. see Gardner, Debra K., 352
Gales, Barry J. see Segars, Larry W., 514
Gardner, Debra K. Simultaneous concentrations of ciprofloxacin in breast milk and in serum in mother and breast-fed infant, 352
Garrelts, James C. White clot syndrome and thrombocytopenia: reasons to abandon heparin i.v. lock flush solution, 797
Golembiewski, Julie A. see Donnelly, Andrew J., 435
Goodwin, S. Diane Criteria for use of zidovudine in adult and pediatric inpatients and outpatients, 63
Gora, Mary Lea Pharmacokinetics of intraperitoneal metoclopramide in a patient with renal failure, 174
Greene, Stan A. see Wermeling, Daniel P., 342
Grimsley, Sara R. Paroxetine, sertraline, and fluvoxamine: new selective serotonin reuptake inhibitors, 930
Guglielmo, B. Joseph see Barriere, Steven L., 223

H

Haas, Curtis E. Book review, 565
Hardin, Thomas C. Who should receive antiendotoxin monoclonal antibody therapy? (editorial), 255
Harter, Chris see Gardner, Debra K., 352
Haykal, Radwan F. see Marken, Patricia A., 851
Healy, Daniel P. Book review, 900
Hecker, Earl T. see Wetmore, Robert W., 958
Henderson, Lisa M. see Parr, Michael D., 1026
Herfindal, Eric T. Complications of home parenteral nutrition, 543
Herzfeld, Jeff see Nee, Chris, 13
Hill, Malcolm R. Regularly scheduled versus as-needed use of inhaled β agonists in the treatment of asthma, 877
Hirokawa, William T. see Babamoto, Kenneth S., 415
Hirsch, Jan D. see Benson, John M., 965
Hogue, Valerie W. see Herfindal, Eric T., 543
Holman, Jonathan S. Influence of sucralfate on the detection of occult blood in simulated gastric fluid by two screening tests, 625
Holmes, Gregory B. see Kozloski, Gary D., 539
Hsu, Van Doren Criteria for use of sumatriptan in adult inpatients and outpatients, 972
Hsu, Van Doren Sumatriptan: a new drug for vascular headache, 919
Huber, Steven see Ippoliti, Cindy, 1022
Hunt, Thomas L. see Kozloski, Gary D., 539

I

Ignoffo, Robert J. Self-study materials review, 568
Ippoliti, Cindy Toxicity of rapidly infused concentrated intravenous immune globulin, 1022
Ishisaka, Denis Y. see Marquardt, Eric D., 1030
Ito, Matthew K. Ticlopidine: a new platelet aggregation inhibitor, 603

J

Jacobson, Pamala A. see Montgomery, Patricia A., 809
Jann, Michael W. see Grimsley, Sara R., 930
Johnson, Jerry B. see Kozloski, Gary D., 539
Jones, Daniel W. see Sands, Charles D., 168
Joubert, Dennis W. Value of transdermal fentanyl (letter), 584
Jung, Kyung M. see Sands, Charles D., 168
Jungnickel, Paul W. Pravastatin: a new drug for the treatment of hypercholesterolemia, 677

K

Kalt, Mark A. see Wetmore, Robert W., 958
Kane, Bud J. Book review, 901
Kennedy, L. Douglas see Littrell, Robert A., 57
Kim, Hyun Jong see Sands, Charles D., 168
Kohler, David R. Value of transdermal fentanyl (letter), 584
Kohler, David R. see also Calis, Karim Anton, 22
Koren, Gideon see Taddio, Anna, 347
Korones, Sheldon B. see Prevost, Rebecca Rogers, 357
Kowalsky, Steven F. see Figge, Helen L., 432
Kozloski, Gary D. Bioequivalence of verapamil hydrochloride extended-release pellet-filled capsules when opened and sprinkled on food and when swallowed intact, 539
Kuhn, John G. see Kane, Bud J., 901

L

Lafin, Suzanne M. see Frenia, Maureen L., 37
Lajoie, Caroline Criteria for use of omeprazole in adult patients and outpatients, 177
Leak, W. David see Littrell, Robert A., 57
Lee, Marisa L. see Ito, Matthew K., 603
Lehman, Mark E. see Wermeling, Daniel P., 342
Lindley, Celeste Book review, 92
Ling, Frank W. see Prevost, Rebecca Rogers, 529
Littrell, Robert A. Muscle spasms associated with intrathecal morphine therapy: Treatment with midazolam, 57

M

MacDonald, John S. see Parr, Michael D., 1026
Maloley, Pierre A. see Jungnickel, Paul W., 677
Mann, Katherine V. Use of succimer (letter), 388
Marcus, Steven M. Use of succimer (letter), 387
Marken, Patricia A. Criteria for use of agents for extrapyramidal adverse effects in adult, adolescent, and child inpatients and outpatients, 553
Marken, Patricia A. Management of psychotropic-induced hyperprolactinemia, 851
Marquardt, Eric D. Removal of ethosuximide and phenobarbital by peritoneal dialysis in a child, 1030
Martin, Emory S. III Danger of epidural use of ionic contrast media (letter), 105
Martin, Emory S. III Seizures after intraventricular cefazolin administration (letter), 104
Mason, Nancy A. see O'Brien, Maureen A., 246
Mauro, Laurie S. see Mauro, Vincent F., 897
Mauro, Vincent F. Book review, 897
McCauley, Dayna L. Treatment of adult acute leukemia, 767
McCollam, Patrick L. see Morales, Enid, 727
McCombs, Janet Treatment of preeclampsia and eclampsia, 236
McIntyre, William J. see Parr, Michael D., 1026
McMahon, Teresa Diabetes control during bowel cleansing with PEG–electrolyte solution (Therapy Consultation), 751
Miller, Donald R. Treatment of nonsteroidal anti-inflammatory drug-induced gastropathy, 690
Miller, Kenneth B. Safety and tolerability of an intravenous immune globulin at various concentrations in 5% dextrose injection or sterile water for injection, 628
Miller, Lucinda G. Oxaprozin: a once-daily nonsteroidal anti-inflammatory drug, 591
Min, David I. Sucralfate-associated aluminum toxicity in a patient with renal failure: treatment with deferoxamine, 636
Mirro, Robert see Prevost, Rebecca Rogers, 357
Montgomery, Patricia A. Criteria for use of amphotericin B bladder irrigation in adult inpatients, 809
Morales, Enid Criteria for use of adenosine in adults with paroxysmal supraventricular tachycardia, 727
Mowatt-Larssen, Christine A. Working group issues report on aluminum contamination of parenteral nutrient solutions (News), 6
Murphy, Christine M. see Coonce, Shannon L., 14
Murphy, Christine M. see also Simon, Pamela A., 387
Murray, William E. see Bradley, John S., 961

N

Nazari, José see Tworek, Deborah A., 48
Nee, Chris Beta-adrenergic agonists in asthma (letter), 13
Nix, David E. see Symonds, William T., 753

O

O'Brien, Maureen A. Systemic absorption of intraperitoneal antimicrobials in continuous ambulatory peritoneal dialysis, 246

P

Parr, Michael D. Pharmacokinetics of ondansetron in patients receiving cisplatin therapy, 1026
Patterson, Larry E. Book review, 901
Phelps, Stephanie J. see Drwal-Klein, Laureen A., 1005
Phillips, Marjorie Shaw Criteria for use of theophylline (aminophylline) in inpatients and outpatients with pulmonary disease, 1033
Pickworth, Kerry K. Long-term dobutamine therapy for refractory congestive heart failure, 618
Pinson, Julianne B. New considerations for *Haemophilus influenzae* type b vaccination, 332
Piscitelli, Stephen C. Clarithromycin and azithromycin: new macrolide antibiotics, 137
Prevost, Rebecca Rogers Criteria for use of beractant (Survanta) in neonates, 357
Prevost, Rebecca Rogers Methotrexate for treatment of unruptured ectopic pregnancy, 529

R

Rasch, Deborah K. see Chan, C. Y. Jennifer, 880
Reitberg, Donald P. see Sanders, Steven W., 533
Renger, Harvey Jr. see Martin, Emory S. III, 104
Restino, Maryann S. Reynolds see Elder, Cheryl A., 337
Robieux, Isabelle see Taddio, Anna, 347
Rodvold, Keith A. see Piscitelli, Stephen C., 137
Ruck, Bruce see Marcus, Steven M., 387

S

Sagraves, Rosalie Transdermal scopolamine for hyperemesis gravidarum (Therapy Consultation), 830
Sahn, Steven A. see Shalansky, Karen F., 428
Sanders, Steven W. Effect of a single dose of lactase on symptoms and expired hydrogen after lactose challenge in lactose-intolerant subjects, 533
Sands, Charles D. Effect of phenylpropanolamine hydrochloride on blood pressure in Korean patients with hypertension controlled by hydrochlorothiazide, 168
Sawyer, William T. see Avent, Minyon L., 632
Schenkein, David P. see Miller, Kenneth B., 628
Schoenbrun, Karen J. Book review, 373
Schumacher, Robert E. see Bhatt-Mehta, Varsha, 355
Segars, Larry W. Mesalamine and olsalazine: 5-aminosalicylic acid agents for the treatment of inflammatory bowel disease, 514
Seifert, Charles F. see Vondracek, Thomas G., 672
Seth, Shiv see Gora, Mary Lea, 174
Shalansky, Karen F. Absolute bioavailability of aminophylline liquid administered enterally in adults requiring mechanical ventilation, 428
Shepherd, Michele F. Criteria for use of antiendotoxin monoclonal antibodies (HA-1A and E5) in adult and pediatric inpatients, 257
Shields, Brenda see Gora, Mary Lea, 174
Shipp, Kenneth W. see Goodwin, S. Diane, 63
Shwed, Jill A. see Holman, Jonathan S., 625
Simon, Pamela A. Asthma in children (letter), 387
Simon, Pamela A. see also Coonce, Shannon L., 14
Skupski, Richard see Donnelly, Andrew J., 435
Slimowitz, Richard Book review, 565
Smith, Alden R. see Ito, Matthew K., 603
Snydman, David R. Use of cytomegalovirus immune globulin (letter), 674
Spivey, J. Michael The postantibiotic effect, 865
Stanfield, Johnny A. see Benson, John M., 965
Stegman, Mary see Stoukides, Cheryl A., 222
Stoukides, Cheryl A. Diffuse rash associated with transdermal fentanyl (letter), 222
Stovall, Thomas G. see Prevost, Rebecca Rogers, 529
Sybert, John W. see Wetmore, Robert W., 958
Symonds, William T. Lomefloxacin and temafloxacin: two new fluoroquinolone antimicrobials, 753

T

Taddio, Anna Effect of lidocaine–prilocaine cream on pain from subcutaneous injection, 347
Taeubel, Mary A. see Bolinger, Ann M., 834
Tisdale, James E. Are antiarrhythmic drugs obsolete? 714
Tisdale, James E. Book review, 277
Tolman, Keith G. see Sanders, Steven W., 533
Torre, Michael see Etzel, Joseph V., 705
Travers, John D. see Mann, Katherine V., 388
Tsu, Gloria L. see Bradley, John S., 961
Tweeddale, Martin G. see Shalansky, Karen F., 428
Tworek, Deborah A. Interference by antiarrhythmic agents with function of electrical cardiac devices, 48

U

Ustad, Cristina see Shalansky, Karen F., 428

V

Vance-Bryan, Kyle Book review, 742
Vaughan, Leigh M. see Shalansky, Karen F., 428
Visconti, James A. see Gora, Mary Lea, 174
Vondracek, Thomas G. Use of ursodiol in a patient with biliary cirrhosis (Therapy Consultation), 672

W

Wasserman, Richard L. see Miller, Kenneth B., 628
Weart, C. Wayne see Pinson, Julianne B., 332
Webb, Charles R. see Tisdale, James E., 714
Weibert, Robert T. Oral anticoagulant therapy in patients undergoing dental surgery, 857
Wermeling, Daniel P. Multicenter evaluation of a patient-controlled analgesia device for the treatment of postoperative pain, 342
West, Dennis see Flynn, Patrice L., 308
Wetmore, Robert W. Intrathecal administration of morphine followed by patient-controlled intravenous administration for postoperative analgesia, 958
Williams, Dennis M. Asthma in children (letter), 386
Williams, Loretta Ann see Ippoliti, Cindy, 1022
Wilson, Dean C. Fluconazole failure in a child with burns and candidemia, 883
Wojtynek, Jeffrey E. see Donnelly, Andrew J., 435
Wong, Alvin F. see Herfindal, Eric T., 543
Woster, Patricia S. see Montgomery, Patricia A., 809

Y

Yurkowski, Peter J. Erythromycin, motilin, and gastroparesis (Therapy Consultation), 917

Z

Zola, Elizabeth M. Use of surfactant products (letter), 583

Advertising Index

A

Abbott Laboratories –Hospital Products Division
Biaxin, 193-196
Adria Laboratories
Adriamycin, 199-200
Alpha Therapeutic Corporation
Venoglobulin-I, 15-16, 379-380
American Lung Association
Institutional, 578
American Society of Hospital Pharmacists
AHFS Drug Information 92, 56, 389, 548, 656, 796
AHFS Drug Information 93, 988
Aseptic Preparation of Parenteral Products, 560
ASHP Databases, 569
ASHP Membership, 647-648, 733-734
ASHP Software, 466, 653, 891
Basic Skills in Interpreting Laboratory Data, 479, 585, 799, 975
Clinical Pharmacy, 221, 470, 586, 671, 904
Concepts in Clinical Pharmacokinetics, 202, 443, 558
Concepts in Immunology and Immunotherapeutics, 91
Concepts in Immunology and Immunotherapeutics, 2nd Edition, 664, 864, 911
Concepts in Oncology Therapeutics, 279, 331, 453, 470, 675
Criteria for Drug Use Evaluation, Volumes 1 and 2, 68, 188, 359, 441, 556
Criteria for Drug Use Evaluation, Volumes 1, 2, and 3, 656, 730, 1042
Drug Information on CD, 578
The Elements of Quality in Pharmaceutical Care, 732, 820, 995
Handbook of Institutional Pharmacy Practice, 979
Handbook on Injectable Drugs, Sixth Edition, 59
Handbook on Injectable Drugs, 7th Edition, 676, 821, 986
IV-Ease, 14
Medication Teaching Manual, 349, 447, 463, 643, 808
MedTeach, 389, 528
Pocket Guide to Injectable Drugs, 1991 Edition, 296
Publications Catalogue, 579
QARx 3.0, 726
Resource Book on Progressive Pharmaceutical Services, 741
Rx Triage, 9, 374, 631
Safe Handling of Cytotoxic and Hazardous Drugs, 414, 624
Understanding Medical Terms, A Guide for Pharmacy Practice, 890, 957
Amgen Inc.
Epogen, 3, 95, 207, 283, 377, 468-469, 573, 659, 748-749, 902-903, 984-985, 992-993
Neupogen, 69-76, 109-116, 265-272, 291-294, 449-452, 459-462, 737-740, 907-910, 1001-1004
ASHP Research and Education Foundation
Anticoagulation Clinic Traineeship Program, 563, 651
Awards Program, 192, 278
Fellowships, 983
Grants Programs, 180
Institutional, 475

B

Bristol-Myers Squibb Oncology
Pravachol, 297-307
Burroughs Wellcome Company
Exosurf Neonatal, 17-21, 181-185, 213-217, 363-367, 471-474, 587-590, 665-668, 913-916

C

Critical Care America
Position Available, 385

E

Egleston Children's Hospital
Position Available, 752
Eisenhower Medical Center
Position Available, 219, 980
Elsevier Science Publishers
Pharmacotherapy: A Pathophysiologic Approach, 673
Enzon, Inc.
Institutional, 390, 465, 577
Epilepsy Foundation of America
Instutitional, 80

H

Health Infusion
Position Available, 995

I

Idaho State University
Positions Available, 81, 204
Immunex Corporation
Position Available, 1038
International Pharmaceutical Federation (F.I.P.)
Institutional, 464

J

Jackson Memorial Hospital
Position Available, 995

L

Eli Lilly and Company
Hospital Division, 7, 203, 209, 457, 575

M

Monongalia General Hospital
Position Available, 829

N

National Council on Patient Information and Education
Institutional, 814
National Easter Seal Society
Institutional, 105
National Osteoporosis Foundation
Institutional, 977

O

Ohio State University
Positions Available, 103, 987

P

Plan International, USA
Childreach Sponsorship, 264

R

Roche Laboratories, Division of Hoffmann-La Roche, Inc.
Rocephin, Feb IBC, OBC, Apr IBC, OBC, Jun IBC, OBC, Aug IBC, OBC, 745-746, Oct IBC, OBC, 981-982, Dec IBC, OBC
Roerig, A Division of Pfizer Pharmaceuticals
Cefobid, 97-98, 557-558, 663-664, 831-832
Diflucan, 10-12, 370-372, 826-828, 996-998
Unasyn, 186-188, 288-290, 566-568, 898-900
Ross Laboratories
Survanta, 5-6, 201-202

S

Saint Barnabas Medical Center
Position Available, 987
Scientific Therapeutics Information
Positions Available, 829, 977
SmithKline Beecham
Timentin, Jan IBC, OBC, Mar IBC, OBC, May IBC, OBC, Jul IBC, OBC, Sep IBC, OBC, Nov IBC, OBC

T

The Toledo Hospital
Positions Available, 81

U

UMI Article Clearinghouse
Microform Reproductions, 221, 585
University of Toronto
Position Available, 671
The Upjohn Company
Zefazone, 88-90, 106-108, 210-212, 360-362, 382-384, 480-482, 580-582

V

VHA of Southern New England
Position Available, 671
Virginia Mason Medical Center
Positions Available, 191, 219

W

Wyeth-Ayerst Laboratories, Inc.
Ativan Injection, 82-84, 100-102, 274-276, 284-286, 444-446, 476-478, 644-646, 660-662, 816-818
Tubex, Jan IFC, Feb IFC, Mar IFC, Apr IFC, May IFC, Jun IFC, Jul IFC, Aug IFC, Sep IFC, Oct IFC, Nov IFC, Dec IFC